BURKET'S
ORAL
MEDICINE

ELEVENTH EDITION

BURKET'S
ORAL MEDICINE

ELEVENTH EDITION

MARTIN S. GREENBERG, DDS, FDS RCS
Professor and Chairman Oral Medicine
Associate Dean Hospital Affairs
School of Dental Medicine
University of Pennsylvania
Chief of Oral Medicine
University of Pennsylvania Medical Center
Philadelphia, Pennsylvania

MICHAEL GLICK, DMD, FDS RCS
Professor of Oral Medicine
Arizona School of Dentistry & Oral Health
Associate Dean for Oral-Medical Sciences
College of Osteopathic Medicine-Mesa
A.T. Still University
Mesa, Arizona

JONATHAN A. SHIP, DMD, FDS RCS
Professor, Department of Oral & Maxillofacial Pathology, Radiology, and Medicine
Director, Bluestone Center for Clinical Research
New York University College of Dentistry
Professor, Department of Medicine
New York University School of Medicine

2008
BC Decker Inc
Hamilton

BC Decker Inc
P.O. Box 620, L.C.D. 1
Hamilton, Ontario L8N 3K7
Tel: 905-522-7017; 800-568-7281
Fax: 905-522-7839; 888-311-4987
E-mail: info@bcdecker.com
www.bcdecker.com

08 09 10/BCD/9 8 7 6 5 4 3 2 1

ISBN 978-1-55009-345-2

Printed in India
Production Editor: Petrice Custance; Typesetter: Charlesworth; Cover Designer: Alex Wheldon

Sales and Distribution

United States
BC Decker Inc
P.O. Box 785
Lewiston, NY 14092-0785
Tel: 905-522-7017; 800-568-7281
Fax: 905-522-7839; 888-311-4987
E-mail: info@bcdecker.com
www.bcdecker.com

Canada
BC Decker Inc
50 King St. E.
P.O. Box 620, LCD 1
Hamilton, Ontario L8N 3K7
Tel: 905-522-7017; 800-568-7281
Fax: 905-522-7839; 888-311-4987
E-mail: info@bcdecker.com
www.bcdecker.com

Foreign Rights
John Scott & Company
International Publishers' Agency
P.O. Box 878
Kimberton, PA 19442
Tel: 610-827-1640
Fax: 610-827-1671
E-mail: jsco@voicenet.com

Japan
Igaku-Shoin Ltd.
Foreign Publications Department
1-28-23 Hongo
Bunkyo-ku, Tokyo, Japan 113-8719
Tel: 3 3817 5611
Fax: 3 3815 4114
E-mail: fd@igaku-shoin.co.jp

UK, Europe, Middle East
McGraw-Hill Education
Shoppenhangers Road
Maidenhead
Berkshire, England SL6 2QL
Tel: 44-0-1628-502500
Fax: 44-0-1628-635895
www.mcgraw-hill.co.uk

Singapore, Malaysia, Thailand, Philippines, Indonesia, Vietnam, Pacific Rim, Korea
Elsevier Science Asia
583 Orchard Road
#09/01, Forum
Singapore 238884
Tel: 65-737-3593
Fax: 65-753-2145

Australia, New Zealand
Elsevier Science Australia
Customer Service Department
Locked Bag 16
St. Peters, New South Wales 2044
Australia
Tel: 61 02-9517-8999
Fax: 61 02-9517-2249
E-mail: customerserviceau@elsevier.com
www.elsevier.com.au

Mexico and Central America
ETM SA de CV
Calle de Tula 59
Colonia Condesa
06140 Mexico DF, Mexico
Tel: 52-5-5553-6657
Fax: 52-5-5211-8468
E-mail: editoresdetextosmex@prodigy.net.mx

Brazil
Tecmedd Importadora E Distribuidora De Livros Ltda.
Avenida Maurílio Biagi, 2850
City Ribeirão, Ribeirão Preto — SP — Brasil
CEP: 14021-000
Tel: 0800 992236
Fax: (16) 3993-9000
E-mail: tecmedd@tecmedd.com.br

India, Bangladesh, Pakistan, Sri Lanka
Elsevier Health Sciences Division
Customer Service Department
17A/1, Main Ring Road
Lajpat Nagar IV
New Delhi – 110024, India
Tel: 91 11 2644 7160-64
Fax: 91 11 2644 7156
E-mail: esindia@vsnl.net

CONTENTS

PREFACE

The first edition of this pioneering text titled *Oral Medicine: Diagnosis and Treatment*, was published in 1946 just after World War II. The text was written entirely by one man, Dr. Lester W. Burket, with the exception of a small section on "Oral Aspects of Aviation Medicine" written by a major in the Dental Corps, Dr. Alvin Goldhush. In this preface, Dr. Burket wrote that "Oral Medicine discusses the many important relationships between oral and systemic disease and it suggests opportunities for a more universal and intimate cooperation between medical and dental practitioners in giving the best possible health service to our common patients."

We believe that the 11th edition of this text follows the example set by Dr. Burket and provides the clinician with an up-to-date description of all major aspects of the science and practice of modern Oral Medicine, with the goal to enable the clinician to provide the best health service to their patients.

During the past decade, the field of Oral Medicine has expanded in both scope and complexity and it is no longer possible for one author or even one editor to have the expertise to write or oversee a majority of a book such as *Burket's Oral Medicine*. In order to accommodate the new knowledge, a third editor, Dr. Jonathan Ship, was added and four entirely new chapters and 27 new authors of international prominence and expertise were invited to coauthor chapters.

The first chapter of this text presents a basic but also an innovative approach to the evaluation and assessment of patients. It provides the necessary tools to properly evaluate and treat patients with acute and chronic health conditions, which is imperative when considering our aging and more medically complex population

Several chapters have been entirely rewritten by new authors including the chapters on Red and White Lesions, Pigmented Lesions, Neuromuscular Diseases, Renal Disease, Hematologic Disease, and Immunology.

For the first time in *Burket's Oral Medicine*, a comprehensive guide to the use of pharmacotherapeutics is available. This chapter provides the entire scope of medical management of major disorders in Oral Medicine for practicing clinicians with detailed information on prescribing drugs in accompanying tables.

The chapters on Ulcerative, Vesicular and Bullous lesions as well as the chapters on Benign Tumors and Oral Cancer have been extensively rewritten with the addition of a new group of color photos and a more clinician-friendly format for the evaluation, diagnosis, and treatment of these common oral diseases.

An increasingly important discipline in Oral Medicine is the diagnosis and management pain syndromes, and this portion of the text has been enhanced with the addition of a chapter devoted to Headache. There is also a major revision of advances in Orofacial Pain syndromes and Temporomandibular disorders.

The chapter on Salivary Diseases has also been revised and provides a state-of-the-art overview of this growing field. Details are provided on clinical presentation, diagnosis including imaging using new multimodal techniques, and treatment. A new section has been added on siallorhea and its pharmacological and surgical treatment options.

The medical chapters of this new text have been updated to reflect recent advances and how these changes alter guidelines and recommendations for safe effective dental care. One major rationale for rewriting these chapters was to add more focus on the provision of dental care for patients with complex medical conditions.

We have combined all of the information on endocrine diseases including diabetes mellitus into one comprehensive chapter that provides the reader with an updated, review of the major endocrinological diseases, their treatment, and head/neck/intraoral manifestations.

A new chapter is dedicated to Genetic Diseases. Increasingly our understanding of disease is enhanced by genetic sciences, and this chapter details the craniofacial genetic diseases of interest to the Oral Medicine and dental practitioner.

The illustrations have been redone and are all in color. The vast majority of references are also updated. The accompanying CD contains supplementary material including the complete bibliography and an expanded section on Principles of Diagnosis. This text reflects the expertise, experience and hard work of clinical scholars from many institutions, countries and specialties. We believe the eleventh edition of this classic text provides the student, resident as well as the experienced practitioner the information required to master the complex field of diagnosis and medical management of maxillofacial diseases as well as provide dental treatment for patients with complex medical disorders.

Martin S. Greenberg, DDS, FDS RCS

Michael Glick, DMD, FDS RCS

Jonathan A. Ship DMD, FDS RCS

July 2007

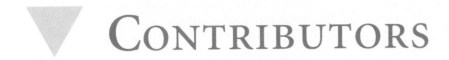

CONTRIBUTORS

Sunday O. Akintoye, BDS, DDS, MS
Department of Oral Medicine
University of Pennsylvania
Philadelphia, Pennsylvania

Faizan Alawi, DDS
Department of Pathology
University of Pennsylvania
Philadelphia, Pennsylvania

Robert Anolik, MD
Allergy and Asthma Specialists
Blue Bell, Pennsylvania

Jane C. Atkinson, DDS
Center for Clinical Research
National Institute of Dental and Craniofacial Research
Bethesda, Maryland

Bruce Blasberg, DMD, FRCD(C)
Department of Oral Medicine and Biological Sciences
University of British Columbia
Vancouver, Canada

Michael T. Brennan, DDS, MHS
Department of Oral Medicine
Carolinas Medical Center
Charlotte, North Carolina

Stephen Challacombe, PhD, FDS RCS, FRCPath
Department of Oral Medicine
Kings College Dental Institute
London, England

Debbie L. Cohen, MD
Department of Medicine
University of Pennsylvania
Philadelphia, Pennsylvania

Michael T. Collins, MD
Department of Craniofacial and Skeletal Diseases
National Institutes of Health
Bethesda, Maryland

Scott S. DeRossi, DMD
Department of Oral Diagnosis
Medical College of Georgia
Augusta, Georgia

Sandhya Desai, MD
Allergy and Asthma Specialists
Blue Bell, Pennsylvania

John A. Detre, MD
Center for Functional Imaging
University of Pennsylvania
Philadelphia, Pennsylvania

Eli Eliav, DMD, PhD
Department of Diagnostic Sciences
New Jersey Dental School
Newark, New Jersey

Michael T. Brennan, DDS, MHS
Department of Oral Medicine
Carolinas Medical Center
Charlotte, North Carolina

Joel Epstein, DMD, MSD
Interdisciplinary Program in Oral Cancer
Chicago Cancer Center
Chicago, Illinois

Philip C. Fox, DDS, FDS RCS
Department of Oral Medicine
Carolinas Medical Center
Charlotte, North Carolina

Michael Glick, DMD, FDS RCS
Department of Oral Medicine
Arizona School of Dentistry
A.T. Still University
Mesa, Arizona

Martin S. Greenberg, DDS, FDS RCS
Department of Oral Medicine
University of Pennsylvania
Philadelphia, Pennsylvania

Palle Holmstrup, DDS, PhD
Department of Periodontology
Copenhagen University
Copenhagen, Denmark

Michaell A. Huber, DDS
Department of Dental Diagnostic Science
University of Texas
San Antonio, Texas

Matin M. Imanguli, DDS
Center for Clinical Research
National Institute of Dental and Craniofacial Research
Bethesda, Maryland

Mats Jontell, DDS, PhD, FDS RCS
Clinic of Oral Medicine
Göteborg University
Göteborg, Sweden

A. Ross Kerr, DDS, MSD
Department of Oral & Maxillofacial Pathology,
    Radiology and Medicine
New York University
New York, New York

Mark LePore, MD
Allergy and Asthma Specialists
Blue Bell, Pennsylvania

Laszlo Littmann, MD
Department of Internal Medicine
Carolinas Medical Center
Charlotte, North Carolina

Peter B. Lockhart, DDS, FDS RCS
Department of Oral Medicine
Carolinas Medical Center
Charlotte, North Carolina

Ali Naji, MD, PhD
Department of Surgery
University of Pennsylvania
Philadelphia, Pennsylvania

Mahvash Navazesh, DMD
Department of Diagnostic Sciences
University of Southern California
Los Angeles, California

Pragna Patel, PhD
Department of Biochemistry and Molecular Biology
University of Southern California
Los Angeles, California

Lauren L. Patton, DDS, FDS RCS
Department of Dental Ecology
University of North Carolina
Chapel Hill, North Carolina

Joan A. Phelan, DDS
Department of Oral & Maxillofacial Pathology,
    Radiology and Medicine
New York University
New York, New York

Andres Pinto, DMD, MPH
Department of Oral Medicine
University of Pennsylvania
Philadelphia, Pennsylvania

David L. Porter, MD
Department of Medicine
University of Pennsylvania
Philadelphia, Pennsylvania

Spencer W. Redding, DDS, MEd
Department of Dental Diagnostic Science
University of Texas
San Antonio, Texas

Vidya Sankar, DMD, MHS
Department of Dental Diagnostic Science
University of Texas
San Antonio, Texas

Lakshman Samaranayake, DSc, FDS RCS, DDS
Department of Oral Biosciences
University of Hong Kong
Hong Kong, China

Frank A. Scannapieco, DMD, PhD
Department of Oral Biology
University at Buffalo
Buffalo, New York

Jonathan A. Ship, DMD, FDS RCS
Department of Oral & Maxillofacial Pathology,
    Radiology, and Medicine
Department of Medicine
Bluestone Center for Clinical Research
New York University
New York, New York

Michael A. Siegel, DDS, MS, FDS RCS
Department of Diagnostic Sciences
Nova Southeastern University
Fort Lauderdale, Florida

David A. Sirois, DMD, PhD
Department of Oral & Maxillofacial Pathology,
    Radiology, and Medicine
Department of Neurology
New York University
New York, New York

Harold C. Slavkin, DDS
Department of Health Promotion and Epidemiology
University of southern California
Los Angeles, California

Thomas P. Sollecito, DMD
Department of Oral Medicine
University of Pennsylvania
Philadelphia, Pennsylvania

Eric T. Stoopler, DMD
Department of Oral Medicine
University of Pennsylvania
Philadelphia, Pennsylvania

Isaac Van der Waal, DDS, PhD
Department of Oral & Maxillofacial Surgery
VU Medical Center
Amsterdam, the Netherlands

Sook Bin Woo, DMD, MMSc
Department of Dental Services
Brigham and Women's Hospital
Boston, Massachusetts

David Wray, BDS, MD, FDS RCS
Department of Oral Medicine
Glasgow University
Glasgow, Scotland

This book is dedicated

With love to my wife Patti, granddaughters Rachel, Hannah, Jade and Peytan and in memory of my mother Pearl.
Martin S. Greenberg

With love and affection to my wife Patricia and children, Noa, Jonathan and Gideon.
Michael Glick

With love and gratitude to my wife Shari and children Nina, Zachary and Maxwell.
Jonathan A. Ship

1

INTRODUCTION TO ORAL MEDICINE AND ORAL DIAGNOSIS: EVALUATION OF THE DENTAL PATIENT

MICHAEL GLICK, DMD, FDS RCS

MARTIN S. GREENBERG, DDS, FDS RCS

JONATHAN A. SHIP, DMD, FDS RCS

Over the past several decades, the need for oral health care professionals to understand basic principles of medicine and diagnosis has grown exponentially.[1] This is due, in part, to changing characteristics of patients seeking oral health services. The population is aging, and an increasing number of patients seeking oral health services are living with chronic illnesses, are taking multiple medications, and have undergone surgical procedures (eg, cardiac surgery, organ transplantation) that prolong life but have a profound effect on craniofacial health and function, as well as on the provision of dental care. Oral health is an integral part of total health, and oral health care professionals must adapt to demographic changes and medical advances and shoulder the responsibility of being part of the patient's overall health care team.

Oral medicine is a specialty within dentistry that focuses on the diagnosis and management of complex diagnostic and medical disorders affecting the mouth and jaws. Clinicians with advanced training in this discipline manage oral mucosal disease, salivary gland disorders, and facial pain syndromes and also provide dental care for patients with complicating medical disease. However, all general dentists and dental specialists must be more aware of oral medicine and the

1

medical status of their patients in order to provide a high level of oral heath care.

Patients consult all oral health care professionals for management of problems related to orofacial structures, and the opportunity and the need to evaluate and assess patients' overall medical status become part of the responsibility of the dentist. This chapter addresses the rationale and method for gathering relevant medical and dental information, including the examination of the patient, and the use of this information to provide safe and appropriate oral health care. This process is divided into five parts:

1. Obtaining and recording the patient's medical history
2. Examining the patient
3. Establishing a differential diagnosis
4. Acquiring the additional information required to make a final diagnosis, such as relevant laboratory and imaging studies and consultations from other clinicians
5. Formulating a plan of action, including oral health care modifications and necessary medical referrals

▼ MEDICAL HISTORY

Obtaining a medical history is an information-gathering method for assessing a patient's health status that will facilitate the diagnostic process for the patient's orofacial complaint and substantiate the institution of necessary modifications for the provision of oral health care. The medical history comprises a systematic review of the patient's chief or primary complaint, a detailed history related to this complaint, information about past and present medical conditions, pertinent social and family histories, and a review of symptoms by organ system. A medical history also includes biographic and demographic data used to identify the patient. An appropriate interpretation of the information collected through a medical history achieves several important objectives; it affords an opportunity for

(1) gathering the information necessary for establishing the diagnosis of the patient's chief complaint
(2) monitoring known medical conditions
(3) detecting underlying systemic conditions that the patient may or may not be aware of
(4) providing a basis for determining whether dental treatment might affect the systemic health of the patient
(5) assessing the influence of the patient's systemic health on patient's oral health
(6) providing a basis for determining necessary modifications to routine dental care

There is no one universally accepted method for gathering the pertinent information that constitutes the medical history; rather, individual approaches are tailored to specific needs. The nature of the patient's dental visit (ie, initial dental visit, complex diagnostic problem, emergency, elective

continuous care, or recall) often dictates how the history is obtained. The different formats include self-administered preprinted forms filled out by the patient, direct interview of the patient by the clinician, or a combination of both. All of these methods have benefits and drawbacks.

The use of self-administered screening questionnaires is the most commonly used method in dental settings (Figure 1). This technique can be useful in gathering background medical information, but the accurate diagnosis of a specific oral complaint requires a history of the present illness, which is obtained verbally. The challenge in any health care setting is to use a questionnaire that has enough items to cover the essential information but is not too long to deter a patient's willingness and ability to fill it out. Preprinted self-administered health questionnaires are readily available, standardized, and easy to administer and do not require significant "chair time." They give the clinician a starting point for a dialogue to conduct more in-depth medical queries but are restricted to the questions chosen on the form and are therefore limited in scope. The questions on the form can be misunderstood by the patient, resulting in inaccurate information, and they require a specific level of reading comprehension. Preprinted forms cover broad areas without necessarily focusing on particular problems pertinent to an individual patient's specific medical condition. Therefore, the use of these forms requires that the provider has sufficient background knowledge to understand why the questions on the forms are being asked. Furthermore, the provider needs to realize that a given standard history form necessitates timely and appropriate follow-up questions, especially when positive responses have been elicited. An established routine for performing and recording the history and examination should be followed conscientiously.

The oral health care professional has a responsibility to obtain all relevant medical and dental health information, yet the patient cannot be held accountable to know this information and cannot always be relied upon to provide an accurate and comprehensive assessment of his or her medical or dental status.

All medical information obtained and recorded in an oral health care setting is considered confidential and constitutes a legal document. Although it is appropriate for the patient to fill out a history form in the waiting room, any discussion of the patient's responses must take place in a safeguarded setting. Furthermore, access to the written or electronic (if applicable) record must be limited to office personnel who are directly responsible for the patient's care. Any other release of private information should be approved, in writing, by the patient and retained by the dentist as part of the patient's medical record.

Changes in a patient's health status or medication regimen should be reviewed at each office visit prior to initiating dental care. This is important as many medical conditions are associated with slow and gradual changes, medication regimens frequently change, and the monitoring of patients' compliance with medical treatment guidelines and

Date _____
Chart Number _____

Name _____   Male _____ Female _____
Address _____   Date of Birth _____
City _____   State _____ Zip Code _____
Occupation _____   Home Phone _____
Social Security No _____   Work Phone _____
    Mobile Phone _____
    E-mail _____

Emergency contact _____
Relationship to patient _____   Phone No _____

Physician's Name _____
Physician's Telephone No _____   Date of Last Visit _____
Reason for Last Visit to a Physician _____

Why are you seeking dental treatment at this time? _____

General Questions. This questionnaire will be used by your dentist to help treat you safely.
Please answer all questions as accurately as possible.
Do you have, or have you had an history of the following?

	Yes	No	Do not know		Yes	No	Do not know
High blood pressure				Kidney disease			
Angina / Chest pain				Renal dialysis			
Heart attack				Organ transplant			
Prosthetic heart valve				Cancer			
Pacemaker/Defibrillator				Radiation therapy			
Heart disease/ surgery				Chemotherapy			
Stroke/TIA				Epilepsy / Seizure			
Emphysema/Bronchitis				Stomach/Intestinal problems			
Asthma				Arthritis			
Diabetes				Artificial joint			
Thyroid disease				Sexually transmitted disease			
Autoimmune disease/Lupus				AIDS/ HIV			
Liver disease				Tuberculosis (TB)			
Hepatitis				Psychiatric treatment			
Anemia				Allergies			
Bleeding disorder				Osteoporosis			

Medications
Please list all medications that you are presently taking, including herbal medications or nutritional supplements.
_____
_____

Allergies
Please list all medications that have caused an allergic, adverse, or untoward reaction after taking.
Please include any previous adverse reactions to latex or local anesthesia.
_____
_____

Social History
Do you smoke tobacco? _____ How much do you smoke? _____ How long have you been smoking? _____
Do you use alcohol? _____ How many drinks per week? _____

Do you use recreational drugs? _____ What type? _____
Last recreational drug use? _____

For women only: Do you believe you are presently pregnant? _____

Please list all major surgeries or hospitalizations
_____
_____

FIGURE 1   Health history questionnaire.

medications and possible drug interactions is part of the oral health care professional's responsibilities.[2]

Consultations with other health care professionals are initiated when additional information is necessary to assess a patient's medical status. Evaluations from other specialists may also be required to make an accurate diagnosis of an orofacial complaint. For example, a patient with facial pain may require a consultation from an otolaryngologist to rule out sinus or ear pathology, whereas a patient with oral mucosal disease and skin lesions would benefit from an evaluation by a dermatologist.

Any verbal and written consultation should be documented in the patient's record. A consultation letter should identify the patient and contain a brief overview of the patient's pertinent medical history and a request for specific medical information (Figure 2). A physician cannot "clear" a patient for treatment. A physician's advice and recommendation may be helpful in managing a dental patient, but the responsibility to provide safe and appropriate care lies ultimately with the oral health care provider.

For an overview of the medical history components, see the attached disc.

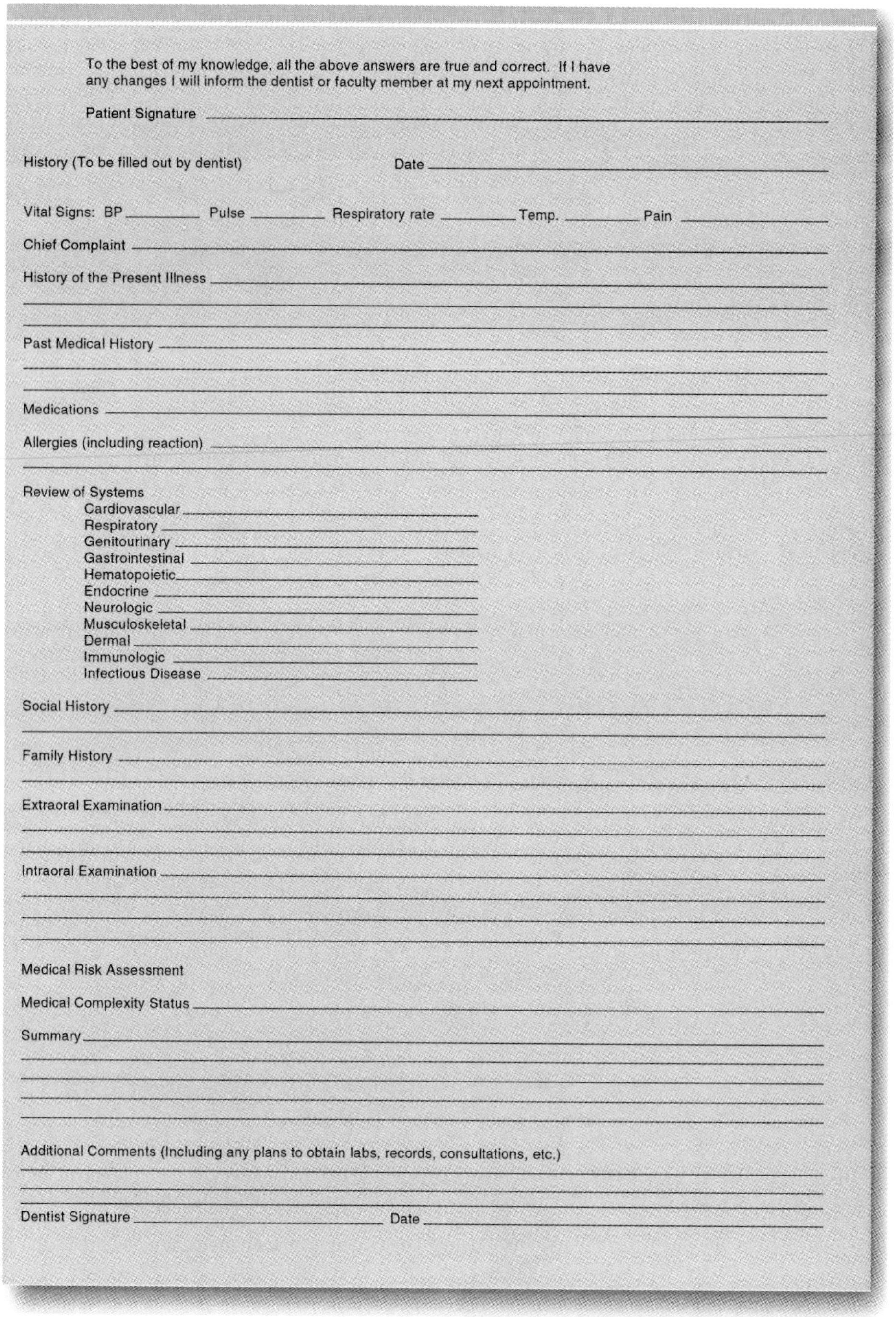

To the best of my knowledge, all the above answers are true and correct. If I have any changes I will inform the dentist or faculty member at my next appointment.

Patient Signature _____

History (To be filled out by dentist)   Date _____

Vital Signs: BP _____ Pulse _____ Respiratory rate _____ Temp. _____ Pain _____

Chief Complaint _____

History of the Present Illness _____
_____
_____

Past Medical History _____
_____
_____

Medications _____

Allergies (including reaction) _____
_____

Review of Systems
  Cardiovascular _____
  Respiratory _____
  Genitourinary _____
  Gastrointestinal _____
  Hematopoietic _____
  Endocrine _____
  Neurologic _____
  Musculoskeletal _____
  Dermal _____
  Immunologic _____
  Infectious Disease _____

Social History _____
_____

Family History _____
_____

Extraoral Examination _____
_____

Intraoral Examination _____
_____
_____
_____

Medical Risk Assessment

Medical Complexity Status _____

Summary _____
_____
_____
_____
_____

Additional Comments (Including any plans to obtain labs, records, consultations, etc.)
_____
_____

Dentist Signature _____ Date _____

FIGURE 1 Continued.

Review of Systems

The review of systems (ROS) is a comprehensive and systematic review of subjective symptoms affecting different bodily systems (Figure 1). The value of performing a ROS together with the physical examination has been well established.[3–5]

The clinician records both negative and positive responses. Direct questioning of the patient should be aimed at collecting additional data to assess the severity of a patient's medical conditions, monitor changes in medical conditions, and assist in confirming or ruling out those disease processes that may be associated with patient's symptoms. The design of the ROS is aimed at categorizing each major system of the body so as to provide the clinician with a framework that incorporates many different anatomic and physiologic expressions reflective of the patient's medical status. The ROS includes general categories to allow for completeness of the review.

Numerous examples can be provided to underscore the importance of the ROS. The ROS may help establish the primary diagnosis by uncovering important symptoms involving other parts of the body. For example, a patient with

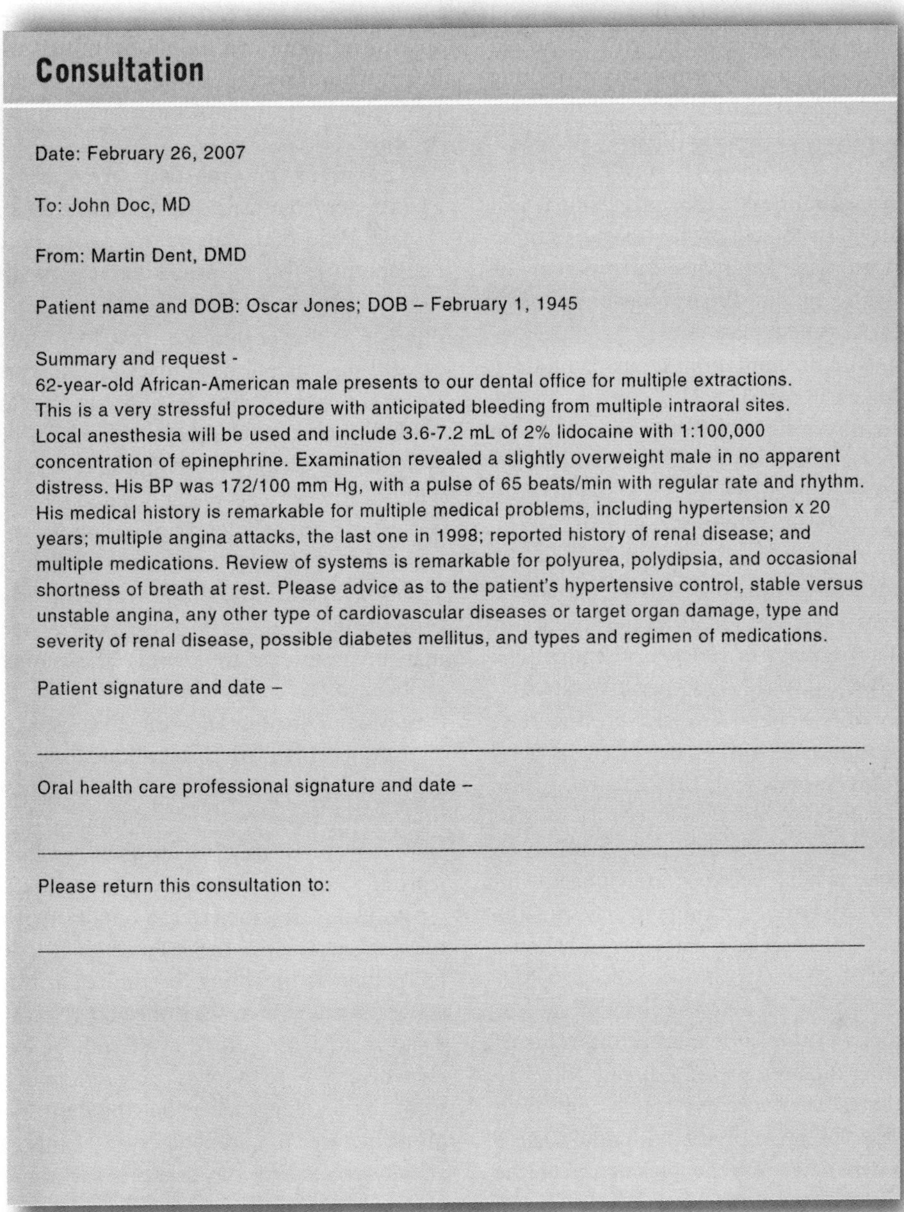

Consultation

Date: February 26, 2007

To: John Doc, MD

From: Martin Dent, DMD

Patient name and DOB: Oscar Jones; DOB – February 1, 1945

Summary and request -
62-year-old African-American male presents to our dental office for multiple extractions.
This is a very stressful procedure with anticipated bleeding from multiple intraoral sites.
Local anesthesia will be used and include 3.6-7.2 mL of 2% lidocaine with 1:100,000
concentration of epinephrine. Examination revealed a slightly overweight male in no apparent
distress. His BP was 172/100 mm Hg, with a pulse of 65 beats/min with regular rate and rhythm.
His medical history is remarkable for multiple medical problems, including hypertension x 20
years; multiple angina attacks, the last one in 1998; reported history of renal disease; and
multiple medications. Review of systems is remarkable for polyurea, polydipsia, and occasional
shortness of breath at rest. Please advice as to the patient's hypertensive control, stable versus
unstable angina, any other type of cardiovascular diseases or target organ damage, type and
severity of renal disease, possible diabetes mellitus, and types and regimen of medications.

Patient signature and date –

_____

Oral health care professional signature and date –

_____

Please return this consultation to:

_____

FIGURE 2 Consultation.

facial pain may also have complaints such as paresthesia, anesthesia, or weakness, indicating that the facial pain may be a symptom of a neurologic disorder. In addition, seemingly unrelated systemic disorders that significantly affect a patient's dental care may be disclosed.

The ROS may also allow the dentist to detect an undiagnosed medical disease, which may require modification of dental treatment. For example, the dentist may suspect undiagnosed or poorly controlled congestive heart failure in a patient with orthopnea, a bleeding disorder in a patient with recent severe nose bleeds and easy bruising, or diabetes in a patient with polyuria and polydipsia.

Supplementary Examination Procedures

With the information obtained from the history and the routine physical examination, a diagnosis can usually be made,

or the information can at least provide the clinician with direction for subsequent diagnostic procedures. Additional questioning of the patient or more specialized examination procedures may still be required to confirm a diagnosis or distinguish between several possible diagnoses. Examples of more specialized physical examination procedures are dental pulp vitality testing; detailed evaluation of salivary gland function (see Chapter 8, "Salivary Gland Diseases"); and assessment of occlusion, masticatory muscles, and temporomandibular joint function (see Chapter 9, "Temporomandibular Disorders"). Radiography of the teeth and jaws, computer-assisted scanning (computed tomography), and magnetic resonance imaging of the temporomandibular joint, salivary glands, and other soft tissue structures of the head and neck can provide visible evidence of suspected physical abnormalities. Furthermore, a variety of laboratory tests (serology, biopsy, blood chemistry, hematologic and microbiologic procedures) can be used to confirm a suspected diagnosis or to identify a systemic abnormality contributing to the patient's signs and symptoms.

Laboratory Studies

There are times when an oral health care professional will want to order laboratory tests to help make a diagnosis of an oral disease, rule out an underlying medical problem, or determine if a patient with a specific disease is healthy enough for the proposed dental treatment plan.

It is important to realize the limitations of any laboratory test. There are no tests that can detect "health"; rather, laboratory tests are used to discriminate between the presence or absence of disease or are used as a predictor or marker of disease. The frequency with which a test indicates the presence of a disease is called sensitivity; specificity is the frequency with which a test indicates the absence of the disease.[6,7] A test that identifies a disease every time has a sensitivity of 100%, whereas a test that identifies the absence of disease every time has a specificity of 100%. Consequently, a test with a sensitivity of 98% has a 2% false-negative rate, and a test with a specificity of 98% has a 2% false-positive rate. The significance of choosing a test with a particular sensitivity or specificity usually corresponds with the outcome of the test result. For instance, it is highly desirable to use a human immunodeficiency virus (HIV) test with a high sensitivity to minimize false-negative results because individuals who believe they are HIV negative may continue to transmit the disease and may not seek medical care. However, sensitivity improves at the expense of specificity, and vice versa.

Another important aspect of a test is its efficacy, or predictive value. Predictive value is defined as the value of positive results indicating the presence of a disease (positive predictive value) or the value of negative results indicating the absence of a disease (negative predictive value). These predictive values are dependent on the prevalence of the particular condition in the population, as well as on the sensitivity and specificity of the test.

Even normal values in tests used to screen asymptomatic populations for disease fall within two standard deviations of the mean. Consequently, a single test will produce an abnormal result 5% of the time. For a "panel" of tests, the percentage of abnormal results increases significantly. Thus, for any decision (or even diagnosis) based on any laboratory test, many different criteria need to be considered.

Laboratory studies are an extension of the physical examination; tissue, blood, urine, or other specimens are obtained from the patient and are subjected to microscopic, biochemical, microbiologic, or immunologic examination. A laboratory test alone rarely establishes the nature of an oral lesion, but when interpreted in conjunction with information obtained from the history and the physical examination, the results of laboratory tests will frequently establish or confirm a diagnostic impression. Specimens obtained directly from the oral cavity (eg, scrapings of oral mucosal cells, tissue biopsy specimens, and swabs of exudates), as well as the specimens more commonly submitted to the clinical diagnostic laboratory (eg, blood), may provide information that is of value in the diagnosis of oral lesions, such as herpes virus infection.

Lesions of the oral cavity may also be complicated by coexistent systemic disease or may be the direct result of such disease. Many of the laboratory studies needed in dental practice are those that are widely used in medicine. The systemic disease suspected by an oral health care professional may often be of greater significance to the patient's health than the presenting oral lesion. By investigating a problem of this type, the oral health care professional is, in effect, investigating a medical problem. It has been argued that the patient in whom systemic disease is suspected should be referred to a physician without further tests being ordered by the dentist. This procedure is clearly the correct one under some circumstances, and professional judgment is required. However, in many situations, laboratory studies made by the oral health care professional prior to medical referral are appropriate and may be necessary to identify the nature of the patient's problem or to assess the severity of an underlying medical condition. Diseases affecting the oral cavity often exhibit features peculiar to this region, and an oral health care professional trained in the management of diseases of the oral cavity may be better equipped to select appropriate laboratory tests and evaluate their results than is a physician with no specific knowledge of the region.

A diagnostic problem can be solved by referral only when the patient accepts the referral. If a lesion is minor or if the patient is unwilling to admit that the lesion may be of systemic origin, then she or he may reject the dentist's advice, delay in following up the referral, or even seek treatment elsewhere. Failure to follow up a referral may sometimes stem from the patient's belief that the dentist is straying beyond his or her area of competence but is more often the result of anxiety created by the dentist's suggesting that the patient may have an undiagnosed medical problem. Referral to a physician is possible only when confidence is firmly established between dentist and patient. Patients who seem unwilling to accept referral to a physician often agree to a screening laboratory test carried out through the oral health care professional's office. When the results of such tests are positive, they strengthen the oral health care professional's recommendation and often achieve the desired referral.

Clinical and laboratory procedures, such as blood pressure measurement, complete blood cell count, blood chemistry screening, throat culture for infections with beta-hemolytic streptococci, and detection of antibodies to hepatitis viruses and HIV, have also been used for epidemiologic purposes in dentistry.[8–12] Except in limited situations, however, the cost of standard screening tests such as a complete blood count or plasma glucose determination has discouraged their routine use in oral health care professional offices and clinics, even though the detection of elevated blood pressure has become customary.

The results of screening tests of this type—and, in fact, the majority of studies carried out by oral health care professionals for the detection of systemic diseases—do not themselves constitute a diagnosis. For example, an oral health care professional who finds elevated plasma glucose levels (ie, from a glucometer) should not tell the patient that he or she has diabetes but should inform the patient that the results of the test indicate an abnormality and advise the patient to seek medical consultation. Reports of abnormal results with systemic implications should be sent directly to the patient's physician, and the diagnosis of diabetes, hypertension, or other disease should be made by the physician on the basis of the physical examination, history, and (possibly) further laboratory tests. The management of medical disorders of the mouth and jaws is within the scope of dentists and dental specialists, whereas systemic medical diseases are within the domain of physicians. The dentist should not consider prescribing medication or other treatment for a systemic disease, even though he or she might be required to provide local care for the oral manifestations.

The success of all screenings for systemic disease, whether carried out by public health authorities or by oral health care professionals, depends on the availability of physicians who are willing to accept such referrals. When ordering or carrying out a laboratory test for the detection of a systemic disease, always consider what can practically be done with the results of the test. Laboratory testing without follow-up is not only futile but can lead to serious anxiety in the patient.

Specialized Examination of Other Organ Systems

The compact anatomy of the head and neck and the close relationship between oral function and the contiguous nasal, otic, laryngopharyngeal, gastrointestinal, and ocular structures often require that evaluation of an oral problem be combined with evaluation of one or more of these related organ systems. For detailed evaluation of these extraoral systems, the oral health care professional should request that the patient consult the appropriate medical specialist, who must be informed of the reason for the consultation. The usefulness of this consultation will usually depend on the dentist's knowledge of the interaction of the oral cavity with adjacent organ systems, as well as the dentist's ability to recognize symptoms and signs of disease in the extraoral regions of the head and neck. Superficial inspection of these extraoral tissues is therefore a logical part of the dentist's examination for the causes of certain oral problems.

Disorders of the temporomandibular joint, referred pain, oropharyngeal and skin cancer screening, dysgeusia, salivary gland disease, postsurgical oropharyngeal and oronasal defects, and various congenital syndromes affecting the head and neck are all conditions that are frequently brought to the attention of oral health care professionals and that require them to look beyond the oral cavity when examining the head and neck. The details of special examinations of the ears, nose, eyes, pharynx, larynx, and facial musculature and integument are beyond the scope of this chapter, and the

reader is advised to consult texts that describe the physical examination of these organs[13] and to obtain training in the use of the headlamp, the otoscope, and the ophthalmoscope, as well as in techniques such as indirect laryngoscopy and the inspection of the nasal cavity. Knowledge of disease processes that affect these organ systems is desirable.

The oral health care professional's initial evaluations of extraoral tissues neither infringe on the rights of other medical specialists nor reduce their professional activities. These evaluations can contribute significantly to the collaboration of dentist and physician in the management of many craniofacial and oral problems. More important, information gathered during these examinations will provide invaluable diagnostic information that is necessary to ensure a proper referral to a medical specialist. Provided that the patient's permission is obtained before these nonsurgical procedures are carried out, there appears to be no legal restriction to the examination of these extraoral organ systems by the dentist. However, this may vary according to local laws and regulations, which should be consulted before initiating procedures that are perceived as outside the realm of dentistry. For example, the dentist may be prohibited by law from specifically diagnosing and treating problems outside the maxillofacial region. In all cases in which there is any concern about the presence of disease in any of these organ systems, referral and treatment for the patient must be sought from the appropriate medical service.

▼ EXAMINATION OF THE PATIENT

The examination of the patient represents the second stage of the evaluation and assessment process. An established routine for the examination is mandatory. A thorough and systematic inspection of the oral cavity and adnexal tissues minimizes the possibility of overlooking previously undiscovered pathologies. The examination is most conveniently carried out with the patient seated in a dental chair, with the head supported. When dental charting is involved, having an assistant record the findings saves time and limits cross-contamination of the chart and pen. Before seating the patient, the clinician should pay attention to the patient's general appearance and gait and should note any physical deformities or handicaps.

The routine oral examination should be carried out at least once annually or at each recall visit. This includes a thorough inspection and, when appropriate, palpation, auscultation, and percussion of the exposed surface structures of the head, neck, and face and a detailed examination of the oral cavity, dentition, oropharynx, and adnexal structures. Laboratory studies and additional special examination of other organ systems may be required for the evaluation of patients with orofacial pain, oral mucosal disease, or signs and symptoms suggestive of otorhinologic or salivary gland disorders or pathologies suggestive of a systemic etiology. A less comprehensive but equally thorough inspection of the face and oral and oropharyngeal mucosae should be carried out at each dental visit. The tendency for the dentist to focus on only the tooth or jaw quadrant in question should be strongly resisted.

Each visit should be initiated by a deliberate inspection of the entire face and oral cavity prior to the scheduled or emergency procedure. The importance of this approach in the early detection of head and neck cancer and in promoting the image of the dentist as the responsible clinician of the oral cavity cannot be overemphasized (see Chapter 7, Oral Cancer).

Examination carried out in the dental office is traditionally restricted to that of the superficial tissues of the oral cavity, head, and neck and the exposed parts of the extremities. On occasion, evaluation of an oral lesion logically leads to an inquiry about similar lesions on other skin or mucosal surfaces or about the enlargement of other regional groups of lymph nodes. Although these inquiries can usually be satisfied directly by questioning the patient, the dentist may also quite appropriately request permission from the patient to examine axillary nodes or other skin surfaces provided that the examination is carried out competently and there is adequate privacy for the patient. A male dentist should have a female assistant present in the case of a female patient. Female dentists should have a male assistant present in the case of a male patient. Similar precautions should be followed when it is necessary for a patient to remove tight clothing for accurate measurement of blood pressure. A complete physical examination should not be attempted when facilities are lacking or when custom excludes it.

The degree of responsibility accorded to the dentist in carrying out a complete physical examination varies from hospital to hospital, from state to state, and from country to country. The oral health care professional's involvement may range from permission to examine extraoral structures for educational purposes only, to permission to carry out certain parts of the complete physical examination under the supervision of a physician who reviews and certifies the findings, to full privileges and responsibility for conducting necessary physical examinations before and after general anesthesia or surgical procedures.

The examination procedure in dental office settings includes five areas: (1) registration of vital signs (respiratory rate, temperature, pain level, pulse, and blood pressure); (2) examination of the head, neck, and oral cavity, including salivary glands, temporomandibular joints, and head and neck lymph nodes; (3) examination of cranial nerve function; (4) special examination of other organ systems; and (5) requisition of laboratory studies.

For an overview of the examination process, see the attached disc.

▼ ESTABLISHING THE DIAGNOSIS

When establishing a diagnosis in the orofacial region, the oral health care professional should establish a differential diagnosis based on the medical history and physical examination and order the necessary laboratory tests, such as biopsies

or imaging studies, required to reach the final diagnosis only after a differential diagnosis has been determined. In other circumstances, when the patient's symptoms suggest the presence of a general medical disease and the clinical data are more complex, the diagnosis may be established using four steps: (1) reviewing the patient's medical history, physical, radiographic, and laboratory findings; (2) listing those items that either clearly indicate an abnormality or that suggest the possibility of a significant health problem requiring further evaluation; (3) grouping these items into primary versus secondary signs and symptoms, acute versus chronic problems, and high versus low priority for treatment; and (4) categorizing and labeling these grouped items according to a standardized system for the classification of disease.

The rapidity and accuracy with which a diagnosis or set of diagnoses can be achieved depends on the history and examination data that have been collected and on the clinician's knowledge and ability to match these clinical data with a conceptual representation of one or more disease processes. Experienced clinicians who have an extensive knowledge of human physiology, disease etiology, and a broad knowledge of the relevant literature can usually rapidly establish a correct diagnosis. Such "mental models" of disease syndromes also increase the efficiency with which experienced clinicians gather and evaluate clinical data and focus supplemental questioning and testing at all stages of the diagnostic process.

For effective treatment, as well as for health insurance and medicolegal reasons, it is important that a diagnosis (or diagnostic summary) is entered into the patient's record after the detailed history and physical, radiographic, and laboratory examination data. When more than one health problem is identified, the diagnosis for the primary complaint (ie, the stated problem for which the patient sought medical or dental advice) is usually listed first, followed by subsidiary diagnoses of concurrent problems. Previously diagnosed conditions that remain as actual or potential problems are also included, with the qualification "by history," "previously diagnosed," or "treated" to indicate their status. Problems that were identified but not clearly diagnosed during the current evaluation can also be listed with the comment "to be ruled out." Because oral medicine is concerned with regional problems that may or may not be modified by concurrent systemic disease, it is common for the list of diagnoses to include both oral lesions and systemic problems of actual or potential significance in the etiology or management of the oral lesion. Items in the medical history that do not relate to the current problem and that are not of major health significance usually are not included in the diagnostic summary. For example, a diagnosis might read as follows:

1. Alveolar abscess, mandibular left first molar
2. Rampant generalized dental caries secondary to radiation-induced salivary hypofunction
3. Carcinoma of the tonsillar fossa, by history, excised and treated with 65 Gy 2 years ago

4. Cirrhosis and prolonged prothrombin time, by history
5. Hyperglycemia; R/O (rule out) diabetes

A definite diagnosis cannot always be made, despite a careful review of all history, clinical, and laboratory data. In such cases, a descriptive term (rather than a formal diagnosis) may be used for the patient's symptoms or lesion, with the added word "idiopathic," "unexplained," or (in the case of symptoms without apparent physical abnormality) "functional" or "symptomatic." The clinician must decide what terminology to use in conversing with the patient and whether to clearly identify this diagnosis as "undetermined." Irrespective of that decision, it is important to recognize the equivocal nature of the patient's problem and to schedule additional evaluation, by referral to another consultant, additional testing, or placement of the patient on recall for follow-up studies.

Unfortunately, there is no generally accepted system for identifying and classifying diseases, and diagnoses are often written with concerns related to third-party reimbursement and to medicolegal and local peer review, as well as for the purpose of accurately describing and communicating the patient's disease status.[14] Within different specialties, attempts have been made to achieve conformity of professional expressions and language.[16]

Some standardization of diagnoses has been achieved in the United States as a result of the introduction in 1983 of the diagnosis-related group (DRG) system as an obligatory cost-containment measure for the reimbursement of hospitals for inpatient care.[14] Most recently, in August 2006, the Centers for Medicare and Medicaid Services (CMS) issued a final ruling that will initiate a transition plan for replacing the current CMS DRGs with a classification methodology that more accurately reflects a patient's severity of disease. Beyond cost containment, patient grouping classifications also are used for epidemiologic monitoring, clinical management, and comparison of hospital activity and as a prospective payment system. Yet groupings are mostly based on medical diagnoses, such as the *International Classification of Diseases, Tenth Revision* (ICD-10).[15]

Although scientifically derived, the DRG system is designed for fiscal use rather than as a system for the accurate classification of disease. It also emphasizes procedures rather than diseases and has a number of serious flaws in its classification and coding system. The ICD system, by contrast, was developed from attempts at establishing an internationally accepted list of causes of death and has undergone numerous revisions in the past 160 years, related to the various emphases placed on clinical, anatomic, biochemical, and perceived etiologic classification of disease at different times and different locations. There is still no official set of operational criteria for assigning the various diagnoses included in the ICD. In addition, the categories for symptoms, lesions, and procedures applicable to oral cavity conditions are limited and often outdated. Medicare and other third-party reimbursers are usually concerned only with diagnoses of those conditions that were actively diagnosed or treated at a given visit; concurrent problems not specifically addressed at that visit are omitted from the reimbursement diagnosis, even if they are of major health significance. The clinician, therefore, must address a number of concerns in formulating a diagnosis, selecting appropriate language for recording diagnoses on the chart, and documenting requests for third-party reimbursement.

The patient (or, when appropriate, a responsible family member or guardian) should also be informed of the diagnosis, as well as the results of the examinations and tests carried out. Because patients' anxieties frequently emphasize the possibility of a potentially serious diagnosis, it is important to point out (when the facts allow) that the biopsy specimen revealed no evidence of a malignant growth, the blood test revealed no abnormality, and no evidence of diseases, such as diabetes, anemia, leukemia, or other cancer, was found. Equally important is the necessity to explain to the patient the nature, significance, and treatment of any lesion or disease that has been diagnosed.

▼ MEDICAL REFERRAL (CONSULTATION) PROCEDURE

Patients for whom a dentist may need to obtain medical consultation include (1) the patient with known medical problems who is scheduled for either inpatient or outpatient dental treatment and cannot adequately describe all of his or her medical problems; (2) the patient in whom abnormalities are detected during history taking or on physical examination or laboratory study of which the patient is not aware; (3) the patient who has a high risk for the development of particular medical problems; and (4) the patient for whom additional medical information is required that may impact the provision of dental care or assist in the diagnosis of an orofacial problem.

When there is a need for a specific consultation, the consultant should be selected for appropriateness to the particular problem, and the problem and the specific questions to be answered should be clearly transmitted to the consultant in writing. Adequate details of the planned dental procedure, with an assessment of time, stress to the patient, and expected period of post-treatment disability, should be given, as well as details of the particular symptom, sign, or laboratory abnormality that gave rise to the consultation. The written request should be brief and should specify the particular items of information needed from the consultant. Importantly, requests for "medical clearance" should be avoided.

Medical risk assessment of patients before dental treatment offers the opportunity for greatly improving dental services for patients with compromised health. It does require considerably more clinical training and understanding of the natural history and clinical features of systemic disease processes than have been customarily taught in pre-doctoral dental education programs[1]; however, a partial solution to this problem has been achieved through undergraduate assignments in hospital dentistry and (most important) through hospital-based dental general practice dentistry, oral medicine, and oral and maxillofacial surgery residency programs. It is hoped that revisions in dental pre-doctoral curricula will recognize this need and provide greater emphasis on both the pathophysiology of systemic disease and the practical clinical evaluation and management of medically complex patients in the dental student's program.

▼ FORMULATING A PLAN OF TREATMENT AND ASSESSING MEDICAL RISK

The diagnostic procedures (obtaining and recording the patient's medical history, examining the patient, establishing a differential diagnosis, acquiring the additional information required to make a final diagnosis, such as relevant laboratory and imaging studies and consultations from other clinicians) outlined in the preceding pages are designed to assist the oral health care professional in establishing a plan of treatment directed at those disease processes that have been identified as responsible for the patient's symptoms. A plan of treatment of this type, which is directed at the causes of the patient's symptoms rather than at the symptoms themselves, is often referred to as rational, scientific, or definitive (in contrast to symptomatic, which denotes a treatment plan directed at the relief of symptoms, irrespective of their causes).

The plan of treatment (similar to the diagnostic summary) should be entered in the patient's record and explained to the patient in detail. This encompasses the procedure, chances for cure (prognosis), complications and side effects, and required time and expense. As initially formulated, the plan of treatment usually lists recommended procedures for the control of current disease as well as preventive measures designed to limit the recurrence or progression of the disease process over time. For medicolegal reasons, the treatment that is most likely to eradicate the disease and preserve as much function as possible (ie, the ideal treatment) is usually entered in the chart, even if the clinician realizes that compromises may be necessary to obtain the patient's consent to treatment. It is also unreasonable for the clinician to prejudge a patient's decision as to how much time, energy, and expense should be expended on treating the patient's disease or how much discomfort and pain the patient is willing to tolerate in achieving a cure.

The plan of treatment may be itemized according to the components of the diagnostic summary and is usually written prominently in the record to serve as a guide for the scheduling of further treatment visits. If the plan is complex or if there are reasonable treatment alternatives, a copy should also be given to the patient to allow consideration of the various implications of the plan of treatment he or she has been asked to agree to. Modifications of the ideal plan of treatment, agreed on by patient and clinician, should also be entered in the chart, together with a signed disclaimer from the patient if the modified plan of treatment is likely to be significantly less effective or unlikely to eradicate a major health problem.

Medical Risk Assessment

The diagnostic procedures described above are also designed to help the dentist (1) recognize significant deviations from normal general health status that may affect dental treatment; (2) make informed judgments on the risk of dental procedures; and (3) identify the need for medical consultation to provide assistance in diagnosing or treating systemic disease that may be an etiologic factor in oral disease or that is likely to be worsened by the proposed dental treatment. The end point of the diagnostic process is thus complex, and an evaluation of any special risks posed by a patient's compromised medical status under the circumstances of the planned anesthetic, diagnostic, or medical or surgical treatment procedures must also be entered in the chart, usually as an addendum to the plan of treatment. This process of medical risk assessment is the responsibility of all clinicians prior to any anesthetic, diagnostic, or therapeutic procedure and applies to outpatient as well as inpatient situations.

A routine of initial history taking and physical examination is essential for all dental patients as even the apparently healthy patient may on evaluation be found to have a history or examination findings of sufficient significance to cause the dentist to reevaluate the plan of treatment, modify a medication, or even defer a particular treatment until additional diagnostic data are available. To respect the familiar medical axiom *primum non nocere* (first, do no harm), all procedures carried out on a patient and all prescriptions given to a patient should be preceded by the dentist's conscious consideration of the risk of the particular procedure. Medical risk assessment, by establishing a formal summary in the chart of the specific risks that are likely to occur in treating a patient, ensures that continuous self-evaluation will be carried out by the clinician.

The dentist traditionally arrives at a decision for or against dental treatment for a medically complex patient by requesting the patient's physician to "clear the patient for dental care." Unfortunately, in many cases, the physician is provided with little information about the nature of the proposed dental treatment (type of treatment, amount of local anesthetics, use of epinephrine, etc.) and may have little (other than personal experience with dental care) on which to judge the stress (physical, psychological) likely to be associated with the proposed dental treatment. The response of a given patient to specific dental treatment situations may also be unpredictable, particularly when the patient has a number of disease processes and is taking multiple medications. In addition, the practitioner identified by the patient as his or her physician may not have adequate or complete data from all previous medical evaluations—requisite information to make an informed judgment on the patient's likely response to dental care. All too frequently, the dentist receives the brief comment "OK for dental care," which suggests that clearances are often given casually and subjectively rather than being based on objective physiologic data.

More importantly, the practice of having the patient "cleared" for dental care confuses the issue of responsibility for untoward events occurring during dental treatment. Although the dentist often must rely on the physician or a consultant for expert diagnostic information and for an opinion about the advisability of dental treatment or the need for special precautions, the dentist retains the primary responsibility for the procedures actually carried out and for the immediate management of any unexpected or unfavorable complication, that is, the safety of the patient. The dentist is most familiar with the procedures he or she is carrying out, as well as with their likely complications, but the dentist must also be able to assess patients for medical or other problems that are likely to set the stage for the development of complications. Therefore, physicians can only advise on what type of modifications are necessary to treat a patient; it is ultimately the responsibility of the treating dentist to ensure a patient's safety.

Several protocols have been developed to facilitate efficient and accurate preoperative assessment of medical risk.[17–21] Many of the earlier guides were developed for the assessment of risks associated with general anesthesia or major surgery and focus on mortality as the dependent variable; guides for the assessment of hazards associated with dental or oral surgical procedures performed under local or regional anesthesia usually take the same approach. Of these, the most commonly used is the American Society of Anesthesiologists (ASA) Physical Scoring System (Table 2).[22] Although scores such as the ASA classification are commonly included in the preoperative evaluation of patients admitted to hospitals for dental surgery, they use relatively broad risk categories, and their applicability to both inpatient and outpatient dental procedures is limited. The validity of preanesthetic risk assessment has also been questioned by several authors in light of data suggesting that the "demonstrable competence" of the anesthetist can also be a significant factor in anesthetic outcome.[23]

TABLE 1 Medical Complexity Status Classification and Protocol

Major categories
  MCS 0 Patients with no medical problems
  MCS 1 Patients with controlled or stable medical conditions
  MCS 2 Patients with uncontrolled or unstable medical conditions
  MCS 3 Patients with medical conditions associated with acute exacerbation, resulting in high risk of mortality

Subcategories
  A   No anticipated complications
  B   Minor complications are anticipated. "Minor complications" are defined as complications that can be successfully addressed in the dental chair.
  C   Major complications are anticipated. "Major complications" are defined as complications that should be addressed by a medical provider and may sometimes require a hospital setting.

Examples of different MCS categories
MCS–0
  A healthy patient

MCS–1A
  A patient with controlled hypertension
  (No modifications to routine dental care are necessary.)

MCS–1B
  A patient with epilepsy (petite mal) that is controlled with medications
  (The patient's epilepsy status is controlled, but if the patient has a seizure, it will pass without any interventions from the oral health care practitioner. It would be pertinent to avoid any dental treatment that may bring about a seizure.)

MCS–1C
  A patient with a penicillin allergy
  (The allergy will not change a stable condition, but if penicillin is given, a major complication may ensue.)

MCS–2A
  A patient with hypertension and a blood pressure of 150/95 mm Hg but without any target organ disease (see Chapter 13, "Diseases of the Cardiovascular System")
  (The patient's hypertension is by definition not controlled, ie, above 140/90 mm Hg. Yet this level of blood pressure, in an otherwise healthy patient, does not justify instituting any dental treatment modifications.)

MCS–2B (see Chapter 21, Diabetes Mellitus and Endocrine Diseases)
  A patient with diabetes mellitus and a glycosylated hemoglobin of 11%
  (Because of the patient's poor long-term glycemic control, the patient may be more susceptible to infections and poor wound healing. Dental modifications, such as possible antibiotics before a surgical procedure, may be indicated.)

MCS–2C
  A patient with uncompensated congestive heart failure
  (Because of the patient's compromised medical condition, it is important to avoid placing the patient in a supine position in the dental chair as this may induce severe respiratory problems for the patient.)

MCS–3
  A patient with unstable angina

TABLE 2   American Society of Anesthesiologists' Physical Status Classification

P1	A normal healthy person
P2	A patient with a mild disease
P3	A patient with a severe systemic disease that limits activity but is not incapacitating
P4	A patient with an incapacitating systemic disease that is a constant threat to life
P5	A moribund patient who is not expected to survive without the operation
P6	A declared brain-dead patient whose organs are being removed for donor puposes

In the event of an emergency, precede the number with an "e."
Adapted from American Society of Anesthesiologists.[22]

A more appropriate medical assessment, the Medical Complexity Status (MCS), was specifically developed for dental patients and has been used successfully for patients with medical problems ranging from nonsignificant to very complex diseases and conditions.[21] The MCS protocol is based on the premise that very few complications will arise during provision of routine dental care in an outpatient setting to patients with stable or controlled medical conditions. However, modification of dental care may still be necessary and should be based on the level of the anticipated complication. The MCS classification and protocol, with examples, are described in more detail in Table 1.

Modification of Dental Care for Medically Complex Patients

In this book, many different medical conditions are discussed, and protocols for the modification of dental care are suggested. Yet the assessment of risk to any medically complex patient follows similar guidelines. It is helpful to focus on the following three questions, which will change according to the severity of the underlying disease or condition:

(1) What is the likelihood that the patient will experience an adverse event due to dental treatment?
(2) What is the nature and severity of the potential adverse event?
(3) What is the most appropriate setting in which to treat the patient?

Each of these questions can be subdivided into smaller entities, which will facilitate the assessment of the patient.

The four major concerns that must be addressed when assessing the likelihood of the patient experiencing an adverse event are:

1. Possible impaired hemostasis
2. Possible susceptibility to infections
3. Drug actions and drug interactions

4. The patient's ability to withstand the stress and trauma of the dental procedure

Patients are designated to a MCS category at their initial dental visit, which may be modified during subsequent visits according to patients' changing medical status. Based on several critical items (MCS category, experience of the oral health care professional, the patient's ability to tolerate dental care, adequacy of the dental facility), a determination of where the patient is best treated should be made: (1) a non–hospital-based outpatient setting; (2) a hospital-based outpatient setting; (3) an inpatient short-procedure unit setting; or (4) an inpatient operating room setting. Most medically complex patients can be safely treated when the factors mentioned above have been addressed.

Monitoring and Evaluating Underlying Medical Conditions

Several major medical conditions can be monitored by oral health care personnel. Signs and symptoms of systemic conditions, the types of medications taken, and the patient's compliance with medications can reveal how well a patient's underlying medical condition is being controlled. Signs of medical conditions are elicited by physical examination, which includes measurements of blood pressure and pulse, or laboratory or other diagnostic evaluations. Symptoms are elicited through a ROS, whereby subjective symptoms that may indicate changes in a patient's medical status are ascertained. A list of the patient's present medications, changes in medications and daily doses, and a record of the patient's compliance with medications usually provide a good indicator of how a medical condition is being managed.[24] The combined information on signs, symptoms, and medications is ultimately used to determine the level of control and status of the patient's medical condition.

Oral Medicine Consultations

Both custom and health insurance reimbursement systems recognize the need of individual practitioners to request the assistance of a colleague who may have more experience with the treatment of a particular clinical problem or who has received advanced training in a medical or dental specialty pertinent to the patient's problem. However, this practice of specialist consultation is usually limited to defined problems, with the expectation that the patient will return to the referring primary care clinician once the nature of the problem has been identified (diagnostic consultation) and appropriate treatment has been prescribed or performed (consultation for diagnosis and treatment).

TYPES OF ORAL MEDICINE CONSULTATIONS

There are three categories of oral medicine consultations:

1. Diagnosis and nonsurgical treatment of orofacial problems. This includes oral mucosal disease, temporomandibular and myofascial dysfunction, chronic jaw and facial pain, dental anomalies and jaw

bone lesions, salivary hypofunction and other salivary gland disorders, and disorders of oral sensation, such as dysgeusia, dysesthesia, and glossodynia.

2. Dental treatment of patients with medical problems that affect the oral cavity or for whom modification of standard dental treatment is required, to avoid adverse effects

3. Opinion on the management of dental disease that does not respond to standard treatment, such as rampant dental caries or periodontal disease in which there is a likelihood that systemic disease is an etiologic cofactor

RESULTS OF THE CONSULTATION

In response to a consultation request, the diagnostic procedures outlined in this chapter are followed, with the referral problem listed as the chief complaint and with supplementary questioning (ie, history of the present illness) directed to the exact nature, mode of development, prior diagnostic evaluation/treatment, and associated symptomatology of the primary complaint. A thorough examination of the head, neck, and oral cavity is essential and should be fully documented, and the ROS should include a thorough exploration of any associated symptoms. When pertinent, existing laboratory, radiographic, and medical records should be reviewed and documented in the consultation record and any additional testing or specialized examinations should be ordered.

A comprehensive consultation always includes a written report of the consultant's examination, usually preceded by a history of the problem under investigation and any items from the medical or dental history that may be pertinent to the problem. A formal diagnostic summary follows, together with the consultant's opinion on appropriate treatment and management of the issue. Any other previously unrecognized abnormalities or significant health disorder should also be communicated to the referring clinician. When a biopsy or initial treatment is required before a definitive diagnosis is possible, and when the terms of the consultation request are not clear, a discussion of the initial findings with the referring clinician is often appropriate before proceeding. Likewise, the consultant usually discusses the details of his or her report with the patient unless the referring dentist specifies otherwise. In community practice, patients are sometimes referred for consultation by telephone or are simply directed to arrange an appointment with a consultant and acquaint him or her with the details of the problem at that time; a written report is still necessary to clearly identify the consultant's recommendations, which otherwise may not be transmitted accurately by the patient.

In hospital practice, the consultant is always advisory to the patient's attending dentist or physician, and the recommendations listed at the end of the consultation report are not implemented unless specifically authorized by the attending physician, even though the consultation report becomes a part of the patient's official hospital record. For some oral lesions and mucosal abnormalities, a brief history and examination of the lesion will readily identify the problem, and only a short written report is required; this accelerated procedure is referred to as a limited consultation.

The Dental/Medical Record: Organization, Confidentiality, and Informed Consent

The patient's record is customarily organized according to the components of the history, physical examination, diagnostic summary, plan of treatment, and medical risk assessment described in the preceding pages. Test results (diagnostic laboratory tests, radiographic examinations, and consultation and biopsy reports) are filed after this, followed by dated progress notes recorded in sequence. Separate sheets are incorporated into the record for the following: (1) summary of medications prescribed for or dispensed to the patient, (2) description of surgical procedures, (3) the anesthetic record, and (4) a list of the patient's problems and the proposed and actual treatment. This pattern of organization of the patient's record may be modified according to local custom and to varying approaches to patient evaluation and diagnostic methodology taught in different institutions.

ORGANIZATION

In recent years, educators have explored a number of methods for organizing and categorizing clinical data, with the aim of maximizing the matching of the clinical data with the "mental models" of disease syndromes referred to earlier in this chapter. The problem-oriented record (POR) and the condition diagram are two such approaches; both use unique methods for establishing a diagnosis and also involve a reorganization of the clinical record.

PROBLEM-ORIENTED RECORD

The POR focuses on problems requiring treatment rather than on traditional diagnoses.[25] It stresses the importance of complete and accurate collecting of clinical data, with the emphasis on recording abnormal findings rather than on compiling the extensive lists of normal and abnormal data that are characteristic of more traditional methods (consisting of narration, checklists, questionnaires, and analysis summaries). Problems can be subjective (symptoms), objective (abnormal clinical signs), or otherwise clinically significant (eg, psychosocial) and need not be described in prescribed diagnostic categories. Once the patient's problems have been identified, priorities are established for further diagnostic evaluation or treatment of each problem. These decisions (or assessments) are based on likely causes for each problem, risk analysis of the problem's severity, cost and benefit to the patient as a result of correcting the problem, and the patient's stated desires. The plan of treatment is formulated as a list of possible solutions for each problem. As more information is obtained, the problem list can be updated, and problems can be combined and even reformulated into recognized disease categories. The POR is helpful in organizing a set of complex clinical data about an individual patient, maintaining an up-to-date record of both acute and chronic problems, ensuring that all of the patient's problems are addressed, and ensuring that preventive as well as active therapy is provided. It is also adaptable to computerized patient-tracking programs. However, without any scientifically based or accepted nomenclature and operational criteria for the formulation of the problem list, data cannot be compared across patients or clinicians.

Despite these shortcomings, two features of the POR have received wide acceptance and are often incorporated into more traditionally organized records: the collection of data and the generation of a problem list. In dentistry, the value of the POR has been documented in orthodontics and hospital dentistry but otherwise appears to have attracted little attention in dental education. The value of a problem list for individual patient care is generally acknowledged and is considered a necessary component of the hospital record in institutions accredited by the Joint Commission on Accreditation of Healthcare Organizations.

THE SOAP NOTE

The four components of a problem—subjective, objective, assessment, and plan (SOAP)—are referred to as the SOAP mnemonic for organizing progress notes or summarizing an outpatient encounter.[26] The components of the SOAP mnemonic are as follows:

- S or Subjective: the patient's complaint, symptoms, and medical history (a brief review)
- O or Objective: the clinical examination, including a brief generalized examination, and then a focused evaluation of the chief complaint or the area of the procedure to be undertaken
- A or Assessment: the diagnosis (or differential diagnosis) for the specific problem being addressed
- P or Plan: the treatment either recommended or performed

The SOAP note is a useful tool for organizing progress notes in the patient record for routine office procedures and follow-up appointments. It is also quite useful in a hospital record when a limited oral medicine consultation must be documented.

For examples of SOAP notes, see the attached disc.

CONDITION DIAGRAM

The condition diagram uses a standardized approach to categorizing and diagramming the clinical data, formulating a differential diagnosis, prevention factors, and interventions (treatment or further diagnostic procedures).[27] It relies heavily on graphic or non-narrative categorization of clinical data and provides students with a concise strategy for summarizing the "universe of the patient's problems" at a given time. Although currently used in only a limited number of institutions, the graphic method of conceptualizing a patient's problems is supported by both educational theory and by its proven success with medical students.

CONFIDENTIALITY OF PATIENT RECORDS

Patients provide dentists and physicians with confidential dental, medical, and psychosocial information with the understanding that the information (1) may be necessary for effective diagnosis and treatment, (2) will remain confidential, and (3) will not be released to other individuals without the patient's specific permission. This information may also be entered into the patient's record and shared with other clinical personnel involved in the patient's treatment unless the patient specifically requests otherwise. Patients are willing to share such information with their dentists and physicians only to the extent that they believe that this contract is being honored.

There are also specific circumstances in which the confidentiality of clinical information is protected by law and may be released to authorized individuals only after compliance with legally defined requirements for informed consent (eg, psychiatric records and confidential HIV-related information). Conversely, some medical information that is considered to be of public health significance is a matter of public record when reported to the local health authorities (eg, clinical or laboratory confirmation of reportable infectious diseases such as syphilis, hepatitis, or acquired immune deficiency syndrome [AIDS]). Courts may also have the power to subpoena medical and dental records under defined circumstances, and records of patients participating in clinical research trials may be subject to inspection by a pharmaceutical sponsor or an appropriate drug regulatory authority. Dentists are generally authorized to obtain and record information about a patient to the extent that the information may be pertinent to the diagnosis of oral disease and its effective treatment. The copying of a patient's record for use in clinical seminars, case presentations, and scientific presentations is a common and acceptable practice provided that the patient is not identified in any way.

Conversations about patients, discussion with a colleague about a patient's personal problems, and correspondence about a patient should be limited to those occasions when information essential to the patient's treatment has to be transmitted. Lecturers and writers who use clinical cases to illustrate a topic should avoid mention of any item by which a patient might be identified and should omit confidential information. Conversations about patients, however casual, should never be held where they could possibly be overheard by unauthorized individuals, and discussion of patients with nonclinical colleagues, friends, family, and others should always be kept to a minimum and should never include confidential patient information.

INFORMED CONSENT

Prior consent of the patient is needed for all diagnostic and treatment procedures, with the exception of those considered necessary for treatment of a life-threatening emergency in a comatose patient.[28] In dentistry, such consent is more often implied than formally obtained, although written consent is generally considered necessary for all surgical procedures (however minor), for the administration of general anesthetics, and for clinical research.

Consent of the patient is often required before clinical records are transmitted to another dental office or institution. In the United States, security control over electronic transmission of patient record has since 1996 been governed by the Health Insurance Portability and Accountability Act (HIPAA). The creation and transmission of electronic records are an evolving process that is mainly dependent on technological advances and fast movement of the integration of electronic patient information. For timely updates on the HIPAA, see <http://www.cms.hhs.gov/HIPAAGenInfo/>. There may also be specific laws that discourage discrimination against individuals infected with HIV by requiring specific written consent from the patient before any HIV-related testing can be carried out and before any HIV-related information can be released to insurance companies, other practitioners, family members, and fellow workers.[29] Dentists treating patients whom they believe may be infected with HIV must therefore be cognizant of local law and custom when they request HIV-related information from a patient's physician, and they must establish procedures in their own offices to protect this information from unauthorized release. In response to requests for the release of psychiatric records or HIV-related information, hospital medical record departments commonly supply the practitioner with the necessary additional forms for the patient to sign before the records are released. Psychiatric information that is released is usually restricted to the patient's diagnoses and medications.

▼ SELECTED READING

American Society of Anesthesiologists. ASA Physical Status Classification System. Available at: http://www.asahq.org/clinical/physicalstatus.htm (accessed July 19, 2007)

Baum BJ. Inadequate trainging in the biological sciences and medicine for dental students. Impending crisis for dentistry. J Am Dent Assoc 2007;138:16–25.

Bewick V, Cheek L, Ball J. Statistics review 13: receiver operating characteristic curves. Crit Care 2004;8:508–12.

Bickley LS, Szilagyi PG. Bate's guide to physical examination and history taking. 9th ed. Philadelphia: Lippincott Williams and Wilkins; 2005.

Boland BJ, Wollan PC, Silverstein MD. Review of systems, physical examination, and routine tests for case-finding in ambulatory patients. Am J Med Sci 1995;309:194–200.

Burris S. Dental discrimination against the HIV-infected: empirical data, law and public policy. Yale J Regul 1996;13:1–104.

Exstrom S, Gollner ML. There is more than one use of SOAP. Subjective data, objective data, assessment and plan. Nurs Manage 1990;21:12.

Feinstein AR. ICD, POR, and DRG. Unsolved scientific problems in the nosology of clinical medicine. Arch Intern Med 1988;148:2269–74.

Findler M, Galili D, Meidan Z, et al. Dental treatment in very high risk patients with ischemic heart disease. Oral Surg Oral Med Oral Pathol 1993;76:298–300.

Glick M. Screening for traditional risk factors for cardiovascular disease: a review for oral health care providers. J Am Dent Assoc 2002;133:291–300.

Glick M. Rapid HIV testing in the dental setting. J Am Dent Assoc 2005;136:1206–8.

Glick M. Medical considerations for dental practice [CD-ROM]. Carol Streams (IL): Quintessence Publishing; 2005.

Glick M, Greenberg BL. The potential role of dentists in identifying patients' risk of experiencing coronary heart disease. J Am Dent Assoc 2005;136:1541–6.

Glick M. Did you take your medications? The dentist's role in helping patients adhere to their drug regimen. J Am Dent Assoc 2006;137:1636–8.

Glick M. Did you take your medications? The dentist's role in helping patients adhere to their drug regimen. J Am Dent Assoc 2006;137:1636–8.

Glick M. Informed consent—a delicate balance. J Am Dent Assoc 2006;137:1060–2.

Goodchild JH, Glick M. A different approach to medical risk assessment. Endod Top 2003;4:1–8.

Gortzak RA, Abraham-Inpijn L, ter Horst G, Peters G. High blood pressure screening in the dental office: a survey among Dutch dentists. Gen Dent 1993;41:246–51.

Hershey SE, Bayleran ED. Problem-oriented orthodontic record. J Clin Orthod 1986;20:106–10.

International Statistical Classification of Diseases and Health Related Problems: The ICD-10 Second Edition. World Health Organization, WHO Press. 2005. Geneva, Switzerland.

McCarthy FM, Malamed SF. Physical evaluation system to determine medical risk and indicated dental therapy modifications. J Am Dent Assoc 1979;99:181–4.

Michota FA, Frost SD. The preoperative evaluation: use the history and physical rather than routine testing. Cleve Clin J Med 2004;71:63–70.

Patton LL, Shugars DC. Immunologic and viral markers of HIV-1 disease progression: implications for dentistry. J Am Dent Assoc 1999;130:1313–22.

Prause G, Ratzenhofer-Comenda B, Pierer G, et al. Can ASA grade or Goldman's cardiac risk index predict peri-operative mortality? A study of 16,227 patients. Anaesthesia 1997;52:203–6.

Russell IJ, Hendricson WD, Harris GD, Gobert DV. A comparison of two methods for facilitating clinical data integration by medical students. Acad Med 1990;65:333–401.

Saah AJ, Hoover DR. "Sensitivity" and "specificity" reconsidered: the meaning of these terms in analytical and diagnostic settings. Ann Intern Med 1997;126:91–4.

Smeets EC, de Jong KJM, Abrahim-Inpijn L. Detecting the medically compromised dental patient in dentistry by means of the medical risk-related history. Prev Med 1998;27:530–5.

Vandersall DC. Concise encyclopedia of periodontology. Ames (IA): Blackwell Munksgaard; 2007.

Verdon ME, Siemens K. Yield of review of systems in a self-administered questionnaire. J Am Board Fam Pract 1997;10(1): 20–7.

For the full reference list, please refer to the accompanying CD ROM.

2

PHARMACOLOGY

JONATHAN A. SHIP, DMD
MICHAEL T. BRENNAN, DDS, MHS
MARTIN GREENBERG, DDS
PETER B. LOCKHART, DDS
SPENCER REDDING, DDS, MEd
VIDYA SANKAR, DMD, MHS
DAVID SIROIS, DMD, PhD
DAVID WRAY, BDS, MD

Pharmacotherapeutic interventions are frequently needed for the vast array of head, neck, and oral diseases encountered in oral medicine. The purpose of this chapter is to provide an overview of the conditions and diseases requiring drug therapies and an outline of drugs used for these conditions. The pharmacologic interventions are not intended to be an exhaustive list of all modalities for the condition described but rather a description of the most commonly used and clinically accepted medications available to the oral medicine practitioner. The categories for pharmacologic intervention are salivary gland disorders, pain, oral mucosal lesions, antibiotic prophylaxis for infective endocarditis and orthopedic joint replacements, antibiotics for the immunocompromised patient, and fungal and viral infections. Delivery of these medications is multimodal, including topical, injectable, and oral. Pharmacokinetic and pharmacodynamic characteristics and the side-effect profile of these medications dictate the circumstances under which they are prescribed and must be used in conjunction with other factors in selecting the appropriate drug: clinical diagnosis, age of the patient, dose, delivery format (eg, injectable vs topic vs oral), frequency of use, and concurrent other medical conditions (eg, liver or renal failure, allergies, history of gastrointestinal [GI] disorders, pregnancy or breast-feeding). All of these factors must be considered seriously by the prescribing practitioner. This chapter is not intended to provide all of the details on these pharmacotherapeutic options; for these details, the reader is referred to a drug textbook.

The vast majority of medications described in this chapter have not undergone extensive phase III US Food and Drug Administration (FDA)-sanctioned controlled clinical trials using hundreds of patients with the index condition and are not FDA approved for the index condition. Therefore, these drug interventions are considered to be "off-label" yet within the scope of practice of oral medicine and general dentistry. Although these oral-medical conditions cause significant impairment of oral and general quality of life and are commonplace, they have not attracted sufficient interest from drug companies for FDA-approved interventions. Importantly, these interventions are not considered experimental and are commonly used by oral medicine practitioners from around the world, and many have undergone scientific investigation with subsequent publication in peer-reviewed journals. They are accepted for use by oral health practitioners delivering oral-medical care and are part of the armamentarium necessary for care of both healthy and medically complex patients of all ages.

▼ MEDICATIONS FOR SALIVARY GLAND DISORDERS

Salivary Gland Infections

Acute and chronic bacterial salivary gland infections can develop when salivary function is diminished or completely reduced.[1] This occurs secondary to concurrent use of multiple medications (polypharmacy-induced salivary hypofunction), head and neck radiotherapy, chemotherapy, or the effects of certain medical problems (eg, Sjögren's syndrome). For more details, see Chapter 8, "Salivary Gland Diseases." Amoxicillin alone or in combination with clavulanate (Augmentin) is the drug of choice when the diagnosis of the salivary infection is bacterial (Table 1). Virally induced sialadenitis occurs less frequently and can be differentiated from bacterial sialadenitis by the lack of suppuration from the salivary gland duct and by constitutional symptoms of viral infections. Viral sialadenitis frequently occurs bilaterally (eg, mumps caused by cytomegalovirus), whereas bacterial sialadenitis is more often unilateral. Viral sialadenitis is treated with an antiviral drug (eg, acyclovir [ACV]; Table 2).

Salivary Gland Hypofunction

The treatment of salivary hypofunction, regardless of etiology, is with the use of nonpharmacologic topical sugar-free gums, mints, and lozenges; nonsugared beverages and salivary substitutes; and pharmacologic cholinergic agonists.[2,3] Sugar-free topical agents aid in salivary stimulation and can assist in augmenting existing salivary glands to produce saliva. Sipping fluids during the day and using salivary substitutes will help keep the mouth from becoming desiccated and will assist in speaking, chewing, and swallowing. The two

TABLE 1 Amoxicillin and Clavulanate for Salivary Gland Infections

Generic name	Amoxicillin and clavulanate potassium
Brand name	Augmentin
Indications	Treatment of bacterial salivary gland infections
Administration	Tablets
Prescription/OTC	Prescription
Dosage	500 mg tid for 5–7 d
Contraindications	Allergy to any penicillin, history of cephalosporin allergies, history of cholestatic jaundice/hepatic dysfunction, modify dosages in renal impairment, infectious mononucleosis
Common side effects	Rash, urticaria, diarrhea, nausea, vomiting, vaginitis
Unusual but important side effects	Hepatic dysfunction in elderly and after prolonged treatment, pseudomembranous colitis
Drug interactions	Cephalosporins: low incidence of cross-allergy Oral contraceptives: efficacy may be reduced Probenacid: decreases renal excretion and increases levels of Augmentin
Monitoring	Monitor for signs of anaphylaxis after first dose; monitor for renal, hepatic, and hematologic dysfunction after prolonged use. If severe diarrhea develops, stop immediately and consider pseudomembranous colitis.

TABLE 2 Systemic Antiviral Drugs for Recurrent Oral Herpes

Generic name	Acyclovir	Valacyclovir	Famciclovir
Brand name	Zovirax	Valtrex	Famvir
Indications	Herpes labialis, herpes zoster, mucocutaneous HSV, varicella-zoster, salivary viral infection		Herpes zoster, recurrent HSV in immunocompromised patients
Administration	Tablets	Tablets	Tablets
Prescription/OTC	Prescription	Prescription	Prescription
Dosage	RHL: 400 mg qid for 5 d HZV: 800 mg q4h for 7–10 d Mucocutaneous: 400 mg qid for 7–14 d HSV prevention: 200 mg tid or 400 mg bid Salivary viral infection: 400 mg qid for 7 d	RHL: 2 g bid for 1 d (separate doses by 12 h) HZV: 1 g tid for 7 d Salivary viral infection: 1 g tid for 7 d	HZV: 500 mg tid for 7 d Recurrent HSV in immunocompromised patients: 125 mg bid for 5 d
Contraindications	Hypersensitivity to acyclovir, valacyclovir	ANC < 500/mm^3, hemoglobin < 8 g/dL	Hypersensitivity to famciclovir
Common side effects	Lightheadedness; anorexia; hives; itching; rash; nausea; vomiting; increased liver enzymes, BUN, creatinine	Headache, dizziness, arthralgia, abdominal pain, vomiting, nausea	Headache, diarrhea, abdominal pain, nausea
Unusual but important side effects	Abdominal pain, erythema multiforme, toxic epidermal necrolysis	Hypersensitivity reactions, aggression, agitation, aplastic anemia, ataxia, erythema multiforme, hepatitis, leukocytoclastic vasculitis, photosensitivity, psychosis, renal failure, thrombocytopenia purpura	Arthralgia, rigors, upper respiratory infection
Drug interactions	Zidovudine, probenecid		Cimetidine, digoxin, probenecid, theophylline
Monitoring		Urinary analysis, BUN, creatinine, liver enzymes, CBC	CBC

RHL = recurrent herpes labialis. HZV = herpes zoster virus

pharmacologic agents most commonly used to stimulate salivary output are cholinergic agonists (pilocarpine, cevimeline), which increase salivary output through stimulation of major salivary gland cholinergic receptors (Table 3). Pilocarpine is a nonselective muscarinic agonist that can increase salivary output and reduce complaints of dry mouth.[4–6] Cevimeline is also a salivary stimulant[7,8] that has selective affinity for the M1 and M3 muscarinic receptors,[9] which are the prevailing subtypes in human salivary glands.[10] Both drugs are ineffective for the patient who has lost all major salivary gland tissue as a result of non–salivary gland–sparing head and neck radiotherapy.

Salivary Gland Hyperfunction (Sialorrhea)

Neurologic and neuromuscular conditions (eg, CVA, Down syndrome, central neurologic infections) can produce neuromuscular incompetence in swallowing function, resulting in salivary pooling in the anterior floor of the mouth and salivary spillage from the oral cavity, termed "drooling."[11] One mechanism for treating these patients is with medications that cause salivary hypofunction due to anticholinergic effects (see also Chapter 8, "Salivary Gland Diseases"). They must be used with caution as anticholinergic effects may adversely interfere with other concurrent medications, and excessive dry mouth may occur, predisposing the patient to the plethora of oral and pharyngeal complications of a dry mouth.

Several drugs to be considered are a scopolamine transdermal patch, propantheline, benztropine, atropine,

glycopyrrolate, and diphenhydramine hydrochloride.[12] Glycopyrrolate is a very commonly used drug for causing dry oral, nasal, and pharyngeal secretions prior to and during general anesthesia. Atropine is also readily available for sialorrhea (Table 4).

Protection of Salivary Glands during Head and Neck Radiotherapy

In addition to improvements in the planning and delivery of radiation therapy,[13–15] radioprotective agents may help limit radiation therapy–induced salivary gland damage. Amifostine, a cytoprotective agent, is FDA approved for xerostomia prevention in patients undergoing radiation treatment for head and neck cancers when the radiation port includes a substantial portion of the parotid glands (Table 5).[16–19] Amifostine is administered intravenously or subcutaneously 15 to 30 minutes prior to each fractionated radiation treatment.[20,21] In combination with intensity-modulated radiotherapy (IMRT), amifostine may provide even more effectiveness in preventing permanent salivary gland destruction. Major side effects include hypotension, nausea, vomiting, and dermatologic reactions.[22] Prevention of significant side effects include preemptive use of fluids and antiemetics and close supervision of vitals and evidence of skin reactions.[23–26] Cancer recurrence rates have not been greater in patients treated with amifostine compared with patients who did not receive cytoprotective agents, which suggests that the therapy may preferentially save healthy tissue.[20]

TABLE 3 Pilocarpine and Cevimeline for Salivary Hypofunction

Generic name	Pilocarpine hydrochloride	Cevimeline hydrochloride
Brand name	Salagen	Evoxac
Indications	1. Symptoms of dry mouth from salivary gland hypofunction caused by radiotherapy for cancer of the head and neck 2. Symptoms of dry mouth in patients with Sjögren's syndrome	
Administration	Tablets	Tablets
Prescription/OTC	Prescription	Prescription
Dosage	5 mg tid, adjusted to therapeutic response and tolerability. Usual dosage range is 15–30 mg daily, not to exceed 10 mg/dose. 12 weeks of uninterrupted therapy is recommended.	30 mg tid
Contraindications	Uncontrolled asthma, hypersensitivity to drug, acute iritis, narrow-angle (angle closure) glaucoma, acute hepatic impairment, uncontrolled asthma	
Common side effects	Sweating, nausea, rhinitis, diarrhea, chills, flushing, urinary frequency, dizziness, asthenia, headache, dyspepsia, lacrimation	
Unusual but important side effects	Visual disturbance, atrioventricular block, biliary contractions and obstruction, precipitation of renal colic	
Drug interactions	Beta-adrenergic antagonists: use with caution All drugs with parasympathomimetic effects Drugs intended to cause anticholinergic effects	
Monitoring	Monitor for significant side effects	

TABLE 4 Glycopyrrolate and Atropine for Sialorrhea

Generic name	Glycopyrrolate	Atropine
Brand name	Robinul	Sal-Tropine
Indications	Sialorrhea (drooling)	Sialorrhea (drooling)
Administration	Tablets	Tablets
Prescription/OTC	Prescription	Prescription
Dosage	1 mg 30–60 min before dental procedures 1 mg every 4–6 h as needed to inhibit drooling	0.4 mg 30–60 min before dental procedures 0.4 mg every 4–6 h as needed to inhibit drooling
Contraindications	Glaucoma, chronic constipation, ulcerative colitis, acute hepatic impairment	
Common side effects	Dry skin, constipation, dry throat, xerostomia, dry nose, dysphagia, drowsiness	
Unusual but important side effects	Fast/irregular heart beat, heatstroke in hot weather, difficulty urinating	
Drug interactions	Increased toxicity with antacids, effects of other anticholinergic agents may be increased with these drugs	
Monitoring	Monitor for significant side effects	

TABLE 5 Amifostine for Reduction of Xerostomia in Patients Undergoing Head and Neck Radiotherapy for Cancer

Generic name	Amifostine
Brand name	Ethyol
Indications	1. To reduce the incidence of moderate to severe xerostomia in patients undergoing postoperative radiation treatment for head and neck cancer, where the radiation port includes a substantial portion of the parotid glands 2. Can be used off-label to reduce the incidence of moderate to severe xerostomia in patients undergoing radiation treatment for head and neck cancer in combination with chemotherapy
Administration	IV infusion Subcutaneous injection
Prescription/OTC	Prescription
Dosage	200 mg/m^2 administered once daily as a 3 min IV infusion, starting 15–30 min prior to radiation treatment 500 mg reconstituted with 2.5 mL normal saline given subcutaneously in one or two injections, once daily, 15 min prior to radiation treatment
Contraindications	Sensitivity to aminothiol compounds, hypotension, dehydration
Common side effects	Transient hypotension, nausea, vomiting, flushing, chills, fever, dizziness, somnolence, hiccups, sneezing
Unusual but important side effects	Acute allergic reaction and anaphylaxis, hypocalcemia, short-term reversible loss of consciousness
Drug interactions	Amifostine should be used with caution in patients taking antihypertensive drugs or other drugs that could cause or potentiate hypotension
Monitoring	Adequate hydration prior to administration Blood pressure during and after administration Nausea and vomiting—antiemetic medication should be given prior to and in conjunction with amifostine (oral 5HT$_3$ receptor antagonists) Serum calcium levels in patients at risk of hypocalcemia (nephritic syndrome)

▼ MEDICATIONS FOR OROFACIAL PAIN

Overview

Orofacial pain is a common experience that can result from two general pathologic mechanisms, tissue injury and inflammation (ie, nociceptive pain), or from a primary lesion or dysfunction of the nervous system (ie, neuropathic pain). The first step in management of orofacial pain is the determination if the pain is primarily nociceptive or neuropathic or a combination of the two. This determination is critical to select the appropriate medication(s) whose mechanisms of action address the underlying pathologic process. Although this determination is often straightforward in instances of acute pain such as toothache or mucosal pain with proximate physical findings (tenderness, signs of injury and inflammation), the determination can be more challenging when there is persistent pain without a clear local cause (myofascial pain, neuropathic pain).

The two most common classes of analgesic medication are nonsteroidal anti-inflammatory drugs (NSAIDs) and opiate analgesics (or a combination of both classes), and these drugs represent the first line of treatment for acute orofacial pain. Chronic orofacial pain may require the use of additional analgesic medications (eg, muscle relaxants) and adjuvant analgesics (eg, anticonvulsants, antidepressants).

Nociceptive Orofacial Pain

There are three major categories of nociceptive orofacial pain: odontogenic conditions (eg, pulpitis, apical periodontitis), mucosal conditions (eg, ulcers, lichen planus, herpes simplex), and musculoskeletal conditions (eg, myofascial pain, temporomandibular joint capsulitis, and arthritis). With the limited exception of myofascial pain, these conditions result from an identifiable source of tissue injury and inflammation and nociceptor sensitization. Pain due to inflammation may also have an underlying infectious etiology; therefore, both anti-inflammatory analgesics and antimicrobial medications may be required. Myofascial pain may involve mechanisms that are both inflammatory and neuropathic and therefore may be treated with more than one class of medication. Nociceptive pain can play a role in the initiation and maintenance of persistent neuropathic orofacial pain, and treatment may require analgesics (for nociceptive pain), alone or in combination with medications for neuropathic pain.

Relief of nociceptive pain is achieved by the use of medications in two broad classes: NSAIDs and opiate analgesics. In each class, there are many medications to choose from, and most have similar mechanisms, pharmacokinetics, adverse effects, and drug interactions.

Neuropathic Orofacial Pain

Neuropathic pain results from a primary lesion or dysfunction[27–29] of the nervous system and does not require nociceptor activity. Neuropathic orofacial pains include the classic cranial neuralgias (trigeminal and glossopharyngeal) and postherpetic neuralgia. Other forms of neuropathic orofacial pain include stomatodynia (burning mouth), phantom tooth pain (atypical odontalgia), and traumatic nerve injuries. Neuropathic pain may follow inappropriate healing after tissue and/or nerve injury, yet local signs of injury often are not present. The hallmark signs of neuropathic pain are mechanical hyperalgesia and allodynia, constant burning or paroxysmal shooting pain, and, less commonly, constant aching or pressure pain. A minority of patients may not have pain as the primary manifestation of neuropathy but instead experience dysmorphic symptoms, paresthesia, and/or altered taste. Primary neuropathic pain may also have an inflammatory component, and effective management may require medications in multiple classes (ie, anti-inflammatory medications). The two major classes of adjuvant analgesics for neuropathic pain are the anticonvulsants and the antidepressants. Figure 1 illustrates a general approach to management of the major orofacial neuropathic pain conditions.

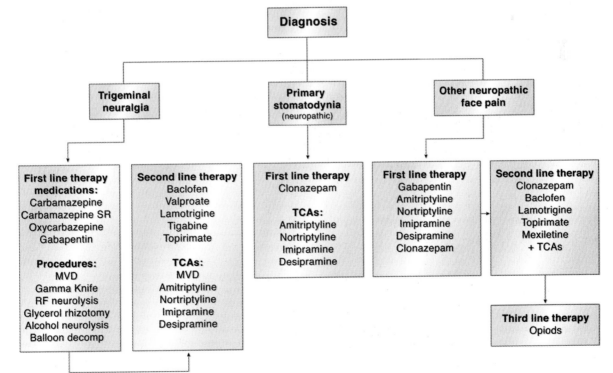

MVD = microvascular decompression , RF = radiofrequency, TCA = tricyclic antidepressants

FIGURE 1 Treatment Guidelines for Neuropathic Face Pain.

Specific Classes of Analgesics for Orofacial Pain

NONSTEROIDAL ANTI-INFLAMMATORY DRUGS

All NSAIDs block cyclooxygenase and prostaglandin synthesis, thereby reducing inflammation and pain due to nociceptor sensitization. The COX-2 isoform is induced at the site of injury and is chiefly responsible for inflammatory pain, yet nonselective NSAIDs (ibuprofen as the prototype) block both isoforms of cyclooxygenase. Inhibition of COX-1 isoforms is associated with the common side effects of NSAIDs: altered hemostasis and GI irritation. Tables 6 and 7 summarize common systemic NSAIDs used for mild to

TABLE 6 Systemic Nonsteroidal Anti-inflammatory Drugs

Generic name	Ibuprofen	Naproxen	Flurbiprofen	Ketoprofen	Celecoxib
Brand name	Advil Motrin	Naprosyn Aleve	Ansaid	Oruvail	Celebrex
Indications	Mild to moderate nociceptive pain				
Administration (many available in liquid form)	Tablets Liquid	Tablets Liquid	Tablets	Tablets	Tablets
Prescription/OTC	OTC and prescription	OTC and prescription	Prescription	Prescription	Prescription
Dosage	Tablets: 200–400 mg q4–6h Liquid: 20–40 mg/cc solution q4–6h	Tablets: 250–500 mg q8–12h Liquid: 125 mg/5 mL solution q8–12h	50–100 mg q8–12h	25–50 mg q6–8h	100–200 mg q12h
Contraindications	Allergy, renal or liver impairment, combination with anticoagulant or antiplatelet medications				
Common side effects	Dyspepsia, nausea, abdominal pain, headache, dizziness, somnolence, rash, elevated liver enzymes, constipation, fluid retention, peripheral edema, tinnitus, ecchymosis				
Unusual but important side effects	GI bleed and ulcers, myocardial infarction, dermatitis, stroke, thromboembolism, hypertension, congestive heart failure, nephrotoxicity, hepatotoxicity, bronchospasm, anemia, blood dyscrasias, Stevens Johnson syndrome, toxic epidermal necrolysis				
Drug interactions	Acetaminophen: increases risk of nephrotoxicity Aspirin: increases risk of bleeding, reduces cardioprotective effects Mycophenolate mofetil: increases risk of bleeding and nephrotoxicity Gabapentin: somnolence SSRIs: increase risk of bleeding Tacrolimus: increases risk of nephrotoxicity				
Monitoring	With chronic use: CBC, metabolic panel with liver enzymes				

TABLE 7 Systemic Nonsteroidal Anti-inflammatory Drugs

Generic name	Naproxen sodium	Diflunisal	Ketorolac	Meloxicam	Nabumetone
Brand name	Anaprox	Dolobid	Toradol	Mobic	Relafen
Indications	Mild to moderate nociceptive pain		Moderate to severe pain	Arthritis (TMD)	
Administration	Tablets	Tablets	Tablets IM injection	Tablets	Tablets
Prescription/OTC	Prescription	Prescription	Prescription	Prescription	Prescription
Dosage	Tablets: 550 mg bid	500 mg bid	Tablets: 10 mg q4–6h IM: 30 mg q6h (limit 5 d)	7.5–15 mg qd	1,000–2,000 mg q12–24h
Contraindications	Allergy, renal or liver impairment, combination with anticoagulant or antiplatelet medications				
Common side effects	Dyspepsia, nausea, abdominal pain, headache, dizziness, somnolence, rash, elevated liver enzymes, constipation, fluid retention, peripheral edema, tinnitus, ecchymosis				
Unusual but important side effects	Gastrointestinal bleeding or ulcer, myocardial infarction, dermatitis, stroke, thromboembolism, hypertension, congestive heart failure, nephrotoxicity, hepatotoxicity, bronchospasm, anemia, blood dyscrasias, Stevens-Johnson syndrome, toxic epidermal necrolysis				
Drug interactions	Acetaminophen: increases risk of nephrotoxicity Aspirin: increases risk of bleeding, reduces cardioprotective effects Mycophenolate mofetil: increases risk of bleeding and nephrotoxicity Gabapentin: somnolence SSRIs: increase risk of bleeding Tacrolimus: increases risk of nephrotoxicity				
Monitoring	With chronic use: CBC, metabolic panel with liver enzymes				

moderate orofacial pain. Unlike opiates, NSAIDs have an analgesic ceiling, and opiates may be required for more severe pain (see below).

Continuous or prolonged NSAID use for chronic orofacial pain should be considered carefully. NSAIDs are metabolized in the liver and can be nephrotoxic and hepatotoxic, with some producing blood dyscrasias. There is also a risk for bleeding and GI ulceration/irritation. Thus, routine complete blood count and metabolic panel should be ordered and monitored for signs of drug-related adverse effects. Finally, recent reports have shown that prolonged use of NSAIDs may reduce the cardioprotective effect of aspirin,[30] and alternate antiplatelet drugs, such as the ADP (adenosine diphosphate) inhibitors, should be considered if NSAID use cannot be discontinued.

OPIATE AND COMBINATION OPIATE-NSAID ANALGESICS

Nociceptive pain in the moderate to severe range may require additional analgesia by combining an opiate analgesic with an NSAID. The use of opiates alone for acute nociceptive pain is

TABLE 8 Opiate Analgesic Medications: Regular/Immediate Release

Generic name	Oxycodone	Codeine sulfate	Hydromorphone	Meperidine	Tramadol
Brand name	Roxicodone	Generic	Dilaudid	Demerol	Ultram
Indications	Moderate to severe nociceptive pain				
Administration	Tablets Liquid	Tablets	Tablets Liquid	Tablets IM/SC	Tablets
Prescription/OTC	Prescription	Prescription	Prescription	Prescription	Prescription
Dosage	Tablets: 5–30 mg q4h prn Liquid: 5 mg/5 mL, 20 mg/mL q4h prn	Tablets: 15–60 mg q4–6h prn	Tablets: 8 mg q3–4h prn Liquid: 1 mg/mL; 5–10 mL q4h prn	Tablets, IM, SC: 50–150 mg q3–4h	Tablets: 50–100 mg q4–6h prn
Contraindications	Allergy; watch combination with other opiates and sedatives; impaired renal or liver function; history of seizure disorder				
Common side effects	Hypotension, sedation and mental clouding, dizzy, constipation, nausea, urinary retention, itching, asthma, respiratory depression, palpitations, xerostomia; dependency with prolonged use, abuse potential				
Unusual but important side effects	Respiratory or CNS depression, shock, cardiac arrest, paralytic ileus, bradycardia				
Drug interactions	Alcohol: increases sedation Anticholinergics: increase constipation CNS depressants: increase sedation				
Monitoring	Therapeutic drug levels in chronic use, addiction behavior, functional and cognitive assessment with chronic use				

TABLE 9 Opiate Analgesic Medications: Extended Release

Generic name	Morphine sulfate ER	Oxycodone ER	Oxymorphone ER	Fentanyl
Brand name	MS Contin Oromorph	OxyContin	Opana ER	Duragesic Actiq
Indications	Continuous/chronic moderate to severe pain; extended release form			
Administration	Tablets	Tablets	Tablets	Transdermal Transmucosal
Prescription/OTC	Prescription	Prescription	Prescription	Prescription
Dosage	Tablets: 15–30 mg q8–12h	Tablets: 10–160 mg q12h	Tablets: start 5 mg PO q12h and titrate to effect	Transmucosal: 200 μg, titrate to effect Transdermal: 25–100 μg/h patch q72h
Contraindications	Allergy; watch combination with other opiates and sedatives; watch impaired renal or liver function; watch seizure disorder			
Common side effects	Hypotension, sedation and mental clouding, dizzy, constipation, nausea, urinary retention, itching, asthma, respiratory depression, palpitations, xerostomia; dependency with prolonged use, abuse potential			
Unusual but important side effects	Respiratory or CNS depression, shock, cardiac arrest, paralytic ileus, bradycardia			
Drug interactions	Alcohol induces sedation, anticholinergics induce constipation, most CNS depressants induce sedation.			
Monitoring	Therapeutic drug levels in chronic use, addiction behavior, functional and cognitive assessment with chronic use			

TABLE 10 Combination NSAID-Opiate Analgesic Medications

Generic name	Acetaminophen + codeine	Hydrocodone + acetaminophen	Hydrocodone + acetaminophen	Hydrocodone + ibuprofen
Brand name	Tylenol #3	Vicodin Lorcet Lortab Norco	Vicodin ES	Vicoprofen
Indications	Moderate to severe nociceptive pain			
Administration	Tablets and liquid			
Prescription/OTC	Prescription			
Dosage	Acetaeminophen: 300 mg Codeine: 30 mg q4–6h prn; 2 tablets q4–6h prn	Acetaminophen: 500 mg Hydrocodone: 5 mg q4–6h prn; 2 tablets q4–6h prn	Acetaminophen: 750 mg Hydrocodone: 7.5 mg q4–6h prn; 1 tablet q4–6h prn	Ibuprofen: 200 mg Hydrocodone: 7.5 mg q4–6h prn; 1 tab q4–6h prn
Contraindications	See contraindications for each drug in Tables 6–9			
Common side effects	See side effects for each drug in Tables 6–9			
Unusual but important side effects	See side effects for each drug in Tables 6–9			
Drug interactions	See interactions for each drug in Tables 6–9			
Monitoring	See monitoring for each drug in Tables 6–9			

TABLE 11 Combination NSAID-Opiate Analgesic Medications

Generic name	Oxycodone + acetominophen	Aspirin + codeine	Acetaminophen + propoxyphene napsylate	Ibuprofen + oxycodone
Brand name	Percocet Roxicet Endocet Tylox	Empirin #3	Darvocet	Combunox
Indications	Moderate to severe nociceptive pain			
Administration	Systemic tablets and liquid forms available			
Prescription/OTC	Prescription			
Dosage	Acetaminophen: 325–500 mg Oxycodone: 2.5–7.5 mg; 2 tablets q4–6h prn PO	Aspirin: 325 mg Codeine: 30 mg; 1–2 tablets q4–6hr prn PO	Acetaminophen: 500 mg Propoxyphene: 100 mg; 1 tablet q4h prn PO	Ibuprofen: 400 mg Oxycodone: 5 mg; 1 tablet PO qd–qid prn
Contraindications	See contraindications for each drug in Tables 6–9			
Common side effects	See side effects for each drug in Tables 6–9			
Unusual but important side effects	See side effects for each drug in Tables 6–9			
Drug interactions Monitoring	See interactions for each drug in Tables 6–9 See monitoring for each drug in Tables 6–9			

not recommended since its use would not address the underlying cause of the pain: inflammation. Opiate analgesics alone or in combination are routinely used for chronic, intractable pain. A variety of combination NSAID-opiate medications are effective for relief of moderate to severe nociceptive pain (Tables 8 to 11).

Opiate analgesics commonly used for orofacial pain share the common mechanism of agonist activity principally at the mu receptor and mimicking the effect of the endogenous pain-relieving chemicals dynorphin, enkephalin, and β-endorphin. Standard preparations have short half-lives and require repeat dosing every 3 to 4 hours; controlled-release formulations allow twice-daily dosing with improved compliance and baseline pain relief for chronic pain. Unlike NSAIDs, opiates do not have an analgesic ceiling, and increased pain relief can always be achieved by increased dose. However, side effects are also dose-dependent and can limit the maximum tolerated dose. Finally, one unique medication with mu-receptor actions and norepinephrine reuptake inhibition (similar to adjuvant tricyclic antidepressant analgesics for neuropathic pain) is tramadol (see Table 8). Due to the high abuse potential, most opiates are controlled substances with increased surveillance by regulatory agencies (eg, FDA).

ADJUVANT ANALGESICS: ANTICONVULSANT AND ANTIDEPRESSANT MEDICATIONS

This category of medications includes three major classes of medication: the anticonvulsants (Tables 12 and 13), antidepressants and anxiolytics (Tables 14 and 15), and muscle relaxants (Table 16).[7–11] Anticonvulsant and antidepressant classes generally affect conductance of ions that reduce neuronal excitability (Na, K, Ca, Cl). In these two classes, most clinical trials have used postherpetic neuralgia or diabetic neuropathy as index conditions, with a smaller number of studies investigating trigeminal neuralgia, fibromyalgia, and stomatodynia.[31–43] Muscle relaxants are generally centrally acting agents (ie, not at the neuromuscular junction). For most chronic orofacial pain conditions, the use of these medications is considered off-label, although there is considerable biomedical literature supporting their use.

TOPICAL ANALGESICS

Topical medications from several different drug classes can be very effective in providing local analgesia and can be mixed with mucosal adherent formulations for improved analgesia (Table 17). Few clinical trials have been conducted with these drugs, but there are minimal risks from topical use.[44–46] Nearly any drug that can have a local action can be formulated for topical use by a compounding pharmacy. There has been recent interest in using compounded anticonvulsants (gabapentin), antidepressants, NSAIDs, NMDA antagonists (N-methyl-D-aspartate), opioids, and α_2-adrenergic agonists, yet no standardized dosing guidelines are available.

▼ ANTIBIOTIC THERAPIES FOR IMMUNOCOMPROMISED PATIENTS

Overview

Numerous medical conditions are associated with suppression of the immune system either directly from an underlying disease or from medications used to manage the disease. A primary concern for an immunocompromised patient is the risk of poor healing and systemic involvement from a dental-alveolar infection. Therefore, consideration for appropriate antibiotics to treat an active dental infection is vital to avoid a systemic infection and enhance healing of an oral infection. In addition to treatment of active infections, prophylactic antibiotics prior to invasive dental procedures have been suggested for numerous medical conditions.[47]

TABLE 12 Anticonvulsant Medications for Chronic Orofacial Pain

Generic name	Carbamazepine	Gabapentin	Pregabalin
Brand name	Tegretol Carbatrol ER	Neurontin	Lyrica
Indications	Cranial neuralgias, traumatic neuropathy, neuropathic pain of undetermined origin, less commonly for stomatodynia (burning mouth)		
Administration	Tablets Suspension	Tablets Solution	Tablets
Prescription/OTC	Prescription	Prescription	Prescription

Dosage	Tablets: 200–600 mg bid Slow escalation
	Suspension: 100 mg/5 cc;
	    dosed as needed 200–600 mg bid
		Tablets: 300–1,200 mg tid Slow escalation
		Solution: 250 mg/5 mL;
		    dosed as needed 300–1,200 mg tid
			100 mg bid–tid Slow escalation

Contraindications	Allergy, hypersensitivity to TCAs, recent MAO
	    inhibitor use, marrow depression, impaired
	    liver or renal function, cardiac disease
		Allergy, congestive heart failure, impaired renal function, careful use in elderly	

Common side effects	Dizziness, drowsiness, nausea/vomiting, blurred
	    vision, allergic rash, cognitive impairment,
	    elevated liver enzymes, hyponatremia, ataxia
		Dizziness, somnolence, ataxia, peripheral edema,
		    nystagmus, nausea/vomiting, tremor, blurred
		    vision, dry mouth, headache, constipation,
		    rhinitis, cognitive impairment, dyspepsia
			Dizziness, somnolence, ataxia, peripheral
			    edema, weight gain, blurred vision,
			    cognitive impairment, dry mouth,
			    tremor, headache, constipation,
			    neuropathy, decreased platelets

Unusual but important side effects	Withdrawal seizures, arrhythmias, syncope,
	    anemia, pancytopenia, hepatitis, hyponatremia,
	    Stevens-Johnson syndrome (rare), erythema
	    multiforme (rare)
		Leukopenia, status epilepticus, withdrawal
		    syndrome, dyskinesia, depression, fractures
			Severe skin reactions, CHF exacerbation,
			    severe myalgia, thrombocytopenia

Drug interactions	CNS depressants: additive sedation Azole antifungals Doxycycline	CNS depressants: additive sedation	CNS depressants: additive sedation
Monitoring	Drug levels, CBC, metabolic panel, liver function	Drug levels, CBC	Drug levels, CBC

TABLE 13   Anticonvulsant Medications for Chronic Orofacial Pain

Generic name	Lamotrigine	Oxcarbazepine	Topirimate
Brand name	Lamictal	Trileptal	Topamax
Indications	Cranial neuralgias, traumatic neuropathy, neuropathic pain of undetermined origin, less commonly for stomatodynia (burning mouth)		
Administration	Tablets	Tablets	Tablets
Prescription/OTC	Prescription	Prescription	Prescription
Dosage	50–200 mg bid Slow escalation	300–600 mg bid Slow escalation	50–100 mg bid Slow escalation
Contraindications	Allergy, impaired renal or liver function, hypersensitivity to Tegretol (oxcarbazepine only)		
Common side effects	Dizziness, headache, ataxia, nausea, blurred vision, somnolence, rhinitis, rash, pharyngitis, vomiting, cough, insomnia, diarrhea, constipation, anxiety, seizures, weight loss, photosensitivity	Dizziness, somnolence, nausea, vomiting, ataxia, abnormal vision, dyspepsia, abnormal gait, hyponatremia, rash, confusion, nervousness, elevated liver enzymes, acne, alopecia, impaired concentration	Metabolic acidosis, dizziness, somnolence, fatigue, nervousness, paresthesias, cognitive impairment, ataxia, anorexia, nausea, depression, diarrhea, mood disturbances, tremor, taste changes, weight loss, insomnia
Unusual but important side effects	Stevens-Johnson syndrome, angioedema, multiple organ failure, pancytopenia, anemia, status epilepticus, sudden death, hepatic failure, pancreatitis	Leukopenia, thrombocytopenia, Stevens-Johnson syndrome	Metabolic acidosis, osteomalacia, osteoporosis, growth suppression (pediatrics), diabetes mellitus, leukopenia, anemia, psychosis, skin reaction, hepatotoxicity, fatal pancreatitis, deep vein thrombosis, pulmonary embolism
Drug interactions	CNS depressants (additive sedation), oral contraceptives, carbamazepine, azole antifungals		
Monitoring	Drug level, CBC, metabolic panel		

TABLE 14   Antidepressant and Anxiolytic Medications for Chronic Orofacial Pain

Generic name	Amitriptyline	Nortriptyline	Imipramine
Brand name	Elavil	Pamelor	Tofranil
Indications	Adjuvant for cranial neuralgias, primary for generalized neuropathic pain, stomatodynia (burning mouth)		
Administration	Tablets	Tablets	Tablets
Prescription/OTC	Prescription	Prescription	Prescription
Dosage	10–100 mg qhs	10–75 mg qhs	10–50 mg qhs
Contraindications	Allergy, recent MAO inhibitor use, myocardial infarction, cardiovascular disease, gastrointestinal/gastrourinary obstruction, urinary retention, narrow-angle glaucoma, seizure disorder, diabetes mellitus, asthma, impaired liver function, alcohol abuse, suicide risk, elderly patients		
Common side effects	Drowsiness, dry mouth, dizziness, constipation, blurred vision, palpitations, incoordination, increased appetite, nausea/vomiting, sweating, cognitive impairment, weakness, restlessness, insomnia, anxiety/agitation, urinary retention, rash, weight gain, libido changes/impotence, tremor, hypo-/hyperglycemia, paresthesias, photosensitivity		
Unusual but important side effects	Orthostatic hypotension, hypertension, syncope, arrhythmia, AV block, myocardial infarction, stroke, seizures, tardive dyskinesia (rare), pancytopenia, hallucinations, suicidality, hepatitis (rare), angioedema, hyperthermia		
Drug interactions	CNS depressants: additive depression; carbamazepine; erythromycin; pregabalin; tramadol		
Monitoring	Drug level, CBC, metabolic panel, ECG		

Dental-Alveolar Infections in Immunocompromised Patients

Patients with an underlying medical condition or receiving medical therapy that suppresses the immune system are at increased risk for a dental-alveolar infection. An important measure to quantitate the severity of suppression is the absolute neutrophil count (ANC). The ANC can be determined by adding the percentage of neutrophils and bands (immature neutrophils) and determining the absolute number of neutrophils from the total white blood cell (WBC) count. Therefore, if a patient had 2,000/μL WBCs with 45% neutrophils and 5% bands, then 50% of all WBCs are neutrophils, providing an ANC of $2,000/\mu L \times 0.5 = 1,000/\mu L$. An ANC < 500 μL represents a severe neutropenia with an increased incidence and severity of infection. It is important to recognize that the ANC is not an appropriate measure of

TABLE 15   Antidepressant and Anxiolytic Medications for Chronic Orofacial Pain

Generic name	Clonazepam	Doxepin	Duloxetine
Brand name	Klonopin	Generic	Cymbalta
Indications	Adjuvant for cranial neuralgias, primary medication for generalized neuropathic pain, stomatodynia (burning mouth)		
Administration	Tablets Transmucosal wafer	Tablets Topical (Table 17)	Tablets
Prescription/OTC	Prescription	Prescription	Prescription
Dosage	Tablets: 0.5–4 mg qhs or divided during day Wafer: 0.25 mg q6h prn	10–50 mg qhs	30–60 mg QD
Contraindications	Allergy, impaired liver function, impaired respiratory function	See Table 14	Allergy, recent use of MAO inhibitors, liver disease, chronic alcohol abuse, history of seizures and suicides, creatinine clearance < 30
Common side effects	Withdrawal syndrome, drowsiness, ataxia, cognitive impairment, constipation, diarrhea, dry mouth, headache, sleep changes, hypotension, rash	See Table 14	Nausea, diarrhea, constipation, dry mouth, insomnia, dizziness, somnolence, decreased appetite, sweating, decreased libido, higher blood pressure, elevated liver enzymes
Unusual but important side effects	Respiratory depression, neutropenia, hepatotoxicity, seizures	See Table 14	Suicidality, worse depression, seizures, hepatotoxicity, glaucoma (rare), hyponatremia, Stevens-Johnson syndrome
Drug interactions	CNS depressant: additive depression; azole antifungals; carbamazepine; erythromycin; opiates, pregabalin	See Table 14	CNS depressant: additive depression
Monitoring	CBC, metabolic panel	See Table 14	CBC, metabolic panel

TABLE 16   Muscle Relaxant Medications for Chronic Orofacial Pain

Generic name	Baclofen	Cyclobenzaprine	Carisoprodol	Tizanidine	Metaxalone
Brand name	Lioresal	Flexeril	Soma	Zanaflex	Skelaxin
Indications	Myofascial pain with muscle tension component				
Administration	Tablets	Tablets	Tablets	Tablets	Tablets
Prescription/OTC	Prescription	Prescription	Prescription	Prescription	Prescription
Dosage	10–20 mg bid	5–10 mg tid	350 mg tid–qid	8 mg q6–8h prn	800 mg tid/qid
Contraindications	Allergy, impaired renal function, seizure, stroke, diabetes, elderly patients	Allergy, recent MAO inhibitor use within 14 d, myocardial infarction, hyperthyroidism, arrhythmias, congestive heart failure, impaired liver function, elderly patients	Allergy, impaired renal and liver function	Allergy, impaired renal and liver function	Allergy, impaired renal and liver function, anemia
Common side effects	Drowsiness, dizziness, dry mouth, fatigue, hypotension, nausea, vomiting, nervousness, confusion, headache rash, pruritis				
Unusual but important side effects	CNS and respiratory depression, ataxia, seizures, hallucinations	Arrhythmias, seizures, myocardial infarction, hepatitis, anaphylaxis	Erythema multiforme, anaphylaxis	Hepatotoxicity, bradycardia, hypotension, hypertension	Anemia, leukopenia, hepatotoxicity
Drug interactions	CNS depressants: additive depression	CNS depressants: additive depression	CNS depressants: additive depression	CNS depressants: additive depression, oral contraceptives	CNS depressants: additive depression
Monitoring	None	None	None	Liver function	CBC, liver function

immunocompromise for many medications that impact the immune system (eg, prednisone and cyclosporine).

The use of appropriate antibiotics for the treatment of an oral infection (eg, periapical, periodontal, mucosal) is vital, particularly in an immunocompromised patient. The timing of definitive therapy (eg, endodontic therapy, extraction) is complicated in patients being treated with cytotoxic cancer therapy since the definitive treatment should be

TABLE 17 Topical Analgesic Medications for Orofacial Pain

Generic name	Lidocaine	Diphenhydramine	Benzocaine	Dexamethasone	Capsaicin	Doxepin
Brand name	Lidoderm patch Xylocaine Xylocaine Viscous	Benadryl	Topicale Hurricane Orajel	Generic	Zostrix	Zonalon
Indications	Mucosal pain Superficial facial pain	Mucosal pain	Mucosal pain Superficial facial pain	Mucosal pain	Stomatodynia Superficial neuropathic facial pain	Superficial neuropathic facial pain
Administration	Topical patch Topical gel Solution	Elixir	Topical gel	Elixir	Topical cream	Topical cream
Prescription/OTC	Prescription	Prescription	Prescription	Prescription	OTC Prescription	Prescription
Dosage	Patch: apply up to 12 h/d Gel 2.5%, 5%: apply q3–4h prn Solution: 2% (20 mg/mL); rinse and expectorate 10 cc q4–6h prn	12.5 mg/5 cc; rinse and expectorate 10 cc q4–6h prn	10%, 15%, 20% gel: apply qd–qid	0.5 mg/5 cc; rinse and expectorate 10 cc q4–6h prn Limited duration use	0.025%, 0.075% cream: apply tid/qid	5% cream, apply q3–4h, limit duration of use
Contraindications	Allergy	Allergy	Allergy	Allergy	Allergy	Allergy
Common side effects	Local erythema, edema, burning					
Unusual but important side effects	Anaphylaxis	Sedation if swallowed in large amounts	Methemoglobinemia	Limited with expectoration	Neurotoxicity	ECG abnormality CNS depression
Drug interactions	Acetaminophen	Limited with expectoration	Acetaminophen	Limited with expectoration	None	None
Monitoring	None	None	None	None	None	None

A 50:50 mixture of an elixir in Kaopectate, Maalox, or Carafate can be used to enhance local analgesia.

timed prior to chemotherapy-associated neutropenia or after WBC counts return to an appropriate level. The development of a dental-alveolar infection during chemotherapy-associated neutropenia is uncommon, which may be partly related to a decreased inflammatory response from deficient WBCs. Use of antibiotics and a delay of definitive dental treatment until WBC counts increase is a rational treatment plan for cancer patients with chemotherapy-associated neutropenia.

Topical antibiotics such as chlorhexidine (Table 18) are appropriate for localized gingival disease during neutropenia. The use of broad-spectrum antibiotics is appropriate for the treatment of active dental-alveolar infections in neutropenic patients. The antibiotic regimen should be based on appropriate susceptibility of bacterial isolates as aerobic and anaerobic bacterial culturing of draining pus should be completed in areas of infection in immunocompromised patients. Outpatient cancer patients or patients without severe neutropenia may respond well to oral antibiotics such as penicillin VK or amoxicillin, clindamycin, azithromycin, tetracycline, or Augmentin (Table 19). Hospitalized cancer patients with severe neutropenia should be placed on appropriate intravenous (IV) antibiotics for management (Table 20). Consultation is recommended with infectious

TABLE 18 Chlorhexidine for Treatment of Gingivitis

Generic name	Chlorhexidine rinse
Brand name	Peridex
Indications	Gingivitis
Administration	Rinse
Prescription/OTC	Prescription
Dosage	10 mL swish and expectorate bid
Contraindications	Allergy
Common side effects	Dental staining, calculus build-up, taste changes
Drug interactions	None
Monitoring	Clinical efficacy

TABLE 20 Intravenous Antibiotics for Intraoral Bacterial Infections

Generic name	Vancomycin HCl	Imipenem/cilastatin
Brand name	Vancocin HCl, Vancoled	Primaxin
Indications	Bacterial infection	Bacterial infection
Administration	IV	IM or IV
Prescription/OTC	Prescription	Prescription
Dosage	500 mg IV q12h	250–1,000 mg q6–8h
Contraindications	Documented hypersensitivity, impaired renal function	Documented hypersensitivity
Common side effects	Hypotension, fever, nausea, chills, eosinophilia, rash	Thrombocytosis, diarrhea, rash, phlebitis, elevated liver function tests, elevated BUN and creatinine
Drug interactions	Cidofovir, clofarabine, gallium nitrate	Ganciclovir
Monitoring	Efficacy, serum levels of vancomycin	Efficacy, renal and hepatic function

TABLE 19 Oral Antibiotics for Intraoral Bacterial Infections

Generic name	Penicillin VK	Amoxicillin	Clindamycin	Tetracycline	Azithromycin
Brand name	V-Cillin K, Veetids	Amoxil Trimox	Cleocin		Zithromax
Indications			Bacterial infection		
Administration			Tablets		
Prescription/OTC			Prescription		
Dosage	500 mg every 6–8 h × 7–10 d	250–500 mg every 8 h × 7 d	300 mg qid × 7 d	250–500 mg q 6 h × 7 d	500 mg day 1, then 250 mg for days 2–5
Contraindications			Documented hypersensitivity		
Common side effects			Rash, nausea, abdominal pain, diarrhea, photosensitivity (tetracycline)		
Unusual but important side effects			Acute allergic reaction and anaphylaxis		
Drug interactions	Chloroquine phosphate, exenatide, methotrexate	Probenecid, chloramphenicol, macrolides, sulfonamides, tetracylines	Exenatide, contraceptives, mycophenolate, neuromuscular blockers	Acitretin, retinoids, aminolevulinic acid, hydroquinone, methoxsalen	Warfarin, macrolides, fluconazole, efavirenz
Monitoring			Clinical efficacy		

disease or oncology specialists regarding the appropriateness of monotherapy (eg, vancomycin or imipenem) or the necessity of multiple antibiotics to manage multiple infections that neutropenic patients may be experiencing.

Prophylactic Antibiotics in Immunocompromised Patients

The use of antibiotics prior to an invasive dental procedure has been proposed for a variety of immunocompromised conditions, including neutropenic cancer patients, patients with end-stage renal disease treated with hemodialysis, organ transplant patients, and poorly controlled diabetes (see Chapter 21, "Diabetes Mellitus and Endocrine Diseases"). The evidence to support the practice of antibiotic prophylaxis prior to invasive dental procedures in these populations is frequently lacking, and recommendations are often based on medicolegal concerns by the clinician. Additionally, the negative consequences of repeated antibiotic use, such as increased antibiotic resistance, costs, and potential allergic reactions, must be weighed against the perceived benefit of infection prevention.

NEUTROPENIC CANCER PATIENTS

Patients with cancer may be neutropenic from the underlying cancer or the chemotherapeutic regimen. Studies have shown that viridans group streptococci (VGS) can cause approximately 60% of bacteremia, with a mortality rate of ≈20%.[48–50] The primary locations for VGS include the GI tract, skin, and oral cavity. Despite the lack of substantial scientific evidence, it is generally recommended that prophylactic antibiotics be used before an invasive dental procedure for an ANC < 1,000 μL.[51] The rationale for this recommendation is that the oral cavity is a common source of bacteremia. Furthermore, chronic gingival and periodontal diseases may place a patient at greater risk of bacteremia than infrequent invasive dental procedures. A delay in elective dental procedures while a patient is neutropenic should be considered. Additionally, cancer patients receiving chemotherapy often have a central venous catheter in place for delivery of chemotherapeutic agents. Antibiotic prophylaxis prior to invasive dental procedures is controversial and likely of no value. This should be discussed with the patient's oncologist.[47] The use of the American Heart Association (AHA) recommendations for antibiotic prophylaxis for cardiac conditions is reasonable (Table 21).

HEMODIALYSIS

Vascular access sites are used for patients receiving hemodialysi, and are at increased risk of becoming infected. Treatment may require hospitalization, systemic antibiotics, and possible shunt removal. The most common infectious agents are gram-positive bacteria, followed by gram-negative and polymicrobial bacteria. Bacteria of oral origin can infrequently be the etiology of vascular access site infections.[52] Infective endocarditis can also result from vascular access

infection, with up to 25% requiring heart valve replacement. The need for antibiotic prophylaxis for the prevention of shunt infections is controversial, and, currently, there are no guidelines. AHA guidelines do not discuss whether antibiotic prophylaxis is recommended for hemodialysis shunts, whereas other dental references give conflicting recommendations.[47,53–55] No well-designed clinical trials have been published in these patients to provide further guidance. Therefore, the best strategy is to consult with the patient's nephrologist to determine if prophylactic antibiotics are deemed necessary.

ORGAN TRANSPLANTATION

To prevent rejection of organ transplants, patients are routinely placed on immunosuppressive medications. These medications may include long-term prednisone, mycophenolate mofetil, cyclosporine, or azathioprine, which function by moderating the T-cell response of the patient to prevent graft rejection. An increased risk of infection is one side effect of these immunosuppressive medications. The use of antibiotic prophylaxis for invasive dental procedures in these patients is controversial.[47] Discussion with the patient's transplant physician regarding the use of antibiotics is recommended. It is reasonable to use prophylactic antibiotics in the first few months after transplantation, when the patient has the highest risk of infection and acute graft rejection. The use of antibiotics recommended by the AHA for prevention of infective endocarditis is reasonable (see Table 21).

TABLE 21   Regimens for a Dental Procedure[37]

Situation	Agent	Regimen—Single Dose 30–60 minutes before procedure	
Oral	Amoxicillin	Adults 2 gm	Children 50 mg/kg
Unable to take oral medication	Ampicillin or	2 g IM or IV*	50 mg/kg IM or IV
	Cefazolin or ceftriaxone	1 g IM or IV	50 mg/kg IM or IV
Allergic to penicillins or ampicillin Oral	Cephalexin**† or	2 g	50 m/kg
	Clindamycin	600 mg	20 mg/kg
	Azithromycin or clarithromycin	500 mg	15 mg/kg
Allergic to penicillins or ampicillin and unable to take oral medication	Cefazolin or ceftriaxone†	1 g IM or IV	50 mg/kg IM or IV
	Clindamycin phosphate	600 mg IM or IV	20 mg/kg IM or IV

*IM – intramuscular; IV – intravenous.
**or other first or second generation oral cephalosporin in equivalent adult or pediatric dosage.
†Cephalosporins should not be used in an individual with a history of anaphylaxis, angioedema, or urticaria with penicillins or ampicillin.[78a]

▼ ANTIBIOTIC PROPHYLAXIS FOR INFECTIVE ENDOCARDITIS AND PROSTHETIC JOINTS

Overview

Bacteria commonly enter the circulation from the oral cavity, and there is a long-standing concern about the potential for pathogenic species to cause distant site infections such as infective endocarditis (IE). Early reports led to the 1955 AHA recommendations for prophylactic antibiotics to prevent IE, which set the standard of care for the past 50 years in the United States. However, controversy surrounds this practice because of the lack of a definitive clinical trial or other scientific data to support these recommendations.[34]

There is evidence demonstrating a benefit from the short-term use of antibiotics at the time of device placement (referred to as primary antibiotic prophylaxis).[56,57] However, there is increasing awareness of a lack of evidence to support the practice of secondary prophylaxis—the use of antibiotic prophylaxis to reduce a procedure-related bacteremia that could result in IE. Dental procedures have been the central focus of the issue of secondary antibiotic prophylaxis since the initial AHA recommendations, but there has never been a prospective, randomized, clinical trial to assess efficacy. As a result, journals and textbooks continue to focus on dental procedures, with or without an emphasis on dental disease and poor oral hygiene.[58–62] The AHA recommendations have been sustained for several reasons: (1) the Focal Infection Theory, which was particularly popular in North America in the early 1900s; (2) the universal mortality from IE in the preantibiotic era and the current levels of morbidity and mortality today; (3) data from early animal studies attempting to replicate IE in humans; (4) the high incidence of VGS, a common component of the oral flora, as the cause of IE; (5) the high frequency of VGS bacteremia following dental office procedures;[63,64] and (6) hundreds of poorly documented case reports of IE that implicated dental procedures. The prognosis for patients with IE has improved dramatically in the antibiotic era, yet a high morbidity and mortality remain for some cardiac patient populations.

In recent decades, there has been a proliferation of non–evidence-based use of the AHA antibiotic regimen as prophylaxis for a wide variety of patient populations who are felt to be at risk for distant site infections in the dental office setting.[47,65,66] For example, it is a common clinical practice to prophylax patients with a variety of disorders (eg, renal dialysis shunts, central nervous system catheters,[67] systemic lupus erythematosus, poorly controlled diabetes) with antibiotics due to an unsubstantiated concern about bacteremia from dental procedures.[68–73] In addition, oral bacteria have been reported to cause infection of vascular grafts and cardiac pacemakers and put immunosuppressed patients at risk as well. Antibiotic prophylaxis prior to dental procedures has been proposed for over 20 patient populations, yet a thorough review of this practice suggests that it is of little or no value, with the possible exception of AHA-defined high-risk cardiac patients.[47,74,75] Accordingly, the AHA recommendations are aimed specifically at the prevention of IE and are not intended for other medical conditions. The AHA has reviewed the issue of antibiotic prophylaxis for nonvalvular cardiovascular devices and, in general, does not support the use of prophylaxis in these situations.[76] Currently, there are official recommendations for only two patient populations: cardiac abnormalities[74,77] and prosthetic joints.[78]

Cardiac Patients

The AHA recommendations for the dental management of patients with cardiac abnormalities are universally recognized in the United States and referred to by virtually all publications on the subject. These guidelines define patients at risk (Table 22), the dental procedures most likely to put patients at risk (Table 23), and the appropriate antibiotic regimen (see Table 21). All previous AHA recommendations have contained changes from previous versions, suggesting that there is still uncertainty as to which dental procedures and which patients should be covered. The 2007 recommendations contain significant changes over the 1997 document in both the dental procedures and patients recommended for coverage. These new guidelines are not intended for other medical conditions such as prosthetic joints.[47]

Prosthetic Joint Patients

Since the mid-1970s, over 90 cases have been reported of joint infection from dental procedures in patients who have prosthetic joints, but an analysis of these case reports suggests that these infections arise from nonoral bacteria and from nonoral sites. Over 60% of late joint infections are caused by *Staphylococcus epidermidis* or *Staphylococcus aureus*.[79] It has

---

TABLE 22 Cardiac Conditions Associated with the Highest Risk of Adverse Outcome from Endocarditis for Which Prophylaxis with Dental Procedures Is Recommended[37]

- Prosthetic cardiac valve
- Previous IE
- Congenital heart disease (CHD)#
    - o Unrepaired cyanotic CHD, including palliative shunts and conduits
    - o Completely repaired congenital heart defect with prosthetic material or device, whether placed by surgery or by catheter intervention, during the first 6 months after the procedure*
    - o Repaired CHD with residual defects at the site or adjacent to the site of a prosthetic patch or prosthetic device (which inhibit endothelialization)
- Cardiac transplantation recipients who develop cardiac valvulopathy

#Except for the conditions listed above, antibiotic prophylaxis is no longer recommended for any other form of CHD.
*Prophylaxis is recommended because endothelialization of prosthetic material occurs within 6 months after the procedure.[78a]

TABLE 23 Dental Procedures for which Endocarditis Prophylaxis is Recommended for Patients in Table 22[37]

All dental procedures that involve manipulation of gingival tissue or the periapical region of teeth or perforation of the oral mucosa*

*The following procedures and events do not need prophylaxis: routine anesthetic injections through noninfected tissue, taking dental radiographs, placement of removable prosthodontic or orthodontic appliances, adjustment of orthodontic appliances, placement of orthodontic brackets, shedding of deciduous teeth and bleeding from trauma to the lips or oral mucosa.[78a]

TABLE 24 Patients at Potential Increased Risk of Hematogenous Total Joint Infection

Immunocompromised/immunosuppressed patients
- Inflammatory arthropathies: rheumatoid arthritis, systemic lupus erythematosus
- Disease-, drug-, or radiation-induced immunosuppression

Other patients
- Insulin-dependent (type 1) diabetes
- First 2 years following joint placement
- Previous prosthetic joint infections
- Malnourishment
- Hemophilia

Adapted from reference 76.

been proposed that oral bacteria cause between 6 and 13% of cases of prosthetic joint infections, but few, if any, of the case reports are well documented.[47]

In 1997, an advisory statement was agreed upon by the American Dental Association (ADA) and American Academy of Orthopedic Surgeons (AAOS), which attempted to define specific orthopedic populations at risk and the dental procedures that put these patients at risk.[76] This document states that "it is advisable to consider" antibiotic coverage for several groups of patients (Table 24). It also gives a list of dental procedures of concern and suggested antibiotic regimens that were adopted from the 1997 AHA recommendations for cardiac patients (Table 25). This statement was intended to reduce the number of patients who were receiving prophylactic antibiotics and focus attention on those patients most likely to benefit. The issue is still controversial, with some authors emphasizing the ADA/AAOS guidelines and others reporting the absence of scientific evidence and the potential greater risk of life-threatening drug reactions outweighing any benefit. To further complicate the issue, case reports exist for both cardiac and hip prosthesis infections following dental procedures, despite appropriate antibiotic prophylaxis.

General Considerations

Oral bacterial pathogens may be responsible for ≈50% of cases of IE and some cases of prosthetic joint infections, yet it is unclear to what extent this results from dental office procedures versus bacteremia from routine daily activities such as tooth brushing and chewing food.[80–82] There is very little evidence demonstrating that dental office procedures cause distant site infections. Therefore, the driving force behind the practice of antiobiotic prophylaxis is the devastating impact of a bacteremia-induced infection of a cardiac valve, prosthetic joint, or indwelling medical device.[83] Given the high frequency of bacteremias from 'natural' causes, the likelihood of distant site infections occurring in the dental office setting is remote.

There are several concerns with the practice of antibiotic prophylaxis, aside from the cost to the health care system and the lack of substantiating scientific evidence. There is a risk of a fatal allergic reaction, albeit small, and the concern for ongoing emergence of resistant bacterial pathogens from the inappropriate use of antibiotics in general.[84] Other issues include the problem of determining who is at risk for

TABLE 25 Suggested Antibiotic Prophylaxis Regimens for Orthopedic Joint Patients

Patients not allergic to penicillin: cephalexin, cephradine, or amoxicillin
    2 g orally 1 hour prior to dental procedure

Patients not allergic to penicillin and unable to take oral medications: cefazolin or ampicillin
    Cefazolin 1 g or ampicillin 2 g IM or IV 1 hour prior to the procedure

Patients allergic to penicillin: clindamycin
    600 mg orally 1 hour prior to the dental procedure

Patients allergic to penicillin and unable to take oral medications: clindamycin
    600 mg IV 1 hour prior to the procedure

Adapted from reference 76.

distant site infections, which dental procedures and bacteria are of concern, and the reported low compliance rate on the part of physicians and dentists. Clearly, much of what drives this practice is long-standing dogma, practice habit, and medicolegal concerns.[66]

▼ MEDICATIONS FOR ORAL LESIONS

Ulcerations

RECURRENT APHTHOUS STOMATITIS

The goal of the management of recurrent aphthous stomatitis (RAS) is chiefly to reduce pain and decrease the size and healing time of the lesions with topical medication.[85] These drugs are generally placed into two categories: analgesics (see Table 17) and corticosteroids (Table 26).[86] Injectable corticosteroids are also referred to as intralesional corticosteroids (Table 27) and are useful for large and painful lesions. In severe minor RAS or major RAS, use of systemic drugs may be considered to prevent lesion formation or at least to reduce the number of lesions.[87] Systemic corticosteroids are usually prescribed in short courses and are reserved for severe outbreaks or after ulcers have not responded to regular use of topical or injectable drugs (Table 28). Continuous use of systemic corticosteroids can lead to the development of significant side effects and should be avoided in managing localized diseases such as RAS. Drugs for preventive therapy include colchicine (Table 29),[88] pentoxifylline (see Table 29),[89] and thalidomide (Table 30).[90] Thalidomide has severe side effects, including deforming birth defects, and must only be reserved for the most severe cases, which do not respond to any other therapy. Thalidomide may only be prescribed under the carefully regulated conditions of the STEPS (System for Thalidomide Education and Prescribing Safety) program.[90] In severe cases, azathioprine can also be used as an adjunct to systemic corticosteroid therapy (Table 31).

BEHÇET'S SYNDROME

The treatment of Behçet's syndrome is similar to the treatment of severe or major RAS. Topical corticosteroids (see Table 26) are used to manage oral lesions. Colchicine (see Table 29), pentoxifylline (see Table 29), thalidomide (see Table 30), and dapsone (Table 32) are helpful to treat both mucocutaneous lesions and systemic manifestations of the disease.[91,92] Immunosuppressive drugs such as azathioprine (see Table 31) are used to manage severe cases.[93]

Vesiculobullous Conditions

PEMPHIGUS VULGARIS

The principal treatment for pemphigus vulgaris is systemic corticosteroids at doses of 1 to 2 mg/kg/d (see Table 28). Adjuvant therapy is frequently required with immuno-

suppressive drugs, such as azathioprine (see Table 31), mycophenolate mofetil (see Table 32), or cyclophosphamide (see Table 32), to reduce corticosteroid dosages and to reduce mortality from the side effects of systemic corticosteroids.[94] Maintenance of remission can often be achieved with topical corticosteroids (see Table 26), allowing reduction of

TABLE 27 Injectable Corticosteroids for Ulcerative and Vescul obullous Oral Mucosal Diseases

Generic name	Triamcinolone	Dexamethasone
Brand name	Kenalog	Decadron
Indications	Severe recurrent aphthous stomatitis Major aphthous stomatitis Erosive lichen planus	
Administration	Intralesional injection	
Prescription/OTC	Prescription	
Dosage	10 mg/mL Inject 0.1 cc/1 cm lesion	4 mg/mL Inject 0.1 cc/1 cm lesion
Contraindications	Hypersensitivity to corticosteroids, systemic fungal infection, live vaccines, active tuberculosis	
Common side effects	Candidiasis, hyperglycemia	
Unusual but important side effects	Peptic ulceration with perforation, osteoporosis, impaired wound healing, mucosal atrophy	
Drug interactions	Increased insulin requirement	
Monitoring	Blood pressure Bone density before and during prolonged treatment	

TABLE 26 Topical Corticosteroids for the Treatment of Ulcerative and Vesiculobullous Oral Mucosal Diseases

Generic name	Beclomethasone	Betamethasone	Clobetasol	Halobetasol	Fluocinonide
Brand Name	QVAR oral inhaler	Diprolene	Temovate	Ultravate	Lidex
Indications		Severe recurrent aphthous stomatitis Behçet's syndrome Pemphigus vulgaris Pemphigoid			
Administration	Metered inhaler spray topically to mucosal lesions	Topical intraoral cream or gel; soluble tablets as a mouthwash	Topical intraoral cream or gel	Topical intraoral cream or ointment	Topical intraoral cream
Prescription/OTC	Prescription	Prescription	Prescription	Prescription	Prescription
Dosage	50–100 µg sprayed bid onto oral lesion	0.1% cream or 0.05% gel applied thinly bid; 0.5 mg 2-4 times daily as a mouthwash	0.05% cream or gel applied thinly bid	0.05% cream or ointment applied thinly bid	0.05% cream applied thinly bid
Contraindications		Untreated infections			
Common side effects		Oral candidiasis			
Unusual but important side effects		Adrenal suppression if doses exceeded			
Drug interactions		Unusual with topical preparations			
Monitoring		Monitor for superinfection, especially candidiasis			

TABLE 28 Systemic Corticosteroids for Ulcerative and Vesiculobullous Oral Mucosal Diseases

Generic name	Prednisone
Brand name	Deltasone
Indications	Severe recurrent aphthous stomatitis Behçet's syndrome Pemphigus vulgaris Pemphigoid Erythema multiforme
Administration	Tablets
Prescription/OTC	Prescription
Dosage*	1. 30–40 mg daily after breakfast for 4–5 d 2. 1–2 mg/kg/d after breakfast until disease controlled 3. 1–2 mg/kg/d, then maintenance of 2.5–15 mg daily 4. 20–40 mg daily for 7–10 d at onset of lesions or until lesions resolve 5. 60 mg daily for 2 d, 50 mg daily for 2 d, 40 mg daily for 2 d, 30 mg daily for 2 d, 20 mg daily for 2 d, 10 mg daily for 2 d
Contraindications	Hypersensitivity to corticosteroids Systemic infection (unless specific antimicrobial therapy given) Peptic disease (unless proton pump inhibitor given) Live vaccines
Common side effects	Dyspepsia, candidiasis, myopathy, osteoporosis, adrenal suppression, Cushing's syndrome, euphoria, depression
Unusual but important side effects	Peptic ulceration with perforation Cushingoid side effects increasingly likely with doses above 7.5 mg daily
Drug interactions	Avoid live vaccines (decreased response to inactivated vaccines) Increased risk of GI ulceration and bleeding with aspirin and NSAIDS Increased insulin and oral hypoglycemic requirements in diabetes mellitus Decreased response to warfarin, potentiated by ketoconazole
Monitoring	Blood pressure, bone density before and during prolonged treatment HPA axis suppression

*Every other day dosing, particularly for longer-term therapy, will reduce hypothalamic-pituitary-adrenal (HPA) axis suppression. After 2 weeks of therapy, gradual tapering is required.

TABLE 29 Colchicine and Pentoxifylline for the Prevention of Severe Recurrent Aphthous Stomatitis

Generic name	Colchicine	Pentoxifylline
Brand name		Trental, Pentoxil
Indications	Treatment of severe recurrent aphthous stomatitis Treatment of Behçet's syndrome	
Administration	Systemic tablets	Systemic tablets
Prescription/OTC	Prescription	Prescription
Dosage	500 µg three times daily	400 mg three times daily
Contraindications	Pregnancy	Cerebral hemorrhage, myocardial infarction, pregnancy, breast-feeding, porphyria
Common side effects	Nausea, vomiting, abdominal pain	Gastrointestinal disturbances dizziness, allergic reactions
Unusual but important side effects	Anorexia	Decreased blood pressure in patients taking antihypertensives
Drug interactions	Clarithromycin Erythromycin Cyclosporine	Analgesics Theophylline
Monitoring	Blood tests for agranulocytosis, aplastic anemia	Blood pressure in patients taking antihypertensives

TABLE 30 Thalidomide for the Treatment of Severe Ulcerative and Vesiculobullous Oral Mucosal Diseases

Generic name	Thalidomide
Brand name	Thalomid
Indications	Severe recurrent aphthous stomatitis unresponsive to other therapy Major aphthous stomatitis in patients with AIDS Behçet's syndrome Erythema multiforme
Administration	Tablets
Prescription/OTC	Prescribable only by those registered in the STEPS program
Dosage	100–300 mg daily with water at bedtime
Contraindications	Pregnancy, unprotected intercourse if risk of pregnancy
Common side effects	Severe birth defects, peripheral neuropathy, drowsiness, malaise, dizziness, headache, rash
Unusual but important side effects	Thrombotic events, neutropenia, increased HIV viral load
Drug interactions	Barbiturates, alcohol, chlorpromazine, reserpine
Monitoring	Baseline nerve conduction studies and after every 10 g of drug Monthly pregnancy testing in women Follow STEPS program (888-423-5436; <www.thalomid.com>)

Users must be registered in STEPS program.

systemic drugs. Isolated lesions can be treated with injectable corticosteroids (see Table 27).

BULLOUS PEMPHIGOID AND MUCOUS MEMBRANE PEMPHIGOID

Pharmacotherapeutic interventions for all subepithelial bullous disorders are similar. Successful treatment of mild or localized oral lesions can be achieved with topical corticosteroids (see Table 26) or intralesional corticosteroids (see Table 27). Tetracycline alone or combined with nicotinamide (Table 33) is beneficial for many patients who do not respond

TABLE 31 Azathioprine for Severe Ulcerative and Vesiculobullous Oral Mucosal Diseases

Generic name	Azathioprine
Brand name	Imuran
Indications	Severe recurrent aphthous stomatitis Behçet's syndrome Pemphigus vulgaris Pemphigoid Erythema multiforme
Administration	Tablets
Prescription/OTC	Prescription
Dosage	1–3 mg/kg/d (modified regimes based on TPMT activity) usually combined with systemic corticosteroids
Contraindications	Hypersensitivity to azathioprine; pregnancy or hope to become pregnant; breast-feeding; unknown, very low, or absent TPMT* levels; concurrent allopurinol treatment; concurrent malignant disease; renal or hepatic insufficiency; live vaccines
Common side-effects	Hypersensitivity reactions, nausea, vomiting, liver impairment, susceptibility to infections
Unusual but important side effects	Pancreatitis
Drug interactions	Allopurinol
Monitoring	TPMT activity before commencing treatment Blood tests for signs of myelosuppression Liver function

TPMT = thiopurine methyltransferase.

to topical therapy alone.[95] Severe cases usually respond to a combination of systemic corticosteroids (see Table 28) and adjuvant immunosuppressive agents (see Tables 31 and 32). Patients with lesions involving the conjunctiva, larynx, or esophagus may require immunosuppressive agents combined with systemic corticosteroids.[96,97]

ERYTHEMA MULTIFORME

The primary causative agent for erythema multiforme is variable, and pharmacotherapeutic intervention must be designed for the etiopathogenesis of the disease. Systemic corticosteroids are used for severe cases (1–2 mg/kg/d; see Table 28), and intermittent cases can be aborted with early use of short courses of systemic corticosteroids. Many cases are associated with herpes simplex reactivation and can be controlled by the use of continuous prophylactic antiviral therapy (see Table 2). Intermittent cases can be aborted by early use of short courses of systemic corticosteroids (see Table 28). Therapy for severe recurrent cases that do not respond to antiviral therapy may require the use of dapsone (see Table 32), thalidomide (see Table 30), or other immunosuppressive drug therapy (see Tables 31 and 32).[98,99]

▼ ANTIVIRAL MEDICATIONS

Overview

Herpes simplex virus 1 (HSV-1), an alphaherpesvirus, is a large DNA virus that causes primary herpetic gingivostomatitis, mucocutaneous orofacial disease, and ocular disease. Recurrent lesions are common on the face and on the lips and less common intraorally. HSV transmission is from direct contact with infected secretions, and the majority of primary infections are subclinical. Data through the US National Health and Nutrition Examination Survey (NHANES) III revealed that 40% of those under 20 years old are antibody seropositive for HSV-1, increasing to 65% in those older than 70 years.[100,101]

After primary infection, the virus ascends sensory axons via retrograde axonal flow, replicates, and establishes latency within the trigeminal ganglion.[102] When an appropriate trigger occurs (such as illness, sunlight, trauma, emotional stress, or menses), the virus reactivates, replicates in the ganglion, and travels centrifugally along the axon to the skin or mucosal site. There it is directly cytopathic to the epithelial cells that consequently become destroyed, resulting in vesicles and ulcers. Reactivation of HSV can occur as asymptomatic shedding in secretions such as saliva or the development of clinical lesions that should more appropriately be termed recrudescent HSV.[100]

Recrudescent HSV-1 in immunocompromised patients (eg, HIV+, AIDS) and those undergoing cytoreductive therapy or those on immunosuppressive drugs (especially after organ transplantation) may develop anywhere in the oral cavity as single or multiple ulcers.[103,104] For example, ulcers that developed during chemotherapy for hematologic malignancies were positive for HSV by culture in 48 to 61% of cases.[103,105,106] Oral recrudescent HSV is dangerous in immunocompromised patients as it may lead to HSV viremia and life-threatening disseminated disease[107] and, accordingly, requires aggressive therapy.[100]

Recurrent herpes labialis (RHL) occurs in 20 to 40% of the general population[108–110] and is probably much higher in immunocompromised patients. Infectivity is highest within the first 24 hours of the appearance of lesions, with 80% of vesicles and 34% of ulcer/crust lesions yielding positive HSV cultures.[111] Because lesions are very short-lived (unless the patient is immunocompromised), the treatment window using topical antivirals (Table 34) is correspondingly short.[100]

Primary infection with HSV-1 may result in gingivostomatitis. These patients may have fever, pain, and oral and perioral ulcerations. If administered within the first 72 hours of the onset of signs and symptoms, ACV has been shown to decrease the number of days the patient has pain and fever as well as the amount of oral lesions.[112] Reactivation is usually typified by a prodromal tingling, vesicle formation, and then crusting. Patients with compromised immune response, such as those with AIDS, leukemia, lymphoma, or altered

TABLE 32 Alternative Drugs for Severe Ulcerative and Vesiculobullous Oral Mucosal Diseases

Generic name	Dapsone	Cyclophosphamide	Mycophenolate mofetil
Brand name		Cytoxan	CellCept
Indications		Pemphigus vulgaris Pemphigoid Erythema multiforme	
Administration		Tablets	
Prescription/OTC		Prescription	
Dosage	1–2 mg/kg/d	1–1.5 mg/kg/d	1 g bid
Contraindications	Porphyria, anemia (treat severe anemia before starting), glucose-6-phosphate dehydrogenase (G6PD) deficiency (requires reduced dose), pregnancy, breast-feeding	Porphyria Pregnancy Breast-feeding	Pregnancy, breast-feeding
Common side effects	Hemolysis, methemaglobinemia, agranulocytosis, skin reactions	Thinning hair Darkened skin Blistering skin Loss of appetite/weight	Gastrointestinal effects, susceptibility to infection
Unusual but important side effects	Dapsone syndrome (rash, fever, eosinophilia)	Hemorrhagic cystitis	Malignancy
Drug interactions	Plasma levels increase with trimethoprim	Increased absorption of phenytoin Clozapine Cytotoxics Suxamethonium	Antacids Antivirals Colestyramine
Monitoring	Measure G6PD levels before treatment	Blood count Liver function	CBC, liver function tests, creatinine

T-lymphocyte response, as well as those taking immunosuppressive drugs, are susceptible to aggressive HSV lesions. HSV reactivation in these individuals is more severe, causing larger ulcers that can take up to several weeks to resolve. Current practice for patients undergoing hematopoietic stem cell transplantation who are seropositive for HSV is prophylaxis with oral or IV ACV (400 mg oral or IV three times a day) during the early transplantation period, although optimum dosing is not well defined.[113] Patients with recrudescence after hospital discharge are treated with ACV as appropriate based upon signs and symptoms. Patients undergoing solid organ transplantation are typically not given antiviral prophylaxis, but all recrudescent lesions are treated with courses of systemic antiviral drugs (see Table 2). Patients who undergo head and neck radiation may also show recrudescence of HSV intraorally and are treated when lesions develop.[100,114,115]

Acyclovir

OVERVIEW

ACV is a synthetic acyclic analogue of 2′-deoxyguanosine with inhibitory activity against HSV-1 and other herpesviruses.[116] After three phosphorylations (the first by thymidine kinase produced by the HSV), the ACV triphosphate inhibits the synthesis of viral DNA by competing with

2′-deoxyguanosine triphosphate as a substrate on the viral DNA polymerase. Once ACV triphosphate is inserted into the viral DNA, synthesis stops, terminating chain elongation and HSV replication.[116] ACV is primarily active in virally infected cells and has high selectivity and minimal toxicity in other tissues. ACV is available in topical, oral, and IV preparations (see Tables 2 and 34). After oral administration, the bioavailability of ACV is only 20%.[100,117]

TOPICAL ACV

Due to poor penetration, 5 or 10% ACV in an ointment base has not been demonstrated to be efficacious for treating RHL in healthy patients.[118–121] ACV 5% in a cream base may be efficacious in reducing the duration of lesions (see Table 34), especially if applied early during the prodrome, but it has little effect on reducing pain. Topical ACV will reduce the duration of lesions by only 1 to 2 days; therefore, it will not be beneficial for patients who have more severe and longer episodes. It may be more helpful to control trigger factors that activate the virus since this is an earlier event.

ORALLY ADMINISTERED ACV

Oral ACV 200 to 400 mg five times a day will shorten healing time, suppress delayed lesions, reduce lesion size and duration of pain, and diminish viral shedding (see Table 2).[122] ACV prophylaxis may be beneficial in patients with

TABLE 33 Nicotinamide and Tetracycline for Severe Ulcerative and Vesiculobullous Oral Mucosal Diseases

Generic name	Nicotinamide or niacinomide	Tetracycline
Brand name	Nicomide	Sumycin
Indications	Pemphigoid	Pemphigoid
Administration	Tablets	Capsules dissolved as a mouthwash Capsules or tablets
Prescription/OTC	Prescription	Prescription
Dosage	1.5–2 g daily with tetracycline	1–2 g daily with nicotinamide
Contraindications	Hypersensitivity to nicotinamide, pregnancy, breast-feeding	Pregnancy, breast-feeding, children less than 12 years, renal disease
Common side effects	Nausea, bloating, flatulence, dizziness	Nausea, diarrhea, vomiting, esophagitis
Unusual but important side effects	Hepatic damage Avoid high dose in patients with diabetes, liver disease	Staining of teeth after prolonged therapy, hepatotoxicity, thrombophlebitis, pseudomembranous colitis
Drug interactions	Decreased clearance of carbamazepine and prednisone	Antacids, anticoagulants, calcium, iron, oral contraceptives, zinc
Monitoring	Hepatic function	Monitor renal function, anecdotal reports of decreased contraceptive efficacy

known triggers such as sunlight or menses or patients who experience erythema multiforme following episodes of recurrent HSV infection.[99,123] Importantly, sunscreen alone reduces the incidence of recurrent RHL in patients with sunlight as a trigger.[100]

Valacyclovir

Valacyclovir is the L-valyl ester and prodrug of ACV that is well absorbed after oral administration. The rapid and almost complete conversion (99%) to ACV in the GI tract and liver results in a three- to five-fold increase in bioavailability.[122] The plasma ACV level following oral administration of valacyclovir is similar to that achieved with IV ACV.[124,125] Valacyclovir at 500 to 2,000 mg/d can suppress RHL. Two grams once a day shortens the duration of episodes and pain, and 1 g twice a day can abort lesions (see Table 2). In patients undergoing dental treatment, taking 2 g twice on the day of dental treatment and 1 g taken twice the next day resulted in fewer clinical lesions, decreased HSV-1-positive specimens, and decreased time to pain cessation.[126] In a case of HSV-induced recurrent erythema multiforme, valacyclovir (500 mg twice daily) completely suppressed HSV and recurrent erythema multiforme after ACV (400 mg twice a day) was ineffectual.[100,127]

Penciclovir

Penciclovir is an acyclic nucleoside analogue similar to ACV. It is phosphorylated by viral thymidine kinase (a different enzyme as the one for ACV) and inhibits viral DNA polymerase.[128] Penciclovir has specific action against virally

TABLE 34 Topical Antiviral Drugs for Recurrent Oral Herpes

Generic name	Acyclovir	Penciclovir	Docosanol
Brand name Indications	Zovirax Herpes labialis	Denavir Herpes labialis	Abreva Herpes labialis
Administration	Cream, ointment	Cream	Cream
Prescription/OTC	Prescription	Prescription	OTC
Dosage	5% cream; qid for 4 d 5% ointment; qid for 4 d	1% cream: q2h for 4 d	10% cream: qid until healed
Contraindications	Hypersensitivity to acyclovir, valacyclovir	Hypersensitivity to penciclovir; previous adverse reaction to famciclovir	Hypersensitivity to docosanol
Common side effects	Pain, burning, stinging	Mild erythema Occasionally headache	Tingling at application site
Unusual but important side effects	None	Local anesthesia, local edema, urticaria, pain, pruritus, paresthesia, skin discoloration, erythematous rash, oropharyngeal edema, parosmia	Headache
Drug interactions	None	None	None
Monitoring	None	None	None

infected cells and has a prolonged half-life in HSV-infected cells, which allows for less frequent dosing.[116,129] However, it is poorly absorbed when given orally and is therefore formulated for IV and topical use. The prodrug of penciclovir, famciclovir (see below), has better bioavailability (41% vs 9%). Topical penciclovir cream 1% is FDA approved for the treatment of RHL (see Table 34). It should be applied every 2 hours from the first prodrome for 4 days to reduce healing time and duration of pain.[100,129,130]

Famciclovir

Famciclovir is a diacetyl-6-deoxy analogue and prodrug of penciclovir. It is rapidly absorbed after oral administration and metabolized by deacetylation in the GI tract, blood, and liver to penciclovir. It has activity against HSV but is only approved to treat herpes zoster virus or shingles (varicella-zoster virus). A dose of 500 mg three times daily is recommended for the quickest healing time (see Table 2).[100,131]

Docosanol

n-Docosanol is a saturated 22-carbon alcohol that inhibits HSV replication by interfering with early intracellular events surrounding viral entry into target cells. Its mechanism of action is still poorly understood.[132] It is a highly lipophilic compound and targets viruses with lipid-containing envelopes such as HSV. It probably inhibits fusion of the HSV envelope with the plasma membrane and therefore blocks subsequent viral replicative events.[133] Docosanol does not act via thymidine kinase or DNA polymerase; therefore, it is active against ACV-resistant HSV strains. It is the only over-the-counter drug that is FDA approved for the treatment of RHL. Docosanol is only available in a topical formulation (see Table 34) and reduces healing time of RHL by 1.6 to 4.6 days when initiated during the prodrome and erythema stage.[134] It may also shorten the duration of pain and other symptoms.[100,135]

▼ ANTIFUNGAL MEDICATIONS

Overview

Oral candidiasis has three common oral variants (pseudomembraneous candidiasis, erythematous candidiasis, angular cheilitis) and several less common variants (hyperplastic candidiasis, linear gingival erythema associated with HIV infection).[138–140] Oral fungal infections can manifest in up to 60% of healthy persons.[137] They are even more common in immunocompromised patients where oral-pharyngeal candidiasis can lead to life-threatening systemic dissemination,[139] which substantiates the aggressive treatment and prophylaxis of this infection.[136]

The risk of developing oropharyngeal candidiasis in the immunocompromised host is dependent on the disease underlying the immunocompromised status and its related local and systemic consequences. For cancers, the increased incidence of oropharyngeal candidiasis is dependent upon both the systemic disease and the therapeutic measures used (eg, cytotoxic drugs, immunosuppressive drugs, radiotherapy).[138,140] The concurrent administration of broad-spectrum antibiotics for the management of infections and

TABLE 35   Topical Antifungal Drugs for the Management of Oral Candidiasis

Generic name	Nystatin	Clotrimazole	Ketoconazole
Brand name	Nystat, Mycostatin	Mycelex, Gyne-Lotrimin	Nizoral
Indications	Oropharyngeal candidiasis	Oropharyngeal candidiasis	Oropharyngeal candidiasis
Administration	Oral suspension, powder, cream, lozenge	Troche	Cream
Prescription/OTC	Prescription	Prescription and OTC	Prescription
Dosage	Oral suspension (100,000 U/mL): 400,000–600,000 units 4–5 times daily (swish and swallow) Troche (200,000 U): 200,000–400,000 U 4–5 times/d 100,000 U/g cream and ointment: apply to affected area 4–5 times/d Powder (50 million U): sprinkle on tissue contact area of denture	10 mg troche: dissolve slowly over 15–30 minutes 5 times daily: apply to affected area bid for 7 d Cream can be applied to the tissue contact areas of the denture	2% cream: rub gently into the affected area 1–2 times daily
Contraindications	Hypersensitivity to nystatin	Hypersensitivity to clotrimazole	Hypersensitivity to ketoconazole; administration with ergot derivatives or cisapride
Common side effects	Nausea, vomiting, diarrhea, stomach pain, contact dermatitis	Abnormal liver function tests, nausea, vomiting, local mild burning, irritation, stinging	Irritation, pruritus, stinging
Unusual but important side effects	Hypersensitivity	Avoid contact with eyes	
Drug interactions	None	None	None
Monitoring	Liver function tests	Liver function tests	Liver function tests

TABLE 36   Systemic Antifungal Drugs for the Management of Oral Candidiasis

Generic name	Fluconazole	Itraconazole	Ketoconazole
Brand name	Diflucan	Sporanox	Nizoral
Indications	Oral and esophageal candidiasis	Oral and esophageal candidiasis	Oral and esophageal candidiasis
Administration	Tablets Powder	Solution	Tablets
Prescription/OTC	Prescription	Prescription	Prescription

Dosage	Tablets: 200 mg on day 1 then 100 mg daily for 7–14 d
	Powder for oral suspension (10 mg/mL);
	    dosing is the same as for tablets
		Solution (10 mg/mL): 100–200 mg/10 mL once
		    a day for 1–2 wk; if refractory to fluconazole:
		    100 mg q12h
			200–400 mg/d as single dose for 7–14 d

	Left ventricular dysfunction, congestive	Contraindications
		Hypersensitivity to ketoconazole;
		    heart failure
			Hypersensitivity to azole drugs
			
			    administration with ergot derivatives or
			    cisapride

Common side effects	Headache, nausea, abdominal pain, vomiting, rash,
	    diarrhea, taste perversion, dyspepsia
		Nausea, edema, hypertension, headache,
		    fatigue, malaise, fever, dizziness, rash, pruritus,
		    decreased libido, hyperkalemia, abdominal pain,
		    anorexia, vomiting, diarrhea, increased liver
		    enzymes, hepatitis
			Pruritus, nausea, vomiting, abdominal pain

Important side effects: rare events	Anaphylactic reactions, liver failure	Adrenal suppression, allergic reactions, arrhythmia,
		    congestive heart failure, Stevens-Johnson
		    syndrome
			Bulging fontanelles, chills, depression,
			    diarrhea, dizziness, fever,
			    gynecomastia, headaches, hemolytic
			    anemia, hepatotoxicity, impotence,
			    leukopenia, photophobia, somnolence,
			    thrombocytopenia

Drug interactions	Cisapride	Inhibits certain cytochrome P-450 substrates. Check drug references for individual drug-drug interactions.	
Monitoring	Liver and renal function tests, potassium	Liver function tests after 1 mo of treatment	Liver function tests

the condition of salivary hypofunction may further predispose these patients to oropharyngeal candidiasis.[136,138,140] Reduced salivary output due to advanced HIV infection or head and neck radiotherapy has been correlated with enhanced recovery of *Candida* from saliva.[139–142] Other conditions increase the risk of developing oral-pharyngeal candidiasis: immunocompromising medical conditions (eg, HIV infection, diabetes mellitus, nutritional deficiencies) and the use of certain medications (eg, broad-spectrum antibiotics, corticosteroids, cytotoxics).[138] For example, over 90% of HIV-infected patients develop oropharyngeal candidiasis at some time during their disease progression,[137,139] and at least 75% of HIV-infected patients with oropharyngeal candidiasis have concurrent AIDS-associated esophageal candidiasis.[136,139]

Topical Treatment of Oral Candidiasis

There are a variety of topically administered antifungal agents that can be used to treat oral candidiasis (Table 35). Nystatin and clotrimazole have traditionally been the initial therapies. Nystatin pastilles have greater efficacy, although the pastilles may not be readily available in some areas. Assuming that predisposing factors that contribute to the development of

candidal infections are eliminated, many of the topically available agents are capable of resolving acute oral infections. These agents should be given multiple times throughout the day at the appropriate dose (7–14 days). Topical agents offer the advantage of having fewer systemic side effects, less likelihood for developing drug-drug interactions, and ability to target specific areas of involvement such as the commissures of the mouth.[136]

Systemic Treatment of Oral Candidiasis

Systemic antifungal drugs are effective in treating both oral mucocutaneous and systemic candidal infections. They may be even more effective than topically applied antifungals due to enhanced patient compliance. When these medications are used for a short period of time, systemic side effects, such as elevated liver enzymes, abdominal pain, and pruritis, are less common.

Systemic fluconazole is as effective as clotrimazole and superior to nystatin. The next choice, itraconazole solution, is as efficacious as fluconazole but should be used only in patients refractory to fluconazole. Ketoconazole and itraconazole capsules are less effective than fluconazole because of variable absorption.[143]

Azole Resistance

Treatment of oropharyngeal candidiasis is complicated by the development of resistance to azole drugs. This resistance is particularly problematic in HIV-infected and AIDS patients, especially patients with (1) low CD4 cell counts, (2) a history of a previous relapse of oral candidiasis, and (3) requirements for long-term suppressive antifungal therapy.[137,144] Certain non-*albicans* species, such as *Candida glabrata* and *Candida krusei*, are less susceptible to fluconazole than *Candida albicans* and are being isolated with increased frequency in HIV-infected patients.[145] Patients from whom fluconazole-resistant yeasts were isolated required longer courses of therapy and higher doses of fluconazole for response, but, overall, excellent responses to fluconazole were observed in patients with advanced HIV infection.[146] Fluconazole-refractory oropharyngeal candidiasis will respond to oral itraconazole therapy (≥ 200 mg/d, preferably in solution form) approximately two-thirds of the time. Intravenous caspofungin (50 mg/d) and intravenous amphotericin B deoxycholate (≥ 0.3 mg/kg/d) are usually effective and may be used in patients with refractory disease.

Treatment of Fungus-Infected Removable Prostheses

Removable prostheses are a risk for developing oral candidiasis, particularly those patients who are immunocompromised.[147] An association exists between the prevalence of denture stomatitis and an unhealthy lifestyle, wearing dentures at night, and poor oral hygiene.[148,149] Xerostomic denture wearers are also more prone to recurrent candidal infections. Denture-related fungal infections accordingly require appropriate disinfection of the denture for definitive cure.[143] When the infection is confined to removable denture-supporting tissues, treatment of the tissues can be accomplished effectively by placing an antifungal cream (eg, clotrimazole 1% cream, nystatin powder; see Table 35) on the surface of the denture prior to placement. This should be done daily until the tissue appears to be clinically healthy and then for an additional 2 weeks. When the candidal infection involves other oral or pharyngeal soft tissues, the patient should be treated with a systemic agent (Table 36). Additionally, the denture should be treated with either a daily 30-minute soak in 0.12% chlorhexidine solution or diluted sodium hypochlorite solution (10 mL/2 teaspoons of 5% bleach in 250 mL or 1 cup of water).[150]

▼ SELECTED READINGS

Akintoye SO, Greenberg MS. Recurrent aphthous stomatitis. Dent Clin North Am 2005;49:31–47, vii–iii.

Baddour LM, Bettmann MA, Bolger AF, et al. Nonvalvular cardiovascular device-related infections. Circulation 2003;108:2015–31.

Balfour HH Jr. Antiviral drugs. N Engl J Med 1999;340:1255–68.

Dworkin RH, Backonja M, Rowbotham MC, et al. Advances in neuropathic pain: diagnosis, mechanisms, and treatment recommendations. Arch Neurol 2003;60:1524–34.

Faver IR, Guerra SG, Su WP, el-Azhary R. Thalidomide for dermatology: a review of clinical uses and adverse effects. Int J Dermatol 2005;44:61–7.

Finnerup NB, Jensen TS. Mechanisms of disease: mechanism-based classification of neuropathic pain—a critical analysis. Nat Clin Pract Neurol 2006;2:107–15.

Grisius MM. Salivary gland dysfunction: a review of systemic therapies. Oral Surg Oral Med Oral Pathol Oral Radiol Endod 2001;92:156–62.

Harman KE, Albert S, Black MM. Guidelines for the management of pemphigus vulgaris. Br J Dermatol 2003;149:926–37.

Koukourakis MI. Amifostine in clinical oncology: current use and future applications. Anticancer Drugs 2002;13:181–209.

Lockhart PB, Loven B, Brennan MT, Fox PC. The evidence base for the efficacy of antibiotic prophylaxis in dental practice. J Amer Dent Assoc 2007;138:458-74.

National Cancer Institute. Oral and dental management prior to cancer therapy [Web site]. 2006 July 14 [cited 2006 November 1]. Available from: http://www.cancer.gov/cancertopics/pdq/supportivecare/oralcomplications/HealthProfessional/page3. This website was accessed on June 12, 2007.

Pappas PG, Rex JH, Sobel JD, et al. Guidelines for treatment of candidiasis. Clin Infect Dis 2004;15;38:161–89.

Reisner L, Pettengill CA. The use of anticonvulsants in orofacial pain. Oral Surg Oral Med Oral Pathol Oral Radiol Endod 2001;91:2–7.

Saarto T, Wiffen PJ. Antidepressants for neuropathic pain. Cochrane Database Syst Rev 2005;(3):CD005454.

Sami N, Yeh SW, Ahmed AR. Blistering diseases in the elderly: diagnosis and treatment. Dermatol Clin 2004;22:73–86.

Ship JA, Hu K. Radiotherapy-induced salivary dysfunction. Semin Oncol 2004;31(6 Suppl 18):29–36.

Ship JA, Vissink A, Challacombe SJ. Use of prophylactic antifungals in the immunocompromised host. Oral Surg Oral Med Oral Pathol Oral Radiol Endod. 2007 Mar;103(Suppl 1):S6-S11.

Spruance SL. The natural history of recurrent herpes simplex labialis: implications for antiviral therapy. N Engl J Med 1977;297:69.

Wilson W, Taubert KA, Gewitz M, Lockhart PB, et al. Prevention of Infective Endocarditis. Guidelines from the American Heart Association. A guide from the American Heart Association Rheumatic Fever, Endocarditis, and Kawasaki Disease e Committee, Council on Cardiovascular Disease in the Young, and the Council on Clinical Cardiology, Council on Cardiovascular Surgery and Anesthesia, and the Quality of Care and Outcomes Research Interdisciplinary Working Group. Circulation published online Apr 19, 2007. Accessed on July 19, 2007 at: http://circ.ahajournals.org/).

Woo SB, Challacombe SJ. Management of recurrent oral herpes simplex infections. Oral Surg Oral Med Oral Pathol Oral Radiol Endod. 2007 Mar;103 Suppl 1:S12-S8.

For the full reference list, please refer to the accompanying CD ROM.

3

ULCERATIVE, VESICULAR, AND BULLOUS LESIONS

SOOK BIN WOO, DMD, MMSc
MARTIN S. GREENBERG, DDS

Many ulcerative or vesiculobullous disease of the mouth have a similar clinical appearance. The oral mucosa is thin, causing vesicles and bullae to break rapidly into ulcers; ulcers are easily traumatized from teeth and food, and they become secondarily infected by the oral flora. These factors may cause lesions that have a characteristic appearance on the skin to have a nonspecific appearance on the oral mucosa.

Mucosal disorders may occasionally be correctly diagnosed from a brief history and rapid clinical examination, but this approach is most often insufficient and leads to incorrect diagnosis and improper treatment. When a careful and detailed history is taken, it provides as much information as the clinical examination and guides the clinician during the clinical examination. Three pieces of information in particular help the clinician rapidly categorize a patient's disease and simplify the diagnosis: the length of time the lesions have been present (acute or chronic lesions), the past history of similar lesions (primary or recurrent disease), and the number of lesions present (single or multiple). In this chapter, the diseases are grouped according to the information just described. This information serves as an excellent starting point for the student who is just learning to diagnose these disorders, as well as the experienced clinician who is aware of the potential diagnostic pitfalls.

A complete review of systems should be obtained for each patient, including questions regarding the presence of skin, eye, genital, and rectal lesions. Questions should also be included regarding symptoms of diseases associated with oral lesions; that is, each patient should be asked about the presence of symptoms such as joint pains, muscle weakness, dyspnea, diplopia, and chest pains. The clinical examination should include a thorough inspection of the exposed skin surfaces. The diagnosis of oral lesions requires knowledge of basic dermatology because many disorders occurring on the oral mucosa also affect the skin.

Dermatologic lesions are classified according to their clinical appearance and include the following frequently used terms that are also applicable in the oral mucosa:

1. *Macules.* These are well-circumscribed, flat lesions that are noticeable because of their change from normal skin or mucosa color. They may be red due to increased vascularity or inflammation, or pigmented due to the presence of melanin, hemosiderin, and foreign material or ingestion of medications. A good example in the oral cavity is the melanotic macule.

2. *Papules.* These are solid lesions raised above the skin or mucosal surface that are smaller than 1 cm in diameter. Papules may be seen in a wide variety of diseases, including erythema multiforme, rubella, lupus erythematosus, and sarcoidosis. In the oral cavity, hyperplastic candidiasis often presents as yellow-white papules.

3. *Plaques.* These are solid raised lesions that are greater than 1 cm in diameter; they are large papules.

4. *Nodules.* These lesions are present deeper in the dermis or mucosa. The lesions may also protrude above the skin or mucosa but are generally wider than they are high. A good example of an oral mucosal nodule is the irritation fibroma.

5. *Vesicles.* These are elevated blisters containing clear fluid that are less than 1 cm in diameter.

6. *Bullae.* These are elevated blisters containing clear fluid that are greater than 1 cm in diameter.

7. *Erosions.* These are red lesions often caused by the rupture of vesicles or bullae or trauma and are generally moist on the skin.

8. *Pustules.* These are blisters containing purulent material.

9. *Ulcers.* These are well-circumscribed, often depressed lesions with an epithelial defect that is covered by a fibrin clot, causing a yellow-white appearance. A good example is an aphthous ulcer.

10. *Purpura.* These are reddish to purple bruises caused by blood from vessels leaking into the connective tissue. These lesions do not blanch when pressure is applied and are classified by size as petechiae (less than 0.5 cm) or ecchymoses.

The first section of this chapter describes acute multiple lesions that tend to occur only once, the second portion of the chapter covers recurring oral mucosal lesions, and the third portion presents the patient with chronic, continuous multiple lesions. The final section describes diseases that present as chronic single lesions. It is hoped that classifying the disorders in this way will help the clinician avoid the common diagnostic problem of confusing viral infections with recurrent oral conditions, such as recurrent aphthous stomatitis, or disorders that present as chronic progressive disease, such as pemphigus and pemphigoid.

▼ THE PATIENT WITH ACUTE MULTIPLE LESIONS

The major diseases that cause acute multiple oral lesions include viral and bacterial stomatitis, allergic reactions (particularly erythema multiforme and contact allergic stomatitis), and lesions caused by cancer chemotherapy or blood dyscrasias (see Chapter 16, "Hematologic Diseases").

Herpes Simplex Virus (HSV) Infection

ETIOLOGY AND PATHOGENESIS

The Herpesviridae family of viruses contains nine different viruses that are pathogenic in humans (Table 1). This chapter discusses only herpes simplex virus (HSV)-1, varicella-zoster virus (VZV), and cytomegalovirus (CMV) infections. Lesions caused by Epstein-Barr virus (EBV) are discussed in Chapter 20, "Infectious Diseases." Herpes viruses have a common structure: an internal core containing the viral genome, an icosahedral nucleocapsid, the tegument, and an outer lipid envelope containing viral glycoproteins on its surface that are derived from host cellular membranes.[1] Nonetheless, each of the herpesviruses is distinct.

HSV-1, an α-herpesvirus, is a ubiquitous virus, and 65% of adults in the United States over age 70 are seropositive for it.[2] In general, infections above the waist are caused by HSV-1 and those below the waist by HSV-2, although with changing sexual practices, it is not uncommon to culture HSV-2 from oral lesions and vice versa.[3] The primary infection, which occurs on initial contact with the virus, is acquired by inoculation of the mucosa, skin, and eye with infected secretions. The virus then travels along the sensory nerve axons and establishes chronic, latent infection in the sensory ganglion (such as the trigeminal ganglion).[4] Extraneuronal latency (ie, HSV remaining latent in cells other than neurons such as the epithelium) may play a role in recurrent lesions of the lips.[5] Recurrent HSV results when HSV-1 reactivates at latent sites and travels centripetally to the mucosa or the skin, where it is directly cytopathic to epithelial cells, causing recrudescent HSV infection in the form of localized vesicles or ulcers.[6]

The most common sites of infection are the oral and genital mucosa and the eye. HSV infection of the cornea (keratitis) is a major cause of blindness in the world. HSV-1 or -2 may cause herpes whitlow, an infection of the fingers when virus is inoculated into the fingers through a break in the skin (Figure 1). This was a common occupational hazard (including within the dental profession) before the widespread use of gloves.[7,8] Other HSV-1 infections include herpes gladiatorum (infections of the skin spread through the sport of wrestling),[9] herpes encephalitis, HSV esophagitis, and HSV pneumonia.[6]

HSV is an important etiologic agent in erythema multiforme, which is discussed below.[10,11] HSV has been recovered in the endoneurial fluid of 77% of patients with Bells palsy.[12] Treatment with antiviral therapy resulted in better outcomes, further supporting the concept of HSV involvement in the pathogenesis of Bells palsy.[13]

TABLE 1 Herpesviridae that Are Pathogenic in Humans

Type of Virus	Primary Infection	Recurrent Infection	Immunocompromised Hosts
Herpes simplex virus 1	Gingivostomatitis, Keratoconjunctivitis, Genital and skin lesions	Herpes labialis ("cold sores"), Intraoral ulcers, Keratoconjunctivitis, Genital and skin lesions	Unusual ulcers at any mucocutaneous site, usually large and persistent
Herpes simplex virus 2	Genital and skin lesions, Gingivostomatitis, Keratoconjunctivitis, Neonatal infections, Aseptic meningitis	Genital and skin lesions Gingivostomatitis, Aseptic meningitis	Unusual ulcers at any mucocutaneous site, usually large and persistent; disseminated infection
Varicella-zoster virus	Varicella (chickenpox)	Zoster (shingles)	Disseminated infection
Cytomegalovirus	Infectious mononucleosis, Hepatitis, Congenital disease		Retinitis, gastroenteritis hepatitis, severe oral ulcers
Epstein-Barr virus	Infectious mononucleosis, Hepatitis Encephalitis		Hairy leukoplakia; lymphoproliferative disorders
Human herpesvirus 6	Roseola infantum, Otitis media, Encephalitis		Fever; bone marrow suppression
Human herpesvirus 7	Roseola infantum		
Human herpesvirus 8	? Infectious mononucleosis, Febrile exanthema		Kaposi's sarcoma; lymphoproliferative disorders; bone marrow suppression
Simian herpesvirus B	Mucocutaneous lesions, Encephalitis		

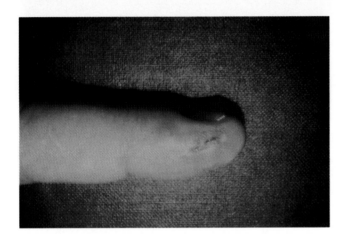

FIGURE 1   Primary herpetic whitlow on the finger of a dentist.

CLINICAL MANIFESTATIONS

Primary Gingivostomatitis.   Most cases of primary HSV-1 infections are subclinical and generally occur in children and teenagers.[6,13] There is a 1- to 3-day viral prodrome of fever, loss of appetite, malaise, and myalgia that may also be accompanied by headache and nausea. Oral pain leads to poor oral intake, and patients may require hospitalization for hydration. The disease is self-limiting in otherwise normal patients and resolves within 10 to 14 days, typical for a viral illness.

Oral Findings.   Within a few days of the prodrome, erythema and clusters of vesicles and/or ulcers appear on the keratinized mucosa of the hard palate, attached gingiva and dorsum of the tongue, and the nonkeratinized mucosa of the buccal and labial mucosa, ventral tongue, and soft palate (Figure 2). Vesicles break down to form ulcers that are usually 1 to 5 mm and coalesce to form larger ulcers with scalloped borders and marked surrounding erythema. The gingiva is often fiery red, and the mouth is extremely painful, causing difficulty with eating (Figure 3). Pharyngitis causes swallowing difficulties. Primary HSV infection in adults follows a similar pattern (Figure 4).[14]

Recrudescent Oral HSV Infection.   Reactivation of HSV may lead to asymptomatic shedding of HSV, in the saliva and oral secretions, an important risk factor for transmission; it may also cause ulcers to form. Asymptomatic shedding of HSV is not associated with systemic signs and symptoms and occurs

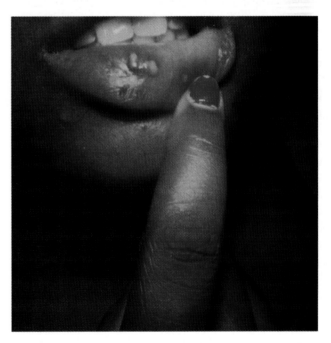

FIGURE 2   A 12-year-old female with primary herpetic gingivostomatitis causing discrete vesicles and ulcers surrounded by inflammation.

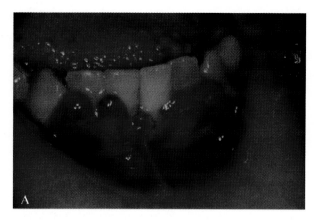
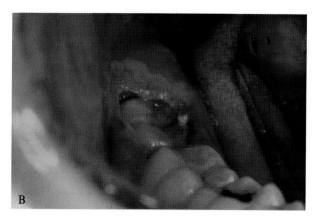

FIGURE 3   Acute marginal gingivitis characteristic of primary herpes simplex virus infection. *A*, Mandibular anterior gingiva; *B*, vesicles and inflammation around mandibular molars.

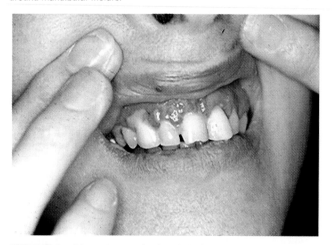

FIGURE 4   Primary herpes simplex of gingiva in an adult.

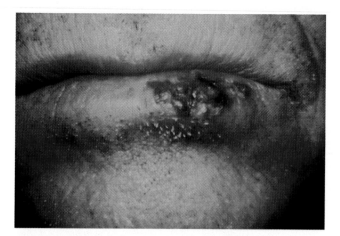

FIGURE 5   Crusted lesions of recurrent herpes labialis.

in 8 to 10% of patients following dental treatment.[15] The term *recrudescent HSV* should be used to refer to the actual ulcerations caused by reactivated virus. Fever, ultraviolet radiation, trauma, stress, and menstruation are important triggers for reactivation of HSV.

Recrudescent HSV on the lips is called recurrent herpes labialis (RHL) and occurs in 20 to 40% of the young adult population.[16,17] These are associated with a prodrome of itching, tingling, or burning approximately 50% of the time, followed in succession by the appearance of papules, vesicles, ulcers, crusting, and then resolution of lesions (Figure 5).[18] Pain generally is present only within the first 2 days. There is a suggestion that patients who do not experience a prodrome develop lesions from extraneural latent HSV within the epithelium and these lesions are less responsive to topical therapy.[19]

Intraoral recrudescent HSV in the immunocompetent host occurs chiefly on the keratinized mucosa of the hard palate, attached gingiva, and dorsum of the tongue.[20] Such lesions are called recurrent intraoral HSV (RIH) infection. They present as 1 to 5 mm single or clustered painful ulcers with a bright erythematous border (Figure 6). One common presentation is the complaint of pain in the gingiva 1 to 2 days after a scaling and prophylaxis or other dental treatment.

Lesions appear as 1 to 5 mm painful vesicles but more often ulcers on the marginal gingiva.

HSV in Immunocompromised Patients.   In immunocompromised patients (such as those undergoing chemotherapy, who have undergone organ transplantation, or who

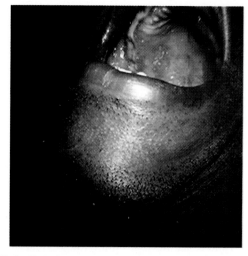

FIGURE 6   Typical lesions of recurrent intraoral herpes simplex virus infection in an immunocompetent patient are clusters of small vesicles and ulcers on the heavily keratinized oral mucosa.

have acquired immune deficiency syndrome [AIDS]), RIH infection may occur at any site intraorally and may form atypical-appearing ulcers that may be several centimeters in size and may last several weeks or months if undiagnosed and untreated (Figures 7 and 8).[21,22] In one study, 50% of patients with leukemia and 15% of patients who had undergone renal transplantation developed recrudescent oral HSV infections.[23] Single RIH ulcers are indistinguishable from recurrent aphthous ulcers if they occur on a nonkeratinized site.[24] These ulcers are painful and similar to those seen in immunocompetent patients except that they may be larger. They appear slightly depressed with raised borders. The presence of 1 to 2 mm vesicles or satellite ulcers at the edges of the main ulcer is a helpful sign.

If undiagnosed and left untreated, RIH infection may disseminate to other sites and cause severe infections in this population.[25] This is a particular problem in patients undergoing hematopoietic stem cell transplantation, where reactivation of HSV occurs in approximately 70% of patients.[26,27]

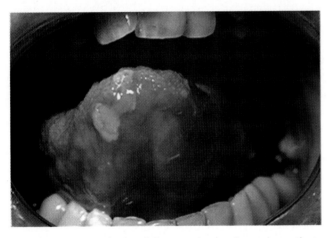

FIGURE 7   Herpes simplex of the tongue in a renal transplant patient.

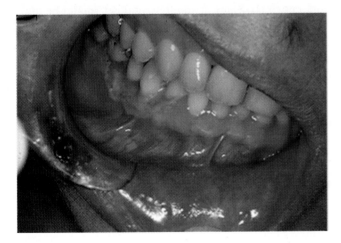

FIGURE 8   Herpes simplex of the gingiva in a patient with leukemia receiving chemotherapy.

DIFFERENTIAL DIAGNOSIS

Coxsackievirus infections (especially hand-foot-and-mouth disease) may present with widespread ulcerations of the oral cavity mimicking primary herpetic gingivostomatitis, but ulcers are generally not clustered and the gingiva is not involved. A viral culture or a cytology smear (see laboratory tests below) differentiates between the two.

RIH infection in the immunocompetent patient on the gingiva may resemble a localized area of necrotizing ulcerative gingivitis (see below), but there is usually a precipitating cause, such as dental treatment. Cultures are positive for HSV, and lesions of necrotizing ulcerative gingivitis are widespread and diffuse rather than localized, as is often seen in RIH. HSV ulcers on the palate may resemble traumatic lesions, such as pizza burns. RIH infection in the immunocompromised host may occur anywhere intraorally and can be differentiated from aphthous ulcers when necessary with a cytology specimen or culture. In the immunocompromised population, ulcers secondary to CMV infection, fungal infection, and neutropenia must also be considered. Differentiation from these entities is accomplished by biopsy, culture, and blood tests.

LABORATORY DIAGNOSIS

HSV isolation by cell culture is the gold standard test for the diagnosis for HSV-1 infections since it grows readily in tissue culture. A swab of the oral ulcers is performed, and the specimen should be refrigerated while awaiting pick-up since the virus is temperature sensitive. The advantage of a culture is that it has high sensitivity and specificity and allows for amplification of virions, subtyping, and testing for sensitivity to antiviral drugs. The disadvantage is that it needs specialized equipment, is expensive, and may take up to several days for a final result. HSV that reactivates in the saliva (asymptomatic shedding) will also grow in culture and may lead to an incorrect diagnosis of HSV of a coincidental lesion.

More recently, polymerase chain reaction (PCR) from swabs has been shown to detect HSV antigen three to four times more often than culture.[28] However, it is expensive and detects antigen and not whole infectious particles, so a positive PCR test for HSV does not equate with active infection.

HSV can be identified from scrapings from the base of lesions (especially vesicles) smeared onto glass slides. These can be stained with Wright, Giemsa (Tzanck preparation), or Papanicolaou stain to demonstrate the characteristic multinucleated giant cells or intranuclear inclusions as seen on histopathology (Figure 9). However, this does not distinguish between HSV or VZV. A similar smear preparation can be used for the direct fluorescent antigen detection test using a monoclonal antibody against HSV conjugated to a fluorescent compound such as fluorescein. Direct fluorescent antigen testing is more accurate than routine cytology.

Primary HSV infection is associated with elevated immunoglobulin (Ig)M titers followed several weeks later by permanent IgG titers (seroconversion) that indicate previous infection but confer no protection against reactivation.

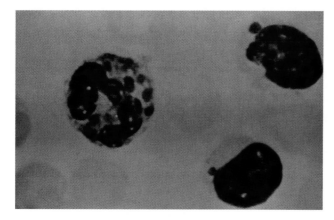

FIGURE 9 Cytology smear stained with Giemsa, demonstrating multinucleated giant cells.

TABLE 2   Pain Control and Supportive Care Measures
2% viscous lidocaine (swish and spit out 5 mL 4–5 times/d)
Liquid diphenhydramine (swish and spit out 5 mL 4–5 times/d)
Combination of viscous lidocaine, diphenhydramine, and a covering agent (such as Kaopectate or Maalox) in 1:1:1 ratio
0.1% diclonine hydrochloride
Benzydamine
Systemic analgesia
Supportive care
Hydration
Ice chips or popsicles
Soft bland diet
Antipyretics such as ibuprofen as needed (avoid aspirin products)*

*The use of aspirin products in children who have a viral illness (especially varicella infection, influenza, or coxsackievirus infection) has been associated with Reye's syndrome, a potentially fatal condition characterized by fatty degeneration of the liver and encephalopathy.

Recurrent infection is associated with a rise in IgG antibody titer in acute and convalescent sera, but a fourfold rise (a criterion that indicates active infection) is seen in only 5% of patients. The assay for HSV IgM is not particularly reliable for diagnostic purposes and overall, the use of serology to diagnose recurrent infection is not advised.

HSV lesions are not generally biopsied because the clinical appearance and history are characteristic, and infection is readily confirmed with a culture or cytologic specimen when necessary. However, if a biopsy is obtained, it will show the presence of multinucleated giant epithelial cells at the edge of the ulcer. The nuclei exhibit typical molding and have a ground-glass appearance. Since intact epithelium is necessary for the diagnosis, a biopsy for a lesion suspicious for HSV must always include epithelium adjacent to the ulcer.

MANAGEMENT

Primary HSV Infection.   Management is directed toward pain control, supportive care, and definitive treatment (Table 2). In the past, healthy patients with primary herpetic gingivostomatitis were treated only with hydration and supportive measures. However, since the acyclovir family of drugs is inexpensive, safe, and readily available, it is appropriate to treat even primary infections definitively because it reduces viral shedding and infectivity.

Acyclovir inhibits viral replication and is activated by virally produced thymidine kinase. As such, it has little activity against non–virally infected cells.[29] The use of acyclovir at 15 mg/kg five times a day in children reduces the duration of fever, reduces HSV shedding, halts the progress of lesions, improves oral intake, and reduces the incidence of hospital admissions.[30] Valacyclovir, the prodrug of acyclovir, has three to five times the bioavailability of acyclovir and, together with famciclovir, is now available.[29]

Recurrent HSV.   RHL can often be suppressed by reducing trigger factors, such as by using sunscreen.[31] Although

RHL is self-limiting, the use of topical antiviral medications reduces shedding, infectivity, pain, and the size and duration of lesions. Topical antiviral medications such as 5% acyclovir cream,[32,33] 3% penciclovir cream,[34,35] and 10% docosanol cream are efficacious[36,37] if applied three to six times a day at the first prodrome or sign of a lesion. Systemic therapy with valacyclovir or famciclovir (500–1,000 mg three times a day) is effective in treating active lesions or for suppression of HSV infection in patients who develop frequent episodes, large lesions, or EM.[38–42] Similar suppressive regimens can be used for patients susceptible to recrudescent HSV after dental procedures.[43]

HSV in Immunocompromised Patients.   In general, HSV infections in immunocompromised hosts should be treated with systemic antivirals to prevent dissemination to other sites (eg, HSV esophagitis) or systemically. The primary pathogen for herpes encephalitis and herpes pneumonitis is HSV-1. For patients undergoing hematopoietic stem cell transplantation, antiviral therapy at suppressive doses should be initiated for all patients who are HSV seropositive. Acyclovir and valacyclovir suppress HSV reactivation in such patients.[26,44] Acyclovir-resistant HSV is most frequently seen in this group of patients, where the virally derived thymidine kinase that activates acyclovir is mutated. In such cases, foscarnet is the drug of choice. The dosage of the acyclovir family of drugs should be adjusted for age and renal health.

A number of vaccines against HSV are currently under development.[45]

Varicella Zoster Virus (VZV) Infection

ETIOLOGY AND PATHOGENESIS

Primary infection with VZV, an α-herpesvirus, leads to varicella (chicken pox). As with all herpesviruses, the virus then becomes latent, usually in the dorsal root ganglia or ganglia of the cranial nerves.[46] Reactivation produces herpes zoster infection (HZI), commonly called shingles. The incidence of HZI increases with age and the degree of immunosuppression.[47] There are 1.5 to 3 cases of HZI per 1,000 subjects; this increases to 10 per 1,000 in those over age 75 years.[48] Therefore, it is not uncommon to see HZI in the elderly, in patients undergoing cancer chemotherapy, in patients on chronic immunosuppressive drug therapy (such as those who have received organ transplants), and in patients with AIDS.[47,49] As with HSV, this virus is cytopathic to the epithelial cells of the skin and mucosa, causing blisters and ulcers. Transmission is usually by the respiratory route, with an incubation period of 2 to 3 weeks.[50]

Postherpetic neuralgia, a morbid sequela of HZI, is a neuropathia resulting from peripheral and central nervous system injury and altered central nervous system processing.[51]

CLINICAL FINDINGS

Primary VZV infection generally occurs in the first two decades of life. The disease begins with a low-grade fever, malaise, and the development of an intensely pruritic, maculopapular rash, followed by vesicles that have been described as "dewdrop-like." These vesicles turn cloudy and pustular, burst, and scab, with the crusts falling off after 1 to 2 weeks. Lesions begin on the trunk and face and spread centrifugally. Central nervous system involvement may result in cerebellar ataxia and encephalitis. Other complications of varicella include pneumonia, myocarditis, and hepatitis.[50]

Immunocompromised hosts usually experience more severe disease with more blisters, a protracted course, and, not infrequently, involvement of the lungs, central nervous system, and liver; there is a significantly higher mortality rate.[52] Secondary bacterial infection by gram-positive cocci may have severe septic consequences.

HZI of the skin (shingles) is more common in adults and starts with a prodrome of deep, aching, or burning pain. There is usually little to no fever or lymphadenopathy. This is followed within 2 to 4 days by the appearance of crops of vesicles in a dermatomal or "zosteriform" pattern. This pattern describes the unilateral, linear, and clustered distribution of the vesicles, ulcers, and scabs in a dermatome supplied by one nerve. Thoracic/lumbar dermatomes are the most frequently involved, followed by the craniofacial area.[47] Lesions heal within 2 to 4 weeks, often with scarring and hypopigmentation. Occasionally, HZI may occur without the appearance of dermatomal lesions (zoster sine eruptione or zoster sine herpete), which makes the diagnosis of this condition challenging; these patients often present with facial palsy. A serious and occasional side effect of HZI is acute retinal necrosis.[49]

One of the most important complications of HZI is postherpetic neuralgia, defined as pain that lingers for 30 days[51] or 120 days[53] after the onset of the acute rash (see Chapter 10). Postherpetic neuralgia affects approximately 8 to 70% of patients over age 50; up to 50% of patients over age 50 have debilitating pain lasting more than 1 month.[49,54] Some unfortunate patients experience pain for years.[51]

Predisposing factors include older age, prodromal pain, and more severe clinical disease during the acute rash phase.[55,56]

Immunocompromised patients often experience more severe VZI that may appear atypical, be bilateral, and involve multiple dermatomes; retinitis, pneumonitis, and encephalitis have been reported as complications in this patient population. On rare occasions, HZI may involve not just the dorsal root ganglion but also the anterior horn cells, leading to paralysis.[49]

ORAL MANIFESTATIONS

Primary VZV infection presents as minor acute ulcerations in the mouth that pale in clinical significance when compared with the skin lesions.

In recurrent VZV infection, the ophthalmic division of the trigeminal nerve is the cranial nerve most often affected (herpes zoster ophthalmicus); corneal involvement may lead to blindness.[49] Involvement of this nerve (V) leads to lesions on the upper eyelid, forehead, and scalp with V1; midface and upper lip with V2; and lower face and lower lips with V3 (Figures 10 and 11). With involvement of V2, patients experience a prodrome of pain, burning, and tenderness, usually on the palate on one side. This is followed several days later by the appearance of painful, clustered 1 to 5 mm ulcers (rarely vesicles, which break down quickly) on the hard palate or even buccal gingiva, in a distinctive unilateral distribution (Figure 12). Ulcers often coalesce to form larger ulcers with a scalloped border. These ulcers heal within 10 to 14 days, and postherpetic neuralgia in the oral cavity is uncommon. Involvement of V3 results in blisters and ulcers on the mandibular gingiva and tongue.

An uncommon complication of HZI involving the geniculate ganglion is Ramsay Hunt syndrome. Patients develop Bells palsy, vesicles of the external ear, and loss of taste sensation in the anterior two-thirds of the tongue.[50] HZI has been reported to cause resorption and exfoliation of teeth and osteonecrosis of the jawbones, especially in patients with HIV disease.[57–60]

DIFFERENTIAL DIAGNOSIS

The pain that is often experienced in the prodrome before the onset of vesicles and ulcers may lead to an incorrect diagnosis of pulpitis, leading to unnecessary dental treatment such as endodontic therapy.

HSV infection appears in a similar fashion and if mild and localized to one side may be mistaken for HZI; cultures differentiate between the two. Other blistering/ulcerative conditions such as pemphigus or pemphigoid are chronic and/or progressive diseases that do not present unilaterally.

In severe cases of localized necrosis of the soft tissues and bone, acute necrotizing ulcerative periodontitis should be considered, particularly in the HIV population. Coinfection with CMV is often noted in immunocompromised patients.[61] Bisphosphonate-associated and radiation-associated osteonecrosis of the jaws will have a history of exposure to bisphosphonate and radiation, respectively, and often is precipitated by dentoalveolar trauma in the absence of clustered ulcers.

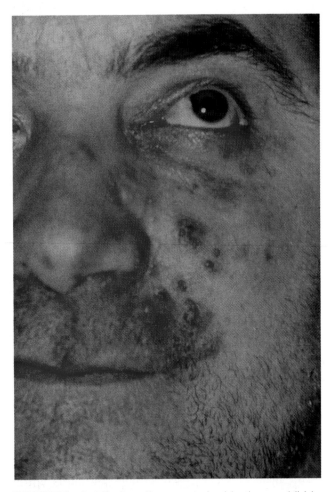

FIGURE 10   Facial lesions of herpes zoster involving the second division of the trigeminal nerve.

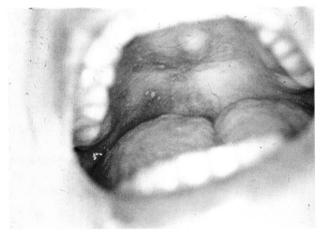

FIGURE 11   Palatal lesions of herpes zoster of second division of the trigeminal nerve.

In this age of bioterrorism, clinicians should be familiar with the signs of infection with vaccinia (smallpox virus), which presents with characteristic skin blisters and pustules.

LABORATORY FINDINGS

As with HSV infection, viral isolation using cell culture is still the best way to confirm a diagnosis of VZV infection, although

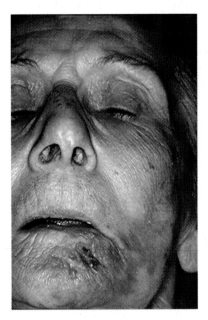

FIGURE 12   Herpes zoster of third division of trigeminal nerve.

VZV is more fastidious and difficult to culture. A simple smear stained with a standard laboratory stain would reveal the presence of multinucleated epithelial cells, but this does not distinguish between HSV and VZV. Direct fluorescent antibody testing using a smear may have greater sensitivity.[62] This test uses a smear obtained by scraping the lesion and staining it with antibody against VZV conjugated to a fluorescent compound. The use of PCR to detect viral antigen is expensive and highly sensitive, but the presence of VZV antigen does not always equate with active infection.[63]

After primary infection, the patient seroconverts and IgG against VZV is detectable in the serum. HZI causes a transient rise in IgM and an increase in levels of IgG, but these are not reliable for diagnostic purposes.[64]

Biopsy is usually not required and not the diagnostic test of choice since the clinical presentation is usually characteristic. If one should be performed, tissue should always include the intact epithelium since that is where the cytopathic effect is best seen. VZV and HZI are cytopathic to the epithelial cells and result in the formation of multinucleated epithelial cells with viral inclusions, similar to HSV infection.

In HZI, there is inflammation of peripheral nerves leading to demyelination and wallerian degeneration, as well as degeneration of the dorsal horn cells of the spinal cord.[51]

MANAGEMENT

As with HSV infection, management of oral lesions of varicella and HZI is directed toward pain control (particularly the prevention of postherpetic neuralgia), supportive care and hydration (see Table 2), and definitive treatment to minimize the risk for dissemination, particularly in immunocompromised patients. Aspirin use, especially in patients with VZV infection or influenza, is associated with the development of Reye syndrome, which is potentially fatal, and is contraindicated; ibuprofen is the preferred analgesic.[65]

Treatment of primary VZV infection includes the use of acyclovir (800 mg five times a day).[66,67] This reduces infectivity, the severity of lesions, and hospitalizations for complications. However, acyclovir has poor bioavailability.

Valacyclovir (1,000 mg three times a day) or famciclovir (500 mg three times a day) for 7 days is effective in treating HZI and should be started within 72 hours of disease onset.[54,55] These drugs also reduce the incidence of postherpetic neuralgia when compared with acyclovir.

The first line of treatment for postherpetic neuralgia is gabapentin[68] and 5% lidocaine patch,[69] and the second line of treatment is with opioid analgesics and tricyclic antidepressants.[53] The use of corticosteroids and antiviral therapy together in an attempt to reduce postherpetic neuralgia has not proved effective.[51,56,70] Other modalities of treatment have been reviewed.[51] Case reports suggest that botulinum toxin may provide relief.[71] For a more detailed description of management of postherpetic neuralgia, see Chapter 10.

A live, attenuated vaccine for the prevention of VZV infection has been shown to reduce the incidence of varicella outbreaks.[72] Vaccination of older adults with this vaccine causes an increase in antibody levels, boosts cell-specific immunity, and reduces the incidence and/or severity of subsequent HZI and postherpetic neuralgia.[73,74]

Cytomegalovirus (CMV) Infection

ETIOLOGY AND PATHOGENESIS

CMV is a β-herpesvirus, and 60 to 70% of the adult population has been exposed.[75] Primary infection may be asymptomatic or cause an infectious mononucleosis–like disease. Manifestations of infection and disease are most evident in the immunocompromised population, such as patients who have received organ transplants or those who have AIDS. It is the most common cause of pneumonia within the first 120 days after hematopoietic stem cell transplantation.[76] Once exposed to CMV, this virus establishes latency within the connective tissue cells, such as the endothelium of blood vessels, mononuclear cells, white blood cells, and epithelial cells.[77] CMV within endothelial cells may contribute to vascular inflammation, vascular occlusion, and end-organ damage.[78] Transmission is by direct transfer of infected white blood cells through intimate contact and through blood products.[77] In organ transplant recipients, CMV in the donor organ leads to CMV infection in the recipient.[79] There is growing evidence that CMV infection is associated with Guillain-Barré syndrome, as well as polyradiculopathy and myopathy in patients with AIDS.[80,81]

A recent study on mucocutaneous CMV infection (mostly perianal) revealed that CMV infection of mucocutaneous sites was usually part of a polymicrobial infection with HSV or VZV.[82] The authors suggest that CMV in such cases is not the pathogenic agent for these ulcers since the presence of those two α-herpesviruses alone could account for the ulceration and tissue damage. These authors also noted that CMV was often found in nonlesional skin.

CLINICAL FINDINGS

Primary CMV infection presents similarly to infectious mononucleosis with marked lymphocytosis; 20% of patients with infectious mononucleosis–like symptoms have CMV rather than EBV infection.[83] Unlike the more common EBV-associated infectious mononucleosis, there is fever but little lymphadenopathy or splenomegaly.[77] Serious complications include meningoencephalitis, myocarditis, and thrombocytopenia.

Approximately 90% of patients with AIDS have circulating antibodies against CMV.[84] In these patients, CMV tends to involve the eye (CMV retinitis that may result in blindness if untreated), gastrointestinal tract (CMV enteritis), and mucocutaneous sites, especially perianal and perigenital areas.

ORAL MANIFESTATIONS

CMV infection in the mouth in the immunocompromised patient tends to present as a single large necrotic ulcer and less often as multiple ulcers. They are usually painful and may have been present for weeks or months. Any site may be involved. Up to one-third of such ulcers are coinfected with other viruses of the herpes family, especially HSV and VZV.[85,86]

There have been occasional reports of mandibular osteomyelitis and tooth exfoliation associated with CMV and VZV infection.[61,87] Both viruses are associated with vasculopathy and thrombosis, which may be the underlying etiopathogenesis.[58,60,88]

DIFFERENTIAL DIAGNOSIS

As indicated earlier, CMV is often seen in association with HSV or VZV infections and, in such situations, may be a bystander rather than pathogenic. Therefore, evaluation for these other two viruses is essential for single or multiple ulcers in the immunocompromised population. In patients with human immunodeficiency virus (HIV)/AIDS, infections with mycobacteria, fungi, and other organisms must be ruled out.

Single ulcers of acute onset present for weeks or months should be evaluated for squamous cell carcinoma or other malignancies. Since patients who develop such ulcers caused by opportunistic pathogens are often immunocompromised, one should have a high index of suspicion for a malignancy.

Benign or malignant salivary gland tumors or soft tissue tumors may also become secondarily ulcerated from trauma. Single ulcers on the tongue may also represent traumatic ulcerative granuloma (see below).

LABORATORY TESTS

CMV infections of the oral cavity presenting as ulcers tend to be deep with viral particles residing in endothelial cells and tissue monocytes. As such, a culture of an ulcer infected by CMV is unlikely to be positive unless there is associated viremia with shedding of CMV from the ulcer surface, an uncommon scenario. Systemic infection is generally identified by blood culture using "shell vials" of cultured cells in which

CMV antigens are detected through the use of monoclonal antibodies; CMV is fairly difficult to grow in culture.[89]

Deoxyribonucleic acid (DNA) hybrid capture using the serum buffy coat is also used to identify the presence of DNA, but this does not equate with active infection. Small amounts of CMV DNA can be identified using PCR or nucleic acid probes and hybridization techniques. CMV matrix protein PP65 is also often found in neutrophils, and these can be assayed.[77] Antibody titers against CMV are unreliable for the diagnosis of active infection.

Biopsy for microscopic examination and/or to obtain tissue for culture is the test of choice for identification of CMV in such ulcers.[86] CMV infection produces large intranuclear inclusions (representing nucleoprotein cores) within endothelial cells and monocytes within the connective tissue, with an associated nonspecific chronic inflammation.[90] The use of immunohistochemical staining helps identify CMV if there are only a few infected cells. A biopsy has the advantage of also ruling out any of the other differential diagnoses discussed. It is important to make sure that the biopsy includes normal epithelium because if the ulcer is coinfected with HSV or VZV, these would be identified on the biopsy in the intact epithelium adjacent to the ulcer.

MANAGEMENT

As with all ulcerative lesions, patients should have pain managed with topical anesthetics and systemic analgesics as needed, with appropriate dietary modifications and good hydration (see Table 2). CMV infection is treated with ganciclovir, valganciclovir (a valine ester of ganciclovir with approximately 10-fold bioavailability of ganciclovir), or cidofovir.

Coxsackievirus (CV) Infection

CV, a ribonucleic acid (RNA) virus, is a member of the genus *Enterovirus* and family Picornaviridae and has features in common with poliovirus.[91] More than 90% of infections caused by the nonpolio enteroviruses are either asymptomatic or result in nonspecific febrile illness. There are 23 CV type A (CVA) and 6 CV type B (CVB) viruses.[92] The viruses replicate first in the mouth and then extensively in the lower gastrointestinal tract, where they shed. Transmission is therefore primarily by the fecal-oral route, although some shedding occurs in the upper respiratory tract.

CVA infection is implicated in paralytic disease, a cold-like illness and upper respiratory tract infection that is usually febrile, and pleurodynia.[91] CVB (in particular CVB4) infection is associated with the development of aseptic meningitis, sometimes complicated by encephalitis, carditis, and disseminated neonatal infection.[93] More recently, it has been implicated in the pathogenesis of type 1 insulin-dependent diabetes mellitus.[91] One theory suggests direct destruction of the pancreatic islets by the virus, whereas another focuses on the viral infection triggering an autoimmune destruction of islet cells because of similarity between viral and islet cell antigens. CVB4 has also been implicated in the pathogenesis of primary

Sjögren syndrome. Enteroviral capsid protein VP1 was identified via immunoperoxidase staining in the salivary gland samples of most patients with primary but, interestingly, not secondary Sjögren syndrome. Furthermore, a 94-base-pair fragment of CVB4, the *p2A* gene found in CVB4 and CVA13, was also found within salivary gland tissue in patients with primary Sjögren syndrome.[94] Cross-reactivity between antibodies to a major B-cell antigen and CV antigen has been demonstrated, and this may play a role in autoantibody generation in patients with primary Sjögren syndrome.[95]

In the oral cavity, CV infections lead to three disease entities: HFM disease, herpangina, and lymphonodular pharyngitis.

HAND-FOOT-AND-MOUTH DISEASE (HFM)

Of all the CVs, CVA16 is the most common cause of this vesicular exanthem, although CVA4–7, CVA9, CVA10, CVA24, CVB2, and CVB5, as well as echovirus 18, have also been implicated.[91] Enterovirus (EV)71 (related to CVA16) is a common cause of HFM disease and has been seen in large outbreaks in Southeast Asia. HFM disease, as with many CV infections, including herpangina, tends to be seasonal (usually summer), occurs in epidemic clusters, and has high transmission rates.

In comparing cases of HFM disease caused by EV71 with those caused by CVA16, EV71 is much more likely to be associated with severe central nervous system disease (such as meningitis and brainstem encephalitis), paralysis, pulmonary edema, and death.[96] In one study of patients with HFM disease and herpangina, 83% of cases were caused by EV71 and only 8% by CVA or CVB.[97] In another study of EV71 infections, 87% of cases manifested with HFM disease and 13% with herpangina.[98]

Clinical Findings. HFM disease usually afflicts children younger than 10 years in summer. Patients have a low-grade fever and sore mouth; 75 to 100% of patients have a skin rash, especially on the hands and feet (dorsa, palms and soles) and 30% on the buttocks.[99,100] The rash is first red and macular and then becomes vesicular.

Oral Manifestations. Patients are febrile and complain of a sore mouth and throat. Lesions begin as erythematous macules that become vesicles and quickly break down to ulcers. Lesions are usually located on the tongue, hard and soft palate, and buccal mucosa but can present on any oral mucosal surface.[99,100]

HERPANGINA

The word *herpangina* derives from *herpes*, meaning "vesicular eruption," and *angina*, meaning "inflammation of the throat." CVA (serotypes 1–10, 16, and 22) are the most common viruses isolated from this disease.[91,101] But CVB1–5,[91,102] echoviruses, and EV71 have also been identified in this condition.[96]

Clinical Findings. As with all CV infections, children under 10 are usually afflicted and outbreaks usually occur in epidemics in summer. Patients develop fever, headache, and myalgia that usually last only 1 to 3 days.

Oral Manifestations. The first oral symptoms of herpangina are sore throat and pain on swallowing. There may be erythema of the oropharynx, soft palate, and tonsillar pillars. Small vesicles form, but these rapidly break down to 2 to 4 mm ulcers. These persist for 5 to 10 days (Figure 13).[91]

Lymphonodular pharyngitis is considered a variant of herpangina[91] and is associated with CVA10. Patients report a sore throat, but rather than presenting with vesicles that break down to ulcers, patients develop diffuse small nodules in the oropharynx.[103]

DIFFERENTIAL DIAGNOSIS

Lesions of both HFM disease and herpangina may resemble primary herpetic gingivostomatitis. However, lesions on the palms and soles are typical for HFM disease, and ulcers in the posterior oral cavity are typical for herpangina. Bright red and painful gingiva also characterize primary HSV infection, and this is uncommon in CV infections. Primary HSV infection also tends to cause more severe constitutional symptoms and signs. Chickenpox presents with generalized vesicular skin lesions, but ulcers are not prominent in the oral cavity; patients also appear more ill.

Streptococcal infections of the throat generally do not produce vesicles or ulcers seen in HFM disease or herpangina but rather a purulent exudate, although the two may appear similar; cultures distinguish between the two. Infectious mononucleosis (primary EBV infection) may also present with sore throat and purulent exudates, but serology distinguishes this from CV infections.

LABORATORY TESTS

CVB infections may be diagnosed by culture (usually from the throat or feces), but only CVA9 and CVA16 grow readily

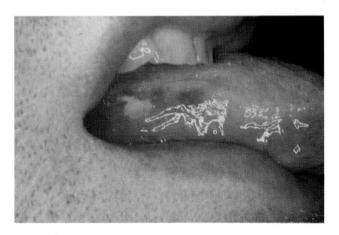

FIGURE 13 A cluster of ulcers on the tongue of a patient with herpangina. The patient also had lesions of the palate and posterior pharyngeal wall.

and CVA is best identified by inoculation into newborn mice.[92] Serum IgM to CVB can be detected early on but is not serotype specific. Reverse transcriptase PCR is another sensitive and rapid way of identifying viral RNA in clinical specimens.[92]

Diagnosis is usually made on clinical findings, and culture and biopsies are rarely necessary for diagnosis. Nevertheless, skin biopsies of HFM disease and herpangina show intraepidermal vesicles with a mixed lymphocytic and neutrophilic infiltrate, degeneration of epidermal cells, and dermal edema. Eosinophilic nuclear inclusions and intracytoplasmic picornavirus particles are seen in the surrounding dermal vessels.[104,105] Biopsy of lymphonodular pharyngitis shows hyperplastic lymphoid nodules.

MANAGEMENT

CV infections are self-limiting (unless complications arise or the patient is immunocompromised), and management is directed toward control of fever and mouth pain, supportive care, and limiting contact with others to prevent spread of the infection. Effective antiviral agents for CV are not available.

Necrotizing Ulcerative Gingivitis (NUG) and Periodontitis (NUP)

NUG, formerly known as acute necrotizing ulcerative gingivitis (ANUG), and its more severe counterpart, necrotizing ulcerative periodontitis (NUP), were reclassified in 1999 by the American Academy of Periodontics under the category of "Necrotizing Periodontal Disease."[106] These are acute ulcerative-inflammatory conditions of the gingiva and periodontium, respectively, that are associated with polymicrobial infection. During World War I, NUG was dubbed "trench mouth" since it was frequent among the soldiers in the trenches. NUG and NUP have strong associations with immune suppression (especially AIDS), debilitation, smoking, stress, poor oral hygiene, local trauma, and contaminated food supply. Diabetes may also be a risk factor.[107] It is unclear if NUG is a forerunner of NUP, but they are often seen in patients with AIDS. Both NUP and noma thrive in communities characterized by a large low socioeconomic class and extreme poverty.[108, 109]

ETIOLOGY AND PATHOGENESIS

The more important and constant of the microbes involved include *Treponema* species, *Prevotella intermedia*, *Fusobacteria nucleatum*, *Peptostreptococcus micros*, *Porphyromonas gingivalis*, *Selenomonas* species, and *Campylobacter*.[110–112] Since some of these fusospirochetal organisms are common in the periodontal tissues, many believe that it is the permissive environment of an immunocompromised host that allows these microbes to proliferate. The tissue destruction is most probably a result of the production of endotoxins and/or immunologic activation and subsequent destruction of the gingiva and adjacent tissues. In addition, patients show reduced neutrophil chemotaxis and phagocytosis, resulting in poor control of infection.[110] Some have identified herpesviruses within the crevicular fluid,[111] but such viruses shed readily in oral secretions, particularly in areas where there is tissue destruction and therefore maybe nonpathogenic bystanders.

If there is underlying systemic illness, NUG and NUP can spread rapidly from the gingiva to the periodontium and into the soft tissues, giving rise to cancrum oris, noma, or orofacial gangrene. This is particularly devastating in children who are malnourished and live in poverty and is seen not infrequently in Africa. *Fusobacterium necrophorum* is likely to play an important role in the progression of NUP to cancrum oris because this organism produces a dermonecrotic toxin, hemolysin, leukotoxin, and proteolytic enzymes, all leading to extensive tissue destruction.[111] It may also stimulate the growth of *P. intermedia*.

CLINICAL FINDINGS

NUG and NUP may or may not be associated with fever and malaise, although submandibular lymphadenopathy is usually present. This may be more prominent in patients with an underlying immunodeficiency.

However, noma generally is accompanied by fluctuating fever, marked anemia, high white cell count, general debilitation, and a recent history of some other systemic illness, such as measles.[109]

ORAL MANIFESTATIONS

NUG has a rapid and acute onset. The first symptoms include excessive salivation, a metallic taste, and sensitivity of the gingiva. This rapidly develops into extremely painful and erythematous gingiva with scattered punched-out ulcerations, usually on the interdental papillae, although any part of the marginal gingiva may be affected (Figure 15). There is accompanying malodor, and there may be gingival bleeding. Because of the pain associated with the gingivitis, there is usually abundant build-up of dental plaque around the teeth because it may be too painful to perform effective oral hygiene.

In patients with AIDS, the prevalence of NUP is approximately 6% and is strongly predictive of a CD4 count below 200 cell/mm³.[113] In this population, these areas of

necrosis may also occur primarily on the soft tissues (Figure 15).[114]

In patients in whom there is severe immunodeficiency or malnutrition, NUG and NUP may progress to noma (Figure 16). The overlying skin becomes discolored, and perforation of the skin ensues. The orofacial lesions are cone-shaped, with the base of the cone within the oral cavity and the tip at the skin aspect. There is sloughing of the oral mucosa followed by sequestration of the exposed, necrotic bone and teeth. Without treatment, the mortality rate is 70 to 90%.[111]

DIFFERENTIAL DIAGNOSIS

The acute onset of erythematous and ulcerated gingiva of NUG may suggest a diagnosis of primary herpetic gingivostomatitis. Desquamative gingivitides (such as mucous membrane (cicatricial) pemphigoid, pemphigus vulgaris, lichen planus, and hypersensitivity reaction) may present primarily on the gingiva, with no skin findings. However, these conditions are not of acute onset but rather chronic and/or progressive over months and years and are characterized by inflammation rather than necrosis.

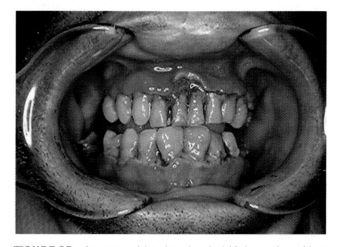

FIGURE 15 Acute necrotizing ulcerative gingivitis in a patient without an underlying medical disorder.

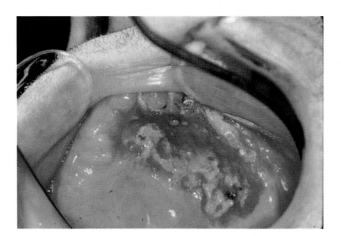

FIGURE 14 Fuzospirochetal palatal lesions in a neutropenic patient.

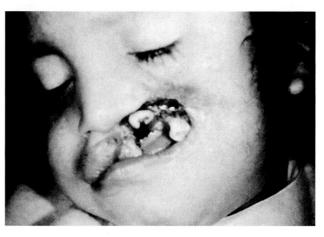

FIGURE 16 Cancrum oris or noma. Courtesy of Dr. Gustavo Berger, Guatemala City, Guatemala.

Single large necrotic ulcers of noma suggest deep fungal infections or infections with the herpes family of viruses, especially in immunocompromised patients. Squamous cell carcinoma is also a consideration in this group of patients.

LABORATORY TESTING

Secretions from the gingival sulcus grow mixed flora but in particular will be culture positive for *Treponema species*, *P. intermedia*, *F. nucleatum*, and other bacteria as indicated above. Necrotizing gingival lesions may also be caused by microbes other than fusospirochetes, such as *Pseudomonas aeruginosa*.[115]

A biopsy usually is not helpful in making a diagnosis, although biopsies may be performed to rule out some other condition that may have a similar clinical presentation. The lesions demonstrate ulceration, extensive necrosis, leukocytoclasia, histiocytic vasculitis with luminal fibrin clots, and a prominent infiltrate of large atypical cells, a histologic picture resembling extranodal Kikuchi disease. More than half of the cases were immunoreactive for HIV p24 within focal histiocytes, whereas EBV RNA was identified in 1 (6%) of 17 cases.[116]

MANAGEMENT

This is directed toward supportive care and pain control (see Table 2), definitive treatment, and identification of underlying predisposing factors. In patients who are malnourished, nutritional rehabilitation is essential to halt the progress of gingival lesions to noma.

Definitive treatment of NUG and NUP consists of gentle débridement to remove as much of the debris and plaque as possible; this is best accomplished with topical anesthesia during the first few visits. The use of chlorhexidine digluconate mouthrinse led to resolution in >90% of cases.[117] Patients with more extensive disease and/or systemic symptoms may require antibiotics active against gram-negative anaerobes, such as β-lactams.[114] Interestingly, metronidazole, which has little activity against spirochetes, also is effective, suggesting that resolution can occur without treatment of the entire microbial complex.

Once the acutely painful episodes have resolved, scaling and root planing to completely remove all residual plaque and calculus are indicated. Periodontal surgery may be necessary to correct gingival and periodontal defects. It may be appropriate to test the patient for HIV or other immunosuppressive conditions, such as blood dyscrasia.

Cases of noma need aggressive treatment with nutritional supplementation, antibiotics, and tissue débridement. Nevertheless, survivors exhibit significant disfigurement and functional impairment from tissue loss and scarring.[111]

Erythema Multiforme (EM)

EM is an acute, self-limited, inflammatory mucocutaneous disease that manifests on the skin and often oral mucosa, although other mucosal surfaces, such as the genitalia, may also be involved.[118–120] There is still controversy over how best to classify EM. In general, EM is classified as EM minor if there is less than 10% of skin involvement and there is minimal to no mucous membrane involvement, whereas EM major has more extensive but still characteristic skin involvement, with the oral mucosa and other mucous membranes affected.[118, 119] Historically, fulminant forms of EM were labeled Stevens-Johnson syndrome (SJS) and toxic epidermal necrolysis [TEN (Lyell disease)]. However, more recent data suggest that EM is etiopathogenetically distinct from those two latter conditions, and they are discussed separately below.

ETIOLOGY AND PATHOGENESIS

EM is a hypersensitivity reaction, and the most common inciting factors are infection, particularly with HSV, or drug reactions to NSAIDS or anticonvulsants.[118,119] Cases of oral EM precipitated by benzoic acid, a food preservative, have been reported.[121] Other viral, bacterial, fungal, and protozoal infections and medications may also play a role. Because it is a hypersensitivity reaction, HSV is not cultured from lesions.

Some studies show that recurrent EM is associated with HSV infection in 65 to 70% of cases, both by history of HSV infection 1 to 3 weeks before onset of EM, seropositivity for HSV antibodies, and identification of HSV antigens.[122–124] Approximately 87% had concurrent RHL (Figure 17).[124] Using PCR techniques, HSV gene products have been identified in 71 to 81% of cases of recurrent EM.[10,11] For nonrecurrent EM, this falls to 27%.[11] It is postulated that HSV antigens incite a T cell–mediated delayed-type hypersensitivity reaction that generates interferon-γ, with the amplified immune system recruiting more T cells to the area. Cytotoxic T cells, natural killer cells, and/or cytokines destroy the epithelial cells.[120]

CLINICAL FINDINGS

EM generally affects those between ages 20 and 40 years, with 20% occurring in children.[118] Patients with recurrent EM have an average of 6 episodes a year (range 2–24), with a mean duration of 9.5 years; remission occurred in 20% of cases.[124] Episodes usually last several weeks.[118,119] There is often a prodrome of fever, malaise, headache, sore throat, rhinorrhea, and cough.[118] These symptoms suggest a viral (especially

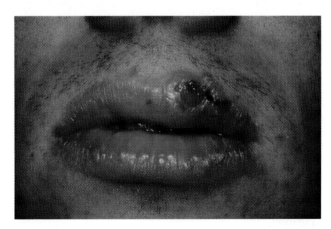

FIGURE 17 Early vesicular lesions in a patient who develops erythema multiforme after each episode of recurrent herpes labialis.

respiratory tract) infection, and this is not surprising since infectious agents are known to trigger EM.

Skin lesions appear rapidly over a few days and begin as red macules that become papular, starting primarily in the hands and moving centripetally toward the trunk in a symmetric distribution. The most common sites of involvement are the upper extremities, face, and neck.[118] The skin lesions may take several forms—hence the term *multiforme*. The classic skin lesion consists of a central blister or necrosis with concentric rings of variable color around it called typical "target" or "iris" lesion that is pathognomonic of EM; variants are called "atypical target" lesions (Figures 18 and 19). The skin may feel itchy and burnt. Postinflammatory hyperpigmentation is common in dark-skinned individuals and may be worsened by sun exposure.[118]

ORAL FINDINGS

The oral findings in EM range from mild erythema and erosion to painful ulcerations (Figure 20).[118] When severe, ulcers may be large and confluent, causing difficulty in eating, drinking, and swallowing, and patients with severe EM may drool blood-tinged saliva.

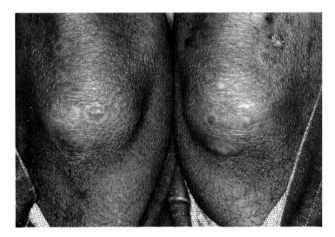

FIGURE 18   Target lesions of the skin of the leg.

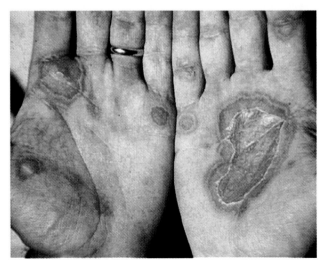

FIGURE 19   Erythema multiforme with target lesions of the skin of the hand.

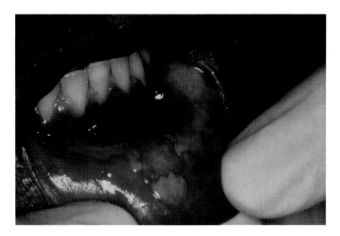

FIGURE 20   Intraoral lesions of erythema multiforme in an 18-year-old male.

Oral lesions are present in 23 to 70% of patients with recurrent EM.[122–125] The most commonly affected sites are the lips (36%), buccal mucosa (31%), tongue (22%), and labial mucosa (19%).[125] Genital and ocular sites are affected in 25 and 17% of cases, respectively.[124]

The concept of pure oral EM is controversial and not universally accepted since some dermatologists believe that the characteristic appearance and distribution of skin lesions are the sine qua non for the diagnosis of EM.[118] Nevertheless, cases of oral EM without skin involvement have been reported. Lesions may present intraorally only or also involve the lips and skin. Intraoral lesions are irregular bullae, erosions, or ulcers surrounded by extensive areas of inflammation. Severe crusting and bleeding of the lips are common.[121,126–129]

DIFFERENTIAL DIAGNOSIS

Primary HSV gingivostomatitis with its viral prodrome and erosions and ulcerations may resemble EM, but these lesions are culture positive for HSV and do not usually present with the typical skin rash. Lesions of HSV are usually smaller and well circumscribed, whereas EM lesions are larger. Autoimmune vesiculobullous disease such as pemphigus and pemphigoid may have oral ulcers and skin lesions, although skin lesions are bullous in nature and not maculopapular, with a centripetal progress such as is seen in EM. They are chronic, slowly progressive diseases that usually persist for months, whereas EM heals within weeks.

Recurrent oral EM in the absence of skin findings may be confused with recurrent aphthous ulcers (see below), but aphthous ulcers present as discrete lesions, whereas lesions of EM are more diffuse.

Some cases of severe EM causing hemorrhagic crusts to form on the lips may resemble paraneoplastic pemphigus (discussed below). These lesions are usually present for months and are associated with malignancy and with severe conjunctival and skin lesions.

LABORATORY FINDINGS

There are no specific laboratory tests that are useful, and the diagnosis is made primarily on clinical findings.

Early lesions show lymphocytes and histiocytes in the superficial dermis around superficial dermal vessels. This is followed by hydropic degeneration of basal cells, keratinocyte apoptosis and necrosis, subepithelial bulla formation, and a lymphocytic infiltrate.[130] Leukocyte exocytosis is also usually noted. Similar changes are seen in the biopsies of patients with oral EM.[131]

MANAGEMENT

Mild EM can be managed with systemic or topical analgesics for pain and supportive care since the disease is self-limiting and resolves within a few weeks. More severe cases are usually managed with systemic corticosteroids. Topical steroids may also help resolve lesions. Cases suspected of being HSV-associated should be treated with antiviral medications. Treatment with acyclovir at the first sign of disease in recurrent EM controls disease in approximately half of patients.[124] Continuous acyclovir at 400 mg twice a day prevents development of EM in most patients with HSV-associated disease, whereas EM not related to HSV responded well to azathioprine (100–150 mg/d).[124] Other studies have also shown good suppression of recurrent HSV-associated EM using 400 mg of acyclovir twice a day or 500 mg of valacyclovir twice daily.[42,132]

Dapsone (100–150 mg/d) and antimalarials are partially successful in suppressing recurrent outbreaks but may be associated with significant side effects.[124]

Stevens Johnson Syndrome (SJS) and Toxic Epidermal Necrolysis (TENS)

Studies done within the last 10 to 15 years now support the concept that SJS is a less severe variant of TEN and separate clinically and etiopathogenetically from EM. Although all three are hypersensitivity reactions and give rise to oral bullae, erosions, ulcers, and crusted lips, the skin lesions of SJS and TEN are different from EM. They are more severe and tend to arise on the chest rather than the extremities on erythematous and purpuric macules; these lesions are called "atypical targets." SJS is much more likely to be associated with medication use and *Mycoplasma pneumoniae* infection and rarely with HSV infection, whereas EM is much more likely to be associated with HSV infection.[133–136] The more common inciting drugs include antibacterial sulfonamides, anticonvulsants, oxicam NSAIDs, and allopurinol.[137] Some believe that SJS in children usually is not associated with a medication hypersensitivity but mainly with infectious agents.[138]

The mucosal surfaces of the eye, genitalia, and mouth are almost always severely affected by SJS/TEN, always with skin involvement. The typical oral manifestation is extensive oral ulceration with hemorrhagic crusts on the vermilion (Figure 21). These lesions resemble oral lesions of paraneoplastic pemphigus, which are long-standing and associated with malignancy (see below).

Histopathologically, most of the disease is localized in the epidermis, presumably this being the site where the drug or its metabolite is bound, with less inflammation in the dermis as is usually seen in EM. The primary cytokine involved is tumor necrosis factor (TNF)-α.

Because of the severity of this condition, treatment is generally with high doses of systemic corticosteroids, intravenous immunoglobulin, and thalidomide[138,139]

Plasma Cell Stomatitis and Oral Hypersensitivity Reactions

ETIOLOGY AND PATHOGENESIS

This is a group of conditions that have protean manifestations. Oral hypersensitivity reactions may take the following forms:

1. Acute onset of ulcers such as in oral EM (discussed above)
2. Red and white reticulated lesions of a lichenoid hypersensitivity reaction (discussed in Chapter 4, "Red and White Lesions of the Oral Mucosa")
3. Fixed drug eruption
4. Marked erosions and erythema with or without ulceration called plasma cell stomatitis (PCS)
5. Swelling of the lips/angioedema (see Chapter 18, "Immunologic Diseases")
6. Oral allergy syndrome that presents mainly with symptoms of itching with or without swelling of the oral structures and oropharynx

This discussion concentrates on lesions of PCS.

PCS is a hypersensitivity reaction that was first described in the late 1960s and early 1970s and was likely a contact stomatitis to a component of chewing gum.[140] Since then, sporadic cases have continued to be reported, and these are all likely caused by a sensitizing contactant, whether or not the contactant is identified. These include khat (*Catha edulis*),[141] components of toothpaste,[141] mint candies,[142] and household cleaners.[143] Sometimes, the terms *mucous membrane plasmacytosis* and *plasma cell orificial mucositis* are used because there may be involvement of the upper respiratory tract.[144] Because of the intense plasma cell infiltration, it is believed that this is a B cell–mediated disorder, with T cells augmenting the response. Some believe that this is caused by components of plaque bacteria, although this is not a universally accepted concept.[145]

CLINICAL FINDINGS

PCS occurs within days of exposure to the contactant, with most signs and symptoms limited to the oral cavity. Some lesions may affect the periorificial tissues or the oropharynx, leading to upper airway symptoms of hoarseness, dysphagia, and mild airway obstruction.[144] Endoscopy may reveal erythematous and thickened mucosa, often with a cobblestoning pattern from the edema. An obvious allergen/contactant is not always identified.[144,146]

ORAL MANIFESTATIONS

PCS occurs within a few days of exposure. It presents as brightly erythematous macular areas of the oral cavity, almost always involving the marginal and attached gingiva or alveolar mucosa and often involving other soft tissues, such as the maxillary and mandibular sulcus or buccal mucosa (Figures

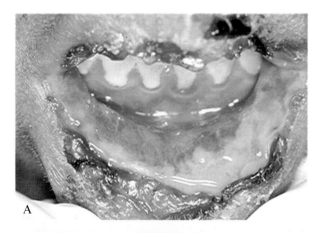

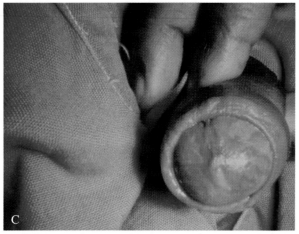

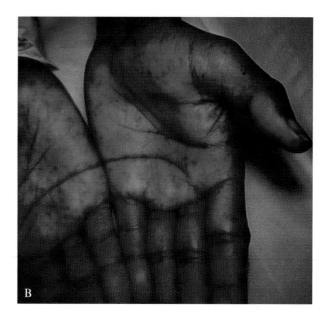

FIGURE 21 Lips and labial mucosa (*A*), skin (*B*), and penile (*C*) lesions in a 17-year-old male with Stevens-Johnson syndrome. The lesions began to arise less than 12 hours before the pictures were taken.

22, 23, and 24). Ulcers may be present, and there may be epithelial sloughing and desquamation. The gingiva may also be swollen and edematous. Patients may complain of pain and sensitivity and bleeding of the gingiva on brushing. Angular cheilitis with fissuring and dry, atrophic lips have been reported.[140,147]

Some cases reported as PCS consisted of a very localized area of erythematous gingiva, usually around a single tooth and measuring usually <1 cm.[145] Interestingly, two adults in this series also demonstrated plasma cell balanitis. It is unclear if this represented classic PCS since most cases of PCS tend to be diffuse.

DIFFERENTIAL DIAGNOSIS

The differential diagnosis for PCS includes any of the desquamative gingivitides, such as erythematous/erosive lichen planus, and the autoimmune vesiculobullous disorders, such as MMP and PV. The biggest difference is the rapid onset of PCS and the presence of generalized gingival inflammation without desquamation, ulceration, or blistering. The lesions

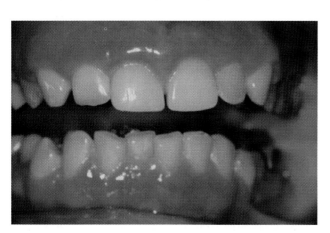

FIGURE 22 Plasma cell gingivitis of unknown etiology.

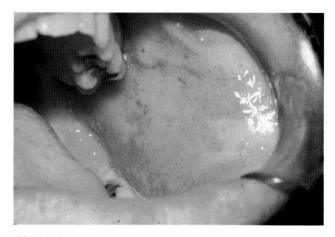

FIGURE 23 Contact allergy of the buccal mucosa due to cinnamon.

will be chronic if the patient continues to be exposed to an undetected allergen. A biopsy for both routine histology and direct immunofluorescence studies to rule out pemphigoid and pemphigus is necessary to make the diagnosis.

Another condition that PCS can mimic is pubertal or pregnancy-induced gingivitis and plaque-associated gingivitis. The difference in the histopathology is in the density of plasma cells since nonspecific gingivitis generally is associated with a plasma cell infiltrate. The clinical appearance of the diffuse red gingiva with a history of a topical irritant helps make the diagnosis. Some of the cases reported by Hedin and colleagues may constitute such plaque-associated and pubertal gingivitis.[145] Chronic granulomatous gingivitis caused by components of polishing agents such as pumice also often present with sensitive or painful erythematous gingiva. A biopsy will show the presence of particulate matter in the gingival connective tissue.

Mouth-breathers often present with erythematous and sometimes edematous gingiva, usually around the upper anterior teeth. A good history and correlation with the histopathologic findings help differentiate this from PCS.

Erythematous candidiasis may present with marked gingival erythema without the usual white curdy papules of "thrush" or pseudomembranous candidiasis. *Candida* may also secondarily infect an area of PCS.

Fixed drug eruptions are rare in the oral cavity, but there have been cases presenting as acute ulcers on the vermilion after exposure to drug such as levocetirizine, an antihistamine, resolution on withdrawal, and reulceration on rechallenge.[148]

PCS should not be confused with a direct toxic irritation of the tissues such as from strongly flavored foods.[149] This would occur in any individual and does not represent a hypersensitivity reaction because ulcers are caused by the noxious and caustic nature of the chemical in question.

LABORATORY FINDINGS

Patch testing to identify an allergen may be helpful. A biopsy is the most useful diagnostic test for this condition.

A biopsy of the gingiva in PCS shows parakeratosis, epithelial hyperplasia, neutrophilic exocytosis, and numerous spongiotic pustules in the absence of *Candida*.[140,150] The most significant finding is a dense infiltrate of plasma cells in the lamina propria; many dilated capillaries lie close to the surface, accounting for the marked erythema. Eosinophils are not seen usually.[144] Immunoperoxidase stains will invariably show the plasma cell infiltrate to be polyclonal, typical for a reactive/inflammatory process, and not monoclonal, which typifies neoplastic lesions.[71]

MANAGEMENT

PCS is self-limiting and will generally, but not always, regress if the contactant is identified and removed. Nevertheless, pain control and anti-inflammatory agents may be helpful during the healing process (see Table 2). Topical steroids may help reduce inflammation and speed healing (see Table 3).[151] Some

lesions have resolved with intralesional triamcinolone injections, although the gingiva is a particularly difficult location for such injections.[152] Cases have also responded well to prednisone.[146] Gingivectomies may be needed to recontour lesions that are long-standing and more fibrotic. One case showed improvement with 2% fusidic acid.[153]

▼ THE PATIENT WITH RECURRING ORAL ULCERS

Recurring oral ulcers are among the most common problems seen by clinicians who manage diseases of the oral mucosa. There are several diseases that should be included in the differential diagnosis of a patient who presents with a history of recurring ulcers of the mouth, including recurrent aphthous stomatitis (RAS), Behçet syndrome, recurrent HSV infection, and recurrent EM. HSV infection and EM were discussed earlier in this chapter.

Recurrent Aphthous Stomatitis (RAS)

RAS is a disorder characterized by recurring ulcers confined to the oral mucosa in patients with no other signs of disease. RAS is considered a diagnosis of exclusion since hematologic deficiencies, immune disorders, and connective tissue diseases may cause oral lesions clinically similar to RAS.

RAS affects approximately 20% of the general population, but when specific ethnic or socioeconomic groups are studied, the incidence ranges from 5 to 50%.[154] RAS is classified according to clinical characteristics: minor ulcers, major ulcers (Sutton disease, periadenitis mucosa necrotica recurrens), and herpetiform ulcers. Minor ulcers, which comprise over 80% of RAS cases, are less than 1 cm in diameter and heal without scars. Major ulcers are over 1 cm in diameter take longer to heal and often scar. Herpetiform ulcers are considered a distinct clinical entity that manifests as recurrent crops of dozens of small ulcers throughout the oral mucosa. There are cases in which a clear distinction between minor and major ulcers is blurred, particularly in patients who experience severe discomfort from continual episodes of over 10 multiple lesions, although each lesion is under 1 cm in diameter. These lesions have been referred to as "severe" minor ulcers.

ETIOLOGY AND PATHOGENESIS

It was once assumed that RAS was a form of recurrent HSV infection, and there are still clinicians who mistakenly call RAS "herpes." Many studies done during the past 40 years have confirmed that RAS is not caused by HSV.[155] This distinction is particularly important at a time when there is specific effective antiviral therapy available for HSV that is ineffective for RAS. "Herpes" is an anxiety-producing word, suggesting a sexually transmitted disease among many lay persons, and its use should be avoided when it does not apply. There have been theories suggesting a link between RAS and a number of other microbial agents, including oral streptococci, *Helicobacter pylori*, VZV, CMV, and human herpesvirus (HHV)-6 and HHV-7, but there are presently no conclusive data linking RAS to a specific microorganism.

The major factors presently linked to RAS include genetic factors, hematologic deficiencies, immunologic abnormalities, and local factors, such as trauma and smoking. There is increasing evidence linking local immune dysfunction to RAS, although the specific defect remains unknown. During the past 30 years, research has suggested a relationship between RAS and lymphocytotoxicity, antibody-dependent cell-mediated cytotoxicity, defects in lymphocyte cell subpopulations, and an alteration in the CD4 to CD8 lymphocyte ratio.[156]

More recent research has centered on dysfunction of the mucosal cytokine network. The work of Buno and colleagues suggests that an abnormal mucosal cytokine cascade in RAS patients leads to an exaggerated cell-mediated immune response, resulting in localized ulceration of the mucosa.[157] The best documented factor is heredity. Miller and colleagues studied 1,303 children from 530 families and demonstrated an increased susceptibility to RAS among children of RAS-positive parents.[158] A study by Ship showed that patients with RAS-positive parents had a 90% chance of developing RAS, whereas patients with no RAS-positive parents had a 20% chance of developing the lesions.[159] Further evidence for the inherited nature of this disorder results from studies in which genetically specific human leukocyte antigens (HLAs) have been identified in patients with RAS, particularly in certain ethnic groups.[160] There have been recent studies by Bazrafshani and colleagues linking minor RAS to genetic factors associated with immune function, particularly genes controlling release of the proinflammatory cytokines interleukin (IL)-1B and IL-6.[161] This work, as well as the work of Buno and colleagues cited above, links the evidence of the hereditary nature of RAS with specific immune abnormalities.

Hematologic deficiency, particularly of serum iron, folate, or vitamin B_{12}, appears to be an etiologic factor in a small subset of patients with RAS.[162] The size of the subset is controversial, but most estimates range from 5 to 10% (Figure 24). Studies of RAS populations from the United Kingdom show a higher level of nutritional deficiency than studies performed in the United States. One study reported clinical improvement in 75% of patients with RAS when a specific hematologic deficiency was detected and corrected with replacement therapy.[163] Some cases of nutritional deficiency, such as celiac disease, are reported to be secondary to malabsorption syndrome.

It was initially reported in the 1960s that there is a negative correlation between RAS and a history of smoking, and many clinicians have reported that RAS is exacerbated when patients stop smoking. A recent study measuring a nicotine metabolite present in the blood of smokers confirmed that the incidence of RAS is significantly lower among smokers.[164]

Other factors that have been reported associated with RAS include anxiety, periods of psychological stress, localized trauma to the mucosa, menstruation, upper respiratory infections, and food allergy.

ORAL FINDINGS

The first episodes of RAS most frequently begin during the second decade of life. The lesions are confined to the oral mucosa and begin with prodromal burning any time from 2 to 48 hours before an ulcer appears. During this initial period, a localized area of erythema develops. Within hours, a small white papule forms, ulcerates, and gradually enlarges over the next 48 to 72 hours. The individual lesions are round, symmetric, and shallow (similar to viral ulcers), but no tissue tags are present from ruptured vesicles, which helps distinguish RAS from diseases that start as vesicles, such as pemphigus, and pemphigoid. Multiple lesions are often present, but the number, size, and frequency vary considerably (Figures 25 and 26). The buccal and labial mucosae are most commonly involved. Lesions are less common on the heavily keratinized palate or gingiva. In mild RAS, the lesions reach a size of 0.3 to 1.0 cm and begin healing within a week. Healing without scarring is usually complete in 10 to 14 days.

Most patients with RAS have between two and six lesions at each episode and experience several episodes a year. The disease is an annoyance for the majority of patients with mild RAS, but it can be disabling for patients with severe frequent lesions, especially those classified as major aphthous ulcers. Patients with major ulcers develop deep lesions that are larger than 1 cm in diameter and last for weeks to months. In the most severe cases, large portions of the oral mucosa may be covered with large deep ulcers that can become confluent, which are extremely painful and disabling, interfering with speech and eating, and these patients may require hospitalization for intravenous feeding and treatment with high doses of corticosteroids. The lesions may last for months and sometimes be misdiagnosed as squamous cell carcinoma, chronic granulomatous disease, or pemphigoid. The lesions heal

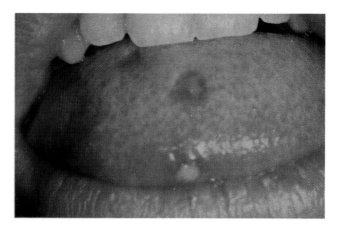

FIGURE 24 A 42-year-old woman with a recent increase in severity of recurrent aphthous ulcers. Iron deficiency was detected, and the ulcers resolved when this deficiency was corrected.

slowly and leave scars that may result in decreased mobility of the uvula and tongue.

The least common variant of RAS is the herpetiform type, which tends to occur in adults. The patient presents with small punctate ulcers scattered over large portions of the oral mucosa.

DIFFERENTIAL DIAGNOSIS

RAS is the most common cause of recurring oral ulcers and is essentially diagnosed by exclusion of other diseases. A detailed history and examination by a knowledgeable clinician should distinguish RAS from primary acute lesions such as viral stomatitis or from chronic multiple lesions such as pemphigus or pemphigoid, as well as from other conditions associated with recurring ulcers, such as connective tissue disease, drug reactions, and dermatologic disorders. The history should emphasize symptoms of blood dyscrasias, HIV, connective tissue disease such as lupus, gastrointestinal complaints suggestive of inflammatory bowel disease, and associated skin, eye, genital, or rectal lesions (Figures 27 and 28).

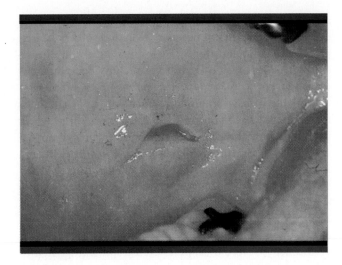

FIGURE 27   Ulcer of the buccal mucosa secondary to Crohn's disease.

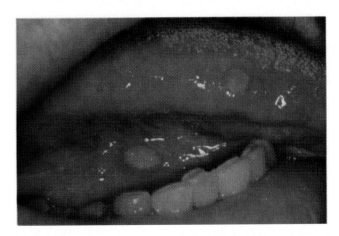

FIGURE 25   Recurrent aphthous stomatitis of the tongue and floor of the mouth.

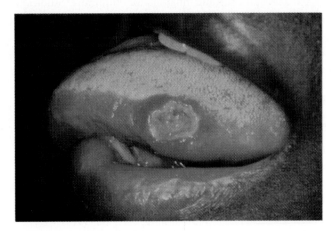

FIGURE 28   Major aphthous ulcer in an HIV-infected patient.

LABORATORY FINDINGS

Laboratory investigation should be ordered when patients do not follow the usual pattern of RAS, for example, when episodes of RAS become more severe, begin past the age of 25, or

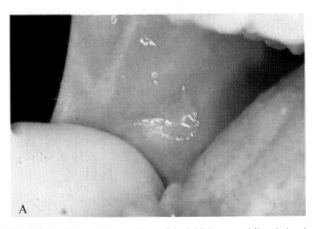

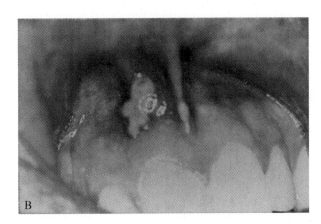

FIGURE 26   Major aphthous ulcers of the labial mucosa (*A*) and alveolar mucosa (*B*).

are accompanied by other signs and symptoms. Biopsies are only indicated when it is necessary to exclude other diseases, particularly granulomatous diseases such as Crohn disease, sarcoidosis, or blistering diseases such as pemphigus or pemphigoid.

Patients with severe minor aphthae or major aphthous ulcers should have known associated factors investigated, including connective tissue diseases and hematologic abnormalities, such as reduced levels of serum iron, folate, vitamin B_{12}, and ferritin. Patients with abnormalities in these values should be referred to an internist to rule out malabsorption syndromes and to initiate proper replacement therapy. HIV-infected patients, particularly those with CD4 counts below $100/mm^3$, may develop major aphthous ulcers, and, occasionally, severe oral ulcers are the presenting sign of AIDS.

Biopsies reveal only a superficial ulcer covered by a fibrinous exudate with granulation tissue at the base and a mixed acute and chronic inflammatory infiltratre. Studies of early lesions of RAS demonstrate an infiltration of large granular lymphocytes and helper-induced CD4 lymphocytes with focal degeneration of basal cells and the formation of small intraepithelial vesicles. The appearance of the ulcer is associated with the appearance of cytotoxic suppressor lymphocytes.[80,89]

MANAGEMENT

Medication prescribed should relate to the severity of the disease. In mild cases with two or three small lesions, use of a protective emollient such as Orabase (Bristol-Myers Squibb, Princeton, NJ) or Zilactin (Zila Pharmaceuticals, Phoenix, AZ), a topical anesthetic is all that is necessary. Pain relief of minor lesions can be obtained with use of a topical anesthetic agent or topical diclofenac, an NSAID frequently used topically after eye surgery. In more severe cases, the use of a high-potency topical steroid preparation, such as fluocinonide, betamethasone, or clobetasol, placed directly on the lesion, shortens healing time and reduces the size of the ulcers. The effectiveness of the topical steroid is partially based upon good instruction and patient compliance regarding proper use. The steroid gel can be carefully applied directly to the lesion after meals and at bedtime two to three times a day or mixed with an adhesive such as Orabase prior to application. Larger lesions can be treated by placing a gauze sponge containing the topical steroid on the ulcer and leaving it in place for 15 to 30 minutes to allow for longer contact of the medication. Other topical preparations that have been shown to decrease the healing time of RAS lesions include amlexanox paste and topical tetracycline, which can be used either as a mouthrinse or applied on gauze sponges. Intralesional steroids can be used to treat large indolent major RAS lesions. It should be emphasized that no available topical therapy reduces the frequency of new lesions.

When patients with major aphthae or severe cases of multiple minor aphthae do not improve sufficiently with topical therapy, use of systemic therapy should be considered. Drugs that have been reported to reduce the number of ulcers in selected cases of major aphthae include colchicine, pentoxifylline, dapsone, short bursts of systemic steroids, and thalidomide.[166–170] Each of these drugs has the potential for side effects, and the clinician must weigh the potential benefits versus the risks.

Thalidomide, a drug originally marketed as a nonaddicting hypnotic in the 1950s, was withdrawn from the market in the early 1960s due to its association with multiple, severe, deforming, and life-threatening birth defects. Further investigation demonstrated that thalidomide has significant anti-inflammatory and immunomodulatory properties and is useful in treating a number of diseases, including erythema nodosum leprosum, discoid lupus erythematosus, graft-versus-host disease, multiple myeloma, and Behçet syndrome. The drug has also been shown to reduce both the incidence and severity of major RAS in both HIV-positive and HIV-negative patients. The use of thalidomide for RAS should be reserved for management of severe major RAS where other less toxic therapies, including high-potency topical steroids, colchicine, and pentoxifylline, have failed to control the disease. Thalidomide must be used with extreme caution in women during childbearing years owing to the potential for severe life-threatening and deforming birth defects. All clinicians prescribing thalidomide in the United States must be registered in the STEPS (System for Thalidomide Education and Prescribing Safety) program, and patients receiving the drug must be thoroughly counseled regarding effective birth control methods that must be used whenever thalidomide is prescribed. For example, two methods of birth control must be used, and the patient must have a pregnancy test monthly. Other side effects of thalidomide include peripheral neuropathy, gastrointestinal complaints, and drowsiness. Monitoring patients taking long-term thalidomide for the development of subclinical peripheral neuropathy with periodic nerve conduction studies is also recommended.

Behçet Disease [BD (Behçet Syndrome)]

Behçets disease (BD) was initially described by the Turkish dermatologist Hulusi Behçet as a triad of symptoms including recurring oral ulcers, recurring genital ulcers, and eye involvement. BD is now understood to be a multisystem disorder with many possible manifestations. The highest incidence of BD has been reported in eastern Asia, the Middle East, and the eastern Mediterranean, particularly Turkey and Japan, where BD is a leading cause of blindness in young males; however, cases have been reported worldwide, including Europe and North America.

ETIOLOGY AND PATHOGENESIS

The cause of BD is unknown, but immune dysregulation, including circulating immune complexes, autoimmunity, cytokines, and heat shock proteins, is a major factor in the pathogenesis of BD.[172] The HLA-B51 genotype is most frequently linked to BD, especially in patients with severe forms of the disease in Asia, but the exact nature of genetics in the etiology of BD is unclear. It is theorized that BD results when a bacteria or virus triggers an immune reaction in a genetically predisposed individual.[173,174]

CLINICAL MANIFESTATIONS

The highest incidence of BD is in young adults between the ages of 25 and 40, with the oral mucosa as the most common site of involvement. The genital area is the second most common site of involvement and presents as ulcers of the scrotum and penis in males and ulcers of the labia in females. The eye lesions consist of uveitis, retinal vasculitis, vascular occlusion, optic atrophy, and conjunctivitis. Blindness is a common complication of the disease, and periodic evaluation by an ophthalmologist is necessary.

Generalized involvement occurs in over half of patients with BD. Skin lesions resembling erythema nodosum or large pustular lesions occur in over 50% of patients with BD. These lesions may be precipitated by trauma, and it is common for patients with BD to have a cutaneous hyperreactivity to intracutaneous injection or a needlestick (pathergy). Arthritis occurs in greater than 40% of patients and most frequently affects the knees, ankles, wrists, and elbows. The affected joint may be red and swollen, as in rheumatoid arthritis, but involvement of small joints of the hand does not occur, and permanent disability does not result.[175]

In some patients, central nervous system involvement is the most distressing component of the disease. This may include brainstem syndrome, involvement of the cranial nerves, or neurologic degeneration resembling multiple sclerosis that can be visualized by magnetic resonance imaging of the brain.[176] Other reported signs of BD include thrombophlebitis, intestinal ulceration, venous thrombosis, and renal, cardiac, and pulmonary disease. Both pulmonary involvement and cardiac involvement are believed to be secondary to vasculitis. Involvement of large vessels is life threatening because of the risk of arterial occlusion or aneurysms.

BD in children, which most frequently presents between the ages of 9 and 10 years, has similar manifestations as does the adult form of the disease, but oral ulcers are a more common presenting sign in children, and uveitis is less common. Oral lesions are the presenting symptom in over 95% of children with BD. A variant of BD, MAGIC syndrome, has been described. It is characterized by mouth and genital ulcers with inflamed cartilage.[177]

ORAL FINDINGS

The most common site of involvement of BD is the oral mucosa. Recurring oral ulcers appear in over 90% of patients; these lesions cannot be distinguished either clinically or histologically from RAS (Figure 29). Some patients experience mild recurring oral lesions; others have the deep, large,

scarring lesions characteristic of major RAS. These lesions may appear anywhere on the oral or pharyngeal mucosa.

DIFFERENTIAL DIAGNOSIS

Because the signs and symptoms of BD overlap with those of several other diseases, particularly the connective tissue diseases, it has been difficult to develop criteria that meet with universal agreement. Five different sets of diagnostic criteria have been in use during the past 20 years. In 1990, an international study group reviewed data from 914 patients from seven countries.[178] A new set of diagnostic criteria was developed that includes recurrent oral ulceration occurring at least three times in one 12-month period plus two of the following four manifestations:

1. Recurrent genital ulceration
2. Eye lesions, including uveitis or retinal vasculitis
3. Skin lesions, including erythema nodosum, pseudofolliculitis, papulopustular lesions, or acneiform nodules in postadolescent patients not receiving corticosteroids
4. A positive pathergy test, which is performed by placing a 20-gauge needle 5 mm into the skin of the forearm. The test is positive if an indurated papule or pustule greater than 2 mm in diameter forms within 48 hours.[1]

LABORATORY FINDINGS

BD is a clinical diagnosis based upon the criteria described above. Laboratory tests are used to rule out other diseases, such as connective tissue diseases (e.g. lupus erythematosus) and blood dyscrasias.

MANAGEMENT

The management of BD depends on the severity and the sites of involvement. Patients with sight-threatening eye involvement or central nervous system lesions require more aggressive therapy with drugs, with a higher potential for serious side effects. Azathioprine and other immunosuppressive drugs combined with prednisone have been shown to reduce ocular disease as well as oral and genital involvement.[179] Pentoxifylline, which has fewer side effects than do immunosuppressive drugs or systemic steroids, has also been reported to be effective in decreasing disease activity, particularly of oral and genital lesions.[180,181] Dapsone, colchicine, and thalidomide have also been used effectively to treat mucosal lesions of BD.[182,183] Agents that are active against the cytokine TNF-α, such as infliximab and ethanercept, have demonstrated potential effectiveness against the mucocutaneous and ocular manifestations of BD.[184,185]

▼ THE PATIENT WITH CHRONIC MULTIPLE LESIONS

Patients with an oral mucosal disease characterized by chronic multiple lesions, which are continuously present, are

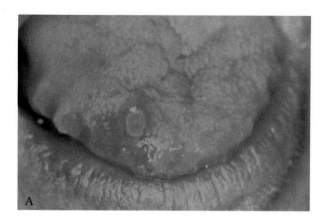
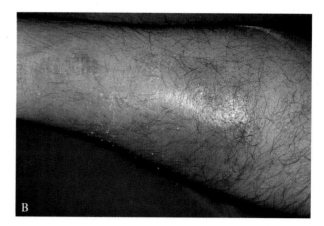

FIGURE 29   Aphthous ulcer (A) and skin lesion (B) in a patient with Behçets disease.

frequently misdiagnosed for weeks to months since their lesions are frequently confused with recurring oral mucosal disorders such as RAS and HSV-associated lesions. The clinician can avoid misdiagnosis by carefully questioning the patient on the initial visit regarding the natural history of the lesions. In recurring disorders such as severe aphthous stomatitis, the patient may experience continual new episodes of ulceration of the oral mucosa, but individual lesions heal and new ones form. In the category of disease described in this section, the same lesions are present for weeks to months. The major diseases in this group are pemphigus vulgaris, pemphigus vegetans, bullous pemphigoid (BP), mucous membrane pemphigoid, linear IgA disease, and erosive lichen planus. Lichen planus is discussed in Chapter 4. Herpes simplex infections in immunocompromised patients are discussed earlier in this chapter.

Pemphigus

Pemphigus includes a group of autoimmune, potentially life-threatening diseases that cause blisters and erosions of the skin and mucous membranes. The susceptibility to develop the autoantibodies that cause pemphigus is genetically determined, but the triggering mechanism that initiates the immune response is unknown.

There are 0.1 to 0.5 cases reported each year per 100,000 population, with the highest incidence occurring in the fifth and sixth decades of life, although rare cases have been reported in children and the elderly. Pemphigus occurs more frequently among Ashkenazi Jews, in whom studies have shown a strong association with HLA-DR4 and DQ8 haplotypes. The DR6 and DQ5 haplotypes are more common in non-Jewish patients.

Desmoglein 1 (DSG1), a glucoprotein adhesion molecule, is primarily found in the skin, whereas desmoglein 3 (DSG3) is chiefly detected in mucosal epithelium. The immune reaction against these glycoproteins causes a loss of cell-to-cell adhesion, resulting in the separation of cells and the formation of intraepithelial bullae.[186]

The major variants of pemphigus are PV, pemphigus foliaceus, paraneoplastic pemphigus (PNPP), and drug-related pemphigus. Pemphigus vegetans is a variant of PV, and pemphigus erythematosus is a variant of pemphigus foliaceus. In pemphigus foliaceus, the blister occurs in the superficial granular cell layer, whereas in PV, the lesion is deeper, just above the basal cell layer. Mucosal involvement is not a feature of the foliaceus and erythematous forms of the disease, where the antibodies are only directed against DSG1.

Drugs associated with drug-induced pemphigus include D-penicillamine and captopril. Discontinuation of the drug frequently results in spontaneous recovery.

Pemphigus Vulgaris (PV)

ETIOLOGY AND PATHOGENESIS

PV is the most common form of pemphigus, accounting for over 80% of cases. The underlying mechanism responsible for causing the intraepithelial lesion of PV is the binding of IgG autoantibodies to DSG3, a transmembrane glycoprotein adhesion molecule present on desmosomes. This glycoprotein strengthens the intercellular connection, and the loss of this connection due to the antibody antigen reaction weakens and finally breaks the connection between epithelial cells, resulting in blisters and desquamation. Patients with PV mainly involving the mucosa have antibodies primarily against DSG3, but patients with PV involving both the skin and mucosa will have antibodies against both DSG3 and DSG1.[187] Evidence for the relationship of the IgG autoantibodies to PV lesion formation includes studies demonstrating the formation of blisters on the skin of mice after passive transfer of IgG from patients with PV.

Pemphigus has been reported coexisting with other autoimmune diseases, particularly myasthenia gravis. Patients with thymoma also have a higher incidence of pemphigus. Several cases of pemphigus have been reported in patients with multiple autoimmune disorders or those with neoplasms such as lymphoma. Death occurs most frequently in elderly patients and in patients requiring high doses of corticosteroids who develop infections and bacterial septicemia, most notably from *Staphylococcus aureus*.

CLINICAL MANIFESTATIONS

The classic lesion of pemphigus is a thin-walled bulla arising on otherwise normal skin or mucosa. The bulla rapidly breaks but continues to extend peripherally, eventually leaving large areas denuded of skin. A characteristic sign of the disease may be obtained by application of pressure to an intact bulla. In patients with PV, the bulla enlarges by extension to an apparently normal surface (Figure 30). Another characteristic sign of the disease is that pressure to an apparently normal area results in the formation of a new lesion. This phenomenon, called the Nikolsky sign, results from the upper layer of the skin pulling away from the basal layer. The Nikolsky sign is most frequently associated with pemphigus but may also occur in other blistering disorders.

Some patients with pemphigus develop acute fulminating disease, but, in most cases, the disease develops more slowly, usually taking months to develop to its fullest extent (Figure 31).

Any mucosal and skin surface may be involved, and in severe cases, the conjunctival, pharyngeal, and laryngeal mucosa may all be involved, along with extensive skin lesions. Patients with oral lesions of pemphigus frequently also have esophageal lesions, and if esophageal symptoms are present, endoscopic examination should be performed to determine the severity of the lesions.

ORAL FINDINGS

Eighty to 90% of patients with PV develop oral lesions sometime during the course of the disease, and in 60% of cases, the oral lesions are the first sign. The oral lesions may begin as the classic bulla on a noninflamed base; more frequently, the clinician sees shallow irregular ulcers because the bullae rapidly break. A thin layer of epithelium peels away in an

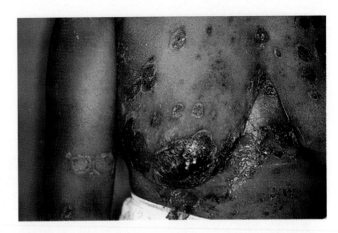

FIGURE 31 Bullae of the skin in a patient with pemphigus vulgaris.

irregular pattern, leaving a denuded base (Figure 32). The edges of the lesion continue to extend peripherally over a period of weeks until they involve large portions of the oral mucosa. Most commonly, the lesions start on the buccal mucosa, often in areas of trauma along the occlusal plane. The palate and gingiva are other common sites of involvement.

It is common for the oral lesions to be present for months before the skin lesions appear (Figure 33). If treatment is instituted during this time, the disease is easier to control, and the chance for an early remission of the disorder is enhanced. Frequently, however, the initial diagnosis is missed, and the lesions are misdiagnosed as herpes infection or candidiasis. The average time from onset of the disease to diagnosis may often take over 5 months, and coexisting candidiasis may mask the typical clinical picture of the pemphigus lesions. There is a small subgroup of pemphigus patients whose disease remains confined to the oral mucosa. These patients often have negative results on indirect and direct immunofluorescence testing.

DIFFERENTIAL DIAGNOSIS

If a proper history is taken, the clinician should be able to distinguish the lesions of pemphigus from those caused by acute viral infections or EM because of the acute nature of the latter diseases. It is also important for the clinician to distinguish pemphigus lesions from those in the RAS category. RAS lesions may be severe, but individual lesions heal and recur. In pemphigus, the same lesions continue to extend peripherally over a period of weeks to months. Lesions of pemphigus are not round and symmetric like RAS lesions but are shallow and irregular and often have detached epithelium at the periphery. In early stages of the disease, the sliding away of the oral epithelium resembles skin peeling after a severe sunburn. In some cases, the lesions may start on the gingiva as desquamative gingivitis. It should be remembered that desquamative gingivitis is not a diagnosis in itself; these lesions **must be** biopsied to distinguish PV from subepithelial **blistering** diseases such as mucous membrane pemphigoid (see below) and erosive lichen planus.

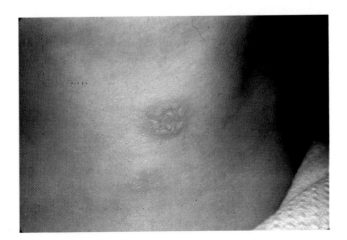

FIGURE 30 Early skin lesion of pemphigus vulgaris.

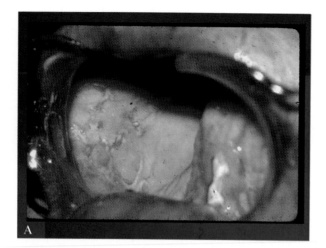 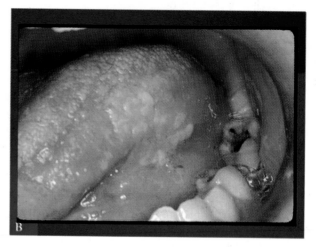

FIGURE 32 Shallow, irregular ulcers of the buccal mucosa (*A*) and tongue in a patient with pemphigus vulgaris (*B*).

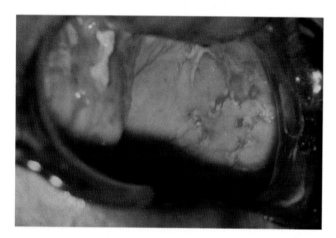

FIGURE 33 Pemphigus vulgaris of the buccal mucosa.

LABORATORY FINDINGS AND PATHOLOGY

PV is diagnosed by biopsy. Biopsies are best done on intact vesicles and bullae less than 24 hours old; however, because these lesions are rare on the oral mucosa, the biopsy specimen should be taken from the advancing edge of the lesion, where areas of characteristic suprabasilar acantholysis may be observed by the pathologist. Specimens taken from the center of a denuded area are nonspecific histologically as well as clinically. Sometimes more than one biopsy is necessary before the correct diagnosis can be made. If the patient shows a positive Nikolsky sign, pressure can be placed on the mucosa to produce a new lesion; biopsy may be done on this fresh lesion, taking care to include the blister base.

The separation of cells, called acantholysis, takes place in the lower layers of the stratum spinosum (Figure 34). Electron microscopic observations show the earliest epithelial changes as a loss of intercellular cement substance; this is followed by a widening of intercellular spaces, destruction of desmosomes, and, finally, cellular degeneration. This progressive acantholysis results in the classic suprabasilar bulla, which involves increasingly greater areas of epithelium, resulting in loss of large areas of skin and mucosa.

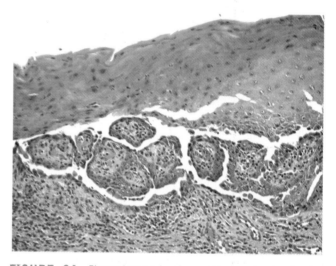

FIGURE 34 Photomicrograph of pemphigus vulgaris showing suprabasilar bulla with acantholysis.

A second biopsy, to be studied by direct immunofluorescence (DIF), should be performed whenever pemphigus is included in the differential diagnosis. This study is best performed on a biopsy specimen that is obtained from clinically normal-appearing perilesional mucosa or skin, which should be placed in Michel's transport medium. In the laboratory, fluorescein-labeled antihuman immunoglobulins are placed over the patient's tissue specimen. In cases of PV, the technique will detect antibodies, usually IgG and complement, bound to the surface of the keratinocytes (Figure 35).

Indirect immunofluorescent (IIF) antibody tests performed on a patient's serum are helpful in distinguishing pemphigus from pemphigoid and other chronic oral lesions and in following the progress of patients during treatment of pemphigus. In this technique, serum from a patient with bullous disease is placed over a prepared slide of a mucosal structure (usually monkey esophagus), and autoantibodies present in the serum will bind to the target antigen in the mucosa. The slide is then overlaid with fluorescein-tagged antihuman gammaglobulin. Patients with PV have antikeratinocyte antibodies

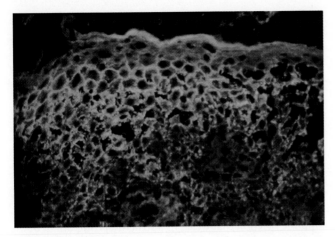

FIGURE 35 Direct immunofluorescence study of pemphigus vulgaris showing intercellular deposition of IgG.

against intercellular substances that show up under a fluorescent microscope. The titer of the antibody has been related to the level of clinical disease and may be repeated periodically during treatment to determine disease activity. An enzyme-linked immunosorbent assay has been developed that can distinguish anti-DSG1 antibodies from anti-DSG3 in serum samples of patients with PV.[188,189]

MANAGEMENT

An important aspect of patient management is early diagnosis, when lower doses of medication can be used for shorter periods of time to control the disease. Management varies according to several factors, including the severity of the disease and the speed at which the disease progresses.

The mainstay of treatment remains high doses of systemic corticosteroids, usually given in dosages of 1 to 2 mg/kg/d. When substantial doses of steroids must be used for long periods of time, adjuvant therapy is recommended to reduce the steroid dose and their potential serious complications. The most commonly used adjuvants are immunosuppressive drugs such as mycophenolate mofetil, azathioprine, or cyclophosphamide. Prednisone is used initially to bring the disease under control, and once this is achieved, the dose of prednisone is decreased to the lowest possible maintenance levels. Patients with only oral involvement also may need lower doses of prednisone for shorter periods of time, so the clinician should weigh the potential benefits of adding adjuvant therapy against the risks of long-term immunosuppression, such as blood dyscrasias and an increased risk of malignancy.

There is no one accepted treatment for pemphigus confined to the mouth, but one 5-year follow-up study of the treatment of oral pemphigus showed no additional benefit of adding cyclophosphamide or cyclosporine to prednisone versus prednisone alone, and it showed a higher rate of complications in the group taking the immunosuppressive drug.[190] Most studies of pemphigus of the skin show a decreased mortality rate when adjuvant therapy is given along with prednisone.[191] The need for systemic steroids may be lowered further in cases of oral pemphigus by combining topical with systemic steroid therapy, either by allowing the prednisone

tablets to dissolve slowly in the mouth before swallowing or by using potent topical steroid creams. Other therapies that have been reported as beneficial are parenteral gold therapy and dapsone.[192] Severe recalcitrant cases may be treated with intravenous immunoglobulins, extracorporeal photophoresis, or plasma exchange.[193–195]

Paraneoplastic Pemphigus (PNPP)

PNPP is a severe variant of pemphigus that is associated with an underlying neoplasm—most frequently non-Hodgkin's lymphoma, chronic lymphocytic leukemia, or thymoma. Castleman disease and Waldenström macroglobulinemia are also associated with cases of PNPP. The damage to the epithelium in PNPP is due to both an autoimmune reaction with epithelial cells and cell-mediated cytotoxicity.[196]

CLINICAL FINDINGS

Patients with PNPP develop severe blistering and erosions of the mucous membranes and skin. The onset of the disease is often rapid, and oral and conjunctival lesions are both common and often severe. These lesions may resemble the inflammatory lesions of a drug reaction, lichen planus, or EM, as well as the blisters seen in pemphigus (Figure 36). In severe cases, the lesions may mimic TEN and often also involve the respiratory epithelium. Unlike EM or TEN, the lesions of PNPP continue to progress over weeks to months. Progressive pulmonary involvement occurs in up to 40% of patients with PNPP.[197]

ORAL MANIFESTATIONS

Oral lesions are the most common manifestation of PNPP, and the oral disease is frequently extensive and painful. The lesions are frequently inflamed and necrotic, with large erosions covering the lips, tongue, and soft palate (Figure 37).

LABORATORY FINDINGS

Histopathology of lesions of PNPP includes changes suggestive of EM, lichen planus, pemphigoid and pemphigus. There is inflammation at the dermal-epidermal junction and

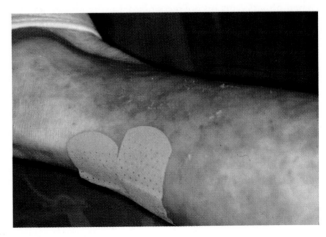

FIGURE 36 Paraneoplastic pemphigus in a patient with non-Hodgkin's lymphoma.

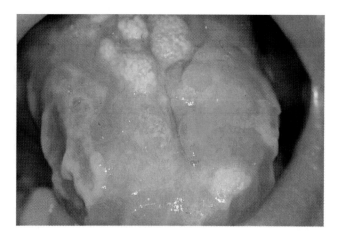

FIGURE 37 Extensive lesions of the tongue in a patient with paraneoplastic pemphigus.

keratinocyte necrosis in addition to the characteristic acantholysis seen in PV. The results of direct and indirect immunofluorescence also differ from those in PV. DIF shows deposition of IgG and complement along the basement membrane as well as on the keratinocyte surface in an intercellular location. IIF demonstrates antibodies that not only bind to epithelium but to liver, heart, and bladder tissue as well.

MANAGEMENT

Patients with PNPP secondary to localized tumors such as Castleman disease improve with the surgical removal of the tumor. Patients with PNPP resulting from lymphoma, however, have a poor prognosis and usually die within 2 years from a combination of the underlying disease, respiratory failure, and extensive mucocutaneous involvement.

Use of a combination of prednisone and immunosuppressive drug therapy may help control the severity of the skin lesions, but the oral, conjunctival, and pulmonary disease is frequently resistant to treatment.

Pemphigus Vegetans

Pemphigus vegetans, which accounts for 1 to 2% of pemphigus cases, is a relatively benign variant of PV because the patient demonstrates the ability to heal the denuded areas. Two forms of pemphigus vegetans are recognized: the Neumann type and the Hallopeau type. The Neumann type is more common, and the early lesions are similar to those seen in PV, with large bullae and denuded areas. These areas attempt healing by developing vegetations of hyperplastic granulation tissue. In the Hallopeau type, which is less aggressive, pustules, not bullae, are the initial lesions. These pustules are followed by verrucous hyperkeratotic vegetations.

Biopsy results of the early lesions of pemphigus vegetans show suprabasilar acantholysis. In older lesions, hyperkeratosis and pseudoepitheliomatous hyperplasia become prominent. Immunofluorescent study shows changes identical to those seen in PV.

ORAL FINDINGS

Oral lesions are common in both forms of pemphigus vegetans and may be the initial sign of disease.[198] Gingival

lesions may be lace-like ulcers with a purulent surface on a red base or have a granular or cobblestone appearance. Oral lesions that are associated with inflammatory bowel disease and resemble pemphigus vegetans both clinically and histologically are referred to as pyostomatitis vegetans (Figure 38).[199]

MANAGEMENT

Treatment is the same as that for PV.

Subepithelial Bullous Dermatoses

The subepithelial bullous dermatoses are a group of mucocutaneous blistering diseases that are characterized by an autoimmune reaction that weakens a structural component of the basement membrane. The diseases in this group include bullous pemphigoid, mucous membrane pemphigoid, linear IgA disease, epidermolysis bullosa aquisita, and chronic bullous dermatosis of childhood. There is significant overlap among these diseases, and the diagnosis is based upon clinical manifestations combined with routine histopathology and, when available, the newer techniques of molecular biology that identify the specific antigen. When one of these diseases is included in the differential diagnosis, a biopsy for DIF should be obtained. Recent research into pathologic mechanisms is defining the specific antigens in the basement membrane complex involved in triggering the autoantibody response. Subsets of patients diagnosed with a subepithelial bullous disease have been found to have an underlying malignancy, and this should be considered during the initial phases of management.

Bullous Pemphigoid (BP)

ETIOLOGY AND PATHOGENESIS

BP, which is the most common of the subepithelial blistering diseases, occurs chiefly in adults over the age of 60 years; it is self-limited and may last from a few months to 5 years. BP may be a cause of death in older debilitated individuals.[200] BP has occasionally been reported in conjunction with other diseases, particularly multiple sclerosis and malignancy, or drug therapy, particularly diuretics.[201]

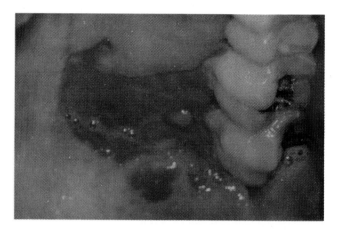

FIGURE 38 Chronic palatal lesions of pemphigus vegetans.

BP is an autoimmune disease caused by the binding of autoantibodies to specific antigens found in the lamina lucida region of the basement membrane on the hemidesmosomes of epithelial basal cells. These antigens are glycoproteins referred to as bullous pemphigoid antigens, BP 180 and BP 230.[202] Binding of antibody to antigen activates both leukocytes and complement, causing localized damage to the basement membrane, resulting in vesicle formation in the subepithelial region.

CLINICAL MANIFESTATIONS

The characteristic skin lesion of BP is a blister on an inflamed base that chiefly involves the scalp, arms, legs, axilla, and groin (Figure 39). Pruritis is a common feature of the skin lesions, which may initially present as macules and papules. The disease is self-limiting but can last for months to years without therapy. Patients with BP may experience one episode or recurrent bouts of lesions. Unlike pemphigus, BP is rarely life threatening since the bullae do not continue to extend at the periphery to form large denuded areas, although death from sepsis or cardiovascular disease secondary to long-term steroid use has been reported to be high in groups of sick elderly patients.[203]

ORAL FINDINGS

Oral involvement is common in BP, occurring in 30 to 50% of patients. The oral lesions of BP are smaller, form more slowly, and are less painful than those seen in PV, and the extensive labial involvement seen in pemphigus is not present. Desquamative gingivitis has also been reported as the most common oral manifestation of BP and the gingival lesions may be the only site of oral involvement. The gingival lesions consist of generalized edema, inflammation, and desquamation with localized areas of discrete vesicle formation. The oral lesions are clinically and histologically indistinguishable from oral lesions of mucous membrane pemphigoid, but early remission of BP is more common.

DIFFERENTIAL DIAGNOSIS

The major diseases that appear clinically similar to BP are the erosive form of lichen planus, pemphigus, and the other

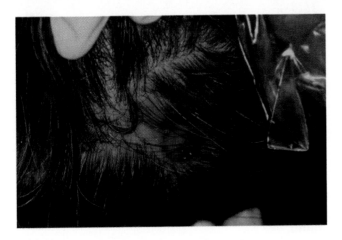

FIGURE 39 Bullous pemphigoid lesion of the scalp.

subepithelial bullous dermatoses. The erosive (ulcerative) form of LP frequently has white lesions and Wickham's striae (Chapter 4), along with ulcerations and erosions. Pemphigus usually has more extensive erosion of mucosa as well as skin involvement, and the lesions do not have the inflammation associated with mucous membrane pemphigoid. The other subepithelial bullous dermatoses (described below) appear clinically similar to mucous membrane pemphigoid and can only be distinguished by immunofluorescent and molecular techniques.

LABORATORY FINDINGS

Routine histology of a biopsy specimen demonstrates separation of the epithelium from the connective tissue at the basement membrane zone and an inflammatory infiltrate that is usually rich in eosinophils, particularly in skin biopsies.

DIF study of a biopsy specimen taken from perilesional inflamed tissue demonstrates deposition of IgG and C3 bound in a linear band to the basement membrane. IIF study of serum obtained from patients with BP demonstrates IgG antibodies bound to the epidermal side of salt-split skin. The salt-split skin test is particularly useful in distinguishing BP from EBA that has IgG antibodies localized to the dermal side of the salt-split skin (floor of the blister). IIF is not a reliable test for BP.

MANAGEMENT

Patients with localized oral lesions of BP may be treated with high-potency topical steroids, such as clobetasol or betamethasone, whereas patients with more extensive disease require use of systemic corticosteroids alone or combined with immunosuppressive drugs such as azathioprine, cyclophosphamide, or mycophenolate. Patients with moderate levels of disease may avoid use of systemic steroids by use of dapsone or tetracycline, doxycycline, or minocycline, which may be combined with niacinamide.[204]

Mucous Membrane Pemphigoid [MMP (Cicatricial Pemphigoid)]

ETIOLOGY AND PATHOGENESIS

MMP is a chronic autoimmune subepithelial disease that primarily affects the mucous membranes of patients over the age of 50, resulting in mucosal blistering, ulceration, and subsequent scarring. The disease occurs twice as frequently in women. The primary lesion of MMP occurs when autoantibodies directed against proteins in the basement membrane zone, acting with complement (C3) and neutrophils, cause a subepithelial split and subsequent vesicle formation. Ten different basement membrane antigens have been identified in cases of MMP.[205] The antigens associated with MMP are most frequently present in the lamina lucida portion of the basement membrane, but an identical antigen is not involved in all cases, and the lamina densa may be the primary site of involvement in some cases. The circulating autoantibodies are also not identical in all cases, and subsets of MMP have been identified by the technique of immunofluorescent staining of skin that has been split at the basement membrane zone with the use of sodium chloride.[206] The majority of cases of MMP demonstrate IgG directed against antigens on the epidermal side of the salt-split skin, which have been identified as BP 180 (also called type XVII collagen); however, cases of MMP have also been identified where the antigen is present on the dermal side of the split. This latter antigen has been identified as epiligrin (laminin 5), an adhesion molecule that is a component of the anchoring filaments of the basement membrane.[206,207] MMP associated with epiligrin has been reported to carry a higher risk of association with an underlying malignancy, but the evidence for this is not conclusive. Further research is required regarding the possible association of pemphigoid with malignancy, and clinicians should consider a referral to rule out a possible underlying malignancy in newly diagnosed MMP patients.[208]

CLINICAL MANIFESTATIONS

MMP generally affects patients over the age of 50 and is twice as common in women than men. The subepithelial lesions of MMP may involve any mucosal surface, but they most frequently involve the oral mucosa. The conjunctiva is the second most common site of involvement and can lead to scarring and adhesions developing between the bulbar and palpebral conjunctiva called symblepharon (Figure 40). Corneal damage is common, and progressive scarring leads to blindness in close to 15% of patients. Lesions may also affect the genital mucosa, causing pain and sexual dysfunction. Laryngeal involvement causes pain, hoarseness, and difficulty in breathing, whereas esophageal involvement may cause dysphagia, which can lead to debilitation and death in severe cases. Skin lesions, usually of the head and neck region, are present in 20 to 30% of patients.

ORAL FINDINGS

Oral lesions occur in over 90% of patients with MMP. Desquamative gingivitis is the most common manifestation and may be the only manifestation of the disease appearing bright red (Figure 41). Since these desquamative lesions resemble the lesions of erosive lichen planus and pemphigus, all cases of desquamative gingivitis should be biopsied and studied with both routine histology and DIF to determine the

correct diagnosis. Lesions may present as intact vesicles of the gingival or other mucosal surfaces, but more frequently they appear as nonspecific-appearing erosions (Figures 42 and 43). The erosions typically spread more slowly than pemphigus lesions and are more self-limiting.

LABORATORY FINDINGS

Patients with MMP included in the differential diagnosis should have biopsy specimens taken for both routine and DIF study. The specimen for routine histology should be taken from the edge of an ulcer or vesicle and a specimen for DIF taken from intact perilesional tissue. Routine histology demonstrates a lesion in the subepidermal basement membrane, which is frequently accompanied by an inflammatory infiltrate (Figure 44). Using the DIF technique (see "Laboratory Tests" under "Pemphigus Vulgaris" for description), biopsy specimens taken from MMP patients demonstrate positive fluorescence for immunoglobulin (IgG) and complement (C3) in the basement membrane zone in 50 to 80% of patients. Splitting the biopsy specimen at the basement membrane zone with 1 M NaCl prior to DIF, the

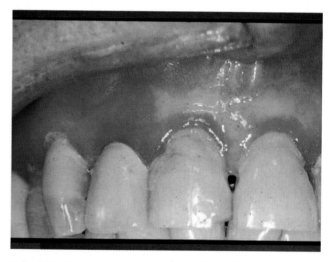

FIGURE 41 Chronic desquamative gingival lesions of mucous membrane pemphigoid.

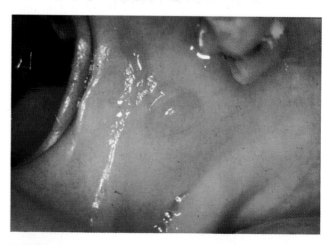

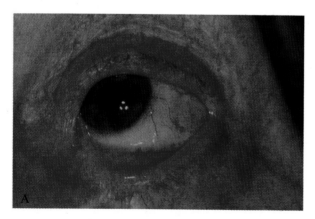

FIGURE 40 Mucous membrane pemphigoid of the conjunctiva with symplepheron formation.

FIGURE 42 Intact vesicle of buccal mucosa in a patient with mucous membrane pemphigoid.

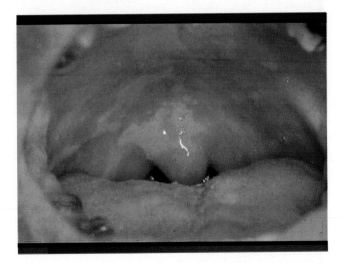

FIGURE 43 Mucous membrane pemphigoid causing lesions of the soft palate.

salt-split skin technique, increases the sensitivity of the test. Only 10% of MMP patients demonstrate positive IIF for circulating antibasement membrane zone antibodies; however, use of salt-split skin as a substrate increases the sensitivity of this test. The conclusions of an international consensus conference published in 2002 concluded that both routine histology and DIF are essential when MMP is suspected.[208]

MANAGEMENT

Management of MMP depends on the severity of symptoms and site of involvement. When the lesions are confined to the oral mucosa, use of systemic corticosteroids should only be considered for short periods of time for severe outbreaks until less toxic forms of therapy can be substituted. Unlike pemphigus, MMP is rarely a fatal disease, and long-term use of systemic steroids for oral lesion involvement alone is seldom indicated.

Patients with mild oral disease should be treated with topical and intralesional steroids. Desquamative gingivitis can often be managed with topical steroids in a soft dental splint that covers the gingiva, although the clinician using topical steroids over large areas of mucosa must closely monitor the patient for side effects such as candidiasis and effects of systemic absorption (Figure 45). When topical or intralesional therapy is not successful, use of tetracycline, doxycycline, or minocycline is often helpful in controlling desquamative gingivitis and other oral lesions. When there are severe oral lesions, conjunctival or laryngeal involvement, dapsone therapy is recommended as the next choice before considering long-term systemic steroids or immunosuppressive drug therapy.[209,210] Since dapsone causes hemolysis and methemoglobinemia, glucose-6-phosphate dehydrogenase deficiency must be ruled out, and the patient's hemoglobin must be closely monitored. Another rare side effect of dapsone is dapsone hypersensitivity syndrome, an idiosyncratic disorder characterized by fever, lymphadenopathy, skin eruptions, and occasional liver involvement. Patients resistant to dapsone should be treated with a combination of systemic corticosteroids and immunosuppressive drugs, particularly when there is risk of blindness from conjunctival involvement or significant laryngeal or esophageal damage. High-dose intravenous immunoglobulin therapy has been shown in several series of cases to be effective adjuvant therapy in patients resistant to less conventional therapy, although controlled trials have not yet been completed.

Linear IgA Disease (LAD)

ETIOLOGY AND PATHOGENESIS

LAD is a subepithelial disease characterized by the deposition of IgA rather than IgG in the basement membrane. The clinical manifestations may resemble either dermatitis herpetiformis or pemphigoid. The cause of the majority of cases is unknown, but some reported cases have been drug induced or associated with systemic diseases, including hematologic malignancies, or connective tissue diseases, such as dermatomyositis.[211] As in MMP, the antigens associated with LAD are heterogeneous and may be found in either the lamina lucida or lamina densa portions of the basement membrane.[212,213]

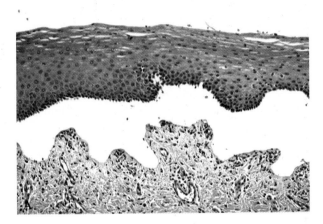
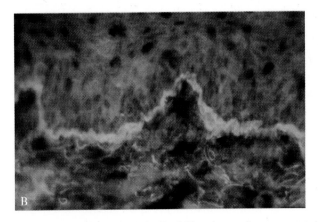

FIGURE 44 *A,* Photomicrograph of mucous membrane pemphigoid showing intact basal cells and subepithelial bulla. *B,* Direct immunofluorescence study of mucous membrane pemphigoid showing positive IgG deposition in the basement membrane zone.

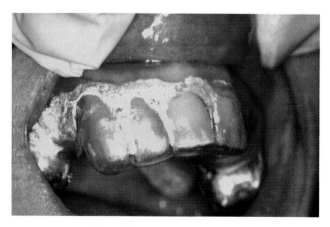

FIGURE 45 Soft medication splint used to treat desquamative gingivitis secondary to mucous membrane pemphigoid.

CLINICAL MANIFESTATIONS

The skin lesions of LAD may resemble those observed in patients with dermatitis herpetiformis, which are characterized by pruritic papules and blisters at sites of trauma such as the knees and elbows. Other patients have bullous skin lesions similar to those seen in patients with BP. The oral mucosa and conjunctiva are also commonly involved.

ORAL FINDINGS

Oral lesions are common in LAD and may be seen in up to 70% of patients. These lesions are clinically indistinguishable from the oral lesions of MMP, with blisters and erosions of the mucosa frequently accompanied by desquamative gingivitis, which cannot be clinically distinguished from lesions of MMP. Similar to MMP, cases have been reported presenting with desquamative gingivitis only.[214] Some investigators believe that there is insufficient evidence to separate mucosal LAD from MMP.[208]

LABORATORY FINDINGS

Routine histology demonstrates a subepithelial lesion in the basement membrane similar to MMP, but DIF study will show deposition of IgA rather than IgG. IIF is usually negative, but when positive, it will demonstrate circulating IgA antibodies against a basement membrane antigen.

MANAGEMENT

As with any subepithelial blistering disease, the clinician should consider the possibility of an underlying drug reaction or malignancy.

The oral lesions of LAD may be managed with the use of topical steroids but characteristically do not respond as well as MMP to either topical or systemic steroid therapy alone. Dapsone is often effective when topical steroids alone are insufficient. Sulfapyridine or tetracycline, which may be combined with niacinamide, is also effective. Severe cases may require a combination of systemic corticosteroids and immunosuppressive drug therapy.

Epidermolysis Bullosa Aquisita (EBA)

Patients with EBA have IgG autoantibodies directed against type VII collagen, a component of the anchoring fibrils of the basement membrane. There are two forms of EBA: the classic form, which results in a lesion of the basement membrane with little inflammation, or the inflammatory form, which includes a significant infiltration of neutrophils.

The clinical course of EBA can resemble BP or MMP with widespread skin lesions or primary involvement of the oral mucosa, genital mucosa, conjunctiva, and larynx.

MANAGEMENT

The treatment is similar as described for MMP and LAD, with the therapy depending upon the extent and severity of the clinical lesions. The classic form of the disease tends to be resistant to treatment, whereas the inflammatory form often responds well to dapsone. Some patients with an inadequate response to dapsone have obtained remission with colchicine. Systemic corticosteroids and immunosuppressive drugs are often required to control the lesions in severe widespread EBA.

Chronic Bullous Disease of Childhood (CBDC)

CBDC is a subepithelial blistering disorder, which chiefly affects children below the age of 5 years. It is characterized by the deposition of IgA antibodies in the basement membrane zone, which are detected by DIF on the epidermal side of salt-split skin or mucosa.

CLINICAL MANIFESTATIONS

The onset of the disease may be precipitated by an upper respiratory infection or drug therapy.[185] The characteristic lesion of CBDC is a cluster of vesicles and bullae on an inflamed base. The genital region is commonly involved, and conjunctival, rectal, and oral lesions may also be present. CBDC is self-limiting and resolves prior to puberty.[215]

ORAL FINDINGS

Oral mucosal involvement is present in up to 50% of cases, and the oral lesions are similar to those observed in patients with MMP. Lesions of the perioral skin are common in CBDC.

DIAGNOSIS AND PATHOLOGY

Diagnosis is made by biopsy demonstrating a subepithelial lesion on routine histology and by deposition of IgA in the basement membrane zone on DIF. IIF demonstrates circulating IgA in 80% of cases.[216] This disease is self-limiting, and the lesions characteristically heal within 2 years. As with LAD, the lesions are responsive to sulfapyridine or dapsone therapy. Systemic corticosteroids may be required for severe cases.

▼ THE PATIENT WITH SINGLE ULCERS

The most common cause of single ulcers on the oral mucosa is trauma.

The diagnosis is usually based on the history and physical findings. However, it is always vital to distinguish traumatic lesions from squamous cell carcinoma. The dentist must re-examine all patients with single ulcers for significant healing in 1 to 2 weeks; if healing is not evident in this time, a biopsy should be taken to rule out cancer or, in immunocompromised patients, the possibility of a deep fungal infection. (Oral cancer is discussed in detail in Chapter 7)

Infections that may cause a chronic oral ulcer include the deep mycoses histoplasmosis, blastomycosis, mucormycosis, aspergillosis, cryptococcosis, and coccidioidomycosis, as well as a chronic herpes simplex infection. Syphilis, another infection that may cause a single oral ulcer in the primary and tertiary stages, is described in Chapter 20, "Infectious Diseases."

The deep mycoses were rare causes of oral lesions prior to HIV infection, myelosuppressive cancer chemotherapy, and immunosuppressive drug therapy. The dentist must consider this group of diseases in the differential diagnosis whenever isolated ulcerative oral lesions develop in known or suspected immunosuppressed patients. Biopsy of suspected tissue, accompanied by a request for appropriate stains, is necessary for early diagnosis.

Traumatic Injuries Causing Solitary Ulcerations

ETIOLOGY AND PATHOGENESIS

Single mucosal ulcers may be caused by direct physical/mechanical, thermal, or chemical trauma to the mucosa or even vascular compromise, causing tissue damage and ulceration. Acute bite injuries, an example of direct physical/mechanical trauma, occur often in the oral mucosa and may be particularly severe if this occurs when the mucosa is numb after local anesthesia has been given for dental procedures. Traumatic injuries may also result from malocclusion, ill-fitting dental prostheses, overzealous toothbrushing and flossing, self-injurious habits, and oral piercings (Figure 46).[217, 218]

Thermal injuries include electrical burns, especially in children who inadvertently chew on electrical wiring. More commonly, thermal burns occur on the palate from ingesting hot foods and beverages (such as hot pizza or coffee).[219] The use of a microwave oven to reheat foods often results in differential heating so that cheese and pastry fillings may be overheated compared with other parts of the food, leading to burns.[220] An iatrogenic cause of thermal injury is from a heated dental instrument inadvertently contacting the mucosa. The burn is usually more serious if the mucosa has been anesthetized and there is prolonged contact.[218,221]

Chemical trauma is caused by patients or dentists placing noxious and caustic substances directly on the mucosa either as a therapeutic measure or unintentionally.[222] A common example is aspirin placed directly on the mucosa to treat a toothache.[223] Mouthwashes or other over-the-counter oral care products with high alcoholic content, hydrogen peroxide, or phenols used too frequently or undiluted can cause mucosal ulcerations.[224] Some over-the-counter medications for

treating aphthous ulcers contain high concentrations of silver nitrate, phenols, or sulfuric acid and should be used with caution. Sucking on or chewing medications formulated to be swallowed (such as aspirin or oral bisphosphonates) may also lead to severe oral ulcers.[225–227] Ulcers have also resulted in the use of denture cleansers as an oral rinse.[228] Prolonged contact of methacrylate monomer on the mucosa may also lead to necrosis of the mucosa. Necrosis of the bone and mucosa has been reported from chemicals used in endodontics if these are pushed past the apices of teeth.[229] Vascular compromise may result from the vasoconstrictors used in dental local anesthetics. The temporary vasoconstriction may be sufficient to lead to infarction necrosis of the tissue.[217]

ORAL FINDINGS

These present as acute ulcerations and necrosis of the mucosa with a clear antecedent history of injury. The extent of the ulceration depends on the agent involved and the site depends on the activity involved.

Electrical burns in particular are caused by high heat, are generally fairly extensive, involve the lips, and are generally seen in young children and toddlers.[217] The initial lesions are charred and dry-appearing. However, after a few days, this charred crust sloughs, and there may be excessive bleeding when the underlying vital structures are exposed.

Burns from hot foods and beverages are generally small and localized to the hard palate or lips and are usually seen in teenagers and adults. The area usually presents as an area of tenderness and erythema that develops into ulcers within hours of the injury. It may take several days to heal depending on the extent of the injury.

DIFFERENTIAL DIAGNOSIS

Careful history taking and identification of the causative agent clinch the diagnosis. However, in all cases, patients should be carefully monitored to ensure that a secondary infection does not develop, particularly involving opportunistic agents such as HSV or Candida.

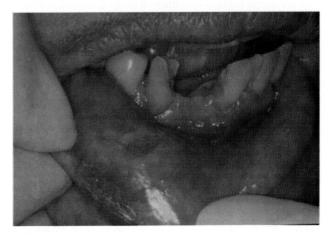

FIGURE 46 Figure 46 Traumatic ulcer of the labial mucosa caused by a sharp tooth..

LABORATORY TESTING

None is required if there is a clear history of injury to the site. Culture may be needed if the areas do not heal well or if suppuration develops, suggesting a secondary infection. A biopsy should be performed if the ulcer does not heal within a reasonable period of time (a few weeks). If leakage of an endodontic filler is suspected, periapical films should be taken.

Biopsy is not necessary if the etiology is obvious. However, if a biopsy is done, the mucosa will show ulceration with acute and chronic inflammation. The epithelium adjacent to the ulcer shows varying degrees of coagulation and necrosis.[230] Care must be taken to rule out the presence of infectious agents that may secondarily infect the site (such as HSV on the hard palatal mucosa).

MANAGEMENT

Electrical burns are generally deep and more extensive, and healing often results in scarring and contracture. If the corners of the mouth are involved, microstomia may result. Children benefit from the use of microstomia prevention devices during this healing period, although surgical correction may still be required to restore function and esthetics. Antibiotics may be necessary to prevent a secondary infection since these burns often take several weeks to heal.[217]

Smaller lesions caused by less severe thermal or chemical injury heal on their own once the irritant is removed. Pain control can be achieved with topical anesthetics (such as viscous lidocaine). Topical steroids may be useful.[220,221] Avoidance of reinjury is also important, and this may be effected by counseling patients regarding the avoidance of use of caustic substances and the correct use of medications. Dentists also should be more aware of taking protective measures when using caustic substances and heated instruments.

Traumatic Ulcerative Granuloma, Eosinophilic Ulcer of Tongue

ETIOLOGY AND PATHOGENESIS

This ulcerative condition of the oral cavity is considered traumatic in nature, although less than 50% of patients recall a history of trauma. These lesions have been experimentally induced in animals by inflicting crush injury on the tongue, the most common site of these lesions.[231] It is likely that the penetrating nature of the inflammation results in myositis that leads to chronicity. As such, other acute or chronic ulcerative conditions left untreated may become deep and penetrating, even if they began initially as an infectious ulcer, for instance. Similar lesions are seen on the ventral tongue in infants caused by the tongue rasping against newly erupted primary incisors, a condition known as Riga-Fede disease.[232] Patients with familial dysautonomia and other conditions, such as Riley-Day syndrome and Lesch-Nyhan syndrome, who have congenital incapacity to sense pain often also develop similar ulcerative and necrotic ulcers because they are unaware of the self-inflicted injury.[233]

CLINICAL MANIFESTATIONS

There is a bimodal age distribution with one group in the first 2 years of life, where lesions are associated with erupting primary dentition.[232] The second group is in adults in the fifth and sixth decades.[234]

ORAL FINDINGS

In children, the ulcers are always on the anterior ventral or dorsal tongue associated with erupting mandibular or maxillary incisors, respectively.[232] The tongue is the site of involvement in approximately 60% of adult cases, usually on the posterior and lateral aspects.[232,234]

An ulcer develops that may not be painful in two-thirds of cases and may persist for months. A history of trauma is elicited in only 20 to 50% of cases. These generally appear cleanly punched out, with surrounding erythema and some whiteness if present for weeks or months. They range from 0.5 cm to several centimeters in size. The surrounding tissue is usually indurated. Other sites that may be involved include the buccal mucosa and labial mucosa, floor of the mouth, and vestibule, all sites where there is abundant underlying skeletal muscle. Five percent are multifocal, and recurrences are not uncommon. In some cases, the lesions present as an ulcerated, mushroom-shaped, polypoid mass on the lateral tongue.[235,236]

DIFFERENTIAL DIAGNOSIS

In children, the diagnosis is usually obvious because of the presence of newly erupted dentition and the location of the ulcers.

The long duration of these lesions, presence of induration, lack of pain, and lack of surrounding erythema readily distinguish them from recurrent aphthous ulcers, although major aphthous ulcers are often associated with scarring. The presence of a single, chronic, painless ulcer with induration raises the suspicion for squamous cell carcinoma (especially if it is on the tongue) or other malignancy of salivary gland or lymphoid origin. Some cases that had been diagnosed as traumatic ulcerative granuloma have subsequently been shown to represent T-cell lymphomas.[237] An infectious etiology should also be considered, especially deep fungal infection, particularly in immunocompromised hosts.

LABORATORY FINDINGS

A biopsy is almost always needed to make the diagnosis and to rule out other conditions. Excision of the lesion often results in complete resolution of the ulcer.

The mucosa is ulcerated, but unlike an aphthous ulcer, the inflammation is deeply penetrating, with chronic inflammatory cells infiltrating the underlying skeletal fibers. There is muscle degeneration associated with variable numbers of eosinophils and mononuclear histiocyte-like cells.[232,234] Immunoperoxidase staining is important to rule out a lymphoma, especially the CD30-positive type.

MANAGEMENT

A careful history is important to rule out continued trauma to the site, although this is sometimes difficult to elicit and sometimes to prevent, especially if trauma occurs during sleep. Intralesional steroid injections performed regularly will often resolve these lesions. Wound débridement also often leads to complete resolution, although up to one-third of cases recur. The use of a nightguard on the lower teeth may help reduce nighttime trauma.

Histoplasmosis

ETIOLOGY AND PATHOGENESIS

Histoplasmosis is caused by the fungus *Histoplasma capsulatum*, a dimorphic fungus with both yeast and mycelial forms that grows in the yeast form in infected tissue. Infection results from inhaling dust contaminated with droppings, particularly from infected birds or bats. An African form of this infection is caused by a larger yeast, which is considered a variant of *H. capsulatum* and is called *Histoplasma duboisii*.

Histoplasmosis is the most common systemic fungal infection in the United States; in endemic areas such as the Mississippi and Ohio River valleys, serologic evidence of previous infection may be found in 75 to 80% of the population. Outbreaks of occupationally acquired histoplasmosis continue to be reported among agricultural workers and laborers in endemic areas. Particularly at risk are individuals working with aerolized topsoil or dust with bat or bird droppings.[238]

CLINICAL MANIFESTATIONS

In most cases, particularly in otherwise normal children, primary infection is mild, manifesting as a self-limiting pulmonary disease that heals to leave fibrosis and calcification similar to tuberculosis. In a small percentage of cases, progressive disease results in cavitation of the lung and dissemination of the organism to the liver, spleen, adrenal glands, and meninges. Patients with the disseminated form of the disease may develop anemia and leukopenia secondary to bone marrow involvement. Immunosuppressed or myelosuppressed patients are more likely to develop the severe disseminated form of the disease, and disseminated histoplasmosis is one of the infections that characterize AIDS.[239]

ORAL FINDINGS

Most cases of oral lesions of histoplasmosis reported during the past two decades have been detected in HIV-infected individuals who live in or have visited endemic areas.

Oral involvement is usually secondary to pulmonary involvement and occurs in a significant percentage of patients with disseminated histoplasmosis. In one study, 3% of HIV-positive patients in an endemic area had oral lesions of histoplasmosis, and oral histoplasmosis has been reported as the first sign of AIDS.[240] Patients diagnosed with histoplasmosis should be tested for HIV infection.

Oral mucosal lesions begin as an area of erythema that becomes a papule and eventually forms a painful, granulomatous-appearing ulcer. The cervical lymph nodes are often enlarged and firm. The clinical appearance of the lesions, as well as the accompanying lymphadenopathy, often resembles that of squamous cell carcinoma, other chronic fungal infections, or lymphoma.

The most common oral lesion of histoplasmosis in patients with HIV is an ulcer with an indurated border, which is most commonly seen on the gingiva, palate, or tongue.[241] These oral histoplasmosis lesions in patients with HIV may occur alone or as part of a disseminated infection.[242]

DIFFERENTIAL DIAGNOSIS

Long-standing chronic ulcers may represent lesions of of infectious etiology (especially deep fungal or mycobacterial in nature), traumatic ulcerative granuloma, squamous cell carcinoma, lymphoma or other malignancy.

LABORATORY FINDINGS

Diagnosis of disseminated histoplasmosis occurs with use of serology, antigen detection procedures, and culture.

A rapid diagnosis may be made with use of a smear of the lesion stained with methenamine silver read by an experienced cytopathologist and a biopsy of the lesion stained with periodic acid–Schiff or methenamine silver, which will reveal the presence of the fungi. Cultures should be performed on a portion of tissue removed during the biopsy. Improved diagnosis of tissue specimens using PCR and DNA probes is under investigation.[243]

MANAGEMENT

Immunocompromised patients with disseminated histoplasmosis should receive treatment with intravenous amphotericin B. AIDS patients can often be switched to itraconazole after 10 weeks and require maintenance therapy for life. Immunocompetent individuals are treated with itraconazole or ketoconazole for 6 to 12 months.

Blastomycosis

ETIOLOGY AND PATHOGENESIS

Blastomycosis is a fungal infection caused by *Blastomyces dermatitidis*. This dimorphic organism can grow in either a yeast or as a mycelial form. The organism is found as a normal inhabitant of soil; therefore, the highest incidence of this infection is found in agricultural and construction workers, particularly in the middle Atlantic and southeastern portions of the United States. This geographic distribution of the infection has led to the designation by some as "North American blastomycosis." Infection by the same organism, however, has also been found in Mexico and Central and South America, Africa, and Asia. In the United States, the endemic area is chiefly in states bordering the Mississippi River. Blastomycosis is not commonly associated with HIV infection.[244]

CLINICAL MANIFESTATIONS

Infection with *Blastomyces* begins in a vast majority of cases by inhalation; this causes a primary pulmonary infection. Although an acute self-limiting form of the disease exists and some cases remain asymptomatic, the infection commonly follows a chronic course beginning with mild symptoms such as malaise, low-grade fever, and mild cough. If the infection goes untreated, the symptoms worsen to include shortness of breath, weight loss, and production of blood-tinged sputum. Infection of the skin, mucosa, and bone may also occur, resulting from metastatic spread of organisms from the pulmonary lesions through the lymphatic system. The skin and mucosal lesions start as subcutaneous nodules, slowly progressing to well-circumscribed indurated ulcers. The skin lesions are most commonly found on exposed skin surfaces.[245,246]

ORAL FINDINGS

Oral lesions are rarely the primary site of infection. When oral lesions have been reported as a first sign of blastomycosis, they have occurred in patients with mild pulmonary symptoms that have been overlooked by the patient or physician. Most cases of oral involvement demonstrate concomitant pulmonary lesions on chest radiographs.

The most common appearance of the oral lesions of blastomycosis is a nonspecific, painless, verrucous ulcer with indurated borders, often mistaken for squamous cell carcinoma. Occasionally, this mistake is perpetuated by an inexperienced histopathologist who confuses the characteristic pseudoepitheliomatous hyperplasia with malignant changes.

Other oral lesions that have been reported include hard nodules and radiolucent jaw lesions. Page and colleagues reported two cases of painless oral mucosal ulcers as the first sign of blastomycosis; in both cases, a careful history taking revealed mild respiratory symptoms.[248]

Bell and colleagues reported seven cases of oral lesions occurring in patients with blastomycosis; four presented as chronic oral ulcers and three as radiolucent bone lesions. Chest radiographs showed concomitant pulmonary involvement in all cases.[249]

DIFFERENTIAL DIAGNOSIS

Dentists should include the diagnosis of blastomycosis in the differential diagnosis of a chronic oral ulcer. The diagnosis cannot be made on clinical grounds alone. The index of suspicion should increase when a chronic painless oral ulcer appears in an agricultural worker or when the review of systems reveals pulmonary symptoms.

LABORATORY FINDINGS

Diagnosis is made on the basis of biopsy and on culturing the organism from tissue obtained at biopsy. The histologic appearance shows pseudoepitheliomatous hyperplasia with a heavy infiltrate of chronic inflammatory cells and microabscesses.[250]

Unlike histoplasmosis, a reliable commercially available skin test does not exist, but serology using an enzyme immunoassay is available, which has a specificity of greater than 90%, although false-positive results have been reported.

Diagnosis is most frequently made from sputum, cytology, or biopsy specimens demonstrating the presence of multinucleated yeast cells with dark cytoplasm and colorless cell walls characteristic of *B. dermatitidis*.[247]

TREATMENT

Treatment for disseminated or progressive blastomycosis includes use of ketoconazole, fluconazole, or itraconazole for mild to moderate disease and amphotericin B for severe disease.

Mucormycosis (Phycomycosis)

ETIOLOGY AND PATHOGENESIS

Mucormycosis (phycomycosis) is caused by an infection with a saprophytic fungus that normally occurs in soil or as a mold on decaying food. The fungus is nonpathogenic for healthy individuals, representing an opportunistic rather than a true pathogen, and is regularly cultured from the human nose, throat, and oral cavity of healthy asymptomatic individuals.

CLINICAL MANIFESTATIONS

Infection occurs in patients with decreased host resistance, such as those with poorly controlled diabetes or hematologic malignancies or those undergoing cancer chemotherapy or immunosuppressive drug therapy. In the debilitated patient, mucormycosis may appear as a pulmonary, gastrointestinal, disseminated, or rhinocerebral infection.[251]

The rhinomaxillary form of the disease, a subdivision of the rhinocerebral form, begins with the inhalation of the fungus by a susceptible individual. The fungus invades arteries and causes damage secondary to thrombosis and ischemia. The fungus may spread from the oral and nasal region to the brain, causing death in a high percentage of cases. The most common symptoms of the rhinomaxillary form include proptosis, loss of vision, nasal discharge, sinusitis, and palatal necrosis.

ORAL FINDINGS

The most common oral sign of mucormycosis is ulceration of the palate, which results from necrosis due to invasion of a palatal vessel (Figure 47).[252,253] The lesion is characteristically large and deep, causing denudation of underlying bone. Ulcers from mucormycosis have also been reported on the gingiva, lip, and alveolar ridge. The initial manifestation of the disease

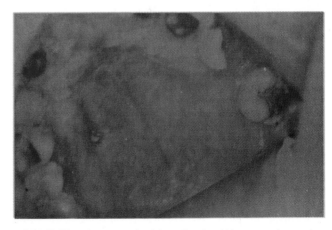

FIGURE 47 Mucormycosis of the palate in a kidney transplant patient taking immunosuppressive drugs.

may be confused with dental pain or bacterial maxillary sinusitis caused by invasion of the maxillary sinus. The clinician must include mucormycosis in the differential diagnosis of large oral ulcers occurring in patients debilitated from diabetes, chemotherapy, or immunosuppressive drug therapy.

LABORATORY FINDINGS

Early diagnosis is essential if the patient is to be cured of this infection. Negative cultures do not rule out mucormycosis because the fungus is frequently difficult to culture from infected tissue; instead, a biopsy must be performed when mucormycosis is suspected. The biopsy specimen should be split so that one portion is sent for culture and the other for histopathology. The histopathologic specimen shows necrosis and nonseptate hyphae, which are best demonstrated by a periodic acid–Schiff stain or the methenamine silver stain. Necrosis and occlusion of vessels are also frequently present.

MANAGEMENT

When diagnosed early, mucormycosis may be cured by a combination of surgical débridement of the infected area and systemic administration of amphotericin B for up to 3 months. Proper management of the underlying disorder is an important aspect affecting the final outcome of treatment. All patients given amphotericin B must be closely observed for renal toxicity by repeated measurements of the blood urea nitrogen and creatinine. Posaconazole, a newly developed oral antifungal agent, shows promise for patients unable to tolerate the toxicity of amphotericin.[254]

▼ SELECTED READINGS

Akintoye, SO, Greenberg MS. Recurrent aphthous stomatitis. Dent Clin North Am 2005;49:31–47.

Chan LS, Ahmed AR, Anhalt GJ, et al. The first international consensus on mucous membrane pemphigoid: definition, diagnostic criteria, pathogenic factors, medical treatment, and prognostic indicators. Arch Dermatol 2002;138:370–9.

Chayakulkeeree M, Ghannoum MA, Perfect JR. Zygomycosis: the re-emerging fungal infection. Eur J Clin Microbiol Infect Dis 2006;25:215–29.

Ciarrocca KN, Greenberg MS. A retrospective study of the management of oral mucous membrane pemphigoid with dapsone. Oral Surg Oral Med Oral Pathol Oral Radiol Endod 1999;88:159–63.

Corey L. Herpes simplex virus. In: Mandell GL, Bennett JE, Dolin R, editors. Mandell, Douglas and Bennett's principles and practice of infectious diseases. 6th ed. Philadelphia: Elsevier, Churchill, Livingstone; 2005. p. 1762–80.

Farthing P, Bagan JV, Scully C. Mucosal disease series. Number IV. Erythema multiforme. Oral Dis 2005;11:261–7.

Flaitz CM, Nichols CM, Hicks MJ. Herpesviridae-associated persistent mucocutaneous ulcers in acquired immunodeficiency syndrome. A clinicopathologic study. Oral Surg Oral Med Oral Pathol Oral Radiol Endod 1996;81:433–41.

Gnann JW Jr, Whitley RJ. Clinical practice. Herpes zoster. N Engl J Med 2002;347:340–6.

Greenberg MS, Friedman H, Cohen SG, et al. A comparative study of herpes simplex infections in renal transplant and leukemic patients. J Infect Dis 1987;156:280–7.

Harman KE, Albert S, Black MM. Guidelines for the management of pemphigus vulgaris. Br J Dermatol 2003;149:926–37.

Jones AC, Gulley ML, Freedman PD. Necrotizing ulcerative stomatitis in human immunodeficiency virus-seropositive individuals: a review of the histopathologic, immunohistochemical, and virologic characteristics of 18 cases. Oral Surg Oral Med Oral Pathol Oral Radiol Endod 2000;89:323–32.

Oxman MN, Levin MJ, Johnson GR, et al. A vaccine to prevent herpes zoster and postherpetic neuralgia in older adults. N Engl J Med 2005;352:2271–84.

Williams PM, Conklin RJ. Erythema multiforme: a review and contrast from Stevens-Johnson syndrome/toxic epidermal necrolysis. Dent Clin North Am 2005;49:67-76, viii.

Woo SB, Lee SF. Oral recrudescent herpes simplex virus infection. Oral Surg Oral Med Oral Pathol Oral Radiol Endod 1997;83: 239–43.

Yazici H, Yurdakul S, Hamuryudan V. Behçet's syndrome. Curr Opin Rhematol 1999;1:53–7.

Sami N, Yeh SW, Ahmed AR. Blistering diseases in the elderly: diagnosis and treatment. Dermatol Clin 2004;22:73–86.

Yancey KB, Egan CA. Pemphigoid: clinical, histologic, immunopathologic, and therapeutic considerations. JAMA 2000;284:350–6.

For the full reference list, please refer to the accompanying CD ROM.

4

RED AND WHITE LESIONS OF THE ORAL MUCOSA

MATS JONTELL, DDS, PHD, FDSRCSED

PALLE HOLMSTRUP, DDS, PHD

▼ RED AND WHITE TISSUE REACTIONS

▼ INFECTIOUS DISEASES
Oral Candidiasis
Hairy Leukoplakia

▼ PREMALIGNANT LESIONS
Oral Leukoplakia and Erythroplakia
Oral Submucous Fibrosis

▼ IMMUNOPATHOLOGIC DISEASES
Oral Lichen Planus
Drug-Induced Lichenoid Reactions
Lichenoid Reactions of Graft-versus-Host Disease
Lupus Erythematosus

▼ ALLERGIC REACTIONS
Lichenoid Contact Reactions
Reactions to Dentifrice and Chlorhexidine

▼ TOXIC REACTIONS
Reactions to Smokeless Tobacco
Smoker's Palate

▼ REACTIONS TO MECHANICAL TRAUMA
Morsicatio

▼ OTHER RED AND WHITE LESIONS
Benign Migratory Glossitis (Geographic Tongue)
Leukoedema
White Sponge Nevus
Hairy Tongue

▼ RED AND WHITE TISSUE REACTIONS

Oral mucosal lesions may be classified according to different characteristics. This chapter describes disorders of the oral mucosa that clinically appear either red or white.

A white appearance of the oral mucosa may be caused by a variety of factors. The oral epithelium may be stimulated to an increased production of keratin (hyperkeratosis, Composition 1) or an abnormal but benign thickening of stratum spinosum (acanthosis, Composition 2). Intra- (Composition 3) and extracellular accumulation of fluid in the epithelium may also result in clinical whitening. Necrosis of the oral epithelium, which may also be perceived as a white lesion, may occur when the oral mucosa is exposed to toxic chemicals. Microbes, particularly fungi, can produce whitish pseudomembranes consisting of sloughed epithelial cells, fungal mycelium, and neutrophils, which are loosely attached to the oral mucosa (Composition 4).

A red lesion of the oral mucosa may develop as the result of atrophic epithelium (Composition 5), characterized by a reduction in the number of epithelial cells (Composition 6) or increased vascularization.

Oral mucosal lesions also present with different tissue textures, which will affect the clinical appearance of the lesions. Thus, it is important to discriminate between reticular, plaque-like, papular, or pseudomembranous structures and to observe if the lesion has a sharp or diffuse demarcation or is raised relative to the normal epithelial surface.

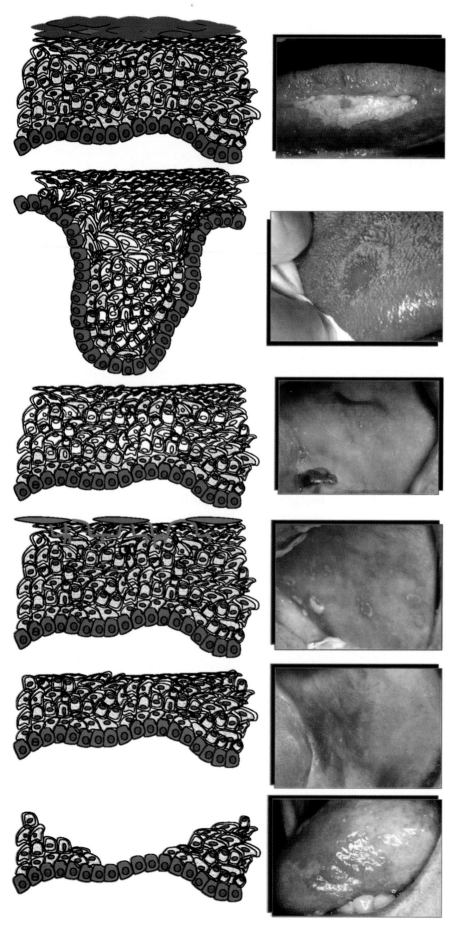

▼ INFECTIOUS DISEASES

Oral Candidiasis

Oral candidiasis is the most prevalent opportunistic infection affecting the oral mucosa. In the vast majority of cases, the lesions are caused by the yeast *Candida albicans*. The pathogenesis is not fully understood, but a number of predisposing factors have the capacity to convert *Candida* from the normal commensal flora (saprophytic stage) to a pathogenic organism (parasitic stage). *C. albicans* is usually a weak pathogen, and candidiasis is said to affect the very young, the very old, and the very sick.[1] Most *Candida* infections only affect mucosal linings, but the rare systemic manifestations may have a fatal course.

Oral candidiasis is divided into primary and secondary infections (Table 1).[1] The primary infections are restricted to the oral and perioral sites, whereas secondary infections are accompanied by systemic mucocutaneous manifestations.

ETIOLOGY AND PATHOGENESIS

C. albicans, C. tropicalis, and *C. glabrata* comprise together over 80% of the species isolated from human *Candida* infections.[1] To invade the mucosal lining, the microorganisms must adhere to the epithelial surface; therefore, strains of *Candida* with better adhesion potential are more pathogenic than strains with poorer adhesion. The yeasts' penetration of the epithelial cells is facilitated by their production of lipases, and for the yeasts to remain within the epithelium, they must overcome constant desquamation of surface epithelial cells.

There is an apparent association between oral candidiasis and the influence of local and general predisposing factors. The local predisposing factors (Table 2) are able to promote growth of *Candida* or to affect the immune response of the oral mucosa. General predisposing factors are often related to the patient's immune and endocrine status (see Table 2).

TABLE 1 Classification of Oral Candidiasis

Primary Oral Candidiasis	Secondary Oral Candidiasis	
The "Primary Triad"	Condition	Subgroup
Acute	Familial chronic mucocutaneous candidiasis	1
Pseudomembranous	Diffuse chronic mucocutaneous candidiasis	2
Erythematous	Candidiasis endocrinopathy syndrome	3
	Familial mucocutaneous candidiasis	4
Chronic	Severe combined immunodeficiency	5a
Pseudomembranous	DiGeorge syndrome	5b
Erythematous	Chronic granulomatous disease	5c
Plaque-like	Acquired immune deficiency syndrome (AIDS)	6
Nodular		
Candida-associated lesions		
Denture stomatitis		
Angular cheilitis		
Median rhomboid glossitis		

TABLE 2

Local predisposing factors for oral candidiasis and *Candida*-associated lesions

  Denture wearing

  Smoking

  Atopic constitution

  Inhalation steroids

  Topical steroids

  Hyperkeratosis

  Imbalance of the oral microflora

  Quality and quantity of saliva

General predisposing factors for oral candidiasis

  Immunosuppressive diseases

  Impaired health status

  Immunosuppressive drugs

  Chemotherapy

  Endocrine disorders

  Hematinic deficiencies

The immune status can be affected by drugs as well as a disease, which suppresses the adaptive or the innate immune system. Pseudomembranous candidiasis is also associated with fungal infections in young children, who do not have a fully developed immune system.

Denture stomatitis, angular cheilitis, and median rhomboid glossitis are referred to as *Candida*-associated infections as these lesions may, in addition to *Candida*, be caused by bacteria.

EPIDEMIOLOGY

The prevalence of *Candida*, as part of the normal oral flora, shows large geographic variations, but an average figure of 35% has been calculated from several studies.[2] With improved detection techniques, a prevalence as high as 90% has been proposed.[3] *Candida* is more frequently isolated from women, and seasonal variations have been observed, with an increase during the summer months. Hospitalized patients have a higher prevalence of *Candida*.[4] In healthy subjects, blood group O and nonsecretion of blood group antigens are separate and cumulative risk factors for oral carriage of *C. albicans*.[5]

In denture-wearers, the prevalence of denture stomatitis varies, but in population studies, it has been reported to be approximately 50%.[6]

CLINICAL FINDINGS

Pseudomembranous Candidiasis.   The acute form of pseudomembranous candidiasis (thrush) is grouped with the primary oral candidiasis (see Table 1) and is recognized as the classic *Candida* infection (Figure 1). The infection predominantly affects patients medicated with antibiotics, immunosuppressant drugs, or a disease that suppresses the immune system.

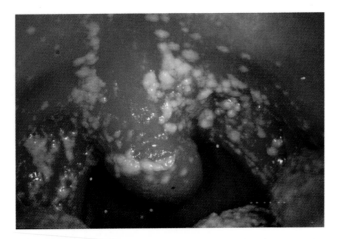

FIGURE 1 Pseudomembranous candidiasis during the immunosuppressive phase following heart transplantation.

The infection typically presents with loosely attached membranes comprising fungal organisms and cellular debris, which leaves an inflamed, sometimes bleeding area if the pseudomembrane is removed. Less pronounced infections sometimes have clinical features that are difficult to discriminate from food debris. The clinical presentations of acute and chronic pseudomembranous candidiasis are indistinguishable.[7] The chronic form emerged as a result of human immunodeficiency virus (HIV) infections as patients with this disease may be affected by a pseudomembranous *Candida* infection for a long period of time. However, patients treated with steroid inhalers may also acquire pseudomembranous lesions of a chronic nature. Patients infrequently report symptoms from their lesions, although some discomfort may be experienced from the presence of the pseudomembranes.

Erythematous Candidiasis. The erythematous form of candidiasis was previously referred to as atrophic oral candidiasis.[8] An erythematous surface may not just reflect atrophy but can also be explained by increased vascularization. The lesion has a diffuse border (Figure 2), which helps distinguish it from erythroplakia, which has a sharper

demarcation. Erythematous candidiasis may be considered a successor to pseudomembranous candidiasis but may also emerge *de novo*.[1] The infection is predominantly encountered in the palate and the dorsum of the tongue of patients who are using inhalation steroids. Other predisposing factors that can cause erythematous candidiasis are smoking and treatment with broad-spectrum antibiotics. The acute and chronic forms present with identical clinical features.

Chronic Plaque-Type and Nodular Candidiasis. The chronic plaque type of oral candidiasis replaces the older term, *candidal leukoplakia*. The typical clinical presentation is characterized by a white plaque, which may be indistinguishable from an oral leukoplakia (Figure 3).

A positive correlation between oral candidiasis and moderate to severe epithelial dysplasia has been observed,[9] and both the chronic plaque-type and nodular candidiasis (Figure 4) have been associated with malignant transformation, but the probable role of yeasts in oral carcinogenesis is

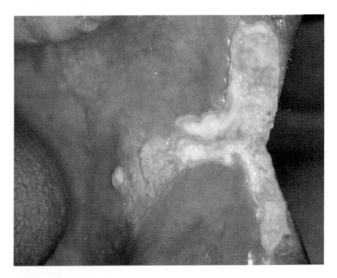

FIGURE 3 Chronic plaque-type candidiasis.

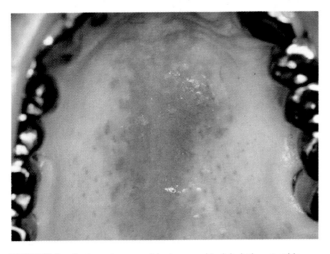

FIGURE 2 Erythematous candidosis caused by inhalation steroids.

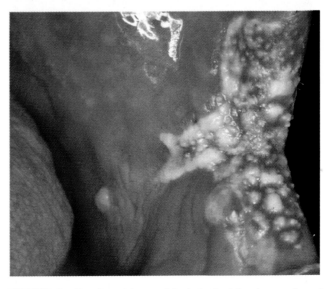

FIGURE 4 Chronic nodular candidiasis in the left retrocommissural area.

unclear.[10] It has been hypothesized that it acts through its capacity to catalyze nitrosamine production.[11]

Denture Stomatitis. The most prevalent site for denture stomatitis is the denture-bearing palatal mucosa (Figure 5). It is unusual for the mandibular mucosa to be involved. Denture stomatitis is classified into three different types.[12] Type I is localized to minor erythematous sites caused by trauma from the denture. Type II affects a major part of the denture-covered mucosa. In addition to the features of type II, type III has a granular mucosa in the central part of the palate. The denture serves as a vehicle that protects the microorganisms from physical influences such as salivary flow. The microflora is complex and contains, in addition to *Candida*, bacteria from several genera, such as *Streptococcus, Veillonella, Lactobacillus, Prevotella* (formerly *Bacteroides*), and *Actinomyces*.[13] It is not known to what extent these bacteria participate in the pathogenesis of denture stomatitis.[8]

Angular Cheilitis. Angular cheilitis is infected fissures of the commissures of the mouth, often surrounded by erythema (Figure 6).[14,15] The lesions are frequently coinfected with both *Candida* and *Staphylococcus aureus*. Vitamin B_{12}, iron deficiencies, and loss of vertical dimension have been associated with this disorder. Atopy has also been associated with the formation of angular cheilitis.[16] Dry skin may promote the development of fissures in the commissures, allowing invasion by the microorganisms. Thirty percent of patients with denture stomatitis also have angular cheilitis, which only affects 10% of denture-wearing patients without denture stomatitis.[17]

Median Rhomboid Glossitis. Median rhomboid glossitis is clinically characterized by an erythematous lesion in the center of the posterior part of the dorsum of the tongue (Figure 7).[18] As the name indicates, the lesion has an oval configuration. This area of erythema resulting from atrophy of the filiform papillae and the surface may be lobulated. The etiology is

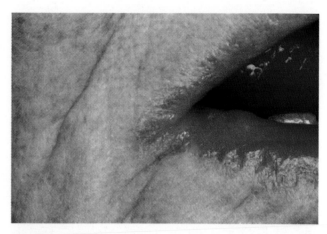

FIGURE 6 Angular cheilitis.

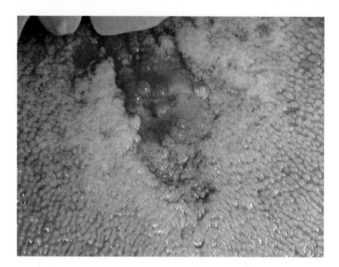

FIGURE 7 Median rhomboid glossitis.

not fully clarified, but the lesion frequently shows a mixed bacterial/fungal microflora. Biopsies yield *Candida* hyphea in more than 85% of the lesions.[19] Smokers and denture-wearers have an increased risk of developing median rhomboid glossitis as well as patients using inhalation steroids. Sometimes a concurrent erythematous lesion may be observed in the palatal mucosa (kissing lesions). Median rhomboid glossitis is asymptomatic, and management is restricted to a reduction in predisposing factors. The lesion does not entail any increased risk for malignant transformation.

Oral Candidiasis Associated with HIV. More than 90% of acquired immune deficiency syndrome (AIDS) patients have had oral candidiasis during the course of their HIV infection, and the infection is considered a portent of AIDS development (Figure 8). The most common types of oral candidiasis in conjunction with HIV are pseudomembranous candidiasis, erythematous candidiasis, angular cheilitis, and chronic hyperplastic candidiasis. As a result of the highly active antiretroviral therapy (HAART), the prevalence of oral candidiasis has decreased substantially. Oral candidiasis associated with HIV infection is presented in more detail in Chapter 20, "Infectious Diseases."

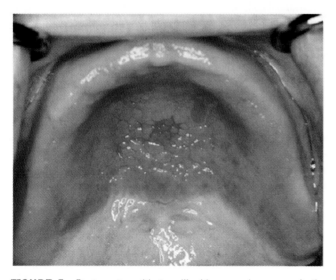

FIGURE 5 Denture stomatitis type III with a granular mucosa in the central part of the palate.

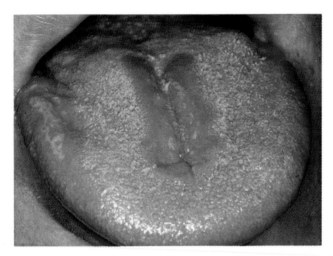

FIGURE 8 Erythematous candidiasis at the central part of the tongue in an AIDS patient. Hairy leukoplakia can be seen at the right lateral border.

CLINICAL MANIFESTATIONS

Secondary oral candidiasis (see Table 1) is accompanied by systemic mucocutaneous candidiasis and other immune deficiencies.[20] Chronic mucocutaneous candidiasis (CMC) embraces a heterogeneous group of disorders, which, in addition to oral candidiasis, also affect the skin, typically the nail bed and other mucosal linings, such as the genital mucosa.[21] The face and scalp may be involved, and granulomatous masses can be seen at these sites. Approximately 90% of the patients with CMC also present with oral candidiasis. The oral affections may involve the tongue, and white hyperplastic lesions are seen in conjunction with fissures. CMC can occur as part of endocrine disorders as hyperparathyroidism and Addison's disease. Impaired phagocytic function by neutrophilic granulocytes and macrophages caused by myeloperoxidase deficiency has also been associated with CMC. Chediak-Higashi syndrome, an inherited disease with a reduced number of impaired neutrophilic granulocytes, lends further support to the role of the phagocytic system in *Candida* infections as these patients frequently develop candidiasis. Severe combined immunodeficiency syndrome is characterized by a defect in the function of the cell-mediated arm of the immune system. Patients with this disorder frequently contract disseminated *Candida* infections. Thymoma is a neoplasm of thymic epithelial cells that also entails systemic candidiasis. Thus, both the native and adaptive immune systems are critical to prevent development of systemic mucocutaneous candidiasis.

DIAGNOSIS AND LABORATORY FINDINGS

The presence of *Candida* as a member of the commensal flora complicates the discrimination of the normal state from infection. It is imperative that both clinical findings and laboratory data (Table 3) are balanced in order to arrive at a correct diagnosis. Sometimes antifungal treatment has to be launched to assist in the diagnostic process.

Smear from the infected area, which comprises epithelial cells, creates opportunities for detection of the yeasts.[22] The

material obtained is fixed in isopropyl alcohol and air-dried before staining with periodic acid–Schiff (PAS). The detection of yeast organisms is considered a sign of infection. This technique is particularly useful when pseudomembranous oral candidiasis and angular cheilitis are suspected. To increase the sensitivity, a second scrape can be transferred to a transport medium followed by cultivation on Sabouraud agar. To discriminate between different *Candida* species, an additional examination can be performed on Pagano-Levin agar. Imprint culture technique can also be used where sterile plastic foam pads (2.5 × 2.5 cm) are submerged in Sabouraud broth and placed on the infected surface for 60 seconds. The pad is then firmly pressed onto Sabouraud agar, which will be cultivated at 37°C. The result is expressed as colony forming units per cubic millimeter (CFU/mm^2). This method is a valuable adjunct in the diagnostic process of erythematous candidiasis and denture stomatitis as these infections consist of fairly homogeneous erythematous lesions. Salivary culture techniques are primarily used in parallel with other diagnostic methods to get an adequate quantification of *Candida*. Patients who display clinical signs of oral candidiasis usually have more than 400 CFU/mL.[23]

In chronic plaque-type and nodular candidiasis, cultivation techniques have to be supplemented by a histopathologic examination. This examination is primarily performed to identify the possible presence of epithelial dysplasia and to identify invading *Candida* organisms by PAS staining. However, for the latter, there is a definitive risk of false-negative results.

MANAGEMENT

Before starting antifungal medication, it is necessary to identify any predisposing factor. Local factors are often easy to identify but sometimes not possible to reduce or eradicate. Antifungal drugs have a primary role in such cases. The most commonly used antifungal drugs belong to the groups of polyenes or azoles (Table 4). Polyenes such as nystatin and amphotericin B are the first alternatives in treatment of primary oral candidiasis and are well tolerated. Polyenes are not absorbed from the gastrointestinal tract and are not associated with development of resistance.[24] They exert the action through a negative effect on the production of ergosterol, which is critical for the *Candida* cell membrane integrity. Polyenes can also affect the adherence of the fungi.[25]

Although rarely realistic, permanent removal of the denture is an effective treatment for denture stomatitis. However, elimination or reduction of predisposing factors should always be the first goal for treatment of denture stomatitis as well as other opportunistic infections. This involves improved denture hygiene and a recommendation not to use the denture while sleeping. The denture hygiene is important to remove nutrients, including desquamated epithelial cells, which may serve as a source of nitrogen. Denture cleaning also disturbs the maturity of a microbial environment beneath the denture. As porosities in the denture harbour microorganisms that may not be accessible to physical cleaning, the denture should

TABLE 3 *Candida* Isolation in the Clinic and Quantification from Oral Samples

Method	Main Steps	Advantages	Disadvantages
Smear	Scraping, smearing directly onto slide	Simple and quick	Low sensitivity
Swab	Taken by rubbing cotton-tipped swabs over lesional tissue	Relatively simple	Selecting sampling sites critical
Imprint culture	Sterile plastic foam pads dipped into Sabouraud (Sab) broth, placed on lesion for 60 s; pad pressed on Sab agar plate and incubated; colony-counter used	Sensitive and reliable; can discriminate between infected and carrier states	Reading above 50 CFU/cm^2 can be inaccurate; selection of sites difficult if no clinical signs present
Impression culture	Maxillary and mandibular alginate impressions; casting in agar fortified with Sab broth; incubation	Useful to determine relative distributions of the yeasts on oral surfaces	Useful mostly as a research tool
Salivary culture	Patient expectorates 2 mL saliva into sterile container; vibration; culture on Sab agar by spiral plating; counting	As useful as imprint culture	Considerable chairside time; not useful for xerostomics; cannot identify site of infection
Oral rinse	Subject rinses for 60 s with PBS at pH 7.2, 0.1 M, and returns it to the original container; concentrated by centrifugation; cultured and counted as in previous methods	Comparable in sensitivity with imprint method; better results if CFU >50/cm^2; simple method	Recommended for surveillance cultures in the absence of focal lesions; cannot identify site of infection

PBS = phosophate-buffered saline
Adapted from.[10]

TABLE 4 Antifungal Agents Used in the Treatment of Oral Candidiasis

Drug	Form	Dosage	Comments
Amphotericin B	Lozenge, 10 mg	Slowly dissolved in mouth 3–4 × /d after meals for 2 wk minimum	Negligible absorption from gastrointestinal tract. When given IV for deep mycoses may cause thrombophlebitis, anorexia, nausea, vomiting, fever, headache, weight loss, anemia, hypokalemia, nephrotoxicity, hypotension, arrhythmias, etc.
	Oral suspension, 100 mg/mL	Placed in the mouth after food and retained near lesions 4 × /d for 2 wk	
Nystatin	Cream	Apply to affected area 3–4 × /d	Negligible absorption from gastrointestinal tract. Nausea and vomiting with high doses.
	Pastille, 100,000 U	Dissolve 1 pastille slowly after meals 4 × /d, usually for 7 d	
	Oral suspension, 100,000 U	Apply after meals 4 × /d, usually for 7 d, and continue use for several days after postclinical healing	
Clotrimazole	Cream	Apply to the affected area 2–3 times daily for 3–4 wk	Mild local effects. Also has antistaphylococcal activity.
	Solution	5 mL 3–4 times daily for 2 wk minimum	
Miconazole	Oral gel	Apply to the affected area 3–4 times daily	Occasional mild local reactions. Also has antibacterial activity. Theoretically the best antifungal to treat angular cheilitis. Interacts with anticoagulants (warfarin), terfenadine, cisapride, and astemizole. Avoid in pregnancy and liver disease.
	Cream	Apply twice per day and continue for 10–14 d after the lesion heals	
Ketoconazole	Tablets	200–400-mg tablets taken once or twice daily with food for 2 wk	May cause nausea, vomiting, rashes, pruritus, and liver damage. Interacts with anticoagulants, terfenadine, cisapride, and astemizole. Contraindicated in pregnancy and liver disease.
Fluconazole	Capsules	50–100 mg capsules once daily for 2–3 wk	Interacts with anticoagulants, terfenadine, cisapride, and astemizole. Contraindicated in pregnancy and liver and renal disease. May cause nausea, diarrhea, headache, rash, liver dysfunction.
Itraconazole	Capsules	100 mg capsules daily taken immediately after meals for 2 wk	Interacts with terfenadine, cisapride, and astemizole. Contraindicated in pregnancy and liver disease. May cause nausea, neuropathy, rash.

Adapted from Ellepola, 2000.[26]
IV = intravenously.

be stored in antimicrobial solutions. Different solutions, including alkaline peroxides, alkaline hypochlorites, acids, disinfectants, and enzymes, have been suggested.[14] The latter seems to be most effective against *Candida*. Chlorhexidine may be used but can discolor the denture and counteracts the effect of nystatin.[26]

Type III denture stomatitis may be treated with surgical excision if it is necessary to eradicate microorganisms present in the deeper fissures of the granular tissue. If this is not sufficient, continuous treatment with topical antifungal drugs should be considered. Patients with no symptoms are rarely motivated for treatment, and the infection often persists without the patient being aware of its presence. However, the chronic inflammation may result in increased resorption of the denture-bearing bone.

Topical treatment with azoles such as miconazole is the treatment of choice in angular cheilitis often infected by both *S. aureus* and *Candida*. This drug has a biostatic effect on *S. aureus* in addition to the fungistatic effect to *Candida*.[27] Fusidic acid (2%) can be used as a complement to the antifungal drugs. If angular cheilitis comprises an erythema surrounding the fissure, a mild steroid ointment may be required to suppress the inflammation. To prevent recurrences, patients have to apply a moisturizing cream, which will prevent new fissure formation.[28]

Systemic azoles may be used for deeply seated primary candidiasis, such as as chronic hyperplastic candidiasis, denture stomatitis, and median rhomboid glossitis with a granular appearance, and for therapy-resistant infections, mostly related to compliance failure. There are several disadvantages with the use of azoles. They are known to interact with warfarin, leading to an increased bleeding propensity. The adverse effect is also valid for topical application as the azoles are fully or partly resorbed form the gastrointestinal tract. Development of resistance is particularly compelling for fluconazole in HIV patients.[29] In such cases, ketoconazole and itraconazole have been recommended as alternatives. However, cross-resistance has been reported between fluconazole on the one hand and ketoconazole, miconazole, and itraconazole on the other.[27] The azoles are also used in the treatment of secondary oral candidiasis associated with systemic predisposing factors and for systemic candidiasis.

The prognosis of oral candidiasis is good given that predisposing factors associated with the infection are reduced or eliminated. Persistent chronic plaque-type and nodular candidiasis have been suggested to entail an increased risk for malignant transformation compared with leukoplakias not allied with a *Candida* infection.[11,30] Patients with primary candidiasis are also at risk if systemic predisposing factors arise. For example, patients with severe immunosuppression as seen in conjunction with leukemia and AIDS may encounter disseminating candidiasis with a fatal course.[31]

Hairy Leukoplakia

Hairy leukoplakia (HL) is the second most common HIV-associated oral mucosal lesion. HL has been used as a marker of disease activity since the lesion is associated with low CD4+ T-lymphocyte counts.[32,33] The lesion is not pathognomonic for HIV since other immune deficiencies, such as immunosuppressive drugs and cancer chemotherapy, are also associated with HL.[34–36] Rarely, individuals with a normal immune system may have HL.[37,38]

ETIOLOGY AND PATHOGENESIS

HL is strongly associated with Epstein-Barr virus (EBV) and with low levels of CD4+ T lymphocytes. Antiviral medication, which prevents EBV replication, is curative[39] and lends further support to EBV as an etiologic factor. There is also a correlation between EBV replication and a decrease in the number of CD1a+ Langerhans' cells, which, together with T lymphocytes, are important cell populations in the cellular immune defense of the oral mucosa.[40]

EPIDEMIOLOGY

The prevalence figures for HL depend on the type of population investigated. Prior to the HAART era, the prevalence was 25%,[41] a figure that has decreased considerably after the introduction of HAART. In patients who develop AIDS, the prevalence may be as high as 80%.[42] The prevalence in children is lower compared with adults and has been reported to be in the range of 2%.[43] The condition is more frequently encountered in men, but the reason for this dependence on gender is not known. A correlation between smoking and HL has also been observed.[44]

CLINICAL FINDINGS

The disorder is frequently encountered on the lateral borders of the tongue but may also be observed on the dorsum and in the buccal mucosa (Figure 9).[45,46] The typical clinical appearance is vertical white folds oriented as a palisade along the borders of the tongue. The lesions may also be displayed as white and somewhat elevated plaque, which cannot be scraped off. As HL may present itself in different clinical forms, it is important to always consider this mucosal lesion whenever the border of the tongue is affected by white lesions, particularly in immunocompromised patients. HL is asymptomatic,[47] although symptoms may be present when the lesion is superinfected with *Candida*.

DIAGNOSIS

The diagnosis of HL is based on clinical characteristics, a histopathologic examination, and detection of EBV (Table 5).

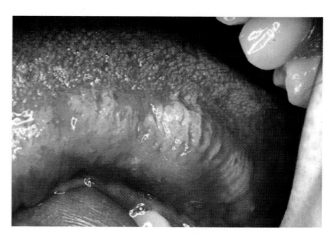

FIGURE 9   Hairy leukoplakia at the left lateral border of the tongue in an AIDS patient.

TABLE 5   Features of the Diagnosis of Oral Hairy Leukoplakia

Provisional diagnosis
   Characteristic gross appearance, with or without nonresponsiveness to antifungal therapy

Presumptive diagnosis
   Light microscopy of histologic sections revealing hyperkeratosis, koilocytosis, acanthosis, and absence of inflammatory cell infiltrate or light microscopy of cytologic preparations demonstrating nuclear beading and chromatin margination

Definitive diagnosis
   In situ hybridization of histologic or cytologic specimens revealing positive staining for EBV DNA or electron microscopy of histologic or cytologic specimens showing herpesvirus-like particles

Adapted from Triantos D et al.[45]
DNA = deoxyribonucleic acid; EBV = Epstein-Barr virus.

It may most easily be confused with chronic trauma to the lateral borders of the tongue.

PATHOLOGY

The histopathology of HL is characterized by hyperkeratosis and acanthosis.[45] Hairy projections are common, which is reflected in the name given to this disorder. Koilocytosis, with edematous epithelial cells and pyknotic nuclei, is also a characteristic histopathologic feature. The complex chromatin arrangements may mirror EBV replication in the nuclei of koilocytic epithelial cells. *Candida* hyphae surrounded by polymorphonuclear granulocytes are also a common feature. The number of immunostained Langerhans' cells is considerably reduced.[48] Mild subepithelial inflammation may also be observed. EBV can be detected by *in situ* hybridization or by immunohistochemistry. Exfoliative cytology may be of value and can serve as an alternative to biopsy.[45]

MANAGEMENT

HL can be treated successfully with antiviral medication,[39] but this is not often indicated as this disorder is not associated with subjective symptoms. In addition, the disorder has also been reported to show spontaneous regression. HL is not related to increased risk of malignant transformation.

▼ PREMALIGNANT LESIONS

Oral Leukoplakia and Erythroplakia

ETIOLOGY AND PATHOGENESIS

The development of oral leukoplakia and erythroplakia as premalignant lesions involves different genetic events. This notion is supported by the fact that markers of genetic defects are differently expressed in different leukoplakias and erythroplakias.[49–51] Activation of oncogenes and deletion and injuries to suppressor genes and genes responsible for DNA repair will all contribute to a defective functioning of the genome that governs cell division. Following a series of mutations, a malignant transformation may occur. For example, carcinogens such as tobacco may induce hyperkeratinization, with the potential to revert following cessation, but at some stage, mutations will lead to an unrestrained proliferation and cell division.

EPIDEMIOLOGY

The prevalence of oral leukoplakia varies among scientific studies. A comprehensive global review points at a prevalence of 2.6%.[52] Most oral leukoplakias are seen in patients over the age of 50 and infrequently encountered below the age of 30. In population studies, leukoplakias are more common in men,[53] but a slight majority for women was found in reviews of referred materials.[54,55]

Oral erythroplakia is not as common as oral leukoplakia, and the prevalence has been estimated to be in the range of 0.02 to 0.1%.[56] The gender distribution is reported to be equal.

CLINICAL FINDINGS

Oral leukoplakia is defined as a predominantly white lesion of the oral mucosa that cannot be characterized as any other definable lesion.[57] This disorder can be further divided into a homogeneous and a nonhomogeneous type. The typical homogeneous leukoplakia is clinically characterized as a white, well-demarcated plaque with an identical reaction pattern throughout the entire lesion (Figure 10). The surface texture can vary from a smooth thin surface to a leathery appearance with surface fissures sometimes referred to as "cracked mud." The demarcation is usually very distinct, which is different from an oral lichen planus (OLP) lesion, where the white components have a more diffuse transition to the normal oral mucosa. Another difference between these two lesions is the lack of a peripheral erythematous zone in homogeneous oral leukoplakia. The lesions are asymptomatic in most patients.

The nonhomogeneous type of oral leukoplakia may have white patches or plaque intermixed with red tissue elements (Figure 11A). Due to the combined appearance of white and red areas, the nonhomogeneous oral leukoplakia has also been called erythroleukoplakia and speckled leukoplakia. The clinical manifestation of the white component may vary from

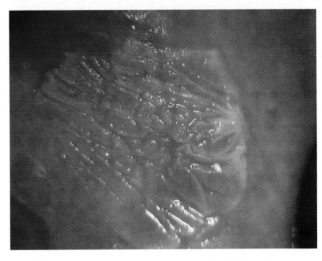

FIGURE 10   A homogeneous leukoplakia at the left buccal mucosa.

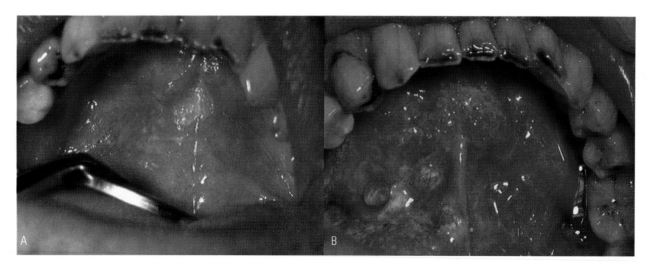

FIGURE 11   *A,* A nonhomogeneous leukoplakia in a heavy smoker. The left part of the lesion has a speckled appearance. *B,* The patient did not attend the follow-up visits for 3 years and developed a squamous cell carcinoma.

large white verrucous areas to small nodular structures. If the surface texture is homogeneous but contains verrucous, papillary (nodular), or exophytic components, the leukoplakia is also regarded as nonhomogeneous. Both homogeneous and nonhomogeneous leukoplakias may be encountered in all sites of the oral mucosa.

Oral leukoplakias, where the white component is dominated by papillary projections, similar to oral papillomas, are referred to as verrucous or verruciform leukoplakias.[58] Oral leukoplakias with this clinical appearance but with a more aggressive proliferation pattern and recurrence rate are designated as proliferative verrucous leukoplakia (PVL) (Figure 12).[59] This lesion may start as a homogeneous leukoplakia but over time develop a verrucous appearance containing various degrees of dysplasia. PVL is usually encountered in older women, and the lower gingiva is a predilection site.[60] The malignant potential is very high, and verrucous carcinoma or squamous cell carcinoma may be present at the primary

examination. As the common surface reaction pattern is similar to what is seen in oral papillomas, the PVL has been suspected to have a viral etiology, although no such association has been confirmed.[61]

Oral leukoplakia may be found at all sites of the oral mucosa. Nonsmokers have a higher percentage of leukoplakias at the border of the tongue compared with smokers.[54] The floor of the mouth and the lateral borders of the tongue are high-risk sites for malignant transformation (Figure 11B). These sites have also been found to have a higher frequency of loss of heterozygosity compared with low-risk sites.[50] However, the separation into high- and low-risk sites has recently been questioned.[55,62]

Oral erythroplakia has not been studied as intensively as oral leukoplakia.[56] Erythroplakia is defined as a red lesion of the oral mucosa that cannot be characterized as any other definable lesion (Figure 13). The lesion comprises an eroded red lesion that is frequently observed with a distinct

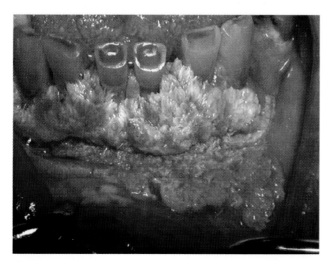

FIGURE 12   A proliferative verrucous leukoplakia in an 80-year-old woman.

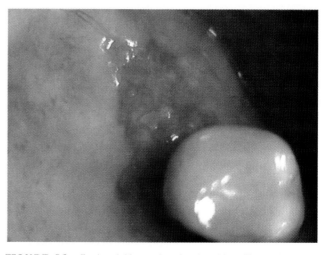

FIGURE 13   Erythroplakia at the alveolar ridge. The patient later developed a squamous cell carcinoma.

demarcation against the normal-appearing mucosa. Clinically, erythroplakia is different from erythematous OLP as the latter has a more diffuse border and is surrounded by white reticular or papular structures. Erythroplakia is usually nonsymptomatic, although some patients may experience a burning sensation in conjunction with food intake.

A special form of erythroplakia has been reported that is related to reverse smoking of *chutta*, predominantly practiced in India.[63] The lesion comprises well-demarcated red areas in conjunction with white papular tissue structures. Ulcerations and depigmented areas may also be a part of this particular form of oral lesion.

DIAGNOSIS

The diagnostic procedure of oral leukoplakia and erythroplakia is identical (Figure 14).[57,64] The provisional diagnosis is based on the clinical observation of a white or red patch that is not explained by a definable cause, such as trauma. If trauma is suspected, the cause, such as a sharp tooth cusp or restoration, should be eliminated. If healing does not occur in 2 weeks, biopsy is essential to rule out malignancy.

PATHOLOGY

The biopsy should include representative tissue of different clinical patterns. Hyperkeratosis without any other features of a definable diagnosis is compatible with homogeneous oral leukoplakia. If the histopathologic examination leads to another definable lesion, the definitive diagnosis will be changed accordingly. However, there is no uniform depiction of an oral leukoplakia and the histopathologic features of the epithelium may include hyperkeratosis, atrophy, and hyperplasia with or without dysplasia. When dysplasia is present, it may vary from mild to severe. Dysplasia may be found in homogeneous leukoplakias but is much more frequently encountered in nonhomogeneous leukoplakias[55,65–67] and in erythroplakias.[68] Epithelial dysplasia is defined in general terms as a precancerous lesion of stratified squamous epithelium characterized by cellular atypia and loss of normal maturation short of carcinoma in situ (Figure 15). Carcinoma in situ is defined as a lesion in which the full thickness of squamous epithelium shows the cellular features of carcinoma without stromal invasion.[69] A more detailed description of

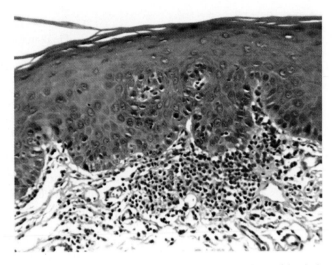

FIGURE 15 An oral epithelium with several characteristics of dysplasia (see Table 6).

TABLE 6 Criteria Used for Diagnosing Epithelial Dysplasia

Loss of polarity of basal cells

The presence of more than one layer of cells having a basaloid appearance

Increased nuclear-cytoplasmic ratio

Drop-shaped rete ridges

Irregular epithelial stratification

Increased number of mitotic figures

Mitotic figures that are abnormal in form

The presence of mitotic figures in the superficial half of the epithelium

Cellular and nuclear pleomorphism

Nuclear hyperchromatism

Enlarged nuclei

Loss of intercellular adherence

Keratinization of single cells or cell groups in the prickle cell layer

Adapted from Pindborg JJ et al.[69]

epithelial dysplasia is presented in Table 6. The prevalence of dysplasia in oral leukoplakias varies from 1 to 30%, whereas the majority of erythroplakias display an atrophic epithelium with dysplastic features.[68]

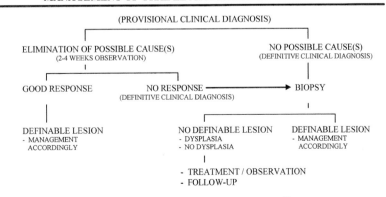

MANAGEMENT OF ORAL LEUKOPLAKIA/ERYTHROPLAKIA

(PROVISIONAL CLINICAL DIAGNOSIS)

ELIMINATION OF POSSIBLE CAUSE(S)
(2-4 WEEKS OBSERVATION)

NO POSSIBLE CAUSE(S)
(DEFINITIVE CLINICAL DIAGNOSIS)

GOOD RESPONSE

NO RESPONSE
(DEFINITIVE CLINICAL DIAGNOSIS)
→ BIOPSY

DEFINABLE LESION
- MANAGEMENT
  ACCORDINGLY

NO DEFINABLE LESION
- DYSPLASIA
- NO DYSPLASIA

DEFINABLE LESION
- MANAGEMENT
  ACCORDINGLY

- TREATMENT / OBSERVATION
- FOLLOW-UP

FIGURE 14 Management of oral leukoplakia/erythroplakia. Adapted from van der Waal I et al.[64]

MANAGEMENT

Oral leukoplakia is a lesion with an increased risk of malignant transformation, which has great implications for the management of this oral mucosal disorder. Since alcohol and smoking are well-established risk factors for the development of oral squamous cell carcinomas, measures should be taken to influence the patients to discontinue such habits. Cold-knife surgical excision, as well as laser surgery, is widely used to eradicate leukoplakias and erythroplakias but will not prevent all premalignant lesions from malignant development.[70–74] On the contrary, surgery has been strongly questioned as squamous cell carcinomas are almost equally prevalent in non–surgically treated patients as in patients subjected to surgery.[55] This may be explained by genetic defects in clinically normal mucosa and is supported by a concept referred to as field cancerization.[75] Field cancerization is caused by simultaneous genetic instabilities in the epithelium of several extralesional sites that may lead to squamous cell carcinomas. However, in the absence of evidenced-based treatment strategies for oral leukoplakias, surgery will remain the treatment for oral leukoplakias and erythroplakias.

Malignant transformation of oral leukoplakias has been reported in the range of 1 to 20% over 1 to 30 years.[62,76,77] Based on a recent review of available European epidemiologic data, the incidence has been calculated not to exceed 1% per year.[78] Sixteen to 62% of oral carcinomas have been reported to be associated with leukoplakia at the time of the diagnosis,[79–81] and in an Indian house-to-house survey, 80% of oral cancers were reported to be preceded by oral precancerous lesions or conditions.[82] Until biomarkers are developed, management of oral leukoplakias and erythroplakias has to rely on traditional clinical and histopathologic criteria. Homogeneous oral leukoplakia entails less risk for malignant transformation than do nonhomogeneous leukoplakias and erythroplakias.

Presently, no consensus has been developed regarding management and follow-up of oral leukoplakias and erythroplakias. A general recommendation may be to reexamine the premalignant site irrespective of surgical excision every 3 months for the first year. If the lesion does not relapse or change in reaction pattern, the follow-up intervals may be extended to once every 6 months. New biopsies should be taken if new clinical features emerge. Following 5 years of no relapse, self-examination may be a reasonable approach.

Oral Submucous Fibrosis

is a chronic disease that affects the oral mucosa as well as the pharynx and the upper two-thirds of the esophagus.[84] There is substantial evidence that lends support to a critical role of areca nuts in the etiology behind submucous fibrosis.[85]

ETIOLOGY AND PATHOGENESIS

There is a dose dependence between areca quid chewing habit and the development of this oral mucosal disorder. Areca nuts contain alcaloids, of which arecoline seems to be a primary etiologic factor.[86] Arecoline has the capacity to modulate matrix metalloproteinases, lysyl oxidases, and collagenases, all affecting the metabolism of collagen, which leads to an increased fibrosis.[87] During the development of fibrosis, a decrease in the water-retaining proteoglycans will occur in favor of an increased collagen type I production.[88] There is also evidence of a genetic predisposition of importance for the etiology behind submucous fibrosis. Polymorphism of the gene, which is coding for tumor necrosis factor α (TNF-α), has been reported to promote the development of the disorder. Fibroblasts are stimulated by TNF-α, thereby participating in the development of fibrosis.[89] Aberrations of other cytokines of importance are transforming growth factor β and interferon-γ, which may lead to increased production and decreased degradation of collagen. A genetic predisposition is also supported by association-specific human leukocyte antigen (HLA) molecules, such as HLA-A10, -B7, and -DR3.[90]

EPIDEMIOLOGY

Areca nut–derived products have several hundred million consumers in the southern parts of Asia. Regional variations exist regarding the preference of the areca nut use, which also accounts for variation in the affected sites. Oral complications are most commonly observed on the lips, buccal mucosa, retromolar area, and soft palatal mucosa.[91] The habit of chewing betel quid, containing fresh, dried, or cured areca nut, and flavoring ingredients is widespread in India, Pakistan, Bangladesh, and Sri Lanka and in immigrants coming from these regions.[92] Tobacco is often used in conjunction with betel quid. The habit is more common among women in some geographic areas, which is also reflected in the gender distribution of submucous fibrosis.

The global incidence of submucous fibrosis is estimated at 2.5 million individuals.[93] The prevalence in Indian populations is 5% for women and 2% for men.[90] It seems as if age groups below 20 years of age more often contract submucous fibrosis. This is reflected in the advertisement of areca nut products, which is directed against younger age groups. Following the introduction of this marketing strategy, the incidence of submucous fibrosis has increased 10 times between 1980 and 1993.[87]

CLINICAL FINDINGS

The first sign is erythematous lesions sometimes in conjunction with petechiae, pigmentations, and vesicles.[85] These initial lesions are followed by a paler mucosa, which may comprise white marbling (Figure 16). The most prominent clinical characteristics will appear later in the course of the disease and include fibrotic bands located beneath an atrophic epithelium. Increased fibrosis eventually leads to loss of resilience, which interferes with speech, tongue mobility, and a decreased ability to open the mouth. The atrophic epithelium may cause a smarting sensation and inability to eat hot and spicy food. More than 25% of the patients exhibit also oral leukoplakias.[94]

DIAGNOSIS

The diagnosis of submucous fibrosis is based on the clinical characteristics and on the patient's report of a habit of betel quid chewing. An international consensus has been reached

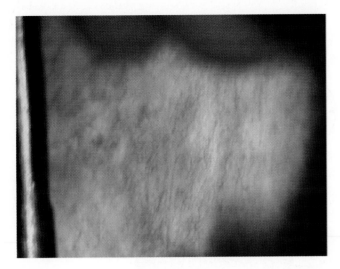

FIGURE 16   A patient with submucous fibrosis with restricted ability to open her mouth. The buccal mucosa has a marbling appearance.

where at least one of the following characteristics should be present[95]:

- Palpable fibrous bands
- Mucosal texture feels tough and leathery
- Blanching of mucosa together with histopathologic features consistent with oral submucous fibrosis (atrophic epithelium with loss of rete ridges and juxtaepithelial hyalinization of lamina propria)

PATHOLOGY

The early histopathologic characteristics for submucous fibrosis are fine fibrils of collagen, edema, hypertrophic fibroblasts, dilatated and congested blood vessels, and an infiltration of neutrophilic and eosinophilic granulocytes.[96] This picture is followed by a down-regulation of fibroblasts, epithelial atrophy, and loss of rete pegs, and early signs of hyalinization occur in concert with an infiltration of inflammatory cells. Epithelial dysplasia in submucous fibrosis tissues appeared to vary from 7 to 26% depending on the study population.[97–99]

MANAGEMENT

Products derived from areca nuts are carcinogenic, regardless of tobacco use as an adjunct. Thus, treatment of submucous fibrosis should be focused on cessation of the chewing habits. If this is successfully implemented, early lesions have a good prognosis as they may regress.[94] A plethora of treatment strategies have been tried, such as topical and systemic steroids, supplement of vitamins and nutrients, repeated dilatation with physical devices, and surgery.[100] None of these treatments have reached general acceptance as the long-term results are dubious.

Malignant transformation of oral submucous fibrosis has been estimated in the range of 7 to 13%[87] and the incidence over a 10-year period at approximately 8%.[98]

▼ IMMUNOPATHOLOGIC DISEASES

Oral Lichen Planus

Lichenoid reactions represent a family of lesions with different etiologies with a common clinical and histologic appearence.[101] Histopathologic examination does not enable discrimination between different lichenoid reactions but may be used to distinguish lichenoid reactions from other pathologic conditions of the oral mucosa. Oral lichenoid reactions include the following disorders:

- Lichen planus
- Lichenoid contact reactions
- Lichenoid drug eruptions
- Lichenoid reactions of graft-versus-host disease (GVHD)

Oral lichenoid contact reactions (LCRs) are included with allergic reactions since these lesions represent a delayed hypersensitivity reaction to constituents derived from dental materials or flavoring agents in foods.

ETIOLOGY AND PATHOGENSIS

The etiology of OLP is not known.[101] During recent years, it has become more evident that the immune system has a primary role in the development of this disease.[102] This is supported by the histopathologic characteristics of a subepithelial band–formed infiltrate dominated by T lymphocytes[103] and macrophages and the degeneration of basal cells known as liquefaction degeneration (Figure 17). These features can be interpreted as an expression of the cell-mediated arm of the immune system being involved in the pathogenesis of OLP through T-lymphocyte cytotoxicity directed against antigens expressed by the basal cell layer.

Autoreactive T lymphocytes may be of primary importance for the development of oral lichen planus (Composition 7).[104] These cells cannot discriminate between inherent molecules of the body and foreign antigens. Activation of the autoreactive T lymphocyte is a process that may arise in other parts of the body than the oral mucosa and may not

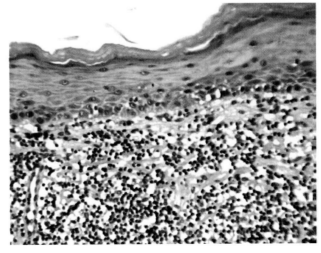

FIGURE 17   Lichenoid reaction with a subepithelial infiltrate of inflammatory cells and liquefaction degeneration in the basal cell layer.

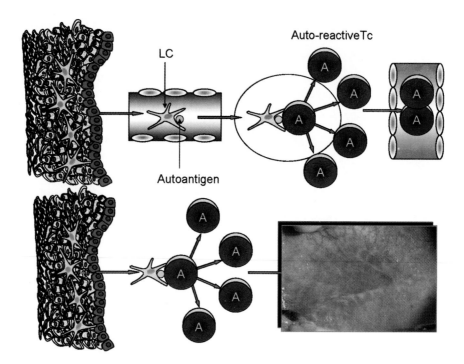

COMPOSITION 7

even occur in concert with the onset of the mucosal lesion. Most likely, it is not one single peptide that has the potential to evoke the inflammatory response but several depending on the specificity of the autoreactive T lymphocyte. The conclusion that follows from this reasoning is that it is complicated to identify a single etiologic factor behind OLP.[104] Other factors, such as stress, may also be of importance to establish the inflammatory process. It is not unusual that patients report that they have been exposed negative social events some months before to the onset of the disease. Altogether, this makes the etiology behind OLP a multifactorial process comprising events that may take place at different time points.

During recent years, an association between OLP and hepatitis C virus (HCV) has been described in populations from Japan and some Mediterranean countries. This association has not been observed in northern European countries or the United States. Furthermore, no association has been reported from Egypt and Nigeria,[105] which are countries with a very high HCV prevalence. It has been postulated that the association may be related to a genetic variability between countries. This is in part supported by the observation that specific alleles of the major histocompatibilty complex, such as HLA-DR6, are more prevalent in Italian patients with HCV-related OLP. However, no comprehensive explanation has been provided regarding the association between OLP and HCV.

EPIDEMIOLOGY

In the literature, different prevalence figures for OLP have been reported and vary from 0.5 to 2.2%.[106–109] These figures may represent an underestimation as minor lesions may easily be overlooked. Among referred patients, the proportion of women is higher than that of men, but this may not be the case in the general population. The mean age at the time of diagnosis is approximately 55 years.

CLINICAL FINDINGS

OLP may contain both red and white elements and provide, together with the different textures, the basis for the clinical classification of this disorder. The white and red components of the lesion can be a part of the following textures:

- Reticulum
- Papules
- Plaque-like
- Bullous
- Erythematous
- Ulcerative

To establish a clinical diagnosis of OLP, reticular or papular textures have to be present.[110] If, in addition, plaque-like, bullous, erythematous, or ulcerative areas are present, the OLP lesion is designated accordingly. OLP confined to the gingiva may be entirely erythematous, with no reticular or papular elements present, and this type of lesion has to be confirmed by a histopathologic examination.

The explanation of the different clinical manifestations of OLP is related to the magnitude of the subepithelial inflammation. A mild degree of inflammation may provoke the epithelium to produce hyperkeratosis, whereas more intense inflammation will lead to partial or complete deterioration of the epithelium, histopathologically perceived as atrophy, erosion, or ulceration. This corroborates with the fact that most erythematous and ulcerative lesions are surrounded by white reticular or papular structures. An inflammatory gradient may be formed where the central part comprises an intense inflammatory process, whereas the periphery is less affected and the epithelial cells are able to respond with hyperkeratosis.

The reticular form of OLP is characterized by fine white lines or striae (Figure 18). The striae may form a network but can also show annular (circular) patterns. The striae often display a peripheral erythematous zone, which reflects the subepithelial inflammation. Although reticular OLP may be encountered in all regions of the oral mucosa, most frequently this form is observed bilaterally in the buccal mucosa and rarely on the mucosal side of the lips. Reticular OLP can sometimes be observed at the vermilion border.

The papular type of OLP is usually present in the initial phase of the disease (Figure 19).[107] It is clinically characterized by small white dots, which in most occasions intermingle with the reticular form. Sometimes the papular elements merge with striae as part of the natural course.

Plaque-type OLP shows a homogeneous well-demarcated white plaque often, but not always, surrounded by striae (Figure 20). Plaque-type lesions may clinically be very similar to homogeneous oral leukoplakias. The difference between these two mucosal disorders is the simultaneous presence of reticular or papular structures in the case of plaque-like OLP. This form is most often encountered in smokers,[107,111] and following cessation, the plaque may disappear and convert into the reticular type of OLP. Some scientific reports lend support to the premise that plaque-like OLP is overrepresented among OLP lesions transforming into oral squamous cell carcinomas.[112]

Typically, the reticular, papular, and plaque-like forms of OLP are asymptomatic, although the patient may experience a feeling of roughness. The bullous form is very unusual but may appear as bullous strucures surrounded by a reticular network.

Erythematous (atrophic) OLP is characterized by a homogeneous red area. When this type of OLP is present in the buccal mucosa or in the palate, striae are frequently seen in the periphery. Some patients may display erythematous OLP exclusively affecting attached gingiva (Figure 21A).[113] This form of lesion may occur without any papules or striae and presents as desquamative gingivitis. Therefore, erythematous OLP requires a histopathologic examination in order to arrive at a correct diagnosis.

Ulcerative lesions are the most disabling form of OLP (Figure 22A). Clinically, the fibrin-coated ulcers are surrounded by an erythematous zone frequently displaying radiating white striae. This appearance may reflect a gradient of the intensity of subepithelial inflammation that is most prominent at the center of the lesion. As for the erythematous form of OLP, the affected patient complains of a smarting sensation in conjunction with food intake.

CLINICAL MANIFESTATION

Cutaneous lesions may be encountered in approximately 15% of patients with OLP.[114] The classic appearance of skin lesions consists of pruritic erythematous to violaceous papules that are flat topped that have a predilection for the trunk and flexor surfaces of arms and legs (Figure 23). The papules may

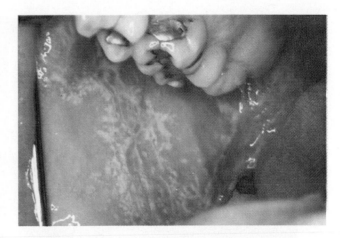

FIGURE 18 A reticular form of oral lichen planus.

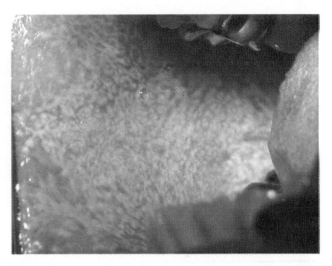

FIGURE 19 Papular oral lichen planus with dense cover of papules. In the upper left corner, the lesion has started to form a more reticular structure.

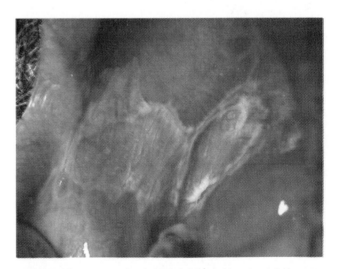

FIGURE 20 A plaque-like oral lichen planus with a plaque in the anterior part. In the posterior part, the lesion has features that are compatible with the reticular form.

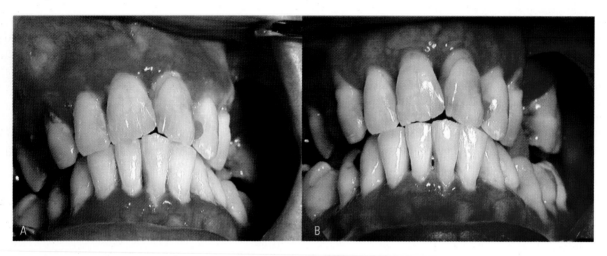

FIGURE 21   *A*, Erythematous oral lichen planus. *B*, Improvement of the lesion following optimal oral hygiene.

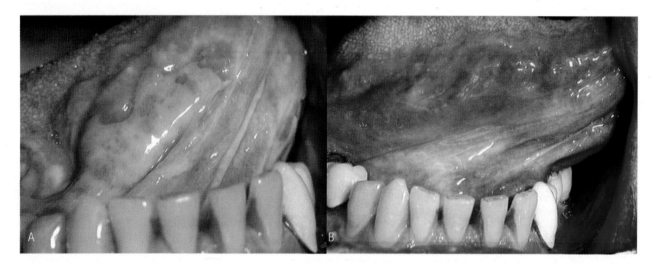

FIGURE 22   *A*, Ulcerative oral lichen planus. *B*, Complete epithelialization following 3 weeks of treatment with 0.025% clobetasol propionate gel, twice daily.

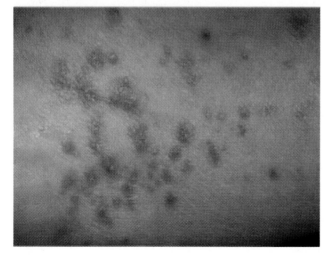

FIGURE 23   Cutaneous lichen planus on the flexor side of the fore arm.

be discrete or coalesce to form plaques. The patients report relief following intense scratching of the lesions, but trauma may aggravate the disease, which is referred to as a Koebner phenomenon.[115] This phenomenon may also be of relevance for OLP, which is continuously exposed to physical trauma during mastication and toothbrushing.

The most frequent extraoral mucosal site involved is the genital mucosa. Close to 20% of women presenting with OLP also have genital involvement.[114] Symptoms including burning, pain, vaginal discharge, and dyspareunia are frequently noted in patients with erythematous or ulcerative disease. No relationship seems to exist between the degree of severity of the oral and genital site. Genital lichen planus has also been reported in males, but the association with OLP is not as frequent as for women. Esophageal OLP has been described to occur simultaneously with OLP in some patients, the main complaint being dysphagia.[114]

DIAGNOSIS

Papules or reticular components have to be present in order to establish a correct clinical diagnosis. These pathognomonic components may exist together with plaque-like, erythematous, or ulcerative lesions. In patients with gingival erythematous lesions, it may be difficult to find striae or papules. A biopsy for histopathologic examination is usually required for an accurate diagnosis of this type of OLP, but it is important that the biopsy is taken as far as possible from the gingival pocket to avoid inflammatory changes secondary to periodontal disease.

OLP can often be separated from LCRs to dental materials, which are most often detected on the buccal mucosa and the lateral borders of the tongue. OLP, on the other hand, usually displays a more general involvement.[116]

Oral lichenoid drug eruptions[117] have the same clinical and histopathologic characteristics as OLP. The patient's disease history may give some indication as to which drug may be involved, but OLP may not start when the drug was first introduced. Withdrawal of the drug and rechallenge are the most reliable way to diagnose lichenoid drug eruptions but may not be possible. Testing for contact allergy with patch testing may be required in some cases.

Oral GVHD has the same clinical appearance as OLP, but the lesion is usually more generalized. The lichenoid reactions are frequently seen simultaneously with other characteristics, such as xerostomia and the presence of localized skin involvement and liver dysfunction, even if an oral lichenoid reaction may emerge as the only clinical sign of GVHD.

Oral mucosal lesions that do not belong to the group of lichenoid reactions may sometimes comprise a differential diagnostic problem. Discoid lupus erythematosus (DLE) shows white radiating striae sometimes resembling those of OLP. The striae present in DLE are typically more prominent, with a more marked hyperkeratinization, and the striae may abruptly terminate against a sharp demarcation (Figure 24). Histopathologic criteria for lupus erythematosus (LE) have been reported to discriminate against OLP with a sensitivity

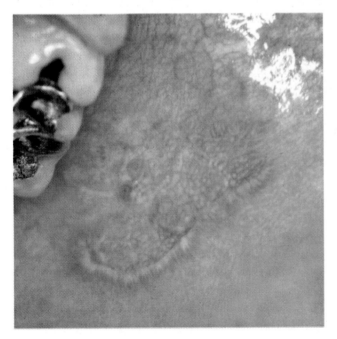

FIGURE 24 Discoid lupus erythematous of the left buccal mucosa.

of 92% and a specificity of 96%.[118] Direct immunofluorescence for immunoglobulin (Ig)M on biopies of the clinically normal oral mucosa (lupus band test) may also be used, although they are only positive in less than 50% of the SLE cases.[119] Plaque-like OLP is discriminated from homogeneous oral leukoplakia as the latter is not featured with papular or reticular elements.

Erythematous OLP of the gingiva exhibits a similar clinical presentation as mucous membrane pemphigoid.[101] In pemphigoid lesions, the epithelium is easily detached from the connective tissue by a probe or a gentle searing force (Nikolsky's phenomenon). A biopsy for routine histology and direct immunofluorescence are required for an accurate differential diagnosis. Ulcerating conditions such as erythema multiforme and adverse reactions to nonsteroidal anti-inflammatory drugs (NSAIDs) may be difficult to distinguish from ulcerative OLP.[102] The former lesions, however, do not typically appear with reticular or papular elements in the periphery of the ulcerations.

PATHOLOGY

To differentiate between the four types of lichenoid reactions, that is, OLP, LCR, lichenoid drug eruptions, and lichenoid reactions related to GVHD, a histopathologic examination is of modest diagnostic value. The reason is that the four lesions display the same histopathologic features. Undoubtedly, histopathology is a valuable tool when lichenoid reactions are to be discriminated from other mucosal lesions. The necessity of a biopsy to arrive at an accurate diagnosis of OLP has been discussed, but explicit guidelines have not been universally approved. When the diagnosis is uncertain, biopsies should always be taken.

The histopathologic features of OLP are (1) areas of hyperparakeratosis or hyperorthokeratosis, often with a thickening of the granular cell layer and a saw-toothed appearance to the rete pegs, and (2) "liquefaction degeneration," or necrosis of the basal cell layer; (3) an eosinophilic band may be seen just beneath the basement membrane and represent fibrin covering the lamina propria.[101] A dense subepithelial band–shaped infiltrate of lymphocytes and macrophages is also characteristic of the disease (see Figure 17). Deposition of antibodies and complement can be observed but is not pathognomonic for OLP; therefore, this technique is not routinely used.[101]

MANAGEMENT

Since the etiology behind OLP is unknown, basic conditions are lacking for development of preventive therapies. Thus, all current treatment strategies are aiming at reducing or eliminating symptoms. Several topical drugs have been suggested, including steroids, calcineurin inhibitors (cyclosporine and tacrolimus), retinoids, and ultraviolet phototherapy.[104] Among these, topical steroids are widely used and accepted as the primary treatment of choice (Figure 22b). Some reports have advocated very potent steroids as clobetasol propionate in favor of intermediate steroids such as triamcinolone acetonide. However, no randomized clinical trials exist where different formulas, strengths, and classes of topically applied steroids have been compared. Topical application of cyclosporine, tacrolimus, and retinoids has been suggested as a second-line therapy for OLP. Cyclosporine has been reported to be less effective than clobetasol propionate and not significantly better than 1% triamcinolone paste. No adverse effects related to these two drugs have been reported except for a temporary burning sensation following the use of cyclosporine.[120] In a comparison of topical application of clobetasol and cyclosporine, the former has been found to be more effective in inducing clinical improvement, but the two drugs have comparable effects on symptoms. Clobetasol was found to give less stable results than cyclosporine when therapy ended and was ascribed a higher incidence of side effects, but none of these were severe enough to require discontinuation of therapy. Topical tacrolimus 0.1% ointment has been reported to have a better initial therapeutic response than triamcinolone acetonide 0.1% ointment.[121,122] However, this drug has been labeled with the US Food and Drug Administration's Black Box Warning: "Possibility of increased risk of malignancy (squamous cell carcinoma and lymphoma) in patients using topical tacrolimus/pimecrolimus for cutaneous psoriasis. These agents should be used in limited circumstances, and patients made aware of these concerns."[123] In conclusion, topical steroids should be used as the primary therapeutic choice for symptomatic OLP. Cyclosporine may be considered a second choice, although the efficacy has been questioned. Tacrolimus should only be used by experts when symptomatic OLP lesions are recalcitrant to topical steroids.

Topical steroids are preferably used as a mouthrinse or a gel. These formulas are often easier for the patient to administer than a paste. Although no systematic studies have compared different frequencies of application, a reasonable approach may be to apply the drug two to three times a day during 3 weeks followed by tapering during the following 9 weeks until a maintenance dose of two to three times a week is reached. There are no consistent results that lend support to decreased levels of endogenous cortisol. Relapses are common, and the general approach should be to use steroids at the lowest level to keep the patient free of symptoms. This approach necessitates an individual amendment of the steroid therapy to each patient. When potent topical steroids are used, a fungal infection may emerge. A parallel treatment with antifungal drugs may be necessary when the number of applications exceeds once a day.

Although topical steroids are usually able to keep OLP patients free of symptoms, systemic steroids are justified to be able to control symptoms from recalcitrant lesions. One milligram per kilogram daily for 7 days has been suggested, followed by a reduction of 10 mg each subsequent day.[115] A maintenance dose with topical steroids may be commenced during the tapering of the systemic steroids.

Erythematous OLP of the gingiva constitutes a therapeutic challenge. To be successful, it is critical to remove both sub- and supragingival plaque and calculus (Figure 21B).[124] If a microbial plaque–induced gingivitis is present, it seems to work in concert with gingival lichen planus and make the latter more resistant to pharmacologic treatment. Thus, oral hygiene should be optimized prior to the beginning of steroid treatment. Once the hygiene treatment is complete, some patients experience a decrease in or even elimination of symptoms and steroid treatment is no longer justified. If symptoms persist, steroid gels in prefabricated plastic trays may be used for 30 minutes at each application to increase the concentration of steroids in the gingival tissue.

As part of OLP lesions, ulcerative areas may be found in close contact with dental materials similar to what is observed in LCRs. The difference is the extension of the LCR, which is limited to such contacts. When symptomatic ulcerations of this kind are present as part of the OLP lesion, replacement of the dental material, usually amalgams, may convert a symptomatic to a nonsymptomatic lesion.[116]

OLP is considered to be a premalignant condition (Figure 25). Premalignant conditions are disorders that entail an increased risk of malignant transformation at some site of the oral mucosa, not necessarily associated with a preexisting lesion. A premalignant lesion, on the other hand, is a lesion that has an inherent increased risk to develop carcinomas compared with the surrounding tissues. Oral leukoplakia and erythroplakia are examples of premalignant lesions.

It is widely accepted that patients with OLP are predisposed to develop oral carcinomas, although it should be emphasized that the risk is low and presumably does not exceed an incidence of 0.2% per year.[104] It may be ambiguous to relate the increased risk to patients with a definite type of OLP lesions. In some studies, plaque-like lesions have been overrepresented, but ulcerative lesions are also suspected to be associated with malignant transformation.[112] Albeit the risk for patients with OLP to contract oral squamous cell carcinomas is low, a minimum of annual monitoring has been suggested.[101] For patients with symptomatic OLP, examination for malignancies will be a part of the evaluation

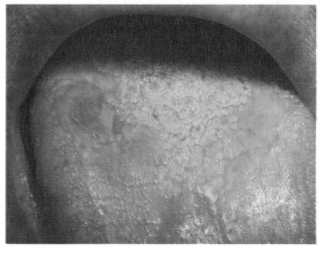

FIGURE 25 A squamous cell carcinoma developed in a plaque-like oral lichen planus.

of symptomatic treatment. In countries with limited health care resources, it may be difficult to conduct annual monitoring, but at the time of diagnosis, patients need to be properly educated on the subject of the malignant potential of OLP.[110]

Drug-Induced Lichenoid Reactions

ETIOLOGY AND PATHOGENESIS

The mechanisms behind drug-induced lichenoid reactions (DILRs) are poorly understood.[116] As the clinical and histopathologic appearances resemble a delayed hypersensitivity reaction, it has been hypothesized that drugs or their metabolites with the capacity to act as haptens trigger a lichenoid reaction. Penicillin, gold, and sulfonamides are examples of drugs that have been related to the development of DILRs.[125] Penicillin and gold may bind directly to self-proteins, which will be presented by antigen-presenting cells (APCs) and perceived as foreign by specific T lymphocytes, similar to a delayed hypersensitivity reaction.[126] Drugs such as sulfonamides haptenate self-proteins indirectly, through formation of reactive metabolites, which will covalently bind to proteins present in the oral mucosa. It has been postulated that DILRs may result from poor drug metabolism because of genetic variation of the major cytochrome P-450 enzymes.[127]

EPIDEMIOLOGY

No prevalence figures are available for DILRs; most likely, DILRs are unusual and constitute a minority of the cases diagnosed as OLP.

CLINICAL FINDINGS

Our knowledge about oral DILRs is limited and primarily based on case reports. It has been suggested that DILRs are predominantly unilateral[128] and present with an ulcerative reaction pattern.[129] These characteristics are far from consistent and are not useful to discriminate between OLP and DILRs (Figure 26A). At present, these two conditions should be considered clinically indistinguishable.[117]

CLINICAL MANIFESTATIONS

Lichenoid drug eruptions appear similar to lichen ruber planus and may be severely pruritic (see Clinical Manifestations of OLP).

DIAGNOSIS

Although diagnostic testing methods exist, they are in general of limited clinical value. One major problem that affects the use of diagnostic tests for drug hypersensitivity is that the immune pathogenesis for most drugs, except for penicillin and gold, is virtually unknown. To be clinically classified as a DILR, the oral lesions should comprise a white reticulum or papules. These characteristics may be observed concurrently with erythematous and ulcerative lesions. DILRs are often a diagnostic challenge as the condition has been associated with a large number of drugs (Table 7). A correct diagnosis is easier to establish when a patient develops DILR after starting a new drug (see Figure 26). For practical reasons, it is difficult to conduct withdrawal unless a patient has a severe symptomatic case.

A DILR may not develop for several months after a new drug is started. It may also take several weeks before DILRs disappear following withdrawal.[117]

MANAGEMENT

DILRs are not usually seen in conjunction with severe life-threatening reactions such as toxic epidermal necrolysis. Discontinuance of the drug and symptomatic treatment with topical steroids are often sufficient. The patient should be properly educated about the responsible drug to prevent future DILRs.

Lichenoid Reactions of GVHD

ETIOLOGY AND PATHOGENESIS

The major cause of GVHD is allogeneic hematopoietic cell transplantation, even if an autologous transplantation may also entail GVHD.[129] In GVHD, it is the transplanted immunocompetent tissue that attempts to reject the tissue of the host.[131] As the first step, conditioning of the host by chemotherapy and radiation will generate host cell damage, release of cytokines, and up-regulation of adhesion and major histocompatibility complex (MHC) molecules, which all facilitate recognition of alloantigens by donor T lymphocytes. A second step comprises an interaction between the recipient's APCs and the donor's T lymphocytes, which will perceive the histocompatibility antigens, expressed by APCs as foreign. This interaction may, in fact, be considered as the donor T lymphocytes recognizing the recipient's APCs as self-APCs expressing nonself-peptides. This interaction resembles the interaction between autoreactive T lymphocytes and APCs, hypothesized to play a role in the development of OLP. In a third step, the inflammatory cascade that follows the APC–T-lymphocyte reaction will stimulate proliferation of stromal cells, resulting in clinical features compatible with a lichenoid reaction.

EPIDEMIOLOGY

Chronic GVHD occurs in 15 to 50% of patients who survive 3 months after transplantation and varies in incidence from 33% of HLA-identical sibling transplants to 64% of unrelated donor transplants. The risk for GVHD increases with the age of the marrow recipient.[130] Chronic GVHD is defined as occurring more than 100 days post-HCT, most commonly as a transition from acute GVHD. In 20 to 30% of the patients, chronic GVHD may occur de novo.

CLINICAL FINDINGS

Oral lichenoid reactions as part of GVHD may be seen both in acute and chronic GVHD, although the latter more often are associated with typical lichenoid features. The clinical lichenoid reaction patterns are indistinguishable from what is seen in patients with OLP, that is, reticulum, erythema, and ulcerations, but lichenoid reactions associated with GVHD

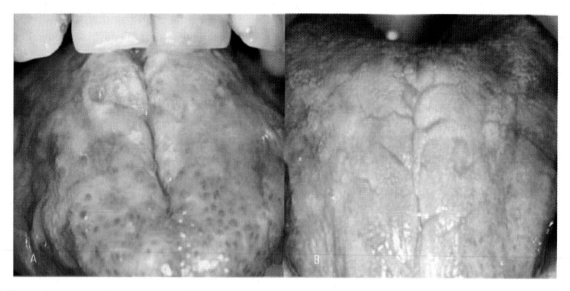

FIGURE 26 A, Drug-induced lichenoid reaction following 1 month of medication with a cholestyramine-containing drug. B, Three weeks following withdrawal of the drug.

TABLE 7 Drug-Related Lichenoid Reactions	
ACE inhibitors	Metformin
Allopurinol	Methyldopa
Amiphenazole	Metronidazole
Antimalarials	Niridazole
Barbiturates	NSAIDs
BCG vaccine	Oral contraceptives
Captopril	Oxpronolol
Carbamazepine	Para-aminosalicylate
Carbimazole	Penicillamine
Chloral hydrate	Penicillins
Chloroquine	Phenindione
Chlorpropamide	Phenothiazines
Cholera vaccine	Phenylbutazones
Cinnarizine	Phenytoin
Clofibrate	Piroxicam
Colchicine	Practolol
Dapsone	Prazosin
Dipyridamole	Procainamide
Ethionamide	Propranolol
Flunarizine	Propylthiouracil
Gaunoclor	Protease inhibitors
Gold	Prothionamide
Griseofulvin	Quinidine
Hepatitis B vaccine	Quinine
Hydroxychloroquine	Rifampicin
Interferon-{157}	Streptomycin
Ketoconazole	Sulfonamide
Labetalol	Tetracycline
Levamisole	Tocainide
Lincomycin	Tolbutamide
Lithium	Triprolidine
Lorazepam	
Mepacrine	Adapted from Scully C and Bagan JV.[124]
Mercury (amalgam)	ACE = angiotensin-converting enzyme; BCG = bacille Calmette-Guérin; NSAIDs = nonsteroidal anti-inflammatory drugs.

are typically associated with a more widespread involvement of the oral mucosa (Figure 27).

CLINICAL MANIFESTATIONS

The skin lesions often present with pruritic maculopapular and mobilliform rash, primarily affecting the palms and soles. Violaceous scaly papules and plaques may progress to a generalized erythroderma, bulla formation, and, in severe cases, a toxic epidermal necrolysis–like epidermal desquamation.[130]

DIAGNOSIS

The presence of systemic GVHD facilitates the diagnosis of oral mucosal changes of chronic oral GVHD. However, the oral cavity may, in some instances, be the primary or even the only site of chronic GVHD involvement. The lichenoid eruptions are important in the diagnostic process of oral GVHD and have the highest positive predictive value of all reaction patterns.[132] It is not possible to distinguish between OLP and oral GVHD based on clinical and histopathologic features.

MANAGEMENT

The same treatment strategy as for OLP may be used for chronic oral GVHD, that is, topical steroid preparations, such as fluocinonide and clobetasol gel. Opportunistic infections such as candidiasis should always be considered in immunosuppressed patients. The development of secondary malignancies has been recognized as a potentially serious complication of GVHD. Patients with a history of oral GVHD should be examined for oral malignancies as part of the medical follow-up procedure.

Lupus Erythematosus

ETIOLOGY AND PATHOGENESIS

LE represents the classic prototype of an autoimmune disease involving immune complexes. Both the natural and the adaptive parts of the immune system are participating, with the latter involving both B and T lymphocytes.[133,134] Environmental factors are of importance as sun exposure, drugs, chemical substances, and hormones which all have been reported to aggravate the disease. A genetic predisposition is supported by an elevated risk for siblings to develop LE and by an increased disease concordance in monozygotic twins. More than 80 different drugs have been associated with the onset of systemic lupus erythematosus (SLE), including hydralazine, methyldopa, chlorpromazine, isoniazid, quinidine, and procainamide.[135]

EPIDEMIOLOGY

SLE predominantly affects women of reproductive age, and the prevalence decreases during the menopause. In the interval of 20 to 40 years, as much as 80% has been reported to be women.[136] This predominance has lent support to an involvement of hormones in the pathogenesis of LE as well as the fact that the disease can be precipitated by hormonal drugs. There are large variations in the distribution of the disease between different ethnic groups. In the United Kingdom, the prevalence of SLE among Asian individuals is 40 per 100,000; for Caucasians, it is 20 per 100,000 individuals.

CLINICAL FINDINGS

The oral lesions observed in SLE and DLE are similar in their characteristics, both clinically and histopathologically. The typical clinical lesion comprises white striae with a radiating orientation, and these may sharply terminate toward the center of the lesions, which has a more erythematous appearance (see Figure 24). However, several clinical manifestations of oral LE exist. The most affected sites are the gingiva, buccal mucosa, tongue, and palate. Lesions in the palatal mucosa can be dominated by erythematous lesions, and white structures may not be observed (Figure 28). Oral mucosa lesions compatible with LE may be the first sign of the disease. Approximately 20% of the patients with LE have been reported

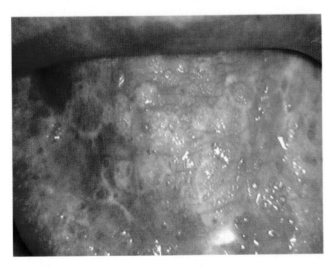

FIGURE 27 Lichenoid reaction in association with graft-versus-host disease following bone marrow transplantation.

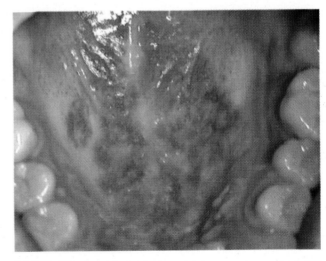

FIGURE 28 Lupus lesion in the palatal mucosa in a patient with systemic lupus erythematosus.

to display oral lesions,[137] although the figures vary from 9 to 45%.[138]

CLINICAL MANIFESTATIONS

The classic categorization of LE into SLE and DLE has during recent years been supplemented with acute cutaneous lupus erythematosus and subacute cutaneous lupus erythematosus.[139] SLE may also occur in concert with other rheumatologic diseases such as secondary Sjögren's syndrome and mixed connective tissue disease. SLE diagnosis requires that four or more of the diagnostic criteria displayed in Table 8 should be present at each time point of the disease. The typical DLE diagnosis comprises well-demarcated cutaneous lesions with round or oval erythematous plaques with scales and follicular plugging. These lesions may form butterfly-like rashes over the cheeks and nose known as malar rash.

LABORATORY FINDINGS

Antinuclear antibodies are frequently found in patients with SLE and can be used to indicate a systemic involvement, but patients with other rheumatologic diseases, such as Sjögren's syndrome and rheumatoid arthritis, may be positive as well. Moderate to high titers of anti-DNA and anti-Smith antibodies are almost pathognomonic of SLE.

PATHOLOGY

The clinical picture of LE varies, which also is reflected in the histopathology. The most common histopathologic features of LE are (1) hyperkeratosis with keratotic plugs, (2) atrophy of the rete processes, (3) deep inflammatory infiltrate, (4) edema in the lamina propria, and (5) thick patchy or continuous PAS-positive juxtaepithelial deposits.[118]

DIAGNOSIS

Oral mucosal lesions seen in conjunction with different types of LE are clinically and histopathologically indistinguishable.

Liquefaction degeneration may also be present, which may result in diagnostic problems in relation to OLP. The criteria mentioned above were tested among clinically atypical cases of DLE and the other groups of mucosal lesions, with a sensitivity of 92% and a specificity of 96% against both OLP and leukoplakia for the presence of two or more of the five criteria.[118] Direct immunohistochemistry is conducted to reveal granular deposition of IgM, IgG, IgA, and C3 (lupus band test).[119] The extralesional oral mucosa in SLE patients has a positive reaction to IgM in 45% of the cases in combination with variable deposits of IgG, IgA, and C3. DLE is accompanied by a positive antibody reaction in as little as 3% of the patients.

MANAGEMENT

Regarding treatment of oral mucosal LE lesions, no randomized clinical trials have been conducted. The oral lesions may respond to systematic treatment used to alleviate the disease and have to be evaluated first. When symptomatic intraoral lesions are present, topical steroids should be considered (Table 9). To obtain relief of symptoms, potent topical steroids such as clobetasol propionate gel 0.05%, betamethasone dipropionate 0.05%, or fluticazone propionate spray 50 µg aqueous solution are usually required. The treatment may begin with applications two to three times a day followed by a tapering during the next 6 to 9 weeks. The overall objective is to use a minimum of steroids to obtain relief. Immunosuppressive drugs used to treat LE may precipitate opportunistic fungal and viral infections. Opportunistic oral infections can also originate the immunologic defects, which are part of the pathogenesis. Another complication of the drugs used in treatment of LE is mucosal ulceration caused by frequent exploitation of NSAIDs.

Oral mucosal lesions often mirror the disease activity. They may regress spontaneously but can also persist for months or even years.

TABLE 8 American College of Rheumatology Criteria for Systemic Lupus Erythematosus*

1. Malar rash
2. Discoid lesions
3. Photosensitivity
4. Presence of oral ulcers
5. Nonerosive arthritis of two joints or more
6. Serositis
7. Renal disorder
8. Neurologic disorder (seizures or psychosis)
9. Hematologic disorder (hemolytic anemia, leukopenia, lymphopenia, or thrombocytopenia)
10. Immunologic disorder (anti-DNA, anti-SM, or antiphospholipid antibodies)

Adapted from Tan 1982.
DNA = deoxyribonucleic acid.
*Systemic lupus erythematosus diagnosis with 4 or more of 11 criteria present at any time.

TABLE 9 Topical Therapy for Oral Lesions of Lupus Erythematosus

Topical Steroid Therapy*	Directions for Use†
0.05% fluocinonide gel	Place on affected area(s) 2 × /d for 2 wk
0.05% clobetasol gel	Place on affected area(s) 2 × /d for 2 wk
Dexamethasone elixir (0.5 mg/mL)	Swish and spit 10 mL 4 × /d for 2 wk
Triamcinolone acetonide 5 mg/mL	Intralesional injection
Topical antifungal therapy, 10 mg clotrimazole troches	Dissolve in mouth 5 × /d for 10 d
Nystatin suspension (100,000 U/mL	Swish and spit 5 mL 4 × /day for 10 d
Chlorhexidine rinse (0.12%)	Swish and spit 10 mL 2 × /day until lesions resolve

Adapted from Brennan 2005.
*Fungal infections are a side effect of topical steroids.
†If lesions do not respond appropriately to topical steroids in 2 weeks, consider systemic therapy such as antimalarials, steroids, thalidomide, clofazimine, and methotrexate.

▼ ALLERGIC REACTIONS

Lichenoid Contact Reactions

LCRs are considered as a delayed hypersensitivity reaction to constituents derived from dental materials. The majority of patients are patch test positive to mercury (Hg), which lends support to LCR being an allergic reaction. Although Hg is usually considered the primary etiologic factor, other amalgam constituents may initiate LCR.

ETIOLOGY AND PATHOGENESIS

The pathogenesis of LCR is not fully elucidated, but based on the knowledge of delayed hypersensitivity, most likely the following will occur (Composition 8). Hg cannot be recognized by the immune system as the T-cell receptor (TCR), expressed by the T lymphocytes, is primarily limited to the identification of peptides. But Hg ions are highly reactive and will bind to self-proteins of the oral epithelium, which will induce transformation changes of the protein. This assembly between Hg and protein will be perceived as nonself, and following pinocytosis by APCs, such as the Langerhans' cells of the oral epithelium, these cells will degrade the protein complex to oligopeptides. The activated APCs will mature through the migration to regional lymph nodes and start to express the Hg-containing peptides together with class II molecules on the cell surface. Class II molecules represent a subset of glycoproteins derived from the MHC, which is critical for the APC–T-lymphocyte interaction. The process of antigen presentation is therefore considered to be class II molecule restricted. Within the lymph node, an interaction between the assembly of class II molecule–Hg-containing peptide on the APC and the TCR expressed on the antigen-specific T lymphocyte will occur. This interaction is known as the first signal in the antigen-presenting process. The second signal comprises further cellular interactions, which is decisive for the clonal expansion of the Hg peptide–specific T lymphocytes to take place. These cells will migrate into the bloodstream to reach and patrol all peripheral tissues of the body. At this state, the patient is considered to be sensitized against Hg.

Once the oral mucosa of a sensitized individual is exposed to Hg, the Langerhans' cells in the oral epithelium are able to present peptide-conjugated Hg to the peripheral T lymphocytes with an appropriate TCR. Thus, in a sensitized individual, the Langerhans' cells are able to fulfil their mission *in situ* and do not have to migrate to the regional lymph node to encounter an appropriate T lymphocyte. The interaction between the cells will instigate a cytokine production, which will lead to an attraction of inflammatory cells necessary to mount a local immune response in the Hg-exposed oral mucosa and eventually also lead to healing once Hg exposure is eliminated. The cytokine profile produced is most likely responsible for the stimulation of inherent cells of the oral mucosa, which gives rise to the clinical reaction pattern of LCR.

EPIDEMIOLOGY

No prevalence figures for LCR have been reported in the literature. The gender distribution seems to be different from OLP, with a higher proportion of women among patients affected by LCR. No significant differences regarding general diseases, drugs, or history of allergy between the LCR and OLP have been reported.

CLINICAL FINDINGS

Oral LCRs are considered to be a type of delayed hypersensitivity reaction to constituents derived from dental materials,

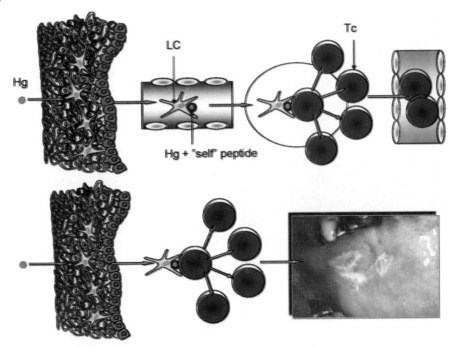

COMPOSITION 8

predominantly amalgam fillings.[140,141] Clinically, LCRs display the same reaction patterns as seen in OLP, that is, reticulum, papules, plaque, erythema, and ulcers (Figure 29A). The most apparent clinical difference between OLP and LCR is the extension of the lesions. The majority of LCRs are confined to sites that are regularly in contact with dental materials, such as the buccal mucosa and the border of the tongue. Lesions are hardly ever observed in sites as the gingiva, palatal mucosa, floor of the mouth, or dorsum of the tongue.[116,142] Most LCRs are nonsymptomatic, but when erythematous or ulcerative lesions are present, the patient may experience discomfort from spicy and warm food constituents. The duration with which the material is in contact with the oral mucosa has a decisive influence on the development of LCR. The clinical implication of this is that some lesions, especially those on the lateral border of the tongue with high mobility, may extend somewhat beyond the direct contact of dental material.

Lichenoid reactions in contact with composites have been observed on the mucosal side of both the upper and lower lips.[143] The majority of this type of LCR resolve following treatment with chlorhexidine. Further studies have to be conducted to substantiate a true lichenoid nature of these lesions.

DIAGNOSIS

The diagnosis is primarily based on the topical relationship to dental materials.[116,144] OLP may display similar clinical characteristics, and replacement of the culprit dental material may assist to discriminate between LCR and OLP (Figure 29B). However, OLP may also improve following the replacement but to a lesser extent compared with LCR.[116,145] The patch test is of minor clinical significance as a substantial number of patients with LCR will test negative to relevant test compounds, although the lesions will resolve following replacement of the dental material.[142] Histopathology will not be of any assistance in the discrimination between OLP and LCR.

MANAGEMENT

Replacement of dental materials in direct contact with LCR will result in cure or considerable improvement in at least 90% of the cases (see Figure 29).[116,140,144,145] Most lesions

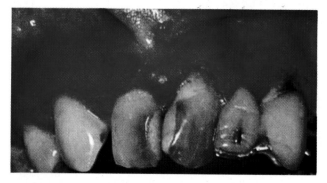

FIGURE 29   An erythematous attached gingiva in a patient allergic to dentifrice.

should be expected to heal within 1 to 2 months. There is no need for replacement of restorative materials that are not in direct contact with the LCR. Healing does not seem to depend on what type of dental material is used for replacement.[116] Although a malignant potential of LCR has been suggested, no prospective studies have been conducted to support this hypothesis.[146]

Reactions to Dentifrice and Chlorhexidine

Delayed hypersensitivity reactions to toothpastes and mouthwashes have been reported, but these reactions are rare.[147–151] The compounds responsible for the allergic reactions may include flavor additives such as as carvone and cinnamon or preservatives. These flavoring constituents may also be used in chewing gum and produce similar forms of gingivostomatitis. The clinical manifestations include fiery red edematous gingiva, which may include both ulcerations and white lesions. Similar lesions may involve other sites, such as the labial, buccal, and tongue mucosae. The clinical manifestations are characteristic and form the basis of the diagnosis, which is supported by healing of the lesions after withdrawal of the allergen-containing agent.

▼ TOXIC REACTIONS

Reactions to Smokeless Tobacco

Smokeless tobacco represents a nonhomogeneous group of compounds and methods of intraoral application. Three different geographic areas are of special interest: South Asia, the United States, and Scandinavia. In India, tobacco is often used in combination with betel leaf, sliced areca nut, and powdered slaked lime, which increases the toxicity of the compound. There is a definitive association between this form of smokeless tobacco and oral cancer (see submucous fibrosis).

Smokeless tobacco in the United States and Scandinavia can be divided into three different groups: chewing tobacco, moist snuff, and dry snuff.[152] All three are different in several respects related to composition, manufacturing procedures, and type of consumers. In Scandinavia, moist snuff is the most popular compound but different in the manufacturing process from moist snuff used in the United States. The latter contains higher concentrations of tobacco-specific nitrosamines and nitrite. This compound has reached an increased attractiveness in favor of dry snuff. Close to 3% of the population in the United States are consumers of smokeless tobacco—6% men and 0.3% women.[153] The prevalences are increased for high school students, of whom 7% are using smokeless tobacco, 11% are males, and 3% are females. With regard to the distribution in different ethnic groups in the United States, the habit is most popular among American Indians and Alaska Natives and the lowest prevalence is found among Asian Americans. There was a significant decrease in smokeless tobacco (snuff and chewing tobacco) use among minor league players from 1998 to 2003.[154] Self-reported past week use rates decreased from 31.7% in 1998 to 24.8% in 2003. No significant changes were observed for major league players. In

Sweden, 22% of the males and 3% of the females are consumers of moist snuff, and the habit doubled between 1970 and 1993 and constitutes a substantial part of the tobacco consumption in this country.[155] As a comparison, 16% of the males in Sweden are smokers compared with 22% of the females.

The clinical picture varies in relation to the type, brand, frequency, and duration of use of moist snuff.[156–158] In its mildest form, the lesion may just be noted as wrinkles at the site of application, whereas high consumers may display a white and leathery lesion (Figure 30), which sometimes contains ulcerations. Hyperkeratinization, acanthosis, and epithelial vacuolizations are common histopathologic features together with different degrees of subepithelial inflammation. Gingival retractions are the most common adverse reaction seen in conjunction with a smokeless tobacco habit. These retractions are irreversible, whereas the mucosal lesion usually regresses within a couple of months. Oral mucosal lesions are less frequently observed in association with chewing tobacco compared with moist snuff.

There is a distinct difference between lesions caused by smokeless tobacco and oral leukoplakia with respect to the presence of epithelial dysplasia, which is more frequently found in the latter.[158] Furthermore, the degree of dysplasia is also of a milder nature. The carcinogenic potential of smokeless tobacco has been a subject of considerable debate, and no global consensus has been reached. However, it is undisputable that smokeless tobacco products contain nitrosamines, polycyclic hydrocarbons, aldehydes, heavy metals, and polonium 210, which all have a potential to cause harm.[159] Some studies conclude that there is a higher risk of oral cancer and pancreas cancer, results that have not been confirmed by others. The World Health Organization International Agency for Research on Cancer established in its report from 2004 that "overall, there is sufficient evidence that smokeless tobacco causes oral cancer and pancreatic cancer in humans, and sufficient evidence of carcinogenicity from animal studies."[160] In a recent comprehensive review, it is concluded that the use of moist snuff and chewing tobacco imposes minimal risks for cancers of the oral cavity and other upper respiratory sites, with relative risks ranging from 0.6 to 1.7 (Figure 31). The use of dry snuff imposes higher risks, ranging from 4 to 13, and the risks from smokeless tobacco, unspecified as to type, are intermediate, from 1.5 to 2.8.[159]

Smoker's Palate

The most common effects of smoking are presented clinically as dark brown pigmentations of the oral mucosa (smoker's melanosis) and as white leathered lesions of the palate, usually referred to as nicotine stomatitis or smoker's palate. In smoker's palate, an erythematous irritation is initially seen, and this lesion is followed by a whitish palatal mucosa reflecting a hyperkeratosis (Figure 32). As part of this lesion, red dots can be observed representing orifices of accessory salivary glands, which can be enlarged and display metaplasia. Histopathologically, smoker's palate is characterized by hyperkeratosis, acanthosis, and a mild subepithelial inflammation.

The prevalence of smoker's palate has been reported in the range of 0.1 to 2.5%.[161–164] Smoker's palate is more prevalent in men and is a common clinical feature in high consumers of pipe tobacco and cigarettes and among individuals who practice inverse smoking.[165,166] The etiology is probably more related to the high temperature rather that the chemical composition of the smoke, although there is a synergistic effect of the two. In a large survey from Saudi Arabia, one-third of all smokers presented with a smoker's palate but increased to two-thirds among pipe smokers.[167]

▼ REACTIONS TO MECHANICAL TRAUMA

Morsicatio

Morsicatio is instigated by habitual chewing (Figure 33). This parafunctional behavior is done unconsciously and is

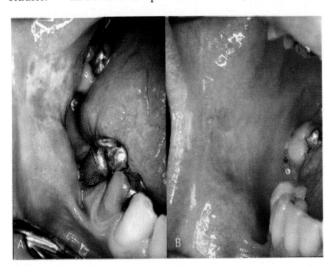

FIGURE 30 *A,* Lichenoid contact reaction associated with an amalgam crown. *B,* Improvement following replacement with a porcelain crown.

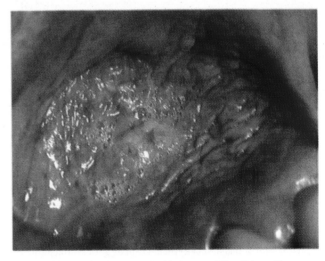

FIGURE 31 Lesion associated with the use of Swedish snuff.

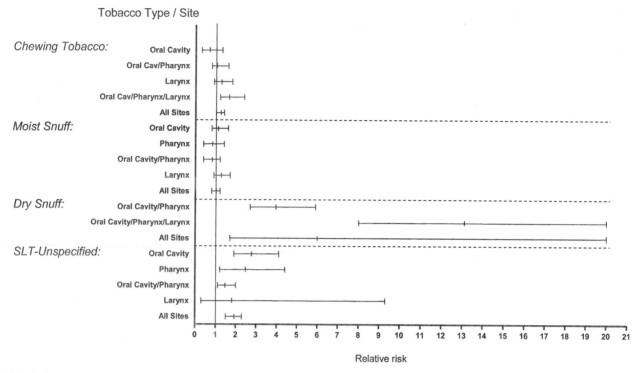

FIGURE 32 Summary relative risk for oral cancer and related sites according to SLT product type. Adapted from.

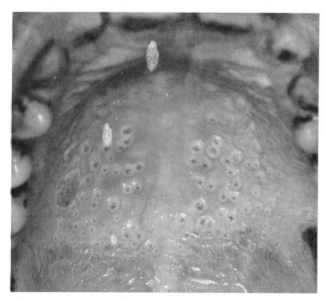

FIGURE 33 Smoker's palate with pronounced orifices of the accessory salivary glands.

therefore difficult to bring to an end. Morsicatio is most frequently seen in the buccal and lip mucosa and never encountered in areas that are not possible to traumatize by habitual chewing. Typically, morsicatio does not entail ulcerations but encompasses an asymptomatic shredded area. In cases of more extensive destruction of oral tissues by habitual chewing, a psychiatric disorder should be suspected. The prevalence has been reported to be in the range of 1.12 to 0.5%.[168–170] The lesion is three times more common among women.

Morsicatio has a very typical clinical appearance, and the diagnosis is relatively easy to establish, with one exception. If the lesion affects the borders of the tongue, it may mimic hairy leukoplakia. This also has bearing for the histopathologic picture, which is characterized by hyperkeratosis and acanthosis. A careful disease history will assist in the discrimination between the two conditions. The management is limited to assurance, and the patient should be informed about the parafunctional behavior. The condition does not involve any negative corollary.

FRICTIONAL HYPERKERATOSIS

Oral frictional hyperkeratosis is typically clinically characterized by a white lesion without any red elements. The lesion is observed in areas of the oral mucosa subjected to increased friction caused by, for example, food intake (Figure 34).

ETIOLOGY AND PATHOGENESIS

Frictional hyperkeratosis is observed in areas subjected to increased abrasion, which stimulates the epithelium to respond with an increased production of keratin. The reaction can be regarded as a physiologic response to minor trauma. Smoking and alcohol consumption have been reported as predisposing factors. Thus, the development of frictional hyperkeratosis is facilitated when the oral mucosa is exposed to these factors.

EPIDEMIOLOGY

In population studies, the prevalence has been reported to be in the range of 2 to 7%.[171] Predisposing factors such as smoking and alcohol will increase the prevalence, and frictional hyperkeratosis is the most common mucosal lesion in individuals with these habits.[172]

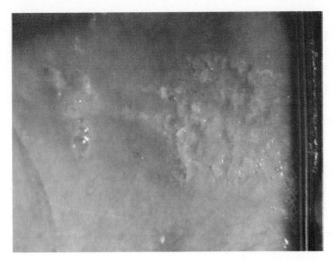

FIGURE 34 Morsicatio of the retrocommissural area of the left buccal mucosa.

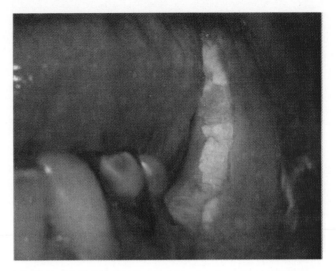

FIGURE 35 Frictional keratosis of the edentulous alveolar ridge.

CLINICAL FINDINGS

Frictional hyperkeratosis is often seen in edentulous areas of the alveolar ridge but may also be observed in other parts of the oral mucosa exposed to increased friction or trauma. The lesion is nonsymptomatic but can cause anxiety to the patient as it can be perceived as a malignant or premalignant lesion. Differential diagnosis against homogeneous leukoplakia is clinically based on a combination of features such as the affected site and a more diffuse demarcation.

DIAGNOSIS

For most lesions, the diagnosis can be established based on clinical features. As frictional hyperkeratosis does not carry any symptoms and is caused by comparatively common habits, it may be difficult to relate the lesions to increased friction. If the diagnosis is doubtful, biopsy is mandatory to exclude premalignant lesions. The histopathologic picture is characterized by hyperkeratosis without dysplasia and no or mild subepithelial inflammation. The ultimate way to differentiate between frictional keratosis and leukoplakia is to reduce or eliminate predisposing factors and await remedy.

MANAGEMENT

No surgical intervention is indicated. Information about the nonmalignant nature of the lesions and attempts to reduce predisposing factors are sufficient.

▼ OTHER RED AND WHITE LESIONS

Benign Migratory Glossitis (Geographic Tongue)

Geographic tongue is an annular lesion affecting the dorsum and margin of the tongue. The lesion is also known as erythema migrans. The typical clinical presentation comprises a white, yellow, or gray slightly elevated peripheral zone (Figure 35).

ETIOLOGY AND PATHOGENESIS

Although geographic tongue is one of the most prevalent oral mucosal lesions, there are virtually no studies available with the objective to elucidate the etiology behind this disorder. Heredity has been reported, suggesting the involvement of genetic factors in the etiology.

EPIDEMIOLOGY

The prevalence for geographic tongue varies considerably between different investigations, which may reflect not only geographic differences but also patient selection procedures and diagnostic criteria. The most frequently reported prevalence is in the range of 1 to 2.5%.[173] The gender distribution appears to be equal.

CLINICAL FINDINGS

Geographic tongue is circumferentially migrating and leaves an erythematous area behind, reflecting atrophy of the filiform papillae. The peripheral zone disappears after some time, and healing of the depapillated and erythematous area starts. The lesion may commence at different starting points, the peripheral zones fuse, and the typical clinical features of a geographic tongue emerge. Depending on the activity of the lesion, the clinical appearance may vary from single to multiple lesions occupying the entire dorsum of the tongue. Disappearance of the peripheral zone may indicate that the mucosa is recovering. Geographic tongue is characterized by periods of exacerbation and remission with different durations over time. The disorder is usually nonsymptomatic, but some patients are experiencing a smarting sensation. In these cases, a parafunctional habit, revealed by indentations at the lateral boarder of the tongue, may be a contributing factor to the symptoms. Patients often report that their lesion is aggravating during periods of stress. Geographic tongue and fissured tongue may be observed simultaneously. Most likely, fissured tongue should be interpreted as an end stage of geographic tongue (Figure 36).[174]

A geographic appearance can be observed at other sites of the oral mucosa than on the dorsum of the tongue and then

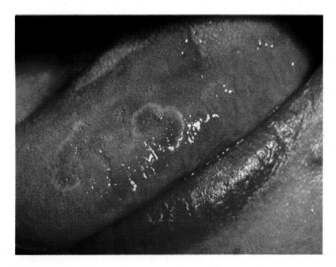

FIGURE 36 Geographic tongue with newly developed lesions on an erythematous area that has just started to recover from a previous lesion.

is denoted as geographic stomatitis.[175–178] The information about geographic stomatitis is sparse and relies on case reports. A similar clinical presentation as for geographic stomatitis may be seen as part of Reiter's disease. This disease is characterized by arthritis, uveitis or conjunctivitis, and urethritis. Reiter's disease is considered to be a reaction that originates from a gastroenteral or urogenital infection.[179,180]

CLINICAL MANIFESTATIONS

An increased prevalence of geographic tongue has been observed in patients with generalized pustular psoriasis.[181–184] In psoriasis in general, no such association has been revealed.[183] No studies have demonstrated that patients with geographic tongue are at increased risk of acquiring psoriasis. An atopic constitution has also been associated with geographic tongue, but this was not confirmed by a recently conducted study in the United States.[185] In this study, a negative relationship with smoking was revealed.

DIAGNOSIS

The clinical features of this mucosal disorder are quite characteristic, and histopathologic confirmation is rarely needed. If biopsy is considered, it should involve the peripheral zone to capture the lesion's typical histopathologic features. These include parakeratosis, acanthosis, subepithelial inflammation of T lymphocytes, and transepithelial migrating neutrophilic granulocytes. These cells may be a part of microabscesses formed near the surface, similar to those found in pustular psoriasis (Munro's microabscesses).[186]

MANAGEMENT

As the etiology is unknown, no causal treatment strategy is available. Symptoms are rarely present, and the management is confined to proper information about the disorder's benign character. When symptoms are reported, topical anesthetics may be used to obtain temporary relief. Other suggested treatment strategies include antihistamines, anxiolytic drugs, or steroids, but none of these have been systematically evaluated.[173]

Geographic tongue may regress, but it is not possible to predict when and to which patient this may happen.[187] The prevalence of the disease seems to decrease with age, which supports spontaneous regression over time.

Leukoedema

ETIOLOGY AND PATHOGENESIS

The etiology of leukoedema is not clear.

EPIDEMIOLOGY

The prevalence of leukoedema in Caucasians has been estimated at 50%.[17,188] The lesion is even more prevalent in the black population. The distribution between genders has been found to be equal.

CLINICAL FINDINGS

Leukoedema is a white and veil-like alteration of the oral mucosa that is merely considered a normal variant. The condition is often encountered bilaterally in the buccal mucosa and sometimes at the borders of the tongue (Figure 37). Leukoedema is less clinically evident after stretching the mucosa but reappears after this manipulation is discontinued. In more pronounced cases, leukoedema

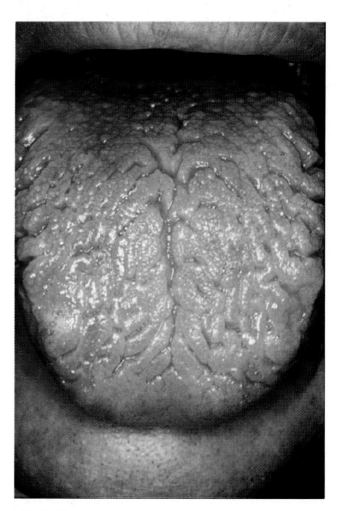

FIGURE 37 Fissured tongue with minor geographic lesions.

is accompanied by mucosal folds. The condition is asymptomatic and has no malignant potential.

DIAGNOSIS

The clinical features of leukoedema are quite different from oral keratosis, such as leukoplakia, as the demarcation is diffuse and gentle stretching results in a temporary disappearance. The histopathology is characterized by parakeratosis and acanthosis together with intracellular edema in epithelial cells of stratum spinosum.

MANAGEMENT

There is no demand for treatment as the condition is nonsymptomatic and has no complications, including premalignant features.

White Sponge Nevus

ETIOLOGY AND PATHOGENESIS

White sponge nevus is initiated following mutations in those genes that are coding for epithelial keratin of the types K4 and K13.[189] In K4-deficient mice, epithelial disturbances have been reported that are compatible with white sponge nevus.[190]

EPIDEMIOLOGY

White sponge nevus has been listed as a rare disorder by the National Institutes of Health, which implicates a prevalence below 1 in 200,000. In a population study of 181,338 males between 18 and 22 years of age, two cases of white sponge nevus were identified.[191] The clinical appearance usually commences during adolescence, and the gender distribution has been reported to be equal.

CLINICAL FINDINGS

White sponge nevus is an autosomal dominant disorder with high penetrans.[192] The typical clinical appearance is a white lesion with an elevated and irregular surface comprising fissures or plaque formations. The most affected sites are the buccal mucosa, but the lesion may also be encountered in other areas of the oral cavity covered by parakeratinized or nonkeratinized epithelium. The disorder may also involve extraoral sites, such as the esophagus and anogenital mucosa.[189,193] Although the lesion does not entail any symptoms, it may cause dysphagia when the esophagus is involved.

DIAGNOSIS

White sponge nevus may constitute a differential diagnostic problem as this disorder may be taken for other oral dyskeratoses, for example, oral leukoplakia and plaque-type candidiasis. The hallmark microscopic feature of this disorder is pronounced intracellular edema of the superficial epithelial cells, predominantly located within the stratus spinosum. Cells with pyknotic nuclei are present, and these cells may imitate koilocytosis observed in viral infections. Deep fissures in the nondysplastic epithelium may reach just above the basal layer, but the lower portions of the epithelium are not involved. No or just mild infiltrations may be seen in the subepithelial tissue.

MANAGEMENT

White sponge nevus does not entail any symptoms, and no treatment is therefore required. Systemic antibiotics have been used in an attempt to resolve the disorder, but with non-consistent results.[194] When a positive effect is obtained, the recurrence rate is considerable. White sponge nevus is a totally benign condition.

Hairy Tongue

ETIOLOGY AND PATHOGENESIS

The etiology of hairy tongue is unknown in most cases.[195] There are a number of predisposing factors that have been related to this disorder, such as neglected oral hygiene, a shift in the microflora, antibiotics and immunosuppressive drugs, oral candidiasis, excessive alcohol consumption, oral inactivity, and therapeutic radiation. The impact of ignored oral hygiene and oral inactivity is supported by the high prevalence of hairy tongue in hospitalized patients, who are not able to carry out their own oral hygiene. Hairy tongue is also associated with smoking habits.[196]

EPIDEMIOLOGY

The reported prevalences vary between different geographic areas, diagnostic criteria, and the frequencies of predisposing factors. In studies from the United States and Scandinavia, the prevalence of hairy tongue is reported below 1%.[17,169]

CLINICAL FINDINGS

Hairy tongue is characterized by an impaired desquamation of the filiform papilla, which leads to the hairy-like clinical appearance (Figure 38). The elongated papillae have to reach lengths in excess of 3 mm to be classified as "hairy," although lengths of more than just 15 mm have been reported in hairy tongue.[196] The lesion is commonly found in the posterior one-third of the tongue but may involve the entire dorsum. Hairy tongue may adopt colors from white to black depending on food constituents and the composition of the oral microflora. Patients with this disorder may experience both physical discomfort and esthetic embarrassment related to the lengths of the filiform papillae.

DIAGNOSIS

The diagnosis is based on the clinical appearance, and microbiologic examinations do not give any further guidance.

MANAGEMENT

The treatment of hairy tongue is focused on reduction or elimination of predisposing factors and removal of the elongated filiform papillae. The patients should be instructed on how to use devices developed to scrape the tongue. The use of food constituents with an abrasive effect may also be used to

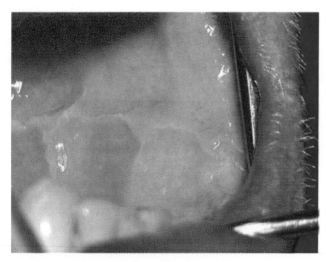

FIGURE 38 Leukoedema associated with parafunctional behavior.

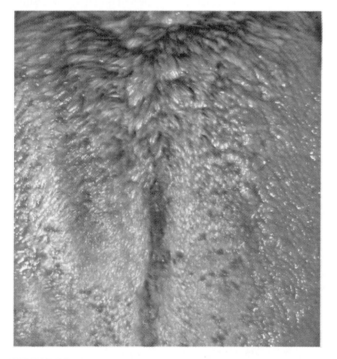

FIGURE 39 Hairy tongue.

prevent recurrences. Attempts have been made with tretinoin, but this treatment has not reached any widespread acceptance. Patients should be informed about the benign and noncontagious nature of hairy tongue.

▼ SELECTED READINGS

Ellepola AN, Samaranayake LP. Oral candidal infections and antimycotics. Crit Rev Oral Biol Med 2000;11:172–98.

Chattopadhyay A, Caplan DJ, Slade GD, et al. Incidence of oral candidiasis and oral hairy leukoplakia in HIV-infected adults in North Carolina. Oral Surg Oral Med Oral Pathol Oral Radiol Endod 2005;99:39–47.

Lodi G, Sardella A, Bez C, et al. Interventions for treating oral leukoplakia. Cochrane Database Syst Rev 2004;(3):CD001829.

Reibel J. Prognosis of oral pre-malignant lesions: significance of clinical, histopathological, and molecular biological characteristics. Crit Rev Oral Biol Med 2003;14:47–62.

Reichart PA, Philipsen HP. Oral erythroplakia—a review. Oral Oncol 2005;41:551–61.

van der Waal I, Schepman KP, van der Meij EH, et al. Oral leukoplakia: a clinicopathological review. Oral Oncol 1997;33: 291–301.

Lodi G, Scully C, Carrozzo M, et al. Current controversies in oral lichen planus: report of an international consensus meeting. Part 1. Viral infections and etiopathogenesis. Oral Surg Oral Med Oral Pathol Oral Radiol Endod 2005;100:40–51.

Lodi G, Scully C, Carrozzo M, et al. Current controversies in oral lichen planus: report of an international consensus meeting. Part 2. Clinical management and malignant transformation. Oral Surg Oral Med Oral Pathol Oral Radiol Endod 2005;100:164–78.

McCartan BE, McCreary CE. Oral lichenoid drug eruptions. Oral Dis 1997;3:58–63.

Woo SB, Lee SJ, Schubert MM. Graft-vs.-host disease. Crit Rev Oral Biol Med 1997;8:201–16.

Brennan MT, Valerin MA, Napenas JJ, et al. Oral manifestations of patients with lupus erythematosus. Dent Clin North Am 2005;49:127–41, ix.

Issa Y, Brunton PA, Glenny AM, et al. Healing of oral lichenoid lesions after replacing amalgam restorations: a systematic review. Oral Surg Oral Med Oral Pathol Oral Radiol Endod 2004;98: 553–65.

Rodu B, Jansson C. Smokeless tobacco and oral cancer: a review of the risks and determinants. Crit Rev Oral Biol Med 2004;15: 252–63.

Shulman J, Carpenter W. Prevalence and risk factors associated with geographic tongue among US adults. Oral Dis 2006;12: 381–6.

Terrinoni A, Rugg EL, Lane EB, et al. A novel mutation in the keratin 13 gene causing oral white sponge nevus. J Dent Res 2001;80: 919–23.

For the full reference list, please refer to the accompanying CD ROM.

5

PIGMENTED LESIONS OF THE ORAL MUCOSA

FAIZAN ALAWI

Oral and perioral pigmentation may be physiologic or pathologic in origin. Physiologic pigmentation is typically brown in appearance. However, in the course of disease, the oral mucosa and perioral tissues can assume a variety of discolorations, including brown, blue, gray, and black. Such color changes are often attributed to the deposition, production, or increased accumulation of various endogenous or exogenous pigmented substances. However, although an area may appear pigmented, the discoloration may not be related to actual pigment but rather to the deposition or accumulation of organic or inorganic substances, including various metals and drug metabolites.

Hemoglobin, hemosiderin, and melanin represent the most common endogenous sources of mucosal color change (Table 1). A submucosal collection of hemoglobin or hemosiderin, produced by lysis of red blood cells, may impart a red, blue, or brown appearance. In contrast, melanin, which is synthesized by melanocytes, may appear brown, blue, or black, and this is often dependent on the amount of melanin and its location within the tissue (ie, superficial vs deep).[1]

Pigmented lesions that are of exogenous origin are usually traumatically deposited directly into the submucosal tissues (Table 2). In some cases, the substances may be ingested, absorbed, and distributed hematogenously, to be precipitated in connective tissues, particularly in areas subject to chronic inflammation, such as the gingiva. In other instances, these ingested substances can actually stimulate melanin production, thus precipitating the color change. Chromogenic bacteria can also produce oral pigmentation, usually resulting in discoloration of the dorsal tongue. Exogenous pigmentation can also be induced by certain foods, drinks, and

confectionaries. However, in most cases, the effect is easily reversed.

The manifestation of oral pigmentation is quite variable, ranging from a focal macule to broad, diffuse tumefactions. The specific hue, duration, location, number, distribution, size, and shape of the pigmented lesion(s) may also be of diagnostic importance.[2] Moreover, in order to obtain an accurate diagnosis, thorough dental, medical, family, and social histories are required, and various diagnostic and laboratory tests, including biopsy, may be necessary. Thus, an understanding of the various disorders and substances that can contribute to oral and perioral pigmentation is essential for the appropriate evaluation, diagnosis, and management of the patient.

Lesions that are associated with mucosal discoloration but are vascular in origin, including developmental, hamartomatous, and neoplastic lesions (eg, hemangioma, lymphangioma, angiosarcoma, Kaposi's sarcoma), are described elsewhere in this textbook and thus are excluded from the current discussion. However, it should be noted that these entities are frequently considered in the differential diagnosis of both macular and mass-forming pigmented lesions. Table 3 lists additional lesions that may be associated with oral mucosal discoloration. Each of these lesions is also discussed in more detail elsewhere in this textbook.

▼ ENDOGENOUS PIGMENTATION

Melanin is found universally in nature.[3,4] Melanin is the pigment derivative of tyrosine and is synthesized by melanocytes, which typically reside in the basal cell layer of

TABLE 1 Common Causes of Endogenous Oral and Perioral Discoloration

Source	Etiology	Examples of Associated Lesion, Condition, or Disease
Vascular	Developmental, hamartomatous, neoplastic, genetic, autoimmune	Varix, hemangioma, lymphangioma, angiosarcoma, Kaposi's sarcoma, hereditary hemorrhagic telangiectasia, CREST syndrome
Extravasated hemorrhage, hemosiderin	Trauma, idiopathic, genetic, inflammatory, autoimmune	Hematoma, ecchymosis, purpura, petechiae, vasculitis, hemochromatosis
Melanin	Physiologic, developmental, idiopathic, neoplastic, reactive, drugs, hormones, genetic, autoimmune, infectious	Melanotic macule, ephelis, actinic lentigo, melanocytic nevus, malignant melanoma, physiologic pigmentation, chloroquine-induced pigment, lichen planus pigmentosus, Laugier-Hunziker pigmentation, smoker's melanosis, oral submucous fibrosis, Peutz-Jeghers disease, adrenal insufficiency, Cushing's syndrome, HIV/AIDS
Bilirubin	Trauma, alcohol, infection, neoplasia, genetic, autoimmune	Jaundice

AIDS = acquired immune deficiency syndrome; HIV = human immunodeficiency virus.

TABLE 2 Sources of Exogenous Oral and Perioral Pigmentation

Source	Etiology	Examples of Associated Lesion, Condition, or Disease
Metal	Iatrogenic, medications, environment	Amalgam tattoo, chrysiasis, black tongue, heavy-metal pigmentation
Graphite/ink	Trauma, factitious, tribal customs	Graphite tattoo
Bacteria	Poor oral hygiene, antibiotics	Hairy tongue
Drug complexes	Medications	Minocycline-induced pigment
Plant derivatives	Factitious, tribal customs	Ornamental tattoo, orange mouth

TABLE 3 Miscellaneous Lesions that May Be Associated with Oral Mucosal Discoloration

Lesion	Color
Pyogenic granuloma	Red, blue
Peripheral ossifying fibroma	Red, blue
Peripheral giant cell granuloma	Red, blue
Mucocele	Blue
Mucoepidermoid carcinoma	Blue
Acinic cell carcinoma	Blue
Lymphoma	Blue, purple
Vascular leiomyoma	Red, blue
Metastatic cancer	Red, blue
Fordyce granule	Yellow
Lipoma	Yellow
Granular cell tumor	Yellow

the epithelium. Investigations into normal melanocyte homeostasis have yielded the discovery that keratinocytes actually control melanocytic growth.[5] Yet the mechanisms by which melanocytes are stimulated to undergo cell division remain poorly understood. Their presence in the skin is thought to protect against the damaging effects of actinic irradiation, as well as to act as scavengers in protecting against various cytotoxic intermediates.[6] The role of melanocytes in oral epithelium is not clear.

In general, native melanocytes are less commonly observed in routine biopsies of oral mucosal epithelium, unless the specimens are derived from individuals of non-Caucasoid descent. Oral melanocytic pigmentation in a Caucasian individual is almost always considered pathologic in origin, although the pathology or pigment in and of itself may be of no significant clinical consequence.

Melanin is synthesized within specialized structures known as melanosomes. Melanin is actually composed of eumelanin, which is a brown-black pigment, and pheomelanin, which has a red-yellow color.[4] Melanin pigmentation may be physiologic or pathologic and focal, multifocal, or diffuse in its presentation. The term *melanosis* is frequently used to describe diffuse hyperpigmentation. Overproduction of melanin may be caused by a variety of mechanisms, the most common of which is related to increased sun exposure. However, intraorally, hyperpigmentation is more commonly a consequence of physiologic or idiopathic sources, neoplasia, medication or oral contraceptive use, high serum concentrations of pituitary adrenocorticotropic hormone (ACTH), postinflammatory changes, and genetic or autoimmune disease. Thus, the presence or absence of other systemic signs and symptoms, including cutaneous hyperpigmentation, is of great importance from the standpoint of diagnosing the cause of oral pigmentation. However, if the etiology of the pigment cannot be ascertained, a tissue biopsy is warranted for definitive diagnosis and is especially critical for the diagnosis of focal pigmentation since malignant melanoma can present in a variety of different configurations.

In addition to biopsy and histologic study, various laboratory and clinical tests, including diascopy, radiography, and blood tests, may be necessary for definitive diagnosis of oral pigmentation.[7] Dermascopy, also known as epiluminescence microscopy, is another increasingly employed clinical test that can be useful in the diagnosis of melanocytic lesions.[8,9] Although current instrumentation is designed primarily for the study of cutaneous pigmentation, several studies have described the use of dermascopy in the evaluation of labial and anterior lingual pigmentation.[10,11] Briefly, this noninvasive technique is performed through the use of a handheld surface microscope using incident light and oil immersion.[10] A more advanced method makes use of binocular stereo microscopes with or without the assistance of digital technology and imaging software. This diagnostic technique has been shown to be effective in discriminating melanocytic from nonmelanocytic lesions and benign versus malignant melanocytic processes.[9] It is recommended that clinicians be appropriately trained in dermascopy prior to including this technique in their armamentarium. Studies have clearly demonstrated the benefits of dermascopy training programs in increasing proper use of the technique and accuracy of diagnosis.[8] Since prospective and controlled studies detailing the predictive value and efficacy of dermascopic diagnosis of oral pigment have not been performed, the practitioner should be wary of its use in common clinical dental practice.

▼ FOCAL MELANOCYTIC PIGMENTATION

Freckle/Ephelis

The cutaneous freckle, or ephelis, is a commonly occurring, asymptomatic, small (1–3 mm), well-circumscribed, tan- or brown-colored macule that is often seen on the sun-exposed regions of the facial and perioral skin.[12] Epheledes are most commonly observed in light-skinned individuals and are quite prevalent in red- or light blond–haired individuals.[13] Although the pigmentation itself is focal in nature, most patients have multiple freckles. Freckles are thought to be developmental in origin. Polymorphisms in the *MC1R* gene are strongly associated with the development of childhood freckles.[13] Another putative freckles-predisposition gene has also been mapped to chromosome 4q32–q34.[14]

Epheledes are usually more abundant in number and darker in intensity during childhood and adolescence. Freckles tend to become darker during periods of prolonged sun exposure (spring, summer) and less intense during the autumn and winter months. Yet the increase in pigmentation is solely related to an increase in melanin production without a concomitant increase in the number of melanocytes. With increasing age, the number of epheledes and color intensity tends to diminish. In general, no therapeutic intervention is required.

Oral/Labial Melanotic Macule

ETIOLOGY AND PATHOGENESIS

The melanotic macule is a unique, benign, pigmented lesion that has no known dermal counterpart.[15,16] Melanotic macules are the most common oral lesions of melanocytic origin. In one large-scale retrospective study, melanotic macules made up over 85% of all solitary melanocytic lesions diagnosed in a single oral pathology laboratory.[17] Although the etiology remains elusive, trauma has been postulated to play a role. Sun exposure is not a precipitating factor.[16]

CLINICAL FEATURES

Melanotic macules develop more frequently in females, usually in the lower lip (labial melanotic macule) and gingiva. However, any mucosal site may be affected. Although the lesion may develop at any age, it generally tends to present in adulthood. Congenital melanotic macules have also been described occurring primarily in the tongue.[18] Overall, melanotic macules tend to be small (<1 cm), well-circumscribed, oval or irregular in outline and often uniformly pigmented (Figure 1). Once the lesion reaches a certain size, it does not tend to enlarge further. Unlike an ephelis, a melanotic macule does not become darker with continued sun exposure. Overall, the oral melanotic macule is a relatively innocuous lesion, does not represent a melanocytic proliferation, and does not generally recur following surgical removal.

PATHOLOGY

Microscopically, melanotic macules are characterized by a normal epithelial layer. However, the basal cells contain an abundance of melanin pigment without an associated increase in the number of melanocytes (Figure 2).[15,16] The pigmentation is often accentuated at the tips of the rete pegs, and melanin incontinence into the submucosa is commonly encountered.

A macular lesion that, histologically, exhibits increased numbers of melanocytes should not be diagnosed as a melanotic macule but rather as melanocytic hyperplasia. A recent report highlighted the importance in making this distinction.[19] The report described a case of malignant melanoma of the palate arising in a patient who, years earlier, had a benign "melanotic macule" removed from the same region. A retrospective review of the original biopsy, which had initially been diagnosed as a melanotic macule, in fact revealed evidence of

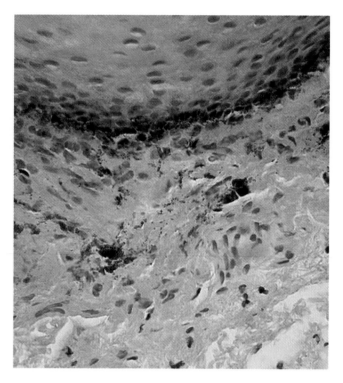

FIGURE 2 Melanotic macule exhibiting increased melanin pigmentation within the basal cell layer with melanin incontinence (hematoxylin and eosin, x400).

melanocytic hyperplasia. Thus, this case illustrates the need to be wary of such lesions and that their biologic potential remains unclear inasmuch as oral melanocytic hyperplasia may potentially herald the development of malignant melanoma.[19]

DIFFERENTIAL DIAGNOSIS

The differential diagnosis may include melanocytic nevus, malignant melanoma, amalgam tattoo, and focal ecchymosis. If such pigmented lesions are present after a 2-week period, ecchymosis can usually be ruled out, and a biopsy specimen should be obtained to secure a definitive diagnosis. Since oral mucosal malignant melanomas have no defining clinical characteristics, a biopsy of any persistent solitary pigmented lesion is always warranted.

Oral Melanoacanthoma

ETIOLOGY AND PATHOGENESIS

Oral melanoacanthoma is another unusual, benign, melanocytic lesion that is unique to the mucosal tissues.[20] Oral melanoacanthoma is an innocuous melanocytic lesion that may spontaneously resolve, with or without surgical intervention.[20–22] Although the term *melanoacanthoma* may imply a neoplastic process, the oral lesion is actually reactive in nature. Most patients report a rapid onset; and acute trauma or a history of chronic irritation usually precedes the development of the lesion. A biopsy is always warranted to confirm the diagnosis, but, once established, no further treatment is required. The biopsy procedure itself may lead to

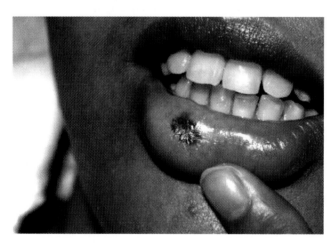

FIGURE 1 Melanotic macule of the lower labial mucosa.

spontaneous regression of the lesion. The underlying source of the irritation should be eliminated in order to minimize recurrence.

CLINICAL FEATURES

Oral melanoacanthoma usually presents as a rapidly enlarging, ill-defined, darkly pigmented macular or plaque-like lesion, and most develop in black females.[20,21] Although lesions may present over a wide age range, the majority occur between the third and fourth decades of life. In rare instances, multiple lesions may present simultaneously.[23]

Oral melanoacanthomas are typically asymptomatic, although pain has been reported.[22] Although any mucosal surface may be involved, the buccal mucosa is the most common site of occurrence. The size of the lesion is variable, ranging from small and localized to large, diffuse areas of involvement, measuring several centimeters in diameter. The borders are typically irregular in appearance, and the pigmentation may or may not be uniform.

Although there is a recognized cutaneous melanoacanthoma,[24] it is clear that the similarities lie solely in the nomenclature. Cutaneous melanoacanthoma represents a pigmented variant of seborrheic keratosis and typically occurs in older Caucasian patients. Dermatosis papulosa nigra is a relatively common facial condition that typically manifests in older black patients, often female, and represents multiple pigmented seborrheic keratoses.[25] These small papules are often identified in the malar and preauricular regions of the face.

PATHOLOGY

Microscopically, oral melanoacanthomas are characterized by a proliferation of benign, dendritic melanocytes throughout the full thickness of an acanthotic and spongiotic epithelial layer (Figure 3).[21] A mild lymphocytic infiltrate with exocytosis is also characteristic. Occasional eosinophils may be observed.

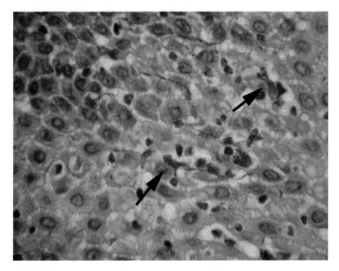

FIGURE 3 Melanoacanthoma. Dendritic-shaped, pigmented melanocytes (*arrows*) are noted throughout the full thickness of a spongiotic and acanthotic epithelium (hematoxylin-eosin stain; × 400 original magnification).

DIAGNOSIS

The clinical presentation, in association with the history, may be disconcerting and should lead the clinician to consider malignant melanoma in the differential diagnosis. Since oral melanoacanthoma may not be distinguishable from other melanocytic lesions, a nevus and melanotic macule could also be given consideration.

Melanocytic Nevus

ETIOLOGY AND PATHOGENESIS

Melanocytic nevi include a diverse group of clinically and/or microscopically distinct lesions.[26,27] Unlike ephelides and melanotic macules, which result from an increase in melanin pigment synthesis, nevi arise as a consequence of melanocytic growth and proliferation.[28] In the oral cavity, the intramucosal nevus is most frequently observed, followed by the common blue nevus.[29,30] Compound nevi are less common, and the junctional nevus and combined nevus (a nevus composed of two different cell types) are infrequently identified. Rare reports of congenital nevus, Spitz nevus, balloon cell nevus, and the cellular, epithelioid, and plaque-type variants of blue nevus have also been described.[31–36] However, the list of morphologically distinct nevi continues to expand.

Relatively little is known about the pathogenesis of the various melanocytic nevi. In fact, there is still debate as to whether "nevus cells" are a distinct cell type derived from the neural crest or if they are simply a unique or immature form of melanocyte.[4,28] Nonetheless, the lesional nevus cells are cytologically and biologically distinct from the melanocytes that colonize the basal cell layer of the epidermis and oral epithelium. Whereas native melanocytes tend to have a dendritic morphology, most nevic melanocytes tend to be round, ovoid, or spindle shaped.[37] Additional differences include the tendency for nevus cells to closely approximate one another, if not aggregate in clusters, and their ability to migrate into and/or within the submucosal tissues.[6]

In general, both genetic and environmental factors are thought to play a role in nevogenesis.[26,28] The effect of sun exposure on the development of cutaneous nevi is well recognized. However, there are also age- and location-dependent differences in the presentation, number, and distribution of nevi. Although most melanocytic nevi are acquired, some may present as congenital lesions (including in the oral cavity). Moreover, there are several examples of increased nevus susceptibility in various inherited diseases, thus confirming the role of genetics. Familial atypical multiple mole and melanoma syndrome is characterized by the formation of histologically atypical nevi,[38] epithelioid blue nevus may be associated with the Carney complex,[39] markedly increased numbers of common nevi are characteristic in patients with Turner's syndrome[40] and Noonan's syndrome,[41] and congenital nevi are typical of neurocutaneous melanosis.[42] Thus, these findings also bring to question whether nevi are true benign neoplasms or hamartomatous or developmental in nature, as they have been historically characterized. A recent study by Pollock and colleagues demonstrated that up to 90% of dermal melanocytic nevi exhibit somatic, activating mutations in the *BRAF* oncogene.[43] Mutations in the *HRAS* and *NRAS* oncogenes have also been identified.[44,45] This lends further credence to the notion that melanocytic nevi are neoplastic. It is currently unknown if oral melanocytic nevi also harbor any of these same mutations.

CLINICAL FEATURES

Cutaneous nevi are a common occurrence. The average Caucasian adult patient may have several nevi; some individuals may have dozens.[26,27] The total number of nevi tends to be higher in males than females. In contrast, oral melanocytic nevi are rare, typically present as solitary lesions, and may be more common in females.

Oral melanocytic nevi have no distinguishing clinical characteristics.[28] Lesions are usually asymptomatic and often present as a small (<1 cm), solitary, brown or blue, well-circumscribed nodule or macule (Figure 4). Up to 15% of oral nevi may not exhibit any evidence of clinical pigmentation.[28] Once the lesion reaches a given size, its growth tends to cease and may remain static indefinitely. In rare cases,

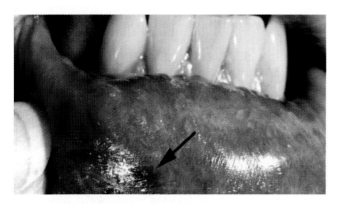

FIGURE 4   Intramucosal nevus of the lower labial mucosa.

multifocal lesions have been described.[46] Whereas some studies suggest a greater prevalence of oral nevi in black patients, other studies have not identified any significant racial predilection. Oral nevi may develop at any age; however, most are identified in patients over the age of 30. The hard palate represents the most common site, followed by the buccal and labial mucosae and gingiva.

PATHOLOGY

In the evolutionary stages of an intramucosal (or intradermal) nevus, the nevus cells initially maintain their localization to the basal layer, residing at the junction of the epithelium and the basement membrane and underlying connective tissue (Figure 5).[28,37] These junctional nevi are usually small (<5 mm), macular or nonpalpable, and tan to brown in appearance. Over time, the clustered melanocytes are thought to proliferate down into the connective tissue, often in the form of variably sized nests of relatively small, rounded cells. Nonetheless, some nevus cells are still seen at the mucosal-submucosal junction. Such nevi often assume a dome-shaped appearance and are referred to as compound nevi. As the lesion further matures, the nevus cells completely lose their association with the epithelial layer and become confined to the submucosal tissue, often with an associated decrease in the amount of pigmentation.[28] At this point, the lesion is given the designation of intramucosal nevus and, clinically, may appear brown or tan or even resemble the color of the surrounding mucosa.

Unlike intramucosal nevi, blue nevi are not derived from the basal layer melanocytes. Blue nevi are characterized by a variety of microscopic appearances.[34–36] The 'common' blue nevus, which is the most frequent histologic variant seen in the oral cavity, is characterized by an intramucosal proliferation of pigment-laden, spindle-shaped melanocytes. The blue nevus is described as such because the melanocytes may reside

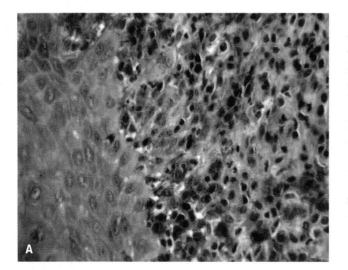

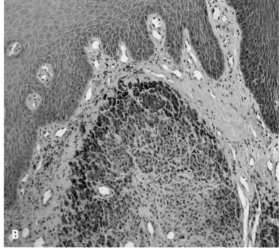

FIGURE 5   *A*, Compound nevus: nevus cells are located at the junction of the epithelium and connective tissue and within the submucosal tissue. The cells are variably pigmented. (hematoxylin-eosin stain; × 400 original magnification). *B*, Intramucosal nevus: the nevus cells are located within the submucosal tissue, with no evidence of any junctional component. The superficial melanocytes are heavily pigmented. Melanin is less evident in the remaining cells (hematoxylin-eosin stain; × 100 original magnification).

deep in the connective tissue and the overlying blood vessels often dampen the brown coloration of melanin, which may yield a blue tint. The less frequently occurring cellular blue nevus is characterized by a submucosal proliferation of both spindle-shaped and larger round or ovoid-shaped melanocytes. It should be noted that histologic differentiation of the two forms is not purely semantic. Whereas the common blue nevus usually has an innocuous clinical course, the cellular blue nevus may behave more aggressively and exhibit a greater rate of recurrence.[47] Rare reports of malignant transformation have also been associated with the cellular cutaneous variant. To date, malignant transformation of an oral nevus has not been well documented in the literature. Nonetheless, it is advised that all oral nevi, regardless of histologic type, be completely removed as they may still represent a potential precursor of malignant melanoma.[6,26,48]

DIAGNOSIS

Biopsy is necessary for diagnostic confirmation of an oral melanocytic nevus since the clinical diagnosis includes a variety of other focally pigmented lesions, including malignant melanoma. Various vascular phenomena may also be considered in the differential diagnosis. Complete but conservative surgical excision is the treatment of choice for oral lesions. Recurrence has only rarely been reported. Laser and intense pulse light therapies have been used successfully for the treatment of cutaneous nevi.[49] However, their value in the treatment of oral nevi is unknown.

Malignant Melanoma

ETIOLOGY AND PATHOGENESIS

Malignant melanoma is the least common but most deadly of all primary skin cancers. Epidemiologic studies suggest that the incidence of melanoma is actually increasing.[50] Similar to other malignancies, extrinsic and intrinsic factors play a role in the pathogenesis of melanoma. A history of multiple episodes of acute sun exposure, especially at a young age; immunosuppression; the presence of multiple cutaneous nevi; and a family history of melanoma are all known risk factors for the development of cutaneous melanoma.[26,51] Melanoma-prone families have a high incidence of germline mutations in the tumor suppressor genes, CDKNA2/p16[INK4a] or, less commonly, CDK4.[38,52] Similar to melanocytic nevi, melanomas also frequently exhibit mutations in the BRAF, HRAS, and NRAS proto-oncogenes.[42] Other recurrent molecular findings, including MC1R polymorphisms and alterations or loss of PTEN function, have also been described.[53,54] This suggests that several distinct genetic changes are required for the molecular evolution of melanoma.

CLINICAL FEATURES

Cutaneous melanoma is most common among white populations that live in the sunbelt regions of the world.[50] However, mortality rates are higher in blacks and Hispanics. Epidemiologic studies suggest that the incidence is increasing in patients, especially males, over the age of 45.[50] In contrast,

the incidence is decreasing in patients under the age of 40. Overall, there is a male predilection, but melanoma is one of the most commonly occurring cancers in women of child-bearing age.[55] However, there is no significantly increased incidence of melanoma in pregnancy, and there is no difference in survival rates between pregnant and nonpregnant women with the disease.[55,56]

Melanomas may develop either de novo or, much less commonly, arise from an existing melanocytic nevus.[26,51] On the facial skin, the malar region is a common site for melanoma since this area is subject to significant solar exposure. In general, the clinical characteristics of cutaneous melanoma are best described by the ABCDE criteria: asymmetry, irregular borders, color variegation, diameter greater than 6 mm, and evolution or surface elevation.[57] These criteria are very useful (although not absolute[58]) in differentiating cutaneous melanoma from other focally, pigmented melanocytic lesions.

There are four main clinicopathologic subtypes of melanoma. These include superficial spreading melanoma, lentigo maligna melanoma, acral lentiginous melanoma, and nodular melanoma.[51] In the first three subtypes, the initial growth is characterized by radial extension of the tumor cells (radial growth phase). In this pattern, the melanocytic tumor cells spread laterally and therefore superficially. These lesions have a good prognosis if they are detected early and treated before the appearance of nodular lesions, which indicates invasion into the deeper connective tissue (ie, a vertical growth phase). The development of nodularity in a previously macular lesion is often an ominous sign.[57]

Melanomas may present with a wide array of histologic and cytologic patterns, and clinical prognosis directly correlates with a number of different microscopic findings. Tumor thickness (Breslow tumor thickness), the level of tumor involvement in the dermis (Clark's level of invasion), surface ulceration, vascular or lymphatic invasion, neurotropism, mitotic index, and absence of tumor infiltrating lymphocytes are all associated with a poor prognosis.[6,26,51] Additionally, various clinical parameters, including tumor site, age of the patient (>60 years), gender (male), and regional or distant metastasis, also are predictive of poor prognosis. The 5-year survival rate of patients with metastatic melanoma is less than 15%.[51]

Increased awareness of the epidemiologic and biologic properties of cutaneous melanoma is necessary for the clinical practitioner. However, a discussion of cutaneous malignant melanoma has little bearing on the clinical, histologic, demographic, and biologic profiles associated with primary mucosal malignant melanoma. In brief, mucosal melanomas are very distinct neoplasms.[59–63]

Primary mucosal melanomas comprise less than 1% of all melanomas. The majority develop in the head and neck, most in the sinonasal tract and oral cavity.[59] The prevalence of oral melanoma appears to be higher among black-skinned and Japanese people than among other populations.[59,60] The tumor presents more frequently in males than females. Unlike the cutaneous variant, which has distinct and well-recognized

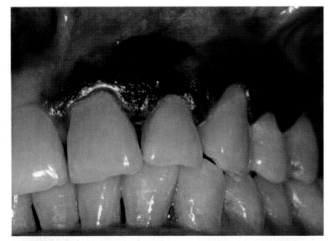

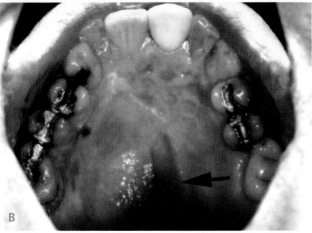

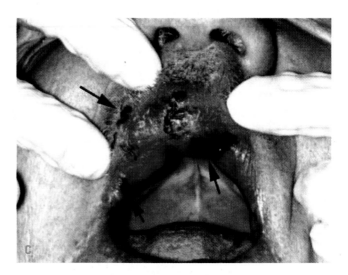

FIGURE 6 *A,* Malignant melanoma exhibiting macular but diffuse involvement of the maxillary gingiva. Courtesy of Dr. Julien Ghannoum. *B,* Malignant melanoma presenting as a mass on the hard palate. One portion of the tumor is heavily pigmented (*arrow*), whereas the opposite side is relatively amelanotic. *C,* Melanoma of the upper lip presenting as an ulcerated mass with multifocal areas of pigmentation (*arrows*). Case courtesy of Dr. Rosalie Elenitsas.

risk factors associated with its development, the etiology of oral melanoma remains unknown. *BRAF* mutations are rarely observed in mucosal melanomas.[62,63]

Oral melanoma may develop at any age, but most present over the age of 50.[60,61] Any mucosal site may be affected; however, the palate represents the single most common site of involvement.[61,64] The maxillary gingiva is the second most frequent site. Oral melanomas have no distinctive clinical appearance. They may be macular, plaque-like or mass-forming, well-circumscribed or irregular and exhibit focal or diffuse areas of brown, blue, or black pigmentation (Figure 6). Up to one-third of oral melanomas may exhibit little or no clinical evidence of pigmentation (amelanosis).[61] In some cases, oral melanomas may present with what appear to be multifocal areas of pigmentation. This phenomenon is often explained by the fact that some tumors may exhibit both melanotic and amelanotic areas.[60,61]

Additional signs and symptoms that may be associated with oral melanoma are nonspecific and similar to those observed with other malignancies. Ulceration, pain, tooth mobility or spontaneous exfoliation, root resorption, bone loss, and paresthesia/anesthesia may be evident. However, in some patients, the tumors may be completely asymptomatic. Thus, the clinical differential diagnosis may be quite extensive and could include melanocytic nevus, oral melanotic macule, and amalgam tattoo, as well as various vascular lesions and other soft tissue neoplasms. It is for this reason that a biopsy of any persistent solitary pigmented lesion is always warranted.

Oral mucosal malignant melanoma is associated with a very poor prognosis. Studies have demonstrated 5-year survival rates of 15 to 40%.[60,65] Regional lymphatic metastases are frequently identified and contribute to the poor survival rates. Less than 10% of patients with distant metastases survive after 5 years.[60]

PATHOLOGY

Microscopically, oral mucosal melanomas (like cutaneous melanomas) may exhibit a radial or a vertical pattern of growth. The radial or superficial spreading pattern is often seen in macular lesions; clusters of pleomorphic melanocytes exhibiting nuclear atypia and hyperchromatism proliferate within the basal cell region of the epithelium, and many of the neoplastic cells invade the overlying epithelium (pagetoid spread) as well as the superficial submucosa (Figure 7). Once vertical growth into the connective tissue is established, the lesions may become clinically tumefactive.

Owing to its rare occurrence, even most renowned clinical cancer centers do not have a large enough cohort of cases to reliably and significantly correlate the histologic findings with prognosis.[60] Thus, apart from tumor thickness greater than 5 mm and the presence of lymphovascular invasion, many of

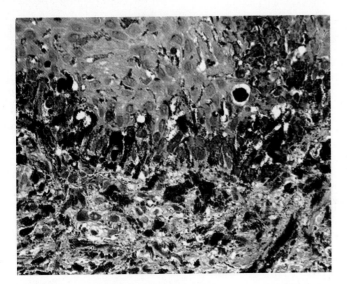

FIGURE 7 Heavily pigmented malignant melanoma exhibiting primarily a radial growth phase with pagetoid spread of tumor cells (hematoxylin-eosin stain; {164}400 original magnification). Photomicrograph courtesy of Dr. Julien Ghannoum.

TABLE 4   Etiology of Multifocal, Diffuse, or Generalized Mucocutaneous Melanosis
Physiologic pigmentation
Laugier-Hunziker pigmentation
Postinflammatory hyperpigmentation
Drug induced
Hormone induced
Adrenal insufficiency
Cushing's syndrome/Cushing's disease
Hyperthyroidism
Primary biliary cirrhosis
Hemochromatosis (early stages)
Genetic disease
Vitamin B$_{12}$ deficiency
HIV/AIDS (late stages)
Malignant melanoma

AIDS = acquired immune deficiency syndrome; HIV = human immunodeficiency virus.

the histologic parameters, including the Breslow classification and Clark's level of invasion, that impart a poor prognosis for cutaneous melanoma generally do not apply to oral melanoma.[6,61,64]

DIAGNOSIS

One of the main clinical and microscopic challenges in diagnosing oral melanoma is determining whether the lesion is a primary neoplasm or a metastasis from a distant site. This is not a semantic distinction since confirming the primary site will dictate the patient's clinical stage and the type of therapy he or she will undergo. A history of a previous melanoma, sparing of the palate and gingiva, amelanosis, and microscopic features, such as a lack of junctional activity and pagetoid spread, are findings that may be more suggestive of a metastatic tumor.[6]

MANAGEMENT

For primary oral melanomas, ablative surgery with wide margins remains the treatment of choice.[60,66] Adjuvant radiation therapy may also be necessary.[65] However, as the sole therapeutic modality, it remains unclear if radiation therapy is beneficial for the treatment of oral mucosal melanoma.[66] Computed tomography and magnetic resonance imaging studies should be undertaken to explore metastases to the regional lymph nodes. A variety of chemo- and immunotherapeutic strategies are often used if metastases are identified or for palliation.[67–69]

Melanoma is one of the most immunogenic cancers, and there are several clinical immunotherapeutic trials currently being conducted to test the effects of various antitumor vaccines.[67] Adjuvant interferon-α-2B therapy has already been approved for the treatment of primary cutaneous melanomas greater than 4 mm in thickness.[67] Unusual side effects of chemo- and immunotherapy may include the onset of diffuse mucocutaneous melanosis and the development of autoimmunity.[70–72] The appearance of autoantibodies and clinical manifestations of autoimmune disease, including vitiligo (see page ??), have been associated with statistically significant improvements in overall survival rates for patients with cutaneous melanoma.[71,72]

▼ MULTIFOCAL/DIFFUSE PIGMENTATION

Physiologic Pigmentation

Physiologic pigmentation is the most common source of multifocal or diffuse oral mucosal pigmentation (Table 4). Dark-complexioned individuals, including blacks, Asians, and South-Americans, frequently show patchy to generalized hyperpigmentation of the oral mucosal tissues.[7] Although in many patients, the pigment is restricted to the gingiva, melanosis of other mucosal surfaces is not uncommon (Figure 8). The pigment is often observed in childhood and usually does not develop de novo in the adult. If there is a sudden or gradual onset of diffuse mucosal pigmentation in adulthood, even in darker-skinned patients, other sources for the melanosis should be given consideration. A differential diagnosis may include idiopathic, drug-induced, or smoking-induced melanosis (discussed below). Hyperpigmentation associated

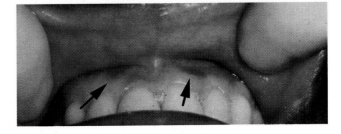

FIGURE 8 Physiologic pigmentation of the maxillary gingiva. Note the patchy distribution of the pigment (*arrows*).

with endocrinopathic and other systemic disease should also be considered. A thorough history and laboratory tests may be necessary to confirm the diagnosis.

Microscopically, physiologic pigmentation is characterized by increased amounts of melanin pigment within the basal cell layer. The pigmentation itself is of no clinical consequence and is considered a variation of normal. Nonetheless, in some patients, the appearance of brown discoloration, even intraorally, can be quite bothersome, even more so if the pigmentation is compromising esthetics. Thus, surgical intervention may be necessary. Gingivectomy and laser therapy have been used to remove pigmented oral mucosa.[73,74] However, with both modalities, the effects may only be temporary since the pigmentation may eventually recur. The cause of the repigmentation remains unclear.

Drug-Induced Melanosis

ETIOLOGY AND PATHOGENESIS

Medications may induce a variety of different forms of mucocutaneous pigmentation, including melanosis. Pigmentation that is caused by the soft tissue deposition of drug metabolites or complexes and pigment associated with deposition of lipofuscin or iron are discussed later in this chapter.

The chief drugs implicated in drug-induced melanosis are the antimalarials, including chloroquine, hydroxychloroquine, quinacrine, and others.[75–79] In the Western world, these medications are typically used for the treatment of autoimmune disease. Other common classes of medications that induce melanosis include the phenothiazines, such as chlorpromazine (Figure 9), oral contraceptives, and cytotoxic medications such as cyclophosphamide and busulfan.[80–87]

TABLE 5 Medications Associated with Mucocutaneous Pigmentation
Amiodarone
Amodioquine
Aziodothymidine
Bleomycin
Chloroquine
Chlorpromazine
Clofazamine
Gold
Hydroxychloroquine
Hydroxyurea
Imipramine
Ketoconazole
Mepacrine
Methacycline
Methyldopa
Minocycline
Premarin
Quinacrine
Quinidine
Tacrolimus

Table 5 lists some of the known melanin-inducing medications.

CLINICAL FEATURES

It has been estimated that 10 to 20% of all cases of acquired melanocytic pigmentation may be drug induced.[75] Intraorally, the pigment can be diffuse yet localized to one mucosal surface, often the hard palate, or it can be multifocal and involve multiple surfaces. Some drugs may even be associated with a specific pattern of pigmentation.[76] Much like other forms of diffuse pigmentation, the lesions are flat and without any evidence of nodularity or swelling. Sun exposure may exacerbate cutaneous drug-induced pigmentation.[75]

PATHOLOGY

Microscopically, there is usually evidence of basilar hyperpigmentation and melanin incontinence without a concomitant increase in the number of melanocytes. Hemosiderin and pigmented, yellow or yellow-red, drug complexes may also be identified.[76] Although the mechanisms by which melanin synthesis is increased remain unknown, one theory is that the drugs or drug metabolites stimulate melanogenesis. Alternatively, some drugs, including chloroquine and chlorpromazine, have been shown to physically bind melanin.[88] This results in retention of the drug within melanocytes, which may contribute to the adverse mucocutaneous effects.

DIAGNOSIS

If the onset of the melanosis can be temporally and accurately associated with use of a specific medication (frequently within several weeks or months before development of the pigmentation), then no further intervention is warranted. In most cases, the discoloration tends to fade within a few months

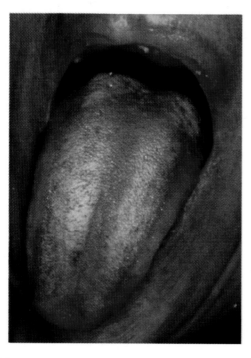

FIGURE 9 Drug-induced pigmentation of the tongue in a patient who was taking chlorpromazine. Courtesy of Dr. Adam Rubin.

after the drug is discontinued.[75,76] Pigmentation associated with hormone therapy may tend to persist for longer periods of time, despite discontinuation of the medications.[84]

A differential diagnosis includes other causes of diffuse mucosal pigmentation. Laboratory tests may be necessary to rule out an underlying endocrinopathy.

Smoker's Melanosis

Diffuse melanosis of the anterior facial maxillary and mandibular gingivae, buccal mucosa, lateral tongue, palate, and floor of the mouth is occasionally seen among cigarette smokers.[89,90] Most smokers (including heavy smokers) usually fail to show such changes. However, it is probable that in certain individuals, melanin synthesis is stimulated by tobacco smoke products. Indeed, among dark-skinned individuals who normally exhibit physiologic pigmentation, smoking stimulates a further increase in oral pigmentation.[91] The pigmented areas are brown, flat, and irregular; some are even geographic or map-like in configuration.

The mechanism by which smoking induces the pigmentation remains unknown. Smokeless tobacco (snuff) does not appear to be associated with an increase in oral melanosis.[92] Thus, it is possible that one or more of the chemical compounds incorporated within cigarettes, rather than the actual tobacco, may be causative. Another possibility is that the heat of the smoke may stimulate the pigmentation.

Epidemiologic studies suggest that oral melanosis increases prominently during the first year of smoking.[92] If there is a reduction in smoking, the pigmentation may eventually resolve.[93] Histologically, basilar melanosis with melanin incontinence is observed. Unlike other smoking-related oral pathologies, smoker's melanosis is not a preneoplastic condition.

Alcohol has also been associated with increased oral pigmentation.[91,94,95] In alcoholics, the posterior regions of the mouth, including the soft palate, tend to be more frequently pigmented than other areas. It has been suggested that alcoholic melanosis may be associated with a higher risk of cancers of the upper aerodigestive tract.[95]

Diffuse or patchy melanotic pigmentation is also characteristically associated with oral submucous fibrosis.[94] Unlike smoker's melanosis, oral submucous fibrosis is a preneoplastic condition caused by habitual chewing of areca (betel) nut. This custom is common in some East Asian cultures. In addition to the melanosis, increased fibrosis of the oral soft tissues is also characteristic. Oral submucous fibrosis is discussed in more detail in Chapter ??.

Postinflammatory (Inflammatory) Hyperpigmentation

Postinflammatory hyperpigmentation is a well-recognized phenomenon that tends to develop more commonly in dark-complexioned individuals.[96] Most cases present as either focal or diffuse pigmentation in areas that were subjected to previous injury or inflammation. The acne-prone face is a relatively common site for this phenomenon.[96] Although unusual, postinflammatory pigmentation may also develop

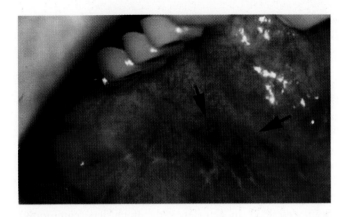

FIGURE 10 Lichen planus–associated pigment. Classic-appearing Wickham's striae and surrounding pigmentation (*arrows*) are seen in this Caucasian patient with biopsy-proven lichen planus. Courtesy of Dr. Scott DeRossi.

in the oral cavity.[97,98] In rare cases, the mucosa overlying a nonmelanocytic malignancy may become pigmented.[99]

Oral pigmentation has also been described in patients with lichen planus (lichen planus pigmentosus).[100] This phenomenon has been described in various races, including Caucasians (Figure 10). In addition to the typical microscopic features associated with lichen planus, there is also evidence of basilar hyperpigmentation and melanin incontinence. Upon resolution of the lichenoid lesion, the pigmentation may or may not disappear. Yet, in most cases, the pigmentation eventually does subside. Although it may be mere semantics, it is unclear whether lichen planus–associated pigment should be appropriately characterized as postinflammatory or inflammatory pigmentation.

Melasma (Chloasma)

Melasma is a relatively common, acquired symmetric melanosis that typically develops on sun-exposed areas of the skin and frequently on the face.[101] The forehead, cheeks, upper lips, and chin are the most commonly affected areas (Figure 11). There is a distinct female predilection, and most

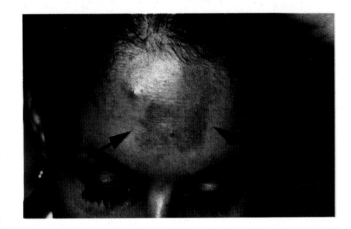

FIGURE 11 Melasma. Pigmentation (*arrows*) developed on the forehead of this female during the second trimester of pregnancy.

cases arise in darker-skinned individuals. Unlike other forms of diffuse melanosis, melasma tends to evolve rather rapidly over a period of a few weeks.[101,102] Sun exposure tends to be an exacerbating, if not precipitating, event.

The term *melasma* has been used to describe any form of generalized facial hyperpigmentation, including those related to postinflammatory changes and medication use. However, the nomenclature is most appropriately used to describe the pigmentary changes associated with pregnancy or ingestion of contraceptive hormones. Both pregnancy and use of oral contraceptives have also been associated with oral mucosal melanosis.[84,102] Rare cases of idiopathic melasma have also been described in females and, much less commonly, males.[103,104] In most cases, it is the combination of estrogen and progesterone that induces the pigment. Estrogen replacement therapy alone, without progesterone, does not precipitate melasma.[101,102] In idiopathic cases, significantly elevated levels of luteinizing hormone have been identified in both sexes, with associated decreases in serum estradiol (in women)[103] and testerone (in males).[104] Various thyroid abnormalities, including hypothyroidism, also may play a role in the pathogenesis of pregnancy-associated melasma.[105]

A biopsy typically reveals basilar melanosis with no increase in the number of melanocytes. However, the melanocytes that are present may be larger than those in the adjacent normally pigmented areas.[106] Melasma may spontaneously resolve after parturition, cessation of the exogenous hormones, or regulation of endogenous sex-hormone levels.

▼ MELANOSIS ASSOCIATED WITH SYSTEMIC OR GENETIC DISEASE

Hypoadrenocorticism (Adrenal Insufficiency, Addison's Disease)

ETIOLOGY AND PATHOGENESIS

Hypoadrenocorticism is a potentially life-threatening disease, as much for its systemic complications as its underdiagnosis.[107] A variety of etiologies may precipitate adrenal insufficiency.[108] In adults, autoimmune disease represents one of the most common causes. However, infectious agents, neoplasia, trauma, certain medications, and iatrogenic causes may lead to adrenal destruction or an impairment of endogenous steroid production. In rare cases, adrenal insufficiency may also be a consequence of genetic disease.[109–111] Regardless of etiology, the end result is essentially the same, that is, a decrease in endogenous corticosteroid levels.

As steroid levels decrease, there is a compensatory activation of ACTH secretion from the anterior pituitary gland.[108] ACTH then acts on the adrenal cortex to stimulate steroid production and ACTH secretion stops. If low steroid levels persist, there is a loss of feedback inhibition, resulting in persistent secretion of ACTH into the serum. Concurrently, the serum levels of α-melanocyte-stimulating hormone (α-MSH) also increase. At the molecular level, this is explained by the fact that the precursor pro-opiomelanocortin gene contains the sequences of both the ACTH and α-MSH genes.[112] During processing of the progenitor hormone, the ACTH and α-MSH genes may be cleaved independently of one another, thus creating two distinct hormones. However, the α-MSH sequence is actually contained within a portion of the ACTH gene; in fact, the first 13 amino acids of the ACTH hormone are identical to α-MSH.[112] Upon cellular processing of the ACTH messenger ribonucleic acid transcript, the sequence containing the α-MSH gene is cleaved and is further processed into its own secretable form. Apart from the wide array of tissues and organs that these hormones act upon, both α-MSH and ACTH are also thought to have stimulatory effects on melanocytes.[112] However, the exact mechanism by which melanin synthesis increases remains unclear.

CLINICAL FEATURES

Weakness, poorly defined fatigue, and depression are some of the typical presenting signs of the illness. However, in some patients, the first sign of disease may be mucocutaneous hyperpigmentation.[108] Generalized bronzing of the skin and diffuse but patchy melanosis of the oral mucosa are hallmarks of hypoadrenocorticism. Any oral surface may be affected. In some patients, oral melanosis may be the first manifestation of their adrenal disease.[113] Diffuse hyperpigmentation is more commonly associated with chronic rather than acute-onset disease.

DIAGNOSIS

The diagnosis of oral addisonian pigmentation requires a clinicopathologic correlation. Endocrinopathic disease should be suspected whenever oral melanosis is accompanied by cutaneous bronzing. An oral biopsy typically shows increased melanin in the basal cell layer with melanin incontinence. Thus, the differential diagnosis includes other causes of diffuse pigmentation, including physiologic and drug-induced pigmentation. Laboratory tests, including the evaluation of serum cortisol and electrolyte levels, are necessary to make a diagnosis of addisonian hyperpigmentation. Hyponatremia and hyperkalemia are frequently associated with adrenal insufficiency.[108] Treatment consists of exogenous steroid replacement therapy. With appropriate therapy, the pigmentation will eventually resolve.

A more detailed discussion of hypoadrenocorticism is included in Chapter ???.

Cushing's Syndrome/Cushing's Disease

ETIOLOGY AND PATHOGENESIS

Cushing's syndrome develops as a consequence of prolonged exposure to relatively high concentrations of endogenous or exogenous corticosteroids.[114] Most cases are iatrogenic in origin and associated with poorly controlled or unmonitored use of topical or systemic steroids. Cushing's syndrome may also arise as a result of various endogenous etiologies, including an activating pituitary tumor (Cushing's disease) and a primary, activating, adrenal pathology (hyperadrenocorticism), as well as ectopic secretion of corticosteroids, ACTH, or corticotropin-releasing hormone by various neoplasms, including small cell carcinoma of the lung.[114–116] Recently, Cushing's syndrome has been described in patients with activating, germline mutations in the ACTH receptor.[117]

CLINICAL FEATURES

Overall, Cushing's syndrome is more prevalent in female patients. However, prepubertal onset is more commonly seen in boys.[118] Apart from the wide array of systemic complications, including weight gain and the characteristic "moon facies," diffuse mucocutaneous pigmentation may be seen in a subset of patients, specifically those whose pathology is associated with increased ACTH secretion. Thus, in most cases, the affected patients have a primary pituitary neoplasm.[114] The pattern of oral pigmentation is essentially identical to that seen in patients with adrenal insufficiency.

DIAGNOSIS

Serum steroid and ACTH determinations will aid in the diagnosis, and the pigment often resolves following appropriate surgical, radiation, or medicinal therapy for the specific source of the endocrinopathy.

Hyperthyroidism (Graves' Disease)

Melanosis is a common consequence of hyperthyroidism (Graves' disease), especially in dark-skinned individuals. Studies suggest that at least 40% of black patients with thyrotoxicosis may present with mucocutaneous hyperpigmentation.[119,120] In contrast, melanosis is very rarely observed in Caucasian patients with the disease. The pigmentation tends to resolve following treatment of the thyroid abnormality.[120] The mechanism by which excessive thyroid activity stimulates melanin synthesis remains unclear.

Primary Biliary Cirrhosis

Diffuse mucocutaneous hyperpigmentation may be one of the earliest manifestations of primary biliary cirrhosis.[121] This uncommon disease is of unknown etiology, although it is thought to be autoimmune in nature. Primary biliary cirrhosis develops mainly in middle-aged women. The disease results from damage to small intrahepatic bile ducts. The mechanism by which melanosis develops is unknown.

Primary biliary cirrhosis may also be a source of generalized nonmelanocytic mucocutaneous discoloration.[121,122] Jaundice is usually an end-stage complication of primary biliary cirrhosis.[122] However, jaundice may also be associated with a variety of other etiologies, including liver cirrhosis, hepatitis, neoplasia, gallstones, congenital disorders, and infection. Jaundice is caused by excessive levels of serum bilirubin (a breakdown product of hemoglobin). Hyperbilirubinemia often induces a yellowish discoloration of the skin, eyes, and mucous membranes. Treatment of the underlying disease will lead to resolution of jaundice. A differential diagnosis should include carotenemia (excessive β-carotene levels) and lycopenemia (excessive lycopene, a compound found within tomatoes and other fruits and vegetables).[123,124] However, the oral mucosal tissues are not affected in either of these latter conditions.

Vitamin B$_{12}$ (Cobalamin) Deficiency

Vitamin B$_{12}$ deficiency may be associated with a variety of systemic manifestations, including megalobastic anemia, various neurologic signs and symptoms, and various cutaneous and oral manifestations, including a generalized burning sensation and erythema and atrophy of the mucosal tissue.[125,126] Diffuse mucocutaneous hyperpigmentation is a rare, and poorly recognized, complication of vitamin B$_{12}$ deficiency.[127–130] The mechanisms by which melanosis develops are unknown. However, the pigmentation resolves following restoration of vitamin B$_{12}$ levels.[128,130]

Peutz-Jeghers Syndrome

Peutz-Jeghers syndrome is an autosomal dominant disease that is associated with mutations in the *STK11/LKB1* tumor suppressor gene.[131] Clinical manifestations include intestinal polyposis, cancer susceptibility, and multiple, small, pigmented macules of the lips, perioral skin, hands, and feet (Figure 12). The macules may resemble ephelides, usually measuring <0.5 cm in diameter. However, the intensity of the macular pigment is not influenced by sun exposure. Although uncommon, similar-appearing lesions may also develop on the anterior tongue and buccal and labial mucosae. The lip and perioral pigmentation is highly distinctive, although not pathognomonic for this disease (see Laugier-Hunziker pigmentation).[132] Histologically, these lesions show increased basilar melanin without an increase in the number of melanocytes.

Other genetic diseases associated with a triad of gastrointestinal disease, cancer susceptibility, and mucocutaneous pigmented macules, among other findings, include Cowden syndrome (and the allelic Bannayan-Riley-Ruvalcaba and Lhermitte-Duclos syndromes) and Cronkhite-Canada syndrome.[133,134]

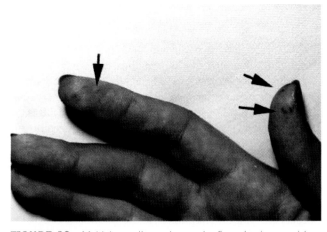

FIGURE 12 Multiple small macules on the fingertips (*arrows*) in a patient with Peutz-Jeghers syndrome. Courtesy of Dr. Rosalie Elenitsas.

TABLE 6 Diseases Commonly Associated with Café au Lait Pigmentation

Ataxia-telangiectasia
Familial café au lait spots
Familial cavernous malformation
Fanconi's anemia
Hereditary nonpolyposis colorectal cancer
Idiopathic epilepsy
Johanson-Blizzard syndrome
McCune-Albright syndrome
Microcephalic osteodysplastic primordial dwarfism
Neurofibromatosis type 1
Neurofibromatosis type 1, Noonan's syndrome
Neurofibromatosis type 2
Nijmegen breakage syndrome
Noonan's syndrome
Ring chromosome 7 syndrome
Ring chromosome 15 syndrome
Ring chromosome 17 syndrome
Russell-Silver syndrome
Tuberous sclerosis
Turcot's syndrome

Café au Lait Pigmentation

Solitary, idiopathic café au lait ("coffee with milk") spots are occasionally observed in the general population, but multiple café au lait spots are often indicative of an underlying genetic disorder.[135] Café au lait pigmentation may be identified in a number of different genetic diseases, including neurofibromatosis type I, McCune-Albright syndrome, and Noonan's syndrome (Table 6).[136–156] Café au lait spots typically present as tan- or brown-colored, irregularly shaped macules of variable size. They may occur anywhere on the skin. Although unusual, examples of similar-appearing oral macular pigmentation have been described in some patients.[137,157]

Neurofibromatosis type I is an autosomal dominant disease that is associated with the development of multiple neurofibromas of various histologic subtypes.[158] In addition, the size, number, and age at onset of the cutaneous café au lait spots are of diagnostic importance for this disease. Axillary and/or inguinal freckling (Crowe's sign) and pigmented lesions of the iris (Lisch nodules) are also highly characteristic of neurofibromatosis type I.[158]

McCune-Albright syndrome and the genetically and phenotypically similar Mazabraud disease[159] are sporadically occurring diseases that are characterized by polyostotic fibrous dysplasia, various endocrinopathies (McCune-Albright), and soft tissue myxomas (Mazabraud disease). In some patients, Addison's disease or Cushing's syndrome may be a potential consequence of McCune-Albright syndrome.[108,136] The café au lait spots in McCune-Albright syndrome appear distinct from those associated with neurofibromatosis. The borders of the pigmented macules are irregularly outlined, whereas in neurofibromatosis, the borders are typically smooth.[160]

Noonan's syndrome and the allelic LEOPARD syndrome (multiple lentigines, electrocardiographic-conduction abnormalities, ocular hypertelorism, pulmonary stenosis, abnormal genitalia, retardation of growth, and sensineural deafness) are autosomal dominant disorders that, among other findings, are also associated with pigmented mucocutaneous macules and multiple melanocytic nevi.[137,161] The classic-appearing café au lait spots are more characteristically seen in patients with the Noonan's phenotype. The LEOPARD phenotype is typically associated with numerous, small, freckle-like macules often involving the facial skin.

Microscopically, when compared with adjacent uninvolved skin, genetic café au lait spots exhibit basilar melanosis without a concomitant increase in the number of melanocytes.[160] The melanocytes that are present demonstrate giant melanosomes (macromelanosomes) that may be visible under light microscopy.[162] In contrast, when compared with similar-appearing lesions in otherwise normal patients, genetic café au lait spots do exhibit increased numbers of melanocytes.[160]

The pathogenesis of genetic café au lait pigmentation remains elusive. It is unclear how the gene mutations that give rise to the various genetic diseases stimulate melanin production. A recent study suggests that the colocalization of neurofibromin (the neurofibromatosis type 1 gene) and amyloid precursor protein in melanosomes may be important for the development of the pigmented lesions in neurofibromatosis patients.[163]

HIV/AIDS-Associated Melanosis

Diffuse or multifocal mucocutaneous pigmentation has been frequently described in human immunodeficiency virus (HIV)-seropositive patients.[164–169] The pigmentation may be related to intake of various medications, including antifungal and antiretroviral drugs,[164] or as a result of adrenocortical destruction by virulent infectious organisms.[170] However, melanosis has also been identified in some patients, including newly diagnosed patients, with no history of adrenocortical disease or medication intake. In these patients, the cause of the hyperpigmentation is undetermined.

Recent studies suggest that melanosis may be an actual, potentially late-stage, clinical manifestation of HIV/AIDS.[165,167,169,171] Goldstein and colleagues demonstrated a significant correlation between mucocutaneous pigment and CD4 counts cells/μL $\leq$ 200.[171] Studies have also shown that the immune dysregulation associated with HIV/acquired immune deficiency syndrome (AIDS) leads to increased secretion of α-MSH from the anterior pituitary gland, which may also stimulate increased melanin synthesis.[172]

HIV/AIDS patients may present with a history of progressive hyperpigmentation of the skin, nails, and mucous membranes. The pigmentation resembles most of the other forms of diffuse melanosis. The buccal mucosa is the most frequently affected site, but the gingiva, palate, and tongue may also be involved. Like all diffuse melanoses, HIV-associated pigmentation is microscopically characterized by basilar melanin pigment, with incontinence into the underlying submucosa.

▼ IDIOPATHIC PIGMENTATION

Laugier-Hunziker Pigmentation

ETIOLOGY AND PATHOGENESIS

Laugier-Hunziker pigmentation (also known as Laugier-Hunziker syndrome) was initially described as an acquired, idiopathic, macular hyperpigmentation of the oral mucosal tissues specifically involving the lips and buccal mucosae.[173] Subsequent reports detailed involvement of other oral mucosal surfaces, as well as pigmentation of the esophageal, genital, and conjunctival mucosae and the acral surfaces.[174–177] Up to 60% of affected patients also may have nail involvement, usually in the form of longitudinal melanotic streaks and without any evidence of dystrophic change.[178] The fingernails are more commonly affected than the toenails.

A relatively limited number of cases have been reported in the literature. This suggests that either this form of pigmentation is exceedingly rare or it is poorly recognized and, thus, underreported. Laugier-Hunziker pigmentation is typically identified in adult patients, with relatively equal sex predilection. This condition more commonly develops in Caucasian or light-skinned individuals. Nonetheless, it remains unclear if this represents a distinct racial predilection or simply an example of clinician bias in the interpretation of the pigmentation.

No systemic abnormalities have been identified in any affected individuals. As a result, some investigators have suggested changing the name of this unusual condition to mucocutaneous lentiginosis of Laugier and Hunziker,[176] idiopathic lenticular mucocutaneous pigmentation,[179] or acquired dermal melanocytosis.[180] Nonetheless, a recent report of Laugier-Hunziker pigmentation occurring in a mother and three of her adult children does suggest the possibility of a genetic predisposition.[175]

CLINICAL FEATURES

Patients typically present with multiple, discrete, irregularly shaped brown or dark brown oral macules. Individual macules are usually no more than 5 mm in diameter.[132] In rare instances, the lesions may coalesce to produce a diffuse area of involvement.[174]

DIAGNOSIS

A differential diagnosis may include physiologic, drug- or heavy metal–induced pigmentation, endocrinopathic disease, and Peutz-Jeghers syndrome.[132] Thus, it is critical to confirm a lack of other systemic signs or symptoms associated with the pigmentation, including gastrointestinal bleeding. If all other potential sources for the pigmentation are ruled out, the clinician may consider the diagnosis of Laugier-Hunziker pigmentation. Hence, in most cases, this is a diagnosis of exclusion.[176,177] Despite the close resemblance of the labial pigmentation to that observed in Peutz-Jeghers syndrome, *STK11/LKB1* gene mutations have not been identified in patients with Laugier-Hunziker pigmentation.[132]

MANAGEMENT

The pigmentation may be esthetically unpleasing, but it is otherwise innocuous. Although treatment is generally not indicated, laser and cryotherapy have been used with some success.[181,182] A biopsy shows findings similar to those seen in other forms of diffuse pigmentation.[177]

▼ TREATMENT OF MUCOCUTANEOUS MELANOSIS

In general, focally pigmented lesions warrant removal, for both diagnostic and therapeutic purposes. However, apart from those cases associated with neoplasia, surgical intervention is less of an option for the treatment of multifocal or diffuse pigmentation. Drug-induced melanosis and other examples of exogenously stimulated generalized pigmentation may spontaneously subside after withdrawal of the offending substance. In other cases, the discoloration may be persistent, if not permanent. In such cases, the cosmetic disfigurement may eventuate in significant social, psychological, and emotional stress.

Laser therapy has proven to be an effective modality for use in the treatment of bothersome oral pigmentation.[74,103] However, the beneficial effects may only be temporary, with recurrence of at least partial pigmentation in upwards of 20% of treated patients.[74] Various types of lasers have been used, including superpulsed CO_2,[74] Q-switched Nd-YAG,[181] and Q-switched alexandrite lasers.[182]

Perioral and facial pigmentation are more challenging to treat since skin type may dictate the occurrence of postoperative complications, including postinflammatory hyperpigmentation.[183] Although laser[184] and cryotherapy[185] have been used to successfully treat such cases, experimental forms of phototherapy have also been employed, including intense pulsed light[186] and fractional photothermolysis.[187] However, first-line therapy remains the application of topical medicaments, that is, bleaching creams.[183] Although single agents such as azelaic acid or hydroquinone have been used, more commonly, dual- or triple-combination therapy is recommended. A combination of 4% hydroquinone–0.05% retinoic acid–0.01% fluocinolone acetonide has proven to be effective in greater than 90% of patients.[188] However, the majority of patients undergoing such therapy may experience immunologic sensitivity or other treatment-related adverse events, including the development of exogenous ochronosis.[189–191]

Exogenous ochronosis is a form of intense cutaneous hyperpigmentation with or without atrophic striae and coarsening of the skin or formation of numerous coalesced, black papules. This phenomenon is more commonly observed in black individuals, usually female, who have undergone long-term bleaching therapy. The intense color changes develop in the areas where the cream was applied (frequently on the face) and are related to the accumulation of a yellow-brown pigmented substance (not melanin) in the dermis.[191] This pigmentation may be permanent.

Finally, there are several substances, including novel tyrosinase inhibitors,[192] that have demonstrable skin-lightening effects in animal models. However, these chemicals remain largely experimental and have not yet been proven to be effective in humans.

▼ DEPIGMENTATION

Vitiligo

ETIOLOGY AND PATHOGENESIS

In some patients, pathologic pigmentation may be cosmetically objectionable. Conversely, areas of depigmentation in patients who have otherwise normal physiologic coloration may be equally bothersome and disfiguring. Vitiligo is a relatively common, acquired, autoimmune disease that is associated with hypomelanosis.[193–195] Epidemiologic studies suggest an incidence of 0.5 to 2% in the general population. Although the etiology and mechanisms remain unknown, the end result is a destruction of the melanocytes.

The pathogenesis of vitiligo is multifactorial, with both genetic and environmental factors likely to play a role in disease pathogenesis. A recent study has identified a single-nucleotide polymorphism in a vitiligo-susceptibility gene that is also associated with susceptibility to other autoimmune diseases, including diabetes type 1, systemic lupus erythematosus, and rheumatoid arthritis.[195,196] Additional putative vitiligo-susceptibility genes have been mapped to various other chromosomal regions.[193]

CLINICAL FEATURES

Vitiligo has a variable clinical presentation. In some individuals, there may only be focal areas of depigmentation. In other patients, an entire segment on one side of the body may be affected. In occasional patients, the skin and hair of most of the body may lose its pigmentation (vitiligo universalis).[197] However, in most cases, vitiligo is characterized by bilateral, symmetric areas of relatively generalized hypomelanosis. The vitiligenous lesions often present as well-circumscribed, round, oval or elongated, pale or white-colored macules that may coalesce into larger areas of diffuse depigmentation. As the disease progresses, additional areas of involvement may become apparent.

The onset of vitiligo may occur at any age, but most patients develop signs of the disease before the third decade of life.[198] The depigmentation is easily apparent in patients who have a darker skin tone. Yet the disease actually occurs in all races. Although many studies suggest a greater prevalence in females, there is actually no significant sex predilection.[193] The reporting bias is probably related to the fact that women are more likely to present with esthetic complaints associated with the disease. Vitiligo may also arise in patients undergoing immunotherapy for the treatment of malignant melanoma.[199] Studies suggest that this phenomenon may be associated with a better prognosis for this group of patients.[72]

Vitiligo rarely affects the intraoral mucosal tissues. However, hypomelanosis of the inner and outer surfaces of

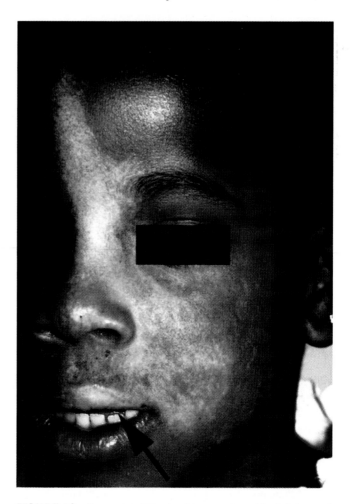

FIGURE 13 Segmental vitiligo involving a portion of the left face and upper lip (*arrow*).

the lips and perioral skin may be seen in up to 20% of patients (Figure 13).[200]

PATHOLOGY

Microscopically, there is a complete loss of melanocytes and melanin pigmentation in the basal cell layer. The use of histochemical stains such as Fontana-Masson will confirm the absence of melanin.

MANAGEMENT

In most cases, the objective of therapeutic intervention is to stimulate repigmentation. Topical corticosteroids and topical or, more commonly, systemic photochemotherapies (psoralen and ultraviolet A exposure) have proven to be effective nonsurgical therapies.[197,201] In rare cases, small foci of normal pigmented skin may be contained within otherwise diffuse areas of hypomelanosis. Thus, to create a unified skin color, medicinal depigmentation may be considered, that is, cutaneous bleaching.

From the standpoint of therapy, labial vitiligo is more resistant to the typical treatments used for cutaneous vitiligo. Due to a lack of hair follicles, the lips do not have a reservoir of melanocytes that can be stimulated to produce pigment.[200] Thus, surgical intervention may be the only option in order to achieve an esthetic result. Autologous epithelial grafts have been used successfully, with patients often reporting a more acceptable cosmetic appearance.[200,202] Punch grafting and micropigmentation (whereby an exogenous brown pigment is injected into the lip, much like a tattoo) have also been described.[201,202] In rare instances, surgical intervention may stimulate spontaneous repigmentation of vitiligenous lesions elsewhere on the body.[201]

▼ HEMOGLOBIN AND IRON-ASSOCIATED PIGMENTATION

Ecchymosis

Traumatic ecchymosis is common on the lips and face yet is uncommon in the oral mucosa, except in cases related to blunt-force trauma and oral intubation.[203] Immediately following the traumatic event, erythrocyte extravasation into the submucosa will appear as a bright red macule or as a swelling if a hematoma forms. The lesion will assume a brown coloration within a few days, after the hemoglobin is degraded to hemosiderin. The differential diagnosis must include other focally pigmented lesions. If the patient recalls an episode of trauma, however, the lesion should be observed for 2 weeks, by which time it should resolve.

When multiple brown macules or swellings are observed and ecchymosis is included in the differential diagnosis, a hemorrhagic diathesis or coagulation disorder should be considered.[204] Certainly, patients taking anticoagulant drugs may present with oral ecchymosis, particularly on the buccal mucosa or tongue, either of which can be traumatized while chewing. Ecchymoses of the oral mucosa may also be encountered in patients with liver cirrhosis, leukemia, and end-stage renal disease undergoing dialysis treatment.[205,206] Laboratory tests, including bleeding time, prothrombin time, partial thromboplastin time, and international normalization ratio (INR), should be obtained in instances of spontaneous ecchymoses to explore defects in the coagulation pathways.

Purpura/Petechiae

Capillary hemorrhages will appear red initially and turn brown in a few days once the extravasated red cells have lysed and have been degraded to hemosiderin. The distinction between purpura and petechiae is essentially semantic and based solely on the size of the focal hemorrhages. Petechiae are typically characterized as being pinpoint or slightly larger than pinpoint and purpura as multiple, small 2 to 4 mm collections of extravasated blood.[204] The same precipitating events can elicit either clinical presentation.

Oral purpura/petechiae may develop as a consequence of trauma or viral or systemic disease (Table 7).[204–218] Petechiae secondary to platelet deficiencies or aggregation disorders are usually not limited to the oral mucosa but may occur concomitantly on the skin. Viral disease is more commonly associated with oral rather than cutaneous petechiae. In most cases, the petechiae are identified on the soft palate, although any mucosal site may be affected. When trauma is suspected, the patient should be instructed to cease whatever activity may be contributing to the presence of the lesions. Within 2 weeks,

TABLE 7   Causes of Oral Purpura/Petechiae
Amyloidosis
Aplastic anemia
Bulimia
Chronic renal failure
Fellatio
Forceful coughing
Hemophilia
Henoch-Schönlein purpura
HIV/AIDS
Infectious mononucleosis
Leukemia
Liver cirrhosis
Nonspecific trauma
Oral intubation
Oral submucous fibrosis
Overexertion
Papular-pupuric "gloves and socks" syndrome
Streptococcal infection
Systemic lupus erythematosus
Thrombocytopenia
von Willebrand's disease

AIDS = acquired immune deficiency syndrome; HIV = human immunodeficiency virus.

the lesions should resolve. Failure to do so should arouse suspicion of a hemorrhagic diathesis, a persistent infectious disease, or other systemic disease, and appropriate laboratory investigations must be undertaken.

Hemochromatosis

Hemochromatosis is a chronic, progressive disease that is characterized by excessive iron deposition (usually in the form of hemosiderin) in the liver and other organs and tissues.[219,220] Idiopathic, neonatal, blood transfusion, and heritable forms of this disease are recognized. Complications of hemochromatosis may include liver cirrhosis, diabetes, anemia, heart failure, hypertension, and bronzing of the skin. Studies also suggest an increased incidence of cancer in patients with hemochromatosis.[221]

The cutaneous pigmentation is seen in over 90% of affected patients, regardless of the etiology of the disease.[219] Although it is less commonly observed, oral mucosal pigmentation is also a well-recognized consequence of hemochromatosis.[222] The oral pigmentation is often diffuse and brown to gray in appearance. The palate and gingiva are most commonly affected.

Early on in the course of disease, the pigmentation may be more commonly a result of basilar melanosis rather than iron-associated pigment.[219] Iron deposition within the adrenal cortex may lead to hypoadrenocorticism and ACTH hypersecretion, with the associated addisonian-type changes. In the later stages of hemochromatosis, the pigmentation is usually a result of hemosiderosis and melanosis.

A lower labial gland biopsy has been shown to be an easy and effective method for the diagnosis of hemochromatosis.[223,224] Increased melanin pigment may be seen in the basal cell layer, whereas golden or brown-colored hemosiderin can be seen diffusely scattered throughout the submucosal and salivary gland tissues. A Prussian blue stain will confirm the presence of iron. Since hemochromatosis can cause a number of serious complications, medical referral is necessary. Hemochromatosis is discussed in greater detail in Chapter ??.

▼ EXOGENOUS PIGMENTATION

Amalgam Tattoo

ETIOLOGY AND PATHOGENESIS

The single most common source of solitary or focal pigmentation in the oral mucosa is the amalgam tattoo.[225] By definition, these are iatrogenic in origin and typically a consequence of the inadvertent deposition of amalgam restorative material into the submucosal tissue.

CLINICAL FEATURES

Some studies suggest that amalgam tattoos may be found in up to 1% of the general population.[226] The lesions are typically small, asymptomatic, macular, and bluish gray or even black in appearance. They may be found on any mucosal surface. However, the gingiva, alveolar mucosa, buccal mucosa, and floor of the mouth represent the most common sites. The lesions are often found in the vicinity of teeth with large amalgam restorations or crowned teeth that probably had amalgams, around the apical region of endodontically treated teeth with retrograde restorations or obturated with silver points, and in areas in and around healed extraction sites (Figure 14).[226,227]

PATHOLOGY

Microscopically, amalgam tattoos often show a fine brown granular stippling of reticulum fibers, with a particular affinity for vessel walls and nerve fibers (Figure 15). In other cases,

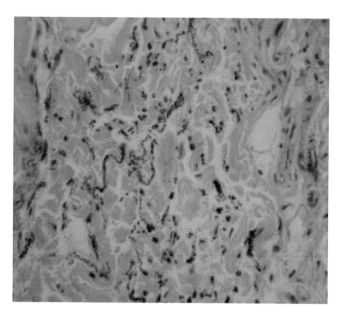

FIGURE 15 Amalgam particles are dispersed throughout the submucosal tissue.

large aggregates of black material may be seen. A foreign body–type giant cell reaction is uncommon; however, a mild to moderate lymphocytic inflammatory infiltrate is often noted.

MANAGEMENT

The amalgam particles are usually quite fine, but in some instances (when large enough), they may be identified on regional radiographs. In some patients, the focal argyrosis may compromise esthetics; thus, surgical removal may be warranted. However, since amalgam tattoos are innocuous, their removal is not always necessary, particularly when they can be documented radiographically. If there is no radiographic evidence of amalgam, the lesion is not in proximity to any restored tooth, or the lesion suddenly appears, a biopsy is necessary. A typical differential diagnosis often includes melanotic macule, nevus, and melanoma.

Pigmentation associated with other dental restorative materials has also been described.[228,229] Studies have demonstrated that metal components from almost all forms of cast alloy material can be detected in the adjacent tissues (Figure 16).[228] Titanium has been associated with pigmentation of the skin, specifically in areas around orthopedic implants.[230] Thus, it is conceivable that dental implants may also be a potential source of exogenous oral pigmentation.

Graphite Tattoos

Graphite tattoos are an unusual source of focal exogenous pigmentation. They are most commonly seen on the palate and represent traumatic implantation of graphite particles from a pencil.[231] The lesions may be indistinguishable from amalgam tattoos, often presenting as a solitary gray or black macule. Since the traumatic event often occurs in childhood, many patients may not report a history of injury. Thus, a biopsy is often warranted. Microscopically, graphite particles

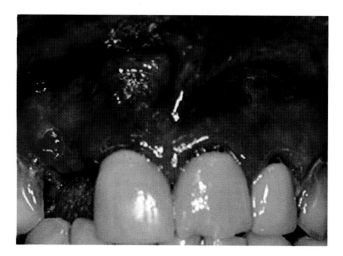

FIGURE 14 Amalgam tattoo of the maxillary alveolar mucosa. The pigment was associated with a retrograde amalgam restoration. Courtesy of Dr. Sunday Akintoye.

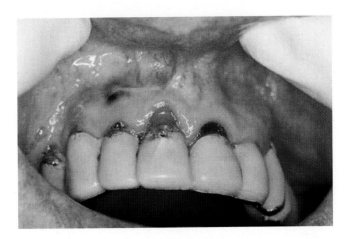

FIGURE 16 Discoloration of the alveolar mucosa associated with extensive crown and bridge restoration. Courtesy of Dr. Scott DeRossi.

resemble those of amalgam. Treatment may be warranted for cosmetic reasons.

Ornamental Tattoos

Mucosal tattoos in the form of lettering or intricate artwork are becoming increasingly common phenomena. In some circles, this type of "art" represents a social statement. Unfortunately, if these patients' philosophical views change over time, a quick look in the mirror will always be a constant reminder of what once was.

Amateur tattoo inks consist of simple, carbon particles originating from a variety of sources, including burnt wood, plastic, or paper, and from a variety of inks, such as India ink, pen ink, and plant-derived matter.[232,233] Laser therapy has been used with some success in the removal of cutaneous tattoos. It is likely that this form of therapy may also be beneficial for the removal of oral tattoos. Without therapy, this type of tattoo is permanent.

In certain tribal cultures, ornamental mucocutaneous tattooing is considered a rite of passage and esthetically pleasing.[234] In most cases, the pigment is plant derived. Female members of certain tribes are more likely to exhibit this form of exogenous pigmentation, usually in an effort to make themselves more attractive or desirable.

An unusual South African female tribal custom includes brushing the teeth and gums with a chewed root of the tree *Euclea natalensis*, with the belief that it promotes oral health.[235] This plant root contains naphthoquinones and other organic substances that have putative antibacterial properties.[236] Naphthoquinones are pigmented, and the mouths of root users are typically bright orange.[236] Unlike ornamental tattoos, this form of pigmentation is usually transient and reversible.

Medicinal Metal-Induced Pigmentation

Historically, a variety of metallic compounds have been used medicinally for the treatment of various systemic diseases. With the exception of gold therapy (for rheumatoid arthritis),[237] such medicaments are rarely or no longer in use.

Colloidal silver is another metal-based substance that has been historically touted for its beneficial health effects.[238] Although its medical use has been significantly curtailed, it remains available as a "nutritional" supplement. Gold and colloidal silver have both been associated with diffuse cutaneous pigmentation. Silver may cause a generalized blue-gray discoloration (argyria), whereas gold-induced pigment may appear blue-gray or purple (chrysiasis). In both cases, the pigmentation may be persistent, if not permanent, even following discontinuation of the substance. Rare examples of diffuse oral argyrosis have been reported.[239] Chrysiasis does not involve the oral mucosal tissues since it is thought that exposure to ultraviolet light or other high-intensity light sources precipitates the pigmentation. However, oral lichenoid eruptions have been associated with systemic gold therapy.[240]

In contrast to the systemic therapies, metal salts remain a component of some topical medications and other substances that are used in clinical practice. Examples include silver nitrate and zinc oxide. Silver nitrate cautery has been used to treat recurrent aphthous stomatitis,[241] and zinc oxide is a common component of sunblock creams.[242] Both substances have been associated with focal mucocutaneous pigmentation. Zinc- and medicinal silver-associated pigment is often gray-black in appearance.[226] Both appear as brown or black particulate matter that is often dispersed throughout the submucosal tissue. A clinicopathologic correlation is necessary since, clinically and microscopically, these forms of pigmentation may be difficult to differentiate from amalgam tattoos.

Generalized black pigmentation of the tongue has been attributed to the chewing of bismuth subsalicylate tablets, a commonly used antacid.[243] This phenomenon is unlike black hairy tongue (see page ??), which is associated with elongation of the filiform papillae, hyperkeratosis, and superficial colonization of the tongue by bacteria. Black tongue induced by bismuth subsalicylate is caused by deposition of actual pigment (bismuth sulfide), without any other lingual changes.[227] Discontinuation of the antacid and cleansing of the tongue are curative. It should be noted that typical black hairy tongue may also be attributed to the use of bismuth subsalicylate.

Heavy-Metal Pigmentation

Diffuse oral pigmentation may be associated with ingestion of heavy metals. Nowadays, this phenomenon is unusually encountered. Yet it remains an occupational and health hazard for some individuals who work in certain industrial plants and for those who live in the environment in and around these types of facilities.[244,245] Other relatively common environmental sources include paints, old plumbing, and seafood.

Lead, mercury, bismuth, and arsenic have all been shown to be deposited in oral tissue if ingested in sufficient quantities or over an extended period of time.[244–247] These ingested metal salts tend to extravasate from vessels in areas of chronic inflammation. Thus, in the oral cavity, the pigmentation is usually found along the free marginal gingiva, where it often dramatically outlines the gingival cuff. This metallic line usually has a gray to black appearance. In some patients, the oral pigmentation may be the first sign of heavy-metal toxicity. Additional systemic signs and symptoms of heavy-metal poisoning may include behavioral changes, neurologic disorders, intestinal pain, and sialorrhea. Diffuse mucocutaneous melanosis may also be observed in some affected individuals.[245]

Drug-Induced Pigmentation

Minocycline, which is a tetracycline derivative and frequently used in the treatment of acne, is a relatively common cause of drug-induced non–melanin-associated oral pigmentation.[248,249] Similar to tetracycline, minocycline can cause pigmentation of developing teeth. However, most patients are prescribed minocycline in early adulthood. When taken chronically, minocycline metabolites may become incorporated into the normal bone. Thus, whereas the teeth may be normal in appearance, the surrounding bone may appear green, blue, or even black.[249] As a result, the palatal and alveolar mucosae may appear similarly and diffusely discolored. As many as 20% of patients may be affected in such a manner.

Minocycline can also induce actual pigmentation of the oral soft tissues, as well as the skin and nails. Minocycline-induced soft tissue pigmentation may appear gray, brown, or black. Often the pigmentation is patchy or diffuse in its presentation. Although a biopsy may reveal basilar melanosis, more commonly, aggregates of fine brown or golden particles are identified within the submucosal tissue.[248,250] The particles are often intracellular and contained within macrophages. Superficially, the submucosal pigment may resemble melanin and does actually stain with what is thought to be a melanin-specific (Fontana-Masson) histochemical stain.[250] However, an iron stain (Prussian blue) also highlights many of the same particles.[248] Thus, it is likely that the particulate substance represents an actual precipitated drug metabolite rather than true melanin.

There is no treatment necessary for minocycline-induced pigmentation. The discoloration often subsides within months after discontinuation of the medication. However, the bone pigment may persist for longer periods of time, if not indefinitely.

Methacycline, another tetracycline derivative that is no longer widely used in clinical practice, can also produce a similar form of pigmentation.[251]

Hairy Tongue

Hairy tongue is a relatively common condition of unknown etiology.[252] The change in oral flora associated with chronic antibiotic therapy may be causative in some patients. The discoloration involves the dorsal tongue, particularly the middle and posterior one-third. Rarely are children affected. The filiform papillae are elongated, sometimes markedly so, and have the appearance of fine hairs.[253] The hyperplastic papillae then become pigmented by the colonization of chromogenic bacteria, which can impart a variety of colors,

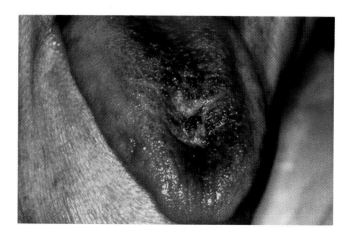

FIGURE 17   Hairy tongue. Courtesy of Dr. Scott DeRossi.

including white, green, brown, or black (Figure 17). Various foods, drinks, and confectionaries can contribute to the diffuse discoloration. Smoking of tobacco or crack cocaine has been associated with black hairy tongue.[253,254] Rare examples of black hairy tongue have also been linked to the use of psychotropic medications.[255]

Microscopically, the filiform papillae are extremely elongated and hyperplastic with hyperkeratosis. External colonization of the papillae by numerous microbial colonies is a prominent feature. There are no additional pathologic findings in the remaining epithelium or in the connective tissue. The condition is so characteristic in its presentation that biopsy is not required, and a clinical diagnosis is usually appropriate. Treatments consist of having the patient brush the tongue, or use a tongue scraper, and limit the ingestion of color-forming foods and drinks until the discoloration resolves. Since the cause is often undetermined, the condition may recur.

▼ SUMMARY

Oral pigmentation may be focal, multifocal, or diffuse. The lesions may be blue, purple, brown, gray, or black. They may be macular or tumefactive. Importantly, some are localized harmless accumulations of melanin, hemosiderin, or exogenous metal; others are harbingers of systemic or genetic disease, and some can be associated with life-threatening medical conditions that require immediate intervention. The differential diagnosis for any given pigmented lesion can be quite extensive and can include examples of endogenous and exogenous pigmentation. Although biopsy is a helpful and necessary aid in the diagnosis of focally pigmented lesions, the more diffuse lesions will require a thorough history and laboratory studies in order to arrive at a definitive diagnosis.

▼ SELECTED READINGS

Abbasi NR, Shaw HM, Rigel DS, et al. Early diagnosis of cutaneous melanoma: revisiting the ABCD criteria. JAMA 2004;292:2771–6.

Adams PC. Review article: the modern diagnosis and management of haemochromatosis. Aliment Pharmacol Ther 2006;23:1681–91.

Blignaut E, Patton LL, Nittayananta W, et al. (A3) HIV phenotypes, oral lesions, and management of HIV-related disease. Adv Dent Res 2006;19:122–9.

Cabrera VP, Rodu B. Differential diagnosis of oral mucosal petechial hemorrhages. Compendium 1991;12:418–22.

De Giorgi V, Massi D, Carli P. Dermoscopy in the management of pigmented lesions of the oral mucosa. Oral Oncol 2003;39:534–5

Dereure O. Drug-induced skin pigmentation. Epidemiology, diagnosis and treatment. Am J Clin Dermatol 2001;2:253–62.

De Schepper S, Boucneau J, Vander HY, et al. Cafe-au-lait spots in neurofibromatosis type 1 and in healthy control individuals: hyperpigmentation of a different kind? Arch Dermatol Res 2006;297:439–49.

Garhammer P, Schmalz G, Hiller KA, Reitinger T. Metal content of biopsies adjacent to dental cast alloys. Clin Oral Investig 2003;7:92–7.

Hicks MJ, Flaitz CM. Oral mucosal melanoma: epidemiology and pathobiology. Oral Oncol 2000;36:152–69.

Hossain MK, Khan MM, Alam MA, et al. Manifestation of arsenicosis patients and factors determining the duration of arsenic symptoms in Bangladesh. Toxicol Appl Pharmacol 2005;208:78–86.

Krengel S. Nevogenesis—new thoughts regarding a classical problem. Am J Dermatopathol 2005;27:456–65.

Mannone F, De Giorgi V, Cattaneo A, et al. Dermoscopic features of mucosal melanosis. Dermatol Surg 2004;30:1118–23.

Mendenhall WM, Amdur RJ, Hinerman RW, et al. Head and neck mucosal melanoma. Am J Clin Oncol 2005;28:626–30.

Mignogna MD, Lo ML, Ruoppo E, et al. Oral manifestations of idiopathic lenticular mucocutaneous pigmentation (Laugier-Hunziker syndrome): a clinical, histopathological and ultrastructural review of 12 cases. Oral Dis 1999;5:80–6.

Newell-Price J, Bertagna X, Grossman AB, Nieman LK. Cushing's syndrome. Lancet 2006;367:1605–17.

ornatora ML, Reich RF, Haber S, et al. Oral melanoacanthoma: a report of 10 cases, review of the literature, and immunohistochemical analysis for HMB-45 reactivity. Am J Dermatopathol 2003;25:12–5.

Passeron T, Ortonne JP. Physiopathology and genetics of vitiligo. J Autoimmun 2005;25 Suppl:63–8.

Ten S, New M, Maclaren N. Clinical review 130: Addison's disease 2001. J Clin Endocrinol Metab 2001;86:2909–22.

Thavarajah R, Rao A, Raman U, et al. Oral lesions of 500 habitual psychoactive substance users in Chennai, India. Arch Oral Biol 2006;51:512–9.

Treister NS, Magalnick D, Woo SB. Oral mucosal pigmentation secondary to minocycline therapy: report of two cases and a review of the literature. Oral Surg Oral Med Oral Pathol Oral Radiol Endod 2004;97:718–25.

For the full reference list, please refer to the accompanying CD ROM.

6

BENIGN LESIONS OF THE ORAL CAVITY

A. Ross Kerr, DDS, MSD
Joan A. Phelan, DDS

This chapter provides an overview of the clinical features, diagnosis, and management of localized nonmalignant growths and tumors of the oral cavity. A variety of lesions of miscellaneous etiologies are discussed, many of which are not true neoplasms. If left untreated, some of the lesions discussed in this chapter will lead to extensive tissue destruction and deformity, whereas others will interfere with mastication and will become secondarily infected following masticatory trauma. Regardless, the major clinical consideration in the management of all of these tumors is to identify their benign nature and to distinguish them from potentially life-threatening malignant lesions. Identification can only be established with certainty by microscopic examination of excised tissue; therefore, biopsy is an essential step in diagnosis and management.

▼ VARIANTS OF NORMAL

Structural variations of the jaw bones and overlying oral soft tissues are sometimes mistakenly identified as tumors, but they are usually easily recognized as within the range of normal variation for the oral cavity, and biopsy in these cases is rarely indicated. Examples of such structural variants are tori; localized nodular connective tissue thickening of the attached gingiva; the papilla associated with the opening of Stensen's duct; a circumvallate papillae on the dorsum of the tongue; and sublingual varicosities in older individuals.

Localized nodular enlargements (exostoses) of the cortical bone of the midline of the palate (torus palatinus), the lingual aspect of the mandible (torus mandibularis), and the buccal aspects of either jaws occur frequently[1] and are considered to be normal structural variants (Figure 1). The lack of obvious irritants for most tori and their negligible growth after an initial slow but steady period of development also suggest that they are usually neither inflammatory hyperplasias nor neoplasms. Histologically, tori consist of layers of dense cortical bone–covered periosteum and an overlying layer of thin epithelium, with minimal rete peg development. Tori may pose a mechanical problem in the construction of dentures; they are frequently traumatized as a result of their prominent position and thin epithelial covering, and the resulting ulcers are slow to heal. Rarely, tori on the palate or lingual mandibular ridge may become sufficiently large to interfere with eating and speaking. Unless a torus is exceptionally large, its surgical removal (when dictated by mechanical concerns) is not a major procedure provided that splints or stents are fabricated beforehand to provide a protective dressing during healing. Similar nodular growths or exostoses arise on the buccal aspect of the maxillary and mandibular alveolae and must be differentiated from bony hyperplasia secondary to a chronic periapical abscess, fibrous dysplasia, or Paget's disease, in which they represent superficial evidence of a more generalized bony dysplasia.

Unencapsulated lymphoid aggregates are normally present in the oral cavity located primarily on the soft palate, the posterolateral aspects of the tongue (Figure 2), the dorsum of the tongue, and the anterior tonsillar pillar. An increase in size as a result of benign (reactive) processes as well as lymphoid neoplasms may represent benign or follicular lymphoid hyperplasia. These may masquerade clinically as a malignancy, principally a lymphoma. Histologic criteria based on architectural, cytologic, and immunologic (leukocyte monoclonal antigen-antibody reactions) features of the lymphoid aggregate have been described in recent years.[2,3]

▼ BENIGN SOFT TISSUE LESIONS

Inflammatory/Reactive Hyperplasia of Soft Tissue

The term *inflammatory hyperplasia* is used to describe a large range of commonly occurring nodular growths of the oral mucosa that histologically represent inflamed fibrous and granulation tissue. The size of these reactive hyperplastic masses may be large or small, depending on the degree to which one or more of the components of the inflammatory

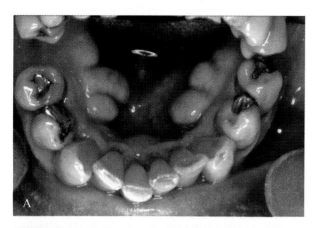

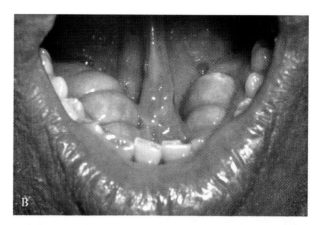

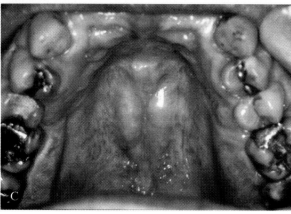

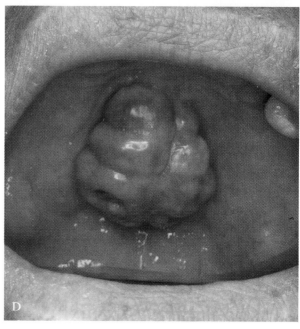

FIGURE 1 *A*, Mandibular tori (tori mandibularis). *B*, Mandibular tori. Note traumatic keratosis on the left side due to the large size of the tori. *C*, Maxillary torus (torus palatinus). *D*, Maxillary torus. Note the large size with a "pedunculated base."

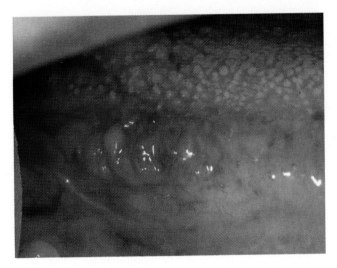

FIGURE 2 Right posterolateral tongue revealing a prominent foliate papilla region containing unencapsulated lymphoid aggregates. A similar presentation was seen on the left side.

reaction and healing response are exaggerated. Some are predominantly epithelial overgrowths with only scanty connective tissue stroma; others are fibromatous, with a thin epithelial covering, and may exhibit either angiomatous, desmoplastic (collagenous), or fibroblastic features. In many lesions, different sections may reveal examples of each of these histologic patterns. Like scar tissue, some inflammatory hyperplasias appear to mature and become less vascular (paler and less friable) and more collagenous (firmer and smaller) with time. Others appear to have a high proliferative ability for exophytic growth until they are excised. This variability of histologic appearance is reflected in the wide range of clinical characteristics exhibited by inflammatory hyperplasias.

The major etiologic factor for these lesions is generally assumed to be chronic trauma from ill-fitting dentures, calculus, overhanging dental restorations, acute or chronic tissue injury from biting, or fractured teeth. With some of these lesions, (eg, pregnancy epulis), the levels of circulating hormones play a role. The majority of lesions occur peripherally on the oral mucosal surface, where irritants are quite common and therefore are subject to continual masticatory trauma. Clinical appearance is swollen, distended, ulcerated, and red to purple lesions due to dilated blood vessels, and they exhibit acute and chronic inflammatory exudates and localized abscesses. Erosion of the underlying cortical bone rarely occurs with peripheral inflammatory hyperplasias; if noted, there should be a strong suspicion that an aggressive process or even malignancy is involved. An excisional biopsy is indicated except when the procedure would produce marked deformity; in such a case, incisional biopsy to establish the diagnosis is mandatory. If the chronic irritant is eliminated when the lesion is excised, the majority of inflammatory hyperplasias will not recur, thus confirming the benign nature of these lesions.

FIBROMAS, COWDEN SYNDROME, TUBEROUS SCLEROSIS

Fibromas may occur as either pedunculated or sessile (broad-based) growths on any surface of the oral mucous membrane. They are also called traumatic or irritation fibromas (Figure 3).[4,5] The majority remain small, and lesions that are > 1 cm in diameter are rare. The giant cell fibroma exhibits a somewhat nodular surface and is histologically distinguished from other fibromas by the presence of stellate-shaped and multinucleated cells in the connective tissue. The etiology of the giant cell fibroma is not known.

Multiple fibromas may indicate Cowden syndrome (multiple hamartoma and neoplasia syndrome)[6] or tuberous sclerosis. Cowden syndrome is inherited as an autosomal dominant trait. Multiple papules on the lips and gingivae are often present, and papillomatosis (benign fibromatosis) of the buccal, palatal, faucial, and oropharyngeal mucosae often produces a "cobblestone" effect on these mucous membranes. The tongue is also pebbly or fissured. Multiple papillomatous nodules (histologically inverted follicular keratoses or trichilemmomas) are often present on the perioral, periorbital, and perinasal skin, and the mucosal surface of the oropharynx often manifests a cobblestone effect on these mucous membranes. Multiple papillomatous nodules are often present also on the pinnae of the ears and neck, accompanied by lipomas, hemangiomas, neuromas, vitiligo, café au lait spots, and acromelanosis elsewhere on the skin. A variety of neoplastic changes occur in the organs exhibiting hamartomatous lesions, particularly an increased rate of breast and thyroid carcinoma and gastrointestinal malignancy. Squamous cell carcinoma of the tongue and basal cell tumors of the perianal skin are also reported.

Tuberous sclerosis[7,8] is an inherited disorder that is characterized by seizures and mental retardation associated with hamartomatous glial proliferations and neuronal deformity

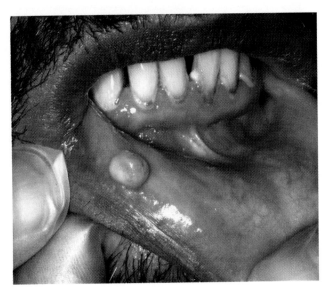

FIGURE 3 Irritation fibroma (traumatic fibroma). Patient reports a daily habit of biting this lesion for several months.

in the central nervous system. Fine wart-like lesions (adenoma sebaceum) occur in a butterfly distribution over the cheeks and forehead (Figure 4A), and histologically similar lesions (vascular fibromas) have been described intraorally (Figure 4B).[9,10] Characteristic hypoplastic enamel defects (pitted enamel hypoplasia) occur in 40 to 100% of those affected.[7,8] Rhabdomyoma of the heart and other hamartomas of the kidney, liver, adrenal glands, pancreas, and jaw[11] are described. The neoplastic transformation of the glial proliferations constitutes the "internal malignancy" of this syndrome.

FIBROUS INFLAMMATORY HYPERPLASIAS

The epulis fissuratum is a reactive inflammatory lesion associated with the periphery of ill-fitting dentures[12] that histologically resembles the fibroma. The growth is often split by the edge of the denture, resulting in a fissure, one part of the lesion lying under the denture and the other part lying between the lip or cheek and the outer denture surface (Figure 5). This lesion may extend the full length of one side of the denture. Many such hyperplastic growths will become less edematous and inflamed following the removal of the associated chronic irritant, but they rarely resolve entirely. In the preparation of the mouth to receive dentures, these lesions are excised to prevent further irritation and to ensure a soft tissue seal for the denture periphery.

Pulp polyps or chronic hyperplastic pulpitis represents an analogous condition. They occur when the pulpal connective tissue proliferates through a large pulpal exposure and fills the cavity in the tooth with a mushroom-shaped polyp that is connected by a stalk to the pulp chamber (Figure 6). Masticatory pressure may lead to keratinization of the epithelium covering these lesions. Pulp polyps contain few sensory nerve fibers and are remarkably insensitive. The crowns of teeth affected by pulp polyps are usually so badly destroyed by caries that endodontic treatment is not feasible.

Inflammatory papillary hyperplasia is a common lesion with a characteristic clinical appearance that develops on the central hard palate in response to chronic denture irritation in approximately 3 to 4% of denture wearers.[13] Old and ill-fitting complete maxillary dentures appear to be the strongest stimuli, but the lesion is also seen under partial maxillary dentures. The exact pathogenesis is unclear, but this palatal lesion is usually associated with denture stomatitis due to chronic candidal infection. The lesion may be red to scarlet with swollen and tightly packed projections resembling the surface of an overripe berry (Figure 7). Such lesions are friable, often bleed with minimal trauma, and may be covered with a thin whitish exudate. When the candidal infection is eliminated, either by removing the denture or by topical administration of an antifungal agent, the papillary surface becomes less erythematous than the rest of the palate and consists of tightly packed nodular projections. If tiny, the nodular projections may even pass unnoticed unless stroked with an instrument or disturbed by a jet of air. Histologic examination of these lesions demonstrates their exophytic nature, and neither epithelial invasion of the submucosa nor resorption of the palatine bone occurs, even under large

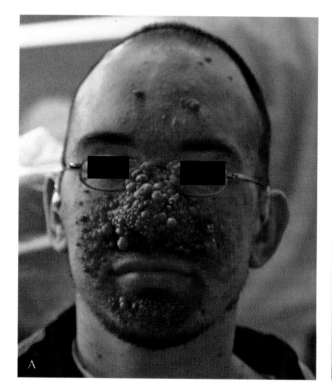
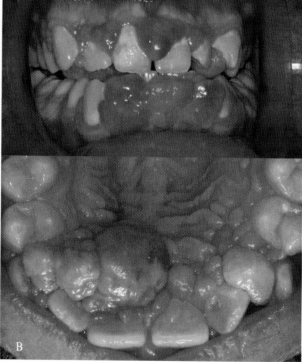

FIGURE 4 *A,* Young male with tuberous sclerosis. There are extensive wart-like lesions (adenoma sebaceum) in a butterfly distribution over the face. *B,* Same patient as in Figure 4A showing intraoral fibromas. Generalized hypoplastic pitted enamel changes are absent.

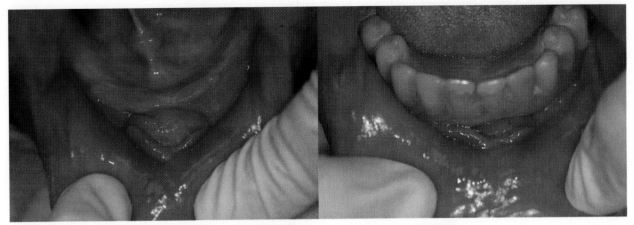

FIGURE 5   Fibrous hyperplasia (epulis fissuratum) secondary to a poorly fitting mandibular complete denture.

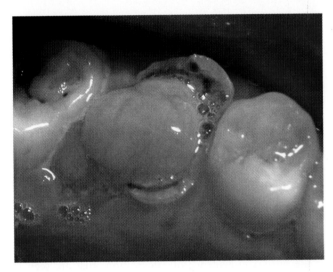

FIGURE 6   Pulp polyp (hyperplastic pulpitis) within a carious maxillary premolar.

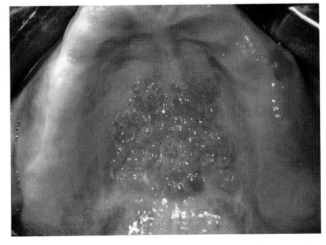

FIGURE 7   Papillary hyperplasia under a poorly fitting maxillary complete denture.

or long-standing lesions, although lesions may exhibit pseudoepitheliomatous hyperplasia. There is no neoplastic potential, a finding that is borne out by the absence of atypia and cellular dysplasia in biopsy specimens and no association with squamous cell carcinoma. Mild cases may be treated successfully by topical or systemic antifungals alone[14]; otherwise, papillary hyperplasia is surgically excised or removed by electrocautery, cryosurgery, or laser surgery. The old denture or a palatal splint can be used as a postoperative surgical dressing, followed by fabrication of a new denture.[15]

Fibrous inflammatory hyperplasias have no malignant potential, and recurrences following excision are almost always a result of the failure to eliminate the source of chronic irritation. The occasional report of squamous cell carcinoma arising in an area of chronic denture irritation, however, underlines the fact that no oral growth, even that associated with an obvious chronic irritant, can be assumed to be benign until proven so by histologic study. Thus, whenever possible, all fibrous inflammatory hyperplasias of the oral cavity should be treated by local excision, with microscopic examination of the excised tissue.

PYOGENIC GRANULOMA, PREGNANCY EPULIS, AND PERIPHERAL OSSIFYING OR CEMENTIFYING FIBROMA

Pyogenic granuloma is a hemorrhagic nodule that occurs most frequently on the gingiva and that has a strong tendency to recur after simple excision if the associated irritant is not removed (Figure 8).[16] It may be difficult on occasion to identify the causative chronic irritation for these lesions, but their close proximity to the gingival margin suggests that calculus, food materials, and overhanging dental restoration margins are important irritants that should be eliminated when the lesion is excised. Their friable, hemorrhagic, and frequently ulcerated appearance correlates with their histologic structure. They are composed of proliferating endothelial tissue, much of which is canalized into a rich vascular network with minimal collagenous support. Neutrophils, as well as chronic inflammatory cells, are consistently present throughout the edematous stroma, with microabscess formation. Histologically, differentiation from a hemangioma is important. Despite the common name for the lesion, a frank discharge of pus is not present; when such a discharge occurs, it is likely a fistula from an underlying periodontal or periapical abscess, the opening of which is often marked by a nodule of granulation tissue (parulis).

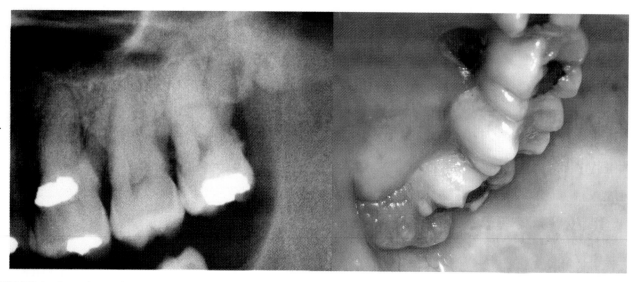

FIGURE 8 Pyogenic granuloma associated with a periodontal defect on the distal aspect of the maxillary left third molar. There is radiographic evidence of subgingival calculus, a likely etiologic factor.

Identical lesions with the same histologic structure occur in association with the florid gingivitis and periodontitis that may complicate pregnancy[17] and are referred to as pregnancy epulis or pregnancy tumor. The prevalence of pregnancy epulides increases toward the end of pregnancy (when levels of circulating estrogens are highest), and they tend to shrink after delivery (when there is a precipitous drop in circulating estrogens). This suggests that hormones play a role in the etiology of the lesion,[18] secondary to an increase in angiogenic factor expression and a reduction in the apoptosis of granulation tissue.[19] Similar to pregnancy gingivitis, these lesions do not occur in mouths that are kept scrupulously free of even minor gingival irritation, and local irritation is clearly also an important etiologic factor. Both pyogenic granulomas and pregnancy epulides may mature and become less vascular and more collagenous, gradually converting to fibrous epu-

lides. Small isolated pregnancy tumors occurring in a mouth that is otherwise in excellent gingival health may sometimes be observed for resolution following delivery, but the size of the lesion or the presence of a generalized pregnancy gingivitis or periodontitis supports the need for treatment during pregnancy.

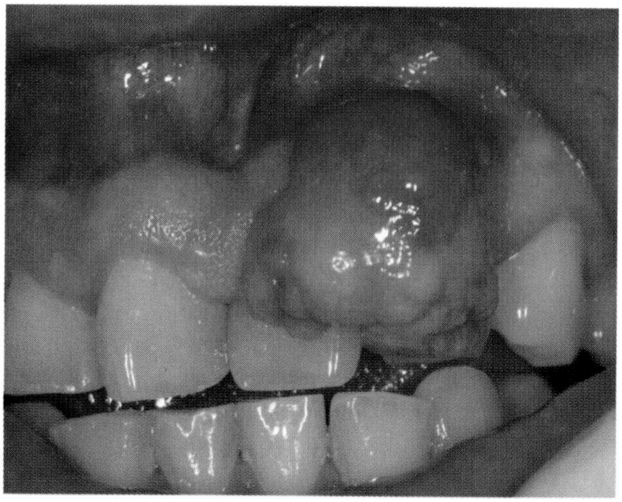

The peripheral ossifying or cementifying fibroma is found exclusively on the gingiva; it does not arise in other oral mucosal locations. Clinically, it varies from pale pink to cherry red and is typically located in the interdental papilla region (Figure 9). This reactive proliferation is named because of the histologic evidence of calcifications that are seen in the context of a hypercellular fibroblastic stroma. Peripheral ossifying or cementifying fibromas occur in teenagers and young adults and are more common in women. The existence of these lesions indicates the need for a periodontal consultation, and treatment should include the elimination of subgingival irritants and gingival pockets throughout the mouth, as well as excision of the gingival growth.

PERIPHERAL GIANT CELL GRANULOMA

Giant cell granuloma occurs either as a peripheral exophytic lesion found exclusively on the gingiva or as a centrally located lesion within the jaw, skull, or facial bones (the central giant cell granuloma is described in the section that includes bone lesions). Peripheral giant cell granulomas are five times as common as the central lesions. Both peripheral and central lesions are histologically similar and are considered to be examples of benign inflammatory hyperplasia in which cells with fibroblastic, osteoblastic, and osteoclastic potential predominate.[20]

NODULAR FASCIITIS AND PROLIFERATIVE MYOSITIS

Nodular fasciitis, a non-neoplastic connective tissue proliferation, usually occurs on the trunk or extremities of young adults. It appears as a rapidly growing nodule that

FIGURE 9 Peripheral ossifying fibroma in a teenage male associated with the maxillary buccal gingiva. The lesion was pedunculated.

histologically imitates a malignant mesenchymal neoplasm but that clinically behaves in a benign fashion. Oral nodular fasciitis occurs at all ages, with the majority during the fourth and fifth decades, with no gender predilection. The most common oral site is the buccal mucosa, most have an exophytic presentation, and growth rates are variable.[21] Nodular fasciitis has distinctive microscopic features that allow for the diagnosis, and the predominant cell type is the myofibroblast. The microscopic features of some of these lesions resemble a sarcoma, and this presents a diagnostic challenge for the pathologist.

Proliferative myositis[22] and focal myositis[23,24] are lesions of skeletal muscle that have similar clinical features and are differentiated by histopathologic findings. Rare cases have been described in the tongue and in other neck and jaw muscles. Proliferative myositis is a reactive fibroblastic lesion that infiltrates around individual muscle fibers. Despite the nomenclature, these lesions do not show histologic signs of inflammation.

GINGIVAL ENLARGEMENT

Gingival enlargement or overgrowth is usually caused by local inflammatory conditions such as poor oral hygiene, food impaction, or mouth breathing. Systemic conditions such as hormonal changes, drug therapy, or tumor infiltrates may also cause or contribute to the severity of gingival enlargement. Histologically, there are a number of explanations for gingival enlargement: hypertrophy (an increase in cell size), hyperplasia (an actual increase in cell number), edema, vascular engorgement, the presence of an inflammatory cell infiltrate, or an increase in dense fibrous connective tissue. One or more of these explanations may predominate depending on the underlying cause.

Inflammatory Gingival Enlargement. Inflammatory gingival enlargement occurs in sites of chronic suboptimal oral hygiene where there is accumulation of plaque, supragingival

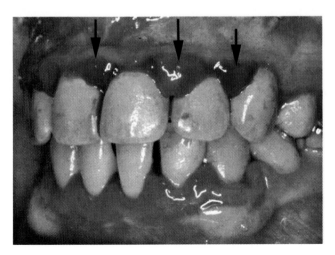

FIGURE 10 Inflammatory gingival enlargement secondary to local factors. Note edematous bright red or purplish-red color and a tendency to hemorrhage upon slight provocation (see *arrows*).

calculus formation, impaction of food, or the presence of aggravating factors such as orthodontic appliances, mouth breathing, hormonal changes, or other systemic diseases. The clinical diagnosis of inflammatory gingival enlargement is straightforward, with tissues exhibiting a glossy edematous bright red or purplish red color and a tendency to hemorrhage on slight provocation (Figure 10). A fetid odor may result from the decomposition of food debris and accumulation of bacteria. In long-standing cases of inflammatory enlargement, there may be an associated loss of periodontal attachment leading to periodontal disease.

Histologically, the exudative and proliferative features of chronic inflammation are seen: a preponderance of inflammatory cells, vascular engorgement, new capillary formation, and associated degenerative changes. Pseudopockets formed by gingival enlargement make the maintenance of good oral hygiene difficult, perpetuating a cycle of inflammation. Long-standing inflammatory gingival enlargement may demonstrate relatively firm, resilient, and pink gingivae that do not bleed readily or demonstrate pitting edema following directly applied pressure with a periodontal probe. This is due to a greater fibrous component with an abundance of fibroblasts and collagen fibers.

Gingival inflammation affecting primarily the maxillary anterior region may be observed in mouth breathers.[25] Hormonal changes (such as during pregnancy or puberty) may exaggerate the local immune response to local factors and contribute to gingival enlargement.[26] The impaired collagen synthesis associated with vitamin C deficiency (scurvy) may also complicate inflammatory gingival enlargement.

Treatment of the inflammatory type of gingival enlargement begins with the establishment of excellent oral hygiene, together with the elimination of all local and/or systemic predisposing factors if possible. This includes a professional débridement (supragingival scaling or subgingival root planing) and prophylaxis and correction of faulty restorations, carious lesions, or food impaction sites. Close follow-up after initial therapy is required to assess improvements in home care and tissue response that will dictate subsequent treatment options. For refractory cases, adjunctive topical or systemic antimicrobials or surgical options may be indicated. The successful treatment of gingival enlargement in mouth breathers depends primarily on the elimination of the habit. Patients should be referred to an otolaryngologist to determine if there is any obstruction of the upper air passages and/or to an orthodontist to assess the potential for treatment to permit the normal closure of the lips during sleep. A tissue biopsy should be considered whenever the cause is unclear, when there is a poor response to local therapy, or to rule out rare systemic diseases that may present with gingival enlargement (eg, acute myelogenous leukemia).

Drug-Induced Gingival Enlargement. Drug-induced gingival enlargement is most commonly associated with the administration of anticonvulsants (principally phenytoin), cyclosporine, and calcium channel blocking agents. The

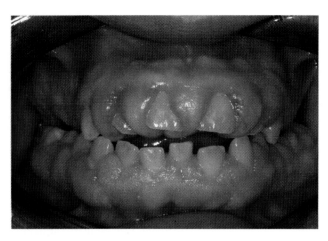

FIGURE 11 Gingival enlargement secondary to long-standing phenytoin use.

extent of inflammation, fibrosis, and cellularity depends on the duration, dose, and identity of the drug; on the quality of oral hygiene; and on individual susceptibility that stems from genetic factors and environmental influences. These drugs likely exert their influence not by direct regulation of extracellular matrix metabolism or proliferation of gingival fibroblasts but due to the dysregulation of cytokines and growth factors.[27]

Phenytoin-induced gingival enlargement (Figure 11) is the most prevalent, affecting approximately 50% of patients who use the drug for longer than 3 months.[28] Although rare, gingival enlargement has also been reported in patients taking other anticonvulsants, namely valproic acid, phenobarbital, and vigabatrin.[28] The immunosuppressant agent cyclosporine causes gingival enlargement in 25 to 30% of adults and, notably, in greater than 70% of children (Figure 12).[28] Nifedipine and dilitiazem are responsible for most cases of calcium channel blocker–induced gingival enlargement, with a prevalence of approximately 5 to 20%.[28] There are also reports of gingival enlargement following use of verapamil, felodipine, and amlodipine.

There is a characteristic clinical appearance of drug-induced gingival hyperplasia, although there is much

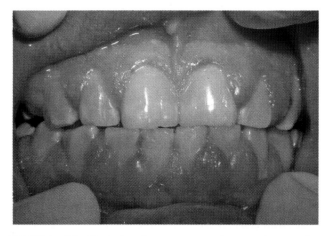

FIGURE 12 Gingival enlargement secondary to long-standing cyclosporine use.

variation predicted by various factors, principally plaque-associated gingival inflammation. After approximately 1 month of drug use, interdental papillae enlargement begins, usually in the anterior regions. The attached gingivae are generally involved, although the enlargement may become more extensive, leading to gingival disfigurement and associated esthetic and functional complications. There are reports that cyclosporine-induced enlargements are less fibrotic compared with those caused by phenytoin or calcium channel blockers.[27] The diagnosis is easily established based on the history of chronic drug use and the clinical appearance.

Prevention through optimal oral hygiene is essential to minimize the severity of enlargement. For patients treated for epilepsy, medications must be reviewed before orthodontic treatment is begun. There are several treatment options for drug-induced gingival enlargement. The most predictable treatment is either the withdrawal or change of medication. However, the control of the underlying medical condition necessitating the use of these medications is not always guaranteed following replacement with a new medication, and physicians may be reluctant to change the patient's regimen. There are, however, a variety of new-generation anticonvulsants, immunosuppressants, and antihypertensives available today. Tacrolimus is a new immunosuppressant that has been shown to be an effective replacement for cyclosporine and does not cause gingival enlargement.[27] Nonsurgical treatments such as professional gingival débridement and topical or systemic antimicrobials may ameliorate gingival enlargement. There are equivocal reports supporting the efficacy of systemic antibiotics, most notably azithromycin to treat renal transplant patients with cyclosporine-induced enlargement.[29] Surgical management is reserved for severe cases and usually does not provide long-term efficacy.[29] Conventional gingivectomy is the most commonly employed, although periodontal flap surgery may be indicated when osseous recontouring is needed, if there are mucogingival considerations, or in pediatric patients in whom tooth eruption is affected. Laser ablation gingivectomy may offer an advantage over conventional surgery since procedures are faster and there is improved hemostasis and more rapid healing.[29]

Hereditary Gingival Fibromatosis. Both autosomal dominant and autosomal recessive patterns of inheritance are recognized. Genetic heterogeneity and variable expressivity contribute to the difficulty encountered in assigning this diagnosis to a specific syndrome. Gingival fibromatosis without other syndrome-associated physical or mental abnormalities is not rare (Figure 13). A putative inherited mutation is in the *sos1* gene.[27] Enlargement may be present at birth or may become apparent only with the eruption of the deciduous or permanent dentitions. The most common problems associated with hereditary gingival fibromatosis are tooth migration, prolonged retention of the primary dentition, and diastemata. Enlargement may completely cover the crowns of the teeth, resulting in difficulty masticating or speaking and poor esthetics. Histologic features include proliferative fibrous overgrowth with a highly collagenized connective tissue stroma sparsely populated with fibroblasts and blood vessels.

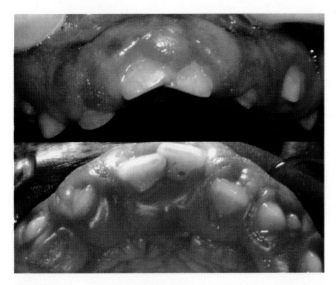

FIGURE 13 Hereditary gingival fibromatosis. Note the severity, with almost complete coverage of teeth in some locations.

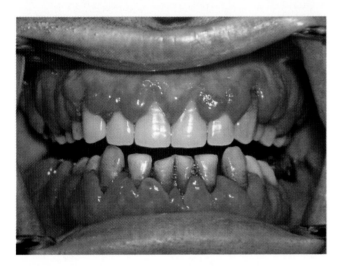

FIGURE 14 Gingival enlargement associated with acute myelogenous leukemia.

Other Causes of Gingival Enlargement. Patients with acute myelogenous leukemia (principally acute monocytic [M4] or acute myelomonocytic [M5] leukemia) may present with gingival leukemic infiltrates (Figure 14).[30] Others include von Recklinghausen's neurofibromatosis (neurofibromatosis 1), Wegener's granulomatosis, sarcoidosis, Crohn's disease, primary amyloidosis, Kaposi's sarcoma, acromegaly, and lymphoma.

Benign Soft Tissue Tumors

Oral mucosal benign tumors comprise lesions that form from fibrous tissue, adipose tissue, nerve, and muscle. Benign proliferations of blood vessels and lymphatic vessels resemble neoplasms but do not have unlimited growth potential and therefore are more appropriately considered hamartomatous proliferations.

EPITHELIAL TUMORS

There are several benign oral epithelial virus–induced growths, principally those caused by the human papillomavirus (HPV).[31,32] Molecular biologic techniques (eg, in situ hybridization, polymerase chain reaction) used to detect HPV[33,34] reveal that viral deoxyribonucleic acid (DNA) can be found in these lesions but may also be present in normal oral mucosa. There are more than 120 HPV strains, of which at least 25 have been detected in oral lesions. Much attention has been focused on the relationship between HPV and oral carcinogenesis (see Chapter 7, "Oral Cancer"). High-risk oncogenic HPV subtypes (primarily HPV 16, but also HPV 18, 31, 33, 35) are commonly detected in oral squamous cell carcinomas (27–47%). They are found to a lesser extent in premalignant lesions and on occasion observed in normal mucosa.[35,36] HPV is more likely to be detected in cancers involving the oropharynx and tonsils compared with the oral cavity.[37]

Of the benign oral epithelial HPV–induced growths (Figures 15), oral squamous papilloma is relatively common. It usually occurs in the third to fifth decades, most commonly as an isolated small growth (< 1 cm diameter) on the palate, ranging in color from pink to white, rugose (ridged or wrinkled), exophytic, and pedunculated. When these lesions occur on the surface of the lips, alveolar gingivae, or palate, they are well keratinized, and on nonkeratinized mucosal surfaces, they appear soft and pink/red. HPV DNA is detected in approximately 50% of squamous papillomas, predominantly HPV 6, followed by HPV 11.[32]

The common wart, verucca vulgaris, is generally found on the skin (sometimes in association with similar skin lesions, often on the fingers) and is caused by the cutaneous HPV subtypes 2 and 57. When involving the oral cavity, these warts are similar in appearance to squamous papillomas and tend to involve the lips, gingivae, and hard palate. Oral papillomas and warts are clinically similar, and local excision is desirable. Care should be exercised when removing HPV-related oral lesions with electrocautery or laser as there exists the possibility of aerosolizing HPV particles. Although these lesions are probably infectious, a history of direct contact with another infected person is unusual, except in the case of multiple and often recurrent oral warts associated with sexual contact or maternal transmission, referred to as condyloma acuminatum (see Chapter 20, Infectious Diseases). HPV 6 and 11 are detected in these lesions.

Focal epithelial hyperplasia (Heck's disease), a condition characterized by numerous soft, well-circumscribed, flat, and sessile (ie, nonpapillomatous) papules that are distributed throughout the oral mucosa, is endemic in some Eskimo and Native American communities but is rare in white people. Recent findings among Puerto Ricans and blacks suggest that further searches for this lesion may show it to be more widespread. Histologically, it is characterized by nondyskeratotic nodular acanthosis, which forms the basis of the papules, and a subepithelial lymphocytic infiltration. HPV DNA 13 and 32 are detected in 75 to 100% of these lesions.[32]

Intraoral papillomatosis, often florid, is common in the HIV-infected population (Figure 16), particularly since the

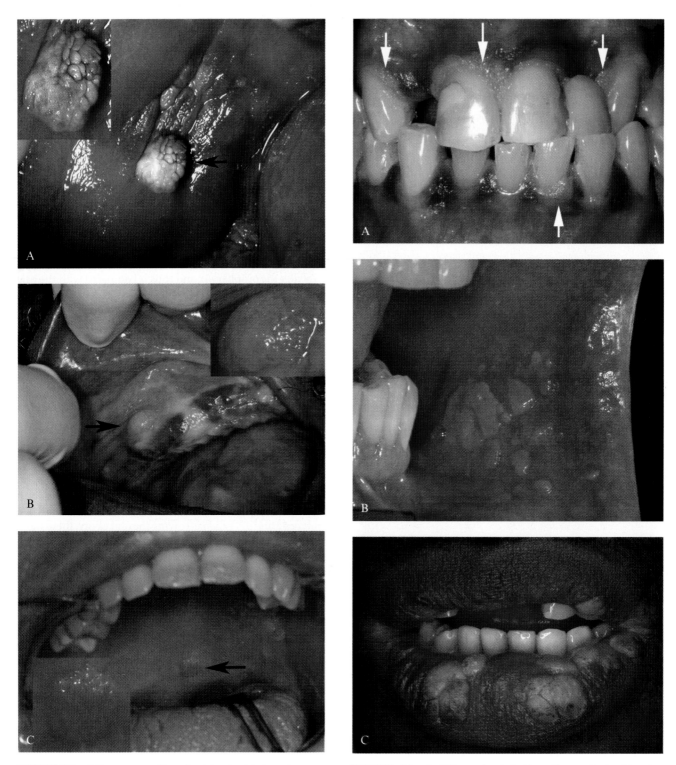

FIGURE 15 *A,* Squamous papilloma involving the right buccal mucosa. Note the papillary and highly keratinized surface, presumably related to the location (see *inset*). *B,* Squamous papilloma with a pebbled surface (*inset*) involving the right maxillary alveolar ridge. *C,* Squamous papilloma with a pebbled surface (*inset*) involving the soft palate.

FIGURE 16 *A,* HIV-associated florid papillomatosis involving free marginal gingivae. *B,* HIV-associated florid papillomatosis involving buccal mucosa. Note coalescing papules, which are flat. *C,* HIV-associated florid papillomatosis involving the lips.

advent of highly active antiretroviral therapy (HAART).[38] Florid papillomatosis may also occur in patients with conditions such as ichthyosis hystrix (a congenitally acquired deforming skin papillomatosis) and Down syndrome.

Molluscum contagiosum is a dermatologic infection acquired by direct skin contact and characterized by clusters of tiny firm nodules that can be curetted from the skin. It is composed of clumps of proliferating epithelial cells with prominent eosinophilic inclusion bodies. This condition is not a neoplasm, but it is included here as one of the spectra of oral epithelial proliferations that result from viral infection. Both intraoral and labial lesions of molluscum contagiosum have been reported,[39,40] principally in human immunodeficiency virus (HIV)-infected patients. It is caused by a poxvirus that infects the skin, where the virus replicates in the stratum spinosum, producing the characteristic and pathognomonic Cowdry type A inclusion bodies that are commonly associated with poxvirus infections but apparently producing only a small number of complete viruses.[41]

Keratoacanthoma[42,43] is a localized lesion that is typically found on sun-exposed skin, including the upper lip. The rapid growth of a keratoacanthoma may be quite frightening, to the point where it is often mistakenly diagnosed as squamous or basal cell carcinoma. These lesions appear fixed to the surrounding tissue (similar to some carcinomas), often grow rapidly, and are usually capped by thick keratin. Occasionally, the lesion matures, exfoliates, and heals spontaneously, but more frequently, block excision is required, and the diagnosis is established from microscopic evaluation. Epithelial tissue adjacent to the lesion is sharply demarcated from that of the lesion, which appears to lie in a cup-shaped depression. The proliferating epithelium constituting this lesion consists of masses of reasonably well-differentiated squamous cells that often produce keratin pearls and show little cellular atypia. The lesion's usual location on the upper lip (where squamous cell carcinoma of actinic etiology is rare, compared with the lower lip) should remind the clinician to consider keratoacanthoma in the differential diagnosis. Intraoral keratoacanthomas are rare.[44,45] Treatment of this lesion is conservative excision, although some believe that it is not clearly separable from squamous cell carcinoma and advocate wide excision to prevent recurrence.

VASCULAR LESIONS

Hemangiomas. Hemangiomas of the head and neck appear a few weeks after birth and grow rapidly. They are characterized by endothelial cell hyperplasia and in most cases undergo involution, with residual telangiectatic, fatty, or scar tissue apparent in approximately 40 to 50% of patients.[46] They have been described in almost all head and neck locations in a variety of presentations: superficial and deep, small and large, most commonly as solitary lesions but also as multiple lesions. Small lesions may be clinically indistinguishable from pyogenic granulomas and superficial venous varicosities. Hemangiomas may be classified as capillary or cavernous types; the former is superficial and the latter is deeper.

Vascular Malformations. Vascular malformations (Figure 17) may be clinically apparent at birth, grow slowly proportional to the growth of the child (characterized by hypertrophy), and never involute. They may be classified depending on the vessel type involved or flow types: arterial and arteriovenous (high flow), capillary, or venous (low flow). Centrally located malformations must be distinguished from the many osteolytic tumors and cyst-like lesions that affect the jaws (see below). Arterial and arteriovenous malformations may first

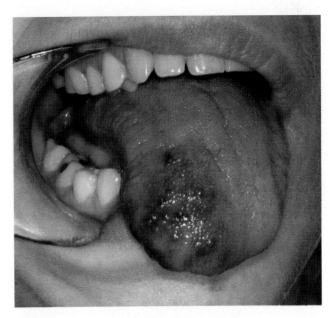

FIGURE 17 Vascular malformation involving the tongue, which developed 2 months previously in a 25-year-old female.

develop following hormonal changes (such as puberty), infections, or trauma, and, clinically, they may be firm, pulsatile, and warm. Venous malformations can sometimes appear first in early adulthood, and, clinically, they are soft and easily compressible.

Diascopy is the technique of applying pressure to a suspected vascular lesion to visualize the evacuation of coloration (Figure 18) and may facilitate the differentiation of a small vascular lesion from a pigmented lesion (see Chapter 5, Pigmented Lesions of the Oral Mucosa). Care should be taken in performing biopsies or excising all vascular lesions: (1) they have a tendency for uncontrolled hemorrhage and (2) the extent of the lesion is unknown since only a small portion may be evident in the mouth. Therefore, identification of the precise anatomic location and depth of tissue extent is warranted before treatment, particularly for the high-flow lesions. Angiography, computed tomography (CT), and magnetic resonance imaging (MRI) are all useful imaging techniques.[47] Treatment modalities (alone or in combination) include superselective intra-arterial embolization (SIAE), sclerotherapy, radiotherapy, or surgical excision/resection using electrocoagulation, cryosurgery, or laser surgery.[48–50]

Angiomatous Syndromes. A number of syndromes are associated with vascular malformations, including Osler-Weber-Rendu syndrome (hereditary hemorrhagic telangiectasia)[51] (Figure 19), blue rubber bleb nevus syndrome, syndrome, Bannayan-Zonana, Sturge-Weber[52] (Figure 20), Klippel-Trénaunay syndrome, Servelle-Martorell syndrome, von Hippel-Lindau syndrome,[53] and Maffucci's syndrome.[54]

Lymphangioma. Lymphangioma is considered to be lymphatic malformation, similar to other vascular malforma-

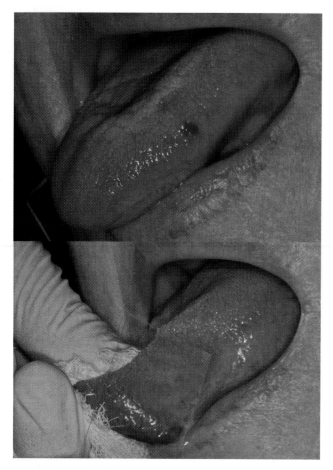

FIGURE 18 Diascopy of a small capillary malformation on the lateral border of the tongue. Note blanching of the lesion.

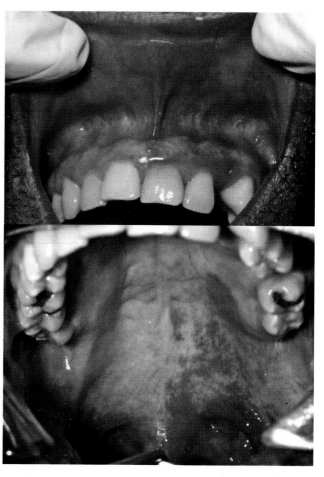

FIGURE 20 Sturge-Weber syndrome. Hypervascular changes are unilateral, which is consistent with a trigeminal nerve distribution, in this case following the second (maxillary) branch of the left trigeminal nerve.

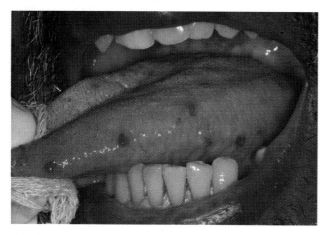

FIGURE 19 Osler-Wendu-Rendu syndrome (hereditary hemorrhagic telangiectasia). Note discrete multiple red papules associated with dilated vessels. Patient has similar papules distributed on his labial mucosae and finger tips.

tions, yet characterized by an abnormal proliferation of lymphatic vessels.[55] The most common extraoral and intraoral sites are the neck (predominantly in the posterior triangle) and tongue, respectively. The vast majority (80–90%) of lymphangiomas arise within the first 2 years of life and are an important cause of congenital macroglossia.[55] Clinically, lymphangiomas are a slow-growing and painless soft tissue mass. This frequently presents without a clear anatomic outline, dissects tissue planes, and can be more extensive than anticipated. Intraosseous lymphangiomas have been reported.[56] Occasionally, they may undergo a rapid increase in size secondary to inflammation from an infection or hemorrhage from trauma. Large lymphangiomas may become life threatening if they compromise the airway or vital blood vessels,[57] and those spreading into and distending the neck are macrocystic and are referred to as cystic hygromas.

Differential diagnoses of lymphangiomas of the tongue include hemangioma, congenital hypothyroidism, mongolism, amyloidosis, neurofibromatosis, various storage diseases (eg, Hurler's syndrome and glycogen storage disease), and primary muscular hypertrophy of the tongue, all of which may cause macroglossia. Abnormalities of the mucosa overlying a lymphangioma may give the appearance of a localized glossitis and may draw attention to the presence of a small lesion buried in the tongue. The typical oral lymphangioma has a racemose or pebbly surface.

The treatment of lymphangiomas is dictated by their type, anatomic site, and extent of infiltration into surrounding structures.[58] Surgical excision is the most common, and sclerotherapy (with chemotherapeutic agents such as picabinil [OK-432] or ethanol) is also advocated.[59,60] Recurrence of oral lymphangiomas has been reported, presumably because the lesion is interwoven between muscle fibers, preventing complete removal.

Glomus Tumor and Other Vascular Endothelial Growths. An unusual abnormality, glomus tumor[61] (glomangioma) develops as a small, painful, unencapsulated nodule. It represents a proliferation of the modified smooth muscle pericytic cells found in the characteristic type of peripheral arteriovenous anastomosis known as the glomus. In addition to having a distinctive histology, these lesions also may secrete various catecholamines. The glomus tumor is rare in the mouth but can occur around the carotid body, in the jugulotympanic region, and in the vagus nerve.[62] Glomus tumors arising in the carotid bodies may produce neck masses and are referred to as chemodectomas or paragangliomas.

NEUROGENIC LESIONS

Traumatic Neuroma. A traumatic neuroma is not a true tumor but a proliferation of nerve tissue that is caused by injury to a peripheral nerve.[63–65] Nerve tissue is encased in a sheath composed of Schwann cells and their fibers. When this sheath is disrupted, the nerve loses its framework. When a nerve and its sheath are damaged, the proximal end of the damaged nerve proliferates into a mass of nerve and Schwann cells mixed with dense fibrous scar tissue. In the oral cavity, injury to a nerve may occur from injection of local anesthesia, surgery, or other sources of trauma.[66] Traumatic neuromas are often painful. The discomfort may range from pain on palpation to severe and constant pain. Most traumatic neuromas occur in adults. Traumatic neuromas in the oral cavity may occur in any location where a nerve is damaged; the mental foramen area is the most common location. The definitive diagnosis is made on the basis of a biopsy and microscopic examination. Traumatic neuromas are treated by surgical excision. Recurrence rates for neuromas are rare.

Oral Mucosal Neuromas and Multiple Endocrine Neoplasia Syndrome. Multiple endocrine neoplasia (MEN) syndromes are a group of disorders that are characterized by tumors or hyperplasias of neuroendocrine tissues.[67] MEN 2B (multiple endocrine neoplasia type 2B or mucosal neuroma syndrome 7) presents with a characteristic phenotype that includes medullary thyroid carcinoma, pheochromocytoma, and neuroma on oral mucosal tissues. MEN 2B is transmitted as an autosomal dominant trait. Identification of mucosal neuromas may precede other components of the syndrome. Management includes prophylactic total thyroidectomy before the age of 4 years.

Palisaded Encapsulated Neuroma. The palisaded encapsulated neuroma[68] is a benign tumor of the peripheral nerve that clinically and histologically resembles the neurofibroma and schwannoma. The lesions are solitary and found in older adults, a feature that distinguishes them from the neuromas in MEN syndrome. The palisaded encapsulated neuroma is a well-circumscribed partially encapsulated nodule composed of spindle-shaped cells exhibiting areas of nuclear palisading often admixed with axons. They contain Schwann cells, perineural cells, and axons and can be distinguished from neurofibromas and schwannomas both by their light microscopic appearance and by immunohistochemical stain that is positive for EMA and S-100.[68] The palisaded encapsulated neuroma is treated by conservative excision, and recurrence is rare.

Neurofibroma and Schwannoma. Neurofibroma and schwannoma (neurilemmoma) are benign tumors derived from the tissue that envelops nerves and includes Schwann cells and fibroblasts.[69,70] Although neurofibroma and schwannoma are distinct tumors microscopically, they are quite similar in their clinical presentation and behavior. The tongue is the most common intraoral location (Figure 21). Neurofibromas and schwannomas may occur at any age, without any sex predilection. Microscopic examination of a neurofibroma reveals a fairly well-delineated but diffuse proliferation of spindle-shaped Schwann cells. A schwannoma is encapsulated and exhibits varying amounts of two different microscopic patterns. One pattern consists of cells in a palisaded arrangement around eosinophilic areas and the other consists of less cellular spindle-shaped cells in a loose myxoid-appearing stroma. For these two lesions, light microscopic examination is generally sufficient to establish the diagnosis. The partial encapsulation of a palisaded encapsulated neuroma may resemble the schwannoma. Differences in immunohistochemical staining have been demonstrated and may be helpful in establishing the definitive diagnosis. The treatment for a neurofibroma or schwannoma is surgical excision. They generally do not recur.

Neurofibromatosis. Multiple neurofibromas occur in a genetically inherited disorder known as neurofibromatosis 1 (NF1) or von Recklinghausen's disease. This disease is transmitted as an autosomal dominant trait, and the *NF1* gene has been identified.[71] Oral neurofibromas are a common feature of the disease. The presence of numerous neurofibromas or a plexiform-type neurofibroma is pathognomonic of NF1.

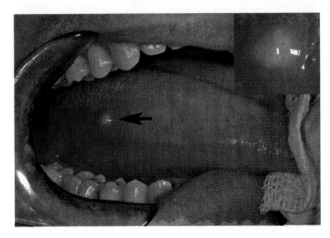

FIGURE 21 Neurogenic tumor involving the right lateral tongue.

Patients with NF1 are at increased risk of the development of malignant tumors, especially malignant peripheral nerve sheath tumor, leukemia, and rhabdomyosarcoma.[71–73]

Granular Cell Tumor. The granular cell tumor is a benign tumor composed of large cells with a granular cytoplasm. The pathogenesis of this tumor has not been established, but most evidence suggests that it arises from Schwann cells or their primitive mesenchymal precursors. The granular cell tumor most often occurs on the tongue (Figure 22A), followed by the buccal and labial mucosa. Other intraoral sites include the palate (Figure 22B), gingiva, and the floor of the mouth. The tumor appears as a painless, nonulcerated nodule. The majority of cases occur in adults with a female predilection. Immunocytochemical staining[74–76] reveals reactivity for S-100 protein and myelin. A report of a granular cell variant of the traumatic neuroma[77] supports further the neurogenic origin of this tumor, as do reports of granular cell tumors associated with neurofibromatosis.[78] Microscopic examination reveals large oval-shaped cells with a granular cytoplasm. The granular cells are found in the connective tissue. The overlying surface epithelium exhibits pseudoepitheliomatous hyperplasia, which is a benign proliferation of epithelium into the connective tissue. This tumor is treated by conservative surgical excision and does not recur.

The congenital epulis, or congenital epulis of the newborn, is a benign neoplasm composed of cells that closely resemble those seen in the granular cell tumor that occurs in adults. The ultrastructural and immunohistochemical features are different from the granular cell tumor that occurs in adults, confirming that this lesion is a completely separate entity. The neoplasm most likely arises from a primitive mesenchymal cell.[79] The congenital epulis is present at birth and presents as a smooth-surfaced, sessile, or pedunculated mass on the gingiva. It usually occurs on the anterior maxillary alveolar ridge and almost always occurs in girls. The congenital epulis is treated by surgical excision and does not recur. Occasionally, the tumors will regress without treatment.[80]

Melanotic Neuroectodermal Tumor of Infancy. Melanotic neuroectodermal tumor of infancy is a benign neoplasm that occurs in young children and almost always occurs during the first year of life. Results of ultrastructural and immunocytochemical studies of this tumor are consistent with its origin from cells of the neural crest. The tumor most commonly occurs in the maxilla, followed by the skull, mandible, and brain. The tumor presents as a rapidly enlarging mass that destroys bone and may exhibit blue-black pigmentation. It has a high recurrence rate, and malignant transformation has been reported rarely. Histologically, the tumor is composed of collections of cells that resemble melanocytes admixed with smaller round cells and variable amounts of melanin. High levels of urinary vanillylmandelic acid are often found in patients with this tumor, and the levels tend to return to normal when the tumor is resected. Conservative surgical removal is usually adequate, but the behavior of this tumor is unpredictable.[81,82]

LIPOMA

The lipoma is a benign tumor of mature fat cells.[83] When occurring in the superficial soft tissue, the lipoma appears as a yellowish mass with a thin surface of epithelium (Figure 23). Because of this thin epithelium, a delicate pattern of blood vessels is usually observed on the surface. Deeper lesions may not demonstrate this finding and therefore are not as easily identified clinically. The majority of oral lipomas are found on the buccal mucosa and tongue and occur in individuals over 40 years of age, without any sex predilection.

There are several microscopic variants of the lipoma. The classic description is of a well-delineated tumor composed of lobules of mature fat cells that are uniform in size and shape. Those tumors with a significant fibrous connective tissue component are designated fibrolipoma, those with numerous small blood vessels angiolipoma, those with a mucoid background myxoid lipomas, and those with an admixture of uniform spindle cells spindle cell lipoma. The pleomorphic lipoma demonstrates spindle cells and bizarre, hyperchromatic giant cells and may be difficult for the pathologist to

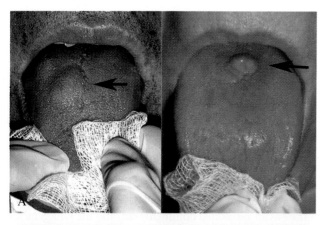

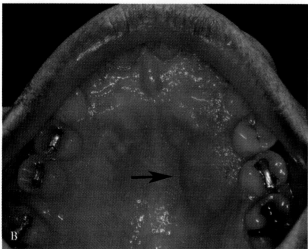

FIGURE 22 *A,* Granular cell tumors of the tongue, the most common site for this benign lesion. *B,* Granular cell tumor involving the palate, an unusual site.

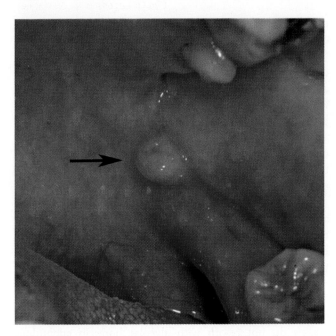

FIGURE 23 Lipoma involving the buccal mucosa. Note yellow color.

clearly distinguish from a pleomorphic liposarcoma. A lipoma that infiltrates among skeletal muscle bundles is called an intramuscular lipoma. It has been reported in the oral soft tissues but is rare.[84] The lipoma is treated by conservative surgical excision and generally does not recur. Intramuscular lipomas have a somewhat higher recurrence rate because they are more difficult to remove completely.

TUMORS OF MUSCLE

Tumors of muscle are extremely uncommon in the oral cavity. The rhabdomyoma, a benign tumor of striated muscle, has been reported to occur on the tongue. The vascular leiomyoma, a benign tumor of smooth muscle cell and vascular endothelium, occasionally occurs in the oral cavity. Treatment is local surgical excision, and recurrence is rare.[85]

▼ BENIGN LESIONS OF BONE

Benign Fibro-osseous Lesions

Benign fibro-osseous lesion is a generic histologic designation for a diverse group of bone lesions that are named for the similarity of their histologic appearance. They are composed of cellular fibrous connective tissue admixed with either osteoid and bone trabeculae or rounded small to large calcified masses that have traditionally been described as cementoid material. Benign fibro-osseous lesions of the jaws include fibrous dysplasia, ossifying and cementifying fibroma, and the cemento-osseous dysplasias. Radiologic imaging is critical for establishing a diagnosis.[86]

Fibrous Dysplasia

Fibrous dysplasia is a disease that is characterized by the replacement of bone with fibro-osseous tissue. The well-vascularized and cellular fibrous tissue contains trabeculae

or spherules (small spheres) of poorly calcified nonlamellar bone that are formed by osseous metaplasia. Fibrous dysplasia starts in childhood, presenting with a slowly progressive enlargement of bone that generally slows or ceases with puberty.[87,88] The pathogenesis is unclear. The most widely accepted theory is that fibrous dysplasia results from an abnormality in the development of bone-forming mesenchyme. Radiographically, fibrous dysplasia classically presents with a "ground glass" appearance and may have varying degrees of radiopacity and lucency depending on the amount of calcified material present. The abnormal bone merges with the adjacent normal bone. CT and technetium 99m bone scans are very useful in the diagnosis of fibrous dysplasia.[89,90]

Biopsy of involved bone reveals a tissue that is often described as "gritty" or "sandy." Several forms of fibrous dysplasia have been described.[86,87] The monostotic form, characterized by the involvement of a single bone, is the most common form. Polyostotic forms are characterized by the involvement of more than one bone and include three different types: (1) craniofacial fibrous dysplasia, in which the maxilla and adjacent bones are involved; (2) Jaffe's type (or Jaffe-Lichtenstein type), in which there is multiple bone involvement along with an irregular macular melanin pigmentation of the skin (café au lait spots); and (3) rare cases in children (McCune-Albright syndrome or Albright's syndrome), in which there is severe, progressive bone involvement with café au lait skin pigmentation and precocious puberty. An elevation in serum alkaline phosphatase may be seen in patients with extensive polyostotic disease.[87] In most cases, once diagnosis has been confirmed, management is appropriate with superficial recontouring of the lesion or curettage of large radiolucent lesions.[91] Radiotherapy is contraindicated in the treatment of fibrous dysplasia. Radiotherapy administered in earlier decades of the twentieth century may have played a role in the rare cases of malignant transformation to fibrosarcoma or osteogenic sarcoma. Attempts at treating advanced cases of the polyostotic form with calcitonin[92] have not been successful.

The clinical problems associated with fibrous dysplasia of bone are related to the site and extent of involvement. In the long bones, deformity and fractures are common complications that often lead to the initial diagnosis. In the jaws and other parts of the craniofacial skeleton, involvement of adjacent structures such as the cranial sinuses, cranial nerves, and ocular contents can lead to serious complications in addition to cosmetic and functional problems. Intracranial lesions arising from the cranial bones may produce seizures and electroencephalographic changes. Extension into and occlusion of the maxillary and ethmoid sinuses and mastoid air spaces are common.[93] Proptosis, diplopia, and interference with jaw function also often prompt surgical intervention.

OSSIFYING FIBROMA AND CEMENTIFYING FIBROMA

Ossifying fibroma and cementifying fibroma are slow-growing, well-circumscribed, benign tumors of bone. They are two very similar and related lesions that probably arise from cells of the periodontal ligament. Radiographically, they both show well-circumscribed margins that are confirmed by subsequent surgery (Figure 24). The cementifying fibroma is usually classified as an odontogenic tumor.[87] The ossifying fibroma is classified as a benign fibro-osseous lesion that is histologically composed of cellular fibrous connective tissue containing varying amounts of osteoid and bone, whereas the cementifying fibroma has rounded cementoid calcifications. Some tumors exhibit combinations of both types of calcification, and these are generally diagnosed as cemento-ossifying fibromas. These benign tumors occur in the mandible more frequently than the maxilla. They are usually diagnosed in the third to fourth decades of age, with a female predilection. Treatment involves conservative surgical excision of the tumor. A variant of the ossifying fibroma is designated as a juvenile ossifying fibroma that appears in younger individuals. This tumor exhibits more aggressive behavior and a greater propensity for recurrence.[94]

CEMENTO-OSSEOUS DYSPLASIAS

Three forms of this dysplastic process involving bone of the jaws are described: periapical cemento-osseous dysplasia, focal cemento-osseous dysplasia, and florid cemento-osseous dysplasia. Periapical and florid types are generally most appropriately diagnosed on the basis of the clinical and radiographic features. The focal type requires a biopsy to establish a definitive diagnosis. The etiology and pathogenesis of these conditions are unknown.[87] These lesions become more

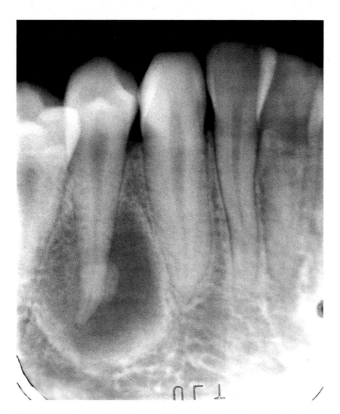

FIGURE 24 Ossifying fibroma. This is well-circumscribed radiolucency surrounding a central radiopacity in a 19-year-old man.

radiopaque with time; large calcified masses become a characteristic histologic feature.

Periapical cemento-osseous dysplasia, previously called cementoma, occurs at the apical aspect of vital mandibular anterior teeth.[95] It is most commonly reported in black women over age 40 years and begins with a radiolucent phase slowly increasing in radiodensity. The condition is asymptomatic and does not require treatment. Differential diagnosis includes dental pulp–related periapical inflammatory disease, and establishment of tooth vitality is critically important.

Focal cemento-osseous dysplasia differs from the periapical form since it occurs at the apical aspect of posterior teeth.[86] It is also reported to occur frequently in white women. Biopsy and histologic examination of the tissue are required to establish the diagnosis.

Florid cemento-osseous dysplasia presents an exuberant form of cemento-osseous dysplasia.[96] It may involve multiple quadrants in the maxilla as well as the mandible. The calcified masses do not resorb with alveolar bone in edentulous patients. In patients with tissue-borne removable dentures, secondary infection may occur from mucosal perforation and subsequent communication between the dysplastic bone and oral cavity.

Langerhans' Cell Histiocytosis (Langerhans' Cell Disease, Histiocytosis X)

Langerhans' cell histiocytosis, formerly called histiocytosis X, comprises a group of conditions that are characterized histologically by a monoclonal proliferation of large mononuclear cells accompanied by a prominent eosinophil infiltrate. The mononuclear cells have been identified as Langerhans' cells (the most peripheral cell of the immune system) by their immunologic staining characteristics and the presence of a cytoplasmic inclusion called the Birbeck granule.[97] Whether these conditions represent a neoplastic process or a non-neoplastic, immunologic, or reactive process remains controversial.

The clinical spectrum of Langerhans' cell histiocytosis includes (1) single or multiple bone lesions with no visceral involvement (eosinophilic granuloma); (2) a chronic disseminated form (Hand-Schüller-Christian disease) that includes a classic triad of skull lesions, exophthalmos, and diabetes insipidus; and (3) an acute disseminated form (Letterer-Siwe disease) that affects multiple organs and has a poor prognosis. Each of these forms tends to affect patients at different ages, with the eosinophilic granuloma affecting older children and young adults, the chronic disseminated form affecting young children, and the acute disseminated form affecting infants and children under the age of 2 years.[98–101]

The single or multiple eosinophilic granulomas with no systemic or visceral involvement are the most common presentation (Figure 25). Both the maxilla and the mandible may be affected in Langerhans' cell histiocytosis, both with and without systemic involvement. The lesions present radiographically as radiolucencies that range from sharply

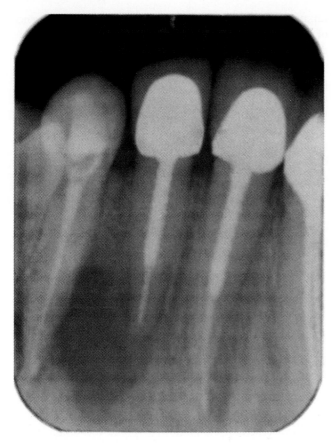

FIGURE 25 Eosinophilic granuloma. The radiolucency seen at the apical region of a mandibular lateral incisor and canine is an eosinophilic granuloma that has the radiographic appearance of a periapical inflammatory lesion.

demarcated, but without a sclerotic rim, to more diffuse radiolucencies. Alveolar bone destruction can mimic periodontal disease. The gingival soft tissues may also be involved, and this may resemble periapical or periodontal inflammatory disease.

The diagnosis of Langerhans' cell histiocytosis is made by biopsy and histologic examination. The treatment varies, based on the clinical presentation of the disease. Solitary eosinophilic granuloma may be treated by surgical curettage. Low-dose radiation therapy has been used successfully for lesions that are multiple, less accessible, or persistent.[100] The older the patient with Langerhans' cell histiocytosis and the less visceral involvement, the better the prognosis. Langerhans' cell histiocytosis is a life-threatening disease in infants and very young children.

Giant Cell Lesions of Bone

Giant cell lesions include the peripheral giant cell granuloma (see soft tissue tumors above) and the central giant cell granuloma, aneurysmal bone cyst, and cherubism discussed here. These conditions are all non-neoplastic lesions that are characterized by a similar histologic appearance. Common to all of them is the presence of numerous multinucleated giant cells in a background of mesenchymal cells that contain round to ovoid nuclei. Extravasated red blood cells and hemosiderin deposits are commonly found in these lesions. The aneurysmal bone cyst contains varying-sized blood-filled spaces frequently admixed with trabeculae of bone. The bone lesions of cherubism are very similar to those of the central giant cell granuloma with eosinophilic deposits surrounding blood vessels throughout the lesion.

CENTRAL GIANT CELL GRANULOMA (CENTRAL GIANT CELL LESION)

Central giant cell granuloma occurs more frequently in the mandible than the maxilla, generally anterior to the first molar, and often cross the midline. The central giant cell granuloma is a lesion of young people, with most cases diagnosed before age 30 years. The radiographic features vary from small lesions mimicking periapical inflammatory disease to large, destructive, multilocular radiolucencies (Figure 26). Complaint of pain is an inconsistent feature of these lesions. Treatment usually involves conservative curettage. Other treatment modalities include systemic calcitonin, intralesional injections of corticosteroids, and subcutaneous α-interferon injections. Recurrence rates ranging from 11 to 49% have been reported.[102–107]

The diagnosis of a central giant cell granuloma requires an evaluation for hyperparathyroidism (see also Chapter 21, Diabetes Mellitus and Endocrine Diseases).[105] Serum calcium, phosphorus, and alkaline phosphatase levels should be obtained prior to surgical removal of a giant cell granuloma, and if abnormal, parathyroid hormone (PTH) levels should be assessed. Lesions radiographically and histologically identical to the giant cell granuloma occur in primary and secondary hyperparathyroidism, and treatment of the lesion in these cases involves treatment of the hyperparathyroidism rather than treatment of the giant cell granuloma. Primary hyperparathyroidism is a result of uncontrolled PTH due to a parathyroid gland abnormality. Secondary hyperparathyroidism develops, usually in patients with chronic renal disease, due to an increase in PTH production in response to chronic low levels of serum calcium.

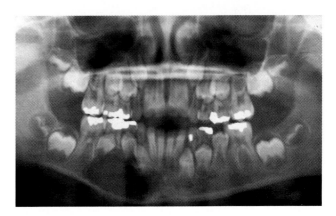

FIGURE 26 Giant cell granuloma. A panoramic radiograph of a giant cell granuloma in a child with a mixed dentition.

ANEURYSMAL BONE CYST

The term *aneurysmal bone cyst* is a misnomer since this lesion is not a cystic lesion and exhibits no epithelial lining. It does contain varying-sized blood-filled spaces. The lesion occurs less frequently in the jaw bones than in the long bones and usually involves the mandible rather than the maxilla.[108–110] Tissue histologically consistent with aneurysmal bone cyst is often seen in association with other bone diseases, such as fibrous dysplasia. Eighty percent of aneurysmal bone cysts occur in patients younger than 30 years of age; both sexes are equally affected.[108] The clinical signs and symptoms are nonspecific. Pain has been reported (however not consistently), and enlargement of the involved bone is common. The radiographic appearance varies from unilocular to multilocular (Figure 27). Treatment depends on the size of the lesions and includes curettage, enucleation, and resection. Recurrence is attributed to incomplete removal.[110]

CHERUBISM

Cherubism is a rare disease of children that is characterized by bilateral painless swellings (mandible and maxilla) that cause fullness of the cheeks; firm, protuberant, intraoral, alveolar masses; and missing or displaced teeth.[111–114] Submandibular lymphadenopathy is an early and constant feature that tends to subside after the age of 5 years and usually has regressed by the age of 12 years. Maxillary involvement can often produce a slightly upward turning of the child's eyes, revealing an abnormal amount of sclera beneath them. It was the upward "looking toward heaven" cast of the eyes combined with the characteristic facial chubbiness of these children that prompted the term *cherubism.* Cherubism is inherited as an autosomal dominant gene, with a penetrance of nearly 100% in males and 50 to 75% in females[115]; however, the exact cause of cherubism remains unknown. Other patterns of inheritance and the occurrence of cherubism in association with other syndromes have been described.[114–116]

The clinical appearance may vary from barely discernible posterior swellings of a single jaw to a grotesque anterior and posterior expansion of both jaws, with concomitant difficulties in mastication, speech, swallowing, and respiration. Disease activity declines with advancing age. Radiographically, the lesions are multiple well-defined multilocular radiolucencies in the mandible and maxilla. They are irregular in size and usually cause marked destruction of the alveolar bone. Numerous displaced and unerupted teeth appear to be floating in radiolucent spaces. Serum calcium and phosphorus are within normal limits, but serum alkaline phosphatase may be elevated. Histologically, the lesions of cherubism closely resemble the central giant cell granuloma. A variety of treatments have been recommended: no active treatment and regular follow-up, extraction of teeth in the involved areas, surgical contouring of expanded lesions, or complete curettage. Long-term longitudinal investigations have reported that the childhood lesions become partially or completely resolved in the adult.[111,113]

Paget's Disease of Bone

Paget's disease of bone (osteitis deformans) is a chronic disease of the adult skeleton characterized by focal areas of excessive bone resorption followed by bone formation.[117–119] Histologically, the involved bone demonstrates prominent reversal lines that result from the resorption and deposition of bone. There is also replacement of the normal bone marrow by vascular fibrous connective tissue. Paget's disease of bone affects about 3% of the population over 45 years of age and is rare in patients younger than 40 years of age. Malignant transformation to osteosarcoma and giant cell tumor occurs in less than 1% of patients.[120–122] The etiology of Paget's disease is not well understood. The possibility of an infective viral etiology is suggested by the ultrastructural demonstration of intranuclear inclusions in the abnormal osteoclasts both in Paget's disease and in the cells of Paget's disease–associated osteosarcoma.[123–125]

Although some patients with Paget's disease have no symptoms, many experience considerable pain and deformity. The narrowing of skull foramina can cause ill-defined neuralgic pains, severe headache, dizziness, and deafness. The bony lesions of Paget's disease produce characteristic deformities of the skull, jaw, back, pelvis, and legs that are readily recognized both clinically and radiographically. Enlargement of the affected bone is common. Irregular overgrowth of the maxilla may lead to the facial appearance described as "leontiasis ossea," and edentulous patients may complain that their dentures no longer fit. Radiographically, there are patchy radiolucent and radiopaque changes that have been described as a "cotton wool" appearance.[119,122] Other radiographic findings of the jaw bones include loss of the lamina dura, root resorption, and hypercementosis. CT and Tc 99m diphosphonate and gallium 67 bone scanning are used to define the extent of bone involvement.[117,119]

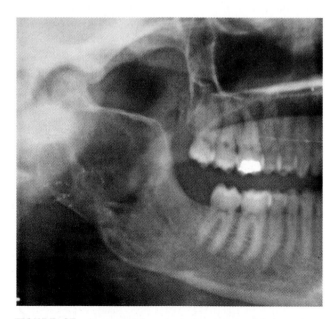

FIGURE 27 Aneurysmal bone cyst. An aneurysmal bone cyst presenting as a multilocular radiolucency in the angle of the mandible of a 31-year-old woman.

Craniofacial disorders, associated medical problems (eg, cardiac failure, hypercalcemia), and the incidence of malignant transformation have encouraged the use of a variety of new treatments.[121,123] These agents include antibiotics (ie, intravenous mithramycin, an effective inhibitor of osteoclastic activity), hormones of human and animal origin (high-dose glucocorticoids and porcine, salmon, and human calcitonin administered subcutaneously or by nasal spray or suppository), salts such as the diphosphonate etidronate (which effectively reduces bone resorption), and cytotoxic agents such as plicamycin and dactinomycin. Urinary levels of calcium and hydroxyproline (a measure of collagen metabolism) and serum alkaline phosphatase levels (a measure of osteoblastic activity) are useful for diagnosing Paget's disease and for monitoring bone resorption and deposition during treatment.

In addition to cosmetic issues, dental concerns include poor healing of dental extraction sites and excessive postsurgical bleeding from the highly vascular bone that is characteristic of this disease. Bone that exhibits unusually rapid change or enlargement suggests the possibility of malignant transformation. In view of the rarity of a giant cell tumor in the jaws except as a complication of Paget's disease,[126] the finding of this lesion in a patient who is older than 40 years of age should raise the possibility of previously undiagnosed Paget's disease.

Cysts of the Jaws and Adjacent Soft Tissues

Cysts are defined as fluid-filled epithelium-lined pathologic cavities. Odontogenic and nonodontogenic cysts occur in the oral soft tissues and in the maxilla and mandible. The cysts included here are those that are most common in the jaws and adjacent soft tissues.

ODONTOGENIC CYSTS

Radicular Cyst (Periapical Cyst). A radicular cyst is a true cyst that occurs in association with the root of a nonvital tooth. It is the most commonly occurring cyst in the oral region.[127] An inflammatory response occurs in the periapical tissue, resulting in resorption of bone and formation of granulation tissue that is infiltrated by acute and chronic inflammatory cells. The epithelial lining for the radicular cyst is thought to develop as a result of proliferation of the rests of Malassez entrapped in the inflamed granulation tissue. Histologically, the radicular cyst appears as a squamous epithelium-lined cyst lumen surrounded by inflamed fibrous connective tissue.[128] Most radicular cysts are asymptomatic and discovered on radiographic examination. They appear as well-circumscribed radiolucencies at the apex or lateral to a tooth root (Figure 28). The radicular cyst is treated by endodontic therapy, apicoectomy, or extraction and curettage of the periapical tissues. A residual cyst forms when the tooth is removed and all or part of a radicular cyst is left behind. Radiographically, the residual cyst appears as a well-circumscribed radiolucency located at the site of a previously extracted tooth. The diagnosis of the residual cyst can only be confirmed on the basis of the radiologic appearance.

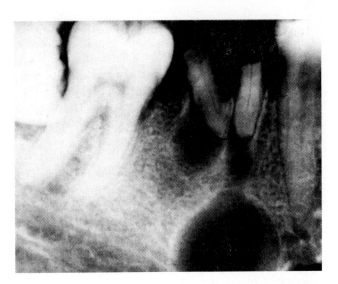

FIGURE 28 Radicular (periapical) cyst.

Therefore, either biopsy or excision of the lesion with histologic examination of the tissue is necessary for diagnosis and the treatment is based on the diagnosis. The treatment of a residual cyst involves conservative surgical excision. The cyst does not recur since the tooth associated with the pathogenesis of the cyst has been removed.

Dentigerous Cyst (Follicular or Eruption Cyst). A dentigerous cyst is diagnosed on the basis of its very specific location. The dentigerous cyst forms around the crown of an unerupted or impacted tooth, which may be part of the regular dentition or a supernumerary tooth. The dentigerous cyst arises from the epithelium of the dental follicle and remains attached to the neck of the tooth, enclosing the crown within the cyst. The epithelial lining varies from cuboidal to squamous and from very thin to hyperplastic. Some unerupted teeth (eg, third molars and canines) appear to be more susceptible than others to the development of such cysts. Dentigerous cysts have the potential for attaining a large size and also tend to resorb the roots of adjacent teeth.[129] Neoplastic changes such as plexiform ameloblastoma[130] and carcinoma[131,132] have been reported to occur within segments of the wall of dentigerous cysts. This potential for neoplastic change, infiltration beyond the cyst wall, and the occasional finding of other odontogenic tumors in association with a dentigerous cyst fully justify the need for histopathologic examination of all material derived from jaw cysts. The eruption cyst is the soft tissue analogue of the follicular cyst; it presents clinically as a bluish gray swelling of the mucosa over an erupting tooth, most commonly first permanent molars and maxillary incisors. These are also referred to as eruption hematomas.[127] If any treatment is needed, excision of a wedge of the mucosa to expose the tooth crown is usually adequate.

Odontogenic Keratocyst. The odontogenic keratocyst is characterized by its unique histologic appearance and frequent recurrence.[133–135] The lumen is lined by epithelium that is generally 8 to 10 cell layers thick and surfaced by para-keratin. The interface between the epithelium and connective tissue is devoid of rete ridges and the basal cell layer is palisaded and prominent. The parakeratin forms a wavy, corrugated surface. Budding of the cyst lining into the connective tissue is also described as a feature of this cyst. The posterior mandible is the most common site of occurrence. However, the odontogenic keratocyst may occur in any location in the maxilla or mandible. Radiographically, the odontogenic keratocyst may present as a small, asymptomatic, unilocular radiolucency. However, larger, multilocular radiolucencies are common presentations of this cyst (Figure 29).

Complete removal of the cyst is necessary to prevent recurrence and may be difficult due to the thin, fragile nature of the cyst wall. Treatment ranges from decompression and enucleation to peripheral ostectomy and chemical cauterization to resection.[134]

The odontogenic keratocyst occurs as an isolated cyst and as a component of nevoid basal cell carcinoma syndrome (Figure 30). Nevoid basal cell carcinoma syndrome is inherited as an autosomal dominant trait that exhibits high penetrance and variable expressivity. In addition to odontogenic keratocysts (usually multiple), components of the syndrome include (among many others) basal cell carcinomas developing at an early age in non–sun exposed skin, mild hypertelorism, enlarged calvarium, calcification of the falx cerebri,

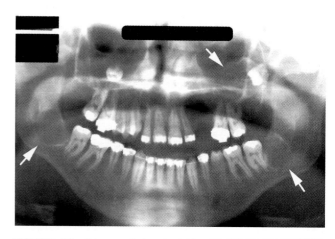

FIGURE 30 Odontogenic keratocyst in nevoid basal cell carcinoma syndrome. The multiple radiolucencies seen in this patient with nevoid basal cell carcinoma syndrome are odontogenic keratocysts.

and rib abnormalities.[136,137] Pitting of the soles and palms (local areas of undermaturation of the epithelial basal cells) is an additional finding in about half of the individuals affected by the syndrome. Despite the syndrome's name, multiple basal cell carcinomas occur in only 50% of cases. Appropriate treatment is simple curettage or marsupialization of the cysts.[138]

Lateral Periodontal Cyst (Botryoid Odontogenic Cyst). Although the lateral periodontal cyst has a distinct and characteristic histologic appearance, the cyst is named for its location.[139] It most often presents as an asymptomatic unilocular (rarely multilocular) radiolucency, lateral to the root of a vital mandibular cuspid or premolar tooth. (Figure 31). Histologically, the lateral periodontal cyst exhibits a very thin lining of stratified squamous epithelium with focal epithelial thickenings. The gingival cyst is the soft tissue analogue of the lateral periodontal cyst. These cysts are treated by conservative surgical excision. A few cases of recurrence of lateral periodontal cysts have been reported.

Calcifying Odontogenic Cyst. The calcifying odontogenic cyst is usually a nonagressive cystic lesion lined by odontogenic epithelium that resembles that of the ameloblastoma, but with characteristic ghost cell keratinization.[140,141] It is usually a well-defined lesion that can present either as a unilocular or multilocular radiolucency. Calcifications are seen radiographically as radiopaque areas within a radiolucent lesion. A solid, noncystic variant histologically resembling the calcifying odontogenic cyst has been described. The calcifying odontogenic cyst is generally treated by surgical enucleation and usually does not recur. The solid variant has been reported to exhibit more aggressive behavior.

NONODONTOGENIC CYSTS

Nasopalatine Canal Cyst. The nasopalatine canal (duct) cyst is derived from remnants of epithelium-lined vestigial oronasal duct tissue.[142,143] The cyst is located within the

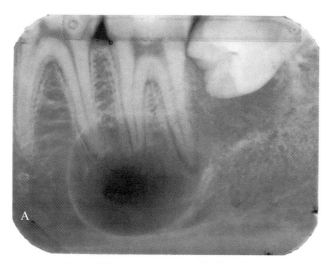

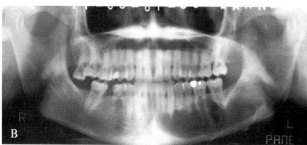

FIGURE 29 Odontogenic keratocyst. *A,* An odontogenic keratocyst presenting as a well-circumscribed radiolucency mimicking a periapical inflammatory lesion. *B,* An odontogenic keratocyst presenting as a large radiolucency in the mandible.

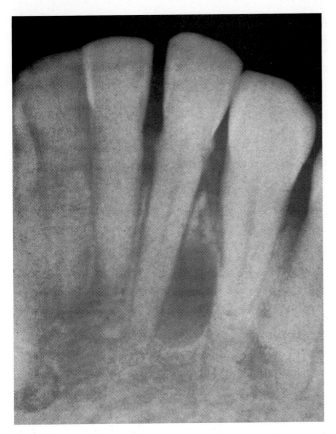

FIGURE 31 Lateral periodontal cyst. A lateral periodontal cyst presenting as a well-circumscribed radiolucency between the roots of a mandibular lateral and cuspid.

nasopalatine canal and presents as a unilocular or heart-shaped radiolucency between the roots of vital maxillary central incisors. The cyst lining varies from squamous to respiratory (pseudostratified ciliated columnar) epithelium. Blood vessels and nerve tissue, contents of the nasopalatine canal, are frequently seen in the connective tissue wall of the cyst. The clinical evaluation involves differentiating this cyst from a normal nasopalatine foramen and a radicular cyst. The cyst of the incisive papilla is the soft tissue analogue of the nasopalatine canal cyst. Both are treated by conservative excision and do not recur.

Nasoalveolar (Nasolabial) Cyst. The nasoalveolar cyst is a soft tissue cyst of uncertain pathogenesis with no alveolar bone involvement.[144,145] The cyst is observed in older adults, with a 4:1 female predilection. Clinically, the cyst presents as a swelling in the mucolabial fold. The cyst lining varies from squamous to respiratory (pseudostratified ciliated columnar) epithelium. Treatment is surgical excision, and recurrence is rare.

Simple (Traumatic, Hemorrhagic) Bone Cyst. The simple bone cyst[146,147] is a pathologic cavity in bone that is not lined with epithelium. The cause is uncertain, although, tradition-ally, an association with trauma has been suggested. The lesion is found most often in young patients, with an equal distribution between males and females. The lesion presents radiographically as a well-defined radiolucency that charac-teristically demonstrates a scalloping pattern around the roots of teeth. The lesion is usually asymptomatic and discovered on routine radiographs. Surgical intervention reveals a void within the bone, and healing generally follows intervention.

Odontogenic Tumors

The classification of odontogenic tumors that is most commonly used divides these tumors into three categories based on the type of cell that forms the tumor: (1) epithelial, (2) mesenchymal, and (3) mixed epithelial and mesenchymal. Odontogenic tumors,[148,149] are derived from tooth-forming tissues, and the developmental stages of tooth formation are emulated in the various odontogenic tumors.

Odontomas are the most commonly occurring odonto-genic tumor, followed by the ameloblastoma. The other odontogenic tumors are much rarer.[150]

EPITHELIAL ODONTOGENIC TUMORS

Ameloblastoma. The ameloblastoma is the best known of the epithelial odontogenic tumors. It is a slow-growing and locally aggressive epithelial odontogenic tumor. The micro-scopic appearance of this tumor includes tumor cells resem-bling ameloblasts, with no formation of calcified material. The ameloblastoma is most commonly seen in the posterior mandible but may also arise in the maxilla and anterior aspect of the jaws. The radiographic appearance ranges from a unilocular to a multilocular radiolucency. Ameloblastomas are rare in children, with most cases occurring in patients between 20 and 50 years of age. Complete removal of the tumor is required to prevent recurrence; the plan for reconstruction often influences the extent of surgery. Rare examples of metastatic foci of an ameloblastoma in lungs or regional lymph nodes have been reported.[151–154]

Microscopically, all ameloblastomas show a fibrous stroma, with islands or masses of proliferating epithelium that resembles the odontogenic epithelium of the enamel organ (ie, palisading of cells around proliferating nests of odontogenic epithelium in a pattern similar to ameloblasts). Follicular, plexiform, and acanthomatous histologic variants of this tumor show basal cells, stellate reticulum, and squa-mous metaplasia. These histologic variants show no correla-tion with either the clinical appearance of the lesion or its behavior, and variation may be seen between different sections of the same tumor. A unicystic variant of the amelo-blastoma tends to occur during teenage years and has been reported to exhibit a less aggressive behavior. Fewer than 20% of unicystic ameloblastomas have been reported to recur after curettage, whereas over 75% of solid ameloblastomas will recur unless treated by resection.[154] Attempts have been made to marsupialize unicystic tumors. Recurrence is associated with incomplete removal of the tumor.

The calcifying odontogenic cyst (Gorlin's cyst, described in the section on odontogenic cysts) exhibits epithelium very similar to that of the ameloblastoma. The calcifying odontogenic cyst has a much less aggressive behavior and is distinguished histologically by the presence of "ghost cell" formation within the epithelium.

Adenomatoid Odontogenic Tumor. Adenomatoid odontogenic tumor (AOT) is a tumor of odontogenic epithelium that exhibits behavior very different from the ameloblastoma. This tumor is characterized histologically by a very distinct capsule surrounding the tumor and structures resembling ducts ("adenomatoid") within the epithelium.[155,156] Approximately 70% of AOTs occur in females younger than 20 years of age and 70% involve the anterior jaw.[155,156] This lesion rarely recurs even with conservative curettage.

Calcifying Epithelial Odontogenic Tumor (Pindborg Tumor). The calcifying epithelial odontogenic tumor differs from other epithelial odontogenic tumors in that the epithelium does not resemble the epithelium of the tooth-forming apparatus. It is composed of sheets of polyhedral epithelial cells with very little stroma. The cells of this tumor may be quite pleomorphic, with large nuclei. Foci of hyalin amyloid material and calcifications exhibiting concentric rings are frequently seen in this tumor. It is important for the pathologist to recognize this distinctive tumor so that it is not misdiagnosed as a squamous carcinoma. The calcifying epithelial odontogenic tumor resembles an ameloblastoma; it is locally invasive and presents as a unilocular or multilocular swelling in the molar-ramus region.[157,158] Treatment is by enucleation or local block excision; the recurrence rate is reported to be 20%.

Squamous Odontogenic Tumor. The squamous odontogenic tumor[159] is an asymptomatic lesion composed of multiple islands of squamous epithelium. The squamous epithelium does not exhibit the ameloblast-like features seen in the ameloblastoma. It is reported to occur equally within the maxilla and mandible. Radiographically, this tumor does not have distinctive features. The radiolucent area may resemble periodontal bone loss or periapical inflammatory disease. Conservative surgical excision is the treatment of choice for this tumor.

MESENCHYMAL ODONTOGENIC TUMORS

Odontogenic Myxoma. Myxomas are tumors composed of very loose cellular connective tissue containing little collagen and large amounts of an intercellular substance that is rich in acid mucopolysaccharide. Myxomas are slow-growing and invasive tumors that can become very large and distend the maxilla or mandible. Since similar lesions are very rare in other bones and since some oral myxomas contain tiny epithelial remnants that resemble inactive odontogenic epithelium, tumors with this histologic appearance that occur in the jaw bone are assumed to be odontogenic in origin. This lesion usually consists of very small rounded and angular cells lying in an abundant mucoid stroma that is reminiscent of dental pulp. Characteristically, it appears radiographically as a unilocular or multilocular lesion and is clinically and radiographically indistinguishable from other lesions that present with a similar radiographic appearance (Figure 32). Treatment is similar to that recommended for ameloblastoma.[87,160]

Central Odontogenic Fibroma. The central odontogenic fibroma is a tumor composed of mature fibroblastic tissue admixed with nests and strands of odontogenic epithelium in varying amounts.[161] It is an uncommon, slow-growing, and nonaggressive lesion. These tumors are usually well-defined unilocular radiolucencies. They are generally small, yet they may cause root resorption. Treatment is conservative excision.[87,161]

Central Cementifying and Ossifying Fibroma. The central cementifying fibroma and the ossifying fibroma are composed of cellular fibrous connective tissue with calcifications that are either rounded or globular or resemble bone trabeculae.[87] Histologically, these tumors are benign fibro-osseous lesions and can be distinguished from other benign fibro-osseous lesions since radiographically and surgically they are well circumscribed. The tumor usually occurs in adults in the third and fourth decades of life, with a greater female predilection; they also occur more frequently in the mandible than the maxilla. Radiographically, these are well-defined lesions that vary from radiolucent to radiopaque depending on the amount of calcified tissue present. These tumors are treated by surgical excision, and recurrence is rare.

Benign Cementoblastoma. The benign cementoblastoma[162] is a cementum-producing lesion that is fused to the roots of a vital tooth. The tumor often occurs in young adults and is associated with a mandibular molar or premolar. Pain is a frequent complaint. Early in its development, this tumor presents as a periapical radiolucency that may be indistinguishable from a periapical inflammatory lesion. Later, the cementoblastoma demonstrates a pathognomonic appearance—a well-defined radiopaque mass surrounded by a radiolucent halo that incorporates the root of the tooth.

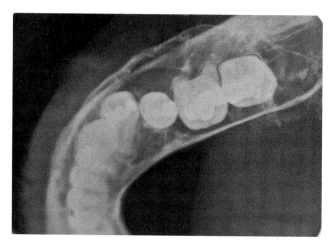

FIGURE 32 Odontogenic myxoma. An occlusal radiograph of an odontogenic myxoma presenting as a multilocular radiolucency.

Treatment involves removing both the tooth and the attached cementoblastoma. The cementoblastoma does not recur.

MIXED ODONTOGENIC TUMORS

Ameloblastic Fibroma. The ameloblastic fibroma[163] is a nonencapsulated tumor that is composed of mesenchymal tissue that resembles the dental papillae and small islands of odontogenic epithelium that resemble the dental lamina. Most cases of this tumor are in patients under 20 years of age, particularly very young children, and congenital cases have been reported.[164] The most common location is the mandibular premolar and molar region. Radiographically, it presents as a radiolucency that may be well defined, poorly defined, unilocular, or multilocular. When tooth formation is associated with this tumor, the tumor is called an ameloblastic fibro-odontoma. The tumor is treated by surgical excision, and the recurrence rate is low.

Compound and Complex Odontomas. Compound and complex odontomas[163,165] are nonaggressive lesions that are more likely to be hamartomatous than neoplastic. Odontogenic cysts and other tumors may also be associated with odontomas. Most odontomas are identified in adolescents and young adults. The compound odontoma is most commonly seen in the anterior maxilla and the complex odontoma in the posterior mandible. A compound odontoma consists of a collection of numerous small teeth. Despite its designation as a hamartoma, the compound odontoma is considered the most common of the odontogenic tumors. It is usually diagnosed by the radiographic identification of multiple small tooth structures. The complex odontoma appears radiographically as a radiopaque mass. It consists of a mass of enamel, dentin, cementum, and pulp that does not morphologically resemble a tooth. Histologic examination of the tissue is generally needed to establish the diagnosis. Treatment of the compound or complex odontoma requires surgical excision. These lesions are not expected to recur.

Benign Non-odontogenic Tumors of the Jaws

OSTEOMAS/GARDNER'S SYNDROME

Osteomas are benign tumors of bone that are composed of mature cancellous or cortical bone. They can form within the bone as a well-circumscribed radiopacity or on the surface of bone as either a sessile or polypoid bony-hard mass. Osteomas are asymptomatic and are generally undetected unless they are discovered on routine radiographic evaluation or cause facial asymmetry. Most are initially diagnosed in young adults. Maxillary and mandibular tori were described earlier in this chapter. Although they are histologically identical to osteomas, they do not have unlimited growth potential and are not considered neoplasms.[166–170]

The most significant feature of osteomas is the association with Gardner's syndrome. Gardner's syndrome is inherited as an autosomal dominant trait with nearly 100% penetrance.[167] A specific gene mutation responsible for Gardner's syndrome has been identified. Polyps of the colon develop in the second and third decades in individuals with Gardner's syndrome. These polyps ultimately exhibit malignant transformation to adenocarcinoma.[167] Patients with Gardner's syndrome develop multiple osteomas of the maxilla and mandible that precede the diagnosis of colonic polyps. Other components of Gardner's syndrome include supernumerary teeth, impacted teeth, skin cysts, and fibrous tumors of the skin.

OSTEOBLASTOMA AND OSTEOID OSTEOMA

Osteoblastoma[171] and osteoid osteoma[172] occur much more commonly in other bones than the jaws. They are clinically, radiographically, and histologically very similar lesions. The size of the lesion is a distinguishing feature: the osteoblastoma is larger than 2 cm, and the osteoid osteoma is smaller than 2 cm. Pain is a presenting feature for both lesions. The pain associated with an osteoid osteoma responds to aspirin and other nonsteroidal anti-inflammatory drugs, whereas the pain associated with an osteoblastoma does not. Most lesions arise before age 30 years, and there is a higher prevalence in males. Radiographically, the osteoblastoma presents as a radiolucency that may be either well or poorly defined, with patchy areas of radiopacity within the lesion. The osteoid osteoma is more likely to present with a surrounding zone of sclerosis. Histologically, they both resemble the cementoblastoma but are not attached to a tooth. They are composed of sheets or irregular trabeculae of bone that exhibit prominent reversal lines. The bone is lined by osteoblast- and osteoclast-like cells that contain multiple and large hyperchromatic nuclei. The central portion of the osteoid osteoma contains a concentration of nerve tissue. Careful evaluation of the radiograph and biopsy specimen by the pathologist is needed to distinguish them from an osteosarcoma. These tumors are generally treated by conservative excision.[173]

CHONDROMA AND CHONDROMYXOID FIBROMA

Cartilaginous tumors of the jaws are very rare, and any tumor-containing cartilage must be evaluated very carefully by the pathologist to rule out a malignant tumor. However, benign tumors of cartilage occurring in the jaws have been reported. The chondromyxoid fibroma[174] is composed of spindle-shaped and stellate-shaped cells in a myxoid and cartilaginous stroma. The major concern with cartilaginous tumors in the jaws is to ensure that the diagnosis is correct. Benign cartilaginous tumors are treated by conservative excision. Multiple chondromas are components of Ollier's disease (multiple enchondromas) and Maffuci's syndrome (multiple enchondromas with soft tissue hemangiomas).

DESMOPLASTIC FIBROMA

The desmoplastic fibroma[175–177] of bone is a rare tumor that has been reported to occur in the jaws. It is composed of uniform-appearing fibroblasts and abundant collagen fibers. The degree of cellularity may vary, but the cells of the desmoplastic fibroma do not show atypia and mitoses are not present. Most tumors have occurred in the mandible in patients under 30 years of age. Painless enlargement of the mandible with an associated unilocular radiolucency is the most common presentation. Radiographically, the tumor may be well or poorly defined and occasionally multilocular. This tumor can behave in an aggressive fashion; accordingly, treatment is based on the extent and rate of tumor growth.

▼ SELECTED READING

Capodiferro S, Maiorano E, Giardina C, et al. Osteoblastoma of the mandible: clinicopathologic study of four cases and literature review. Head Neck 2005;27:616–21.

Dayan D, Nasrallah V, Vered M. Clinico-pathologic correlations of myofibroblastic tumors of the oral cavity: 1. Nodular fasciitis. J Oral Pathol Med 2005;34:426–35.

Fakhry C, Gillison ML. Clinical implications of human papillomavirus in head and neck cancers. J Clin Oncol 2006; 24:2606–11.

Iida S, Fukuda Y, Ueda T, et al. Calcifying odontogenic cyst: radiologic findings in 11 cases. Oral Surg Oral Med Oral Pathol Oral Radiol Endod 2006;101:356–62.

Johann AC, Aguiar MC, do Carmo MA, et al. Sclerotherapy of benign oral vascular lesion with ethanolamine oleate: an open clinical trial with 30 lesions. Oral Surg Oral Med Oral Pathol Oral Radiol Endod 2005;100:579–84.

Ohki K, Kumamoto H, Nitta Y, et al. Benign cementoblastoma involving multiple maxillary teeth: report of a case with a review of the literature. Oral Surg Oral Med Oral Pathol Oral Radiol Endod 2004;97:53–8.

Rawashdeh MA, Bataineh AB, Al-Khateeb T. Long-term clinical and radiological outcomes of surgical management of central giant cell granuloma of the maxilla. Int J Oral Maxillofac Surg 2006;35:60–6.

Roodman GD, Windle JJ. Paget disease of bone. J Clin Invest 2005;115:200–8.

Said-Al-Naief N, Fernandes R, Louis P, et al. Desmoplastic fibroma of the jaw: a case report and review of literature. Oral Surg Oral Med Oral Pathol Oral Radiol Endod 2006;101: 82–94.

Scheper MA, Nikitakis NG, Sarlani E, et al. Cowden syndrome: report of a case with immunohistochemical analysis and review of the literature. Oral Surg Oral Med Oral Pathol Oral Radiol Endod 2006;101:625–31.

Theos A, Korf BR. Pathophysiology of neurofibromatosis type 1. Ann Intern Med 2006;144:842–9.

Wang CP, Chang YL, Sheen TS. Vascular leiomyoma of the head and neck. Laryngoscope 2004;114:661–5.

Whyte MP. Clinical practice. Paget's disease of bone. N Engl J Med 2006;355:593–600.

For the full reference list, please refer to the accompanying CD ROM.

7

ORAL CANCER

JOEL EPSTEIN, DMD, MSD, FRCD(C)
ISAÄC VAN DER WAAL, DDS, PHD

▼ SQUAMOUS CELL CARCINOMA

Epidemiology

Worldwide, oral carcinoma is one of the most prevalent cancers and is one of the 10 most common causes of death. Of the more than one million new cancers diagnosed annually in the United States, cancers of the oral cavity and oropharynx account for approximately 3%.[1] If oral cancers and cancers of the nasopharynx, pharynx, larynx, sinus, and salivary glands are combined, these sites represent more than 5% of total body cancers. In males, oral cancer represents 4% of total body cancers; in females, 2% of all cancers are oral. Oral cancer accounts for 2% of cancer deaths in males and 1% of cancer deaths in females.[1] The statistics are similar throughout North America but vary throughout the world; in French men, the incidence is up to 17.9 cases per 100,000 population, and high rates are reported in India and other Asian countries. Higher rates in these countries also are reported in females, with the highest rate in Singapore (5.8 cases per 100,000 population).[1] The majority of oral cancers are squamous cell cancers. Other malignant diseases that can occur in the head and neck include tumors of the salivary glands, thyroid gland, lymph nodes, bone, and soft tissue. This chapter focuses on squamous cell cancer.

Approximately 95% of oral squamous cell carcinoma (OSCC) occur in people older than 40 years, with an average age at diagnosis of approximately 60 years.[2,3] However, OSCC at a young age has attracted attention in the literature.[4] Oral tongue and base of the tongue and tonsilar malignancies have increased in 20- to 44-year-old adults.[5]

The overall age-related incidence of OSCC suggests that time-dependent factors result in the initiation and promotion of genetic events that result in malignant change. The majority of oral cancers involve the tongue, oropharynx, and floor of the mouth.[1–3] The lips, gingiva, dorsal tongue, and palate are less common sites. Primary squamous cell carcinoma (SCC) of bone is rare; however, a tumor may develop from epithelial rests and from epithelium of odontogenic lesions, including cysts and ameloblastoma. Individuals who have had a previous cancer are at high risk of developing a second oropharyngeal cancer.[6–10] African Americans in the United States have a higher risk of developing oropharyngeal cancer than do Caucasians.[2,11,12] The increased risk appears to be due to environmental factors, although possible genetic factors have not been determined.

Etiology and Risk Factors

The incidence of oral cancer is age related, which may reflect time for the accumulation of genetic changes and duration of exposure to initiators and promoters (these include chemical and physical irritants, viruses, hormonal effects), cellular aging, and decreased immunologic surveillance with aging. Evidence from long-term follow-up of immunosuppressed patients after solid organ and hematopoietic stem cell transplantation shows that immunosuppression increases the risk of the development of SCC.

TOBACCO AND ALCOHOL

Tobacco and alcohol are acknowledged risk factors for oral and oropharyngeal cancer.[2,3,13–15] Tobacco contains potent carcinogens, including nitrosamines, polycyclic aromatic hydrocarbons, nitrosodicthanolamine, nitrosoproline, and polonium. Tobacco smoke contains carbon monoxide, thiocyanate, hydrogen cyanide, nicotine, and metabolites of these constituents. Nicotine is a powerful and addicting drug. Epidemiologic studies have shown that up to 80% of oral cancer patients were smokers.[4,12,14] In addition to the risk of primary cancers, the risk of recurrent and second primary oral cancers is related to continuing smoking after cancer treatment.[6–10,17–19] Of patients who were observed for 1 year, 18% developed a recurrence or a second primary oral cancer, and those who continued to smoke had a 30% risk.[6] The effect of smoking on cancer risk diminishes 5 to 10 years after quitting. Smoking has declined in North America, particularly in adults; approximately 30% of adults smoke. This trend may be emerging worldwide but is not seen in teenagers and young adults. The incidence of oral squamous cell cancer varies worldwide and may be explained partly by differences in the use of tobacco products. In parts of Asia where the use of tobacco, betel nuts, or lime to form a quid is widespread (eg, India, Taiwan), the incidence of oral cancer is high and more commonly involves the buccal mucosa.[2] It has been observed that the tongue is a common site in the nonsmoking group in contrast to the smoking group in which the floor of the mouth is a common location; furthermore, the prevalence and spectrum of TP53 mutations are significantly less than in smokers.[20]

Most studies have focused on cigarette use; however, other forms of tobacco use have been associated with oral cancers. The use of smokeless tobacco products (chewing tobacco and snuff) is of increasing concern due to the increase in their use and to their use at a young age.[21–26] Benign

hyperkeratosis and epithelial dysplasia have been documented after short-term use, and it is likely that chronic use will be associated with an increasing incidence of malignant lesions.[2,14,27] In a population-based case-control study, no association between marijuana use and OSCC has been observed.[28]

All forms of alcohol, including "hard" liquor, wine, and beer, have been implicated in the etiology of oral cancer. In some studies, beer and wine are associated with greater risk than hard liquor.[14,15] The combined effects of tobacco and alcohol result in a synergistic effect on the development of oral cancer.[13–16,18,29–32] The mechanism(s) by which alcohol and tobacco act synergistically may include dehydrating effects of alcohol on the mucosa, increasing mucosal permeability, and the effects of potential carcinogens in alcohol or tobacco. Secondary liver dysfunction and nutritional status also may play a role.

NUTRITIONAL FACTORS

Vitamin A may play a role in oral cancer.[2,33–36] This hypothesis is based on population studies in which deficiency was associated with the risk of SCC, on population studies of vitamin A and carotenoid supplementation, and on studies of reduction in carcinogenesis in animal models. Vitamin A may cause regression of premalignant leukoplakia.

OTHER RISK FACTORS

Factors for which no evidence for a role in oral cancer has been documented include denture use, denture irritation, irregular teeth or restorations, and chronic cheek-biting habits.[2,3,37,38] However, it is possible that chronic trauma, in addition to other carcinogens, may promote the transformation of epithelial cells, as has been demonstrated in animal studies.[39] The findings of a study among 189 head and neck cancer patients suggest that seropositivity to herpes simplex virus, HSV-1 and HSV-2, may modify the risk of head and neck cancer associated with exposure to tobacco, alcohol, or human papillomavirus (HPV) oncogenic subtypes.[40]

High alcohol content in mouthwashes has been implicated in oral cancer. However, it has been suggested that smokers may use mouthwash more frequently; thus, the correlation between regular use of high-alcohol mouthwash and oral cancer may be confounded by alcohol and tobacco use.[15] In contrast with the well-documented risk associated with the use of alcohol and tobacco products, the role of other environmental agents (such as pollution) requires future study.

In lip cancer, sun exposure, fair skin and a tendency to burn, pipe smoking, and alcohol are identified risk factors.[15] The decreasing incidence of lip cancer reflects greater public awareness of the potential damaging effects of the sun and compliance with recommendations for prevention.[2]

The suggested association between sideropenic anemia (Plummer-Vinson disease) and head and neck cancers appears to be more of limited significance in lesions arising in the postcricoid region of the hypopharynx.[41,42] At the same time, it has been demonstrated that hemoglobin levels appear to be associated with locoregional control and overall survival.[43]

Patients undergoing allogenic stem cell transplantation are at high risk of developing secondary neoplasms, particularly leukemias and lymphomas; OSCC has been reported up to a 14-fold increase in risk.[44–46] OSCC is documented after an extended period of immunosuppression post-transplantation and with similar molecular changes, as seen in non–medically induced immunosuppression.[47] Oral, pharyngeal, and laryngeal SCCs were examined in 1,515 patients after liver transplantation who were followed for up to 6 years, and 11 cases (0.86%) were detected, exclusively in smokers.[48]

A review of fluoride use (based on a study conducted by the National Toxicology Program) demonstrated equivocal evidence of carcinogenicity in male rats.[49] The evidence was based on the finding of a few cases of osteosarcoma in male rats, but in female rats and in male and female mice, no malignant disease was seen.[49] Other animal studies have not confirmed these results. There is no epidemiologic evidence of an association between fluoride and osteosarcoma or other malignant disease in humans.[49–51]

Pathogenesis

The molecular pathogenesis of OSCC reflects an accumulation of genetic changes that occur over a period of years. Although it is not known if SCC can occur without premalignant changes in the tissue, at least 20% of OSCCs are documented arising in or are associated with a clinically visible precursor lesion, such as leukoplakia and erythroplakia. There is an ongoing debate about whether oral lichen planus is a premalignant lesion or a disorder. Apparently, the risk for a patient with oral lichen planus to progress to SCC is much lower than in oral leukoplakia or erythroplakia. It is likely that patients with lichen planus who are at increased risk of progression to OSCC are those with dysplasia on biopsy; indeed, similar paterns of allelic loss (loss of heterozygosity [LOH]) to those with dysplastic leukoplakia have been reported in a subset of lichen planus lesions, whereas lichen planus without dysplasia did not harbor allelic loss.[52]

Carcinogenesis is a genetic process that leads to a change in morphology and in cellular behavior. The assessment of molecular change may become the primary means of diagnosis and may guide management. Major genes involved in head and neck squamous cell carcinoma (HNSCC) include proto-oncogenes and tumor suppressor genes (TSGs). Other factors that play a role in the progression of disease may include allelic loss at other chromosome regions, mutations to proto-oncogenes and TSGs, or epigenetic changes such as deoxyribonucleic acid (DNA) methylation or histone deacetylation. Cytokine growth factors, angiogenesis, cell adhesion molecules, immune function, and homeostatic regulation of surrounding normal cells also play a role.

Proto-oncogenes may coding for growth factors, growth factor receptors, protein kinases, signal transducers, nuclear phosphoproteins, and transcription factors. Although proto-oncogenes increase cell growth and differentiation and

are likely involved in carcinogenesis, few have been consistently reported in HNSCC. Proto-oncogenes associated with HNSCC include ras (rat sarcoma), cyclin-D1, myc, erb-b (erythroblastosis), bcl-1, bcl-2 (B-cell lymphoma), int-2, CK8, and CK19.[53]

TSGs negatively regulate cell growth and differentiation. Functional loss of TSGs is common in carcinogenesis.[54] Both copies of a TSG must be inactivated or lost (LOH) for loss of function (the "two-hit" hypothesis). Chromosomes are numbered (1 to 23), and the arms of each chromosome are divided by the centromere into a short arm (designated P) and a long arm (designated Q). These TSGs have been associated with sites of chromosome abnormalities where LOH has been reported to commonly involve chromosome arms 3p, 4q, 8p, 9p, 11q, 13q, and 17p. TSGs involved in HNSCC are *P53*, *Rb* (retinoblastoma), and *p16INK4A*. Other candidates include *FHIT* (fragile histidine triad), *APC* (adenomatous polyposis coli), *DOC1 VHL* (gene for von Hippel-Lindau syndrome), and *TGF- R-II* (gene for transforming growth factor type II receptor).[55–58]

Molecular staging may provide more precise predictions of the malignant potential than conventional clinicopathologic features do as it represents the fundamental biologic characteristics of each tumor. The current model of carcinogenesis is a multistage process, with loss occurring on chromosome arms 3p and 9p early in the lesion's progress from benign to dysplastic, with additional losses later in the disease, often involving 8p, 13q, and 17p. Putative TSGs at these sites of loss are *P16* loss at 9p and *P53* gene loss at 17p (Figure 1). Molecular markers are likely to become important clinical markers in diagnosis and staging and in treatment planning. Chromosome arm 3p may code for *FHIT* and is involved in epithelial cancers. Diadenosine tetraphosphate may accumulate in the absence of FHIT, which may lead to DNA synthesis and cell replication. TSGs at another site of 3p may include the *VHL* gene, which encodes membrane proteins that function in signal transduction and cell adhesion. LOH on 9p is seen in 72% of lesions and may represent the site for *P16*, which encodes a cell cycle protein that inhibits cyclin-dependent kinases and that arrests the cell

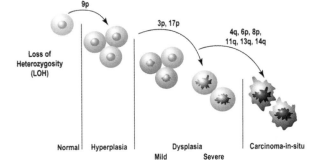

Molecular Model of Dysplasia and Carcinogenesis

FIGURE 1 Molecular model with early and late changes that accumulate over time, leading to cancer.

cycle at the G1–S phase, and loss may lead to cell proliferation. Later changes are seen on chromosomes 13 and 17, which are associated with progression to malignancy. LOH on 13q is identified in more than 50% of HNSCC.[53,59] The putative TSGs are near the interferon locus and are close to the *Rb* locus. LOH on 13q has been associated with lymph node metastasis in HNSCC. LOH on 17p (the region of the *P53* gene) is found in 50% of cases of HNSCC. The p53 protein functions in transcription activation, DNA repair, apoptosis, senescence, and G1 and G2 cell cycle inhibition. Other genetic changes have been identified on chromosomes 4, 8, and 11.[60–64] Loss on chromosome 4 occurs in up to 80% of HNSCC cases; the putative TSG may be the epidermal growth factor (*EGF*) gene. Loss on 8p occurs in up to 67% of HNSCCs and is associated with a higher stage and a poor prognosis; the related TSG is unknown. Loss on chromosome 11 is present in up to 61% of HNSCCs; the common site lost may code the cyclin D1 gene. LOH on 13q correlates with lymph node metastases and recurrence in HNSCC.

LOH has been studied in oral premalignant lesions and predicts the malignant risk of low-grade dysplastic oral epithelial lesions.[53,56,61,62,65–68] The importance of allelic loss has been confirmed in a prospective study of patents with dysplasia, where lesions with allelic loss at 3P, 9P, and 17 P predict risk of progression to SCC, even in histologically benign or tissue with mild dysplasia.[69] This is of importance as the majority of oral premalignant lesions (hyperplasia, mild and moderate dysplasia) do not progress to cancer. Lesions that progress to SCC appear to differ genetically from nonprogressing lesions, although they may not demonstrate different histomorphologic findings. Molecular analysis, therefore, may become necessary in diagnosis. LOH on 3p and/or 9p is seen in virtually all progressing cases. LOH on 3p and/or 9p (but no other chromosome arms) has a 3.8 times relative risk of developing SCC, and if additional sites of LOH are present (4q, 8p, 11q, 13q, or 17p), a 33-fold increase in risk of progression to cancer is seen. Accumulation of allelic loss is seen in progressing lesions, and the majority of progressing dysplasias have LOH on more than one arm (91% vs 31% of nonprogressing dysplasias); 57% have loss on more than two arms (vs 20% of dysplasias without progression). LOH on 4q, 8p, 11q, 13q, and 17p is common in severe dysplasia/carcinoma in situ or SCC.

There is increasing evidence of the prognostic value of LOH in HNSCC.[59,69,70] Molecular changes predate the morphologic criteria for diagnosis, predict tumor behavior and in determining margins. In the future, treatment may be directed at the function of proto-oncogenes or TSGs rather than to current therapies with their associated toxicities. TSG changes may provide tools for prognosis and may serve as intermediate markers in assessing treatment and prevention outcomes.

The role of promotor hypermethylation of CpG islands is being investigated in OSCC as methylation of epigenetic DNA has been shown to result in a loss of function in some genes involved in cell cycle regulation and DNA repair that may lead to loss or change in tumor suppressor genes involved in carcinogenesis.[71,72] Changes in DNA methylation of six genes and a significantly higher frequency of methylation in a number of TSGs, including cyclin A1 and p16 promotor sequences, have been seen.[73,74] Mitochondrial DNA (mtDNA) content increases with oxidative damage as possible compensation to mitochondrial dysfunction. MtDNA as assessed by polymerase chain reaction for specific mitochondrial genes was shown to increase with severity of dysplasia and in SCC.[75,76] These findings support the model of accumaltion of genetic alterations as mucosal disease progresses from dysplasia to SCC and the contention that mtDNA increases with histologic grade.

Matrix metalloproteinase 2 (MMP) and tissue inhibitor of metalloproteinase play an important role in cancer initiation and development, as has been demonstrated in 239 head and neck cancer patients and 250 matched controls in a Thai population.[77] Others have also supported the prognostic significance of tissue inhibitors of MMP.[78–80] ICAM-5 (telencephalin) is an intercellular adhesion molecule reported to be expressed only in the somatodendritic membrane of telencephalin neurons. Maruya and colleagues suggested that ICAM-5 may play a role in tumorigenesis and perineural invasion.[81] The development of malignant epithelial neoplasms is associated with disruption of cell-to-cell and cell-to-matrix adhesion. Syndecans are a family of heparan sulfate proteoglycan receptors that are thought to participate in both cell-to-cell and cell-to-matrix adhesion. In a study of 43 SCCs, a reduction of syndecan 1 correlated to histologic grade, tumor size, and mode of invasion.[82] Alpha(v) beta6 integrin is frequently expressed in SCC and in leukoplakia lesions that progress but not in lesions that did not progress, suggesting that this integrin could be associated with malignant transformation.[83] The initiation or progression of oral cancer may be associated with polymorphism of the vascular endothelial growth factor (VEGF) gene.[84]

Multiple cancers within the upper aerodigestive tract may derive from a common clonal progenitor cell, which is a different explanation than provided by Slaughter and colleagues in their theory of field cancerization.[85–88]

The potential role of viruses in oral cancer is under continuing study. The interaction of viruses with other carcinogens and oncogenes may be an important mechanism of disease. Herpes simplex virus (HSV) has been shown to produce a number of mutations in cells.[89] A cocarcinogenic effect between HSV and chewing tobacco has been demonstrated in animal studies.[90–92] Smokers demonstrate higher antibody titers to HSV, suggesting reactivation.[93,94] Neutralizing antibodies to HSV are present in the serum of patients with oral cancer at higher titers in those who have advanced cancer, and antibody response to HSV antigen is greater in patients than in controls.[93,94] However, HSV has not been detected in human squamous cell carcinoma.[89,95] If HSV is etiologic, it is likely that the virus has an effect that leaves no evidence of its presence after its oncogenic effect (a "hit-and-run" effect).[12,89] The association of HPV with anogenital and cervical dysplasia, carcinoma in situ, and invasive carcinoma has been well established.[50,89,96,97] HNSCCs with transcriptionally active HPV-16 DNA are characterized by occasional chromosomal loss, whereas HNSCCs lacking HPV DNA are characterized by gross deletions that involve whole or large parts of chromosomal arms and that occur early in HNSCC development. These distinct patterns of genetic alterations suggest that HPV-16 infection is an early event in HNSCC development.[98] The sensitivity of methods and the sequences of DNA selected for study may explain the variability of findings in the study of HPV in HNSCC. In some studies, approximately half of OSCCs contain HPV types 16 or 18 (HPV-16 or -18).[50,99–102] In one study, when assessed by polymerase chain reaction, 90% of oral carcinomas were found to contain HPV-16 or HPV-18.[102] HPV is detected with increased frequency in oral dysplastic ($2–3\times$) and malignant epitheilum ($4.7\times$) than in beinign oral mucosa, and the probability of high-risk HPV was increased ($2.8\times$).[103–105] Oropharyngeal SCC, particularly involving the tonsil, base of the tongue, and larynx, has a higher prevalence of high-risk HPV-16 than oral SCC.[106–109] Nonkeratinizing cancer of the base of the tongue and the tonsil associated with HPV appear to have an improved response to radiation sensitivity.[109]

Repair mechanisms of cellular damage may play a role in the understanding of malignant disease and in future therapy.[50,110] Genetic risk and cocarcinogenesis are continuing to be investigated (see above). The role of cytokines, including epidermal and transforming growth factors, may be relevant in OSCC.[50,110,111] Changes in cell surface receptors and major histocompatibility class I and class II antigens have been seen and may indicate that immune surveillance and immune function may be affected in patients with oral cancer.[111] The changes noted in human leukocyte antigen (HLA) expression may be useful in the prognosis of tumor behavior. Other cell surface changes include a loss of cytoplasmic membrane binding of lectins, which has been shown to correlate to the degree of cellular atypia. Cell surface markers are altered in neoplastic dedifferentiation; examples are the loss of ABO blood group antigens, β_2-microglobulin, and involucrin and a loss of reaction to pemphigus antisera. Alterations in cell-bound immunoglobulins and circulating immunocomplexes are detectable, but the importance of these changes is unclear. Carcinoembryonic antigens are elevated in patients with oral cancer. Intracellular enzymes are altered or lost, commensurate with the degree of cellular dysplasia.

The development of malignant disease in immunosuppressed patients indicates the importance of an intact immune response (see above). Mononuclear cell infiltration correlates with prognosis, and more aggressive disease is associated with limited inflammatory response. Total numbers of T cells may be decreased in patients with head and neck cancer and the mixed lymphocyte reaction is reduced in some patients, and a diminished migration of macrophages has been demonstrated. Cluster designation 8 (CD8) lymphocytes (T

suppressor cells) predominate in the infiltrate, suggesting that immunosuppression is associated with progression of disease. Langerhans' cells (intraepithelial macrophages) may be altered in neoplastic epithelium. Further understanding of immune function and the response to SCC may lead to the development of new therapies that modulate the immune response.[110]

SCC primarily spreads by direct local extension and by regional extension via the lymphatics. Regional spread in the oral mucosa may occur by direct extension and sometimes by submucosal spread and result in wide areas of involvement. Production of type I collagenase and other proteinases, prostaglandin E_2, and interleukin-1 may affect the extracellular matrix, and motility of epithelial cells may allow invasion.[50,111,112] Changes in the basement membrane, such as the breakdown of laminin and collagen, occur with invasion. Understanding the biology of invasion by malignant cells may lead to additional approaches to diagnosis and management.

Presenting Signs and Symptoms

Unfortunately, patients are most often identified only after the development of symptoms at advanced stages of disease. Discomfort is the most common symptom that leads a patient to seek care and may be present at the time of diagnosis in up to 85% of patients.[2,113] Patients also may present with an awareness of a mass in the mouth or neck. Dysphagia, odynophagia, otalgia, limited movement, oral bleeding, neck masses, and weight loss may occur with advanced disease.

Head and neck and oral examinations have been shown in a large trial in India to result in earlier identification of OSCC and to translate into improved survival compared with a control group.[114] In this study, subjects over age 35 years were randomized to examination by trained health care workers at 3-year intervals. Head and neck and oral examinations resulted in earlier stage detection of OSCC (37.6% stage I, II vs 18.9% stage I, II) and improved survival compared with the control group (57.5% vs 38.8%; $p < .05$).[114] However, a patient delay–tumor stage relationship has not been documented in all cases, possibly because a proportion of tumors may be silent until advanced stage, and approximately two-thirds present with advanced-stage disease (stages 3 and 4).[115–117] In a study in the United Kingdom, the proportion of patients presenting with advanced disease has not changed in 40 years despite public education.[118] Therefore, the oral cavity should be examined following a careful assessment of the cervical and submandibular lymph nodes. Examination of the oral cavity should not neglect any area, but the high-risk sites for oral carcinoma, including the lower lip, the anterior floor of the mouth, and the lateral borders of the tongue, must be carefully examined. The patient should be assessed for tissue changes that may include a red, white, or mixed red-and-white lesion; a change in the surface texture producing a smooth, granular, rough, or crusted lesion; or the presence of a mass or ulceration (Figure 2 to 6).

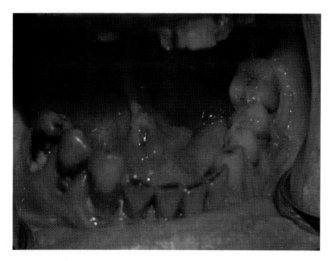

FIGURE 2 Irregular ertyholeukoplakia of the L lateral border of the tongue.

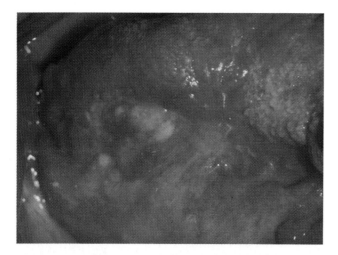

FIGURE 3 Irregular erthroleukoplakia (Figure 2), following application by toluidine blue. Inferior of lesion and supperior stained site, were biopsy proven squamous cell carcinoma.

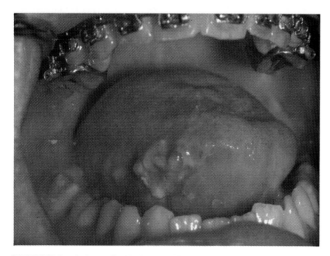

FIGURE 4 Indurated and ulcerated lesion of the R anterior tongue in a 15 year old girl, persisting after removal of orthodontic appliances, proven to be squamous cell carcinoma on biopsy.

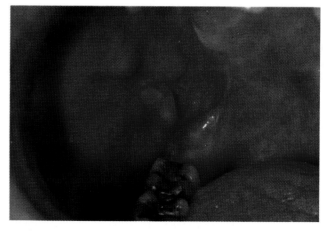

FIGURE 5 Nonpainful, irregular indurated exophytic and ulcerated buccal mass histolpathology revealed squamous cell carcinoma.

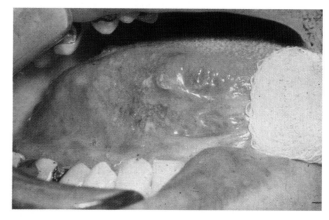

FIGURE 6 Eroded, erythroluekoplakic, indurated lesion in the R posterior third of the lateral border of tongue diagnosed as squamous cell carcinoma.

The lesion may be flat or elevated and ulcerated or nonulcerated and may be minimally palpable or indurated. Loss of function involving the tongue can affect speech, swallowing, and diet.

Lymphatic spread of oral carcinoma usually involves the submandibular and digastric nodes, the upper cervical nodes, and, finally, the remaining nodes of the cervical chain. The nodes most commonly involved are those that are on the same side as the primary tumor, although the closer the tumor is to the midline and the more posterior in the oral cavity or oropharynx, the more common is the involvement of the bilateral and contralateral nodes. Lymph node involvement may not occur in an orderly fashion, and thorough examination is mandatory. Lymph nodes associated with cancer become enlarged and firm to hard in texture. The nodes are not tender unless they are associated with secondary infection or an inflammatory response is present, which may occur after a biopsy. The fixation of nodes to adjacent tissue due to invasion of cells through the capsule is a late occurrence and evidence of aggressive disease. The fixation of the primary tumor to adjacent tissue overlying bone suggests the involvement of the periosteum and possible spread to bone. Spread of tumor is critical for prognosis and for selection of treatment. It is critical that the status of the lymph nodes be carefully assessed before a biopsy is performed. The understaging of nodes by cursory assessment or the over-staging of nodes following a biopsy, when an inflammatory component may be present, impacts the selection of treatment. Therefore, accurate node examination is needed before biopsy, and the individual who is performing the procedure must be experienced in lymph node palpation.

Diagnostic Aids

Early detection of malignant lesions is a continuing goal. Thorough head and neck and intraoral examination is a prerequisite. Aids to oral examination include imaging and light technologies, vital tissue staining using toluidine blue, and computer-assisted cytology of oral brush biopsy specimens.[119]

Toluidine blue can be applied directly to suspicious lesions or used as an oral rinse. A study of the application of toluidine blue to a consecutive series of patients who had prior head and neck cancer and in whom all lesions were examined by biopsy revealed 100% of the carcinomas in situ and SCCs (no false-negatives; sensitivity was 100%), whereas clinical findings would not have led to biopsy being performed on only 28% of these malignant lesions ($p = .02$).[120] The assessment of dye uptake depends on clinical judgment and experience (Figures 7 and 8). Positive retention of toluidine blue (particularly in areas of leukoplakia, erythro-plakia, and uptake in a peripheral pattern of an ulcer) may indicate the need for biopsy. False-positive dye retention may occur in inflammatory and ulcerative lesions, but false-negative retention is uncommon.[120] A return appointment in 14 days, providing time for inflammatory lesions to improve, may lead to a decrease in false-positive results. Toluidine blue rinse has been assessed in a multicenter study that enrolled 668 patients, in which all identified mucosal lesions were biopsied. Twenty-nine of 30 cases of SCC were identified by toluidine blue, whereas only 12 were identified by unaided expert clinical examination ($p = .002$), without the need for an excessive number of unecessary biopsies.[121] A prospective study assessed the risk of progression of oral premalignant lesions to SCC, and it was shown that toluidine blue posi-tiveity identified sites of LOH abnormality and predicted those lesions that progress to cancer.[69] The definitive test remains a biopsy, and any suspicious lesion should not remain undiagnosed. Toluidine blue predicts oral premalignant lesions at risk of progressing to squamous cell cancer, provides guidance for the selection for the biopsy site, and accelerates the decision to biopsy. In postradiotherapy follow-up, the retention of toluidine blue may assist in distinguishing nonhealing ulcers and persistent or recurrent disease.

Computer-assisted analysis of oral brush cytology is completed on Pap-stained exfoliated cells, scanned by computer for abnormal cell morphology and keratinization, and a final diagnosis is made by an examining pathologist on the basis of standard histomorphologic criteria. This approach was evaluated in 945 patients, of whom only approximately one-third underwent biopsy, and true positive results were

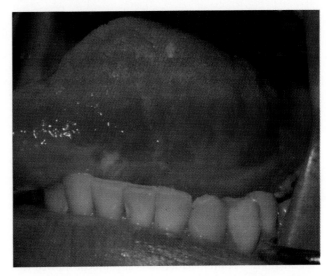

FIGURE 7 Asymptomatic erythroplakia in the floor of the mouth in a patient presenting due to toothache, diagnosed on biopsy as squamous cell carcinoma.

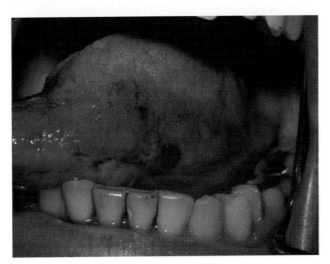

FIGURE 8 Previously treated squamous cell carcinoma, are at risk of recurrent squamous cell carcinoma. This case was treated with surgery and post-operative radiation therapy, and presented with an area of leukoeryth-roplakia that was diagnosed as recurrent squamous cell carcinoma.

reported in 100% of the lesions that were positive by brush cytology (sensitivity 100%; no false-negative results); unfor-tunately, not all patients underwent biopsy, and false-negative results are not evaluable. Of importance, 4.5% of clinically benign lesions that were positive on brush cytology were subsequently evaluated by biopsy and diagnosed as dysplasia or SCC. Brush cytology may be useful and can be used in conjunction with vital staining.[119] Future develop-ments may include studies of exfoliated cells by using molecular markers of dysplasia or carcinoma to improve the diagnostic and prognostic value. Exfoliative oral epithelial cells have the same genetic changes associated with dysplasia and cancer as did paired biopsy specimens.[122] Increased mitochondrial and nuclear DNA have been detected in the saliva of patients with HNSCC independent of age and smoking.[123] Studies have shown that biomarkers of OSCC are present in saliva.[123–126]

Using the methylation-specific polymerase chain reaction in tumor and serum samples of 17 OSCC patients, aberrant p16 methylation was detected in the primary tumor in 11 patients. Six of these 11 patients showed the same alteration in their serum; the aberrancy was also detected in the serum of 3 of 4 patients with recurrence.[127] Despite the great promise of a number of new molecular approaches for cancer detection, much of the current technology limits their implementation into routine clinical use.[128,129]

ViziLite is a disposable chemiluminescent light source, approved by the US Food and Drug Administration (FDA) and used in conjuction with a standard visual examination and toluidine blue. A single-center study of 485 consecutive subjects over 40 years old with a positive tobacco history reported brighter, sharper, and smaller lesions size of lesions with ViziLite illumination compared with incandescent illumination.[130] A multicenter clinical protocol showed that ViziLite enhanced the visibility of oral leukoplakia in 134 patients by increasing the brightness, texture, or margin idenfication in 54% of lesions ($p < .001$), which may allow identification of lesions requiring further assessment.[131]

There is an increasing interest in the use of optical spectroscopy systems to provide tissue diagnosis in real time, noninvasively, and in situ.[132] Oral cavity flouresence using blue light excitation was reported due to interaction with collagen and modified by epithelial cellular metabolism and structure and was felt primarily to be related to collagen breakdown and increased hemoglobin absorption of light. This clinical in vivo flouresence was reported to discriminate normal mucosa from severe dysplasia, and SCC was assessed in patients for whom biopsy decision was based upon clinical features and toluidine blue stain retention assessment of oral premalignant lesions has not been reported.[133]

Imaging

Routine radiology, computed tomography (CT), nuclear scintiscanning, magnetic resonance imaging (MRI), and ultrasonography can provide evidence of bone involvement and can indicate the extent of some soft tissue lesions. Positron emission therapy (PET) using the radiolabeled glucose analog 18-fluorodeoxyglucose (^{18}FDG) offers a functional imaging approach for the entire body. In a pilot study among head and neck cancer patients, this imaging technique was shown to be valuable in a subset of patients who are at substantial risk.[134] Bone involvement is important in staging, selecting therapy, and determining the prognosis. PET fused with computed tomography (PET-CT) was shown to provide additional information for staging and in the evaluation of patients with suspected recurrent squamous cell carcinoma of the head and neck, in whom anatomic imaging is inconclusive due to the locoregional distortions rendered by surgery and radiotherapy.[135]

Imaging to determine bone involvement may include routine radiology (including dental radiographs for alveolar bone involvement), CT, and bone scanning (Figures 9 to 15). Nuclear scintiscanning may provide evidence of bone involvement by tumor and bony necrosis following radiation therapy. MRI is of limited value in determining bone involvement

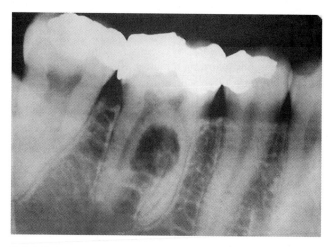

FIGURE 9 Periapical radiograph demonstrating bone destruction in the furcation of the first molar tooth and associated resorption of the root. A subsequent biopsy specimen demonstrated squamous cell carcinoma, which was diagnosed as a primary intra-alveolar lesion.

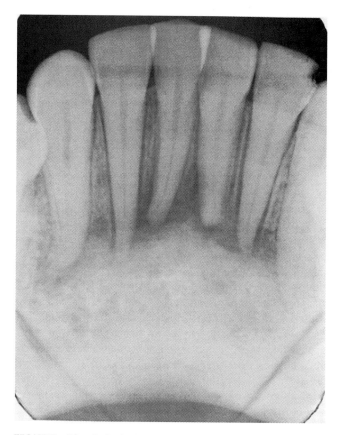

FIGURE 10 Periapical radiograph demonstrating an irregular radiolucency involving the bone of the apical region of the mandibular anterior teeth, without a change in root anatomy. The teeth tested vital. The radiographic finding was the first indication of involvement of the bony adenocarcinoma.

but may show distortion of bony trabeculae. Future developments may include monoclonal antibodies linked to a radiolabel to enhance the sensitivity and specificity of the imaging and combined PET-CT imaging.

Soft tissue involvement of the antrum and nasopharynx can be assessed with CT and MRI. Panoramic radiography of

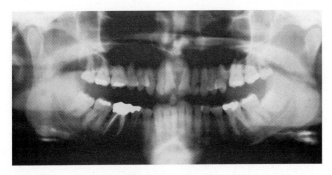

FIGURE 11 Panoramic radiograph taken at the time of diagnosis of adenocarcinoma.

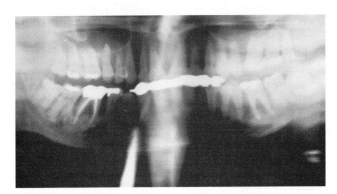

FIGURE 12 Massive bone destruction of the mandible, shown after 5 years of follow-up in a case of adenocarcinoma (see Figures 10 and 11) extending to the molar regions bilaterally. The anterior teeth had been lost due to progressive destruction of the anterior mandible and floor of the mouth.

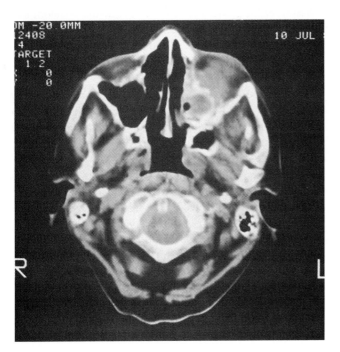

FIGURE 13 Computed tomographic scan demonstrating destruction of the medial wall of the antrum and opacification of the antrum. Additional views suggested that the opacification represented a tissue mass that was consistent with tumor.

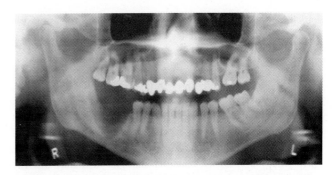

FIGURE 14 Panoramic radiograph showing bony destruction of the molar region of the right mandible due to invasion of contiguous tumor. Paresthesia of the right lip was present at the time of diagnosis.

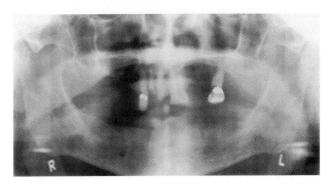

FIGURE 15 Panoramic radiograph demonstrating a destructive lesion of the right mandible overlying the mandibular canal. Anesthesia of the mandibular nerve and jaw pain were present. The bone biopsy specimen was consistent with metastatic colon carcinoma, which was subsequently diagnosed.

patients with antral carcinoma may document the lesion in a large number of such cases. MRI is rapidly replacing CT as the imaging technique of choice for the head and neck.[136] Each MRI image should include T1-weighted images, which demonstrate normal anatomy with detail and soft tissue definition, and T2-weighted images, which demonstrate the tumor in comparison with adjacent muscle and other soft tissues. MRI will allow more accurate distinctions between tumor and benign inflammatory disease than CT. Motion distortion can limit its imaging, particularly in moving tissues, but the continuing development of MRI is resulting in less time required for imaging.

CT and MRI aid in determining the status of the cervical lymph nodes. There is evidence that imaging will enhance the findings of expert clinical examination when positive lymph nodes are being sought.[137] Small-part ultrasonography may also be of value for imaging salivary gland masses and for the assessment of lymph nodes; however, differentiation between benign and malignant nodes may not be possible. The ultrasonographically guided needle biopsy technique may be useful in the assessment of head and neck masses, including lymph nodes.

There may be a place for lymphatic mapping with sentinel node biopsy.[138–141]

In the assessment of metastases to the lung, conventional radiography will detect advanced involvement (>1 cm);

detection of smaller masses or lymph nodes is possible with CT and evaluation by PET can provide additional information.

Acquisition of a Tissue Specimen

In addition to the standard biopsy techniques, tissue can be acquired for histopathology by using fine-needle aspiration (FNA) and exfoliative cytology (see above). Open biopsy of enlarged lymph nodes is not recommended; in such cases, FNA biopsy should be considered. FNA also may aid the evaluation of suspicious masses in other areas of the head and neck, including masses that involve the salivary glands, tongue, and palate.

Exfoliative cytology for morphologic assessment is of limited value in the assessment of cancer because squamous mucosa is difficult to sample to the basal epithelium, which may be overcome using cytology brush collections. An additional means of improving diagnostic value may be the application of molecular markers to exfoliated cells because LOH at sites of putative TSGs in exfoliated cells has been shown to reflect those found on biopsy.[122–124]

Histopathology

Microscopic examination is required for diagnosis. Dysplasia or atypia describes a range of cellular abnormalities that includes changes in cell size and morphology, increased mitotic figures, hyperchromatism, and alteration in normal cellular orientation and maturation. The descriptions of mild, moderate, and severe dysplasia refer to epithelial abnormality of varying severity. When the abnormality involves the full thickness of the epithelium, the diagnosis is carcinoma in situ. When the basement membrane is violated, carcinoma is diagnosed. Well-differentiated carcinoma may retain some anatomic features of epithelial cells and may retain the ability to produce keratin, whereas poorly differentiated carcinoma loses the anatomic pattern and function of epithelium. Tumors may be associated with a mixed inflammatory infiltrate. Inflammatory and reactive lesions can be difficult to differentiate from dysplasia, and the experience of the pathologist becomes important with the need for clinical reassessment and repeat investigation. Recognition of tumor invasion may be assisted by a study of type IV collagen (basement membrane collagen) by immunocytochemistry.[111] Invasion of lymphatics, blood vessels, and perineural spaces is of critical importance but is difficult to determine.[111]

VERRUCOUS CARCINOMA

Verrucous carcinoma is a subtype of SCC with characteristic clinical findings. Verrucous carcinoma can be described clinically as papillary, verrucoid, fungating, or cauliflower-like. Verrucous carcinoma may develop from progression of proliferative verrucous leukoplakia and progress to carcinoma.[142]

Histologically, the first change is a piling up of keratin on the surface, with downgrowth of club-shaped fingers of hyperplastic epithelium pushing rather than infiltrating into the tissue. Only mild dysplasia may be present. Usually, a dense infiltrate of lymphocytes and plasma cells is present. Verrucous carcinoma rarely spreads to lymph nodes and remains locally destructive.[143] The difficulty in diagnosis and treatment is due to mild dysplastic change that may be seen despite progressive and recurent disease. The treatment is surgical excision as verrucous carcinoma is relatively resistant to radiotherapy.

VARIANTS OF SCC OTHER THAN VERRUCOUS CARCINOMA

The term *basaloid squamous carcinoma* (BSC) has been introduced for tumors of which the major portion was composed of solid growth of basaloid cells with small cystic spaces containing periodic acid–Schiff– and alcian blue–positive material. The histologic hallmark of the neoplasm is that of an SCC in intimate relationship with a basaloid component. Immunohistochemical findings may be helpful in distinguishing BSC from the histopathologically similar tumors.[144] It has been suggested that HPV-associated cancers of the oral cavity are more likely to have basaloid features.[104] BSC has a poorer prognosis than the conventional SCC.

Spindle cell carcinomas, also referred to as sarcomatoid SCCs, are rare variants of SCC. The histologic criterion to accept a diagnosis of spindle cell carcinoma is the demonstration of epithelial changes ranging from prominent dysplasia to frank SCC in conjunction with a dysplastic spindle cell element or evidence of direct transition of epithelial cells to dysplastic spindle cells. In a few cases, osteoid-appearing material within the spindle cell component can be found. Surgery is the treatment of choice.

A few cases have been reported of adenoid SCCs of the oral mucosa. The adenoid structure results from loss of cohesion of the epidermoid tumor cells, without sialomucin production. Insufficient data are available to comment on treatment and prognosis. Separation of adenosquamous carcinoma from mucoepidermoid carcinoma may be difficult.

Papillary squamous carcinoma is an exophytic papillary lesion that shows epithelial dysplasia, possibly even carcinoma in situ, and relatively inconspicuous areas of invasive SCC and should be distinguished from verrucous carcinomas.

Rare cases of carcinoma cuniculatum have been reported.[145] Carcinoma cuniculatum is a rare variant of carcinomas usually involving the foot. Histologically, stratified squamous epithelium is observed with keratin filled crypts but without cytologic features of malignancy.[146,147]

Intraoral sebaceous carcinoma probably represents a sebaceous-like differentiation.[148,149] Currently, diagnosis is based on the interpretation of histomorphologic changes.

While histopathology is the gold standard in diagnosis, it is a subjective assessment of tissue, with inter- and intrarater variability.[150] However, phenotypic changes appear following molecular change, and it is possible that when molecular markers become available, they will provide additional information and may ultimately become the gold standard in diagnosis.

Treatment of Oral Cancer

The principal objective of treatment is to cure the patient of cancer. The choice of treatment depends upon cell type and degree of differentiation; the site and size of the primary lesion; lymph node status; the presence of bone involvement; the ability to achieve adequate surgical margins; the presence or absence of metastases, the ability to preserve oropharyngeal function, including speech, swallowing, and esthetics; the medical and mental status of the patient; available support throughout therapy; a thorough assessment of the potential complications of each therapy; the experience of the surgeon and radiotherapist; and the personal preferences and cooperation of the patient. If the lesion is not cured by the initial therapy, the options for treatment may be limited, and the likelihood of cure is reduced.

Surgery and radiation are used with curative intent in the treatment of oral cancer. Chemotherapy is an adjunct to the principal therapeutic modalities of radiation and surgery and is now standard combined therapy in mangement of advanced disease. Either surgery or radiation may be used for many T1 and T2 lesions; however, combined radiation and chemotherapy with or without surgery is usually employed for more advanced disease.

Technical advances such as intensity-modulated radiotherapy (IMRT) reduce the size of the high-dose field of irradiation and limit the exposure of adjacent vital structures, including the salivary glands. Due to poor cure rates in head and neck cancer, particularly at advanced stages of disease, more intensive treatment including hyperfractionation, combined chemoradiotherapy, and reirradiation for recurrence of second primary cancers are provided.[151,152]

SURGERY

Surgery is indicated (1) for tumors involving bone, (2) when the side effects of surgery are expected to be less significant than those associated with radiation, (3) for tumors that lack sensitivity to radiation, and (4) for recurrent tumor in areas that have previously received radiotherapy. Surgery also may be used in palliative cases to reduce the bulk of the tumor and to promote drainage from a blocked cavity (eg, antrum). Surgery may fail due to incomplete excision, tumor seeding in the wound, unrecognized lymphatic or hematogenous spread, neural invasion, or perineural spread. Adequate surgical margins are required but may not be attainable due to the size and location of the tumor and limited information on the molecular status of the margins. Surgery results in a sacrifice of structure, which may have important esthetic and functional considerations. Surgical management of clinically positive cervical nodes is the treatment of choice. Surgery is needed when bone is involved, and radiotherapy alone cannot be considered adequate to produce a cure. In some cases with minimal bone involvement of the alveolar crest, a partial mandibulectomy may allow the continuity of the mandible to be maintained. However, in many cases, mandibulectomy and resection in continuity with the involved nodes are required. There is an ongoing debate about the value of preoperative assessment of mandibular invasion and the consequences on the management, that is, marginal

mandibulectomy versus segmental resection.[153] Neck dissection can be used in salvage treatment of cancer that has recurred in the neck. Tumors with node involvement should be treated aggressively due to the poorer prognosis that is seen with positive nodes. Management of the N0 neck remains a subject of discussion.[154] In a study of 80 patients with a T1/T2N0 SCC of the tongue, significant fewer regional recurrences were seen in patients receiving elective neck dissection, although no statistical differences were found in overall and disease-specific survival.[155]

Surgical excision of dysplastic and malignant lesions can be accomplished with laser therapy. Laser therapy for these lesions is well tolerated and usually decreases the period of hospitalization but has the disadvantage of limiting the assessment of the margins for histopathologic confirmation.

Advances in surgical management include new surgical approaches and new approaches to reconstruction, such as vascularized flaps, free microvascular reconstruction, and neurologic anastomoses of free grafts.[137,152] Reconstruction with the use of osseointegrated implants offers the ability to provide stable prostheses and enhanced esthetic and functional results. The ability to place implants in irradiated bone has increased options for rehabilitation.

RADIATION THERAPY

Radiation therapy may be administered with intent to cure, as part of a combined radiation-surgery and/or chemotherapy management, or for palliation.[151] Radical radiotherapy is intended to cure, the total dose is high, the course of therapy is prolonged, and early and late radiation effects are common. In palliative care, radiation may provide symptomatic relief from pain, bleeding, ulceration, and oropharyngeal obstruction. Hyperfractionation of radiation (usually twice-daily dosing) is being used more extensively as chronic complications appear to be reduced although acute complications are more severe.

Radiation kills cells by interaction with water molecules in the cells, producing charged molecules that interact with biochemical processes in the cells and by causing direct damage to DNA. The affected cells may die or remain incapable of division. Due to a greater potential for cell repair in normal tissue than in malignant cells and a greater susceptibility to radiation due to the higher growth fraction of cancer cells, a differential effect is achieved. To achieve therapeutic effects, radiation therapy is delivered in daily fractions for a planned number of days. The relatively hypoxic central tumor cells are less susceptible to radiotherapy but may become better oxygenated as peripheral cells are affected by radiation and thus become more susceptible to subsequent fractions of radiation.[156] SSCs are usually radiosensitive, and early lesions are highly curable. In general, the more differentiated the tumor, the less rapid will be the response to radiotherapy. Exophytic and well-oxygenated tumors are more radiosensitive, whereas large invasive tumors with small growth fractions are less responsive. SSC that is limited to the mucosa is highly curable with radiotherapy; however, tumor spread to bone reduces the probability of cure with radiation alone. Small cervical metastases may be controlled with radiation therapy alone, although advanced cervical node involvement is better managed with combined therapy.

The biologic effect of radiation depends on the dose per fraction, the number of fractions per day, the total treatment time, and the total dose of radiation. Methods for representing the factors of dose, fraction size, and time of radiation with a single calculation using the time-dose fraction (TDF) and the nominal standard dose (NSD) calculations have been described.[156–158] When comparing studies of radiation effect and when describing the results of studies of cancer patients treated with radiotherapy, reporting the total dose is inadequate because of the importance of fraction size and the time of therapy (which are not available for comparison). The use of the TDF or the NSD will facilitate the understanding of the biologic effect. The tolerance of the vascular and connective tissues to radiation influences both the success of tumor control and the development of treatment complications. The late complications of radiotherapy are due to effects on vascular, connective, and slowly proliferating parenchymal tissues. Late effects are related to the number of fractions, fraction size, total dose, tissue type, and volume of tissue irradiated. An increase in fraction size or a reduction in the number of fractions with the same total dose results in increased late complications, including tissue fibrosis and soft tissue and bone necrosis.[159]

Radiation therapy has the advantage of treating the disease in situ and avoiding the need for the removal of tissue, and it may be the treatment of choice for many T1 and T2 tumors. Radiation may be administered to a localized lesion by using implant techniques (brachytherapy) or to a region of the head and neck by using external beam radiation. External beam therapy can be provided in such a way as to protect adjacent uninvolved tissues, with enhanced effects by using smaller boost fields or by combining external beam and interstitial techniques. Innovations in radiation therapy include IMRT, using radiation beams of varying intensity, which provides the ability to conform the prescription dose to the shape of the target tissues in three dimensions, reducing the dose to surrounding normal tissues.[160] During the optimization process, each beam is divided into small "beamlets" whose intensity can be varied so that the optimal dose and distribution are obtained.[161] The resultant intensity profile of each beam is complex. Rapid dose gradients outside the target result in sparing of normal tissues. IMRT is ideally suited for head and neck malignancies given the proximity of these tumors to critical structures, including the brainstem, optic chiasm, and salivary glands. IMRT has been shown to have comparable disease control as standard radiotherapy in head and neck oncology, with reduced acute and late toxicity.[162–166] Additional ability to modify dose and fields of radiation has been introduced with image-guided radiotherapy (IGRT) in which integrated CT guides changes in radiation throughout the course of treatment as treatment causes change in volume of tumor during treatment.

Concurrent Chemotherapy and Radiotherapy (CCRT) and IMRT are becoming a standard modalities of treatment of head and neck SCC. CCRT has increased cure rates but is associated with a concomitant increase in toxicity. Primary tumors of the posterior third of the tongue, oropharynx, and tonsillar pillar are best treated by external beam radiotherapy, with or without chemotherapy and surgery is reserved for the treatment of tumors with node involvement. Larger radiation fields result in increased patient complications. Smaller fields may be used to boost the dose to the central portion of the tumor since control of peripheral well-oxygenated cells may be possible at a lower dose than that used for the central less well-oxygenated tumor mass.

Radiation Sources. For treatment of superficial tumors, radiation with low penetration may be used. Low-kilovolt radiation (50–300 kV) can be used in the treatment of skin and lip lesions. Electron beam therapy provides superficial radiation and has largely replaced low-kilovolt x-ray machines because electrons produce a rapid dose buildup and falloff of dose; thus, the depth of penetration can be relatively controlled. Electrons are useful in providing radiation to skin lesions, parotid tumors, and cervical nodes. Deep-seated tumors may be treated with heavy-particle irradiation, such as neutron beam radiation, which is considered for salivary gland tumors and central nervous system malignancies.

Megavoltage radiation using cobalt 60 or the use of a linear accelerator of ≥ 4 MeV is reported to be skin and bone sparing. The linear accelerator provides variable penetration due to its ability to vary the energy of the photons. Heavy-particle raditon therapy may have increased effect on electrons in salivary gland tumors and may be combined with gamma knife surgery for local disease with poor prognostic features.[167–169]

Treatment Planning. The radiation treatment plan is determined by the tumor site and size, the volume to be radiated, the number of treatment fractions, the total number of days of treatment, and the tolerance of the patient.[151] The dose to the eye, optic chiasm or spinal cord, salivary glands, alveolar bone, and soft tissue can be limited through the selection of the radiation source, field set-up, and shielding and by moving the uninvolved tissue out of the field. The current approach to treatment with the greatest potential to spare high-dose irradiation to vital tissue adjacent to tumor includes IMRT and IGRT. For repeated doses of radiation to be applied to the site of treatment, the patient and the area of treatment are immobilized, but using various techniques and materials, including head holders; bandages; laser positioning, using head and neck "landmarks"or tattoos; and custom acrylic shells (mold room technique). Custom shells provide the best means of immobilization and positioning of patients that are critical in IMRT and IGRT. These techniques may be combined with an oral device to position the mandible, allowing the maxilla or mandible to be moved into or out of the radiation field (Figures 16 to 18). The oral device can incorporate a tongue depressor to position the tongue in or

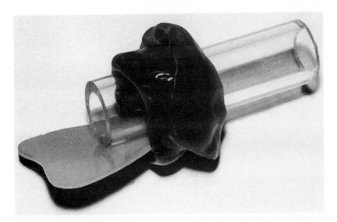

FIGURE 16 Tongue and mandibular positioning device. The tube is clear acrylic; the tongue deflector is acrylic but cut to shape and attached by baseplate wax that has been softened and formed to the dentition or residual alveolar ridge.

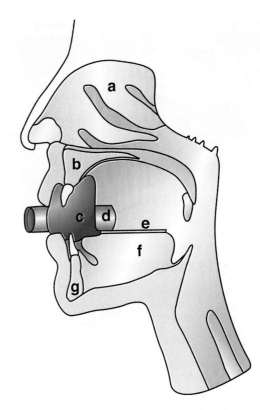

FIGURE 18 Schematic diagram of the positioning device placed intraorally. a = nasal cavity; b = upper alveolus; c = wax impression; d = acrylic tube; e = acrylic tongue depressor; f = tongue; g = lower alveolus.

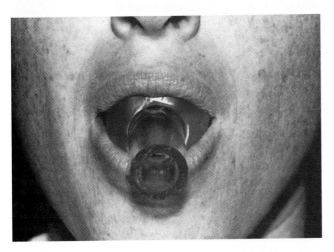

FIGURE 17 Tongue and mandibular positioning device placed intraorally. The wax impression and tube displace the soft tissue minimally to reduce the local irritation that can occur during irradiation.

out of the treatment field. This device can be made by using an acrylic tube around which wax is placed. Impressions in warmed baseplate wax can be readily accomplished with bite pressure. The tube serves as a handle and can facilitate respiration. The device can be left as wax or can be processed in acrylic.

Treatment planning requires localization of the tumor, and tumor margins can be marked with radiopaque gold seeds or lead wire. If a shell is used, markings can be placed on the shell or by a marking on the skin (Figures 19 to 21). The contours of the radiation field as planned by computer modeling and alterations can be made as needed. IGRT provides accurate and ongoing tumor contours and margin delineation during radiotherapy.

For most epithelial malignancies, radiation is commonly delivered in 1.8 to 2.2 Gy per fraction for 6 to 7 weeks to a total dose of 6,500 to 7,500 cGy. Hyperfractionation protocols vary; commonly, 100 to 150 cGy often are delivered twice daily. Therapy can be accelerated to produce a total dose of 5,000 cGy in 3 weeks. In external beam therapy, the principal field arrangements are parallel opposed fields (bilateral) and wedged-pair fields; increasing numbers of fields in more complex models are now used. The wedged-pair field allows a therapeutic dose to unilateral disease while sparing a high dose to the opposite side (Figure 22). When a large tumor or midline lesion is present, a parallel opposed-field set-up or three-field set-up may be needed, which produces relatively uniform exposure for midline disease. More complex set-ups include boost fields and sequential-field set-ups to maximize therapeutic effects and reduce complications (Figure 23). IMRT provides multiple fields with potential for variable dosing, allowing real-time modification of dose and field during each treatment visit. Specific portions of fields such as the orbit, spinal cord, and portions of the alveolus may be blocked with lead (Figure 24) or avoided by use of IMRT. IMRT is becoming the standard of care for head and neck cancer therapy. High-dose reirradiation is now offered in some centers as salvage treatment and may be considered in case of recurrent or second primary head and neck cancer, particularly when salvage surgery is not feasible.[170]

Brachytherapy. Interstitial and intracavitary implants may be used to treat primary cancers in the head and neck. Brachytherapy may be the primary treatment modality for localized tumors in the anterior two-thirds of the oral cavity, for boosted doses of radiation to a specific site, or for

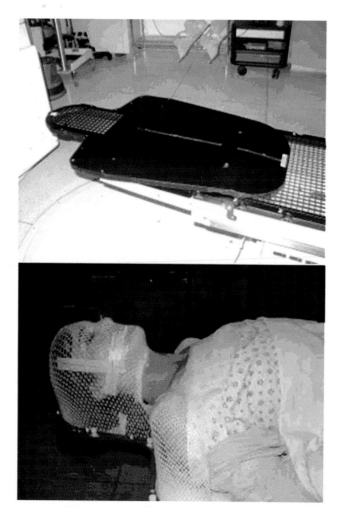

FIGURE 19 A patient positioned on a head support. An oral positioning device is in place, and plaster bandages have been placed to form an impression.

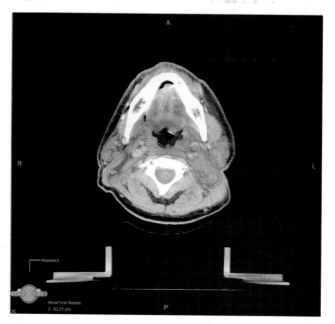

FIGURE 20 The acrylic shell or mold is made following removal of the plaster impression. A plaster facial model is poured, and the shell is formed to the model by means of a vacuform technique. The shell and the oral positioning device are used to place the patient in a reproducible position on the machine.

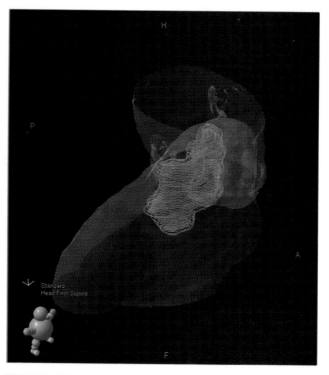

FIGURE 21 The final shell with cutouts, field markings, and identification wedges prior to radiation treatment.

treatment following recurrence. The isotopes used include cesium, iridium, and gold. Directly implanted sources may be used to deliver radiation, or an afterloading technique may be used in which the radiation source is placed by using previously inserted catheters or guide tubes.

The frequency of tissue necrosis is related to the treated volume and to the proximity of the implant to bone. Tissue deflectors can be made to deflect the tongue so that an implant designed to treat a cancer of the tongue does not expose adjacent alveolar bone. These devices can be fabricated by using a double layer of flexible mouthguard material or by using heat-cured acrylic (Figure 25). Lead foil can be added to the surface of the deflector if needed. Similarly, devices can be made to keep radiation from superficial treatment of the lip from affecting the alveolar bone (Figure 26). Lead cutouts can be made and placed on the skin to isolate the lesion; these may be used in combination with an intraoral device that can shield the intraoral tissues (Figure 27).

Future developments in radiotherapy include investigations of radiation sources, radiation fractionation, radiosensitizers, radioprotectors, and combined therapy.[112,171]

Advances in radiotherapy that are currently being studied include the use of heavy particles (ie, neutrons), which may provide a more focused distribution of cellular damage and which are less sensitive to hypoxia than are conventional radiation sources.[169] Methods of protecting tissues from late radiation effects (such as those that compromise the

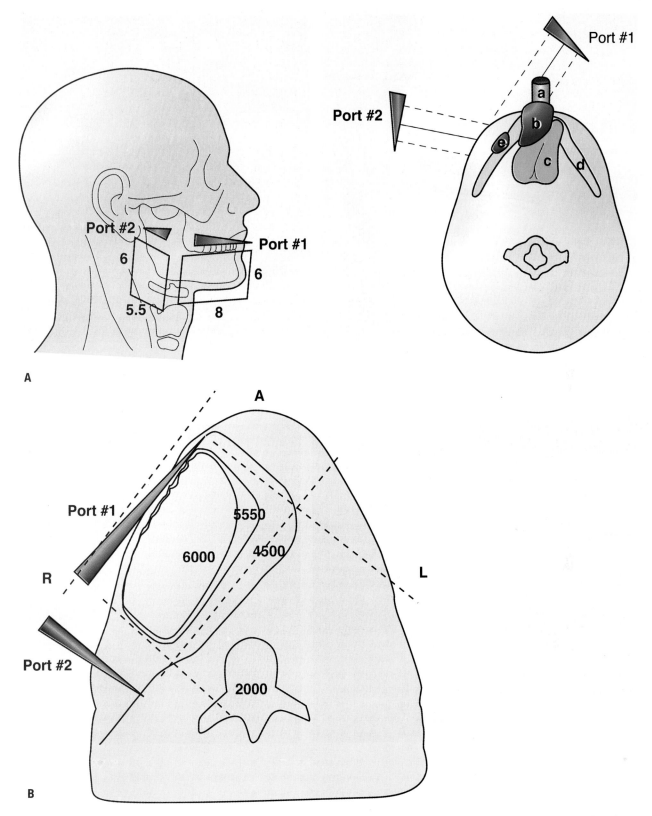

FIGURE 22 *A*, Treatment plan for external beam radiotherapy using a wedged-pair field set-up for squamous cell carcinoma involving the buccal mucosa adjacent to the mandible. The field size and wedges are shown. *B*, The positioning device was designed to displace the tongue laterally away from the high-dose volume, as demonstrated in this figure. a = acrylic tube; b = wax impression; c = tongue; d = mandible; e = tumor. *C*, Radiotherapy treatment plan with detailed representation of the field set-up and isodose calculations.

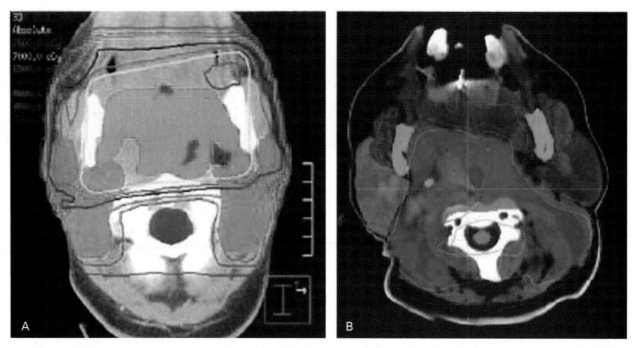

FIGURE 23 *A*, Conventional Radiation is delivered in few fields and may result in high dose exposure across the region of exposure. Exposure to vital structures such as midbrain and optic nerves and salivary gland may be included in the high dose volume. *B*, IMRT allows control of contours of radiation fields and allow tailoring of dose to allow high dose to tumor volumes, and shaping of fields to result in reduced dose to vital tissues such as brain stem, optic nerves, and salivary gland.

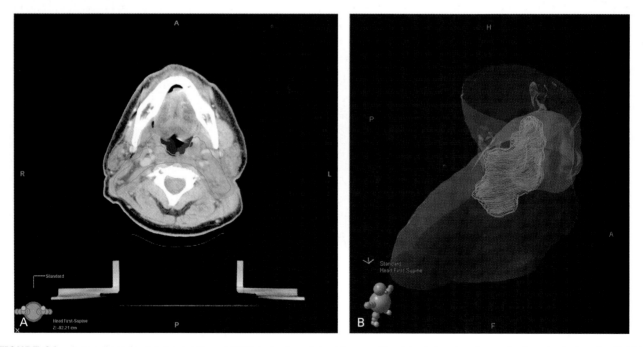

FIGURE 24 *A*, two dimensional representation of IMRT dosing to unilateral tumor, with minimal dose to salivary glands and spinal cord, with high treatment dose to tumor and parapharyngeal lymphnodes. *B*, Three dimensional reconstruction of treatment fields using IMRT, where doses are contoured in three dimensions to maximize tumor dose and minimize dose to vital and uninvolved structions.

vasculature) are under study. Hyperfractionation (ie, the use of more than one fraction of radiation each day of therapy) may result in improved tumor control with a reduction in late complications; however, increased severity of oral mucositis is reported.[156,172] Thus, efforts to prevent or palliate mucositis will reduce one of the treatment-limiting complications associated with hyperfractionation of radiation therapy. The development of in vitro clonagenic assays to determine tumor cell kinetics and susceptibility to therapy may lead to improvements in the selection of treatment.

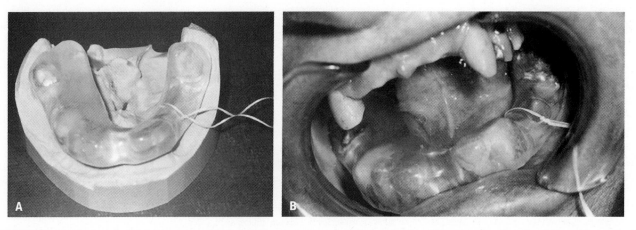

FIGURE 25   *A*, Tongue deflector, fabricated by using three thicknesses of vacuform vinyl on the side of the planned implant. The vinyl provides a smooth soft surface to displace the tongue away from the alveolus. *B*, The appliance in situ.

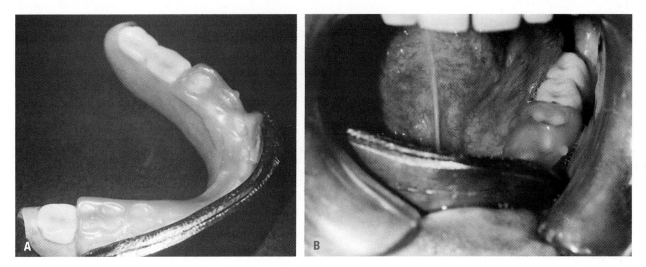

FIGURE 26   *A*, A denture that has been modified with a double thickness of lead shielding attached with baseplate wax. *B*, The modified appliance, shown in situ, prevents exposure of the alveolus to the radiation source.

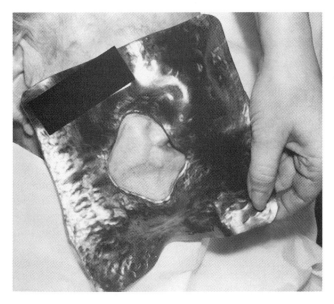

FIGURE 27   Lead cutout designed to shield the tissue adjacent to the tumor from radiation exposure.

CHEMOTHERAPY

Chemotherapy is used as induction therapy prior to local therapies, simultaneous chemoradiotherapy (concurrent CCRT), and adjuvant chemotherapy after local treatment.[112,151,173,174] The objective of induction chemotherapy is to promote initial tumor reduction and to provide early treatment of micrometastases due to the recognition that local control has improved with aggressive combined therapy, but distant failure due to metastatic disease has increased. The potential toxic effects of chemotherapy include mucositis, nausea, vomiting, and bone marrow suppression. The principal agents that have been studied alone or in combination in head and neck cancer are methotrexate, bleomycin, Taxol and derivatives, platinum derivatives (cisplatin and carboplatin), and 5-fluorouracil. The initial tumor response to chemotherapy prior to radiotherapy may predict tumor responsiveness to radiation. Concurrent chemotherapy and radiotherapy protocols are now the standard of care for stage 3 and 4 as primary therapy and following surgery for disease with poor prognostic findings following surgery including

TABLE 1 Staging of Oral Squamous Cell Carcinoma

T	—	Primary tumor
TX	—	Primary tumor cannot be assessed
T0	—	No evidence of primary tumor
Tis	—	Carcinoma in situ
T1	—	Tumor 2 cm or less in greatest dimension
T2	—	Tumor more than 2 cm but not more than 4 cm in greatest dimension
T3	—	Tumor more than 4 cm in greatest dimension
T4a	—	(lip) Tumor invades through cortical bone, inferior alveolar nerve, floor of mouth, or skin (chin or nose)
T4a	—	(oral cavity) Tumor invades through cortical bone, into deep/extrinsic muscle of tongue (genioglossus, hyoglossus, palatoglossus, and styloglossus), maxillary sinus, or skin of face
T4b	—	(lip and oral cavity) Tumor invades masticator space, pterygoid plates, or skull base, or encases internal carotid artery

Note: Superficial erosion alone of bone/tooth socket by gingival primary is not sufficient to classify a tumor as T4.

N	—	Regional lymph nodes
NX	—	Regional lymph nodes cannot be assessed
N0	—	No regional lymph node metastasis
N1	—	Metastasis in a single ipsilateral lymph node, 3 cm or less in greatest dimension
N2	—	Metastasis in a single ipsilateral lymph node, more than 3 cm but not more than 6 cm in greatest dimension; or in multiple ipsilateral lymph nodes, none more than 6 cm in greatest dimension; or in bilateral or contralateral lymph nodes, none more than 6 cm in greatest dimension
	N2a —	Metastasis in a single ipsilateral lymph node, more than 3 cm but not more than 6 cm in greatest dimension
	N2b —	Metastasis in multiple ipsilateral lymph nodes, none more than 6 cm in greatest dimension
	N2c —	Metastasis in bilateral or contralateral lymph nodes, none more than 6 cm in greatest dimension
N3	—	Metastasis in a lymph node more than 6 cm in greatest dimension
M	—	Distant metastasis
MX	—	Distant metastasis cannot be assessed
M0	—	No distant metastasis
M1	—	Distant metastasis

Stage grouping

Stage 0	Tis	N0	M0
Stage I	T1	N0	M0
Stage II	T2	N0	M0
Stage III	T1, T2	N1	M0
	T3	N0, N1	M0
Stage IVA	T1, T2, T3	N2	M0
	T4a	N0, N1, N2	M0
Stage IVB	Any T	N3	M0
	T4b	Any N	M0
Stage IVC	Any T	Any N	M1

Adapted from Sobin LH, Wittekind Ch. TNM classification of malignant tumours. 6th ed. New York: Wiley & Sons; 2002.

close margin, and vascular invasion by tumor.[151,175–185] Induction chemotherapy has not yet become standard in treatment protocols; however, there is evidence of impressive response rates, with survival benefit yet to be established.[186–190] As CCRT becomes more widely used, the morbidities associated with these therapies will become more pronounced.

As with treatment of many other malignancies, new target-directed chemotherapeutic agents are being studied as adjuncts or replacements for older agents. The role of new directed agents, such as EGFR (epidermal growth factor receptor) modulators, are currently being defined in the treatment of HNSCC.[191–194] Trials combining agents that target different pathways, such as bevacizumab and erlotinib, have also been completed with promising results.[195] Agents such as capecitabine offer a method of delivering chemotherapy to patients who, due to the significant side effects with standard agents, may not be candidates for conventional chemotherapy. Interferon alpha 2b may be effective as a tool for adjuvant therapy along with conventional therapies to overcome immunosuppression and cytotoxicity of tobacco-related HNSCC patients.[196] Research will continue and may include investigations into increasing the number of drugs used in combination, increasing the number of courses of chemotherapy provided, using modulators of chemotherapeutics, and modifying administration, such as by intermittent and continuous infusion.

COMBINED RADIATION AND SURGERY

Advantages of radiotherapy include the potential to to eradicate well-oxygenated tumor cells at the periphery of a tumor and to manage subclinical regional disease. Surgery more readily manages tumor masses that may possess relatively radiation-resistant hypoxic cells and tumor that involves bone. Thus, combined therapy can result in improved survival in cases of advanced tumors and tumors that show aggressive biologic behavior.[137] Radiation can be used preoperatively, postoperatively, or with a planned split-course approach, although there is controversy on the best approach. The advantages of preoperative radiation are the destruction of peripheral tumor cells, the potential control of subclinical disease, and the possibility of converting inoperable lesions into operable lesions. The disadvantages include delayed surgery and delayed postsurgical healing. Postoperative chemoradiotherapy can be used to treat cells that remain at the margin of resection and to control subclinical disease. Local control of the primary disease appears to be similar with preoperative or postoperative radiotherapy, but in some series, the incidence of metastases was lower in the postoperative group.[197,198]

GENE THERAPY

One animal study has shown that SCC antigen 1 has potential as a biomarker of tongue cancer and as the potential therapeutic target for gene therapy.[199]

IMMUNOTHERAPY

Based on an analysis of a gene expression profile in matched tumor and normal fibroblast cell lines, a number of proteins were detected that might be potential targets for immunotherapy of head and neck cancer patients.[200]

Prognosis

GENERAL REMARKS

The American Joint Committee on Cancer (AJCC) has developed the tumor, node, and metastasis (TNM) system of cancer classification.[201] The UICC classification is principally a clinical description of the disease but also includes imaging in the classification (Table 1). T is the size of the primary tumor, N indicates the presence of regional lymph nodes, and M indicates distant metastasis. The staging system for SCC combines the T, N, and M to classify lesions as stages 1 to 4. Classification of the cancer by TNM description is more accurate than use of the four staging groups and may reflect the biology of the tumor. For example, there are differences in biology and response to treatment between a stage 3 tumor that is classified as T1N1M0 and a stage 3 tumor that is classed as T3N0M0.

The various aspects related to TNM staging of cancers of the head and neck are discussed by Patel and Shah.[202] It has been suggested that the T4 classification of upper gingival and hard palate carcinomas by defining the boundary between T1–T3 and T4 as extensive invasion of the maxillary sinus, nasal cavity, or external skin.[203] Local or regional spread of oral SSC is common and affects the choice of therapy and prognosis. Metastases to cervical lymph nodes are common, but distant metastases below the clavicle are rare. Oral cancer occurring in the posterior aspect of the oral cavity and oropharynx and inferior in the mouth tends to be associated with a poorer prognosis, which may be explained by diagnosis occurring with advanced disease and a higher incidence of spread to lymph nodes at the time of diagnosis.[204] Ipsilateral lymph node metastases are frequent; however, spread to contralateral nodes also occurs and is more common with midline and posterior lesions.

The most important factor in survival is the stage of disease at diagnosis. Unfortunately, the majority of oral cancers are diagnosed in advanced stages, after becoming symptomatic.[3] Since 1960, some progress has been seen with an increase in 5-year survival rates from 45 to 53%.[1] African Americans have had a poorer 5-year survival rate and continue to have a survival rate of less than one-third compared with Caucasians, who have a 5-year survival rate of 53%.[1,2,11,12] These survival rates may be conditioned by physical and social environment; lack of health knowledge; risk-promoting lifestyle, attitude, and behavior; and limited access to health care. At least half of the difference in survival in the poor has been attributed to late diagnosis.[11,12]

The incidence of spread is influenced by tumor size. Lesions classed as T1 may show regional spread in 10 to 20% of cases, T2 lesions in 25 to 30% of cases, and T3 to T4 tumors in 50 to 75%.[204–206] A 3-year follow-up with no evidence of disease occurs with approximately 75 to 85% of T1 lesions, 50 to 60% of T2 lesions, and 20 to 30% of T3 to T4 lesions.[207] For patients without lymph node involvement, the overall 3-year no-evidence-of-disease rate is approximately 50 to 60%; however, with lymph node involvement, the rate of cure is approximately 33 to 50%.[209]

Review of the report of the National Cancer Data Base indicated that patients with localized tumors of the oral cavity and pharynx had an overall survival rate of 70%.[209] Those treated surgically had an 81% survival rate, those with combined surgery and radiation had a 70% survival rate, and those treated with radiation alone had a 55% survival rate. For patients with regional disease, overall survival was 46%; survival rates were 60% for those treated with surgery alone, 58% for those treated with combined surgery and radiation, and 39% for those treated with radiation alone. For patients with distant metastases, overall survival was 33%. The findings have led to increased aggressive therapy and combining surgery, chemotherapy, and radiation therpy to improve survival. The National Cancer Institute's Surveillance, Epidemiology, and End Results program shows relative survival rates of 51% over a 5-year period and a 10-year survival rate of 41%.[210] Progress in the control of oral and pharyngeal cancer has been seen in years of life lost due to cancer: 23.1 years in 1970 and 19.9 years in 1985.[211]

In an analysis of 621 cases of HNSCC age, T classification, number of positive lymph nodes, and extracapsular spread were shown to be independent prognostic indicators.[212] The reported incidence of extracapsular spread of lymph node metastases varies from 6% to 85%, which is probably due to the degree of accuracy and lack of standardized criteria of histopathologic assessment.[213]

There is rarely a second chance for a cure; therefore, the initial approach to therapy is critical. Locoregional causes of death from head and neck cancer may be due to erosion of major vessels, erosion of the cranial base, cachexia, and secondary infection of the respiratory tract. With more aggressive locoregional tratement, distant failure with metastatic disease is increasingly seen. Probably a high fraction of oral cancer deaths is attributable to heavy alcohol consumption, particularly related to spirit consumption rather than wine and bear.[214] Several articles have discussed the psychological outcome of patients following treatment for oral cancer.[215]

A thorough understanding of each treatment modality, efficacy, and side effects is needed, which has led to the need for a team approach in cancer therapy that include surgeons, radiation oncologists, medical oncologists, dentists, and adjunctive health care workers.

PROGNOSTIC HISTOPATHOLOGIC MARKERS

Size of the primary tumor, specific oral subsite, tumor thickness, mode of invasion, and perineural spread have been shown to be of predictive value of HNSCC.[77,216,217]

PROGNOSTIC MOLECULAR MARKERS

In recent years, numerous markers, commonly using immunohistochemical techniques, have been suggested to be of prognostic value. Examples are a reduced expression of E-cadherin,[218–220] intratumoral expression of thymidylate synthase, P53 mutations, and HPV infection, aberrant catenin expression, Fas and Fas-ligand expression, diffuse expression of laminin gamma 2 chain in the cancer cells, high collagenase 3 expression, p27 expression, and the expression of the proliferative marker Ki-67 (MIB1).[221–229] Expression of cyclin D1 seems to have predictive value of metastastic disease.[230,231] A number of markers have been claimed to be predictive of lymph node involvement in OSCC.[220,232–235] Different chromosomal imbalances, including LOH, have been detected in metastasized and nonmetastasized tongue carcinoma as being identified by comparative genomic hybridization (see above).[237] Although no single marker has emerged as the most critical marker, it appears likely that a panel of markers will be identified that will facilitate prediction of tumor behavior and prognosis.

Prevention

Prevention has focused on to tobacco as a major cause of oral cancers, and attention has been paid to strategies of tobacco cessation.[236–238]

▼ OTHER HEAD AND NECK CANCERS

Malignant Tumors of the Salivary Glands

Tumors of the salivary glands, the majority of which involve the parotid glands, represent less than 5% of all head and neck tumors. Approximately two-thirds of these tumors are benign mixed tumors (pleomorphic adenomas). When tumors involve the submandibular or sublingual glands, there is a high probability that they are malignant. In order of decreasing frequency, the malignant salivary gland tumors are mucoepidermoid carcinoma, adenoid cystic carcinoma, adenocarcinoma, SCC, malignant pleomorphic adenoma, undifferentiated carcinoma, lymphoma, melanoma, and a mixed group of sarcomas. Most salivary gland tumors spread by local infiltration, by perineural or hematogenous spread and, less commonly, via lymphatics. Rarely, metastases from other malignancies may involve the parotid glands. The cause of salivary gland tumors remains obscure, but ionizing radiation has been identified as a risk factor.

Malignant salivary gland tumors most commonly present as a mass that may be ulcerated. Neurologic involvement may lead to discomfort and numbness, and with parotid gland tumors, involvement of the facial nerve may cause facial paralysis. Most small malignant lesions are indistinguishable from benign lesions. The majority of minor salivary gland tumors are malignant. The most common site is the posterior hard palate, but other sites in the oral cavity or upper respiratory tract may be involved. The presentation is usually a painless mass. The staging of salivary gland tumors is shown in Table 2.

Necrotizing sialometaplasia is a self-limiting non-neoplastic inflammatory condition of unknown etiology that

TABLE 2 Staging for Salivary Gland Cancer (Major Salivary Glands Only)

T (Size of Primary Tumor)	N (Lymph Node Involvement)	M (Distant Metastases)
T1: tumor <2 cm	N0: no nodal involvement	M0: no metastases
T2: tumor >2 and <4 cm	N1: ipsilateral lymph node involvement <3 cm	MI: distant metastases
T3: tumor >4 and <6 cm	N2: ipsilateral lymph node involvement >3 cm or multiple ipsilateral nodes	
T4: tumor >6 cm	N2a: single ipsilateral node >3 and <6 cm	
T1–T4a: no local extension	N2b: multiple ipsilateral nodes <6 cm	
T1–T4b: local extension (clinical or macroscopic extension to skin, bone, nerve)	N2c: bilateral or contralateral nodes <6 cm N3: lymph >6 cm	

Adapted from American Joint Committee on Cancer. Manual for staging of cancer. 3rd ed. Philadelphia: J.B. Lippincott; 1988.

affects the palatal salivary glands. The painful lesion occurs in sites of mucus-secreting glands and results in an ulceration with rolled borders. Clinical and histologic differentiation may be difficult, but accurate diagnosis is critical because necrotizing sialometaplasia will resolve spontaneously, usually within 1 to 2 months.

Biopsy of masses in the major glands may be accomplished by FNA, and diagnosis may be made without open biopsy. However, surgical biopsy may be necessary if FNA is not diagnostic. In masses involving minor glands, biopsy can be performed with routine techniques.

TREATMENT OF SALIVARY GLAND TUMORS

Surgery is the principal treatment of the primary tumor. Radiotherapy at a high dose is effective in malignant salivary gland tumors.[171] Postoperative radiation can contribute to cure and to improved local control and is indicated for patients with residual disease following surgery, extensive perineural involvement, lymph node involvement, high-grade malignant disease, tumors with more than one local recurrence after surgery, inoperable tumors, or malignant lymphoma and for those who refuse surgery. Doses and fractionation similar to those used in the treatment of SCC are usually employed. Heavy-particle radiation sources (neutron beam) have been shown to provide effective treatment for salivary gland tumors.[168,169]

PROGNOSIS

The prognosis of salivary gland tumors is related to tumor type, tumor size, lymph node involvement, and extension of disease.[137] Small tumors, acinic cell tumor, low-grade mucoepidermoid carcinoma, and mixed tumors have a high probability of cure. Tumors with a poor prognosis include large tumors, adenocarcinoma, adenoid cystic carcinoma, high-grade mucoepidermoid carcinoma, poorly differentiated carcinoma, and SCC. Histologic findings that correlate with lymph node involvement include deep (>8 mm) and diffuse invasion of stromal tissue and invasion of lymphatics.[239] Adenoid cystic carcinoma has a high incidence of progression with extension along nerves, and 10- and 15-year survivals must be examined due to late progression.

Malignant Lesions of the Jaw

OSTEOSARCOMA/CHONDROSARCOMA

Osteosarcoma is a malignant tumor, characterized by the direct formation of bone or osteoid by the tumor cells. Osteosarcomas are more common in patients between 10 and 25 years of age and occur more often in men than in women. The most common presenting finding of osteosarcomas of the jaws is mass (85–95.5%).[240,241] Pain accompanies the swelling in approximately half of cases, and trigeminal sensory disturbances occur in 21.2% of cases. The etiology is unknown, although trauma has been suggested as a possible trigger. Osteosarcomas may also develop in a patient affected by Paget's disease or in a patient who has been irradiated

either for a benign bone lesion or for adjacent soft tissue disease.[242] The latent time period may vary widely.

Approximately 6% of all osteosarcomas are located in the jaws, the estimated incidence being approximately one per million population per year.[243] Osteosarcomas occur slightly more often in the mandible than in the maxilla. Most osteosarcomas of the jaws are centrally located in the bone. Juxtacortical or parosteal location, a location adjacent to the outer surface of the cortical bone, is unusual. Associated symptoms consist of swelling, mobile teeth, anesthesia or paresthesia, toothache, and nasal obstruction. In many cases, there is patient and doctor delay in diagnosis due to misleading clinical, radiographic, and histologic features.[243]

In the osteoblastic type, the radiograph may show an opaque lesion, with bony trabeculae directed perpendicularly to the outer surface resulting in a "sunray" appearance. Over time, there is expansion and perforation of the cortical bone. The osteolytic type is far less characteristic and appears as an ill-defined lucency that causes expansion and destruction of the cortical bone. In the presence of teeth, a widening of the periodontal ligament may be observed even before changes can be noticed elsewhere in the bone. Loss of follicular cortices of unerupted teeth is highly suggestive of malignancy. Widening of the mandibular canal is another ominous sign. Bone scintigraphy will show a positive picture but is not diagnositic.

Histopathologically, proliferation of atypical osteoblasts is observed and irregular osteoid and bone formation is seen. Sometimes a proliferation of anaplastic fibroblasts appears. Vascular clefts may be encountered, resulting in terms such as *telangiectatic osteogenic sarcoma*. Multinucleated giant cells may be scarce or abundant. Osteosarcomas of the jaws are, in general, better differentiated than similar tumors in the long bones. Even if the tumor largely consists of malignant-looking cartilage, the so-called chondroblastic type, it is still to be considered an osteosarcoma whenever osteoid and bone are being formed in the stroma. Low-grade osteosarcomas may be misdiagnosed as fibrous dysplasia or other benign fibro-osseus lesions.

Osteosarcomas are usually graded according to histopathologic criteria in low-grade (grade I) to high-grade (grade III) malignancies. Disparate histologic responses may be observed in simultaneously resected primary and metastatic osteosarcoma following intravenous neoadjuvant chemotherapy and, in some cases, between two or more metastatic tumor deposits.

Treatment requires aggressive local surgery. Several authors advise the use of (neo)adjuvant chemotherapy. Others report that the introduction of chemotherapy did not dramatically alter the prognosis of osteosarcoma of the jaw.[241] Metastasis is usually via the bloodstream and often occurs within 1 to 2 years. Of the patients who die from osteosarcoma, most do so with uncontrolled local disease. The 5- and 10-year survival rates after treatment are approximately 60% and 50%, respectively.[243,244]

PRIMARY SCC OF THE JAW

Primary SCC of the jaw is a rare disease and may arise from epithelial rests in the jaw or from the epithelium of odontogenic lesions.

METASTASES OF PRIMARY MALIGNANCIES FROM ELSEWHERE IN THE BODY

Tumors metastatic to the jaw most often involve the posterior mandible. Metastases are rare, representing approximately 1% of all oral malignant tumors.[246] Common tumors that metastasize to the jaw are adenocarcinomas (of the breast, prostate, and gastrointestinal tract) and renal carcinoma. Other reported sites of primary tumors that metastasize include the thyroid, testes, bladder, ovary, and uterine cervix.[246–248] Symptoms associated with metastases to the jaw may include pain, paresthesia, anesthesia, mobility of teeth, and swelling. Destruction of bone may be visualized with imaging (see Figure 15). Lesions in periapical regions can be mistaken for dental disease. Gingival masses can occur as signs of metastatic tumor; however, metastases to soft tissue are extremely rare, representing less than 0.1% of oral tumors.[246] Diagnosis requires biopsy.

MULTIPLE MYELOMA

Multiple myeloma may cause radiolucent lesions and pain in multiple bones, including the jaw. Multiple myeloma frequently presents with pain and presents a clinical and radiologic diagnostic challenge when associated with the teeth.[249,250]

Nasopharyngeal Carcinoma

Nasopharyngeal cancer (NPC) presents a number of concerns to dental providers because patients may present with complaints that may mimic temporomandibular disorders (TMDs).[251] In one study, 13.5% of patients with NPC presented with common TMD signs and symptoms, with 44.2% describing their pain as headache, earache, or jaw, midface, or neck pain. Symptoms associated with NPC include pain, limited jaw opening, earache, and other ear complaints. Symptoms that aid in differentiation of TMD and NPC may occur late or concurrently and include nasal stuffiness, nosebleed, and neck mass. Risk factors for NPC include Epstein-Barr virus infection, smoking, childhood consumption of salted fish and other preserved foods that are common in a Cantonese diet, and origin from southern China.[15,110,252–254] Long-term survival is approximately 50% because most patients are identified after the tumor has spread regionally and lymph nodes are involved.[254,255] FNA can provide tissue diagnosis, and the sensitivity can be enhanced by DNA amplification (polymerase chain reaction) of the Epstein-Barr virus genome, which is commonly associated with NPC but is rare in other head and neck cancers.[256]

Treatment requires radiation therapy, which is increasingly combined with chemotherapy and IMRT or a three field set-up for conventional radiotherapy as shown in Figure 23.[254] Surgery may play a role in involved neck nodes but not in the treatment of the primary tumor. Radiation therapy for NPC results in mucositis and includes all major saliva glands, leading to hyposalivation and oral complications post-treatment.

Basal Cell Carcinoma

Basal cell carcinoma (BCC) is a locally destructive cancer that may occur in the head and neck. Sun exposure is considered the principal etiologic factor. BCC presents as persistent keratotic lesions (indurated papules) of the skin that may develop rolled borders and ulcerate. If advanced, they may lead to locoregional tissue necrosis and ulceration. Although BCC rarely metastasizes, recurrence or second primary lesions are common. Dental workers have the opportunity to identify basal cell lesions on the head and neck if routine extraoral examination is conducted with care.[257] Treatment is primarily surgical, although radiotherapy may be required for lesions not amenable to excision or to incompletely excised or recurrent tumors.

Malignant Melanoma

Melanoma may present as an area of altered pigmentation involving the skin. Oral malignant melanoma is extremely rare (2% of all melanomas).[258,259] Among 65 patients with head and neck melanoma, two-thirds of the patients were in their sixth decade, and only 10% of cases involved the oral mucosa.[258] Intraoral melanoma is more common among Japanese people, in whom oral lesions account for 14% of all cases of melanoma.[50] The oral lesions may present as tissue masses or ulceration that may be pigmented, but nonpigmented lesions also are reported. Most intraoral cases occur in the maxillary mucosa, presenting as a mass or flat lesions that may ulcerate and may be associated with bleeding. Melanoma is an aggressive malignant disease; metastasis id through lymphatic and hematogenous routes, and the prognosis is poor. Aggressive therapy of the primary tumor is needed with hypofractionated radiotherapy and CT and careful investigation for metastases.

Non-Hodgkin's Lymphoma

Non-Hodgkin's lymphoma (NHL) may primarily be localized in the oral soft tissues (eg, the gingiva, palate, and tongue). Primary NHL of salivary glands is usually of the mucosa-associated lymphatic tissue (MALT) lymphoma type. Oral NHL may be one of the manifestations of human immunodeficiency virus (HIV) infection. Hodgkin's lymphoma rarely occurs in the mouth, in contrast to NHL.

The usual clinical presentation of oral NHL is a submucosal swelling, sometimes bilaterally, especially at the junction of the hard and soft palate and the gingiva.[260,261] NHL may also be located within the jaw bones, particularly in the mandible. Symptoms may consist of unilateral anesthesia of the lower lip and sometimes swelling of the involved part of the bone. The radiograph may mimic the picture of osteomyelitis.

FNA biopsy or incisional biopsy in conjunction with immunocytochemistry is a useful aid in diagnosing malignant lymphoma, but in most cases, a confirmatory biopsy is required.

The oral NHLs usually involve the B-cell system, less often T cells and infrequently the histiocytic-monocytic system. Natural killer/T-cell lymphomas rarely occur in the mouth, and oral lymphomas usually are of the B-cell type.[262] The World Health Organization (WHO) has published a report on classification in 2000 (Table 3).[263]

A staging procedure must be carried out before instituting treatment. The Ann Arbor staging classification of lymphoma is commonly used (Table 4). Treatment usually consists of a combination of chemotherapy and radiotherapy and hematopoietic stem cell transplantation. The prognosis is largely determined by the histologic type and the stage of the disease.[264] Spontaneous regression is rare.[265] The International Prognostic Index is presented in Table 5.

Sarcomas of the Soft Tissues

Soft tissue sarcomas of the oral cavity are rare and account for approximately 1% of all oral malignancies.[260,261] Subtypes include fibrosarcoma, malignant fibrous histioctyoma, liposarcoma, rhabdomyosarcoma, leiyomyosarcoma, angiosarcoma, and alveolar soft part sarcoma. Soft tissue sarcoma

TABLE 4 Ann Arbor Staging System

Stage	Defining Status
Stage I*	Restricted to single lymph node region (I) or a single extranodal site (I-E).
Stage II*	Two or more areas of nodal involvement on same side of the diaphragm (II) or one or more lymph node regions with an extranodal site (II-E)
Stage III*	Lymphatic involvement on both sides of the diaphragm (III), possibly with an extranodal site (III-E), the spleen* (III-S), or both (III-SE)
Stage IV	Liver, marrow, or other extensive extranodal disease
Substage	
Substage E	Localized, extranodal disease
Substage A	Absence of systemic signs
Substage B	Presence of unexplained weight loss ($\geq$ 10% in 6 months), and/or unexplained fever, and/or night sweats

Adapted from Carbone PP, Kaplan HS, Musshof K, et al. Report of the Committee on Hodgkin's Disease Staging Classification. Cancer Res 1971;31:1860–1.

*The spleen is considered nodal

TABLE 3 World Health Organization REAL classification of Non-Hodgkin's Lymphomas According to Clinical Aggressiveness

Indolent lymphomas
  B-cell neoplasms
    Small lymphocytic lymphoma/B-cell chronic lymphocytic leukemia
    Lymphoplasmocytic lymphoma ($\pm$ Walderström's macroglobulinemia)
    Plasma cell myeloma/plasmacytoma
    Hairy cell leukemia
    Follicular lymphoma (grades I and II)
    Marginal zone B-cell lymphoma
    Mantle cell lymphoma

  T-cell neoplasms
    T-cell large granular lymphocytic leukemia
    Mycosis fungoides
    T-cell prolymphocytic leukemia

  Natural killer cell neoplasms
    Natural killer cell large granular lymphocytic leukemia

Aggressive lymphomas
  Follicular lymphoma (grade III)
  Diffuse large B-cell lymphoma
  Peripheral T-cell lymphoma
  Anaplastic large cell lymphoma, T-null cell

Highly aggressive lymphomas
  Burkitt's lymphoma
  Precursor B lymphoblastic leukemia/lymphoma
  Adult T-cell lymphoma/leukemia
  Precursor T lymphoblastic leukemia/lymphoma

Special group of localized indolent lymphomas
  Extranodal marginal zone B-cell lymphoma of MALT type
  Primary cutaneous anaplastic large cell lymphoma

Adapted from Jaffe ES, Harris NL, Stein H, Vardiman JW, editors. World Health Organization classification of tumours. Pathology and genetics of tumours of the haematopoietic and lymphoid tissue. Lyon: IARC Press; 2001.

MALT = mucosa-associated lymphoid tissue.

TABLE 5 International Prognostic Index for Non-Hodgkin's Lymphoma

Age $\geq$ 60 yr
Advanced stage (III or IV)
Extranodal involvement of > 1 site
Performance status $\geq$ 2
Serum lactate dehydrogenase level raised (above normal)

Risk group stratification (according to total number of above-listed features)
0–1: Low risk
2: Low intermediate risk
3: High intermediate risk
4–5: High risk

Adapted from The International Non-Hodgkin's Lymphoma Prognostic Factors Project. A predictive model for aggressive non-Hodgkin's lymphoma. N Engl J Med 1993;329:987–94.

usually presents as a slow- or rapid-growing swelling of the mucosa involving any part of the oral cavity. Treatment usually consists of surgery with adjuvant radiotherapy for those with high-grade tumors and/or positive margins.[266,267] The efficacy of adjuvant chemotherapy is poorly defined.

Paraneoplastic Syndromes

Neuropathies are commonly reported (1.7–5.5%) in patients with malignancy, comprising direct effects of the tumor, paraneoplasia, and treatment-related toxicity. Of paraneoplastic syndromes, neuropathy is the most common and has been reported in as many as 5% of all cancer patients.[268–271] Paraneoplastic sensory neuropathy is most frequently associated with small cell lung cancer and less often with stomach, colon, breast, and ovarian cancer.[272,273]

Paraneoplastic pemphigoid presents in a similar manner as benign mucous membrane pemphigoid and may present with gingival and mucosal involvement with erythema and ulceration. In patients with paraneoplastic syndromes, the most common clinical picture is that of numbness, paresthesias, and burning pain, which are often accompanied by detectable autoantibodies.

Head and Neck Malignant Disease in AIDS

HIV infection that leads to immunosuppression increases the risk of the development of neoplastic disease.[274] Advances in the management of HIV infection have led to a reduction in the prevalence of manifestations of immunosuppression, but it is anticipated that HIV disease may ultimately progress and that oral findings will be identified. Improved manangement of HIV disease using highly active antiretroviral therapy (HAART) and newer agents has led to a dramatic decrease in the prevalence of oral manifestations, including Kaposi's sarcoma (KS), although lymphoma remains a common malignancy.[275] KS is the most common neoplastic disease of acquired immune deficiency syndrome (AIDS). Lymphoma is the most rapidly increasing malignant disease of AIDS. NHL, most commonly of B-cell origin, may present with central nervous system involvement but also may present with head, neck, or oral lesions. The lymphomas are aggressive and carry a poor prognosis. Oropharyngeal SCC has been reported in patients with HIV disease; however, prevalence rates have not been determined.

KS is a multicentric neoplastic proliferation of endothelial cells. KS was very common prior to HAART, occuring in up to 55% of homosexual males with AIDS and often representing the first sign of progression to AIDS or occurring during the course of the disease. KS is less common in AIDS patients whose risk factor is not sexual transmission, suggesting that KS is associated with a sexually transmitted agent, which has now been identified as human herpesvirus type 8 (HHV-8). Advances in HIV therapy have had a dramatic impact on the prevalence of KS, and as increasing numbers of intravenous drug abusers are affected, the frequency of KS has decreased. KS can involve any oral site but most frequently involves the attached mucosa of the palate, gingiva, and dorsum of the tongue. Lesions begin as blue purple or red purple flat discolorations that can progress to tissue masses that may ulcerate (Figures 28 to 30). The lesions do not blanch with pressure. Initial lesions are asymptomatic but can cause discomfort and interfere with speech, denture use, and eating when lesions progress. The differential diagnosis includes ecchymosis, vascular lesions, and salivary gland tumors. Definitive diagnosis requires biopsy. Because KS is a multicentric neoplastic disease, multiple sites of involvement can occur, including skin, lymph nodes, gastrointestinal tract, and other organ systems.

Intralesional chemotherapy for treatment of oral KS has shown effective palliation.[257,274–277] Intralesional treatment with vinblastine and interferon has been reported. The lesions can be treated with the injection of vinblastine (0.2 mg/mL) under local anesthesia. The effect of treatment may continue

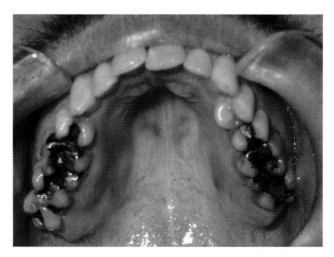

FIGURE 28 Bilateral involvement of the anterior and posterior hard palate with purple discolorations consistent with Kaposi sarcoma.

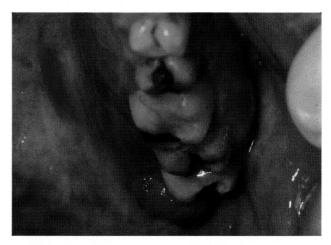

FIGURE 29 Palatal and gingival involvement by Kaposi sarcoma, with discoloration and enlargement and soft tissue mass on the maxillary tuberosity.

for several weeks and may result in palliation for approximately 4 months (see Figure 30). Repeat injection can be completed with similar efficacy. KS is radiosensitive, and radiation can be palliative for regional disease. Fractionated radiotherapy (for a total dose of 25 to 30 Gy over 1 to 2 weeks) may be provided for oral KS. Severe mucositis can follow radiotherapy for oral KS, although this may be less severe with fractionated treatment. If KS progresses at multiple sites, systemic chemotherapy may be needed. Additional approaches to management include drugs that reduce angiogenesis, antiviral agents for HHV-8 infection, and agents that block VEGF.[278,279]

▼ PRETREATMENT ORAL AND DENTAL ASSESSMENT

Detailed oral and dental assessment is necessary prior to cancer treatment.[280] The oral assessment is needed to identify conditions that should be treated prior to cancer therapy to

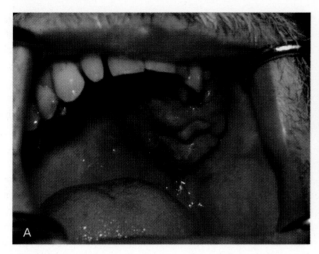
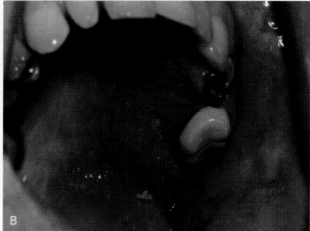

FIGURE 30 *A*, Kaposi sarcoma with mass effect and ulceration involving the maxillary molar resulting in impingement with occlusion and mobility of involved molar teeth. *B*, Kaposi sarcoma treated with intralesional vinblastine, resulting in successful palliation with elimination of discomfort and mobility of the involved teeth, reduction in tissue mass, but persistence of discoloration.

(1) identify oral involvement by cancer, (2) reduce the risk or severity of complications, (3) reduce the risk of infection involving the dentition and mucosa, and (4) minimize and manage the complications of hyposalivation. The assessment also will aid the institution of a program for preventing caries. The acquisition of baseline data will allow assessment of the progress of the patient's oral condition during and following cancer therapy. Pretreatment interventions are directed at the maintenance of mucosal and bony integrity, dental and periodontal health, salivary gland function, and prevention of potential complications of therapy.[281]

The patient history should review past dental care, current oral or dental symptoms, and the presence and condition of prostheses. The assessment must be comprehensive and include head and neck examination (with attention to the presence of lymphadenopathy), intraoral mucosal examination, and periodontal and dental examination. The periodontal examination must include full periodontal probing. Periodontal attachment loss is greater in radiated fields, and this future attachment loss should be considered in preradiotherapy treatment planning.[282] Definitive dental diagnosis and management must be provided prior to radiation therapy because dental and periodontal disease may require periodontal surgery or extractions, which are fraught with risk if the teeth involved were within the high-dose fraction. Radiographic examination should allow detailed evaluation of the teeth and periapical regions and should include imaging of any bone pathosis. Saliva production should be measured prior to therapy to document any change in flow rate, which may predict a risk of oral complications. Study models should be acquired for the provision of custom gel carriers, for construction of surgical prostheses if indicated, and for permanent records. Cultures for patients with suspected infections of the mucosa (eg, *Candida*) are indicated throughout the course of treatment. Culture of cariogenic bacteria in xerostomic patients is important for the diagnosis of cariogenic risk and indicates the need

for therapy (see "Caries," later in this chapter). A shift to cariogenic oral flora occurs due to hyposalivation and is not seen during radiation therapy in patients who are provided with fluoride and maintain plaque control.[283] Dental status, plaque control, and gingivitis at first examination provide evidence of past oral care, and unless it is believed that a true change in habits can be achieved, past practices should be expected to predict future care.

Prior to radiation therapy, teeth to be maintained should be scaled and root planed. Sites of potential mechanical irritation should be eliminated. The prevention of osteonecrosis requires the extraction of nonrestorable or questionable teeth, root tips, and periodontally involved teeth in the planned radiation field (see "Tissue Necrosis," later in this chapter). If time permits, asymptomatic periapical radiolucent lesions can be managed; however, endodontics can be performed following radiation if expert management is accomplished. Detailed review of oral hygiene, oral care during radiation therapy, and oral care following radiotherapy is an important part of long-term care.

▼ COMPLICATIONS OF CANCER TREATMENT

Acute reactions occur during the course of radiotherapy and combined radiochemotherapy because of direct tissue toxicity and possibly secondary bacterial irritation resulting in ulcerative mucositis; these reactions resolve over weeks to months following the completion of therapy. Chronic complications or late radiation reactions occur due to change in the vascular supply, fibrosis in connective tissue and muscle, and change in the cellularity of tissues. These complications develop slowly over months to years following treatment. Chronic effects in the mucosa include epithelial atrophy, altered vascular supply, and fibrosis in connective tissue, resulting in an atrophic and friable and sensitive mucosa. The connective tissue and musculature may demonstrate increased fibrosis, which may result in limited movement and altered function. In salivary glands, loss of acinar cells, alteration in duct epithelium, fibrosis, and fatty degeneration occur. In bone, hypovascularity and hypocellularity lead to the risk of osteoradionecrosis. Surgical treatment of the malignant disease results in acute pain and may result in chronic complications due to structural change, fibrosis, and neurologic changes. Hyperfractionation of radiation therapy may reduce the late complications but increases the severity of the acute reactions.

Mucositis

Ulcerative oral mucositis is a painful and debilitating condition that is a dose- and rate-limiting toxicity of cancer therapy. The potential sequelae of mucositis consist of severe pain, increased risk of local and systemic infection, compromised oral and pharyngeal function, and oral bleeding that affect quality of life; may lead to hospitalization or increase the duration of hospitalization; and increase the cost of care. Mucositis is the most common cause of pain during the treatment of cancer and the most distressing side effect of head and neck radiation therapy and myelosuppressive chemotherapy and stem cell transplantation.[284–286] Pain due to oropharyngeal mucositis frequently requires the use of opioid analgesics, which is associated with increased costs and side effects. The increasing use of more aggressive therapy to improve cancer cure rates has increased the frequency and severity of oral complications. In neutropenic patients, the risk of systemic infection due to oral opportunistic and acquired flora is increased with mucosal ulceration. Increased risk of mucositis has been associated with poor oral hygiene, tobacco use, hyposalivation at baseline, and older age.[287–292] Hyperfractionation, combined chemoradiotherapy, and the use of radiosensitizers cause increased severity of oral mucositis. Risk factors for oral mucositis are related to the cancer therapy, and individual risk factors, for example, the presence of single-nucleotide polymorphisms (SNPs) that detoxify methotrexate, have been associated with the risk of mucositis.[293]

ASSESSMENT

Oral mucositis is virtually a universal complication in patients with head and neck cancer treated with radiotherapy and chemotherapy. The reported incidence and severity of mucositis depend on the methods used for oral assessment, as demonstrated in a study in which a chart review and an interview were conducted and mucositis was identified in 30% and 69%, respectively, of the same patients and is generally thought to be underreported in cancer treatment trials.[294] Clinical examination of tissue change and assessments of symptoms are the principal means of assessing mucositis. The Oral Mucositis Assessment Scale (OMAS) is a semiquantitative tissue score that is a validated, reliable scale, with demonstrated intrarater and interobserver reproducibility and temporal changes with treatment.[295] The WHO and the National Cancer Institutes (NCI) scales provide overall mucositis scores but mixed tissue damage and function

scales.[296] Other markers of mucositis may become available. Current investigations include cell morphology and viability of exfoliated buccal cells; the viability of cells was determined by the trypan blue dye exclusion test, and a shift from mature to immature cells was seen as mucositis developed.[297] Oral symptoms, function scales, and validated measures of tissue damage currently represent the best means of assessing the outcome of treatment interventions.

PATHOGENESIS

Cytotoxic chemotherapy and radiation therapy have direct effects on connective tissue and vascular elements and mucosal epithelial cells, resulting in thinning of the epithelium and ultimately to loss of the barrier. Mucositis begins with an initial inflammatory/vascular and epithelial phase that is followed by an ulcerative/bacteriologic phase and, ultimately, a healing phase.[298,299] In the initial phase, changes in cell surface molecules and epidermal growth factor (EGF) may increase the risk of mucositis, and cytokines that reduce epithelial cell proliferation may decrease the severity of tissue damage.[300,301] Interaction with cytokines produced in the connective tissue affects tissue damage. The oral microflora appear to play a role following the development of the ulcerative phase.[298,302] Shifts in the oral microflora include the development of a flora high in *Streptococcus mutans*, lactobacilli, *Candida*, and gram-negative bacilli, which may result in oral infections and may aggravate mucositis (Figure 31). Resolution of mucositis is dependent on epithelial cell regeneration and angiogenesis and may also be dependent on white blood cell function and the production of growth factors. Pain associated with mucositis is dependent on the degree of tissue damage, the sensitization of pain receptors, and the elaboration of inflammatory and pain mediators. Oral defenses compromised due to irradiation include altered mucosal cell turnover, increased permeability and loss of the mucosal barrier, changes in saliva production, reduced levels of antimicrobial factors in saliva, loss of

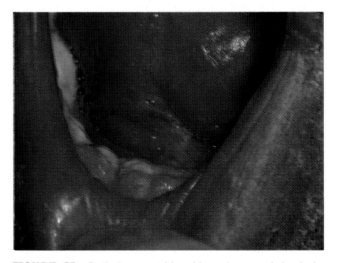

FIGURE 31 Radiation mucositis with erythema and developing ulceration in the floor of the mouth and ventral tongue; angular cheilitis representing a clinical manifestation of candidiasis.

protective mucins, and diluting effects. Impairment of the mobility of oral structures may lead to reduced clearing of local irritants and food products.

The first signs of mucositis may be a white appearance to the mucosa, caused by epithelial hyperplasia/hypertrophy and intraepithelial edema, or a red appearance due to hyperemia and epithelial thinning (Figure 32). Pseudomembrane formation represents ulceration with a fibrinous exudate with oral debris and microbial components (Figures 33 and 34). Radiation has more marked effects on nonkeratinized mucosa. Late changes in the mucosa reflect endarteritis and vascular changes associated with hypovascularity and with hyalinization of collagen (Figure 35).[303] With common fractions of 180 to 220 cGy per day, mucositis with erythema is noted in 1 to 2 weeks and increases throughout the course of therapy (often to a maximum in 4 to 5 weeks), with persistence until healing occurs 2 or more weeks after the completion of therapy.[304] Metal dental restorations, implants, and appliances may block radiation, affecting tumor dose, reflect the beam, and produce secondary radiation, altering the impact of irradiation on adjacent tissue, resulting in

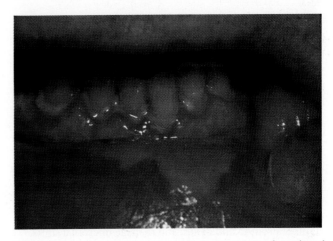

FIGURE 34 Extensive ulceration and pseudomembrane formation of the labial mucosa, compromising oral hygiene which may further aggravate oral mucositis.

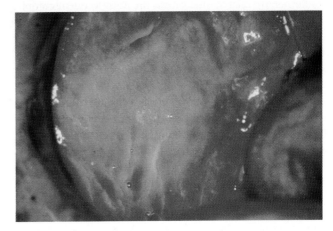

FIGURE 35 Late complications of radiation therapy with atrophy of mucosa, and fibrosis of connective tissue in the field of treatment.

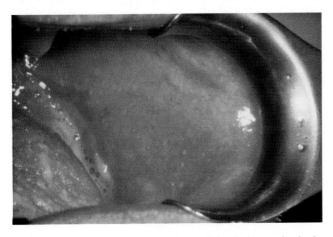

FIGURE 32 Erythema, viscous saliva, and developing erosion in the second week of radio-chemotherapy for head and neck cancer.

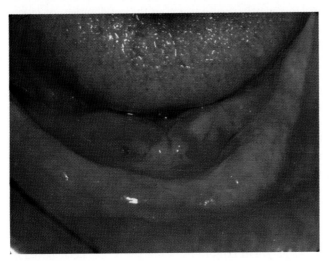

FIGURE 33 Erythema and ulceration increasing in the floor of the mouth in the fourth week of radiation therapy.

increased mucositis and risk of late effects. Thus, removable dental appliances should be removed during radiation; however, metal restorations are not removed, and their significance in complications is not well documented. The increasing use of dental implants will require consideration in future treatment planning for patients with head and neck cancer.

Bilateral exposure of the major salivary glands to radiation therapy will predictably result in hyposalivation. In patients who receive radiotherapy for treatment of Hodgkin's disease (mantle fields), saliva production is affected when the upper limit of the field is at the chin to the mastoid; below this level, minimal long-term effects are seen.[305] Irreversible effects occur at a total dose of greater than 5,000 Gy. Radiation results in acinar cell atrophy and necrosis, changes in the vascular connective tissue, and altered neurologic function. During radiation, the serous acini are affected earlier than the mucinous acini, resulting in a thick viscous secretion that can be upsetting to the patient. Saliva production rapidly decreases and can be reduced by 50% after 1 week of standard fractionated radiation. Depending on the volume of salivary tissue in the field, hyposalivation may improve within 6 months, but in many cases, the loss of function is permanent. A review of patients at 3 years post–radiation therapy that included the major glands in the field showed a 95% reduction in saliva volume.[306] Xerostomia in such patients is lifelong; therefore, prevention of oral complications needs to be continued indefinitely.

Changes in the composition of saliva also occur. Decreases in secretory immunoglobulin A, buffering capacity, and acidity are seen.[307–309] These changes affect the microbial flora and the remineralizing potential of teeth. The goals in the management of hyposalivation are to stimulate the remaining salivary gland function and (if such stimulation is not achieved) to palliate xerostomia, prevent tooth demineralization and caries, and manage microbial shifts.

RADIATION THERAPY–RELATED MUCOSITIS AND FUNGAL AND VIRAL COLONIZATION

Radiotherapy-related mucositis is the most frequent complication in patients receiving irradiation for head and neck cancers. Chronic oral sensitivity frequently continues after treatment, due to mucosal atrophy (33%) and neurologic syndromes (16%).[310,311]

Oral colonization by *Candida* species and candidiasis is common during and following radiotherapy and is related to hyposalivation and to denture and tobacco use.[283,312] The role of fungal colonization and infection in radiation mucositis is not clearly understood. In a group of patients receiving head and neck irradiation, patients who were on fluconazole, one developed mycotic infection and had 14 nonscheduled breaks in radiation therapy compared with 19 infections and 30 breaks in radiation therapy for those not provided fungal prophylaxis.[313] However, an association between candidiasis or oral colonization and mucositis during irradiation has not been confirmed by other studies.[316] The potential role of the reactivation of HSV during head and neck radiation therapy is unclear, and reactivation of HSV infection does not appear to commonly complicate radiation mucositis.[315]

PREVENTION AND MANAGEMENT OF MUCOSITIS

The literature does not provide definitive evidence for direct management of mucositis, but guidelines have been developed and research is continuing.[296,316]

SYSTEMIC APPROACHES TO MANAGEMENT

There are currently no systemic approaches to prevention of mucositis in head and neck radiation therapy, although studies of growth factors are being undertaken.[296,316–319]

Amifostine (Ethyol) is a sulfhydryl compound that acts by scavenging free radicals generated in tissues exposed to radiation and that promotes repair of damaged DNA. Amifostine has been shown to protect a variety of tissues, including mucosa, cardiac tissue, renal tissue, bone marrow, and neuro- and ototoxicity when administered prior to irradiation and chemotherapy. There is reduced uptake of amifostine into tumor, and tumor protection has not been reported. Although amifostine is now indicated for salivary gland protection, trials are under way to assess the impact of amifostine upon mucositis in patients with head and neck cancer who are being treated with chemoradiotherapy.[316,319–324] Side effects include nausea, vomiting, and reversible hypotension with intravenous administration, and intramuscular administration is being assessed. Amifostine has been approved in the United States for reduction of renal toxicity secondary to cisplatin administration and for reduction of xerostomia in patients who are treated with radiotherapy. This agent has potential for reducing the effects of the acute and chronic toxicity of cancer therapy, including mucositis with intravenous, intramuscular, and topical delivery; however, further study including efficacy and cost-benefit analysis is needed.[316,324]

Extensive studies have been conducted on biologic response modifiers. These are molecules that affect cellular function, including growth and tissue repair. Early findings on the effect of granulocyte colony-stimulating factor (G-CSF) upon reducing oral mucositis have been described, although this has not been confirmed in other studies.[325] Granulocyte-macrophage colony-stimulating factor (GM-CSF) has shown benefits in a number of initial clinical trials in patients treated with chemoradiotherapy.[296,318,319,326–329] Keratinocyte growth factor (KGF), a member of the fibroblast growth factor family, binds to KGF receptor, accelerating the healing of wounds.[330] Systemic KGF modifies the proliferation and differentiation of epithelial cells and may protect the cells from damage. Animal studies have shown the potential of KGF to reduce mucositis caused by radiation and chemotherapy.[330–334] Double-blind controlled trials in radiotherapy are in progress.

ORAL CARE AND TOPICAL APPROACHES TO MANAGEMENT

Recommendations for oral care and topical interventions for management of mucositis have been developed.[296,316,317,319,335,336]

The effect of oral hygiene and the elimination of local irritants may have an impact on the development of mucositis. Maintaining good oral hygiene has been shown to reduce the severity of oral mucositis and does not increase the risk of septicemia in neutropenic patients.[337,338]

Mucositis is not reduced with the use of chlorhexidine rinses during radiation therapy.[302,335,339,340] This may be due to the inactivation of chlorhexidine by saliva, the lack of an etiologic role for gram-positive bacteria in mucositis, and a limited effect of chlorhexidine on gram-negative organisms that may be important in the development of ulcerative mucositis. Other studies, using an oral lozenge containing polymyxin, tobramycin, and amphotericin B or similar combinations, have also not shown reduction in mucositis, although an impact on *Candida* colonization and gram-negative bacilli has been shown.[302,335,341]

Palliation of symptoms of mucositis may be achieved by the use of bland oral rinses and topical anesthetic and coating agents; however, controlled studies are lacking (Table 7).

Saline, bicarbonate, dilute hydrogen peroxide, and water also have been suggested for hydrating and diluting by rinsing. Lip applications with water-based lubricants (eg, lubricating jelly, such as K-Y Jelly [Johnson & Johnson]) or preparations that contain lanolin have been suggested rather than the use of oil-based products because the chronic use of oil-based products (eg, Vaseline) results in the atrophy of epithelium and the risk of infection under occlusion of the application. A study comparing saline and hydrogen peroxide rinses in radiation therapy found no significant differences among patients with mucositis, although oral sensitivity was greater in those using peroxide.[342] Coating agents used as oral rinses, such as Milk of Magnesia, liquid Amphogel, and Kaopectate (Pharmacia Corp., Peapack, NJ), are often recommended but have not been subjected to double-blind studies.[335,343] Viscous lidocaine is frequently recommended, although there are no studies that assess its benefit or its potential for toxicity in cancer patients. Lidocaine may cause local symptoms that include burning and that eliminate taste and affect the gag reflex. Potent topical anesthetic agents should be used with caution due to their potential for decreasing the gag reflex, causing central nervous system depression or excitation and causing cardiovascular effects that may follow excessive absorption. Local applications of topical anesthetic creams or gels may be useful for local painful mucosal ulcerations. A combination of agents that may include a coating agent and an analgesic or anesthetic agent also have been suggested, but no randomized controlled studies of mixtures of agents have been reported.

Benzydamine hydrochloride (Tantum, Riker-3M, Canada; Diflam, UK) is a nonsteroidal agent that possesses analgesic anti-inflammatory properties and is mildly anesthetic. Benzydamine may stabilize cell membranes, inhibit the degranulation of leukocytes, affect cytokine production, and alter the synthesis of prostaglandins. A number of studies have shown that signs and symptoms of oral mucositis are reduced when benzydamine is used prophylactically throughout the course of radiation therapy.[302,304,335,340,344-346] However, another study comparing the use of chlorhexidine and benzydamine did not show less severe mucositis in patients using benzydamine rinse.[347] Benzydamine is currently available in Europe and Canada but has not been approved by the FDA.

Sucralfate suspension has not been shown to reduce mucositis, although discomfort may be reduced with use.[296,348-351] Another potential benefit is a reduction in potentially pathogenic oral organisms in patients with mucositis.[349,352,353] Hydroxypropyl cellulose has been applied to isolated ulcers and may form a barrier on the surface, reducing symptoms.[354] Hydroxypropyl cellulose has been combined with topical anesthetic agents (eg, benzocaine), with clinical reports of efficacy.

Chlorhexidine has been assessed in radiotherapy patients, and the majority of studies show no prophylactic impact on mucositis.[340,355-357] The effects of chlorhexidine on plaque levels, gingival inflammation, caries, and oral streptococcal colonization have not been the primary end points in these studies, but they may be valuable during cancer therapy. A prospective study of patients treated with chemoradiotherapy for head and neck cancer showed that mucositis was reduced in those who received oral applications of povidone-iodine compared with those who received sterile water rinses.[357] However, the impact of oral hygiene may be a confounding factor in these studies.

Other topical agents are being assessed in clinical trials and should provide additional treatment options in the future.[317]

Oral capsaicin in a taffy-like candy vehicle produced temporary partial pain reduction in a small single-center study.[358] The findings suggest that some of the pain of mucositis is mediated by substance P.

Radiation shields to protect normal tissue from radiation exposure may be used during radiation therapy. They were shown to be effective, with patients experiencing less weight loss, fewer hospitalizations for nutritional support, and a trend toward fewer treatment interruptions when compared with control patients.[296,359]

Interest in the use of cytokines in the prevention and treatment of mucositis is increasing. An animal model of mucositis has been used to assess the potential of growth factors to affect oral mucositis.[318,360-365] In this model, EGF increased the severity of mucosal damage when given concurrently with chemotherapy.[365] Transforming growth factor β_3, which reduces the proliferation of epithelial cells, reduced the incidence, severity, and duration of mucositis; however, this finding has not been confirmed in human trials to date.[365,368] The use of interleukin-11 (IL-11) resulted in a statistically significant reduction in mucositis.[360,361,364] A rat model of inflammatory bowel disease also showed a reduction in gross and microscopic damage to the colon in animals treated with IL-11.[364] Due to hyposalivation, the quantity of EGF in saliva decreased in people receiving head and neck irradiation, and its concentration in saliva decreased as mucositis increased.[300] EGF may represent a marker for mucosal damage and has the potential to promote the resolution of radiation-induced mucositis. A double-blind trial of EGF mouthwash used in patients treated with chemotherapy showed no differences in the healing of established ulcers, but a delay in onset and reduced severity were seen in recurrent ulceration, suggesting that topical EGF may protect the mucosa from toxicity.[366] Several preliminary studies have assessed the effect of GM-CSF on oral mucositis, and a less severe or reduced duration of mucositis was seen in several trials.[367,368]

Low-energy helium-neon laser has been reported to reduce the severity of oral mucositis in patients receiving head and neck radiation therapy.[336,369] The mechanism of action is unknown but has been suggested to be due to cytokine release following laser exposure.

CURRENT MANAGEMENT

Guidelines for management of oral mucositis have been developed.[296,316,335,336,338,339] Current management of mucositis in radiotherapy patients (see Table 6) includes an

TABLE 6   Management of Mucositis

Diluting agents
Saline, bicarbonate rinses, frequent water rinses, ice chips

Coating agents
Kaolin-pectin, aluminum chloride, aluminum hydroxide, magnesium hydroxide, hydroxypropyl cellulose, sucralfate

Lip lubricants
Wax, water based lubricants, lanolin

Topical anesthetics
Dyclonine HCl, xylocaine HCl, benzocaine HCl, diphenhydramine HCl

Topical anesthetics
Benzydamine HCl; doxepin HCl

Maintain oral hygiene

Systemic analgesics

Maintain nutrition and hydration

TABLE 7   Classification of Postradiation Osteonecrosis

Stage	Description	Treatment
I	Resolved, healed	Prevention of recurrence
Ia	No pathologic fracture	
Ib	Past pathologic fracture	
II	Chronic, nonprogressive	Local wound care; HBO if indicated
IIa	No pathologic fracture	
IIb	Pathologic fracture	
III	Active, progressive	Local wound care
IIIa	No pathologic fracture	HBO and surgery if indicated*
IIIb	Pathologic fracture	

Reproduced with permission from Epstein JB.[250]

HBO = hyperbaric oxygen therapy.

*Combined surgery and HBO described by Marx RE.[391]

emphasis on good oral hygiene, the use of frequent oral rinses for wetting the surfaces and diluting oral contents, avoidance of irritating foods and oral care products, avoidance of tobacco products, and the use of benzydamine (in countries where available). The management of oropharyngeal pain in cancer patients frequently requires systemic analgesics, adjunctive medications, physical therapy, and psychological therapy, in addition to local measures, oral care, and topical treatments.

Biologic response modifiers offer the potential to prevent oral mucositis and to speed the healing of damaged mucosa. Topical antimicrobials, including chlorhexidine and systemic antimicrobials, have little effect in preventing mucositis in radiation patients but may be used for effect upon plaque levels, caries and gingivitis risk, and candidiasis. Amifostine provides salivary gland protection but requires further study to document a potential role in prevention of oral mucositis. Innovative new products are in clinical trials and low-energy lasers and (possibly) anti-inflammatory medications require further study.

Hyposalivation

STIMULATION OF SALIVARY FUNCTION

For patients with residual gland function, high fluid intake and the use of sugarless gum or candies also may assist the stimulation of residual gland function. Systemic sialagogues offer the advantage of stimulating saliva secretion that includes all normal components and protective functions of saliva. Measurement of saliva flow rates to determine the amount of residual function should be conducted before prescribing a sialagogue. If no saliva is collected under resting or stimulated conditions, it is unlikely that a systemic agent will be effective.

Pilocarpine is the best studied sialagogue.[2,370–374] Pilocarpine is a parasympathomimetic agent and has its major effects at the muscarinic cholinergic receptor of salivary gland acinar cells. In doses of 5 to 10 mg tid, increased secretion of saliva occurs, and few cardiovascular side effects have been noted.

Other agents have been studied, including bethanechol and civemiline.[2,371,375]

Bethanechol (75–200 mg/d in divided doses), which stimulates the parasympathetic nervous system, has been reported to have potential benefits without causing gastrointestinal upset. Anetholetrithione (not available in the United States; Paladin Laboratories Inc, Montreal, Canada) has been reported to be beneficial in the management of dry mouth.[372] The mechanism of action may be due to an increase in the number of cell surface receptors on salivary acinar cells. Because pilocarpine stimulates the receptors and because anetholetrithione may act by stimulating the formation of receptor sites, synergistic effects may result with the combined use of these drugs.[372]

Stimulation of the salivary glands during radiation therapy has been suggested as a possible means of reducing damage to the glands. Patients who begin radiation therapy with higher initial flow rates retain more residual flow.[305] Preliminary study of the prophylactic use of pilocarpine (5 mg qid) in patients receiving radiation therapy suggests that parotid gland function may be better preserved; however, this effect was not demonstrated in submandibular and sublingual gland saliva following treatment.[307] Amifostine, administered by the intravenous or intramuscular route prior to radiation exposure, has been approved by the FDA for prevention of salivary gland dysfunction and may reduce the severity of oral mucositis; however, additional study is needed to determine its impact on mucositis and its cost effectiveness.[316,324]

SYMPTOMATIC TREATMENT

Mouth-wetting agents or saliva substitutes may be used when it is not possible to stimulate salivary function.[371] Frequent sipping of water and a moist diet are mandatory. The desired characteristics of saliva substitutes are excellent lubrication, surface wetting, inhibition of overgrowth of pathogenic microorganisms, maintenance of the hardness of dental structure, pleasant taste, long duration of effect, extended shelf life, and low cost. The majority of products currently available are based on carboxymethylcellulose. Complex molecules and animal mucins have been incorporated into some products. Most commercial products are more viscous than saliva and do not simulate the viscoelastic properties of saliva. They also do not contain the complex enzyme systems and antibodies of natural saliva. Many of the commercial products being marketed have not been subjected to controlled clinical study.

Candidiasis

In irradiated patients, the most common clinical infection of the oropharynx is candidiasis. During radiation therapy, the number of patients colonized by *Candida*, quantitative counts, and clinical infection increase (see Figure 31).[280,283,289,339,373,374,376] These changes persist in patients, with continuing hyposalivation. Candidiasis may enhance the discomfort of mucositis and may be associated with discomfort and change in taste after treatment.

Patients who receive radiation therapy can be managed with topical antifungals because oral candidiasis produces oral discomfort but does not lead to systemic infection unless the patient is immunocompromised.[377] Systemic azoles are used for infection that occurs while using topicals and if compliance with topical oral therapy is poor. When prescribing topical antifungal drugs, the presence of sucrose in the product must be known because frequent use of sucrose-sweetened products may promote caries, particularly in patients with dry mouth.

Caries

Caries associated with hyposalivation typically affect the gingival third and the incisal cusp tips of the teeth (Figure 36). The etiology is related to a lack of production of saliva, loss of remineralizing potential, loss of buffering capacity, reduced pH, and change in the bacterial flora. Treatment of each component of the caries process must be addressed to prevent demineralization and rampant caries.

Oral hygiene must be scrupulously maintained. Hyposalivation should be managed, and thorough trials of sialagogues should be considered. The tooth structure may be hardened by the use of fluorides, and remineralization may be enhanced by the use of fluorides and remineralizing products.[302,359,378–381] The effects of topical products may be enhanced by increased contact time on the teeth, which can be achieved by applying them with occlusive vacuform splints or gel carriers, which should extend over the gingival margins of the teeth. Custom vinyl trays are useful for the application of fluoride to prevent and control caries in high-risk patients.[280,302,306,379,380] A comparison of neutral sodium fluoride gel in carriers with a twice-daily fluoride rinse protocol suggested a similar efficacy of the rinse protocol, but this was not a controlled comparative study.[381] Further studies are needed to define the simplest effective protocol. However, until controlled studies are available, treatment should remain fluoride application in gel carriers; for those who do not comply with carrier application, high-potency brush-on fluoride dentrifice may be suggested as it is simpler and may reduce demineralization and caries. Continuing reinforcement of topical fluoride use is needed and will enhance patient compliance.

A shift to a cariogenic flora has been documented in patients following head and neck radiation therapy. A high risk of caries that is associated with *Streptococcus mutans* and *Lactobacillus* speices has been demonstrated in cancer patients.[382,383] Assessment of quantities of cariogenic organisms should be carried out before considering whether antimicrobials are needed. A high risk of caries is reported if more than 10^5 *Streptococcus mutans* and more than 10^4 *Lactobacillus* colony-forming units per milliliter of saliva are present. Topical fluorides and chlorhexidine rinses may reduce levels of *Streptococcus mutans*.[382,383] A 2% chlorhexidine gel applied in mouth guards demonstrated an enhanced ability to control cariogenic flora in cancer patients with xerostomia.[386]

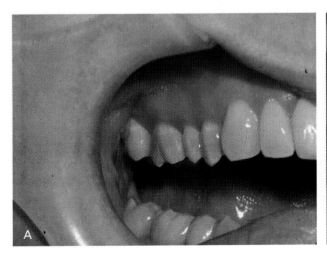
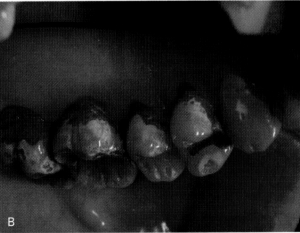

FIGURE 36 *A,* Hyposalivation following cancer therapy with extensive demineralization of incisal/cusp tips and gingival regions of posterior teeth. Intervention may prevent rampant demineralization and cavitation at this stage. *B,* Ravages of hyposalivation involving the dentition with cavitation in gingival surfaces and cusp tip/incisal edges, with extensive demineralization involving all enamel surfaces.

Tissue Necrosis

SOFT TISSUE AND OSTEONECROSIS

Soft tissue necrosis may involve any oral site, including the cheeks and tongue. Involvement of tissue overlying bone that has received high-dose radiation may predispose patients to necrosis of bone (Figure 37). Postradiation osteonecrosis (PRON) may be chronic or progressive. A classification of PRON for identifying stages of the condition for research and clinical purposes and for guiding therapy has been described (Table 7).[385,386] Radiation therapy causes endarteritis that affects vascularity, resulting in hypovascular, hypocellular, and hypoxic tissue that is unable to repair or remodel itself effectively when a challenge occurs (Figure 38). The challenge may take the form of trauma (such as from surgical procedures), active periodontal disease or denture trauma, and idiopathic or spontaneous necrosis for which no known cause is identified. Although PRON may be secondarily infected, the infection is not etiologic. Symptoms and signs may include discomfort or tenderness at the site, bad taste, paresthesia and anesthesia, extraoral and oroantral fistulae, secondary infection causing secondary osteomyletis, and pathologic fracture. The primary risk factor for the development of PRON is radiation therapy, in which dose, fraction, and numbers of fractions result in the biologic effect (eg, a high risk when TDF > 109). The volume of bone included in the field of irradiation increases the risk. The presence of teeth in a high-dose radiation field represents a risk factor for PRON, probably in relation to dental or periodontal disease or irritation. The risk of necrosis is lifelong and may occur many years after irradiation. The risk of developing PRON has been estimated in the last 20 years as between 2.6 and 15%.[385,386] The mandible is most commonly involved, although cases can occur in the maxilla.

BISPHOSPHONATE-ASSOCIATED OSTEONECROSIS

Osteonecrosis and osteomyelitis of the jaws may develop in patients using bisphosphonate.[336,387–389] The clinical presentation is of bone exposure with or without pain, swelling, and fistula formation. The cumulative incidence is rising and has been reported to be 10% after 3 years of drug use of intravenous bisphosphonate use; the risk with oral bisphosphonates are less, and there are no epidemiologic studies available.

The prevention of osteonecrosis begins with the preradiation dental examination and radiotherapy treatment planning. Teeth in the high-dose fraction with questionable prognosis (particularly when due to periodontal disease and when excellent compliance with regular oral care is unlikely) should be extracted prior to radiotherapy. For bisphosphonate-associated osteonecrosis (BON), pretreatment examination is encouraged and teeth with infection or that may require surgery for future care should be extracted. Dental treatment may be without additional risk in the first several months of use of bisphosphonates. If extractions are planned, it is desirable to allow as much healing time as possible; 7 to 14 days and up to 21 days prior to radiotherapy have been

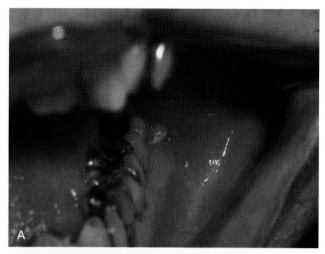

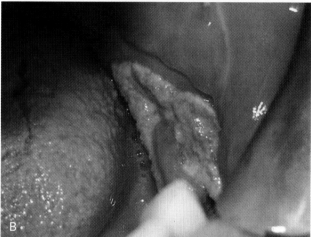

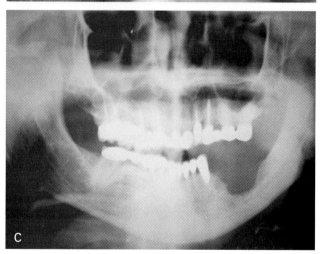

FIGURE 37 *A*, Chronic asymptomatic bone exposure in the buccal aspect of the mandible, within the high dose radiation volume. *B*, Clinical presentation of exposed bone in a patient following radiation therapy associated with mild discomfort, and intermittent swelling due to secondary infection, when pain was increased. *C*, Panoramic radiograph of postradiation osteoncrosis, demonstrating bone destruction approaching the inferior border of the mandible.

suggested.[386,390] The time required may depend on the nature of the extraction, and expert atraumatic extraction will require less healing time.

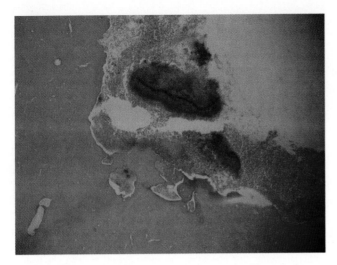

FIGURE 38 Histopathologic appearance of bone with empty lacunae and haversian canals of nonvital bone, in post-radiation osteonecrosis.

Therapy is not defined for BON; however, for BON and PRON, management recommendatons include avoiding mucosal trauma and irritants, discontinuing the use of dental appliances if they contact the area of the lesion, maintaining nutritional status, stopping smoking, and eliminating alcohol consumption. Appropriate analgesics should be provided. Topical antibiotic (ie, tetracycline) or antiseptic (chlorhexidine) rinses may reduce the potential secondary local irritation from the microbial flora. When secondary infection occurs, topical and systemic antimicrobials are needed. For chronic persisting PRON (stage II), this therapy and regular follow-up may be the best approach to treatment. Hyperbaric oxygen (HBO) therapy increases the oxygenation of tissue, increases angiogenesis, and promotes osteoblast and fibroblast function. In PRON cases associated with symptoms of pain and progression (stage III), HBO is a part of therapy. HBO therapy and surgical guidelines have been established for PRON but not for BON.[390–394] HBO therapy is usually prescribed as 30 dives at 100% oxygen and 2 to 2.5 atmospheres of pressure. Sequestra may be managed with limited resection or may require mandibulectomy. If surgery is required, postsurgical HBO therapy of 10 dives is recommended. The mandible can be reconstructed to provide continuity for esthetics and function for PRON because the field of bony change is known; however, in BON, the entire bone is affected. In PRON, vascularized grafts and microvascular surgery has improved outcomes in cases in which affected bone and soft tissue can be replaced with vascularized tissue and good blood supply established. Prophylactic HBO therapy may be considered (1) when surgery is required after radiation therapy, (2) when the patient is felt to be at extreme risk due to high-dose radiation to the bone with a high biologic effect (TDF > 109), and (3) when extensive surgery is required. However, if expert atraumatic extraction is performed, HBO therapy may be considered only if delayed healing occurs. In a selected population of patients referred for HBO therapy and surgery, prophylactic HBO therapy was suggested.[390] In a general cancer clinic, however, extractions were managed with expert surgery, and approximately 5% of extractions were associated with delayed healing; it was recommended that in most cases, HBO therapy should be reserved for those in whom osteonecrosis developed.[386]

Continuing benefits of HBO have been shown in a a long-term follow-up of patients after their first episode of necrosis showed that in patients with a prior episode of PRON and HBO treatment, 10% experienced a recurrence of necrosis.[393] This study supports the potential value of HBO therapy in managing initial episodes of necrosis and in potentially preventing the recurrence or additional episodes. Studies indicate that chronic asymptomatic, nonprogressive necrosis (stage II) may remain stable and without progression over extended periods following initial treatment with HBO.

Speech and Mastication

Abnormal speech may follow surgery or radiation due to removal of structure and because of hyposalivation and fibrosis that affects tongue mobility, mandibular movement, and soft palate function (Figure 39). Maxillectomy that produces a palatal defect must be managed with prostheses to allow function in speech, mastication, and deglutition. Speech therapy and speech prostheses are the principal means of managing these complications.[152]

Nutrition: Taste and Smell Impairment

Radiation therapy produces changes in the patient's perceptions of taste and smell.[395] Taste may be affected directly, due to an effect on the taste buds, or indirectly, due to hyposalivation and secondary infection. A total fractionated dose of >3,000 Gy reduces the acuity of all tastes (ie, sweet, sour, bitter, and salty).[396] Taste often will recover slowly over several months, but permanent alteration may result.[2] Zinc supplementation (zinc sulfate, 220 mg twice daily) may be useful for some patients who experience taste disturbances.[2,397]

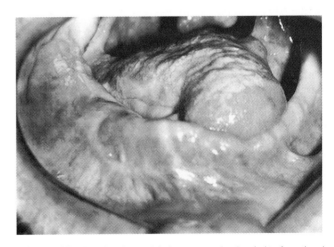

FIGURE 39 Results of a partial glossectomy that has led to func-tional impairment of speech and manipulation of food and to difficulty inretaining the mandibular denture.

Nutritional counseling in which the focus is on the maintenance of caloric and nutrient intake may be required during and following cancer therapy. Long-term complications include hyposalivation, altered ability to chew, difficulty in forming the food bolus, and dysphagia. Consideration must be given to taste, texture, moisture, and caloric and nutrient content.

Mandibular Dysfunction

Musculoskeletal syndromes may arise due to fibrosis of muscles, which may follow radiation and surgery. Limited opening has been related to radiation exposure of the upper head of the lateral pterygoid muscle.[398,399] Mandibular stretching exercises and prosthetic aids (Therabite device or tongue blades) and use of microcurrent electrotherapy and pentoxifylline may increase mouth opening and may reduce the severity of fibrosis and limited mandibular movement when conducted before severe limitation has developed, but few benefits are seen after such limitation has developed. Mandibular discontinuity following surgery and the emotional stress associated with malignant disease and its treatment may influence musculoskeletal syndromes, causing pain. The management of temporomandibular disorders in this population may present additional difficulties due to muscular fibrosis and major discontinuity of the mandible when present, with severe limitation of function and emotional reaction. There is no research that documents the best choices of therapy for these patients. Therapy may include occlusal stabilization appliances, physiotherapy, exercises, trigger point injections and analgesics, muscle relaxants, tricyclic medications, and other chronic pain management strategies.[113] Management of pain is discussed later in this chapter.

Dentofacial Abnormalities

When children receive radiotherapy to the facial skeleton, future growth and development may be affected.[400] Agenesis of teeth, cessation of root formation, abnormal root forms, or abnormal calcification may occur (Figure 40). Despite these dental abnormalities, teeth will erupt even without root formation and may be retained for years. Growth of the facial skeleton in the radiated field may be affected, which can result in micrognathia, retrognathia, altered growth of the maxilla, and asymmetric growth (Figure 41). Altered growth and development may occur if treatment affects the pituitary gland. Trismus may occur in patients secondary to fibrosis of muscles.

Dental abnormalities pose significant management challenges due to these effects on dental development and skeletal growth and impact of radiothearpy on bone remodeling and healing if orthodontics and surgery are planned for orofacial abnormailities.

Pain

Head and neck and oral pain may be due to a number of causes (Table 8) and is particularly challenging as oral function including speech, swallowing, and other motor

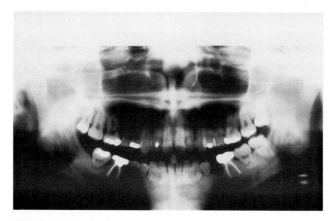

FIGURE 40 Radiograph showing the effects of radiation on thedevelopment of the dentition. Agenesis, shortened root forms, lack of rootdevelopment, and premature closure of apical foramina are seen in teeththat were in the primary radiation field and that were in the process ofdevelopment during radiation therapy.

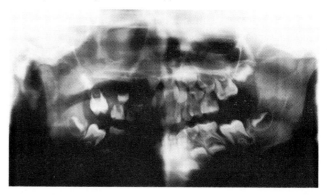

FIGURE 41 Radiograph demonstrating the effect of unilateral radi-ation that was required during dentofacial development. Asymmetricdevelopment of height and width of the ramus and body of the mandibleand dentition resulted.

functions of the head and neck and oropharynx are constant triggers of pain and compound the affective and cognitive impact of the pain experience.[400] Cancer pain causes reduced performance status, increased anxiety and depression, sleep dysfunction, and diminished quality of life (QOL).

In patients with head and neck cancer, pain is reported in up to 85% of cases at diagnosis.[251] Pain may arise due to mucosal ulceration, inflammation, bone destruction, and nerve injury that involve inflammatory and/or neuropathic mechanisms. Pain due to therapy is universal in head and neck cancer, secondary to surgery, radiotherapy, and/or chemotherapy. Pain due to oral mucositis is the most frequently reported patient-related complaint impacting QOL during cancer therapy. Pain in cancer patients may also occur coincidentally due to other conditions unrelated to cancer but may be interpreted by the patient as progression or recurrence of the cancer. This includes common conditions such as toothaches, TMDs, sinusitis, and headaches.

Chronic and Post-Therapy Pain

In cancer patients, the post-treatment pain experience is characterized by acute pain lasting 1 to 2 months with a gradual time-related improvement. However, head and neck cancer survivors (>3 years) may continue to suffer from significantly more pain and functional problems than matched control subjects, although there is a gradual return to general function and mental health.[401]

Pain following surgery involves inflammatory and neuropathic pain mechanisms. Functional consequences are secondary to pain and may involve wound contracture and scarring.[402]

▼ MANAGEMENT OF PAIN IN OROFACIAL CANCER

Pain, whether related to the tumor, recurrence or progression of tumor, tor reatment of tumor or unrelated to the cancer, often is interpreted as being due to the disease and is influenced by an emotional response caused by fear of cancer. The important emotional components of the reaction to pain must be considered in the patient's complaint and in management. Pain at diagnosis of head and neck cancer is common and is usually described as low-grade discomfort.[113] Acute pain following radiotherapy and surgery is universal. Neurologic pain states, including neuropathic pain and neuralgia-like pain, may require the use of centrally acting medications, including antidepressants and anticonvulsants. Chronic pain management approaches, including counseling, relaxation therapy, imagery, biofeedback, hypnosis, and transcutaneous nerve stimulation, may be needed. Pain associated with musculoskeletal syndromes is reviewed in the section entitled "Mandibular Dysfunction."

Health care providers have been criticized for the needless suffering of patients caused by the providers' lack of use of analgesics and adjuvant medications, lack of attention to the emotional and social aspects of pain, and failure to use adjunctive physical and psychological treatment. The management of cancer pain requires attention to the potential multiple causes of pain (see Table 8).

Dental and periodontal disease that causes pain may be controlled with analgesics and antibiotics; however, definitive dental management is needed. Management of mucositis is discussed above. Bacterial, fungal, and viral infections are managed with specific antimicrobial agents. In mucosal infection, topical antifungals and antiseptics may be effective, but if resolution does not occur, systemic medications may be needed.

Management of Pain due to Oral Mucositis

Effective management requires diagnosis and treatment of the cause(s) of pain in cancer patients and symptom management. Impediments to adequate pain management include patients' reluctance to report pain, patients and health care workers preconceived negative ideas, and regulatory barriers to the use of opioids.

Pain in oral mucositis results from tissue injury that causes production of reactive oxygen species, release of proinflammatory cytokines, neurotransmitters, and secondary mucosal

TABLE 8   Head, Neck, and Oral Pain in Cancer Patients
Pain due to tumor
Loss of epithelial barrier; ulceration; exposure of nerves
Tumor necrosis; secondary infection
Chemosensitization of nerves; pressure on nerves
Tumor infiltration of bone, muscle, nerve, blood vessels
Exacerbation of dental or periodontal disease
Pain due to cancer therapy
Pain following surgery
Acute surgical injury
Secondary infection
Myofascial or musculoskeletal syndromes
Neuroma; deafferentation pain
Pain due to radiotherapy
Mucositis
Necrosis of soft tissue or bone
Myofascial or musculoskeletal syndromes
Exacerbation of dental or periodontal disease
Pain due to chemotherapy
Mucositis
Peripheral neuropathy
Infection
Exacerbation of dental or periodontal disease
Pain unrelated to cancer or cancer therapy

infection at the site of injury. Pain experienced is due to the degree of tissue damage and conditioned by the emotional and sociocultural background.

TOPICAL AGENTS

The oral mucosa is accessible for topical medications, but saliva dilutes the preparation and limits contact time. Topical anesthetics are used for mucositis pain, producing a short period of mucosal anesthesia (up to half an hour), but may sting with application on damaged mucosa and affect taste and gag reflex. Topical anesthetics are often mixed with coating and antimicrobial agents such as milk of magnesia, diphenhydramine, or nystatin; however, these mixes have not been subjected to controlled studies, and effectiveness, acceptance, and tolerability are variable. Topical doxepin, a tricyclic antidepressant, produces analgesia for 4 hours or longer following a single application in cancer patients.[403] In addition to extended duration of pain relief, burning does not accompany topical application on damaged mucosa.

Topical morphine has been shown to be effective for relieving pain, although there is concern about dispensing large volumes of the medication.[404]

Topical fentanyl prepared as lozenges provides relief from oral mucositis pain.[405] Topical coating agents have been promoted for use in patients with mucositis. Sucralfate may have a role to play in pain management but has not been shown to reduce oral mucosal damage.[296] Other coating agents, such as antacids and milk of magnesia, may be mixed as discussed above but have not been shown to reduce pain.

Topical benzydamine, an anti-inflammatory and analgesic/anesthetic agent (not FDA approved, but available in many countries), has been shown in a randomized controlled multicenter study to reduce mucosal damage and pain in oral mucositis.[264]

SYSTEMIC AGENTS

The WHO Pain Management Ladder has been recommended for managing pain in cancer patients (Figure 42).[406] Modification of the WHO ladder is recommended to add topical therapy before and during use of systemic agents and to move from nonopioid analgesics to powerful opioids at sufficient dose and frequency to control pain, and with adjuvant therapy.[407–411]

A meta-analysis has challenged the effectiveness of "weak" opioids (step II medications), in which no difference was seen between effectiveness of NSAIDs (step 1) and weak opioids (step 2) and greater side effects are reported in those using weak opioids.[412–414] Therefore, use of lowest does of powerful opioids has been suggested when step 1 medications are not sufficient and previously used step 2 medications (mild opioids) are not recommended. Transdermal fentanyl has become widely used for extended duration therapy in the management of pain in cancer patients. Addiction in opioid therapy has become less of a concern in general and particularly for cancer patients. Tolerance and side effects such as constipation, nausea, vomiting, and mental clouding are a concern with opioid use and should be anticipated and managed. Stool softeners and other approaches to bowel management should be initiated, along with the initial opioid prescription and adequacy of the approach assessed on a regular basis.

Other approaches that may improve pain control include opioid substitution and opioid rotation and adjuvant medications. Frequent assessment of pain levels and modification of management will improve pain control in head and neck cancer patients receiving radiotherapy. Adjuvant medications, such as tricyclic antidepressants and other centrally acting pain medications, such as neurontin, should be considered.[410,415] Gabapentin is a voltage-sensitive sodium and calcium channel blocker that may be used for adjuvant pain management. If sleep is nonrestorative, adequate pain control should include the additional use of medications to promote sound sleep. Tricyclic antidepressants, some of the anxiolytic/hypnotics, and some of the benzodiazepines can be considered (Table 9).

Analgesics, when required, should be provided on a regularly scheduled or time-contingent basis, not on an as-needed basis, as improved pain control can be achieved using lower total doses of analgesics. In general, non-narcotic analgesics should be provided to all patients even if potent opioids are required because this may allow a lower dose of narcotic medication. Adjuvant medications such as tricyclic antidepressants may enhance the analgesic effects of other agents, possess analgesic potential themselves, and promote sleep, which is often disrupted by pain. Adjuvant medications directed at the etiology of the pain should be used whenever possible. For example, for neuralgia-like pain, anticonvulsant medications should be included. Possible side effects, such as constipation due to opioids, should be anticipated and treated. Regular reassessments of the effectiveness of pain control, with an awareness of toxicity and side effects, should be conducted.

ALTERNATIVE AND PHYSICAL THERAPY

Medications should not be used alone but should be part of a pain control strategy that also includes physical therapy, counseling, relaxation therapy, biofeedback, hypnosis, and transcutaneous nerve stimulation. Physical management of orofacial pain includes use of ice chips for oral cooling and cold compresses. Alternative approaches considered to potentially affect pain in cancer patients include biofeedback, hypnosis, relaxation, imagery, cognitive behavioral training, acupuncture, transcutaneous nerve stimulation, and massage therapy.[416]

▼ CONCLUSION

Oral and dental care is important in all phases of the diagnosis and treatment of the patient with head and neck cancer. Early recognition and diagnosis are important for improving

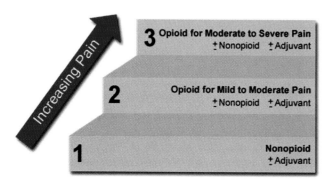

FIGURE 42 World Health Organization's pain ladder.

TABLE 9 Pain Management in Head and Neck Cancer

Category of Medication	Action
Topical anesthetic	Topical anesthesia
Analgesic	Elevate pain threshold
Anti-inflammatory	Reduce inflammation; mild to moderate analgesic
Antimicrobial	Modify pathologic process
Anticonvulsant	Modify pathologic process
Anxiolytic	Antianxiety
Antidepressant	Reduce depression; analgesic effect; promote sound sleep
Muscle relaxant	Reduce muscle tension or spasm

survival and for limiting the complications of therapy. Prevention of the oral complications that arise during or after therapy and management of the complications when they occur require the involvement of a knowledgeable practitioner. Dental providers are a part of the health care team and must be involved in the care of the head and neck cancer patient. Continuing research is needed in the epidemiology, pathogenesis, etiology, prevention, diagnosis, and management of head and neck cancer.

▼ SELECTED READING

American Society of Clinical Oncology; Ganz PA, Kwan L, et al. The role of prevention in oncology practice: results from a 2004 survey of American of Clinical Oncology members. J Clin Oncol 2006;24:2948–57.

Anthony L, Bowen J, Garden A, et al. New thoughts on the pathobiology of regimen-related mucosal injury. Support Care Cancer 2006;14:516–8.

Bensadoun RJ, Schubert MM, Lalla RV, Keefe D. Amifostine in the management of radiation-induced and chem.-induced mucositis. Support Care Cancer 2006;14:566–72.

Chitapanarux I, Lorvidhaya V, Sittitrai P. Oral cavity cancers at a young age: analysis of patient, tumor and treatment characteristics in Chiang Mai University Hospital. Oral Oncol 2006;42:83–8.

Dijkstra PU, Huisman PM, Roodenburg JLN. Criteria for trismus in head and neck oncology. Int J Oral Maxillofac Surg 2006;35:337–42.

Ha PK, Califano JA. Promoter methylation and inactivation of tumour-suppressor genes in oral squamous-cell carcinoma. Lancet Oncol 2006;7:77–82.

Hernández JF, Hernández-Hernández DM, Flores-Díaz R, et al. The number of sentinel nodes identified as prognostic factor in oral epidermoid cancer. Oral Oncol 2005;41:947–52.

Kasperts N, Slotman B, Leemans CR, Langendijk JA. A review on re-irradiation for recurrent and second primary head and neck cancer. Oral Oncol 2005;41:225–43.

Koon HB, Bubley GJ, Pantanowitz L, et al. Imatinib-induced regression of AIDS-related Kaposi's sarcoma. J Clin Oncol 2005;23:982–9.

McGuire DB, Correa MEP, Johnson J, Wienandts P. The role of basic oral care and good clinical practice principles in the management of oral mucositis. Support Care Cancer 2006;14:541–7.

Parker TM, Smith EM, Ritchie JM, et al. Head and neck cancer associated with herpes simplex virus 1 and 2 and other risk factors. Oral Oncol 2006;42:288–96.

Scheifele C, Reichart PA, Hippler-Benscheidt M, et al. Incidence of oral, pharyngeal, and laryngeal squamous cel carcinomas among 1515 patients after liver transplantation. Oral Oncol 2005;41:670–6.

Syrjänen S. Human papillomavirus (HPV) in head and neck cancer. J Clin Virol 2005;32S:S59–66.

Woolgar JA. Histopathological prognosticators in oral and oropharyngeal squamous cell carcinoma. Oral Oncol 2006;42:229–39.

Wu NC, Gorsky M, Bostrom A, et al. Assessment of the use of sialogogues in the clinical management of patients with xerostomia. Spec Care Dentist 2006;26:468–74.

For the full reference list, please refer to the accompanying CD ROM.

8

SALIVARY GLAND DISEASES

PHILIP C. FOX, DDS
JONATHAN A. SHIP, DMD

Patients with salivary gland disease most frequently present with complaints of oral dryness (xerostomia), swelling, or a mass in a gland. This chapter addresses the means of evaluation of the patient who has signs and symptoms that are suggestive of salivary gland dysfunction. The examination of a patient with dry mouth or a salivary mass is described. The major salivary gland disorders are described and current management options are discussed.

▼ SALIVARY GLAND ANATOMY AND PHYSIOLOGY

There are three major salivary glands: the parotid, submandibular, and sublingual (Figure 1). These are paired glands that secrete a complex, protein-rich saliva. Initial water transport (from the serum) is through the acinar cell end pieces, the sole site for water movement in the glands.[1] The saliva is highly modified as it is carried via a branching duct system

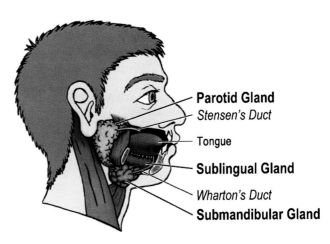

Parotid Gland
Stensen's Duct

Tongue

Sublingual Gland

Wharton's Duct
Submandibular Gland

FIGURE 1 Three major salivary glands.

into the oral cavity. Parotid saliva is secreted through Stensen's duct, the orifice of which is visible on the buccal mucosa adjacent to the maxillary first molars. Sublingual saliva may enter the floor of the mouth via a series of short independent ducts but will empty into the submandibular (Wharton's) duct about half of the time. The orifice of Wharton's duct is located on either side of the lingual frenum. There are also hundreds of minor salivary glands throughout the mouth and extending down the tracheobronchial tree, which are named for their anatomic location (labial, palatal, buccal, etc.). These minor glands are located just below the mucosal surface and secrete onto the mucosa through short ducts. At rest (basal or unstimulated function), it is estimated that the minor glands may produce up to half of the saliva in the oral cavity.[2,3] With stimulation, however, the major glands predominate and minor gland secretions account for less than 10% of the saliva. Stimulation of salivation occurs between 10 and 20% of the day, with the amount of time dependent on habit and dietary preferences.

Saliva is the product of the major and minor salivary glands dispersed throughout the oral cavity. It is a highly complex mixture of water and organic and nonorganic components. Most of the constituents are produced locally within the glands; others are transported from the systemic circulation. The three major salivary glands share a basic anatomic structure. They are composed of acinar and ductal cells arranged much like a cluster of grapes on stems (Figure 2). The acinar cells (the "grapes" in this analogy) make up the secretory end pieces. The acinar cells of the parotid gland are serous, those of the sublingual and minor glands are mucous, and the submandibular gland is composed of mixed mucous and serous types. The duct cells (the "stems") form an extensively branching system that carries the saliva from the acini into the oral cavity. The duct cell morphology changes as it progresses from the acinar junction toward the mouth, and different distinct regions can be identified.

Although fluid secretion occurs only through the acini, proteins are produced and transported into the saliva through both acinar and ductal cells. The primary saliva within the acinar end pieces is isotonic with serum but undergoes extensive resorption of sodium and chloride and secretion of potassium within the duct system. The saliva, as it enters the oral cavity, is a protein-rich hypotonic fluid.[1]

The secretion of saliva is controlled by sympathetic and parasympathetic neural input.[4] The stimulus for fluid secretion is primarily via muscarinic-cholinergic receptors, whereas the stimulus for protein release occurs largely through β-adrenergic receptors. Salivary cells also display an array of additional receptors that influence secretory functions. Activation of these receptors induces a complex signaling and signal transduction pathway within the cells, involving numerous transport systems, resulting in a tightly regulated secretion process.[4,5] Mobilization and regulation of intracellular calcium are a critical component of this process within the secretory cells.

There are aspects of secretory physiology that have implications for the treatment of salivary gland dysfunction. Most importantly, loss of acini will limit the ability of the gland to transport fluid and therefore to produce saliva. Acinar cell loss occurs in a number of clinical conditions, particularly the autoimmune exocrinopathy Sjögren's syndrome. Also, muscarinic agonists (parasympathomimetics) are efficacious as secretogogues as they are the primary stimulus of fluid secretion. Indeed, these agents are now widely used to increase salivary output transiently and relieve xerostomia in dry mouth patients. However, other agonists and receptors can stimulate secretion and represent potential therapeutic approaches. Finally, unstimulated salivary function is very important for both the comfort and protection of the oral cavity as this is the functional state the great majority of the time. It is important to check unstimulated function when evaluating a symptomatic dry mouth patient for salivary gland dysfunction.

▼ DIAGNOSIS OF THE PATIENT WITH SALIVARY GLAND DISEASE

The most common presentation of salivary gland disease is the complaint of dry mouth. The subjective report of oral dryness is termed xerostomia, which is a symptom, not a diagnosis or disease. The term is used to encompass the spectrum of oral complaints voiced by patients with dry mouth. It is important to recognize that a patient complaining of dry mouth should not be assumed immediately to have salivary dysfunction. Although oral dryness is most commonly the result of reduced salivation, it may have other causes.[6,7] Since individuals with salivary gland dysfunction are at risk of a variety of oral and systemic complications due to alterations in normal salivary performance, patients need careful objective examination to identify the basis of their complaint. They should be evaluated fully, and appropriate treatment should be implemented. Further, as salivary gland dysfunction may be the result of a systemic disorder, early recognition and accurate diagnosis may be of great benefit to an individual's general health and well-being. Patients also may present with a salivary mass or gland enlargement, with or without xerostomia. This requires a similar evaluation process.

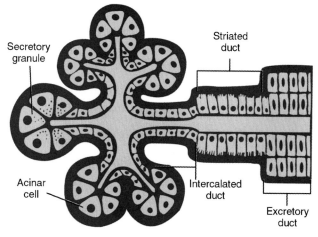

FIGURE 2   Acinar and ductal composition of a major salivary gland.

Salivary and nonsalivary causes of oral dryness complaints are discussed in detail in specific sections of the chapter. Nonsalivary causes include dehydration, central cognitive alterations, and oral sensory disturbances, as well as psychological conditions.[6,7]

Dysfunction of the salivary glands, however, is the most common cause of complaints of dry mouth. It is important to recognize that changes in salivary composition may be as important as a reduction in salivary output in some cases. Therefore, the demonstration of seemingly adequate salivary flow alone is not a guarantee of normal salivary gland function.

The differential diagnosis of xerostomia, salivary masses, and salivary gland dysfunction is lengthy.[6,7] The optimal approach to diagnosis is a systematic plan that first establishes the extent and cause of the complaint, then determines if salivary gland hypofunction is present and its severity, next establishes (if possible) a definitive diagnosis, and finally assesses the potential for treatment. An initial evaluation should include a detailed evaluation of symptoms, a past and present medical history, a head/neck/oral examination, and an assessment of salivary function. Further techniques that may be indicated are analysis of salivary constituents, salivary imaging, biopsy, and clinical laboratory assessment. These are described below in greater detail.

Symptoms of Salivary Gland Dysfunction

Symptoms in the patient with salivary gland hypofunction are related to decreased fluid in the oral cavity and the effects this has on mucosal hydration and oral functions. Patients complain of dryness of all the oral mucosal surfaces, including the lips and throat, and also of difficulty chewing, swallowing, and speaking. Unfortunately, the general complaint of oral dryness is not correlated well with decreased salivary function, although specific symptoms may be.[8] For example, although complaints of oral dryness at night or on awakening have not been found to be associated reliably with reduced salivary function, the complaints of oral dryness while eating, the need to sip liquids to swallow food, or difficulties in swallowing dry food have all been highly correlated with measurable decreases in secretory capacity. These complaints focus on oral activities (swallowing and eating) that rely on stimulated salivary function. Patients should also be questioned concerning dryness at other body sites, especially the eyes. Most will carry fluids at all times for oral comfort and to aid speaking and swallowing. Oral pain is common. The mucosa may be sensitive to spicy or coarse foods, which limits the patient's enjoyment of meals and may compromise nutrition.[9–11]

Past and Present Medical History

A thorough history is essential. If the past and present medical history reveals medical conditions or medications that are known to be associated with salivary gland dysfunction, a diagnosis may be obvious. Examples would be a patient who has received radiotherapy for a head and neck malignancy or an individual who has recently started taking a tricyclic antidepressant. Over 400 drugs are reported to have dry mouth as a side effect.[12] A complete history of all medications being taken (including over-the-counter medications, supplements, and herbal preparations) is critical. Often the temporal association of symptom onset with the treatment is a valuable clue. When the history does not suggest an obvious diagnosis, further exploration of the symptomatic complaint should be undertaken. A patient's report of eye, throat, nasal, skin, or vaginal dryness, in addition to xerostomia, may be a significant indication of a systemic condition, such as Sjögren's syndrome.[13]

Clinical Examination

Most patients with advanced salivary gland hypofunction have obvious signs of mucosal dryness.[6,7] The lips are often cracked, peeling, and atrophic. The buccal mucosa may be pale and corrugated in appearance, and the tongue may be smooth and reddened, with loss of papillation. Patients may report that their lips stick to the teeth, and the oral mucosa may adhere to the dry enamel. There is often a marked increase in erosion and caries, particularly decay on root surfaces and even cusp tip involvement. The decay may be progressive, even in the presence of vigilant oral hygiene. One should look for active caries and determine whether the caries' history and current condition are consistent with the patient's oral hygiene. With diminished salivary output, there is a tendency for greater accumulations of food debris in interproximal regions, especially where recession has occurred. It has not been determined definitively whether increased prevalence or severity of periodontal pathology is associated with salivary gland hypofunction.

Candidiasis, most commonly of the erythematous form, is frequent, appearing as red patches on the mucosa, rather than the more familiar white, curd-like mucocutaneous type (thrush). Angular cheilitis is also common. Two additional indications of oral dryness that have been gleaned from clinical experience are the "lipstick" and "tongue blade" signs. In the former, the presence of lipstick or shed epithelial cells on the labial surfaces of the anterior maxillary teeth is indicative of reduced saliva (saliva would normally wet the mucosa and aid in cleansing the teeth). To test for the latter sign, the examiner can hold a tongue blade against the buccal mucosa; in a dry mouth, the tissue will adhere to the tongue blade as the blade is lifted away. Both signs suggest that the mucosa is not sufficiently moisturized by the saliva.

Enlargement of the salivary glands is seen frequently. In these cases, one must distinguish between inflammatory, infectious, or neoplastic etiologies.[14] The major salivary glands should be palpated to detect masses and also to determine if saliva can be expressed via the main excretory ducts. Normally, saliva can be expressed from each major gland orifice by compressing the glands with bimanual palpation and by pushing toward the orifice. The consistency of the secretions should be examined. The expressed saliva should be clear, watery, and copious. Viscous or scant secretions suggest chronically reduced function. A cloudy exudate may be a sign of bacterial infection, although some patients with very low salivary function will have hazy, flocculated secretions that are sterile. In these cases, there may be mucoid accretions and clumped epithelial cells, which lend the saliva a cloudy appearance. The exudate should be cultured if it does not appear clear, particularly in the case of an enlarged gland.

Normally, palpation of the salivary glands is painless. Enlarged glands that are painful on palpation are indicative of infection or acute inflammation. The consistency of the gland should be slightly rubbery but not hard, and distinct masses within the body of the gland should not be present. Tumors of the parotid gland will typically present as solitary painless mobile masses, most often located at the tail of the gland. It is important to document function of the facial nerve when evaluating parotid tumors because the nerve runs through the gland, and evidence of decreased motor function of the nerve thus has diagnostic significance. Facial nerve paralysis is usually indicative of malignancy. Rarely, benign tumors may cause paralysis by either sudden rapid growth or the presence of an infection. Other findings suggesting malignancy include multiple masses, a fixed mass with invasion of surrounding tissue, and the presence of cervical lymphadenopathy.

Tumors in the submandibular or sublingual glands usually present as painless, solitary, slow-growing mobile masses. Bimanual palpation, with one hand intraorally on the floor of the mouth and the other extraorally below the mandible, is necessary to evaluate the glands adequately. Tumors of the minor salivary glands are usually smooth masses located on the hard or soft palate. Ulceration of the overlying mucosa should raise suspicion of malignancy.

Other lesions may mimic the presentation of salivary gland tumors. Inflammatory diseases, infections, and nutritional deficiencies may present as diffuse glandular enlargement (usually of the parotid gland). Patients who are seropositive for human immunodeficiency virus (HIV) may develop cystic lymphoepithelial lesions that may be confused with tumors.[15] Both melanoma and squamous cell carcinoma can metastasize to the parotid gland and appear similar to a primary salivary tumor.[16] Chronic sialadenitis in the submandibular glands can commonly be confused with a tumor.

Saliva Collection

Salivary flow rates provide essential information for diagnostic and research purposes, and gland function should be determined by objective measurement techniques. Salivary flow rates can be calculated from the individual major salivary glands or from a mixed sample of the oral fluids, termed "whole saliva."

Whole saliva is the mixed fluid contents of the mouth. The main methods of whole saliva collection include the draining, suction, spitting, and absorbent (sponge) methods.[17] The latter two are used most often. In the spitting method, the patient allows saliva to accumulate in the mouth and then expectorates into a preweighed tube, usually once every 60 seconds for 5 to 15 minutes. The absorbent method uses a preweighed gauze sponge that is placed in the patient's mouth for a set amount of time.[18]

If a stimulated whole saliva collection is desired, a standardized method of stimulation should be used. Chewing unflavored gum base or an inert material such as paraffin or a rubber band at a controlled rate (usually 60 times per minute) is a reliable and reproducible means of inducing saliva secretion. For research investigations, 2% citric acid is placed on the tongue at 30-second intervals.

Individual parotid gland saliva collection is performed by using Carlson-Crittenden collectors.[19] Collectors are placed over the Stensen duct orifices and are held in place with gentle suction. Saliva from individual submandibular and sublingual glands is collected with an aspirating device[20] or an alginate-held collector called a segregator.

Flow rates are determined gravimetrically in milliliters per minute per gland, assuming that the specific gravity of saliva is 1 (ie, 1 g equals 1 mL of saliva). Samples to be retained for compositional analysis should be collected on ice and frozen until tested.[6] Flow rates are affected by many factors. Patient position, hydration, diurnal and seasonal variation, and time since stimulation can all affect salivary flow. Whichever technique is chosen for saliva collection, it is critical to use a well-defined, standardized, and clearly documented procedure. This allows meaningful comparisons to be made with other studies and for repeat measures in an individual over time. To ensure an unstimulated sample, patients should refrain from eating, drinking, smoking, or any oral stimulation (such as oral hygiene) for 90 minutes prior to the collection.

For a general assessment of salivary function, unstimulated whole saliva collection is the recommended method of collection. It is easy to accomplish and is accurate and reproducible if carried out with a consistent and careful technique. Ideally, dentists would determine baseline values for unstimulated whole saliva output at an initial examination. This would allow later comparisons if patients begin to complain of oral dryness or present with other signs and symptoms of salivary dysfunction. For research purposes, or if more specific functional information is required for one particular gland, individual gland collection techniques can be used. These are not difficult but require specialized equipment and more time to accomplish.

It is difficult to determine a "normal" value for salivary output as there is a large amount of interindividual variability and consequently a large range of normal values.[21] However, with the collection methods described above, most experts do agree on the minimal values necessary to consider salivary output normal.[22] Unstimulated whole saliva flow rates of <0.1 mL/min and stimulated whole saliva flow rates of <0.7 mL/min are considered abnormally low and indicative of marked salivary hypofunction. It is important to recognize that higher levels of output do not guarantee that function is normal. Indeed, they may represent marked hypofunction for some individuals. These values represent a lower limit of normal and serve as a guide for the clinician.

Sialochemistry

Saliva is a complex exocrine secretion containing more than 60 constituents.[23,24] Numerous changes in salivary chemistries have been described with a variety of salivary gland disorders.[25–27] However, most reported alterations are related more to the reduced gland function than to a specific disorder. Therefore, most salivary constituent changes are nonspecific diagnostically and have minimal utility in determining the cause of the salivary gland dysfunction. In contrast, saliva has recently been shown to be an important medium for diagnosis and monitoring of a number of systemic conditions.[28–30] Saliva is now used routinely to determine viral infections,[31] blood alcohol,[32] and hormone[33,34] levels and to screen for drugs of abuse[35] and shows promise to screen for cancers and other significant systemic diseases.[36]

Salivary Gland Imaging

A number of imaging techniques are useful in evaluation of the salivary glands.[37–39] The following describes specific techniques as they relate to the diagnosis of salivary gland disorders. Depending on the technique used, imaging can provide information on salivary function, anatomic alterations, and space-occupying lesions within the glands. This section discusses plain-film radiography, sialography, ultrasonography, radionuclide imaging, magnetic resonance imaging (MRI), and computed and positron emission tomography (Table 1).

PLAIN-FILM RADIOGRAPHY

Since the salivary glands are located relatively superficially, radiographic images may be obtained with standard dental radiographic techniques. Symptoms suggestive of salivary gland obstruction (acute swelling of the gland and pain; sialoliths – Figure 3A and 3B) warrant plain-film radiography of the major salivary glands in order to visualize possible radiopaque sialoliths. Panoramic or lateral oblique and anteroposterior (AP) projections are used to visualize the parotid glands. Panoramic views overlap anatomic structures that can mask the presence of a salivary stone. A standard occlusal film can be placed intraorally adjacent to the parotid duct to visualize a stone close to the gland orifice. However, this technique will not capture the entire parotid gland. Sialoliths obstructing the submandibular gland can be visualized by panoramic, occlusal, or lateral oblique views.

Smaller stones or poorly calcified sialoliths may not be visible radiographically. If a stone is not evident with plain-film radiography, but clinical evaluation and history are suggestive of salivary gland obstruction, additional images are necessary.

SIALOGRAPHY

Sialography is the radiographic visualization of the salivary gland following retrograde instillation of soluble contrast material into the ducts (Figure 4). Sialography is the recommended method for evaluating intrinsic and acquired abnormalities of the ductal system because it provides the clearest visualization of the branching ducts and acinar end pieces. Ductal obstruction, whether by a sialolith, tumor, or stricture, can be easily recognized by sialography. When patients present with a history of rapid-onset, painful swelling of a single gland (typically brought on by eating), sialography is the indicated imaging technique. Potential neoplasms are better visualized by cross-sectional imaging techniques such as computed tomography (CT) or MRI.

TABLE 1   Salivary Gland Imaging Modalities: Indications, Advantages, and Disadvantages

Imaging Modality	Indications	Advantages	Disadvantages
Ultrasonography	Biopsy guidance; mass detection	Noninvasive; cost-effective	No quantification of function; observer variability; limited visibility of deeper portions of gland; no morphologic information
Sialography	Stone, stricture; R/O autoimmune or radiation-induced sialadenitis	Visualizes ductal anatomy/blockage	Invasive; requires iodine-containing dye; no quantification
Radionuclide imaging	R/O autoimmune sialadenitis; sialosis, tumor	Quantification of function	Radiation exposure; no morphologic information
Computed tomography	R/O calcified structure; tumor	Differentiates osseous structures from soft tissue	No quantification; contrast dye injection; radiation exposure
Magnetic resonance imaging	R/O soft tissue lesion	Soft tissue resolution excellent, with ability to differentiate osseous structures from soft tissue; no radiation burden	Dental scatter; contraindicated with pacemaker or metal implant; no quantification
Positron emission tomography	Identify regional salivary gland functional alterations and inflammation	Highly sensitive to metabolic activity	Radiation exposure; no morphologic information

R/O = rule out.

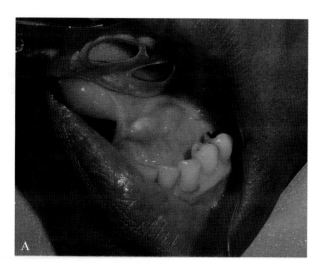

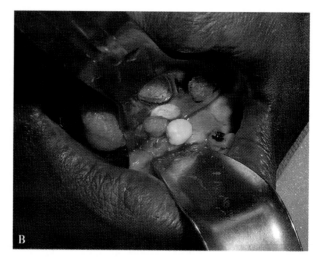

FIGURE 3 *A*, Sialolith within the left submandibular gland duct. Courtesy of Dr. Michael D. Turner, New York University. *B*, Surgical exploration of a sialolith within the left submandibular duct. Courtesy of Dr. Michael D. Turner, New York University.

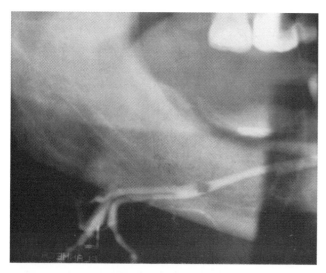

FIGURE 4 This is a sialogram of the submandibular gland demonstrating an uncalcified sialolithiasis in Wharton's duct, which can be visualized where the submandibular duct overlies the inferior alveolar canal. Courtesy of Dr. Elisa Mozaffari, University of Pennsylvania.

The two contraindications to sialography are active infection and allergy to contrast media. Sialography performed during active infection may further irritate and potentially rupture the already inflamed gland. Additionally, the injection of contrast material might force bacteria throughout the ductal structure and worsen the infection. The iodine in the contrast media may induce an allergic reaction and also can interfere with thyroid function tests and with thyroid cancer evaluation by nuclear medicine if these are done concurrently.

Sialography can be performed on both the submandibular and parotid glands. Initial plain-film radiography is recommended for visualizing radiopaque stones and potential bony destruction from malignant lesions, as well as to provide a background for interpreting the sialogram. Oil- and water-based contrast media are available. Both contain iodine and are therefore contraindicated in patients with iodine sensitivity.

Oil-based contrast material is not diluted by saliva or absorbed across the mucosa, which allows for maximum opacification of the ductal and acinar structures. However, if extravasation into the glandular tissue occurs, the residual contrast material will remain at the site and may interfere with subsequent CT images. Inflammatory responses and even the formation of granulomas have been reported following sialography using oil-based contrast.[40,41] Also, injection of oil-based contrast media requires more pressure because of its viscosity and may be more painful for the patient.

Water-based dyes are soluble in saliva and can diffuse into the glandular tissue, which can result in decreased radiographic density and poor visualization of peripheral ducts, compared with oil-based contrast. Higher-viscosity water-soluble contrast agents that allow better visualization of the ductal structures are available and are recommended.

Radiograpic views for sialography include panoramic, lateral oblique, AP, and "puffed-cheek" AP views. The normal ductal architecture has a "leafless tree" appearance (see Figure 4). As the ductal structure branches through the major glands, the submandibular gland demonstrates a more abrupt transition in ductal diameter, whereas the parotid gland demonstrates a gradual decrease in ductal diameter. Ductal stricture, obstruction, dilatation, ductal ruptures, and stones can be visualized by sialography. Nonopaque sialoliths appear as voids. The appearance of focal collections of contrast medium within the gland is termed sialectasis and is seen in cases of sialadenitis and Sjögren's syndrome. Sialography is the imaging technique of choice for delineating ductal anatomy and for identifying and localizing sialoliths. It also may be a valuable tool in presurgical planning prior to the removal of salivary masses.

Following the procedure, the patient should be instructed to massage the gland and/or to suck on lemon drops to promote the flow of saliva and contrast material out of the gland. A postprocedure radiograph is performed approximately 1 hour later. If a substantial amount of contrast material remains in the salivary gland at that time, follow-up visits should be scheduled until the contrast material empties or is fully resorbed. Incomplete clearing can be due to obstruction of salivary outflow, extraductal or extravasated contrast, collection of contrast material in abscess cavities, or impaired secretory function.

ULTRASONOGRAPHY

Due to their superficial locations, the parotid and submandibular glands are easily visualized by ultrasonography (Figure 5), although the deep portion of the parotid gland is difficult to visualize because the mandibular ramus lies over the deep lobe.[42,43] Ultrasonography is best at differentiating between intra- and extraglandular masses, as well as between cystic and solid lesions. In general, solid benign lesions present as well-circumscribed hypoechoic intraglandular masses. Ultrasonography can demonstrate the presence of an abscess in an acutely inflamed gland, as well as the presence of sialoliths, which appear as echogenic densities that exhibit acoustic shadowing. Recent studies have established sonographic diagnostic criteria for Sjögren's syndrome.[44] Ultrasonography is a noninvasive and cost-effective imaging modality that can be used in the evaluation of masses occurring in the submandibular gland and the superficial lobe of the parotid gland.

RADIONUCLIDE SALIVARY IMAGING

Scintigraphy with technetium (Tc) 99m pertechnetate is a dynamic and minimally invasive diagnostic test to assess salivary gland function and to determine abnormalities in gland uptake and excretion.[45] Scintigraphy provides quantitative information on the functional capabilities of the glands (Figure 6).[46] Technetium is a pure gamma ray–emitting radionuclide that is taken up by the salivary glands (following intravenous injection), transported through the glands, and then secreted into the oral cavity. Only the parotid and submandibular glands are visualized distinctly, as well as the thyroid gland, which binds and retains Tc. Uptake and secretion phases can be recognized on the scans. Uptake of Tc 99m by a salivary gland indicates that there is functional epithelial tissue present. The Tc 99m scan has been shown to correlate

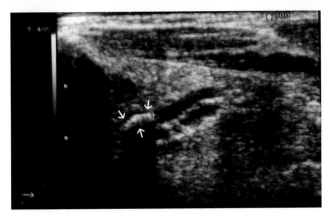

FIGURE 5 Change to: Ultrasound of a salivary gland. A sialolith within the left submandibular gland is visualized (arrows)

well with salivary output[47] and serves as a measurement of fluid movement in the salivary acinar cells.[48] Duct cells can also accumulate Tc 99m. Scintigraphy is indicated for the evaluation of patients when sialography is contraindicated or cannot be performed (such as in cases of acute gland infection or iodine allergy) or when the major duct cannot be cannulated successfully. It has also been used to aid in the diagnosis of ductal obstruction, sialolithiasis, gland aplasia, Bell's palsy, and Sjögren's syndrome.

Several rating scales are used for the evaluation of salivary scintiscans; however, no standard rating method presently exists.[49] Current approaches to functional assessment include visual interpretation, time-activity curve analysis, and numeric indices. Most radiologists interpret Tc 99m scans by visual inspection and clinical judgment. A semiquantitative method exists in which Tc 99m uptake and secretion are calculated by computer analysis of user-defined regions of interest. Recently, normal values for uptake and excretion of Tc 99m in the major salivary glands have been reported.[50]

A normal scintigraphic time-activity curve may be separated into three phases: flow, concentration, and washout. The flow phase is about 15 to 20 seconds in duration and represents the time immediately following radionuclide injection when the iostope is equilibrating in the blood and accumulating in the salivary gland at a submaximal rate. The concentration (or uptake) phase represents the accumulation of Tc 99m pertechnetate in the gland through active transport. With normal salivary function, the radionuclide will be secreted and tracer activity should be apparent in the oral cavity without stimulation after 10 to 15 minutes. Approximately 15 minutes after administration, tracer concentration begins to increase in the oral cavity and decrease in the salivary glands. A normal image should demonstrate uptake of Tc 99m by both the parotid and submandibular glands, and the uptake should be symmetric. The sublingual glands cannot be distinguished reliably.

The last phase is the excretory or washout phase. During this phase, the patient is given a lemon drop, or citric acid is applied to the tongue, to stimulate secretion. Normal clearing of Tc 99m should be prompt, uniform, and symmetric. Activity remaining in the salivary glands after stimulation is suggestive of obstruction, certain tumors, or inflammation.

With few exceptions, neoplasms arising within the salivary glands do not concentrate Tc 99m. The exceptions are Warthin's tumor and oncocytomas, which arise from ductal tissue and are capable of concentrating the tracer. They retain Tc 99m because they do not communicate with the ductal system, and they appear as areas of increased activity on static images.[51] The difference is accentuated during the washout phase, when the glandular signal decreases following stimulation while activity is retained in the tumors. Other salivary tumors may appear as voids or areas of decreased activity on scintiscans.

CT AND MRI

CT and MRI are useful for evaluating salivary gland pathology, adjacent structures, and the proximity of salivary lesions to

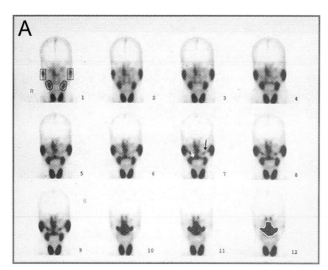

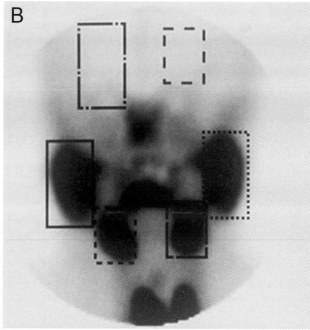

FIGURE 6 *A* (left) Technetium 99m pertechnetate radionuclide image (scintiscan) of the major salivary glands. This sequential salivary scintiscan is an anterior Water's projection of an individual with normal salivary function. The 4 major glands are outlined in frame 1 as regions of interest for further analyses. In frame 7, the dark arrow denotes Stenson's duct and the white arrow Wharton's duct, both emptying into the oral cavity. A secretogogue, usually citric acid, is placed in the oral cavity between frames 9 and 10, inducing a rapid emptying of the salivary glands. In frame 12, 10 minutes following application of the secretogogue, tracer is absent in the salivary glands and concentrated in the oral cavity, which is outlined. Courtesy of Dr. Frederick Vivino, University of Pennsylvania. *B* (right) A single frame of a salivary scintiscan demonstrating significant uptake in both parotid and submandibular glands (4 lower windows) with excretion into the oral cavity. The 2 upper windows represent background activity from the blood flow which is subtracted from the four regions of interest to determine specific salivary activity. Courtesy of Dr. Frederick Vivino, University of Pennsylvania.

the facial nerve.[52,53] The retromandibular vein, carotid artery, and deep lymph nodes also can be identified on CT.

Osseous erosions and sclerosis are better visualized by CT than by MRI. Since calcified structures are better visualized by CT, this modality is especially useful for the evaluation of inflammatory conditions that are associated with sialoliths. Abscesses have a characteristic hypervascular wall that is evident with CT imaging. CT also provides definition of cystic walls, making it possible to distinguish fluid-filled masses (ie, cyst) from abscess.

CT images of salivary glands should be obtained by using continuous fine cuts through the involved gland. Axial-plane cuts should include the superior aspect of the salivary glands, continuing to the hyoid bone and visualizing potentially enlarged lymph nodes in the suprahyoid neck region. Dental restorations may interfere with CT imaging and may require repositioning the patient to a semiaxial position.

Nonenhanced and enhanced CT images are obtained routinely (Figure 7). The initial nonenhanced scans are reviewed for the presence of sialoliths, masses, glandular enlargement and/or asymmetry, nodal involvement, and loss of tissue planes. Glandular damage from chronic disease often alters the density of the salivary glands and makes the identification

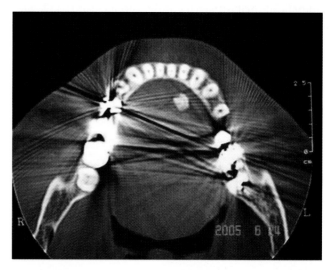

FIGURE 7 Sialolith of the left submandibular duct, on axial computed tomography. Courtesy of Dr. Michael D. Turner, New York University.

of masses more difficult. Contrast-enhanced images are more defined and accentuate pathology. Tumors, abscesses, and inflamed lymph nodes have abnormal enhancement compared with that of normal structures.

Ultrafast CT and three-dimensional–image CT sialography have been reported to be an effective method of visualizing masses that are poorly defined on MRI[54]; ultrafast CT is advocated for patients who are unable to lie still long enough for adequate MRI (pediatric, geriatric, claustrophobic, and mentally or physically challenged patients) and for patients for whom MRI is contraindicated. The disadvantages of CT include radiation exposure, administration of iodine-containing contrast media for enhancement, and potential scatter from dental restorations.

MRI has become the imaging modality of choice for preoperative evaluation of salivary gland tumors because of its excellent ability to differentiate soft tissues and its ability to provide multiplanar imaging (Figure 8).[55] It provides images for evaluating salivary gland pathology, adjacent structures, and proximity to the facial nerve. Recent work has examined MR of salivary glands in Sjögren's syndrome.[56] Structures and conditions that are dark on both T1- and T2-weighted images include calcifications, rapid blood flow, and fibrous tissue. The use of intravenous MRI contrast can improve imaging and aid in defining neoplastic processes, but its uses are specific, and indications should be discussed with the radiologist.

MRI is preferred for salivary gland imaging because (a) patients are not exposed to radiation, (b) no intravenous contrast media are required routinely, and (c) there is minimal artifact from dental restorations. The utility of MRI

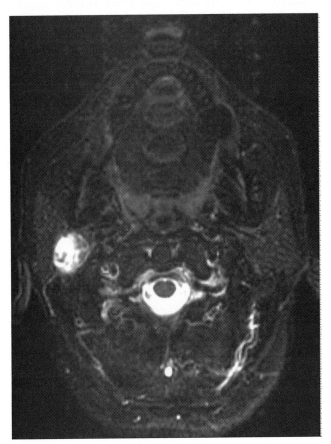

FIGURE 8   MRI image of a salivary gland. The opaque image in the left parotid gland is a pleomorphic adenoma.

has been enhanced by combination with sialography.[57,58] This allows a much finer evaluation of ductal alterations and any filling defects. MRI is contraindicated for patients with pacemakers or implants such as aneurysmal bone clips. If the implant contains magnetic metal, an MRI cannot be performed; however, dental implants are not magnetic and so are not contraindicated. Patients who have difficulty maintaining a still position or patients with claustrophobia may have difficulty tolerating the MRI procedure, which may result in poor image quality.

POSITRON EMISSION TOMOGRAPHY

Positron emission tomography (PET) has been used recently for evaluation of the salivary glands. Preliminary reports suggest that this may be a useful technique for measuring regional salivary gland function and recognizing inflammatory changes.[59] Combination of PET with CT may allow differentiation of salivary gland alterations in Sjögren's syndrome.[60] The advantages and disadvantages of each method of imaging, as well as their indications, are listed in Table 1.

Salivary Gland Biopsy

Definitive diagnosis of salivary pathology may require tissue examination. When Sjögren's syndrome is suspected, the labial minor salivary gland is the most frequently sampled site. This procedure is considered to be the most accurate sole criterion for diagnosis of the salivary component of this disorder.[61] Standardized histopathologic grading systems are used to assess the extent of changes.[62,63] Biopsy of minor glands can also be used to diagnose amyloidosis and sarcoidosis and in diagnosing and monitoring chronic graft-versus-host disease. Minor gland biopsy is a minimal operative procedure that can be done with limited morbidity, using appropriate techniques.[64] The incision is made on the inner aspect of the lower lip, near the midline, so that it is not externally visible. Six to 10 minor gland lobules from just below the mucosal surface are removed and submitted for examination. The incision should be made through normal-appearing tissue, avoiding areas of trauma or inflammation of the lip that could influence the appearance of the underlying minor glands. Care must be exercised to avoid damage to minor glands adjacent to the biopsy site as this can induce formation of a mucocele.

Biopsy of the parotid and submandibular glands usually requires an extraoral approach, although the sublingual glands are often approached intraorally. There is minimal morbidity for parotid biopsy, and it is done routinely as an outpatient procedure. However, biopsy of the parotid gland has not been shown to offer diagnostic superiority to the minor gland procedure in patients with Sjögren's syndrome.[65] When major gland biopsy is indicated for the evaluation of a distinct salivary mass, fine-needle aspiration (FNA) can be attempted. If this does not yield an adequate sample for diagnosis, an open biopsy procedure should be done. In cases of suspected lymphoma, immunophenotyping of the tissue is essential for diagnosis.[66,67]

FNA biopsy is a simple and effective technique that aids the diagnosis of solid lesions.[68] It may be particularly useful for elderly patients who cannot tolerate an excisional biopsy because of medical considerations. A syringe is used to aspirate cells from the lesion for cytologic examination. To establish a diagnosis accurately, it is important to have a well-trained cytopathologist who is familiar with salivary cytology read the specimen. FNA biopsies do not provide a specimen with anatomic structure. The cytologist will examine the individual cells aspirated from the lesion and will offer a diagnosis based on the cellular characteristics of different lesions. Even if an exact diagnosis is not made, it may be possible to determine if a lesion is benign or malignant. Knowing the biologic aggressiveness of the tumor prior to definitive surgery is helpful in planning optimal treatment.

A preoperative surgical biopsy is rarely indicated for salivary masses. In almost all salivary gland tumors, the treatment of choice is an excisional biopsy. In the parotid gland, this most often consists of a superficial parotidectomy, with careful preservation of the facial nerve. In small well-localized tumors of the parotid gland, local excision may be performed. Enucleation of tumors or local excision, however, is associated with a high recurrence rate in the parotid gland and is infrequently recommended. Tumors in the submandibular gland require the total removal of the gland. For tumors in the minor salivary glands, total excision with a margin of normal tissue is required. This approach is both diagnostic and curative in the majority of salivary gland tumors.

Analysis of frozen sections should be performed at the time of surgery to establish a diagnosis and guide the surgical approach. More than 80% of the time, the diagnosis based on the frozen section agrees with the final pathologic diagnosis from fixed and stained tissue. Most errors involve a failure to recognize malignant lesions. Malignant tumors are incorrectly called benign 5 to 24% of the time, but benign tumors are incorrectly diagnosed as malignant only 0 to 2% of the time. If frozen sections reveal a malignant tumor, the surgical margins may require extension.[69,70]

Serologic Evaluation

Laboratory blood studies are helpful in the evaluation of dry mouth, particularly in suspected cases of Sjögren's syndrome. The presence of nonspecific markers of autoimmunity, such as antinuclear antibodies, rheumatoid factors, elevated immunoglobulins (particularly immunoglobulin G [IgG]), and erythrocyte sedimentation rate, and the presence of antibodies directed against the extractable nuclear antigens SS-A/Ro or SS-B/La are important contributors to the definitive diagnosis of Sjögren's syndrome.[13] Approximately 80% of patients with Sjögren's syndrome will display antinuclear antibodies, and about 60% will have antibodies against anti-SS-A/Ro.[13] This latter autoantibody is considered the most specific marker for Sjögren's syndrome, although it may be found in a small percentage of patients with systemic lupus erythematosus or other autoimmune connective tissue disorders. Another serologic marker that may prove useful for the diagnosis of salivary gland disorders is serum amylase.

This is frequently elevated in cases of salivary gland inflammation.[71,72] Determination of amylase isoenzymes (pancreatic and salivary) will allow the recognition of salivary contributions to the total serum amylase concentration.

▼ SPECIFIC DISEASES AND DISORDERS OF THE SALIVARY GLANDS

Developmental Abnormalities

OVERVIEW

Complete absence (aplasia or agenesis) of salivary glands is rare, although it may occur together with other developmental defects, especially malformations of the first and second brachial arch, which manifest with various craniofacial anomalies. Patients with salivary gland aplasia experience xerostomia and increased dental caries. Importantly, rampant dental caries in children who have no other symptoms has led to the diagnosis of congenitally missing salivary glands. Enamel hypoplasia, congenital absence of teeth, and extensive occlusal wear are other oral manifestations of salivary agenesis.[73]

Parotid gland agenesis has been reported alone and in conjunction with several congenital conditions, including hemifacial microstomia, mandibulofacial dysostosis (Treacher Collins syndrome), cleft palate, lacrimo-auriculo-dento-digital (LADD) syndrome, and anophthalmia.[74] It has also been observed in ectodermal dysplasia, whereas hypoplasia of the parotid gland has been associated with Melkersson-Rosenthal syndrome. Congenital fistula formation within the ductal system has been associated with brachial cleft abnormalities, accessory parotid ducts, and diverticuli.[73,75–80] Although heredity is a significant factor, some patients have no familial history of salivary agenesis.

Aberrant salivary glands are salivary tissues that develop at unusual anatomic sites. Aberrant salivary glands have been reported in a variety of locations, including the middle-ear cleft, external auditory canal, neck, posterior mandible, anterior mandible, pituitary, and cerebellopontine angle. These are usually incidental findings and do not require intervention.[52–56]

When the submandibular salivary gland sits within a depression on the lingual posterior surface of the mandible, it is referred to as Staphne's cyst. Staphne's cyst is usually located between the angle of the mandible and the first molar below the level of the inferior alveolar nerve. The gland is usually asymptomatic and appears on radiographs as a round, unilocular, well-circumscribed radiolucency. The characteristic location and radiographic appearance make Staphne's cyst easily recognized. Palpation of the salivary gland can be performed occasionally, and sialography has been used to aid in diagnosis. Surgical intervention is recommended only in atypical situations in which the diagnosis is unclear and a tumor is suspected. Less commonly, anterior lingual submandibular salivary glands have been reported.[81–84]

Aberrant salivary glands occur rarely in the anterior mandible and are difficult to diagnose. They may give rise to radiolucent lesions at the apex of teeth, between tooth roots, and at extraction sites. The differential diagnosis includes the numerous unilocular radiolucent lesions of the mandible, and definitive diagnosis usually requires surgical intervention. FNA biopsy is an accurate, cost-effective diagnostic tool for these and other lesions[82,85,86] and contributes to conservative management in many patients with non-neoplastic conditions.[87]

ACCESSORY SALIVARY DUCTS

Accessory ducts are common and do not require treatment. In a study of 450 parotid glands by Rauch and Gorlin, half of the patients had accessory parotid ducts. The most frequent location was superior and anterior to the normal location of Stensen's duct.[88]

DIVERTICULI

By definition, a diverticulum is a pouch or sac protruding from the wall of a duct. Diverticuli in the ducts of the major salivary glands often lead to pooling of saliva and recurrent sialadenitis. Diagnosis is made by sialography. Patients are encouraged to regularly milk the involved salivary gland and to promote salivary flow through the duct.[89]

DARIER'S DISEASE

Salivary duct abnormalities have been reported in Darier's disease. Sialography of parotid glands in this condition revealed duct dilation, with periodic stricture affecting the main ducts. Symptoms of occasional obstructive sialadenitis have been reported. Progressive involvement of the salivary ducts in Darier's disease may be more common than reported previously.[90]

Sialolithiasis (Salivary Stones)

DESCRIPTION AND ETIOLOGY

Sialoliths are calcified organic matter that forms within the secretory system of the major salivary glands. The true prevalence of sialolithiasis is difficult to determine since many cases are asymptomatic. The etiology of sialolith formation is still unknown, yet several factors that cause pooling of saliva within the duct are known to contribute to stone formation: inflammation, irregularities in the duct system, local irritants, and anticholinergic medications. A nidus of salivary organic material becomes calcified and gradually forms a sialolith. Crystallization inhibitors (eg, *myo*-inositol hexaphosphate or phytate) have also been suggested in the etiopathogenesis of sialoliths.[91] Since the underlying cause is unknown and uncorrected in most patients, the recurrence rate is approximately 20%.[92,93]

The structure of sialoliths is crystalline, and sialoliths are composed primarily of hydroxyapatite.[94] The chemical composition is calcium phosphate and carbon, with trace amounts of magnesium, potassium chloride, and ammonium. Gout can cause salivary calculi composed of uric acid; however,

patients with a history of renal stone formation do not have an increased incidence of salivary gland stone formation. Fifty percent of parotid gland sialoliths and 20% of submandibular gland sialoliths are poorly calcified. This is clinically significant as these sialoliths will not be detected radiographically.[92,93,95,96]

The prevalence of sialoliths varies by location. They are by far most common in the submandibular glands (80–90%), followed by the parotid (5–15%) and then sublingual (2–5%) glands. The higher rate of sialolith formation in the submandibular gland is due to (1) the torturous course of Wharton's duct, (2) higher calcium and phosphate levels, and (3) the dependent position of the submandibular glands, which leaves them prone to stasis.[92,93]

CLINICAL PRESENTATION

Patients with sialoliths most commonly present with a history of acute, painful, and intermittent swelling of the affected major salivary gland. The degree of symptoms is dependent on the extent of salivary duct obstruction and the presence of secondary infection. Typically, eating will initiate the salivary gland swelling. The stone totally or partially blocks the flow of saliva, causing salivary pooling within the gland ductal system. Since the glands are encapsulated, there is little space for expansion, and enlargement causes pain. If the sialolith partially blocks the duct, then the swelling subsides when salivary stimulation ceases and output decreases.[97,98]

Salivary glands with obstructive sialoliths are frequently enlarged and tender. Stasis of the saliva may lead to infection, fibrosis, and gland atrophy. Fistulae, a sinus tract, or ulceration may occur over the stone in chronic cases. An examination of the soft tissue surrounding the duct may show edema and inflammation. Bidigital palpation along the pathway of the duct may confirm the presence of a stone. Suppurative or nonsuppurative retrograde bacterial infections can occur, particularly when the obstruction is chronic. Other complications from sialoliths include acute sialadenitis, ductal stricture, and ductal dilatation.[98]

DIAGNOSIS

Radiographs are helpful to visualize sialoliths; however, poorly calcified stones may not be readily identifiable (see Figure 3). An occlusal radiograph is recommended for submandibular glands. Stones in the parotid gland can be more difficult to visualize due to the superimposition of other anatomic structures; therefore, requesting proper radiographic views is important. An AP view of the face is useful for visualization of a parotid stone. An occlusal film placed intraorally adjacent to the duct may also help. CT images may be used for the detection of sialoliths and have a 10-fold greater sensitivity of plain-film radiography for detecting calcifications. Calcified phleboliths are stones that lie within a blood vessel; they can be easily mistaken radiographically for sialoliths. Phleboliths occur outside the ductal structure, and sialography can therefore aid in differentiating these lesions.

FNA techniques for submandibular sialoliths have been described and may have some utility, particularly when the differential diagnosis may include cysts or benign or malignant tumors.[98] A relatively new technique for visualizing and subsequently removing sialoliths is sialoendoscopy, where a small (<1 mm diameter) probe attached to a specially designed endoscopic unit can explore primary and secondary ductal systems.[99–102] The endoscopic unit also has a surgical tip that can obtain soft tissue biopsies and help remove calcified materials using a minimally invasive technique under local anesthesia.[100,103,104]

TREATMENT

During the acute phase, therapy is primarily supportive. Standard care includes analgesics, hydration, antibiotics, and antipyretics, as necessary. In pronounced exacerbations, surgical intervention for drainage or removal of the stone may be required. Stones at or near the orifice of the duct can often be removed transorally by milking the gland, but deeper stones require removal with surgery or sialoendoscopy. After the acute phase has subsided, surgery can be performed. Location within the duct determines the type of surgery planned. For example, stones located in the intraglandular portion of the duct require complete removal of the gland. Alternatively, if the stone can be removed from the duct without damaging the body of the gland, nearly complete salivary recovery can occur.[105]

Lithotripsy and sialoendoscopy can be helpful as noninvasive or minimally invasive treatments for sialoliths.[101–103,106,107] Ultrasonography will detect stones (diameter >2 mm) and extracorporeal lithotripsy will fragment the stone, although repeat lithotripsy procedures may be needed. Lithotripsy has been reported to be more effective for parotid versus submandibular calculi (57% vs 33%), with a 68% success rate after 10 years.[108] Reported complications from lithotripsy include transient hearing changes, hematoma, and pain. Sialoendoscopy is an endoscopic technique useful for soft tissue biopsies, explorative procedures, and removal of stones.[100,104] Visualization helps the practitioner establish a diagnosis and determine the least invasive treatment of choice, with few complications encountered.[100]

Extravasation and Retention Mucoceles and Ranulas

MUCOCELE

Description and Etiology. Mucocele is a clinical term that describes swelling caused by the accumulation of saliva at the site of a traumatized or obstructed minor salivary gland duct. Mucoceles are classified as extravasation types and retention types.[109] A large form of mucocele located in the floor of the mouth is known as a ranula (see below; Figure 9). The formation of an extravasation mucocele is believed to be the result of trauma to a minor salivary gland excretory duct. Laceration of the duct results in the pooling of saliva in the adjacent submucosal tissue and consequent swelling. The extravasation type of mucocele is more common than the retention form. Although often termed a cyst, the

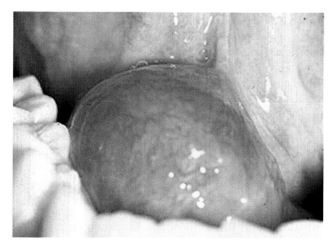

FIGURE 9   Sublingual salivary gland ranula. Courtesy of Dr. Michael D. Turner, New York University.

extravasation mucocele does not have an epithelial cyst wall or a distinct border. In contrast, the retention mucocele is caused by obstruction of a minor salivary gland duct by calculus or possibly by the contraction of scar tissue around an injured minor salivary gland duct. The blockage of salivary flow causes the accumulation of saliva and dilation of the duct. Eventually, an aneurysm-like lesion forms, which can be lined by the epithelium of the dilated duct.

Clinical Presentation. Extravasation mucoceles most frequently occur on the lower lip, where trauma is common. The buccal mucosa, tongue, floor of the mouth, and retromolar region are other commonly traumatized areas where mucous extravasation may be found. Mucous retention cysts are more commonly located on the palate or the floor of the mouth. A common clinical sequence is a history of a traumatic event, followed by the development of the lesion. Mucoceles often present as discrete, painless, smooth-surfaced swellings that can range from a few millimeters to a few centimeters in diameter. Superficial lesions frequently have a characteristic blue hue. Deeper lesions can be more diffuse, covered by normal-appearing mucosa without the distinctive blue color. The lesions vary in size over time; superficial mucoceles are frequently traumatized, allowing them to drain and deflate. In these circumstances, the mucocele will recur (Figure 10). Although the development of a bluish lesion after trauma is highly suggestive of a mucocele, other lesions (including salivary gland neoplasms, soft tissue neoplasms, vascular malformation, and vesiculobullous diseases) should be considered.

Treatment. Surgical excision is the primary treatment for mucoceles, particularly to prevent recurrence. Aspiration of the fluid from the mucocele will not provide long-term benefit. Surgical management is challenging since it could cause trauma to other adjacent minor salivary glands and lead to the development of a new mucocele. Intralesional injections of corticosteroids have been used successfully to treat mucoceles.

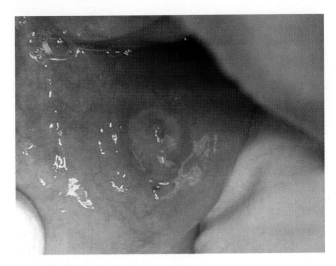

FIGURE 10 Minor salivary gland mucocele of the lower lip. Courtesy of Dr. Michael D. Turner, New York University.

RANULA

Description and Etiology. A ranula is a large mucocele located on the floor of the mouth. Ranulas may present as either a mucous extravasation phenomenon or, when the inflammatory components disappear, a sessile firm mass with a normal mucous membrane.[109] The most common cause of ranula formation is trauma. Other causes include an obstructed salivary gland or a ductal aneurysm. They are most common in the second decade of life and in females.[110]

Clinical Presentation. The term *ranula* is used because this lesion often resembles the swollen abdomen of a frog. The most common presentation is a painless, slow-growing, soft, and movable mass located in the floor of the mouth (see Figure 9). Usually, the lesion forms to one side of the lingual frenum; however, if the lesion extends deep into the soft tissue, it can cross the midline. Like mucoceles, superficial ranulas can have a typical bluish hue, but when the lesion is deeply seated, the mucosa may have a normal appearance. The size of the lesions can vary, and larger lesions can cause deviation of the tongue. A deep lesion that herniates through the mylohyoid muscle and extends along the fascial planes is referred to as a plunging ranula and may become large, extending into the neck.

Diagnosis. Radiography will help rule out a sialolith as a cause of duct obstruction. Radiopaque material instilled into the ranula cavity may be helpful in delineating the borders and full extent of the lesion.

Treatment. Surgical intervention is the treatment of choice for ranulas. A marsupialization procedure that unroofs the lesion is the initial treatment, especially for smaller lesions. Postsurgical complications include lesion recurrence, sensory deficits of the tongue, and damage to Wharton's duct.[111] Frequency of recurrence is related to the surgical technique

selected (marsupialization, 67%; ranula excision, 58%; sublingual gland excision, 1%), and given these results, excision of the lesion and the gland should be considered.[110] Intralesional injections of corticosteroids have been used successfully in the treatment of ranulas.

Inflammatory and Reactive Lesions

NECROTIZING SIALOMETAPLASIA

Description and Etiology. Necrotizing sialometaplasia is a benign, self-limiting, reactive inflammatory disorder of the salivary tissue. Clinically, this lesion mimics a malignancy, and failure to recognize this lesion has resulted in unnecessary radical surgery. The etiology is unknown, although it likely represents a local ischemic event, infectious process, or perhaps an immune response to an unknown allergen.[112]

Clinical Presentation. Necrotizing sialometaplasia has a rapid onset. Lesions occur predominantly on the palate; however, lesions can occur where any salivary gland tissue exists, including the lips and the retromolar trigone region. Lesions initially present as a tender erythematous nodule. Once the mucosa breaks down, a deep ulceration with a yellowish base forms. Even though lesions can be large and deep, patients often describe only a moderate degree of dull pain. Lesions often occur shortly after oral surgical procedures, restorative dentistry, or administration of local anesthesia, although lesions also may develop weeks after a dental procedure or trauma. It is not uncommon for lesions to develop in an individual with no obvious history of trauma or oral habit. Necrotizing sialometaplasia has been reported in connection with vomiting episodes in bulimia.[113–116]

Diagnosis. Diagnosis requires an adequate biopsy specimen and histopathologic diagnosis from a pathologist with expertise in oral lesions. In addition to the specimen, a complete clinical history should be provided to the pathologist to aid in distinguishing this lesion from squamous cell carcinoma. Microscopically, necrosis of the salivary gland, pseudoepitheliomatous hyperplasia of the mucosal epithelium, and squamous metaplasia of the salivary ducts are seen. There is diffuse infiltration of lymphocytes, histiocytes, neutrophils, and eosinophils.[112] Critically, there are no malignant cells and the lobular architecture is preserved even though necrosis is present.[117,118]

Treatment. This is a self-limiting condition lasting approximately 6 weeks, with healing by secondary intention. No specific treatment is required, but débridement and saline rinses may help the healing process. Recurrence and impairment are unusual.

EXTERNAL BEAM RADIATION–INDUCED PATHOLOGY

Description and Etiology. External beam radiation therapy is standard treatment for head and neck cancers, and the salivary glands are often within the field of radiation.[119] Although therapeutic dosages for cancer are typically in excess of 65 Gy, permanent salivary gland damage and symptoms of oral dryness can develop after only 24 to 26 Gy.[120–122] Etiopathogenesis of radiation-induced salivary gland destruction is multifactorial, including programmed cell death (apoptosis), in conjunction with production of reactive oxygen species and other cytotoxic products. Radiation-associated impaired blood flow may also contribute to the destruction of glandular acinar and ductal cells.[123]

Clinical Presentation. Acute effects on salivary function can be recognized within a week of initiating radiotherapy, with symptoms of oral dryness and thick, viscous saliva developing by the end of the second week. Mucositis is a very common consequence of treatment and can become severe enough to alter the radiation therapy regimen.[123,124] By the end of a typical 6- to 7-week course of radiotherapy, salivary function is nearly absent. This can be permanent if the major salivary glands receive more than 24 to 26 Gy. Permanent xerostomia and oral complications of salivary hypofunction impair a patient's quality of life (Figure 11).[125,126] Oral and pharyngeal sequelae of radiation-induced salivary dysfunction are new and recurrent dental caries, candidiasis, microbial infections, plaque retention, gingivitis, difficulty in speaking and tasting, dysphagia, impaired use of removable prostheses, and mucosal pain.[123,125,127,128] *Radiation caries* is the term commonly used to describe rapidly advancing caries, which characteristically occur at the incisal or cervical aspects of the teeth.[129] In spite of meticulous oral hygiene, the caries rate is often difficult to control and poses a diagnostic, preventive, and treatment challenge. Patients are also at risk of developing osteoradionecrosis, a necrotic avascular condition, most commonly occurring in the mandible after more than 60 Gy exposure.[130,131] Risk increases with time after radiotherapy and persists for the remainder of a patient's life. Finally, there is an increased incidence of second primary tumors involving the radiated tissues and increased incidence of salivary gland neoplasms.[132,133]

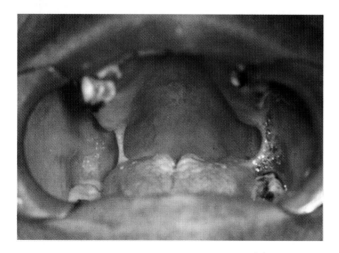

FIGURE 11 Severe salivary hypofunction in a patient who received 65 Gy external beam radiotherapy for a posterior tongue squamous cell carcinoma.

Prevention and Treatment. Radiation planning is critically important for protecting salivary gland tissue from external beam radiotherapy. Intensity-modulated radiotherapy (IMRT) using three-dimensional conformal CT-assisted radiation delivery techniques has proven successful in limiting exposure to salivary glands considered to be at low risk of tumor spread while restricting radiation dosages to tumors and those head and neck regions at risk of tumor spread.[134–138] Recurrence rates have been no different compared with nonsalivary sparing techniques[139,140]; therefore IMRT is recommended depending upon tumor type, location, extension, grade, and radiation treatment plan.[119]

In addition to improvements in the planning and delivery of radiation therapy, radioprotective agents may help limit radiation therapy–induced salivary gland damage. Amifostine, a cytoprotective agent, is approved by the US Food and Drug Administration (FDA) for xerostomia prevention in patients undergoing radiation treatment for head and neck cancers when the radiation port includes a substantial portion of the parotid glands.[141–144] The proposed mechanism of action involves the intracellular scavenging of free oxygen radicals. Following administration, amifostine is dephosphorylated in the circulation by alkaline phosphatase to a pharmacologically active free thiol metabolite. The thiol metabolite scavenges free oxygen species generated by radiation. Healthy, normal tissue is more vascular than the tumor and has higher capillary levels of alkaline phosphatase. Therefore, the concentration of the active thiol metabolite is higher in normal tissue and thus will protect the normal tissue but not the cancer. Amifostine is administered intravenously or subcutaneously 15 to 30 minutes prior to each fractionated radiation treatment.[145,146] In combination with IMRT, amifostine may provide even more effectiveness in preventing permanent salivary gland destruction. Major side effects include hypotension, nausea, vomiting, and dermatologic reactions.[147] Prevention of significant side effects includes preemptive use of fluids and antiemetics and close supervision of vital signs and evidence of skin reactions.[148–151]

Patients experiencing the plethora of oral side effects from external beam radiotherapy require regular follow-up and aggressive treatment for salivary hypofunction (see below and Chapter 2, "Pharmacology"), candidal and other microbial infections (see Chapter 2, "Pharmacology"), dental caries, and gingivitis. Rigorous daily oral hygiene and use of prescription-strength topical fluorides are necessary to prevent dental caries. Prevention of dental disease is important in order to reduce the need for dental-alveolar surgery, which could induce osteoradionecrosis of irradiated bone.

INTERNAL RADIATION-INDUCED PATHOLOGY

Description and Etiology. Disseminated thyroid cancer is treated by the removal of the thyroid gland and frequently postoperative radioactive iodine 131 (^{131}I). Radioactive iodine is taken up by thyroid tissue in addition to the oncocytes in salivary gland tissue. In some circumstances, ^{131}I treatment may lead to glandular fibrosis and permanent salivary gland hypofunction.[152–155]

Clinical Presentation. Patients complain of parotid swelling, pain, mouth dryness (xerostomia), and decreased salivary gland function soon after treatment.[156,157] Importantly,[131]I oral effects are limited to the salivary glands (as opposed to all oral hard and soft tissues with external beam radiotherapy) and will likely cause less destruction to the salivary glands.

Diagnosis. A history of ^{131}I administration will help establish the diagnosis. Salivary gland scintigraphy may be used to determine the extent of parenchymal damage.[158]

Treatment. Following administration of ^{131}I, patients should undergo an aggressive salivary stimulation routine that includes sugar-free lozenges and gums to stimulate salivary flow.[156] This will aid in clearing the ^{131}I from the salivary glands and will potentially decrease salivary gland damage. Other therapeutic protocols should be followed as with any other dry mouth patient to prevent development of further oral-pharyngeal disorders. Amifostine demonstrated some efficacy in protecting rabbit salivary glands during high-dose iodine therapy[142] and is worthy of consideration.

CHRONIC SCLEROSING SIALADENITIS (KUTTNER'S TUMOR)

Description and Etiology. Chronic sclerosing sialadenitis is a rare chronic inflammatory disease of the submandibular salivary gland,[159,160] although it has been reported to occur in parotid and minor salivary glands.[160,161] The etiopathogenesis is unknown, but it has been suggested to be the result of an immune process triggered by intraductal agents.[162]

Clinical Presentation. Patients present with clinical features simulating a salivary tumor with enlarged, firm, and painful unilateral or bilateral submandibular salivary glands.[159,163]

Diagnosis. This condition requires biopsy for histologic diagnosis since, clinically, it cannot be differentiated from a neoplasm.[164] It is characterized by progressive periductal fibrosis, dilated ducts with a dense lymphocyte infiltration, and lymphoid follicle formation, with acinar atrophy.[165] Sonographic findings include duct dilatation and calculi and prominent intraglandular vessels.[163]

Treatment. Surgical excision is successful for this benign condition.

Allergic Sialadenitis

DESCRIPTION AND ETIOLOGY

Enlargement of the salivary glands has been associated with exposure to various pharmaceutical agents and allergens (Table 2). It is unclear whether all of the reported cases are true allergic reactions or whether some represent secondary infections resulting from medications that reduced salivary output.

TABLE 2 Compounds Associated with Allergic Sialadenitis
Ethambutol
Heavy metals
Iodine compounds
Isoproterenol
Phenobarbital
Phenothiazine
Sulfisoxazole

CLINICAL DESCRIPTION

The characteristic feature of such an allergic reaction is acute salivary gland enlargement, often accompanied by itching over the gland. Cases have been reported of salivary gland enlargement without rash or other signs of allergy.

DIAGNOSIS

The diagnosis of allergic reaction should be made judiciously, especially when salivary gland enlargement is not accompanied by other signs of an allergic reaction. The possibility of infection or autoimmune disease should also be considered.

TREATMENT

Allergic sialadenitis is self-limiting. Avoiding the allergen, maintaining hydration, and monitoring for secondary infection are recommended.[166]

Viral Diseases

OVERVIEW

Several viruses have been associated with acute nonsuppurative salivary gland enlargement. The viruses responsible for the majority of virally induced salivary gland enlargement are paramyxovirus, cytomegalovirus (CMV), HIV, and hepatitis C virus (HCV). Echoviruses, Epstein-Barr virus (EBV), parainfluenza virus, and choriomeningitis virus infections have been linked to occasional reports of nonsuppurative salivary gland enlargement.

MUMPS (PARAMYXOVIRUS OR EPIDEMIC PAROTITIS)

Description and Etiology. Mumps is an acute viral infection caused by a ribonucleic acid (RNA) paramyxovirus and is transmitted by direct contact with salivary droplets. The Centers for Disease Control and Prevention (CDC) began recommending measles-mumps-rubella (MMR) vaccination in children in 1977. With current guidelines for an initial vaccination at 12 to 18 months of age and a second dose at 4 to 6 years of age, there has been a steady decline in disease prevalence. Mumps virus vaccine is not recommended for severely immunocompromised children because the protective immune response often does not develop, and risk of complications exists.[167,168] No epidemiologic studies have demonstrated a direct link between the MMR vaccine and autism or inflammatory bowel disease, yet some parents have refused vaccination for their children, raising the possibility of reemergence of the disease.[169] Therefore, this infection must be considered in cases of acute nonsuppurative salivary gland inflammation in unvaccinated patients who have not had mumps.

Clinical Presentation. Mumps typically occurs in children between the ages of 4 and 6 years. The incubation period is 2 to 3 weeks; this is followed by salivary gland inflammation and enlargement, preauricular pain, fever, malaise, headache, and myalgia. The majority of cases involve the parotid glands, but 10% of the cases involve the submandibular glands alone (Figure 12). The salivary gland enlargement is sudden and painful to palpation, with edema in the skin overlying the involved glands. Salivary gland ducts are inflamed but without purulent discharge. If partial duct obstruction occurs, the patient may experience pain when eating. One gland can become symptomatic 24 to 48 hours before another gland does. Swelling is usually bilateral and lasts approximately 7 days. Complications of mumps include mild meningitis and encephalitis. Deafness, myocarditis, thyroiditis, pancreatitis, and oophoritis occur less frequently. Males can experience epididymitis and orchitis, resulting in testicular atrophy and infertility if the disease occurs in adolescence or later.

Diagnosis. The diagnosis is made by the demonstration of antibodies to the mumps S and V antigens and to the hemagglutination antigen. The diagnosis of mumps in adults can be more difficult. A rapid, commercially available oral fluid assay using a mumps-specific immunoglobulin M (IgM) capture enzyme immunoassay has demonstrated good sensitivity and specificity as an alternative to the conventional serologic test.[170] A salivary test using reverse transcriptase–polymerase chain reaction (PCR) and loop-mediated isothermal gene amplification may help in the calculation of viral loads, which can assist in the assessment of disease pathogenesis.[171]

Treatment. The treatment of mumps is symptomatic, and vaccination is important for prevention. Rare fatalities have occurred from viral encephalitis, myocarditis, and neuritis.

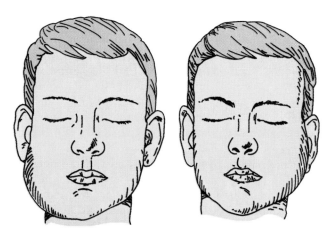

FIGURE 12 *Left*: Typical location and configuration of swelling associated with mumps. *Right*: Usual location and configuration of swelling associated with abscessed mandibular molars.

CMV INFECTION

Description and Etiology. CMV is a beta herpesvirus that infects only humans and is the major cause of non-EBV infectious mononucleosis in the general population. After initial exposure and infection, CMV may remain latent for many years. Reactivation can occur in healthy individuals without clinical illness; however, in immunocompromised individuals, this can be life threatening.[172,173] CMV can be cultured from blood, saliva, feces, respiratory secretions, urine, and other body fluids, and a large percentage of healthy adults have serum antibodies to the virus. Horizontal transmission occurs through blood transfusion, allograft transplants, and sexual contact. High rates of seropositivity are found in homosexual males, intravenous drug users, prostitutes, and individuals who have undergone multiple transfusions.[174–177] Transmission from children to adults or between children occurs through fomites, urine, saliva, and respiratory secretions. Between 11 and 24% of children attending day-care centers have CMV in their saliva.[178,179] Vertical transplacental transmission results in congenital infection and malformations. Perinatal infection occurs in 3% of all live births and is thought to be due to transmission from breast milk, saliva, fomites, or urine. Infection in newborns and young children can be fatal.[175,177]

Clinical Presentation. CMV mononucleosis often occurs in the young adult population and presents as an acute febrile illness that includes salivary gland enlargement. For healthy adults, the prognosis is excellent. Transplacental transmission of CMV can result in prematurity, low birth weight, and various congenital malformations. Infected newborns and young children develop multiple organ disorders, and the disease is often fatal.[174] In adults, infection can occur by reactivation of the latent virus or by primary infection. An impaired immune system allows the virus to replicate and allows disseminated infection to occur. Patients taking immunosuppressive medications and patients with hematologic abnormalities or HIV infection are susceptible to severe CMV infections. CMV is considered a clinical marker for acquired immune deficiency syndrome (AIDS), and the CDC surveillance case definition for AIDS includes CMV infection of the salivary glands that lasts longer than 1 month in adult patients. HIV-infected patients have demonstrated salivary CMV shedding,[180–182] suggesting that these patients could transmit CMV.

Diagnosis. Diagnosis is based on an elevated titer of CMV antibodies, as well as viral culture, antigen detection, and CMV deoxyribonucleic acid (DNA) detection. Diagnosis of primary infection in an immunocompetent patient uses a combination of IgM anti-CMV antibody seropositivity, IgG seroconversion, and viral culture. Antibodies to CMV are less useful diagnostically in immunocompromised individuals. The presence of IgG antibodies against CMV is used to detect past CMV infection in immunocompetent patients who are being screened for blood or organ donation.[183,184]

Histopathologic examination of CMV-infected tissue reveals large atypical cells with inclusion bodies.[185] These cells can be two times the normal size and have eccentrically placed nuclei, resulting in an "owl-like" appearance. Tissue necrosis and nonspecific inflammation may also be seen histologically.

Treatment. Immunocompetent patients are treated symptomatically. Immunocompromised patients require aggressive management and may be treated with intravenous antiviral ganciclovir, foscarnet, cidofovir, or valganciclovir. Salivary gland enlargement will respond to CMV antiviral therapies, which consist of two phases: induction therapy and maintenance therapy. Induction therapy is designed to treat the disease and usually takes 2 to 3 weeks. Maintenance therapy is intended to prevent the virus from causing disease again in the future, and duration depends upon the extent of CMV infections and concurrent immunocompromising conditions.

HIV INFECTION

Description and Etiology. Neoplastic and non-neoplastic salivary gland lesions occur with increased frequency in HIV-infected patients, and a Sjögren's syndrome–like phenomenon is also seen.[186] AIDS-related tumors (Kaposi's sarcoma, lymphoma) can also manifest in salivary gland enlargements. Frequently referred to as "HIV salivary gland disease" (HIV-SGD), it encompasses a range of conditions, including xerostomia and benign (unilateral or bilateral) salivary gland enlargement in HIV-positive patients.[187–189] The prevalence of HIV-SGD is ≈1.0% in adult HIV-infected patients but has been reported to be as high as 19% in pediatric patients. Homosexual persons and intravenous drug users experience gland enlargement more frequently than patients infected by other routes of transmission. The etiology of HIV-SGD is poorly understood, but the reactivation of a latent virus has been hypothesized.[190]

HIV-SGD is associated with a CD8+ cell lymphocytosis of the salivary glands and with the diffuse infiltrative lymphocytosis syndrome. In this condition, lymphocytic infiltration is found in the salivary glands, lungs, gastrointestinal tract, and liver.[185,187] Multiple human herpes viruses, including EBV, CMV, herpes simplex virus (HSV)-1, and HSV-8, have also been found in the saliva of HIV-infected patients, demonstrating that these patients' saliva can be a prominent source of viral contamination.[191]

Clinical Manifestations. The primary sign of HIV-SGD is salivary gland swelling, primarily in the parotid glands and frequently bilateral (Figure 13). Xerostomia is a common symptom. Salivary flow rates may be decreased,[192] which may occur relatively early in HIV infection.[193] HIV-infected women with low CD4 counts and undergoing highly active antiretroviral therapy (HAART) have been demonstrated to be at high risk of developing xerostomia and salivary gland hypofunction.[194] Elevated levels of major salivary gland secretory leukocyte protease inhibitor (SLPI) are found, which

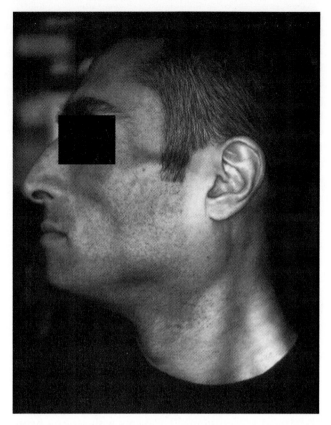

FIGURE 13 Parotid salivary gland enlargement in an HIV-infected patient. Courtesy of Dr. Michael Glick (Arizona School of Dentistry and Oral Health).

is the antimicrobial protein found in saliva with anti-HIV activity.[192] Importantly, one study demonstrated a high prevalence of salivary gland bacterial, fungal, and viral infections in patients who did not have complaints or signs of salivary diseases, which suggests that salivary pathology in these patients may be underestimated.[195]

Diagnosis. HIV-SGD frequently resembles Sjögren's syndrome and therefore must be distinguished from this disorder by appropriate salivary, ophthalmologic, and serologic evaluation.[186] Salivary flow rates may be reduced, and salivary immunoglobulin A (IgA) may be elevated both in patients with Sjögren's syndrome and in patients with HIV-SGD. Peripheral blood changes can resemble the changes seen in cases of Sjögren's syndrome and include hypergammaglobulinemia, circulating immune complexes, and rheumatoid factors. However, anti-SS-A and anti-SS-B autoantibodies are usually negative in the HIV-SGD population. A minor salivary gland biopsy may be indicated, and histologic findings resemble changes seen in cases of Sjögren's syndrome (including focal mononuclear cell infiltration) with routine tissue examination. Using immunohistochemical stains to differentiate the infiltrating cells, there is a preponderance of CD8+ cells in HIV-SGD compared with the CD4+ infiltrates that predominate in Sjögren's syndrome.

Enlarged major salivary glands can be imaged with ultrasonography, CT, or MRI. Multiple cystic masses are characteristic of HIV-associated benign lymphoepithelial hypertrophy. With persistent enlargement of a major gland, a biopsy of the affected tissue may be necessary to exclude neoplasia. Of particular concern are lymphoma and Kaposi's sarcoma, both of which have been reported in the salivary glands of HIV-infected individuals. Furthermore, saliva is the only mucosal fluid in which infectious HHV-8 (the etiologic agent of Kaposi's sarcoma) has been identified.[196] Histopathology of an HIV-SGD–involved major gland demonstrates hyperplastic lymph nodes, lymphocytic infiltrates, and cystic cavities.[180]

Oral fluids are the preferred method for rapid HIV-antibody tests (OraQuick) and were approved by the FDA in 2004.[197] They are commonly used for source-patient testing following occupational exposures.[198] Finally, assessment of the HIV-infected patient who has salivary complaints must consider the possible diagnosis of medication-induced xerostomia. When salivary gland enlargement is present, bacterial infection should be considered also.

Treatment. Treatment of neoplastic lesions is addressed under "Salivary Gland Tumors." Treatment for HIV-SGD is primarily symptomatic. Xerostomia may be relieved by use of sugar-free lozenges, candies, and gums; sipping water and other nonsugared beverages; and using saliva substitutes (see "Treatment of Xerostomia"). Patients with salivary hypofunction must follow a rigorous regimen of daily oral hygiene, and dentate individuals must use fluoride to control caries.

Benign parotid enlargement is an esthetic concern for some patients, and surgery has been performed for cosmetic reasons. Treatment of the enlargement with external radiation therapy (24 Gy in 1.5 Gy doses) has been reported with some success but has the potential for radiation-induced malignancy, and regular follow-up visits are required to monitor for malignant changes.[199,200] Radiation therapy also may increase the degree of xerostomia. It is speculated that systemic anti-HIV treatment may augment radiation therapy. However, antiretroviral treatments alone have shown minimal effects on enlarged parotid glands.[201]

Two other treatment methods include the aspiration of cysts and tetracycline sclerosis. The injection of a tetracycline solution into cystic areas will sometimes induce an inflammatory reaction and eventual sclerosis.[202]

HEPATITIS C VIRUS INFECTION

Description and Etiology. Viruses have been considered potential triggers of autoimmune diseases, and it is known that retroviruses can infect cells of the immune system and disrupt immunoregulation. Sicca symptoms mimicking Sjögren's syndrome have been described in diseases caused by retroviruses (see HIV-SGD, above). HCV DNA has been detected in the saliva of patients with chronic hepatitis C infection, and it has been demonstrated that the saliva of HCV carriers is infective.[203,204] A causal relationship between autoimmune disease and HCV is unlikely, yet salivary gland pathology is observed in HCV-infected patients.[205–208] There are also several reports of an association between HCV and Sjögren's syndrome,[209–212] although other investigators found no association.[213–215] The potential relationship between HCV and autoimmune disease remains an area of continuing debate.

Clinical Manifestations. HCV infection has many extrahepatic manifestations, including sialadenitis, complaints of xerostomia, and chronic major salivary gland enlargement.[205,216] Clinical manifestations and salivary histologic lesions generally are significantly milder in patients with chronic HCV infection than in patients with Sjögren's syndrome.[217,218] Importantly, HCV-infected patients with xerostomia do not commonly experience dry eyes, which can help distinguish this condition from Sjögren's syndrome.

Diagnosis. The diagnosis of HCV infection is established by the serologic detection of anti-HCV antibodies and HCV DNA. Detection of HCV-RNA in saliva has been demonstrated.[203,219]

Treatment. Hepatitis-associated sialadenitis is treated symptomatically.

Bacterial Sialadenitis

Description and Etiology. Bacterial infections of the salivary glands are most commonly seen in patients with reduced salivary gland function.[220] An acute and sudden onset of a swollen and painful salivary gland is termed an acute bacterial sialadenitis, whereas repeated infections are termed chronic bacterial sialadenitis (due to continuing and nonresolved infections). In the past, a retrograde bacterial infection was commonly experienced by patients after general anesthesia due to the markedly decreased salivary flow during anesthesia, often as the result of administered anticholinergic drugs and relative dehydration. More recently, with the administration of prophylactic antibiotics and routine perioperative hydration, this condition occurs much less frequently.[221] Today, the majority of bacterial infections occur in patients with disease- or medication-induced salivary gland hypofunction. Reduced salivary flow results in diminished mechanical flushing, which allows bacteria to colonize the oral cavity and then to invade the salivary duct and cause an acute bacterial infection. Poor oral hygiene contributes to these infections, and older adults are particularly susceptible to bacterial sialadenitis due to the frequent combination of medication-induced salivary hypofunction and poor oral hygiene.

Although sialoliths occur more frequently in the submandibular glands, bacterial sialadenitis occurs more frequently in the parotid glands. It is theorized that the submandibular glands may be protected by the high level of mucin in the saliva, which has potent antimicrobial activity. Anatomy may also play a protective role; tongue movements tend to clear the floor of the mouth and protect Wharton's duct. In contrast, the orifice of Stensen's duct is located adjacent to the molars, where heavy bacterial colonization occurs.[222]

Clinical Presentation. Patients usually present with a sudden onset of unilateral or bilateral salivary gland enlargement. Approximately 20% of the cases present as bilateral infections. The involved gland is painful, indurated, and tender to palpation.[223] The overlying skin may be erythematous.

Diagnosis. A purulent discharge may be expressed from the duct orifice, and samples of this exudate should be cultured for aerobes and anaerobes (Figure 14).[224] A second specimen should be sent for testing with a Gram stain. The predominant aerobes are *Staphylococcus aureus, Haemophilus influenzae, Streptococcus viridans, Streptococcus pneumoniae,* and *Escherichia coli.* Common anaerobes are gram-negative bacilli (including pigmented *Prevotella* and *Porphyromonas* species, *Fusobacterim* species) and *Peptostreptococcus* species.[224] Institutionalized individuals are particularly susceptible to infections caused by methicillin-resistant *Staphylococcus aureus.* Due to the dense capsule surrounding the salivary glands, it is difficult to determine, based on physical examination alone, whether an abscess has formed. Sialography, sialoendoscopy, ultrasonography, and CT are useful in the diagnosis of chronic salivary gland infections, cysts, and obstructions.[101,223,225,226]

Treatment. If a purulent discharge is present, empiric administration of a penicillinase- resistant antistaphylococcal antibiotic is indicated. Patients should be instructed to "milk" the involved gland several times throughout the day. Increased hydration, salivary stimulants (sugar-free candies, gums, mints), and improved oral hygiene are required. With these measures, significant improvement should be observed within 24 to 48 hours. If this does not occur, then incision and drainage should be considered.[223] Intraductal instillation of penicillin or saline is an alternative for the treatment of chronic bacterial parotid or submandibular sialadenitis.[227] The mortality rate for bacterial sialadenitis was once high, but the availability of a selection of broad-spectrum antibiotics has eliminated mortality in non–critically ill patients. Salivary

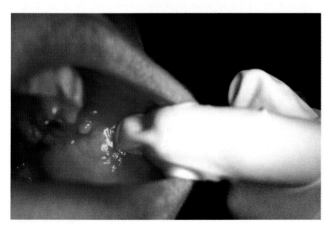

FIGURE 14 Acute bacterial sialadenitis and purulent discharge from Stensen's duct. Culture and sensitivity testing will produce guidance to appropriate antibiotics.

gland enlargement may also be nonbacterial in origin (eg, virally induced swelling, Sjögren's syndrome); therefore, antibiotics should not be started routinely unless bacterial infection is clinically obvious. Under all circumstances, purulent discharge from the salivary gland should be cultured to confirm the diagnosis and determine antibiotic sensitivity.[220]

Systemic Conditions with Salivary Gland Involvement

METABOLIC CONDITIONS

Diabetes. Diabetes mellitus is a common endocrine disease that produces multiple metabolic abnormalities and long-term complications, such as renal hypertension, neuropathies, and ophthalmic disease.

Many patients with uncontrolled diabetes report dry mouth and experience salivary hypofunction.[228–232] It appears that salivary disorders may be related to the efficacy of control of diabetes, with poorly controlled patients experiencing more salivary disorders than well-controlled patients or controls.[228,231] Children with diabetes are also affected by impaired salivary flow rates[233] and salivary compositional changes.[234]

The etiology of diabetic salivary gland dysfunction may be related to multiple problems, including polyuria, poor hydration, or underlying salivary gland pathology, including alterations in the basement membranes of salivary glands.[235] Poor glycemic control,[228–230,233] autonomic nervous system dysfunction,[231] and concomitant medications[236] may also account for salivary dysfunction. Xerostomic complaints in these patients could also be attributed to diabetes-associated thirst, a common manifestation of diabetes.

Anorexia Nervosa/Bulimia. Salivary gland enlargement and dysfunction can occur in patients with anorexia nervosa and bulimia,[237,238] possibly due to nutritional deficiencies and the habit of repeated induced vomiting. One case study reported histopathologic findings of acinar enlargement and reduced interstitial fat.[238] In bulimia, total and salivary specific amylase levels are increased. Salivary amylase tends to increase with the frequency of binge eating,[237,239] and salivary cortisol has been correlated with plasma cortisol demonstrating the overdrive of the hypothalamic-pituitary-adrenal axis in these patients.[240] Salivary gland enlargement usually resolves when patients return to normal weight and discontinue unhealthy dietary habits. However, benign hypertrophy may persist and be a cosmetic concern. Although superficial parotidectomy will reduce salivary hypertrophy, surgical management is contraindicated for patients with an eating disorder due to the increased risk associated with the patient's metabolic imbalance and psychological profile.

Eating disorders are difficult to diagnose because of the secretive nature of the condition. To facilitate early diagnosis and treatment, dentists should be aware of the common oral findings (enamel erosion, xerostomia, salivary gland enlargement, mucosal erythema, and cheilitis). Patients should be questioned directly if an eating disorder is suspected. Eating disorders must be considered in the differential diagnosis of salivary gland hypofunction and hypertrophy.

Chronic Alcoholism. Chronic alcoholism is associated with salivary gland dysfunction and bilateral salivary (usually parotid) gland enlargement. The exact etiology is unclear, but the decreased salivary flow may be attributed to dehydration and poor nutrition.[241] Enlarged salivary glands in alcoholic patients demonstrate fatty tissue changes,[242] acinar hypertrophy and structural changes in the striated ducts,[243] and excessive accumulation of secretory granules in the cytoplasm of acinar cells.[244] The enlargement of lumens within the ductal system could be the principal cause of glandular hypertrophy.[244]

Dehydration. Normal salivary output requires movement of water from the systemic circulation through acinar cells, into the salivary ductal system, and ultimately into the mouth. Dehydration has been demonstrated to result in diminished salivary output and increased symptoms of dry mouth.[245] Interestingly, dehydration causes a greater and more prolonged period of salivary hypofunction in older adults compared with younger adults, probably due to an age-associated diminished secretory reserve in older compared with younger adults.[246]

MEDICATION-INDUCED SALIVARY DYSFUNCTION

There are over 400 medications that are listed as having dry mouth as an adverse event,[12] and medication-induced salivary hypofunction is the most common cause of salivary disorders in the elderly.[7,247–249] When compared with younger adults, older healthy adults experience a greater extent and duration of salivary hypofunction.[250] This may be due to an impaired secretory reserve with aging,[251] which may account for the high incidence of salivary disorders in the elderly.[252–254]

Due to insufficient prospective clinical investigations, relatively few drugs have been shown objectively to reduce salivary function. Some drugs may not actually cause impaired salivary output but may produce alterations in saliva composition that lead to the perception of oral dryness. Table 3 summarizes the drug categories most commonly associated with salivary hypofunction. Medication-induced salivary hypofunction usually affects the unstimulated output, leaving stimulated function intact.

Instead of prescribing xerostomia-associated drugs, substitution with similar types of medications with fewer xerostomic side effects is preferred. For example, serotonin-specific reuptake inhibitors (SSRIs) have been reported to cause less dry mouth than tricyclic antidepressants.[255,256] If anticholinergic medications can be taken during the daytime, nocturnal xerostomia can be diminished since salivary output is lowest at night.[12] Furthermore, if drug dosages can be divided, unwanted side effects from a large single dose can

TABLE 3 Common Medication Categories Associated with Salivary Hypofunction

Anticholinergics
Antihistamines
Antihypertensives
Anti-Parkinson's disease
Antiseizure
Cytotoxic agents
Sedatives and tranquilizers
Skeletal muscle relaxants
Tricyclic antidepressants

be minimized or avoided. Such strategies can assist in diminishing the xerostomic potential of many pharmaceuticals used by patients presenting with xerostomia.

Polypharmacy is a common problem among the elderly, who can be treated concomitantly by multiple health care providers. Occasionally, medications with xerostomic sequelae may no longer be required, but the patient continues to take them. Other times multiple drugs are prescribed for similar medical conditions by different health care providers. Under these conditions, it is advisable to recommend critical review of all medications, and perhaps some can be substituted or even deleted from the daily regimen to diminish unwanted side effects, including xerostomia and salivary hypofunction.

IMMUNE CONDITIONS

Mikulicz's Disease. Mikulicz's disease, previously known as benign lymphoepithelial lesion, is characterized by symmetric lacrimal, parotid, and submandibular gland enlargement with associated lymphocytic infiltrations.[257,258] Mikulicz's disease had at one time been included within the diagnosis of primary Sjögren's syndrome, but the clinical and immunologic presentations warrant consideration of Mikulicz's disease as a distinct autoimmune phenomenon.[259] Histopathologically, Mikulicz's disease is associated with prominent infiltration of IgG4-positive plasmacytes into involved exocrine glands. Mikulicz's disease may be a systemic disease rather than a localized lacrimal and salivary gland disorder. It has been proposed that the entity be termed an IgG4-related plasmacytic exocrinopathy.[258]

The etiology of Mikulicz's disease is unknown. It has been speculated that autoimmune, viral, or genetic factors are involved. This condition predominantly affects middle-aged women. Patients present with unilateral or bilateral salivary gland swelling due to lymphoid infiltration. Reduced salivary flow makes these patients susceptible to salivary gland infections. The differential diagnosis includes Sjögren's syndrome, lymphoma, sarcoidosis, viral infections, and other diseases associated with salivary gland enlargement. Diagnosis is based on findings of salivary gland biopsy and the absence of the alterations in peripheral blood and autoimmune serologies seen in Sjögren's syndrome.

The lesions have been found to be highly responsive to corticosteroids, which are the preferred therapy.[260] Treatment with methylprednisolone pulse therapy and prednisolone has been recommended. An important consideration is the possibility of neoplastic transformation. It is important to differentiate the benign lesions of Mikulicz's disease from an indolent mucosa-associated lymphoid tissue (MALT) lymphoma (arising spontaneously or in the context of Sjögren's syndrome), and examination of the biopsy specimen for a monoclonal lymphocytic infiltrate is indicated.[261]

Sjögren's Syndrome (Primary and Secondary). Sjögren's syndrome is a chronic autoimmune disease characterized by symptoms of oral and ocular dryness, exocrine dysfunction and lymphocytic infiltration, and destruction of the exocrine glands.[13,262] The etiology of Sjögren's syndrome is unknown, and there is no cure. The salivary and lacrimal glands are primarily affected, but Sjögren's syndrome is a systemic disorder, and dryness may affect other mucosal areas (nose, throat, trachea, vagina) and the skin and involve many organ systems (thyroid, lung, kidney, etc.). Sjögren's syndrome patients also frequently experience arthralgias, myalgias, peripheral neuropathies, and rashes.

Sjögren's syndrome primarily affects peri- and postmenopausal women (the female- to-male ratio is 9:1) and is classified as primary or secondary. Patients with secondary Sjögren's syndrome have salivary and/or lacrimal gland dysfunction in the setting of another connective tissue disease (eg, systemic lupus erythematosus, rheumatoid arthritis, scleroderma, primary biliary cirrhosis). Primary Sjögren's syndrome is a systemic disorder that includes both lacrimal and salivary gland dysfunctions without another autoimmune condition.

Clinical Manifestations. Patients with Sjögren's syndrome experience the full spectrum of oral complications that result from decreased salivary function.[262] Virtually all patients complain of dry mouth and the need to sip liquids throughout the day. Oral dryness causes difficulty with chewing, swallowing, and speaking without additional fluids. The mucosa may be painful and sensitive to spices and heat. Patients often have dry, cracked lips and angular cheilitis. Intraorally, the mucosa is pale and dry, friable, or furrowed; minimal salivary pooling is noted; and the saliva that is present tends to be thick and ropy. The tongue is often smooth (depapillated) and painful. Mucocutaneous candidal infections are common, particularly of the erythematous form, in this patient population. Decreased salivary flow results in increased dental caries and erosion of the enamel structure.

Both primary and secondary Sjögren's syndrome patients usually have prominent serologic signs of autoimmunity, including hypergammaglobulinemia, autoantibodies, an elevated sedimentation rate, decreased white blood cells, monoclonal gammopathies, and hypocomplementemia.[13]

Patients with Sjögren's syndrome may experience intermittent or chronic salivary gland enlargement (Figure 15). They are also susceptible to salivary gland infections and/or

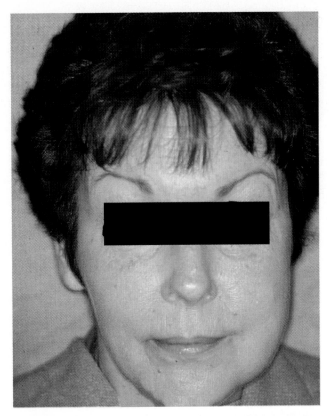

FIGURE 15 Chronic unilateral parotid salivary gland enlargement in a patient with Sjögren's syndrome.

gland obstructions that present as acute exacerbations of chronically enlarged glands. Patients have an increased risk of developing malignant lymphoma, most typically mucosa-associated B-cell lymphomas (MALT lymphomas) involving the salivary glands. It has been estimated that primary Sjögren's syndrome patients have a 20- to 40-fold increased risk of lymphoma.[263,264] Recently, factors have been identified to recognize those Sjögren's syndrome patients at greatest risk of lymphoma. These include vasculitis, low C4, and salivary gland enlargement at initial presentation.[265,266]

Diagnosis. Classification criteria for Sjögren's syndrome were developed and validated between 1989 and 1996 by the European Study Group on Classification for Sjögren's syndrome.[267,268] These criteria were reviewed by the American-European Consensus Group (AECG), which suggested some modification, defined clearer classification rules for primary versus secondary disease, and provided more precise exclusion criteria. The most recent results were published in 2002.[269] The widespread acceptance of these AECG classification criteria in the research community has greatly aided standardization of diagnosis and definition of patients.

There are six criteria: two dealing with symptoms of ocular and oral dryness, one measuring lacrimal function, one quantifying salivary function, another the labial minor salivary gland biopsy, and the last the presence of autoantibodies against anti-SS-A (Ro) and anti-SS-B (La). Four of these six criteria are required for positive case classification of primary Sjögren's syndrome. Critically, either a positive labial minor salivary gland biopsy or the presence of at least one of the autoantibodies is required to establish a definitive case. Alternatively, if three of the four objective criteria are satisfied, classification criteria are met. These criteria were found to have acceptably high sensitivity and specificity, are clinically practical, and greatly aid in evaluation of patients.

The labial minor salivary gland biopsy is considered to be the best sole diagnostic criterion for the salivary component of Sjögren's syndrome.[61] A grading system exists for quantifying the salivary histologic changes seen in the minor glands,[63] as follows: (1) the numbers of infiltrating mononuclear cells are determined, with an aggregate of 50 or more cells being termed a focus; (2) the total number of foci and the surface area of the specimen are determined; and (3) the number of foci per 4 mm^2 is calculated. This constitutes the focus score. The range is from 0 to 12, with 12 denoting confluent infiltrates. A focus score of ≥ 1 is considered positive for salivary involvement consistent with Sjögren's syndrome. Acinar degeneration, with the relative preservation of ductal structures, is also noted (Figure 16).

Imaging of the salivary glands was discussed earlier in this chapter. Sialography shows characteristic changes (sialectasis) and may be useful in the evaluation of Sjögren's syndrome. MRI or CT can be helpful also, particularly in the assessment of enlarged glands and potential lymphadenopathies. MRI is preferable to CT, unless a stone or other calcified structure requires visualization, as MRI provides better resolution of soft tissue. Some clinicians use Tc 99m radionuclide studies to determine salivary gland function.

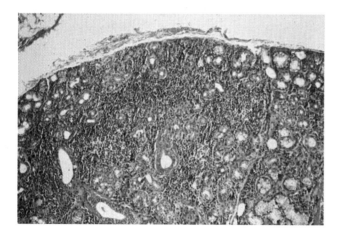

FIGURE 16 Histologic section of a biopsy of a labial minor salivary gland in a patient with Sjögren's syndrome. Chronic sialadenitis affects the entire gland with fatty replacement of some areas, fibrosis and atrophy of the gland parenchyma, and cystic dilatation of ducts.

Treatment. Treatment for Sjögren's syndrome has advanced a great deal in the last decade.[270] Numerous clinical trials have been conducting evaluating systemic agents to treat the underlying exocrinopathy through manipulation of the immune system. However, these remain experimental, and most available treatment modalities are primarily symptomatic. Management of the oral consequences of salivary dysfunction is not different from those in other causes of secretory damage. Symptomatic therapies include artificial saliva, oral rinses and gels, mouthwashes, and water sipping (see "Treatment of Xerostomia").[7,271] Patients with remaining salivary function can also stimulate salivary flow by chewing sugar-free gum or by sucking on sugar-free candies.

Parasympathomimetic secretogogues have shown the most success for xerostomia relief. There are two FDA-approved medications for the relief of dry mouth in Sjögren's syndrome: pilocarpine and cevimeline. Both medications are muscarinic agonists, which induce a transient increase in salivary output and statistically significant improvement in complaints of oral dryness.[272–274] Cevimeline has a reported increased specificity to M1 and M3 muscarinic receptors compared with pilocarpine, which might suggest the potential for fewer side effects.[275,276] However, clinical trials have not confirmed a lower side-effect profile with cevimeline. Common side effects of both medications include sweating, flushing, urinary urgency, and gastrointestinal discomfort. Side effects are frequent but are rarely severe or serious. Parasympathomimetics are contraindicated in patients with uncontrolled asthma, narrow-angle glaucoma, or acute iritis and should be used with caution in patients with significant cardiovascular disease, Parkinson's disease, asthma, or chronic obstructive pulmonary disease. Pilocarpine is currently recommended at a dosage of 5 mg up to four times daily, whereas cevimeline is commonly prescribed at 30 mg three times daily. These medications are widely used and provide significant relief of dryness complaints in many patients. Pilocarpine has also been approved for treatment of xerostomia related to head and neck radiotherapy.[277,278]

In Sjögren's syndrome, there have been substantial efforts to improve salivary function and oral symptoms with systemic therapies directed at the underlying disease process. Therapeutic strategies include hormone modulation, general and targeted anti-inflammatory approaches, blunting of the B-cell response, and treatment of potential viral etiologies.

Sex hormones are known to influence autoimmune activity; however, hormonal treatments have shown limited success in Sjögren's syndrome. A relatively nonvirilizing androgen, dehydroepiandrosterone (DHEA), demonstrated no benefit compared with placebo in a randomized, double-blind trial.[279] A small pilot study did show some benefit with nandrolone decanoate for the relief of xerostomia, although there were no differences in any objective dryness measures when compared with placebo.[280]

Moderation of the inflammatory response in Sjögren's syndrome using antirheumatic agents has shown little success for improvement of dryness symptoms. Trials of prednisone, azathioprine, and hydroxychloroquine have shown minimal benefit for dry mouth.[281–283] These agents do have value in Sjögren's syndrome, primarily for management of extraglandular manifestations such as vasculitis and fatigue.

Recent studies have targeted specific biologic pathways to modify the underlying disease process. The efficacy of very low-dose natural (nonrecombinant) interferon-α, 150 IU/ three times per day, has been studied in primary Sjögren's syndrome. Initial studies showed increases in salivary output and improvement in labial minor salivary gland histopathology.[284,285] A subsequent phase 3 trial demonstrated increased unstimulated salivary function compared with placebo at 24 weeks.[286] However, the coprimary end points of stimulated whole saliva flow and oral dryness were not significantly improved relative to placebo. Further trials will be necessary to determine the efficacy of this agent in Sjögren's syndrome.

Another approach has been to modify the inflammatory cytokine pathway, specifically targeting tumor necrosis factor α (TNF-α). Anti-TNF-α agents, including etanercept, infliximab, and thalidomide, have shown no significant efficacy for dry mouth symptoms or salivary function in randomized controlled trials in Sjögren's syndrome.[287–289]

As there is well-documented B-cell hyperreactivity in Sjögren's syndrome, modulation of B-cell activity may impact the underlying disease and improve salivary performance. Rituximab, a humanized monoclonal antibody, binds to the CD20 antigen, which is present on B cells and involved in activation. In an initial case report and then in an open-label phase 2 study, improvement in dryness symptoms and salivary gland function was demonstrated.[290,291] Serum sickness–like symptoms were found in 20% of patients. A randomized controlled trial is necessary to confirm these promising results. Initial studies have been done testing other agents directed at B cells (such as an anti-CD22 antibody) in Sjögren's syndrome,[292] and preliminary results are positive.

A randomized clinical trial was conducted using an antiretroviral medication for the treatment of primary Sjögren's syndrome, based on the finding of a Sjögren's syndrome–like condition in some cases of HIV infection. Lamivudine, a reverse transcriptase inhibitor, 150 mg two times daily or placebo, was given. No significant clinical improvements were noted.[293]

There is a recognized increased incidence of malignant lymphoma in Sjögren's syndrome.[263,264] These tumors often involve the salivary glands. It has been hypothesized that salivary gland enlargement in Sjögren's syndrome may progress from a benign sialadenitis with polyclonal lymphocytic infiltration to an oligoclonal infiltration and that monoclonal lymphoid malignancy may later develop. Chronic salivary gland enlargement or any lymphadenopathy in Sjögren's syndrome patients should be viewed with caution. Routine monitoring is required and should include regular physical evaluation (including a head and neck examination) and assessment of immunoglobulin levels. Laboratory studies should determine if a monoclonal gammopathy is present.

Suspicious lesions can be assessed by cytologic examination of FNA biopsy specimens for clonality of lymphoid cells. Histologic findings dictate the degree of intervention. An oncologist should be consulted when lymphoma or a monoclonal gammopathy is detected. Often salivary lymphomas in Sjögren's syndrome are indolent and progress very slowly, and the recommended treatment is close monitoring. However, lesions can be aggressive, and this must be considered when exploring treatment options.[265]

GRANULOMATOUS CONDITIONS

Tuberculosis. Tuberculosis (TB) is a chronic bacterial infection, caused by *Mycobacterium tuberculosis*, leading to the formation of granulomas in the infected tissues. The lungs are most commonly affected, but other tissues, including the salivary glands, may be involved.[181,294,295] Patients with TB may experience xerostomia and/or salivary gland swelling, with granuloma or cyst formation within the affected glands.[296] Salivary gland enlargement usually presents as part of a characteristic symptom complex; however, salivary gland changes have been reported in the absence of systemic symptoms. Using PCR-based salivary assays, evidence of *Mycobacterium tuberculosis* was found in 98% of patients, a detection rate significantly better than culture (17%), suggesting that in the future salivary tests may be helpful for the diagnosis of TB.[297]

The worldwide increase in mycobacterial diseases and their association with immunocompromised patients must be considered when developing a differential diagnosis. Diagnosis depends on the identification of the bacterium. Treatment of the salivary involvement involves standard multidrug anti-TB chemotherapy. Chemotherapy and salivary gland surgery occasionally are required to treat persistent salivary gland pathology.[298,299]

Sarcoidosis. Sarcoidosis is a chronic condition in which T lymphocytes, mononuclear phagocytes, and granulomas cause destruction of involved tissue. Parotid gland involvement occurs in approximately 6% of patients with sarcoidosis.[300] Heerfordt's syndrome (uveoparotid fever) is a form of sarcoid that can occur in the presence or absence of systemic sarcoidosis. The syndrome is defined by the triad of inflammation of the uveal tract of the eye, parotid swelling, and facial palsy.[180] Sarcoidosis can also occur in conjunction with Sjögren's syndrome or could mimic Sjögren's syndrome.[301] Sarcoidosis affects the salivary glands in approximately 5% of cases. Clinical presentation is bilateral, painless, and firm salivary gland enlargement, with diminished salivary output from affected glands.[302] Unilateral salivary gland enlargement has been reported. Examination of a minor salivary gland biopsy specimen can confirm the diagnosis of sarcoidosis with classic noncaseating granulomata.[303] Serum laboratory chemistries including calcium level, autoimmune serologies, and angiotensin 1–converting enzyme concentration aid in the diagnosis. Treatment of the salivary component of sarcoidosis is primarily palliative. Depending on the extent of disease affecting other tissues or during exacerbations, corticosteroids and other immunosuppressive and immunomodulatory medications are used.

▼ MANAGEMENT OF XEROSTOMIA

Treatment that is available for the dry mouth patient may be divided into five main categories: (1) preventive therapy, (2) symptomatic (palliative) treatment, (3) local or topical salivary stimulation, (4) systemic salivary stimulation, and (5) therapy directed at an underlying systemic disorder. Each is reviewed below. Based on the current literature and best clinical practice, the overall management strategy for xerostomia and salivary gland hypofunction should include a combination of supplemental fluoride, topical palliative agents, and a secretogogue.[7,14,270,304–307] Clearer evidence of clinical efficacy must be demonstrated before disease-modifying therapies can be recommended routinely. Management approaches are summarized in Table 4.

Preventive Therapy

The use of topical fluorides in a patient with salivary gland hypofunction is absolutely critical to control dental caries. There are many different fluoride therapies available, from low-concentration over-the-counter fluoride rinses to more potent highly concentrated prescription fluorides (eg, 1.0% sodium fluoride) that are applied by brush or in a custom carrier. Oral health care practitioners may also use fluoride varnishes. The dosage chosen and the frequency of application (from daily to once per week) should be determined based on the severity of the salivary dysfunction and the rate of caries development.[308]

It is essential that patients maintain meticulous oral hygiene. Patients will require more frequent dental visits (usually every 3–4 months) and must work closely with their dentist to maintain optimal dental health.[309] Patients should be counseled as to diet, avoiding cariogenic foods and beverages and brushing immediately after meals. Chronic use of alcohol and caffeine can increase oral dryness and should be minimized. When salivary function is compromised, the normal process of tooth remineralization is compromised and demineralization is increased, speeding the loss of tooth structure. Remineralizing solutions may be used to alleviate some of the effects of the loss of normal salivation.[310]

Patients with dry mouth also experience an increase in oral infections, particularly mucosal candidiasis.[7,311] This often takes an erythematous form (without the easily recognized pseudomembranous plaques), and the patient may present with redness of the mucosa and complaints of a burning sensation of the tongue or other intraoral soft tissues. A high index of suspicion should be maintained, and appropriate antifungal therapies should be instituted as necessary (see Chapter 2, Pharmacology). Patients with salivary gland dysfunction may require prolonged treatment periods and periodic retreatment to eradicate oral fungal infections.[262]

Symptomatic Treatment

Several symptomatic treatments are available. Water is by far the most important. Patients should be encouraged to sip water throughout the day; this will help moisten the oral cavity, hydrate the mucosa, and clear debris from the mouth. The use of water with meals can make chewing and forming the food bolus easier, will ease swallowing, and will improve taste perception. Use of sugar-free carbonated drinks is not recommended as the acidic content of many of these beverages is high and may increase tooth demineralization. An increase in environmental humidity is exceedingly important. The use of room humidifiers, particularly at night, may lessen discomfort markedly. As part of the normal diurnal variation, salivary flow drops almost to zero during rest. In individuals who have any degree of secretory hypofunction, the desiccation of the mucosa is particularly troublesome at night, and frequent awakening may interfere with restorative sleep.

There are a number of oral rinses, mouthwashes, and gels available for dry mouth patients.[310] Patients should be cautioned to avoid products containing alcohol, sugar, or strong flavorings that may irritate sensitive dry mucosa. Moisturizing creams are important. The frequent use of products containing aloe vera or vitamin E should be encouraged. Persistent cracking and erythema at the corners of the mouth (angular cheilitis) should be investigated for a fungal or bacterial cause.

There are many commercially available salivary substitutes. However, saliva replacements ('artificial salivas') are not well accepted by most patients. Although there is clearly a role for the use of saliva replacements, particularly in individuals who have no residual salivary gland function, it must be recognized that this is not a highly effective symptomatic therapy.[312]

Salivary Stimulation

LOCAL OR TOPICAL STIMULATION

Several approaches are available for stimulating salivary flow. Chewing will stimulate salivary flow effectively, as will sour and sweet tastes. The combination of chewing and taste, as

TABLE 4	Management of Xerostomia
Management Approach	**Examples**
Preventive therapies	Supplemental fluoride; remineralizing solutions; optimal oral hygiene; noncariogenic diet
Symptomatic (palliative) treatments	Water; oral rinses, gels, mouthwashes; increased humidification; minimize caffeine and alcohol
Local or topical salivary stimulation	Sugar-free gums and mints
Systemic salivary stimulation	Parasympathomimetic secretogogues: cevimeline and pilocarpine
Therapy of underlying systemic disorders	Anti-inflammatory therapies to treat the autoimmune exocrinopathy of Sjögren's syndrome

provided by gums or mints, can be very effective in relieving symptoms for patients who have remaining salivary function. However, patients with dry mouth must be told not to use products that contain sugar as a sweetener due to the increased risk of dental caries. Electrical stimulation has also been examined as a therapy for salivary hypofunction but has been inadequately investigated clinically.[270] A device that delivers a very low-voltage electrical charge to the tongue and palate has been described, although its effect was modest in patients with dry mouth.[313] Recently, a modified device has been tested and has shown promise in initial trials.[314]

Acupuncture, with application of needles in the perioral and other regions, has been proposed as a therapy for salivary gland hypofunction and xerostomia. Further well-controlled trials are necessary to evaluate this treatment modality fully.[315]

Systemic Stimulation

The use of systemic secretogogues for salivary stimulation has long been examined, with the earliest reports dating from the late 1800s. More than 24 agents have been proposed as means of stimulating salivary output systemically. Four have been examined extensively in controlled clinical trials; these are bromhexine, anetholetrithione, pilocarpine HCl, and cevimeline HCl.

Bromhexine is a mucolytic agent used in Europe and the Middle East but not available in the United States. The proposed mechanism of action for salivary stimulation is unknown. No proven benefit to salivary function has been shown in controlled clinical trials. Bromhexine may stimulate lacrimal function in patients with Sjögren's syndrome, although this is controversial.[316,317]

Anetholetrithione is a mucolytic agent that has been shown to increase salivary output in clinical trials with mild adverse effects. The mechanism of action is not known definitively, but it has been suggested that anetholetrithione may up-regulate muscarinic receptors. In patients with mild salivary gland hypofunction, anetholetrithione significantly increased saliva flow.[318] However, it was ineffective in patients with marked salivary gland hypofunction.[319] One study suggested a possible synergistic effect of anetholetrithione in combination with pilocarpine.[320] This agent is unavailable in the United States.

Pilocarpine HCl is FDA approved specifically for the relief of xerostomia following radiotherapy for head and neck cancers and for those with Sjögren's syndrome.[274,277,278] Pilocarpine HCl is a parasympathomimetic drug, functioning as a muscarinic cholinergic agonist, which increases salivary output and stimulates any remaining gland function. The adverse effects of pilocarpine in human studies are common and are usually mild, consistent with the known mechanism of action of the drug. Sweating is the most common side effect, with other frequently reported side effects, including hot flashes, urinary frequency, diarrhea, and blurred vision.

After administration of pilocarpine, salivary output increases fairly rapidly, usually reaching a maximum within 1 hour. The best-tolerated doses are those of 5.0 to 7.5 mg, given three or four times daily.[321] The duration of action is approximately 2 to 3 hours. Pilocarpine is contraindicated for patients with pulmonary disease, asthma, cardiovascular disease, or narrow angle glaucoma. Patients do not appear to develop tolerance to pilocarpine following prolonged use. Pilocarpine has been shown to be a safe and effective therapy for patients with diminished salivation but who have some remaining secretory function that can be stimulated.

Cevimeline HCl is another parasympathomimetic agonist that is FDA approved for the treatment of symptoms of oral dryness in Sjögren's syndrome.[272,273] Cevimeline is prescribed at 30 mg/three times daily. This medication reportedly selectively targets the M1 and M3 muscarinic receptors of the salivary and lacrimal glands.[275,276] However, in clinical use, its side effects are similar to those of pilocarpine, and it still must be used with caution in patients with a history of glaucoma or cardiovascular, respiratory, or gallbladder disease and in patients who use various medications. The duration of secretogogue activity is longer than pilocarpine (3–4 hours), and the onset is somewhat slower. Cevimeline is presently in clinical trials for postradiotherapy xerostomia.

Pilocarpine HCl and cevimeline HCl are the only systemic sialagogues that are available in the United States. Both are effective at transiently relieving symptoms of oral dryness and increasing salivary output. Consultation with the patient's physician prior to prescribing these drugs for patients with significant medical conditions may be indicated, although they have a good safety record in many years of use. Increased understanding of the causes of xerostomia and salivary gland dysfunction undoubtedly will lead to improvement in the available treatments through the design and testing of more specific therapies with alternate mechanisms of action.

Treatment of Underlying Systemic Disorders

Most clinical work has been done in Sjögren's syndrome, and therapeutic trials are discussed in detail in the section on treatment of Sjögren's syndrome. Also, therapies used during head and neck radiotherapy to minimize salivary gland dysfunction are detailed in the section on management of radiation-induced salivary disease.

▼ SIALORRHEA

Description and Etiology

Sialorrhea is defined as an excessive secretion of saliva or hypersalivation.[322] The cause is an increase in saliva production or a decrease in salivary clearance.[323,324] Hypersalivation can be caused by medications (Table 5),[325] hyperhydration, infant teething, the secretory phase of menstruation, idiopathic paroxysmal hypersalivation, heavy metal poisoning, organophosphorous (acetylcholinesterase) poisoning, nausea, gastroesophageal reflux disease, obstructive esophagitis, neurologic changes such as in a cerebral vascular accident (CVA), neuromuscular diseases, neurologic diseases, and central neurologic infections.[326] Minor hypersalivation may

TABLE 5 Conditions that Cause Hypersalivation and Drooling

Medications
 Pilocarpine
 Cevimeline
 Lithium
 Bethanechol
 Physostigmine
 Clozapine
 Risperidone
 Nitrazepam

Neurologic diseases
 Parkinson's disease
 Wilson's disease
 Amyotrophic lateral sclerosis
 Down syndrome
 Fragile X syndrome
 Autism
 Cerebral palsy

Heavy metals
 Iron
 Lead
 Arsenic
 Mercury
 Thallium

result from local irritations, such as aphthous ulcers or an ill-fitting oral prosthesis.

Clinical Presentation

Hypersalivation can cause drooling, which produces social embarrassment, rejection, and a severe impairment in the quality of a person's life.[327] In severe cases, a partial or total blockage of the airway can occur, producing aspiration of oral contents and possibly aspiration pneumonia. Hypersalivation also causes perioral irritations and traumatic ulcerations that can become secondarily infected by fungal or bacterial organisms.

Diagnosis

Since there are a multitude of etiologic causes of hypersalivation, it is essential to obtain the exact history of the hypersalivation as well as a thorough and complete past medical history. A systematic oral evaluation should be performed, focusing on salivary gland enlargements, oral ulcerations, head/neck/oral masses, neuromuscular function, and condition of removable intraoral prostheses. Since most cases of hypersalivation are a secretion clearance issue, a swallowing study should be obtained from a clinician with expertise in speech and swallowing. If it is not a clearance issue, a salivary flow rate should be obtained. The normal rate of unstimulated salivary output from all glands is approximately 2.0 to 3.5 mL per 5 minutes.[17] Collection of unstimulated whole saliva using a drooling technique into a preweighed container that results in more than 5.0 mL in 5 minutes suggests greater than normal production of saliva and can help differentiate between an overproduction of saliva versus a salivary clearance issue. Blood samples should also be obtained and evaluated for heavy metals (see Table 5) and organophosphate pesticides. Premenopausal women should be evaluated for potential pregnancy, and in postmenopausal or male patients, androgen levels should be determined to rule out an androgen-excreting tumor. If the onset is acute, a CT scan of the brain should be obtained to rule out a CVA or a central nervous system mass.

Treatment

Treatment for hypersalivation should take into consideration the etiology of the hypersalivation, the risk versus benefit of the treatment, and, most importantly, the quality of life of the patient.[328] Depending on the etiology, there are three types of treatments for hypersalivation: physical therapy, medications, and surgery.

Physical therapy can be used to improve neuromuscular control, but patient cooperation is essential. Speech and swallowing therapy should be attempted prior to medical or surgical interventions. Unfortunately, studies have shown a low success rate with this therapeutic modality.

Drug-based treatments for hypersalivation are devised based upon etiology. If the patient is experiencing hypersalivation secondary to a pharmaceutical treatment, alternate medications can be evaluated, and if the therapeutic regimen cannot be altered, compatible xerostomic agents (scopolamine transdermal patch, propantheline, benztropine, atropine, glycopyrrolate, diphenhydramine hydrochloride) should be considered.[327] One randomized, double-blind, placebo-controlled, crossover study reported that amisulpride (400 mg/d up-titrated from 100 mg/d over 1 week) produced significant improvements in a hypersalivation rating scale.[329]

Consultations should be made with the patient's physician to help prevent deleterious drug-drug interaction problems or polypharmacy-induced side effects. Hypersalivation that occurs secondary to chronic nausea (eg, during chemotherapy) can be treated with antiemetic medications. Hypersalivation due to gastroesophageal reflux disorder (GERD) is a protective buffering response to acids encountered in the oral cavity. The GERD should be treated, and under most circumstances, the hypersalivation will resolve. Neurologic and neuromuscular conditions (eg, CVA, Down syndrome, central neurologic infections) can result in neuromuscular incompetence in swallowing function, resulting in salivary pooling in the anterior floor of the mouth and salivary spillage from the oral cavity (drooling). Xerostomic medications (see above) can be attempted for these conditions. Based on open-label and controlled studies, intraglandular botulinum toxin injections can be used to improve sialorrhea in patients with Parkinson's disease, parkinsonian syndromes, motor neuron disease, and cerebral palsy.[330–334] Botulinum toxin A (7.5–15 units) can be infiltrated, by trained individuals, into the body of the parotid gland. However, the response is only temporary and necessitates reinfiltration 2 to 3 months later. Possible side effects are xerostomia, pain at the injection site, and temporary facial nerve paralysis if the injections are placed deep within the gland.

There are a multitude of surgical techniques that have been devised to treat hypersalivation, particularly in patients with poor or deficient neuromuscular function. Historically, redirection of the submandibular ducts and parotid ducts posteriorly to the tonsillar pillars has been performed with good success, although patients with poor salivary clearance will not benefit from this technique.[335-337] Bilateral tympanic neuronectomy has also been performed, but this leaves a permanent anesthesia to the anterior portion of the tongue and is not recommended. Other techniques involve redirection of submandibular glands and excision of sublingual glands[338] or ductal ligation of all major submandibular/sublingual ducts.[339] These techniques are successful in reduction of drooling approximately 80% of the time, with occasional postoperative complications such as ranula formation, pain, and numbness.[336] The advantage of the duct ligation technique is that it involves an intraoral surgical approach, thereby reducing the risk of damaging the facial nerve. A final strategy is excision of one or more major salivary glands. Although this does provide a permanent cure for hypersalivation, it subsequently produces salivary hypofunction and severe xerostomia.

▼ SALIVARY GLAND TUMORS

There are nearly 40 different entities of major and minor salivary gland tumors, ranging from benign to extremely malignant.[340-343] The majority of salivary gland tumors (about 80%) arise in the parotid glands.[344-346] The submandibular glands account for 10 to 15% of tumors, and the remaining tumors develop in the sublingual or minor salivary glands. Approximately 80% of parotid gland tumors and approximately half of submandibular gland and minor salivary gland tumors are benign. In contrast, more than 60% of tumors in the sublingual gland are malignant. For minor salivary glands, pleomorphic adenoma is the most common benign tumor, and mucoepidermoid carcinoma is the most common malignant tumor.[347] The risk of malignancy for all salivary tumors increases as the size of the tumor decreases, which supports the importance of early detection.[343,348] Over 85% of salivary gland tumors occur in adults. Salivary tumors in children are most often located in the parotid glands, with more than half being benign.[349] The most common malignant lesions in children are mucoepidermoid carcinoma and acinic cell carcinoma.[350] Treatments for patients of any age involve surgical removal and adjuvant radiotherapy for more advanced cancers.[351-353] Brachytherapy is an effective technique for delivering postoperative radiotherapy to small malignant minor salivary gland tumors.[354] Efficacy of treatment of malignant tumors is dependent upon stage, location, presence of perineural invasion, treatment modality, histologic type, and presence of regional invasion.[355] Clinicians should be cognizant of the possibility of development of salivary gland tumors as second cancers in patients who have previously received radiotherapy for previous cancers.[356]

Benign Tumors

PLEOMORPHIC ADENOMA

Description. The pleomorphic adenoma is the most common tumor of the salivary glands; overall, it accounts for about 60% of all salivary gland tumors. It is often called a mixed tumor because it consists of both epithelial and mesenchymal elements. The majority of these tumors are found in the parotid glands, with less than 10% in the submandibular, sublingual, and minor salivary glands.[340,357,358] Pleomorphic adenomas may occur at any age, but the highest incidence is in the fourth to sixth decades of life.[359] It also represents the most common salivary neoplasm in children.

Clinical Presentation. These tumors appear as painless, firm, and mobile masses that rarely ulcerate the overlying skin or mucosa. In the parotid gland, these neoplasms are slow growing and usually occur in the posterior inferior aspect of the superficial lobe. In the submandibular glands, they present as well-defined palpable masses. It is difficult to distinguish these tumors from malignant neoplasms and indurated lymph nodes. Intraorally, pleomorphic adenomas most often occur on the palate, followed by the upper lip and buccal mucosa. Pleomorphic adenomas can vary in size, depending on the gland in which they are located. One case series reported an infrequent yet clinically significant malignant transformation to carcinoma of 8.5%.[357] In the parotid gland, the tumors are usually several centimeters in diameter but can reach much larger sizes if left untreated. When observed in situ, the tumors are encased in a pseudocapsule and exhibit a lobulated appearance.[360]

Pathology. The gross appearance of pleomorphic adenoma is that of a firm smooth mass within a pseudocapsule. Histologically, the lesion demonstrates both epithelial and mesenchymal elements. The epithelial cells make up a trabecular pattern that is contained within a stroma. The stroma may be chondroid, myxoid, osteoid, or fibroid. The presence of these different elements accounts for the name *pleomorphic tumor* or *mixed tumor*. Myoepithelial cells are also present in this tumor and add to its histopathologic complexity. One characteristic of a pleomorphic adenoma is the presence of microscopic projections of tumor outside of the capsule. If these projections are not removed with the tumor, the lesion will recur.

Treatment. Surgical removal with adequate margins is the principal treatment. Because of its microscopic projections, this tumor requires a wide resection to avoid recurrence. In spite of the capsule, close excision should not be attempted. A superficial parotidectomy is sufficient for the majority of these lesions. A small tumor in the tail of the parotid gland may be removed with a wide margin of normal tissue, sparing the remainder of the superficial lobe.[352,359,361] Lesions that occur in the submandibular gland are treated by the removal of the entire gland.

MONOMORPHIC ADENOMA

A monomorphic adenoma is a tumor that is composed predominantly of one cell type, as opposed to a mixed tumor (pleomorphic adenoma), in which different elements are present. Management is the same as for a pleomorphic adenoma.

PAPILLARY CYSTADENOMA LYMPHOMATOSUM

Description. Papillary cystadenoma lymphomatosum, also known as Warthin's tumor, is the second most common benign tumor of the parotid gland. It represents ≈6 to 10% of all parotid tumors and is most commonly located in the inferior pole of the gland, posterior to the angle of the mandible. The tumor demonstrates a slight predilection toward males, and it usually occurs between the fifth and eighth decades of life. These tumors occur bilaterally in about 6 to 12% of patients.[340,343,344,361]

Clinical Presentation. This tumor presents as a well-defined, slow-growing mass in the tail of the parotid gland. It is usually painless unless it becomes superinfected. Because this tumor contains oncocytes, it will take up technetium and will be visible on Tc 99m scintiscans.

Pathology. The gross appearance of this tumor is smooth, with a well-defined capsule. Cutting a specimen reveals cystic spaces filled with thick mucinous material. Histologically, the tumor consists of papillary projections lined with eosinophilic cells that project into cystic spaces. The projections are characterized by a lymphocytic infiltrate.

Treatment. Papillary cystadenoma lymphomatosum is easily removed with a margin of normal tissue. Larger tumors that involve a significant amount of the superficial lobe of the parotid gland are best treated by a superficial parotidectomy. Recurrences and malignant degeneration of this tumor are rare.[343,352]

ONCOCYTOMA

Description. Oncocytomas are less common benign tumors that make up less than 1% of all salivary gland neoplasms. The name of the tumor is derived from the presence of oncocytes, which are large granular acidophilic cells. This tumor occurs almost exclusively in the parotid glands and is equally distributed in both men and women. The sixth decade of life is the most common time of presentation.[340,343,344,361]

Clinical Presentation. Oncocytomas are usually solid round tumors that can be seen in any of the major salivary glands but are extremely rare intraorally. Bilateral presentation of this tumor can occur, and it is the second most common salivary gland tumor that occurs bilaterally (after Warthin's tumor).

Pathology. On gross examination, these tumors appear noncystic and firm. Histologically, they consist of brown granular eosinophilic cells. The oncocytes within this tumor

concentrate technetium, and this tumor can be visualized by Tc 99m scintigraphy. Malignant oncocytomas can occur, and these are aggressive lesions.

Treatment. Oncocytomas undergo a benign course, grow very slowly, and are unlikely to undergo recurrences. The treatment of choice for parotid oncocytomas is superficial parotidectomy with preservation of the facial nerve. Removal of the gland is the treatment of choice for tumors in the submandibular gland, and gland removal with a normal cuff of tissue is the treatment of choice for oncocytomas of the minor salivary glands.[362]

BASAL CELL ADENOMAS

Description. Basal cell adenomas are slow-growing and painless masses that account for approximately 1 to 2% of salivary gland adenomas. This lesion has a male predilection (male-to-female ratio is 5:1). Seventy percent of basal cell adenomas occur in the parotid gland, and the upper lip is the most common site for basal cell adenomas of the minor salivary glands.[363]

Pathology. Histologically, three varieties of basal cell adenomas exist: solid, trabecular-tubular, and membranous.[364] The solid form consists of islands or sheets of basaloid cells. Nuclei have a normal size and are basophilic, with minimal cytoplasmic material. The trabecular-tubular form consists of trabecular cords of epithelium. The membranous form is multilocular, and 50% of the lesions are encapsulated. The membranous form tends to grow in clusters interspersed between normal salivary tissue.

Treatment. Lesions are removed, with conservative surgical excision extending to normal tissue. In general, lesions do not recur; however, the membranous form has a higher recurrence rate.[364]

CANALICULAR ADENOMA

Description. Canalicular adenomas predominantly occur in persons older than 50 years of age and occur mostly in women. Eighty percent of cases occur in the upper lip. The lesions are slow growing, movable, and asymptomatic.

Pathology. This lesion is composed of long strands of basaloid tissue, usually arranged in a double row. The supporting stroma is loose, fibrillar, and highly vascular.

Treatment. Treatment is surgical excision with a margin of normal tissue. Recurrence is rare but has been reported; thus, patients should be monitored periodically.

MYOEPITHELIOMA

Description. Most myoepitheliomas occur in the parotid gland and in the minor salivary glands of the palate. No gender predilection exists, and lesions tend to occur in adults, with the average age in the sixth decade of life. Clinical features include a well-circumscribed, asymptomatic, slow-growing mass.

Pathology. Myoepitheliomas consist of spindle-shaped cells, plasmacytoid cells, or a combination of the two.[365] Diagnosis is based on the identification of myoepithelial cells and must be differentiated from other benign and malignant epithelial and mesenchymal tumors for treatment planning purposes.[366] Growth patterns vary from a solid to a loose stroma formation with myoepithelial cells. This tumor is epithelial in origin; however, it functionally resembles smooth muscle and is demonstrated by immunohistochemical staining for actin, cytokeratin, and S-100 protein.

Treatment. Standard surgical excision, including a border of normal tissue, is recommended. Recurrence is uncommon.[343,352]

SEBACEOUS ADENOMA

Sebaceous adenomas are rare. These lesions are derived from sebaceous glands located within salivary gland tissue. The parotid gland is the most commonly involved gland.

Pathology. Cells derived from sebaceous glands are present. Benign forms contain well-differentiated sebaceous cells, whereas malignant forms consist of more poorly differentiated cells.

Treatment. Removal of the involved gland is the treatment of choice. Intraoral lesions are surgically removed with a border of normal tissue.

DUCTAL PAPILLOMA

Description. Ductal papillomas form a subset of benign salivary gland tumors that arise from the excretory ducts, predominantly of the minor salivary glands. The three forms of ductal papillomas are simple ductal papilloma (intraductal papilloma), inverted ductal papilloma, and sialadenoma papilliferum.[367]

Simple Ductal Papilloma. The simple ductal papilloma presents as an exophytic lesion with a pedunculated base. The lesion often has a reddish color. Microscopic examination reveals epithelium-lined papillary fronds projecting into a cystic cavity without proliferating into the wall of the cyst. Local surgical excision is the recommended treatment. A minimal recurrence rate is reported.

Inverted Ductal Papilloma. The inverted ductal papilloma occurs in the minor salivary glands. It presents clinically as a submucosal nodule that is similar to a fibroma or lipoma. The inverted ductal papilloma histologically resembles the sialadenoma. This form of ductal papilloma also consists of projections of ductal epithelium that proliferate into surrounding stromal tissue, forming clefts. The lesion is treated by surgical excision. A low recurrence rate is reported.[367]

Sialadenoma Papilliferum. The sialadenoma papilliferum form of ductal papilloma is analogous to the syringocystadenoma papilliferum of the skin. An adult male predilection exists, and most lesions occur between the fifth to eighth decades of life. This lesion occurs primarily on the palate and buccal mucosa and presents as a painless exophytic mass. Clinically, the lesion resembles a papilloma. Microscopic examination shows epithelium-lined papillary projections supported by fibrovascular connective tissue, forming a series of clefts within the lesion. Local surgical excision is the recommended treatment, and recurrences are rare.

Malignant Tumors

MUCOEPIDERMOID CARCINOMA

Description. Mucoepidermoid carcinoma is the most common malignant tumor of the salivary glands. It is the most common malignant tumor of the parotid gland and the second most common malignant tumor of the submandibular gland, after adenoid cystic carcinoma. Approximately 60 to 90% of these lesions occur in the parotid gland; the palate is the second most common site. Men and women are affected equally by this tumor, and the highest incidence occurs in the third to fifth decades of life. This tumor occurs rarely in children.[368] The mucoepidermoid carcinoma consists of both epidermal and mucous cells, and it is classified as high grade or low grade, depending on the ratio of epidermal cells to mucous cells. The low-grade tumor has a higher ratio and is a less aggressive lesion. Although low-grade tumors have the ability for metastasis and local invasion, they behave more like benign tumors. The high-grade form is a more malignant tumor and has a poorer prognosis.[369]

Clinical Presentation. The clinical course depends on the grade. It is not uncommon for low-grade tumors to undergo a long period of painless enlargement. In contrast, high-grade mucoepidermoid carcinomas often demonstrate rapid growth and a higher likelihood for metastasis. Pain and ulceration of overlying tissue are occasionally associated with this tumor. If the facial nerve is involved, the patient may exhibit a facial palsy.

Pathology. Macroscopically, low-grade mucoepidermoid carcinomas are usually small and partially encapsulated. The high-grade tumors are less likely to demonstrate a capsule because of the more rapid growth and local tissue invasion. After sectioning, the low-grade tumors usually demonstrate a mucinous fluid, but the high-grade lesions are usually solid. Microscopically, the low-grade lesions consist of regions of mucoid cells with interspersed epithelial strands. The high-grade tumors consist primarily of epithelial cells, with very few mucinous cells, and special stains are necessary to differentiate between these high-grade tumors and squamous cell carcinoma. An unusual form of the tumor is the sclerosing variant, characterized by an intense central sclerosis with an inflammatory infiltrate of plasma cells, eosinophils, and lymphocytes in the peripheral regions.[370]

Treatment. A low-grade mucoepidermoid carcinoma can be treated with a superficial parotidectomy if it involves only the superficial lobe. Frequently, the facial nerve can be spared. High-grade lesions should be treated aggressively to avoid recurrence. A total parotidectomy is performed, with facial nerve preservation if possible.[371] If there is any possibility that the tumor involves the facial nerve, the nerve is resected with the tumor. Immediate nerve reconstruction can be performed at the time of tumor extirpation. Neck dissections may be necessary for lymph node removal and staging in high-grade lesions. Postoperative radiation therapy is a useful adjunct in treating the high-grade tumor. Overall, 5-year (79%) and 10-year (65%) survival rates depend upon grade, stage, and margin status.[369] With high-grade lesions, recurrence with metastases can occur in up to 60% of patients. The survival rate for patients with low-grade lesions is about 95% at 5 years; for patients with high-grade lesions, this rate drops to approximately 40%.[371,372]

ADENOID CYSTIC CARCINOMA

Description. Adenoid cystic carcinomas account for approximately 6 to 10% of all salivary gland tumors and are the most common malignant tumors of the submandibular and minor salivary glands.[362,373] They comprise 15 to 30% of submandibular gland tumors, 30% of minor salivary gland tumors, and 2 to 15% of parotid gland tumors. Approximately 50% of all adenoid cystic carcinomas occur in the minor salivary glands. The tumor affects men and women equally and usually occurs in the fifth decade of life.[374] It is characterized by frequent late distant metastases and local recurrences, which account for low long-term survival rates.[373]

Clinical Presentation. Adenoid cystic carcinoma usually presents as a firm unilobular mass in the gland. Occasionally, the tumor is painful, and parotid tumors may cause facial nerve paralysis in a small number of patients. This tumor has a propensity for perineural invasion; thus, tumor tissue often can extend far beyond the obvious tumor margin. Unfortunately, the tumor's slow growth may delay diagnosis for several years, allowing perineural invasion to be advanced at the time of surgical removal. An intraoral adenoid cystic carcinoma may exhibit mucosal ulceration, a feature that helps distinguish it from a benign mixed tumor. Radiographically, the tumor reveals extension into adjacent bone. Metastases into the lung are more common than regional lymph node metastasis.

Pathology. On gross examination, the tumor is unilobular and either partially encapsulated or nonencapsulated. There is often evidence of invasion into adjacent normal tissue. Microscopic evidence of perineural or intraneural invasion is the distinguishing feature of adenoid cystic carcinoma. The individual cells are small and cuboidal. Nuclear atypia and mitotic figures are not seen, but chromatin aggregation is dense. Pseudocystic spaces filled with acellular material are a characteristic feature of this tumor. An update on cytologic criteria for diagnosis was published in 2005.[375]

Treatment. Because of the ability of this lesion to spread along the nerve sheaths, radical surgical excision of the lesion is the appropriate treatment. Even with aggressive surgical margins, tumor cells can remain, leading to long-term recurrence.[376] The site of origin appears to be an important factor in survival, with better survival in tumors originating from the parotid gland compared with minor salivary glands.[376] Frozen pathologic sections of the nerve sheath can help the surgeon achieve a clear margin. Postoperative radiotherapy and chemotherapy have not demonstrated consistent benefit beyond aggressive surgery alone. Patients are more likely to develop metastases rather than local recurrence when careful surgical extirpation has been conducted; therefore, they need to be observed indefinitely.[377] Factors affecting the long-term prognosis are the size of the primary lesion, its anatomic location, the presence of metastases at the time of surgery, and facial nerve involvement.[374,376]

ACINIC CELL CARCINOMA

Description. Acinic cell carcinoma represents about 1% of all salivary gland tumors. Between 90 and 95% of these tumors are found in the parotid gland; almost all of the remaining tumors are located in the submandibular gland. The distribution of acinic cell carcinoma reflects the location of acinar cells within the different glands. This tumor occurs with a higher frequency in women and is usually found in the fifth decade of life. It is the second most common malignant salivary gland tumor in children, second only to mucoepidermoid carcinoma.

Clinical Presentation. These lesions often present as slow-growing masses. Pain may be associated with the lesion but is not indicative of the prognosis. The superficial lobe and the inferior pole of the parotid gland are common sites of occurrence. Bilateral involvement of the parotid gland has been reported in approximately 3% of cases.

Pathology. The gross specimen is a well-defined mass that is often encapsulated. Microscopically, two types of cells are present; cells similar to acinar cells in the serous glands are seen adjacent to cells with a clear cytoplasm. These cells are positive on periodic acid–Schiff staining. Lymphocytic infiltration is often found.

Treatment. Acinic cell carcinomas initially undergo a relatively benign course.[378] Unfortunately, long-term survival is not as favorable, and the 20-year survival rate is about 50%. Treatment consists of superficial parotidectomy, with facial nerve preservation if possible. When these tumors are found in the submandibular gland, total gland removal is the treatment of choice.

CARCINOMA EX PLEOMORPHIC ADENOMA

Description. Carcinoma ex pleomorphic adenoma is a malignant tumor that arises within a preexisting pleomorphic adenoma. The malignant cells in this tumor are epithelial in origin. This tumor represents 2 to 5% of all salivary gland tumors.

Clinical Presentation. These tumors are slow growing and have usually been present for 15 to 20 years before they suddenly increase in size and become clinically apparent. Carcinoma ex pleomorphic adenoma occurs more often in pleomorphic adenomas that have been left untreated for long periods of time; for this reason, early removal of pleomorphic adenomas is recommended.

Pathology. Macroscopically, these tumors are nodular or cystic, without encapsulation. The sectioned tumor appears similar to pleomorphic adenoma except for the presence of necrosis and hemorrhage associated with the malignant tumor. Histologically, the tumor appears as a squamous cell carcinoma, adenocarcinoma, or undifferentiated carcinoma located within a benign mixed tumor. It may appear as a small focus of malignancy within the pleomorphic adenoma, or the malignant cells can almost completely replace the mixed tumor, making its appearance similar to that of a primary malignant tumor. Destructive infiltrative growth is usually seen around the malignancy.

Treatment. This is a malignant salivary gland tumor that has an aggressive course with a very poor prognosis. Local and distant metastases are common. Surgical removal with postoperative radiation therapy is the recommended treatment. Early removal of benign parotid gland tumors is recommended to avoid the development of this lesion.

ADENOCARCINOMA

Any tumors arising from salivary duct epithelium are, by definition, adenocarcinomas. This group of neoplasms has been divided into discrete entities based on structure and behavior. The term *adenocarcinoma* is often used as a catch-phrase to refer to lesions that do not meet the specific criteria for other lesions (such as polymorphous low-grade adeno-carcinoma, epimyoepithelial carcinoma, or salivary duct carcinoma). Clarification of the type of adenocarcinoma with a histologic description should be obtained in order to determine an appropriate treatment approach.

LYMPHOMA

Description. By definition, the term *primary lymphoma* describes a situation in which a salivary gland is the first clinical manifestation of the disease. Primary lymphoma of the salivary glands probably arises from lymph tissue within the glands. However, primary lymphoma of the salivary glands is rare.[379,380] The major forms of lymphoma are non-Hodgkin's lymphoma (NHL) and Hodgkin's disease. NHL is less curable and is often disseminated at diagnosis. There is an increased incidence of NHL in patients with autoimmune disease, including Sjögren's syndrome (see above). The parotid gland is the most commonly involved gland, followed by the submandibular gland.

Clinical Presentation. This lesion commonly presents as painless gland enlargement or adenopathy.

Pathology. Histologic examination demonstrates B-cell lymphoma tissue that originates from lymphoid tissue associated with malignant mucosa,[379] also referred to as lymphoma of MALT.[381] Since these lesions are not typically suspected, results from FNA are often misleading, and parotidectomy is required for a definitive diagnosis.[382]

Treatment. A staging workup is required to determine the treatment plan.[380] For isolated asymptomatic parotid gland masses, a superficial parotidectomy is recommended. An initial phase of observation is not uncommon for patients with asymptomatic low-grade disease. For early-stage primary NHL, radiotherapy alone resulted in overall survival of 90% at 5 years and 71% survival at 10 years.[383] Appropriate treatment includes radiation therapy, chemotherapy, or a combination of the two, depending on the staging of the lymphoma.[381,384,385]

MYOEPITHELIAL CARCINOMA

Description. Myoepithelial carcinoma or malignant myoepi-thelioma is a very rare malignant salivary gland neoplasm with good short-term survival and poor long-term survival.[386] Mean age is the sixth decade of life, with the parotid gland being the most common site.

Clinical Presentation. This is a rapidly growing tumor with extensive local growth, invasion of surrounding tissues, and infrequent cervical node metastasis but high rates of distant metastasis.[387]

Pathology. Due to their morphologic heterogeneity, these neoplasms can be confused easily with other tumors.[388] Aspirates of these neoplasms demonstrate primarily spindle cells,[389] whereas histopathology reveals infiltrative growth with a characteristic multinodular architecture with a cellular periphery and central necrotic/myxoid zones.[388] Necrosis is frequently present with perineural and vascular invasion.

Treatment. Early and aggressive surgery with close follow-up is required, whereas radiotherapy and neck dissection may not be necessary.[387]

▼ SELECTED READINGS

Baum BJ. Principles of saliva secretion. Ann N Y Acad Sci 1993;694:17–23.

Baur DA, Heston TF, Helman JI. Nuclear medicine in oral and max-illofacial diagnosis: a review for the practicing dental professional. J Contemp Dent Pract 2004;5:94–104.

Baurmash HD. Mucoceles and ranulas. J Oral Maxillofac Surg 2003;61:369–78.

Brennan MT, Shariff G, Lockhart PB, Fox PC. Treatment of xero-stomia: a systematic review of therapeutic trials. Dent Clin North Am 2002;46:847–56.

Chavez EM, Taylor GW, Borrell LN, Ship JA. Salivary function and glycemic control in older persons with diabetes. Oral Surg Oral Med Oral Pathol Oral Radiol Endod 2000;89:305–11.

Choo RE, Huestis MA. Oral fluid as a diagnostic tool. Clin Chem Lab Med 2004;42:1273–87.

Jensen SB, Pedersen AM, Reibel J, Nauntofte B. Xerostomia and hypofunction of the salivary glands in cancer therapy. Support Care Cancer 2003;11:207–25.

Kassan SS, Moutsopoulos HM. Clinical manifestations and early diagnosis of Sjogren syndrome. Arch Intern Med 2004;164: 1275–84.

Koukourakis MI, Danielidis V. Preventing radiation induced xerostomia. Cancer Treat Rev 2005;31:546–54.

Malamud D, Abrams WR, Bau H, et al. Oral-based techniques for the diagnosis of infectious diseases. J Calif Dent Assoc 2006;34:297–301.

Nahlieli O, Bar T, Shacham R, et al. Management of chronic recurrent parotitis: current therapy. J Oral Maxillofac Surg 2004;62:1150–5.

Navazesh M, Mulligan R, Barron Y, et al. A 4-year longitudinal evaluation of xerostomia and salivary gland hypofunction in the Women's Interagency HIV Study participants. Oral Surg Oral Med Oral Pathol Oral Radiol Endod 2003;95:693–8.

Pastore L, Fiore JR, Tateo M, et al. Detection of hepatitis C virus-RNA in saliva from chronically HCV-infected patients. Int J Immunopathol Pharmacol 2006;19:217–24.

Rabinov JD. Imaging of salivary gland pathology. Radiol Clin North Am 2000;38:1047–57, x–i.

Shah GV. MR imaging of salivary glands. Neuroimaging Clin N Am 2004;14:777–808.

Ship JA, Hu K. Radiotherapy-induced salivary dysfunction. Semin Oncol 2004;31(6 Suppl 18):29–36.

Ship JA. Xerostomia: aetiology, diagnosis, management and clinical implications. In: Edgar M, Dawes C, O'Mullane D, editors. Saliva and oral health. 3rd ed. London: British Dental Association; 2004. p. 50–70.

Sreebny LM, Schwartz SS. A reference guide to drugs and dry mouth—2nd edition. Gerodontology 1997;14:33–47.

Theander E, Henriksson G, Ljungberg O, et al. Lymphoma and other malignancies in primary Sjogren's syndrome: a cohort study on cancer incidence and lymphoma predictors. Ann Rheum Dis 2006;65:796–803.

Thomson WM, Chalmers JM, Spencer AJ, Slade GD. Medication and dry mouth: findings from a cohort study of older people. J Public Health Dent 2000;60:12–20.

Vissink A, Jansma J, Spijkervet FK, et al. Oral sequelae of head and neck radiotherapy. Crit Rev Oral Biol Med 2003;14:199–212.

Vitali C, Bombardieri S, Jonsson R, et al. Classification criteria for Sjogren's syndrome: a revised version of the European criteria proposed by the American-European Consensus Group. Ann Rheum Dis 2002;61:554–8.

Woo SB, Lee SJ, Schubert MM. Graft-vs.-host disease. Crit Rev Oral Biol Med 1997;8:201–16.

For the full reference list, please refer to the accompanying CD ROM.

9

TEMPOROMANDIBULAR DISORDERS

BRUCE BLASBERG, DMD, FRCD(C)
MARTIN S. GREENBERG, DDS

This chapter focuses on the assessment and management of disorders of the masticatory system. The masticatory apparatus is a specialized unit that performs multiple functions, including those of suckling, speaking, cutting and grinding food, and swallowing. The loss of these functions in association with pain is characteristic of masticatory system disorders and causes significant distress that can be severely disabling.

In the past, disorders of the masticatory system were generally treated as one condition or syndrome, with no attempt to differentiate subtypes of muscle and joint disorders. With increased understanding, the ability to identify different muscle or joint disorders has become possible; this should lead to a better understanding of the natural course, more accurate predictions of prognosis, and more effective treatments. The term *temporomandibular disorders* (TMDs) used in this chapter is a collective term embracing a number of clinical problems that involve the masticatory muscles, the temporomandibular joints (TMJs) and associated structures, or both.[1] These disorders are characterized by (1) facial pain in the region of the TMJs and/or muscles of mastication, (2) limitation or deviation in mandibular movements, and (3) TMJ sounds during jaw movement and function.[2]

The cause of most TMDs remains unknown, although numerous hypotheses have been proposed. The relationship of occlusal disharmony and TMD became a focus after Costen reported that a group of patients with multiple complaints associated with the jaws and ears improved after their occlusal-vertical dimension was altered.[3] The occlusal hypothesis was then expanded to include other occlusal discrepancies in addition to loss of vertical dimension.[4] During the 1950s and 1960s, a muscular cause not directly related to occlusion was proposed.[5–7] In the late 1970s, advances in diagnostic imaging resulted in a better understanding of intracapsular problems of the TMJ.[8,9] The lack of a clear understanding with regard to cause, the existence of multiple hypotheses, and strongly held beliefs by some clinicians have resulted in a wide spectrum of recommended treatments. The lack of standardized methods for assessment, classification, and treatment has diminished the value of the previous TMD literature. This chapter presents a general approach to the diagnostic assessment and nonsurgical management of the most common TMDs.

▼ FUNCTIONAL ANATOMY

Temporomandibular Joint

The TMJ articulation is a joint that is capable of hinge-type movements and gliding movements. The bony components are enclosed and connected by a fibrous capsule. The mandibular condyle forms the lower part of the bony joint and is generally elliptical, although variations in shape are common.[10] The articulation is formed by the mandibular condyle occupying a hollow in the temporal bone (the mandibular or glenoid fossa) (Figures 1 and 2). The S-shaped form of the fossa and eminence develops at about 6 years of

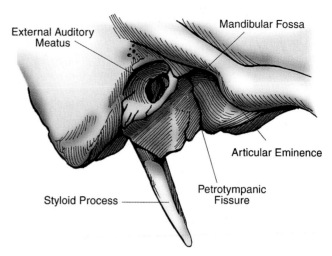

FIGURE 1   The S-shaped form of the fossa and eminence develops at about 6 years and continues into the second decade. The mandibular condyle occupies the space of the fossa, with enough room to both rotate and translate during mandibular movements.

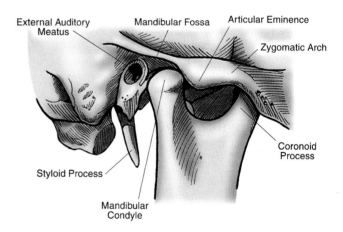

FIGURE 2   The articulation is formed by the mandibular condyle occupying a hollow in the temporal bone (the mandibular or glenoid fossa) during wide mouth opening; the condyle rotates around an axis and glides, causing it to move beyond the anterior border of the fossa, the articular eminence.

age and continues into the second decade.[11] During wide mouth opening, the condyle rotates around a hinge axis and glides, causing it to move beyond the anterior border of the fossa, identified as the articular eminence.[12] The TMJ has a rigid end point determined by tooth contact. Rotation of the condyle contributes more to normal mouth opening than translation.[13]

The capsule is lined with synovium and the joint cavity is filled with synovial fluid. The synovium is a vascular connective tissue lining the fibrous joint capsule and extending to the boundaries of the articulating surfaces. Both upper and lower joint cavities are lined with synovium. The synovial membrane consists of macrophage-like type A cells and fibroblast-like type B cells identical to those in other joints. The macrophage-like type A cells react with antimacrophage and macrophage-derived substances, including the major histocompatibility class II molecule, and show a drastic increase in their number in the inflamed synovial membrane.[14] Synovial fluid is a filtrate of plasma with added mucins and proteins. Its main constituent is hyaluronic acid. Fluid forms on the articulating surfaces and decreases friction during joint compression and motion.[15] Joint lubrication is achieved by mechanisms described as weeping lubrication and boundary lubrication. Weeping lubrication occurs as fluid is forced laterally during compression and expressed through the unloaded fibrocartilage.[16] As the adjacent areas become loaded, the weeping lubrication aids in reducing friction. Boundary lubrication is a function of water that is physically bound to the cartilaginous surface by a glycoprotein.[17]

Distinguishing features include a covering of fibrocartilage rather than hyaline cartilage on the articulating surfaces, and the mandible connecting the right and left joints. Fibrocartilage is less distensible than hyaline cartilage due to a greater number of collagen fibers. The matrix and chondrocytes are decreased because of the larger irregular bundles of collagen fibers. Fibrocartilage derives its nutrition from the diffusion of nutrients into the synovial fluid that then diffuse through the dense matrix to the chondrocytes.

Articular Disc

A fibrocartilage made up primarily of dense collagen of variable thickness and referred to as a disc occupies the space between the condyle and mandibular fossa (Figures 3 and 4).

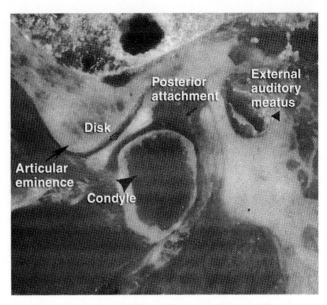

FIGURE 4 A cadaver section through the temporomandibular joint shows the relationship of the condyle, fossa, and articular disc.

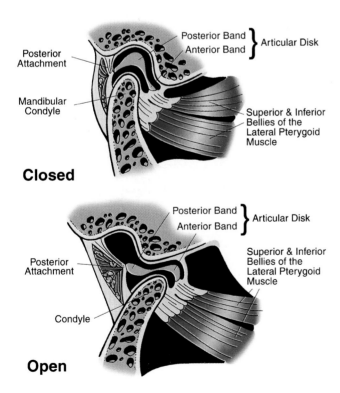

FIGURE 3 The temporomandibular joint is capable of hinge-type movements and gliding movements. The articular disc has ligamentous attachments to the mandibular fossa and condyle. The disc's attachments create separate superior and inferior joint compartments.

The disc consists of collagen fibers, cartilage-like proteoglycans,[18] and elastic fibers.[19] The disc contains a variable numbers of cells that resemble fibrocytes and fibrochondrocytes.[20] Collagen fibers in the center of the disc are oriented perpendicular to its transverse axis. The collagen fibers become interlaced as they approach the anterior and posterior bands, and many fibers are oriented parallel to the mediolateral aspect of the disc. Cartilage-like proteoglycans contribute to the compressive stiffness of articular cartilage.[21] The disc is attached by ligaments to the lateral and medial poles of the condyle. The ligaments consist of both collagen and elasti fibers.[22] These ligaments permit rotational movement of the disc on the condyle during mouth opening and closing. The disc is thinnest in its center and thickens to form anterior and posterior bands. This arrangement is considered to help stabilize the condyle in the glenoid fossa. The disc is primarily avascular and has little sensory nerve penetration.

The disc provides an interface for the condyle as it glides across the temporal bone. The disc and its attachments divide the joint into upper and lower compartments that normally do not communicate. The passive volume of the upper compartment is estimated to be 1.2 mL and that of the lower compartment is estimated to be 0.9 mL.[22] The roof of the superior compartment is the mandibular fossa, whereas the floor is the superior surface of the disc. The roof of the inferior compartment is the inferior surface of the disc and the floor is the articulating surface of the mandibular condyle.[22] At its margins, the disc blends with the fibrous capsule. Muscle attachments inserting into the anterior aspect of the disc have been observed.[23] Fibers of the posterior one-third of the temporalis muscle and deep masseter muscle may attach on the anterolateral aspect.[23] Fibers of the superior head of the lateral pterygoid have been observed to insert into the anteromedial two-thirds of the disc.[23]

Retrodiscal Tissue

A mass of soft tissue occupies the space behind the disc and condyle. It is often referred to as the posterior attachment. The posterior attachment is a loosely organized system of collagen fibers, branching elastic fibers, fat, blood and lymph vessels, and nerves. Synovium covers the superior and inferior surfaces. The attachment has been described as being arranged in two lamina of dense connective tissue,[24] but this has been challenged.[25] Between the lamina, a loose areolar, highly vascular, and well-innervated tissue has been described. The superior lamina arises from the posterior band of the disc and attaches to the squamotympanic fissure and tympanic part of the temporal bone. The superior lamina consists primarily of elastin.[24,26] The inferior lamina arises from the posterior band of the disc and inserts into the inferior margin of the posterior articular slope of the condyle and is composed mostly of collagen fibers.[24]

Temporomandibular Ligaments

CAPSULAR LIGAMENT

The capsular ligament is a thin inelastic fibrous connective tissue envelope that attaches to the margins of the articular surfaces (Figure 5). The fibers are oriented vertically and do not restrain joint movements. The medial capsule is composed of loose areolar connective tissue.[25] The capsule and the lateral discal ligament join and attach to the lateral aspect of the neck of the condyle.[27]

LATERAL TEMPOROMANDIBULAR LIGAMENT

The lateral temporomandibular ligament is the main ligament of the joint, lateral to the capsule but not easily separated from it by dissection. Its fibers pass obliquely from bone lateral to the articular tubercle in a posterior and inferior direction and insert in a narrower area below and behind the lateral pole of the condyle (see Figure 5). In earlier literature, this ligament was identified as an oblique band from the condylar neck to the anterosuperior region on the eminence and as a horizontal band from the lateral condylar pole to an anterior attachment of the eminence.[22] A recent study was unable to confirm a distinct structure separate from the capsule.[27]

ACCESSORY LIGAMENTS

The sphenomandibular ligament arises from the sphenoid bone and inserts on the medial aspect of the mandible at the lingula. It is not considered to limit or affect mandibular movement. The stylomandibular ligament extends from the styloid process to the deep fascia of the medial pterygoid muscle. It is thought to become tense during protrusive movement of the mandible and may contribute to limiting protrusive movement.

Muscles of Mastication

The muscles of mastication are the paired masseter, medial and lateral pterygoid, and temporalis muscles (Figures 6 to 8). Mandibular movements toward the tooth contact position are performed by contraction of the masseter, temporalis, and medial pterygoid muscles. Masseter contraction contributes to moving the condylar head toward the anterior slope of the mandibular fossa. The posterior part of the temporalis contributes to mandibular retrusion. Unilateral

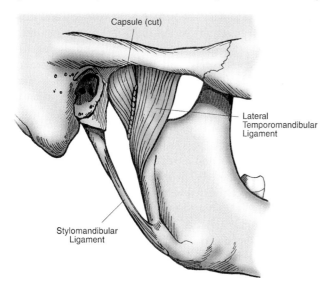

FIGURE 5 The capsular ligament is a thin, inelastic, fibrous connective tissue envelope, oriented vertically, that attaches to the margins of the articular surfaces. The capsular ligament does not restrain condylar movements. The temporomandibular ligament is lateral to the capsule but is not easily separated from it by dissection. Its fibers pass obliquely from bone lateral to the articular tubercle in a posterior and inferior direction to insert in a narrower area below and behind the lateral pole of the condyle.

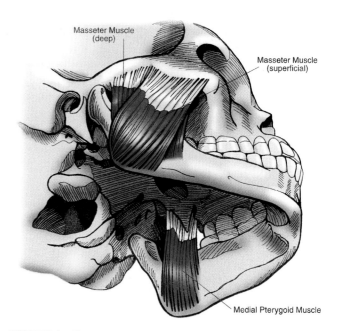

FIGURE 6 The masseter and medial pterygoid muscles have their insertions at the inferior border of the mandibular angle. They join together to form a sling that cradles the ramus of the mandible and produces the powerful forces required for chewing. The masseter muscle has been divided into a deep portion and a superficial portion.

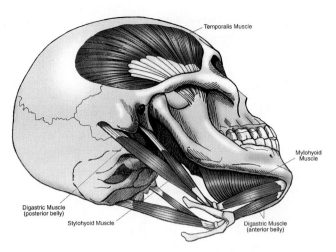

FIGURE 7 The digastric muscle is a paired muscle with two bellies. The anterior belly attaches to the lingual aspect of the mandible at the parasymphysis and courses backward to insert into a round tendon attached to the hyoid bone. Contraction produces a depression and retropositioning of the mandible. The mylohyoid and geniohyoid muscles contribute to depressing the mandible when the infrahyoid muscles stabilize the hyoid bone during mandibular movement. These muscles may also contribute to retrusion of the mandible. The temporalis muscle is broadly attached to the lateral skull. The muscle fibers converge to insert on the coronoid process and anterior aspect of the mandibular ramus. The posterior part traverses anteriorly and then curves around the anterior root of the zygomatic process before insertion. The posterior part of the temporalis contributes to mandibular retrusion.

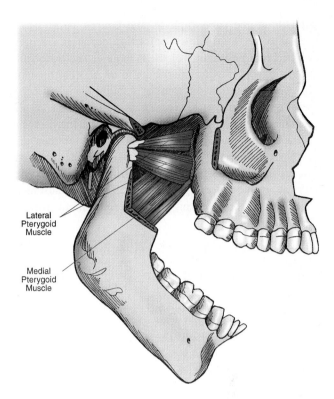

FIGURE 8 The lateral pterygoid muscle is the main protrusive and opening muscle of the mandible. It is arranged in parallel-fibered units that allow for greater displacement and velocity than that of the multipennated closing muscles. The lateral pterygoid muscle is divided into two parts. The inferior part arises from the outer surface of the lateral pterygoid plate of the sphenoid and the pyramidal process of the palatine bone. The superior part originates from the greater wing of the sphenoid and the pterygoid ridge. The fibers of the upper and lower heads course posteriorly and laterally, fusing in front of the temporomandibular joint. They insert into the anteromedial aspect of the condylar neck. Some of the fibers insert into the most anterior medial portion of the disc, but most of the lateral pterygoid fibers insert into the condyle. Translation of the condylar head onto the articular eminence is produced by contraction of the lateral pterygoid.

contraction of the medial pterygoid contributes to a contralateral movement of the mandible. The masseter and medial pterygoid muscles have their insertions at the inferior border of the mandibular angle. They join together to form a sling that cradles the mandible and produces the powerful forces required for chewing. The masseter is divided into deep and superficial parts.

The temporalis muscle is broadly attached to the lateral skull and has been divided into anterior, middle, and posterior parts. The muscle fibers converge into a tendon that inserts on the coronoid process and anterior aspect of the mandibular ramus. The anterior and middle fibers are generally oriented in a straight line from their origin on the skull to their insertion on the mandible. The posterior part traverses anteriorly and then curves around the anterior root of the zygomatic process before insertion.

The lateral pterygoid is the main protrusive and opening muscle of the mandible. The inferior head is the main section responsible for lateral jaw movements when the teeth are in contact.[28] The lateral pterygoid is arranged in parallel-fibered units, whereas the other muscles are multipennated. This arrangement allows greater displacement and velocity in the lateral pterygoid and greater force generation in the elevator muscles.[29]

The lateral pterygoid muscle arises from two heads. The inferior head arises from the outer surface of the lateral pterygoid plate of the sphenoid and the pyramidal process of

the palatine bones. The superior head originates from the greater wing of the sphenoid and the pterygoid ridge. The fibers of the upper and lower heads course posteriorly and laterally, fusing in front of the condyle.[30] They insert into the anteromedial aspect of the condylar neck. Some of the fibers insert into the most anterior medial portion of the disk, but most of the lateral pterygoid fibers insert into the condyle.[30] The superior part of the insertion consists of an identifiable tendon inserting through fibrocartilage. The inferior part of the insertion consists of muscle attached to periosteum.[31] Debate continues about the functional anatomy of the lateral pterygoid. The superior head is thought to be active during closing movements, and the inferior head is thought to be active during opening and protrusive movements.[32–34] Translation of the condylar head onto the articular eminence is produced by contraction of the lateral pterygoid.

The digastric muscle is a paired muscle with two bellies. The anterior belly attaches to the lingual aspect of the mandible at the parasymphysis and courses backward to insert into the hyoid bone. Contraction produces a depression and retropositioning of the mandible. The mylohyoid and geniohyoid muscles contribute to depressing the mandible when the infrahyoid muscles stabilize the hyoid bone. These muscles may also contribute to retrusion of the mandible. The buccinator attaches inferiorly along the facial surface of the mandible behind the mental foramen and superiorly high on the alveolar surface behind the zygomatic process. The fibers are arranged horizontally. Anteriorly, fibers insert into mucosa, skin, and lip. The buccinator helps position the cheek during chewing movements of the mandible.

Vascular Supply of Temporomandibular Structures

The external carotid artery is the main blood supply for the temporomandibular structures. The artery leaves the neck and courses superiorly and posteriorly embedded in the substance of the parotid gland. The artery sends two important branches, the lingual and facial arteries, to the region. At the level of the condylar neck, the external carotid bifurcates into the superficial temporal artery and the internal maxillary artery. These two arteries supply the muscles of mastication and the TMJ. Arteries within the temporal bone and mandible also send branches to the capsule.

Nerve Supply of Temporomandibular Structures

The masticatory structures are innervated primarily by the trigeminal nerve, but cranial nerves VII, IX, X, and XI and cervical nerves 2 and 3 also contribute. The peripheral nerves synapse with nuclei in the brainstem that are associated with touch, proprioception, and motor function. The large spinal trigeminal nucleus occupies a major part of the brainstem and extends to the spinal cord. The spinal trigeminal nucleus is thought to be the main site for the reception of impulses from the periphery involved in pain sensation. The mandibular division of the trigeminal nerve supplies motor innervation to the muscles of mastication and the anterior belly of the digastric muscle. Branches of the auriculotemporal nerve supply the sensory innervation of the TMJ; this nerve arises from the mandibular division in the infratemporal fossa and sends branches to the capsule of the joint (Figure 9). The deep temporal and masseteric nerves supply the anterior portion of the joint. The auriculotemporal nerve, a branch of the mandibular portion (V3) of the trigeminal nerve, provides innervation of the TMJ. About 75% of the time, the masseteric nerve, a branch of the maxillary division of the trigeminal nerve (V2), innervates the anteromedial capsule of the TMJ. In about 33%, a separate branch from V2 comes through the mandibular notch and innervates the anteromedial capsule.[35] These nerves are primarily motor nerves, but they contain sensory fibers distributed to the anterior part of the TMJ capsule. The autonomic nerve supply is carried to the joint by the auriculotemporal nerve and by nerves traveling along the superficial temporal artery.

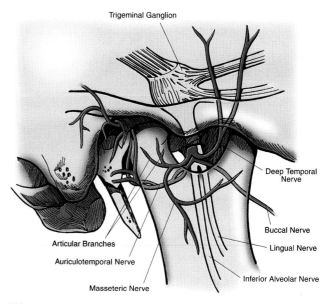

FIGURE 9 Branches of the auriculotemporal nerve supply sensory innervation of the TMJ. This nerve arises from the mandibular division in the infratemporal fossa and sends branches to the capsule of the joint.

▼ ANATOMY OF CLINICAL INTEREST

Jaw Jerk Reflex

The jaw jerk reflex is analogous to the knee jerk reflex. It is a stretch reflex that occurs by applying a downward tap on the chin. The tap produces a reflex contraction. It demonstrates the existence of a feedback loop from the jaw-closing muscles to their own motor neurons in the central nervous system. This reflex is thought to relate to the fine control of jaw movements to take into account different consistencies of food.[36] Neurosensory testing for examination, diagnosis, and classification of orofacial pain disorders has received attention in the research community, but measuring the jaw jerk reflex has not yet become a valuable clinical test.[37]

Jaw-Opening Reflex

Stimulating mechanoreceptors or nociceptors in the mouth triggers the jaw-opening reflex. The pathway is polysynaptic; the first synapse is in either the trigeminal sensory nuclei or the adjacent reticular formation and the final synapse is in the trigeminal motor nucleus. The reflex results in an inhibition of the activity of the jaw-closing muscles. This reflex is thought to help prevent injury when biting or chewing objects that may cause damage.[36]

The jaw-opening reflex has been used to study lingual nerve injuries. Differences in the reflex were found when stimulating tongue mucosa on the injured side, but the difference was not helpful in predicting recovery.[38]

Rest Position

When the mandible is not functionally active, it adopts a rest position in which the condyle occupies a relatively central position in the glenoid fossa with the teeth separated. The rest position is considered to be associated with minimum muscular activity, with the lower teeth a few millimeters from the occlusal contact position.[39] This position varies for a number of reasons (including head posture and levels of muscle activity) and is not an exact position.[40]

Centric Relation

Centric relation is a position that has traditionally relied on guiding the condyles into a position to rotate around a stationary axis in the mandibular fossa. The definition stated in the "The Glossary of Prosthodontic Terms" is "the maxillomandibular relationship in which each condyle articulates with the thinnest avascular portion of the disc in an anterosuperior position against the posterior slope of the articular eminence."[41] This position can be reproduced and transferred to an articulator. Adjusting the maximum intercuspal position to be coincident with centric relation is recommended by some clinicians to treat TMDs. The evidence for this as a standard treatment is lacking.[42]

Range of Mandibular Movement

Mandibular motion is composed of translation and rotation of the condyles. During translation, the disc and condyle move downward and forward along the posterior slope of the articular eminence. Gallo and colleagues calculated the average rotation of the condyle to be 24° and the condylar translation to be between 13 and 15 mm for maximum opening.[43] The articular disc translates with the condyle, but its movement is limited to a range of 5 to 9 mm.[44] At maximum mouth opening, the condyle moves to the crest of the articular eminence or beyond. A wide variation in mandibular movement exists. Incisor displacement remains the most common diagnostic indicator.[45] The temporomandibular, sphenomandibular, and stylomandibular ligaments, together with the articular eminence, have been suggested as the main constraints of jaw opening.[46] Muscular constraint of jaw opening has also been proposed as a significant contributing factor.[47]

Articular Covering

The fibrocartilage found on the articulating surfaces of the TMJ is thought to provide more surface strength against forces in many directions while allowing more freedom of movement than would be possible with hyaline cartilage. Fibrocartilage also forms the articular disc. This covering is thickest on the posterior slope of the articular eminence and on the anterior slope of the condylar head; these are the areas thought to receive the greatest functional load. The thinnest part of the fibrocartilage covering is on the roof of the mandibular fossa. Fibrocartilage has a greater repair capacity than hyaline cartilage. This may affect how the TMJ responds to degenerative changes.[48]

Disc Displacements

Demonstration of the lateral pterygoid's attachment to the anterior articular disc has led to the theory that some anterior disc displacements may be related to lateral pterygoid muscle dysfunction. The theory suggests that hyperactivity of the superior head of the lateral pterygoid is capable of pulling the disc forward from its normal position over the mandibular condyle.[49] Research on cadaver specimens has indicated that muscle fibers inserting into the disc or the condyle are not differentiated into inferior and superior heads.[30,50] The fibers that do insert into the disc are located primarily at the medial portion. Carpentier and colleagues postulated that the two heads did not have distinct independent actions and that the lateral pterygoid was not a significant cause of disc displacement.[30] Clicking has been reported as the most common TMJ irregularity detected during clinical examination and may occur as an isolated finding.[51] An estimated one-third of asymptomatic volunteers on magnetic resonance imaging (MRI) examination of the TMJs had disc displacements.[52]

The angle or steepness of the mandibular fossa has been considered a contributing factor in intra-articular disorders. The steep, vertical form of the fossa has been associated with articular disc displacements (ADDs) in some published reports and not substantiated in others. Osseous changes in response to the disc displacement have been found suggesting that the steepness of the eminence may be a consequence of disc displacement rather than a cause.[53] Chronic subluxation or dislocation of the condyle has been related to the form and steepness of the fossa. Surgical treatments that increase the steepness or flatten the eminence have been recommended.

Nitzan and Etsion proposed that adhesion of the disc in the fossa might cause closed lock.[54] Adhesion occurs when hyaluronic acid and associated phospholipids are degraded. Support for this hypothesis is the improvement of mouth opening after arthrocentesis.[54]

The inferior lamina of the posterior attachment is considered to be the primary restraint preventing the disc from moving forward. Injury to this ligament has been proposed as the cause of disc displacements.[55]

Joint Noises

ADDs are thought to be the most common cause of joint noises, specifically clicking. Clicking can occur in individuals who have a normal disc position on MRI.[56] Other explanations for TMJ clicking include condylar hypermobility, enlargement of the lateral pole of the condyle, structural irregularity of the articular eminence, and loose intra-articular bodies other than the disc.[57]

Nerve Entrapment

Compression of nerves due to decreased occlusal vertical dimension and variations in their course close to the mandibular condyle was an early hypothesis proposed by Costen to explain TMD pain.[3] Close proximity of the auriculotemporal nerve to the medial aspect of the condyle has been described. Medial displacement of the articular disc exposing the auriculotemporal nerve to mechanical irritation has been described as a possible cause.[58] Anatomic study of the condyle and its relationship to the auriculotemporal nerve make this an unlikely cause of TMDs.[59]

Occlusion

The intercuspal position is achieved when maximum intercuspation of opposing teeth occurs.[44] Occlusal stability has been defined as "the equalization of contacts that prevents tooth movement after closure."[60] A physiologic occlusion has been defined as "an occlusion in which a functional equilibrium or state of homeostasis exists between all tissues of the masticatory system."[61] There is general agreement that occlusal forces at the intercuspal position are best directed toward the long axes of teeth.[62,63] A reduced number of contacting teeth in the intercuspal position and loss of posterior teeth have been reported as risk factors for the development of TMDs.[64] The research literature to evaluate occlusal treatment for TMD is limited.[65] Studies examining occlusal characteristics and TMD symptoms have failed to identify a strong association.[66] The loss of occlusal vertical dimension has been considered a cause of TMD, but the evidence for this is lacking.[67]

Ear Symptoms Associated with TMDs

Earache, tinnitus, fullness, and loss of hearing are complaints that occur in patients with TMD.[68,69] A ligament connecting the disc and the malleus has been observed in anatomic specimens.[70] The superior retrodiscal lamina has been considered to be a remnant of the ligament connecting the lateral pterygoid tendon to the malleus through the squamotympanic fissure in the fetus.[71] This anatomic finding has been used to explain the prevalence of auditory symptoms in TMDs, but research has not established that this is a functioning ligament between the TMJ and the middle ear.[72,73] Pressure on the anterior tympanic artery that enters the petrotympanic fissure in the mandibular fossa is an alternative hypothesis. The most common disorders associated with ear pain unrelated to ear disease were cervical spine disorders, TMDs or both.[74]

Injection Sites

Injections to anesthetize sensory innervation of the joint may be a part of the diagnostic assessment or injecting medication such as corticosteroids may be part of therapy. The site of injection should be anterior to the tragus to minimize the risk of intravascular injection of the external carotid artery or the accompanying vein. Because the auriculotemporal nerve enters the capsule from the medial aspect, injections (normally given from the lateral aspect) may not completely anesthetize the joint.[75] Fernandes and colleagues found the auriculotemporal nerve to be between 10 and 13 mm inferior to the superior surface of the condyle and 1 and 2 mm posterior to the neck of the condyle.[59]

Muscle Palpation

Intraoral palpation of the lateral pterygoid muscle has been challenged because of its location and inaccessibility (Figure 10).[76] The examination procedure is likely to cause discomfort in individuals without a TMD, diminishing the value of lateral pterygoid palpation as a diagnostic test.[77] The

fibers of the deep masseter muscle are intimately related to the lateral wall of the joint capsule. This makes differentiating muscle and joint pain in this area difficult.[78,79]

Jaw Jerk Reflex and the Silent Period

Masseter and temporalis muscles exhibit suppressed periods of electromyographic (EMG) activity when subjected to mechanical stimuli or electric shocks.[80] A prolonged period of electrical inactivity on EMG recordings has been observed in TMD patients,[81] but this "silent period" has not been established as a valuable test for the diagnosis of TMDs.

▼ ETIOLOGY, EPIDEMIOLOGY, AND CLASSIFICATION

Etiology

The etiology of the most common TMDs is unknown. Two hypotheses, occlusal disharmony and psychological distress, have dominated the literature, but clear and convincing evidence for either being the primary etiology does not exist.[50] Research studying discrepancies between centric relation and centric occlusion, nonworking side occlusal interferences, and Angle's occlusal classification has not established a strong association in patients with myofascial pain compared with controls.[82–85] Significant differences in occlusion are not found between patients with myofascial pain compared with control subjects, although in some cases, an occlusal problem might be an initiating factor.[86] Overjet and overbite were not found to be predictors of joint clicking, crepitus, pain, or limited opening.[87,88]

A relationship between tooth loss and osteoarthrosis has been found in studies of patients with TMDs[89] but not in nonpatient populations.[90] No difference between a symptomatic and control population was found when attempting to correlate incisal relationships, condylar position, and joint sounds.[91] An observed relationship between severe overbite and TMD symptoms has been reported but has not been consistently observed.[92,93]

Malocclusion, for example, anterior open bite, may be the result of anatomic changes in the TMJs due to inflammation and degenerative changes associated with rheumatoid arthritis (RA).[94] Masseter pain induced by saline injections caused a shift in the apex point of the gothic arch, suggesting that pain might be a factor in producing the occlusal changes that are sometimes reported by patients with TMDs.[95]

Masticatory muscle hyperactivity progressing to a "vicious cycle" has been proposed as the cause of myofascial pain. The diagnostic terms *myospasm*, *muscle spasm*, and *reflex splinting* have been used to describe this condition. The link between muscle hyperactivity and masticatory muscle pain has not been established.[96–100] No difference has been found between resting EMG activity in painful jaw-closing muscles and nonpainful muscles.[101] Tooth attrition signaling dental wear due to bruxing has not been associated with TMJ pain or clicking or tenderness of masticatory muscles.[102] Experimental

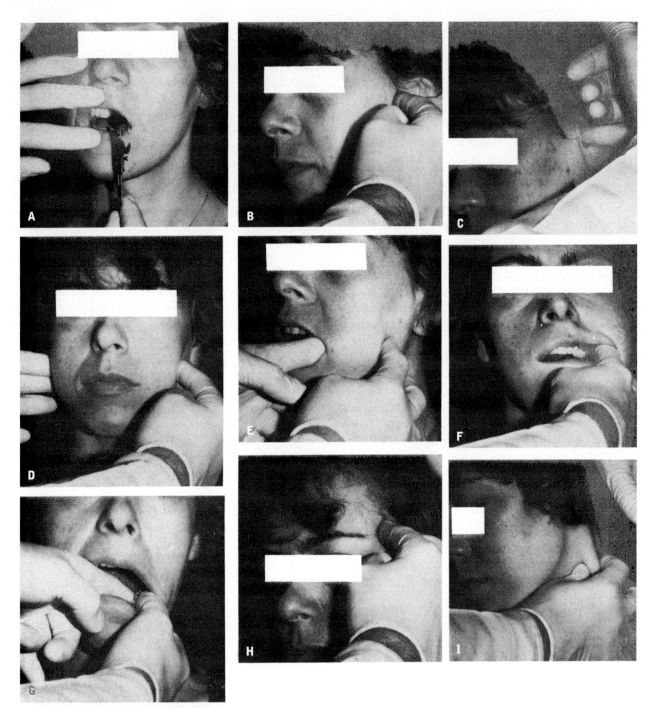

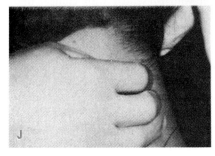

FIGURE 10   The clinical examination. *A*, Measuring maximum interincisal opening. *B*, Palpation of the pretragus area; the lateral aspect of the temporomandibular joint (TMJ). *C*, Intra-auricular palpation; the posterior aspect of the TMJ. *D*, Palpation of the masseter muscles. *E*, Bimanual palpation of the masseter muscle. *F*, Palpation of the lateral pterygoid muscle. *G*, Palpation of the medial pterygoid muscle. *H*, Palpation of the temporalis muscle. *I*, Palpation of the sternocleidomastoid muscle. *J*, Palpation of the trapezius muscle. Note that the lateral and medial pterygoid muscle palpations are from an intraoral approach. Access to these muscles is limited, and the procedure may produce an unacceptable rate of false-positive results (pain on palpation). The results of lateral and medial pterygoid palpation should be interpreted with caution.

evidence suggests that tooth clenching might be a source of pain in some individuals.[103] Positive findings on muscle examination were more frequent in individuals who perform tooth-clenching activities.[104]

The Pain-Adaptation Model has been proposed as an alternative to the "vicious cycle" hypothesis. This model is based on observations that EMG activity and force output of the muscle are lower in patients with musculoskeletal pain.[105] The reduction in muscle activity in this model is thought to be protective to prevent further injury.

The results of a number of experimental studies of myofascial pain are consistent with the hypothesis that the pain is caused by altered central nervous system processing.[106–110] The debate continues as to whether these findings are a consequence of the pain rather than the cause of the pain.

The psychological hypothesis proposes that TMDs evolve as a consequence of psychological distress, usually due to the individual's stressful environment. The psychological distress leads to parafunctional activities (tooth clenching and grinding) that result in muscle pain.[111–113] A challenge that is continually faced in chronic pain disorders is determining how much of the psychological distress is a cause or a consequence of chronic pain.[114] The weight of the evidence suggests that in most cases, the emotional distress is more likely a consequence than a cause of pain.[115]

The lack of a clear single cause of TMDs has resulted in the proposal of a multifactorial etiology.[112] Multiple factors come together contributing to the initiation, aggravation, and/or perpetuation of the disorder. The factors proposed are

1. Parafunctional habits (eg, nocturnal bruxing, tooth clenching, lip or cheek biting)[116–118]
2. Emotional distress[119,120]
3. Acute trauma to the jaw[121,122]
4. Trauma from hyperextension (eg, dental procedures, oral intubations for general anesthesia, yawning, hyperextension associated with cervical trauma)[122,123]
5. Instability of maxillomandibular relationships[124]
6. Laxity of the joint[125,126]
7. Comorbidity of other rheumatic or musculoskeletal disorders[127]
8. Poor general health and an unhealthy lifestyle[128]

The frequency and the importance of these factors as causes are unknown.

Myofascial pain with arthralgia and myofascial pain alone were associated with trauma, clenching, third molar removal, somatization, and female gender.[129] Generalized joint hypermobility has been proposed as a cause of TMDs, but a systematic review found few studies that met the authors' criteria, and the results are not clear.[130] A number of studies have been performed to investigate a possible relationship between orthodontic treatment and the development of TMD, but the results do not support a causal relationship.[131–133]

Epidemiology

Between 65 and 85% of people in the United States experience one or more symptoms of TMD during their lives.[134] Approximately 12% experience prolonged pain or disability that results in chronic symptoms.[134] Although the prevalence of one or more signs of mandibular pain and dysfunction is high in the population, only about 5 to 7% have symptoms severe enough to require treatment.[83,134,135] TMD patients are similar to headache and back pain patients with respect to disability, psychosocial profile, pain intensity, chronicity, and frequency.[136,137] The lower prevalence of TMD signs and symptoms in older age groups supports the probability that a significant portion of TMDs are self-limiting. The natural course of TMDs is still unclear, but there is some evidence to suggest that the course might be different in men and women.[138]

Available evidence indicates that TMDs are most prevalent between the ages of 20 and 40 years and more frequently affect women. The reason why women make up the majority of patients presenting for treatment is still unclear. In a community-based study, a greater likelihood of developing TMD was associated with oral contraceptives and estrogen replacement in women over 40 years of age.[139] Asian, Swedish, and American populations with TMDs shared similar characteristics.[140]

Signs and symptoms of masticatory muscle and TMJ dysfunction are commonly observed in children.[141–143] A study of individuals in Sweden between the ages of 12 and 19 years reported that 4.2% reported TMD pain.[144] Girls reported TMD pain more frequently than boys, 6% compared with 2.7%.[144] Belfer and Kaban reported on a group of 40 children, aged 10 to 16 years, presenting with signs and symptoms of TMD. Fourteen (35%) were diagnosed as having acute reactive depression.[145] In another study, arthrography and computed tomography (CT) were performed on 31 children complaining of TMJ pain and dysfunction.[146] Twelve were diagnosed with disc displacement with reduction, and 17 were found to have disc displacement without reduction. In 12 of the 29 patients with internal derangement, the problem was thought to be due to a previous injury. In a survey of 1,000 12-year-old children, 1% had a maximum mouth opening of less than 40 mm. It was only a small number of children who presented with clinical findings severe enough to warrant treatment.[147]

Classification

Due to the uncertainty about etiology, current diagnostic classifications of TMD are based on signs and symptoms. Earlier classifications characterized disorders as intracapsular (TMJ) or extracapsular (muscle) disorders and were often not versatile enough to allow for multiple diagnoses of masticatory muscle and TMJ abnormalities. More recent classifications allow for more than one diagnosis, and this better reflects the clinical reality.[148,149] Arthrography has provided evidence resulting in more accurate descriptions of intracapsular disorders in relation to presenting clinical features.[97,150]

TABLE 1 Classification for Diagnosing Temporomandibular Disorders

Diagnostic Category	Diagnoses
Muscle and facial disorders	Myalgia; muscle contracture; splinting; hypertrophy; spasm; dyskinesia; forceful jaw closure habit; myositis (bruxism)
TMJ disorders	Disc condyle incoordination; osteoarthritis; disc condyle restriction; inflammatory polyarthritis; open dislocation; traumatic articular disease; arthralgia
Disorder of mandibular mobility	Ankylosis; adhesions (intracapsular); fibrosis of muscular tissue; coronoid elongation-hypermobility of TMJ
Disorders of maxillomandibular growth	Masticatory muscle hypertrophy/atrophy; neoplasia (muscle, maxillomandibular or condylar); maxillomandibular or condylar hypoplasia/hyperplasia

Adapted from Clark GT et al.[151]
TMJ = temporomandibular joint.

Disc disorders are now differentiated on the basis of MRI findings.

In 1989, Clark and colleagues published a classification system that is useful to the practicing clinician (Table 1).[105,151]

The American Academy of Orofacial Pain (AAOP) has published a general classification of disorders that affect the cranial bones, TMJs, and masticatory muscles (Table 2).[152] This classification system is useful because it attempts to define the diagnostic terms and provide diagnostic criteria. This classification has not been subjected to testing for validity. It represents an attempt by experts to apply available knowledge to the development of an acceptable and useful system for clinical practice. Table 3 provides a partial list of the diagnostic terms and their diagnostic criteria. This classification does provide the clinician with an aid in clinical decision-making. Clinical findings accompanying the diagnosis are listed in the latest AAOP publication on orofacial pain guidelines.[1] Supporting signs in disc disorders that may have additional clinical value are listed in Table 3 as "clinical findings that may support the diagnosis."

Interpretation of the TMD literature and advances in knowledge have been impeded by the lack of accepted methods or standards for selecting or describing patients who take part in clinical research. Dworkin and Le Resche developed a classification for the most common TMDs to provide a system for clinical research. The Research Diagnostic Criteria for Temporomandibular Disorders (RDC/TMD) were published as a system "offered to allow standardization and replication of research into the most common forms of muscle and joint-related TMD."[45] The classification scheme is intended to provide a means for standardizing data collection and comparing data between clinical investigators. Because of the chronicity of TMDs, a classification system that reflects psychological, behavioral, and social issues is as important as an accurate description of the physical pathology. The RDC/TMD classification has a separate axis to assess psychosocial status to create profiles of disability, depression, anxiety, and preoccupation with other physical symptoms. The RDC/TMD classification is presently being used in a multicenter study for validation.

TABLE 2 Diagnostic Classification of Temporomandibular Disorders

Diagnostic Category	Diagnoses
Cranial bones (including the mandible)	Congenital and developmental disorders: aplasia, hypoplasia, hyperplasia, dysplasia (eg, first and second branchial arch anomalies, hemifacial microsomia, Pierre Robin syndrome, Treacher Collins syndrome, condylar hyperplasia, prognathism, fibrous dysplasia) Acquired disorders (neoplasia, fracture)
Temporomandibular joint disorders	Deviation in form Disc displacement (with reduction; without reduction) Dislocation Inflammatory conditions (synovitis, capsulitis) Arthritides (osteoarthritis, osteoarthrosis, polyarthritides) Ankylosis (fibrous, bony) Neoplasia
Masticatory muscle disorders	Myofascial pain Myositis spasm Protective splinting Contracture

Adapted from McNeill C.[127]

The classifications published by Clark and the AAOP were designed for clinical practice and are more comprehensive. The RDC/TMD classification was developed for research purposes but is useful in clinical practice for the types of TMD most likely to present to a dentist. The classification does not include the less common conditions. Muscle conditions (such as myositis, contracture, and myospasm) and TMJ conditions involved in rheumatic disease, acute trauma, hyperplasia, and neoplasia are not part of the defined conditions.

The RDC/TMD system allows for multiple TMD diagnoses for each individual but only one muscle diagnosis and for each joint one disc disorder and one articular bone diagnosis. The terms used are clearly defined, and the criteria required to meet the diagnosis are detailed, although the validation of these criteria and the classification system will

TABLE 3   Diagnostic Terms and Clinical Criteria for Temporomandibular Disorders

Diagnostic Terms	Clinical Criteria
Deviation in form (painless mechanical dysfunction or altered function due to irregularities or aberrations in the form of intracapsular soft and hard articular tissues)	Complaint of faulty or compromised joint mechanics Reproducible joint noise, usually at the same position during opening and closing Radiographic evidence of structural bony abnormality or loss of normal shape
Disc displacement with reduction (abrupt alteration or interference of the disc-condyle structural relationship during mandibular translation with mouth opening and closing; from a closed-mouth position, the "temporarily" misaligned disc reduces or improves its structural relationship with the condyle when mandibular translation occurs with mouth opening, which produces joint noise described as clicking or popping)	Pain (when present) is precipitated by joint movement Reproducible joint noise, usually at variable positions during opening and closing mandibular movements Soft tissue imaging reveals displaced disc that improves its position during jaw opening. Clinical findings that may support the diagnosis: pain (when present) precipitated by joint movement; deviation during movement coinciding with a click; no restriction in mandibular movement (episodic and momentary catching of smooth jaw movements during mouth opening [< 35 mm] that self-reduces with voluntary mandibular repositioning)
Disc displacement without reduction (altered or misaligned disc-condyle structural relationship that is maintained during mandibular translation)	Pain precipitated by function Marked limited mandibular opening Uncorrected deviation to the affected side on opening Marked limited laterotrusion to the contralateral side Soft tissue imaging reveals displaced disc without reduction. Clinical findings that may support the diagnosis: pain precipitated by forced mouth opening; history of clicking that ceases with the locking; pain with palpation of the affected joint; ipsilateral hyperocclusion
Synovitis or capsulitis (inflammation of the synovial lining or loading of capsular lining) T2-weighted MRI may show joint fluid	Localized pain at rest exacerbated by function, especially with superior and posterior joint Limited range of motion secondary to pain
Osteoarthrosis (degenerative noninflammatory condition of the joint, characterized by structural changes of joint surfaces secondary to excessive strain on the remodeling mechanism)	Crepitus Limited range of motion with possible deviation to the affected side on opening. Radiographic evidence of structural bony change (subchondral sclerosis, osteophyte formation) and joint-space narrowing
Osteoarthritis (degenerative condition accompanied by secondary inflammation [synovitis] of the TMJ)	Same as for osteoarthrosis, plus pain with function due to inflammation, and point tenderness on palpation
Myofascial pain (regional dull aching pain and presence of localized tender spots [trigger points] in muscle, tendon, or fascia that reproduce pain when palpated and may produce a characteristic pattern of regional referred pain and/or autonomic symptoms on provocation)	Regional pain, usually dull Localized tenderness in firm bands of muscle and/or fascia Reduction in pain with local muscle anesthetic injection or vapocoolant spray and stretch of muscle trigger points
Myositis, delayed onset (painful condition due to intermittent overuse that results in interstitial inflammation) Myositis, generalized (constant, acutely painful, and generalized inflammation and swelling, usually of the entire muscle)	Increased pain with mandibular movement Onset following prolonged or unaccustomed use (up to 48 hours afterward) Pain usually acute in localized area Localized tenderness over entire region of the muscle Increased pain with mandibular movement Moderately to severely limited range of motion due to pain and swelling Onset following injury or infection
Protective muscle splinting (restricted or guarded mandibular movement due to co-contraction of muscles as a means of avoiding pain caused by movement of the parts)	Severe pain with function but not at rest Marked limited range of motion without significant increase on passive stretch
Contracture (chronic resistance of a muscle to passive stretch as a result of fibrosis of the supporting tendon, ligaments, or muscle fibers themselves)	Limited range of motion Unyielding firmness on passive stretch History of trauma or infection

Adapted from McNeill C.[127]

MRI = magnetic resonance imaging; TMJ = temporomandibular joint.

have to await further research. To allow greater application in the research environment, diagnostic imaging is not included. In clinical practice, rigidly adhering to the criteria may not be applicable, but the assessment and classification system serves as a useful method of organizing clinical information for the most commonly presenting TMD (Tables 4 and 5).[45] The reliance on clinical findings for diagnosis is consistent with the research purpose, but diagnostic imaging might be required to establish a disc disorder diagnosis such as "disc displacement without reduction, without limited opening." The clinician should recommend diagnostic imaging as part of the assessment when the diagnosis and choice of treatment

TABLE 4 Research Diagnostic Criteria for Clinical Temporomandibular Disorder Conditions, Axis I[45]

Clinical Location	RDC/TMD Diagnoses
Muscle	Myofascial pain Myofascial pain with limited opening
Disc displacement	Disc displacement with reduction Disc displacement without reduction, with limited opening Disc displacement without reduction, without limited opening
Articular bone	Arthralgia *Osteoarthritis* of the TMJ *Osteoarthrosis* of the TMJ

RDC/TMD = Research Diagnostic Criteria for Temporomandibular Disorders;
TMJ = temporomandibular joint.

might benefit. The reader is referred to the publication by Dworkin and LeResche[45] and the website of the International RDC-TMD Consortium (<http://rdc-tmdinternational.org/index.htm>).

Schiffman and colleagues compared clinical findings and tomographic findings to define criteria for intra-articular disorders and presented criteria for the classification of articular disorders.[152] No single sign or symptom was consistently accurate for establishing a diagnosis, but the patterns listed in Table 6 show 75% agreement when compared with findings by arthrotomography.[152]

The diagnosis of chronic articular disc displacement without reduction may be the most problematic diagnosis without imaging. A clinical history of clicking that stopped with an abrupt limitation of mouth opening that improved gradually may be associated with this specific diagnosis.

▼ ASSESSMENT

Present examination methods do not have the ability to accurately differentiate individuals with a TMD from those without.[153] The most valuable aspects of the diagnostic assessment are a thorough history and physical examination.[154] Most of the tests used to assess TMD patients have not been validated and are not standardized.[155] Diagnostic tests such as ultrasonography of joint sounds, thermography, jaw tracking, and EMG do not offer the assurance of a more accurate diagnosis or better treatment outcomes.[156] These

TABLE 5 Definitions and Clinical Criteria for Temporomandibular Disorders

Definitions*	Clinical Criteria*
Myofascial pain (pain of muscle origin, including complaint of pain associated with localized areas of tenderness to palpation in muscle)	Report of pain or ache in jaw, temples, face, preauricular area, or inside ear at rest or during function and pain on palpation in three or more muscle sites
Myofascial pain with limited opening	Myofascial pain, pain-free unassisted mandibular opening of <40 mm, and a maximum assisted opening of ≥5 mm greater than the pain-free unassisted opening
Disc displacement with reduction (disc is displaced from its position between the condyle and eminence to an anterior and medial or lateral position but is reduced in full opening, usually resulting in a noise)	Click on both vertical opening and closing that occurs at a point at least 5 mm (interincisal opening) greater than on closing, is eliminated on protrusive opening, and is reproducible in two of three consecutive trials or click on opening or closing and click on lateral excursion or protrusion, reproducible in two of three consecutive trials
Disc displacement without reduction, with limited opening (disc is displaced from normal position between condyle and fossa to an anterior and medial or lateral position, associated with limited opening)	History of significant limitation of opening Maximum unassisted opening ≤35 mm, passive stretch increases opening by ≤4 mm and contralateral excursion <7 mm and/or uncorrected deviation to the ipsilateral side on opening Absence of joint sounds or sounds that do not meet criteria for disc displacement with reduction
Disc displacement without reduction without limited opening (disc is displaced from its position between condyle and eminence to an anterior and medial or lateral position, not associated with limited opening)	History of significant limitation of mandibular opening Maximum unassisted opening >35 mm, passive stretch increases opening by ≥5 mm over maximum unassisted opening, contralateral excursion ≥7 mm, and presence of joint sounds not meeting criteria for disc displacement with reduction
Arthralgia (pain and tenderness in joint capsule and/or synovial lining of the TMJ)	Pain in one or both joint sites and self-report of pain in region of joint Pain in joint during maximum opening (assisted or unassisted) Pain in joint during lateral excursion
Osteoarthritis of the TMJ (inflammatory condition within the joint, resulting from a degenerative condition of joint structures)	Arthralgia and coarse crepitus or imaging showing one or more of the following: erosion of normal cortical outlines, sclerosis of parts or all of condyle and articular eminence, flattening of joint surfaces, osteophyte formation
Osteoarthrosis of the TMJ (degenerative joint disorder in which joint form and structure are abnormal)	Absence of arthralgia Coarse crepitus or imaging showing one or more of the following: erosion of normal cortical outlines, sclerosis of parts or all of condyle and articular eminence, flattening of joint surfaces, osteophyte formation

TMJ = temporomandibular joint.
* For the complete description, refer to Dworkin S and LeResche L.[45]

TABLE 6   Clinical Findings of Disc Disorders, Correlating with Arthrotomography

Assessment Procedure	Clinical Findings			
	Normal	ADD with Reduction	Acute ADD without Reduction	Chronic ADD without Reduction
History	None	None	Positive for mandibular limitation	Positive for TMJ noise
Physical examination	Reciprocal click No coarse crepitus Passive stretch ≥ 40 mm Lateral movements ≥ 7 mm If S-curve is present, joint is silent	Reciprocal click or popping No coarse crepitus Passive stretch ≥ 35 mm	No reciprocal click No coarse crepitus Maximum opening ≤ 35 mm Passive stretch < 40 mm Contralateral movement < 7 mm No S-curve deviation	No reciprocal click Coarse crepitus or joint sounds other than reciprocal clicking
Tomography	No decreased translation in ipsilateral condyle No osseous change	None	Decreased translation of ipsilateral condyle	Decreased translation of ipsilateral condyle or positive osseous changes

Adapted from Schiffman E et al.[152]

ADD = articular disc displacement; TMJ = temporomandibular joint.

devices were reviewed for their diagnostic value in assessing patients with temporomandibular complaints.[154] Analysis of TMJ synovial fluid is an active area of research but has not yet become a standard procedure in diagnosis or the selection of treatment. These tests require sophisticated instrumentation that would increase health care costs to the patient that, for the present, are not justified.

In most cases, the correct diagnostic classification can be reached by using the history and examination findings.[152,157] Diagnostic imaging is of value in selected conditions but not as a routine part of a standard assessment. Diagnostic imaging can increase accuracy in the detection of internal derangements[158] and abnormalities of articular bone.[159]

Facial pain similar to the pain of a TMD may be associated with serious undetected disease. Muscle or joint pain may be a secondary feature of another disease or may mimic a TMD. A diagnosis of a more serious condition may be missed or delayed.[160,161] Severe throbbing temporal pain associated with a palpable nodular temporal artery, increasingly severe headache associated with nausea and vomiting, and documented altered sensation or hearing loss are all indications of serious disease requiring timely diagnosis and management.

Behavioral Assessment

Assessment should result in a diagnosis of a TMD and an estimation of psychological distress and pain-related disability. Some TMDs evolve into a chronic pain disorder, resulting in psychological distress and disruption of interpersonal relationships and an inability to perform daily activities, including work. Psychosocial factors are considered more important in predicting treatment outcome than physical factors.[162] The lack of a direct relationship between physical pathology and intensity of pain and subsequent disability emphasizes the need to assess the psychological and behavioral effects of the disorder.

Fricton recommends developing a problem list of the contributing factors associated with TMD.[163] Contributing factors may affect the symptom control and the long-term success of treatment. Table 7 lists the contributing factors discussed by Fricton.[163] No one health care professional can be expected to manage the physical pathology of the temporomandibular structures and the various lifestyle, emotional, cognitive, and social issues that may affect the individual with chronic pain. Chronic TMDs are best managed in a multi- or interdisciplinary setting.

Rudy and colleagues classified TMD patients based on psychosocial and behavioral parameters in three unique subgroups: dysfunctional patients, interpersonally distressed patients, and adaptive copers.[164] TMD patients have been found to have psychosocial and behavioral profiles similar to those of back pain patients.[136,165] Interventions targeting pain and psychological distress are of equal importance to the pathophysiology of temporomandibular structures in managing a chronic TMD. Turner and colleagues showed that TMD patients who catastrophized had higher scores on clinical examination, more activity interference, and greater health care use regarding the TMD than TMD patients who did not.[166]

Psychosocial assessment should provide the clinician with an appreciation of the extent to which pain and dysfunction interfere with or diminish the patient's quality of life. A measure of the severity of limitation in activity will provide a reflection of the magnitude of the condition.[167,168] Korff and colleagues reported that approximately 16% of TMD patients experienced significant activity limitation compared with approximately 3% of controls.[169]

A systematic method of screening is necessary because dentists have been found to be inaccurate in identifying psychological problems in TMD patients.[170] The RDC/TMD uses a questionnaire developed in part from previously used scales to assess pain intensity and disability, depression, and nonspecific physical symptoms. The reader is referred to the publication by Dworkin and LeResche for the full discussion of this assessment[45] and the website of the International RDC-TMD Consortium (<http://rdc-tmdinternational.org/index.htm>).

TABLE 7   Problem List of Contributing Factors Associated with Temporomandibular Disorders

Lifestyle	Emotional Factors	Cognitive Factors	Biologic Factors	Social Factors
Diet	Prolonged anger	Negative self-image	Other illnesses	Work stresses
Sleep	Anxiety	Unrealistic expectations	Past trauma	Unemployment
Alcohol	Excessive worry	Inadequate coping	Past jaw surgery	Family stresses
Smoking	Depression			Litigation
Overwork				Financial difficulty

Adapted from Fricton J.[163]

Clinical circumstances that are indicators of the need for expert psychological evaluation of a TMD patient include the following[171]:

1. When pain persists beyond the expected healing time and no clear physical explanation is identified
2. When the patient displays signs or symptoms of significant psychological distress
3. When the disability greatly exceeds what is expected on the basis of the clinical findings
4. When excessive use of health care services, including tests and treatments, seems inappropriate
5. With prolonged use of opioids, sedatives, minor tranquilizers, antianxiety medications, and alcohol for pain control

History

The most common symptom related to TMD is pain. The pain usually shows some relationship to mandibular function, or an alternative diagnosis should be suspected. Pain severity or intensity is a subjective measure provided by the patient and can be rated in several ways. A visual analogue scale (VAS) using a 10 cm line anchored on the left side with the descriptor of 'no pain' and on the right 'the worst pain ever experienced.' The patient is asked to mark the severity along the line. The VAS can be used to assess present, past, or average pain ratings. A numeric scale asks the patient to rate pain by identifying a number between 0 and 10 that best reflects pain intensity. Verbal descriptors such as no pain, mild pain, moderate pain, severe pain, and intolerable pain can provide an assessment.

A "pain diary" can be a useful tool for identifying events or times of increased and decreased pain; it may also serve to identify behaviors or situations that are contributing to the persistence of symptoms. A pain diagram of the head and neck is helpful in defining the extent of pain and may also be used to assess treatment progress. A diagram that includes the whole body will help identify patients who have multiple sites of pain, which suggests a more systemic disorder. Table 8 lists questions that are useful (as part of the history) for assessing mandibular function.

Miscellaneous symptoms are sometimes reported in association with temporomandibular dysfunction and include dizziness; nausea; fullness or ringing in the ears; diminished

TABLE 8   History: Questions to Ask When Evaluating a Patient for Mandibular Dysfunction*

Do you have pain in the face, front of the ear, and temple areas?

Do you get headaches, earaches, neckache, or cheek pain?

When is pain at its worst (morning [on awakening] or as day progresses [toward evening])?

Do you experience pain when using the jaw (opening wide, yawning, chewing, speaking, or swallowing)?

Do you experience pain in the teeth?

Do you experience joint noises when moving your jaw or when chewing (clicking, popping, or crepitus)?

Does your jaw ever lock or get stuck (locking in the open position or locking in the closed position)?

Does your jaw motion feel restricted?

Have you had an abrupt change in the way your teeth meet together?

Does your bite feel "off" or uncomfortable?

Have you had any jaw injuries?

Have you had treatment for the jaw symptoms? If so, what was the effect?

Do you have any other muscle, bone, or joint problem, such as arthritis or fibromyalgia?

Do you have pain in any other body sites?

*Miscellaneous symptoms are sometimes reported in association with temporo mandibular dysfunction and may include dizziness; nausea; fullness or ringing in the ears; diminished hearing; facial swelling; redness of the eyes; nasal congestion; altered sensation such as numbness, tingling, or burning; altered vision; and muscle twitching.

hearing; earache; facial swelling; redness of the eyes; nasal congestion; altered sensation such as numbness, tingling, or burning; altered vision; muscle twitching; altered occlusion; and jaw misalignment.

Physical Examination

No one physical finding can be relied on to establish a diagnosis, but a pattern of abnormalities may suggest the source of the problem and a possible diagnosis. Masticatory muscle tenderness on palpation (see Figure 10) is the most consistent examination feature present in TMDs.[148] The clinical features studied that distinguish patients from controls are passive mouth opening,[172] masticatory muscle tenderness on palpation and maximal mouth opening,[173] and an uncorrected deviation on maximum mouth opening and tenderness on palpation.[134] Components of the physical examination that are discussed in this section are summarized in Table 9.

Range of Mandibular Movement

Interincisor separation plus or minus the incisor overlap in centric occlusion provides the measure of mandibular movement. Maximum opening should be measured using a ruler, without pain, as wide as possible with pain and after opening with clinician assistance. Mouth opening with assistance is accomplished by applying mild to moderate pressure against the upper and lower incisors with the thumb and index finger. Passive stretching (mouth opening with assistance) is a technique for assessing and differentiating limitation due to a muscle or joint problem.

Assisted opening can be compared with active opening. Performing the procedure also provides the examiner with the quality of resistance at the end of the movement. Muscle restrictions are associated with a soft end-feel and result in an increase of more than 5 mm above the active opening (wide opening with pain). Joint disorders such as acute non-reducing disc displacements are described as having a hard end-feel and characteristically limit assisted opening to < 5 mm. The normal maximum mouth opening is ≥ 40 mm. In a study of 1,160 adults, the mean maximum mouth opening was 52.8 mm (with a range of 38.7 to 67.2 mm) for men and 48.3 mm (with a range of 36.7 to 60.4 mm) for women.[174] Measures of lateral movement are made with the teeth slightly separated, measuring the displacement of the lower midline from the maxillary midline and adding or subtracting the lower-midline displacement at the start of movement. Protrusive movement is measured by adding the horizontal distance between the upper and lower central incisors and adding the distance the lower incisors travel beyond the upper incisors. Normal lateral and protrusive movements are ≥ 7 mm.[96,175–177] Measures of the mandibular range of movement are similarly performed in children. The mean maximum mouth opening recorded in 75 boys and 75 girls aged 6 years was 44.8 mm.[178] A study of 189 individuals with a mean age of 10 years reported similar values (a mean maximum opening of 43.9 mm, with a range of 32 to 64 mm).[179] The means of left, right, and protrusive maximal movements were each approximately 8 mm.

Palpation of Masticatory Muscles

The primary finding related to masticatory muscle palpation is pain. The methods for palpation are not standardized in clinical practice. The amount of pressure to apply and the exact sites that are most likely associated with TMD are unknown. Some clinicians have recommended attempting to establish a baseline (to serve as a general guide or reference) by squeezing a muscle between the index finger and thumb or by applying pressure in the center of the forehead or thumbnail to gauge what pressure becomes uncomfortable. The RDC/TMD guidelines recommend 1 lb of pressure for the joint and 2 lbs of pressure for the muscles.[45] The RDC/TMD pressures have been established for research purposes. In the clinical setting, a greater range of pressures is probably required.

Palpation should be accompanied by asking the patient about the presence of pain at the palpation site, whether palpation produces pain spread or referral to a distant site, and whether palpation reproduces the pain the patient has been experiencing. Reproducing the site and the character of the pain during the examination procedure helps identify the potential source of the pain. The distant origin of referred pain can be identified by palpation.

Palpation of the muscles for pain should be done with the muscles in a resting state. There are no standardized methods of assessing the severity of palpable pain, and the patient should be asked to rate the severity by using a scale (eg, a numeric scale from 1 to 10, a VAS, or a ranking such as none, mild, moderate, or severe). The RDC/TMD recommends using the categories of pressure only, mild pain, moderate pain, and severe pain. These ratings may be useful in assessing treatment progress. Abnormalities such as trigger points and taut bands in muscle have not been sufficiently characterized in the masticatory muscles to enable the clinician to distinguish these sites anatomically from normal muscle. The lateral pterygoid is in a position that does not allow access for adequate palpation examination even though there are examination protocols and descriptions for palpating this muscle.[180]

TABLE 9 Physical Examination Directed toward Mandibular Dysfunction

Examination Component	Observations
Inspection	Facial asymmetry, swelling, and masseter and temporal muscle hypertrophy Opening pattern (corrected and uncorrected deviations, uncoordinated movements, limitations)
Assessment of range of mandibular movement	Maximum opening with comfort, with pain, and with clinician assistance Maximum lateral and protrusive movements
Palpation examination	Masticatory muscles Temporomandibular joints Neck muscles and accessory muscles of the jaw Parotid and submandibular areas Lymph nodes
Provocation tests	Static pain test (mandibular resistance against pressure) Pain in the joints or muscles with tooth clenching Reproduction of symptoms with chewing (wax, sugarless gum)
Intraoral examination	Signs of parafunction (cheek or lip biting, accentuated linea alba, scalloped tongue borders, occlusal wear, tooth mobility, generalized sensitivity to percussion, thermal testing, multiple fractures of enamel and restorations)

Palpation of Cervical Muscles

Patients with TMDs often have musculoskeletal problems in other regions, particularly the neck.[181,182] The upper cervical somatosensory nerves send branches that synapse in the spinal trigeminal nucleus, which is one proposed mechanism to explain referral of pain from the neck to the orofacial region. The sternocleidomastoid and trapezius muscles are often part of cervical muscle disorders and may refer pain to the face and head. Other cervical muscle groups to include in the palpation examination include the paravertebral (scalene) and suboccipital muscles.

Palpation of the TMJ

Palpation of the TMJs will reveal pain and irregularities during condylar movement, described as clicking or crepitus. The lateral pole of the condyle is most accessible for palpation during mandibular movements. Palpating just anterior and posterior to the lateral pole should detect pain associated with the capsular ligament. In addition to joint noises and pain, there may be palpable differences in the form of the condyle comparing right with left. A condyle that does not translate may not be palpable during mouth opening and closing. This may be a finding associated with an ADD without reduction. A click that occurs on opening and closing and is eliminated by bringing the mandible into a protrusive position before opening is most often associated with ADD with reduction.

Provocation Tests

Provocation tests are designed to elicit the described pain. Since pain is often aggravated by jaw use, a positive response adds support for a diagnosis of TMD. The static pain test involves having the mandible slightly open and remaining in one position while the patient resists the slowly increasing manual force applied by the examiner in a lateral, upward, and downward direction. If the mandible remains in a static position during the test, the muscles will be subjected to activation. However, the ability of this test to discriminate between muscle and joint pain is not known. Clenching the teeth or chewing wax or gum is expected to load the joints and muscles. According to one study, approximately 50% of TMD patients who chewed half of a leaf of 28-gauge casting wax for 3 minutes reported increased pain, but 30% reported decreased pain and 20% reported no change.[183]

Assessment of Parafunctional Habits

It is difficult to determine the presence of active oral habits, and only indirect means are generally available. Patients are often unaware of tooth clenching or other behaviors contributing to jaw hyperactivity while awake. Self-report, monitoring daytime jaw activity and tooth position, and reports by sleeping partners of tooth-grinding noises are helpful. Assessing tooth wear, soft tissue changes (lip or cheek chewing, an accentuated occlusal line, and scalloped tongue borders), and hypertrophic jaw-closing muscles may suggest hyperactivity.

Diagnostic Imaging

When the clinical presentation suggests a progressive pathologic condition of the TMJs, imaging should be part of the assessment. Recent injury, sensory or motor abnormality, severe restriction in mandibular motion, and acute alterations of the occlusion are clinical findings for which imaging is indicated. The most frequent abnormalities that are imaged in TMD patients are degenerative changes of the articular bones and disc displacement.

TMJs can be examined by using plain-film radiography, tomography, arthrography, CT, MRI, single-photon emission computed tomography, and radioisotope scanning (Figures 11 and 12). MRI has become the imaging method of choice to assess disc form and position. For the majority of TMDs, diagnostic imaging has not proven to be a valuable test for directing treatment, predicting treatment outcome, and determining long-term prognosis.

A large variation exists in condylar position in plain-film radiographic and tomographic studies, making the condyle-fossa relationship of little value in the diagnosis or treatment of TMD.[184] No differences were found in joint-space narrowing in the centric occlusion position in symptomatic and asymptomatic patients by transcranial plain-film radiography and tomography.[185,186] Using plain films (such as transcranial radiography) to determine condylar position or using the condylar position on these films to assess disc position is not recommended.[185–187]

Tomography and CT are the imaging of choice to document osteodegenerative joint disease. CT provides detail for bony abnormalities and is an appropriate study when considering ankylosis, fractures, tumors of bone, and osteodegenerative joint disease.

MRI is the method of choice for establishing alterations in articular disc form and position in open and closed mouth positions (Figure 13). MRI studies in asymptomatic volunteers have shown disc abnormalities in approximately one-third of subjects.[188] With the use of T2-weighted MRI, a correlation between joint pain and joint effusion has been suggested, but the results are conflicting.[189,190] TMJ

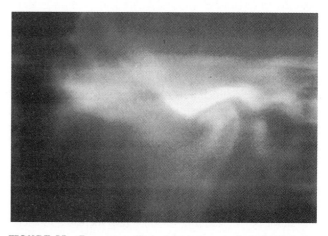

FIGURE 11 Temporomandibular joint tomogram displaying flattening of the condylar head in degenerative joint disease.

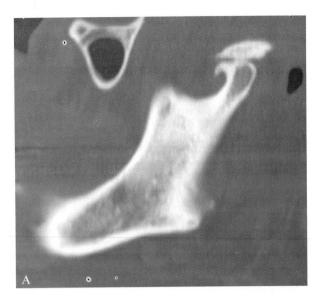

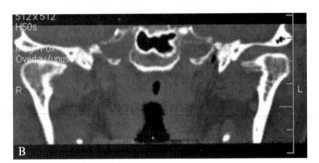

FIGURE 12 Sagittal (*A*) and coronal (*B*) CT images demonstrating flattening and beaking of the mandibular condyles in a patient with degenerative joint disease.

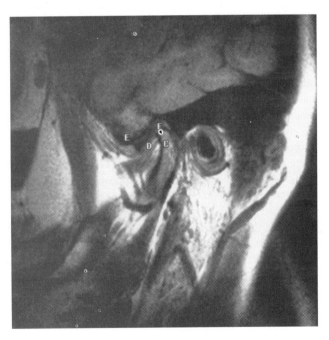

FIGURE 13 MRI image of an anterior disc displacement in the closed mouth position. The disc and critical bone image darker than surrounding tissue. C = condyle, D = disc, F = fossa, E = eminence, MRI = magnetic resonance imaging.

effusion is associated with an elevated concentration of synovial fluid proteins, including proinflammatory cytokines, but the ability to confirm the presence or absence of synovitis in the joint has not been established.[191] It is still not possible to predict the presence of pain based on MRI findings. Individual features on MRI of internal derangement, osteoarthrosis, effusion, and bone marrow edema are not predictive of TMJ pain, but when these features occur together, an increased risk of TMJ pain has been observed.[192]

Radioisotope scanning for detecting increases in metabolic activity has been used to detect condylar hyperplasia. Bone scanning is a sensitive indicator of metabolic bone activity and will show similar activity in a joint that is undergoing physiologic remodeling as well. Scintigraphy is a sensitive test but is not specific for TMJ disease. Bone scintigraphy in combination with other imaging and clinical findings (including findings on periodic examinations) is usually effective in diagnosing continued condylar change due to hyperplasia.

Diagnostic Local Anesthetic Nerve Blocks

Injections of anesthetics into the TMJ or selected masticatory muscles may help confirm a diagnosis. Elimination of or a significant decrease in pain and improved jaw motion should be considered a positive test result.

Diagnostic injections may also be helpful in differentiating pain arising from joints or muscle. In situations in which a joint procedure is being considered, local anesthetic injection of the joint may confirm the joint as the source of pain. Kopp has described a technique for TMJ injection.[193] Injecting trigger points or tender areas of muscle should eliminate pain from the site and should also eliminate referred pain associated with the injected trigger point.[194] These tests, like all others, require interpretation in the context of all the diagnostic information since a positive result does not ensure a specific diagnosis.

Prediction of Chronicity

Whereas most TMD patients respond to nonsurgical management that can be provided or coordinated by a dentist, some individuals evolve into a chronic musculoskeletal pain disorder that results in significant disability. This group experiences great psychological distress and disruption of their normal daily activities and requires ongoing access to health care resources. Predicting cases that are likely to become chronic is important to provide alternative or additional interventions. Psychosocial factors have been better predictors of treatment outcome than physical findings, diagnosis, or how much treatment was pursued.[195]

Psychological factors seem to be more important than peripheral injury or physical disease of the masticatory system in predicting chronicity.[196–199] Epker and colleagues found that the combination of high pain intensity (as measured by RDC/TMD scales) and a myofascial pain diagnosis (reported pain on palpation of muscles) was predictive of persisting TMD symptoms in their population.[200]

Comorbidity with widespread musculoskeletal pain is likely to contribute toward the development of a chronic TMD. Individuals with fibromyalgia, a chronic widespread musculoskeletal pain disorder, have a significantly higher frequency of masticatory myofascial pain than the general population.[201,202] The presence of pain in other body sites in myofascial pain dysfunction (MPD) patients is high[180] and may indicate that a musculoskeletal problem affecting the jaws is part of a more generalized pain disorder. In a follow-up study on MPD patients, the group that self-reported the coexistence of fibromyalgia had a higher frequency of chronic TMD symptoms.[203]

Trauma associated with the onset of TMD has always been considered to be a factor likely to increase severity and extend the course of the disorder. The literature is ambivalent about this since studies have resulted in conflicting conclusions. In a comparison of treatment between groups with TMD associated with trauma and without trauma, there was no difference to the treatment outcome, suggesting that trauma may not be an important factor, but more research is needed to draw conclusions.[204] Post-traumatic TMD patients in another study had a decreased response to treatment and required more treatment than a nontrauma patient group.[205]

Referral to a Pain Specialist

The majority of patients with TMDs respond to available treatments and can be appropriately managed by dental professionals in association with psychologists, physiotherapists, and other health care professionals. Some patients may be more appropriately managed by a pain specialist within a setting of a multidisciplinary pain clinic. This may be indicated when (1) the disability greatly exceeds what is expected on the basis of physical findings, (2) the patient makes excessive demands for tests and treatments that are not indicated, (3) the patient displays significant psychological distress (eg, depression), or (4) the patient displays aberrant behavior, such as continual nonadherence to treatment.[150]

▼ GENERAL PRINCIPLES OF TREATING TMDs

The most important feature of TMD is pain. Pain may be present at rest, may be continuous or intermittent, and characteristically increases with jaw functions such as chewing or opening wide. Other common findings include pain reported during palpation of the TMJ and/or muscles of mastication, a restricted range of mandibular movement or uncoordinated movements, and irregularities in the joints during mouth movements, characterized by clicking or grating sounds. Myofascial pain is the most common TMD[148] and may present with or without restricted mouth opening. Pain causes the jaw-closing muscles to co-contract, so the pain itself may influence the degree of mandibular restriction in cases of MPD.[206,207] Chronic TMD pain (like all chronic pain) results in psychological, behavioral, and social disturbances, and these characteristics may be a dominant part of the problem.

Treatment goals for TMDs are to control pain, improve mandibular motion, and restore function as close to normal as possible. Clinical case studies suggest that the majority of individuals with TMD respond to conservative noninvasive therapy, making the use of invasive procedures unwarranted as initial therapy. No one treatment has emerged as superior, although many of the treatments studied have shown beneficial effect.[208] The symptoms of TMD tend to be intermittent, fluctuate over time, and are often self-limiting.[209–211] Recently, Rammelsberg and colleagues reported on a 5-year study that indicated that only a third of TMD patients studied experienced remission, a third had persisting symptoms, and a third experienced recurring symptoms.[212] The process of deciding whether to treat and how aggressively to treat should take into account the course of symptoms. Patients who are improving at the time of assessment may require a minimum of care and follow-up compared with the individual whose symptoms are becoming progressively more severe and disabling.

The variations in treatment recommended by dentists have been explained by the gap between published information in the medical and dental literature and individual dentist's beliefs and attitudes.[213,214] These observations suggest that the treatment effect may be nonspecific and related more to the therapeutic relationship established between therapist and patient than to the specific treatment.[215]

Patients with irreversible anatomic abnormalities such as disc disorders are still able to regain pain-free jaw function.[216,217] Decreasing pain and improved physical findings are not directly related.[162,218] The presence of joint noises and deviations from the ideal in occlusion, in maxillomandibular relationships, and in the morphology of bony structures such as the condyle are relatively common in the general population. Evidence indicating prophylactic treatment of these anatomic abnormalities when no pain, impairment of function, or disability exists is lacking. Rather, treatment should be based on the severity of pain and disability and should be directed toward those factors that are considered important in initiating, aggravating, or perpetuating the disorder.

Episodes of pain and dysfunction may recur even after successful symptom control. Reinjury or factors that contributed to earlier episodes of symptoms may be responsible. Recurrence should not be considered a treatment failure, and initiating previous treatment that was successful should be considered first. In one study, myogenous disorders required re-treatment more frequently than did articular disorders.[219]

For the smaller group of patients in whom TMD progresses to a chronic pain disorder, treatment becomes more complex. These patients may still benefit from local therapies but will also require more comprehensive management to address the emotional and behavioral disabilities that result from chronic pain. The drug therapy may also be complex, requiring knowledge and experience that are not common in general dental practice. These patients are often at risk for unnecessary investigations or treatments that may be harmful and that may further complicate their problems.[220,221]

A National Institutes of Health conference on TMD therapy produced the following conclusions[222]:

1. Significant problems exist with present diagnostic classifications because these classifications are based on signs and symptoms rather than etiology.
2. No consensus has been developed regarding which TMD problems should be treated and when and how they should be treated.
3. The preponderance of the data does not support the superiority of any method for initial management, and the superiority of such methods to placebo controls or to no treatment controls remains undetermined.
4. Because most individuals will experience the improvement or relief of symptoms with conservative treatment, the vast majority of TMD patients should be initially managed with noninvasive and reversible therapies.
5. The efficacy of most treatment approaches for TMD is unknown because most have not been adequately evaluated in long-term studies and because virtually none have been studied in randomized controlled group trials.
6. Therapies that permanently alter the patient's occlusion cannot be recommended on the basis of current data.
7. Surgical intervention should be considered for the small percentage of patients with persistent and significant pain and dysfunction who show evidence of pathology or evidence that an internal derangement of the TMJ is the source of their pain and dysfunction and for whom more conservative treatment has failed.
8. Relaxation and cognitive-behavioral therapies (CBTs) are effective approaches to managing chronic pain.

▼ SPECIFIC DISORDERS AND THEIR MANAGEMENT

The majority of patients likely to present in a dental practice with a complaint of temporomandibular pain and dysfunction can be broadly categorized into muscle disorders, articular disc disorders, and disorders affecting the articular bones. The most common muscle disorder is myofascial pain. This pain is not associated with an identifiable anatomic muscle abnormality.

Intracapsular disorders affecting the TMJ are divided into two broad categories: osteodegenerative joint disease and articular disc disorders. Either may be present without causing symptoms. It is important for the clinician treating patients with TMDs to distinguish clinically significant disorders that require therapy from incidental findings in a patient with facial pain from other causes. TMJ abnormalities are often discovered on routine examination and may not require treatment. The need for treatment is largely based on the level of pain and dysfunction and the progression of symptoms. The discovery of an anatomic abnormality such as a long-standing joint noise that is otherwise asymptomatic and consistent with a disc displacement is usually not treated given the presently available treatments. Diagnostic imaging using magnetic resonance has identified disc displacements in about 30% of individuals who do not have temporomandibular symptoms or a TMD requiring treatment.[223]

Myofascial Pain of the Masticatory Muscles

The term most commonly used for muscle pain produced on palpation is *myofascial pain*. The term *myofascial pain* has also been characterized by muscle pain that also radiates or is referred when the muscle is stimulated during palpation examination. The ability to diagnose and explain the pathology associated with muscle pain is still a challenge for further research. Since treatment cannot be designed to address a particular cause, multiple therapies for controlling symptoms and restoring range of movement and jaw function are usually combined in a management plan. These therapies are more effective when used together than when used alone.[149,224–227]

Most of the research on the natural course of this disorder suggests that for most individuals, symptoms are intermittent and usually do not progress to chronic pain and disability. The dentist is the appropriate clinician to manage these patients, using conservative methods. The principles of treatment are based on a generally favorable prognosis and an appreciation of the lack of clinically controlled trials indicating the superiority, predictability, and safety of treatments presently available. The literature suggests that many treatments have some beneficial effect, although this effect may be nonspecific and not directly related to the particular treatment.

Treatments that are relatively accessible, not prohibitive due to expense, safe, and reversible should be given priority. Treatments with these characteristics include education, self-care, physical therapy, intraoral appliance therapy, short-term pharmacotherapy, behavioral therapy, and relaxation techniques (Table 10). There is evidence to suggest that combining treatments produces a better outcome.[228] Occlusal therapy continues to be recommended by some clinicians as an initial treatment or as a requirement to prevent recurrent symptoms. Research does not support occlusal abnormalities as a significant etiologic factor.[229] The evaluation of occlusion and correction of occlusal abnormalities are an important part of dental practice but should not be a standard treatment for TMDs.

TABLE 10 Initial Treatment of Myofascial Pain

Treatment Component	Description
Education	Explanation of the diagnosis and treatment
	Reassurance about the generally good prognosis for recovery and natural course
	Explanation of patient's and doctor's roles in therapy
	Information to enable patient to perform self-care
Self-care	Eliminate oral habits (eg, tooth clenching, chewing gum)
	Provide information on jaw care associated with daily activities
Physical therapy	Education regarding biomechanics of jaw, neck, and head posture
	Passive modalities (heat and cold therapy, ultrasound, laser, and TENS)
	Range of motion exercises (active and passive)
	Posture therapy
	Passive stretching, general exercise and conditioning program
Intraoral appliance therapy	Cover all the teeth on the arch the appliance is seated on
	Adjust to achieve simultaneous contact against opposing teeth
	Adjust to a stable comfortable mandibular posture
	Avoid changing mandibular position
	Avoid long-term continuous use
Pharmacotherapy	NSAIDs, acetaminophen, muscle relaxants, antianxiety agents, tricyclic antidepressants
Behavioral/relaxation techniques	Relaxation therapy
	Hypnosis
	Biofeedback
	Cognitive-behavioral therapy

NSAIDs = nonsteroidal anti-inflammatory drugs; TENS = transcutaneous electrical nerve stimulation.

EDUCATION AND INFORMATION

A source of great anxiety for patients is the possibility that their condition is progressive and degenerative and will lead to greater pain and disability in the future. Patients may have sought prior consultations from other physicians and dentists who were not able to establish a diagnosis or explain the nature of the problem. This often leads to fears of a more catastrophic problem, such as a brain tumor or other life-threatening disease. Explaining the nature of the pain, its source, and the varied nature of the symptoms that may occur is an important part of treatment to reduce anxiety that results in an amplification of pain and increased disability. Education is the basis for self-care activities that patients must perform for symptom control. This requires enough time in an unhurried environment for the dentist to provide information and to allow the patient to express his or her concerns and to ask questions. This interaction is the basis for the therapeutic relationship. Education and information provide the patient with an understanding of the condition and the ability to perform activities and make choices that have a direct effect on the symptoms. The patient has to participate in developing strategies to avoid stresses that aggravate symptoms or interfere with the ability to manage therapy.

SELF-CARE AND HABIT REVERSAL

Attention to jaw activities that are unrelated to function (such as tooth clenching, jaw-posturing habits, jaw-muscle tensing, and leaning on the jaw) is a critical beginning. Those behaviors associated with hyperactivity need to be replaced with restful jaw postures, and this should be part of any initial therapy. Habit control was found to be helpful in reducing pain in myofascial pain patients.[230] Dispensing a set of instructions to patients can help focus their attention on habits that are contributing to the aggravation or persistence of symptoms (Table 11). Instructions for habit reversal and for resting the jaw should also be accompanied by physical therapy that can be performed at home without specialized equipment (eg, the application of moist heat to the affected areas for 15 to 20 minutes twice daily, range of motion exercises that stay within the comfort zone, and the occasional use of cold application for pain control or for relief of an acute flare superimposed over a chronic TMD [cold compress 10 minutes every 2 hours during an acute episode]).[231,232]

PHYSIOTHERAPY

Although clinical trials necessary to confirm the effectiveness of physiotherapy are lacking, the clinical literature suggests that physiotherapy is a reasonable part of initial therapy.[233] Physiotherapy has been shown to be better than placebo, but no differences between various physical therapies have been demonstrated.[234] Both passive and active treatments are commonly included as part of therapy. Posture therapy has been recommended to avoid forward head positions that are thought to adversely affect mandibular posture and masticatory muscle activity.

Passive modalities such as ultrasound, laser, and transcutaneous electrical nerve stimulation (TENS) are often used initially to reduce pain. Passive modalities are used in association with joint mobilization and muscle stretching to reduce discomfort associated with these procedures. TENS uses a low-voltage biphasic current of varied frequency and is designed for sensory counterstimulation for the control of pain. It is thought to increase the action of the modulation that occurs in pain processing at the dorsal horn of the spinal cord and (in the case of the face) the trigeminal nucleus of the brainstem. Ultrasound relies on high-frequency oscillations that are produced and converted to heat as they are transmitted through tissue; it is a method of producing deep heat more effectively than the patient could achieve by using surface warming.

Exercises to increase the range of jaw motion in the comfort zone, passive stretching, and isotonic and isometric exercises are exercise programs provided for patients as part of a home program. Mouth-opening and mouth-closing exercises in a straight line in front of a mirror and/or with the tongue in contact with the palate are common controlled

TABLE 11   Instructions to Patients for Self-Care as Part of Initial Therapy

Be aware of habits or patterns of jaw use.

   Avoid tooth contact except during chewing and swallowing.

   Notice any contact the teeth make.

   Notice any clenching, grinding, gritting, or tapping of teeth or any tensing or rigid holding of the jaw muscles.

   Check for tooth clenching while driving, studying, doing computer work, reading, or engaging in athletic activities and also when at work or in social situations and when experiencing overwork, fatigue, or stress.

   Position the jaw to avoid tooth contacts.

   Place the tip of the tongue behind the top teeth and keep the teeth slightly apart; maintain this position when the jaw is not being used for functions such as speaking and chewing.

Modify your diet.

   Choose softer foods and only those foods that can be chewed without pain.

   Cut foods into smaller pieces; avoid foods that require wide mouth opening and biting off with the front teeth or foods that are chewy and sticky and that require excessive mouth movements.

   Do not chew gum.

Do not test the jaw.

Do not open wide or move the jaw around excessively to assess pain or motion.

Avoid habitually maneuvering the jaw into positions to assess its comfort or range.

Avoid habitually clicking the jaw if a click is present.

Avoid certain postures.

   Do not lean on or cup the chin when performing desk work or at the dining table.

   Do not sleep on the stomach or in postures that place stress on the jaw.

Avoid elective dental treatment while symptoms of pain and limited opening are present.

During yawning, support the jaw by providing mild pressure underneath the chin with the thumb and index finger or with the back of the hand.

Apply moist hot compresses to the sides of the face and to the temple areas for 10 to 20 min twice daily.

mouth-opening exercises. A 3-month study of treatment consisting of education only or education plus a home physical therapy program found that education plus home physical therapy was more effective.[231]

Some physiotherapists apply mobilization techniques to increase mandibular motion. These are done passively under the control of the physiotherapist and will usually include distraction and some combination of lateral and protrusive gliding movements. The choice and timing of treatment are individual considerations since the literature is not developed enough to provide specific guidelines.

INTRAORAL APPLIANCES

Intraoral appliances (splints, orthotics, orthopedic appliances, bite guards, nightguards, or bruxing guards) are used in TMD treatment. Their use is considered to be a reversible

part of initial therapy. A number of studies on splint therapy have demonstrated a treatment effect, although researchers disagree as to the reason for the effect.[211,228,235,236] In a review of the literature on splint therapy, Clark found that patients reported a 70 to 90% improvement with splint therapy.[237] A review of the research on splint therapy suggests that using a splint as part of therapy for masticatory myalgia, arthralgia, or both is supported by the literature.[238] A number of studies have reviewed this issue, concluding in general that the use of appliances in TMD treatment is beneficial, but available high-quality evidence is still lacking.[65,239–243]

A decrease in masticatory muscle activity has been associated with splint therapy and might be the reason for the effects of splint therapy.[244] Alternatively, a nonspecific treatment effect has been proposed.[245] Other explanations for the effects of splint therapy include occlusal disengagement, altered vertical dimension, realigned maxillomandibular relationship, mandibular condyle repositioning, and cognitive awareness of mandibular posturing and habits.[246] The nature of treatment effects of appliance therapy will require further research. For the present, however, intraoral appliance therapy is considered to be a reversible treatment that is often included in initial treatment.

The choice of material for the construction of an appliance remains one of individual preference. A study comparing a hard and soft material during a 3-month trial found no difference in outcome when either the hard or the soft appliance was used.[247] Long-term continuous wearing of an occlusal appliance is a risk for a permanent change in the occlusion.[248] This is a greater concern with appliances that provide only partial coverage or that occlude only on selected opposing teeth.[249]

A survey of dentists and dental specialists reported that a flat-plane splint made of hard acrylic was used more frequently than any other design or material.[250] The most common purposes advocated for appliance therapy are to provide joint stabilization, protect the teeth, redistribute forces, relax elevator muscles, and decrease bruxism.[246]

The appliance most commonly used is described as a stabilization appliance or muscle relaxation splint (Figure 14). Such appliances are designed to cover a full arch and are adjusted to avoid altering jaw position or placing orthodontic forces on the teeth. The appliance should be adjusted to provide bilateral even contact with the opposing teeth on closure and in a comfortable mandibular posture. Anterior guidance during excursive movements is preferred and can often be achieved with an appropriate acrylic contour. During the period of treatment as symptoms improve, the appliance should be reexamined periodically and readjusted as necessary to accommodate changes in mandibular posture or muscle function that may affect the opposing tooth contacts on the appliance. At the beginning of appliance therapy, a combination of appliance use during sleep and for periods during the waking hours is appropriate. This should be monitored to determine the most effective schedule for appliance use. Factors such as tooth clenching when driving or

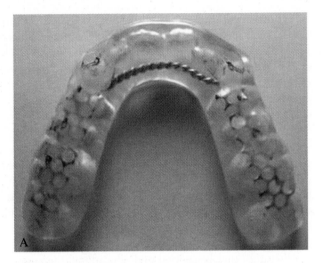

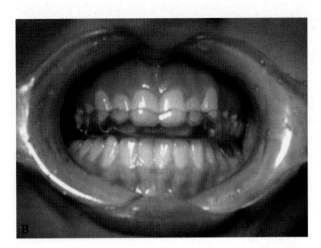

FIGURE 14 Maxillary acrylic full-coverage stabilization splint.

exercising or pain symptoms that tend to increase as the day progresses may be better managed by increasing splint use during these times. To avoid the possibility of occlusal change, the appliance should not be worn continuously (ie, 24 hours per day) over prolonged periods. Many patients continue to wear stabilization splints during sleep with periodic monitoring. Full-coverage appliance therapy during sleep is a common practice to reduce the effects of bruxing and is not usually associated with occlusal change.

The choice of inserting a stabilizing appliance on the upper or lower arch is a clinical judgment related to how the appliance is to be used and the clinical findings. Placing the appliance on the arch with missing teeth allows for an increase in occlusal contact position. For patients who are likely to benefit from daytime wear, a lower appliance is usually less visible and does not interfere with speech as much as an upper appliance. When an appliance is to be used only at night, most clinicians choose the upper arch.

Splints that reposition the mandible anteriorly have been used effectively in treating disc displacements,[251] but they increase the risk of permanently altering the occlusion and should be used with caution. These splints have been made for the upper or lower arch, although the maxillary appliance is better able to maintain a forward mandibular posture by using a ramp extending from the anterior segment that guides the mandible forward during closure. These appliances were used with greater frequency in the past to correct disc position as a step toward more permanently altering mandibular position through permanent changes in the occlusion. This approach was associated with great technical difficulties, and the treatment failed to correct disc displacement in a significant percentage of patients. Repositioning appliances used for short periods intermittently can be useful in controlling symptoms arising from the mechanical instability of the disc-condyle relationship. Short-term intermittent repositioning therapy may be helpful when transient episodes of jaw locking

occur due to disc displacement and are accompanied by pain and dysfunction.

In summary, a stabilizing oral appliance that fully covers one arch and does not reposition the mandible or alter the occlusion is considered a standard part of initial therapy. Continuous appliance wear, appliances that only provide partial coverage, and appliances that reposition the mandible and alter the occlusion have a greater chance of adverse effects.

PHARMACOTHERAPY

Mild analgesics, nonsteroidal anti-inflammatory analgesic drugs (NSAIDs), antianxiety agents, tricyclic antidepressants, and muscle relaxants are medications used as part of initial treatment. All of these drugs may be of use in therapy, especially at the beginning of treatment, to enhance pain control. Because of the adverse effects of all of these drugs, short-term or intermittent use is preferred, but a smaller percentage of patients who evolve into a chronic musculoskeletal pain disorder are usually taking combinations of medications long term. Opioids are usually reserved for complex chronic pain disorders or briefly for acute injuries to the TMJs or muscles where moderate to severe pain is present.

Drug therapy as part of TMD management should follow the general principles of analgesic therapy and be used on a fixed dose schedule rather than as needed for pain. Drug therapy requires a thoughtful assessment of the potential risks relative to the benefits, including the clinician's own professional ability and confidence in using the particular drug or drugs.

NSAIDs are probably the most commonly prescribed medication for pain control in TMD therapy. The promise of the COX-2 inhibitors (eg, rofecoxib) as safer alternatives to other NSAIDs has proven unfulfilled due to the association of cardiovascular incidents. Rofecoxib has been withdrawn as an available drug, and the uncertainty about others makes using these drugs inappropriate for most TMD therapy. There is modest evidence for efficacy of NSAIDs in TMD therapy.[252] In one study, ibuprofen 2,400 mg daily for 4 weeks did not demonstrate a clear analgesic effect due to the drug.[253] Naproxen 500 mg twice daily in a 6-week trial was more effective than placebo or celecoxib.[254] A trial of systemic NSAIDs is a reasonable part of initial therapy. NSAIDs for most TMDs should be short term to supplement the other nondrug therapies that should reduce the need for long-term NSAID therapy. A mild analgesic such as acetaminophen might be a first choice for analgesic drug treatment since it is much less likely to cause adverse side effects when taken in the appropriate dose for short periods.

Topical NSAIDs have demonstrated significant pain-reducing effects in acute and chronic musculoskeletal injuries. NSAIDs can be incorporated in transdermal creams for application on the skin over the painful joint or muscle. Ketoprofen, felbinac, ibuprofen, and piroxicam had significant efficacy. This efficacy held true for chronic conditions such as arthritis. The incidence of local and systemic adverse events was low and no different from placebo.[255] Capsaicin cream (0.025% and 0.075%) has not been studied for TMD therapy but has been recommended as a topical analgesic when applied to the skin over a sore joint or muscle four times daily for at least 2 weeks. Capsaicin is a substance P depleter, a neurotransmitter responsible for increased nerve sensitization. It was originally found to be of value in treating postherpetic neuralgia. Capsaicin therapy is limited due to its burning quality on application, which frequently causes the patient to abandon treatment.

The long-acting benzodiazepine clonazepam was effective in a pilot study of TMD treatment,[256] but more recently, cyclobenzaprine, a muscle relaxant, was found to be superior to clonazepam at managing morning jaw pain.[257] Muscle relaxants are a class of drugs that act in the central nervous system, inhibiting interneurons and depressing motor activity. The study used one tablet (10 mg) of cyclobenzaprine before sleep. Some patients taking 10 mg of cyclobenzaprine experience continued sedation into the day but are able to tolerate lower does by splitting the tablet into two or four sections. Cyclobenzaprine has sedative effects that may contribute to their effect and be of value in promoting sleep. These medications are used before sleep due to their sedative effects.

Tricyclic antidepressants, particularly amitriptyline, have proven to be effective in managing chronic orofacial pain. Amitriptyline is analgesic at low doses, has sedative effects, and promotes restful sleep; all of these effects can be helpful in treatment. It is the anticholinergic effects of the drug (dry mouth, weight gain, sedation, and dysphoria) that often make it intolerable. An effective dose can be as low as 10 mg at night but can be increased gradually to 75 to 100 mg, depending on the patient's tolerance of the side effects. Two clinical studies demonstrated a positive treatment effect using low-dose amitriptyline for TMD treatment.[258,259]

Drug therapy with an NSAID, acetaminophen, amitriptyline, or cyclobenzaprine, along with the other components of initial therapy, may contribute to symptom control.[260] The choice of drugs and their management as a part of a complex chronic pain disorder is different and is not covered in this chapter.

BEHAVIORAL THERAPY AND RELAXATION TECHNIQUES

Integrating behavioral therapy and relaxation techniques in chronic pain management is effective.[261] In some cases, self-care and awareness of habits may not be sufficient to change behaviors that are contributing to symptoms. A more structured program supervised by a clinician who is competent in behavioral therapy offers a greater chance of addressing issues that are contributing factors. There is general agreement in the literature that behavioral and educational therapies are effective in the management of chronic pain disorders, although the existing research is not sufficient to conclude that any one technique is superior. Relaxation techniques, biofeedback, hypnosis, and CBT have all been used to reduce symptoms in patients with TMD.[262] The mechanism of action of these techniques is unclear.

Relaxation techniques generally decrease sympathetic activity and (possibly) arousal. Deep methods include autogenic training, meditation, and progressive muscle relaxation.[261] These techniques are aimed at producing comforting body sensations, calming the mind, and reducing muscle tone. Brief methods for relaxation use self-controlled relaxation, paced breathing, and deep breathing. Hypnosis produces a state of selective or diffuse focus in order to induce relaxation. The technique includes pre- and postsuggestion and is used to introduce specific goals. Individuals vary greatly in their susceptibility to hypnosis and suggestion. Hypnosis does not affect endorphin production, and its affect on catecholamine production is not known.

CBT, which often includes relaxation techniques, changes patterns of negative thoughts. Hypnosis and CBT have been hypothesized to block pain from entering consciousness by activating the frontal limbic attention system to inhibit pain impulse transmission from the thalamic to the cortical structures.[261] A six-session CBT intervention enhanced the treatment effect of usual TMD treatment.[263]

Biofeedback is a treatment method that provides continuous feedback, usually by monitoring the electrical activity of muscle with surface electrodes or by monitoring peripheral temperature. The monitoring instruments provide patients with physiologic information that allows them to reliably change physiologic functions to produce a response similar to that produced by relaxation therapies. The patient performs relaxation exercises that are aimed at either lowering the electrical activity of the muscle or raising peripheral temperature. Repetitive practice using the biofeedback instrumentation provides the training for the patient to achieve a more relaxed state and also a greater sensitivity to the activities that have adverse effects.

Barriers to integrating behavioral and relaxation therapy exist in standard medical and dental care. The biomedical model of disease is emphasized in medical and dental education. The biomedical model emphasizes the anatomic and pathophysiologic aspects of disease and does not stress psychosocial issues or the importance of the patient's experience of disease. Behavioral therapies can be time-intensive and may also not be supported by insurance companies.

For the patient who does not respond to initial treatment and who continues to have significant pain and disability, additional therapies beyond those described above are usually required. These patients are characterized more as having a chronic pain disorder than as having an anatomic abnormality that is unique to the masticatory system. Treatments used in the management of chronic pain are indicated for this group. Multidisciplinary pain clinic management may be required. The use of chronic pain medications, including opioids and the drugs described as adjuvant analgesics (tricyclic antidepressants, anticonvulsants, membrane stabilizers, and sympatholytics), may be part of a long-term management plan. Chronic pain disorders cause psychosocial changes that require management to reduce the associated disability.

A greater focus on behavioral therapies and coping strategies may provide additional benefits. Sleep disorders may require the use of hypnotics or other drug combinations to increase restorative sleep. Depression commonly accompanies chronic pain. Surgery for a chronic muscle pain disorder has no value.

TRIGGER POINT THERAPY

Trigger point therapy has used two modalities: the cooling of skin over the involved muscle and stretching and the direct injection of local anesthetic into the muscle.

'Spray and stretch' therapy is performed by cooling the skin with a refrigerant spray (eg, fluoromethane) and stretching the involved muscle. Cooling allows for stretching without pain that causes a reactive contraction or strain. Travell and Simons described this technique in detail, introducing the method for the treatment of MPD.[194] Patients who respond to this therapy can use a variation at home by first warming the muscle, then briefly icing it, and then gently stretching the jaw passively.

Intramuscular trigger point injections have been performed by injecting local anesthetic, saline, or sterile water or by dry needling without depositing a drug or solution. The choice of solution for injection exists because of the lack of established benefits of any one method.[264] Injection of sterile water was associated with greater injection pain than was injection of saline.[265] In a study in which MPD patients were treated with injection of lidocaine or with dry needling, both groups reported decreased pain immediately after injection, but the group that received dry needling experienced greater soreness 48 hours after the procedure.[266] Procaine diluted to 0.5% with saline has been recommended because of its low toxicity to the muscle,[267] but 1% lidocaine is an alternative.

There are no tested protocols for trigger point injection therapy. Three to five weekly sessions has been recommended,

and this may be continued with modification of the intervals between injections, depending on the response.[268] Injections can be given to a muscle group in a series of five weekly or biweekly treatments. If there is no response to the initial series of injections, treatment should be abandoned. Hopwood and Abram analyzed treatment outcomes for 197 patients who received trigger point injection therapy for myofascial pain.[269] They found that (1) unemployment due to pain increased the odds of treatment failure threefold, (2) a longer duration of pain and greater change in social activity increased the risk of failure twofold, and (3) constant pain (versus intermittent pain) increased the likelihood of treatment failure by 80%. These results emphasize that chronic pain is a multidimensional and complex problem and that a variety of factors will influence treatment outcome.

Other TMD Treatments

The above sections highlight only the most common treatment methods and has not addressed many treatments that have been recommended for the management of TMDs. Acupuncture has been shown to be an effective part of the management of chronic pain. Botulinum toxin has been advocated for the treatment of TMDs,[270] but randomized clinical trials to assess its effectiveness have not been performed to establish the true efficacy of this treatment. Acupressure, different forms of injection therapy using natural substances, massage therapy, naturopathic and homeopathic remedies, and herbal remedies are just a few of the treatments patients may pursue. The Internet has produced treatment programs that even allow patents to evaluate their problem to determine whether the advertised treatment will be of benefit. There is a critical need (which will increase in the future) for dentists to help patients evaluate the treatments and products that are promoted for TMD therapy. Many of these treatments lack publication of articles in the scientific literature that is even descriptive. The large variety of treatments promoted, coupled with the lack of clarity in the scientific research about cause, makes the need to establish a trusting doctor-patient relationship critical.

Restorative Dental Procedures in TMD Patients

Patients who require elective dental treatment should defer such procedures until the TMD symptoms have resolved or are under reasonable control. Patients who develop active dental disease requiring treatment while they are suffering from TMD pain are likely to have increased pain and dysfunction after dental procedures. The dentist should attempt to minimize the effect of a procedure on myofascial pain by using a variety of measures, as outlined in Table 12.

Articular Disc Disorders of the TMJ

ADD is an abnormal relationship between the disc, the mandibular condyle, and the articular eminence, resulting from the elongation or tearing of the attachment of the disc to the condyle and glenoid fossa. ADD may result in abnormal joint sounds, limitation and deviation of mandibular motion, and

TABLE 12　Managing Temporomandibular Disorder Patients Requiring Dental Procedures

Prior to the procedure
　Use hot compresses to masseter and temporalis areas 10 to 20 minutes two to three times daily for 2 days.
　Use a minor tranquilizer or skeletal muscle relaxant (eg, lorazepam, 1 mg; cyclobenzaprine, 10 mg) on the night and day of the procedure (patient must be accompanied by an adult).
　Start a nonsteroidal anti-inflammatory analgesic the day of the procedure, before the procedure.

During the procedure
　Use a child-sized surgical rubber mouth prop to support the patient's comfortable opening; remove periodically to reduce joint stiffness.
　Consider intravenous sedation and/or inhalation analgesia.
　Provide frequent rest periods to avoid prolonged opening.
　Apply moist heat to masticatory muscles during rest breaks.
　Gently massage masticatory muscles during rest breaks.
　Perform the procedure in the morning, when reserve is likely to be greatest.

After the procedure
　Extend the use of muscle relaxant and NSAID medication as necessary.
　Apply cold compresses to the TMJ and muscle areas during the 24 hours after the procedure.

NSAID = nonsteroidal anti-inflammatory drug; TMJ = temporomandibular joint.

pain. The majority of cases of ADD occur without significant pain or joint dysfunction. MRI studies have demonstrated that ADD is present in 25 to 35% of the normal asymptomatic adult population.[271,272] This is similar to the finding of asymptomatic clinically insignificant disc displacement that is well documented in the knee and spine.[273,274] ADD of the TMJ does not appear to affect children below the age of 5 years.[275]

The most common disc displacement is anterior and medial to the condyle.[276] It is theorized that ADD occurs more frequently when the superior head of the lateral pterygoid muscle attaches to the disc. This attachment would pull a loosened disc anterior and medial to the condyle. Posterior disc displacement (when a portion of the disc is found posterior to the top of the condyle) is rare but has been reported in the literature.[277]

A specific etiology in the majority of cases of disc displacement is poorly understood. Some cases result from direct trauma to the joint from a blow to the mandible. It is also generally believed that chronic low-grade microtrauma resulting from long-term bruxism or clenching of the teeth is a major cause of ADD. Studies using arthroscopic examination of the TMJ have demonstrated a relationship between intracapsular disorders and bruxism.[278] There is evidence that ADD may be associated with a generalized laxity of joints.[279] Craniofacial morphology may also play a role in ADD.[280]

Clinicians have also theorized that indirect trauma from cervical flexion extension injuries or certain types of malocclusion may also predispose an individual to disc displacement. These theories are not proven, and the events that result in ADD are unknown. It is likely that a combination of mechanisms related to the anatomy of the joint and the facial skeleton, connective tissue chemistry, and chronic loading of the joint increases the susceptibility of certain individuals to a disturbance of the restraining ligaments and displacement of the disc. ADD results in significant pain or dysfunction when accompanied by capsulitis and synovitis.

CLINICAL MANIFESTATIONS

Disc displacement is divided into stages based on signs and symptoms combined with the results of diagnostic imaging. A simple classification system divides ADD into (1) anterior disc displacement with reduction (clicking joint), (2) anterior disc displacement with intermittent locking, and (3) anterior disc displacement without reduction (closed lock).

Anterior Disc Displacement with Reduction.　This condition is caused by an articular disc that has been displaced from its position on top of the condyle due to elongation or tearing of the restraining ligaments. An alteration in the form of the disc has also been proposed as a possible factor. A reducing disc displacement is common in the general population, and a clicking or popping joint is of little clinical significance unless it is accompanied by pain, loss of function, and/or intermittent locking. An individual may seek professional advice regarding treatment of an audible click that is not accompanied by pain but that may be socially embarrassing.

The clinician must distinguish the patient with myofascial pain and coincidental clicking from the patient whose pain is related directly to disc displacement. Clinicians should also be aware that symptoms of pain and dysfunction associated with anterior disc displacement with reduction usually resolve over time with minimal noninvasive therapy.[281]

Palpation and auscultation of the TMJ will reveal a clicking or popping sound during both opening and closing mandibular movements (reciprocal click). The clicking or popping sound due to anterior disc displacement with reduction is characterized by a click that may occur on opening in the early, middle, or late movement and in the closing movement just before the teeth come in contact. This is due to movement of the disc as the condyle translates. Clinicians examining patients with ADD may observe a deflection of the mandible early in the opening cycle prior to the click with correction to the midline after the click. Tenderness of the joint will be present when ADD is accompanied by capsulitis or synovitis.

Anterior Disc Displacement without Reduction (Closed Lock).　Closed lock may be the first sign of TMD occurring after trauma or severe long-term nocturnal bruxism. It is detected more frequently in patients with clicking joints that progress to intermittent brief locking and then permanent locking. A patient with an acute closed lock will often have a history of a long-standing TMJ click that abruptly disappears followed by a sudden restriction in mandibular opening. This limited mandibular opening occurs due to disc interference with the normal translation of the condyle. Other findings include pain directly over the joint during mandibular opening (especially at maximum opening) and limited lateral movement to the side away from the affected joint. During maximum mouth opening, the mandible will deviate toward the affected side. The condyle on the affected side will not translate normally and will not be as palpable on examination. In chronic closed lock, the disc will deform and maximum mouth opening will gradually improve. The displacement of the disc exposes the posterior attachment to compression by the condyle. The posterior attachment has been shown to react to the change by depositing hyaline in the connective tissue[282] and has been called a "pseudomeniscus."[283]

Posterior Disc Displacement.   Posterior disc displacement has been described as the condyle slipping over the anterior rim of the disc during opening, with the disc being caught and brought backward in an abnormal relationship to the condyle when the mouth is closed. The disc is folded in the dorsal part of the joint space, preventing full mouth closure.[284] The clinical features are (1) a sudden inability to bring the upper and lower teeth together in maximal occlusion, (2) pain in the affected joint when trying to bring the teeth firmly together, (3) displacement forward of the mandible on the affected side, (4) restricted lateral movement to the affected side, and (5) no restriction of mouth opening.[284]

MANAGEMENT

Longitudinal studies demonstrate that most symptoms associated with ADD resolve over time either with no treatment or with minimal conservative therapy.[285] One study of patients with symptomatic anterior disc displacement without reduction experienced resolution without treatment in 75% of cases after 2.5 years.[286] Since symptoms associated with anterior disc displacement with and without reduction tend to decrease with time, the clinician should not treat patients on the assumption that asymptomatic clicking will inevitably progress to painful clicking or locking. Painful clicking or locking should initially be treated with conservative therapy

Recommended treatments for symptomatic ADD include splint therapy, physical therapy including manual manipulation, anti-inflammatory drugs, arthrocentesis, arthroscopic lysis and lavage, arthroplasty, and vertical ramus osteotomy. Many of these nonsurgical and surgical techniques are effective in decreasing pain and in increasing the range of mandibular motion, although the abnormal position of the disc is not usually corrected.[287]

Anterior Disc Displacement with Reduction.   Patients with TMJ clicking or popping that is not accompanied by pain do not require therapy. Flat-plane stabilization splints that do not change mandibular position and anterior repositioning splints have both been used to treat painful clicking. Anterior repositioning splints maintain the mandible in an anterior position, preventing the condyle from closing posterior to the disc. One meta-analysis that summarized the results of previous studies concluded that repositioning splints were

more effective than stabilization splints in eliminating both clicking and pain in patients with ADD.[288] Clinicians must weigh the potential benefits of using repositioning splints against the potential adverse effects that include tooth movement and open bite. Clinicians have advocated techniques that are designed to "recapture" the disc to its normal position, but splint therapy, arthrocentesis, or arthroscopy rarely corrects disc position and function. Painful symptoms resolve, although the disc remains displaced.

Anterior Disc Displacement without Reduction.   Some patients with closed lock may present with little or no pain, whereas others have severe pain during mandibular movement. Treatment options should depend on the degree of pain and limitation associated with the ADD. Management of a locked TMJ may be nonsurgical or surgical. The goals of successful therapy are to eliminate pain, restore function, and increase the range of mandibular motion. Correcting the disc position is not necessary to achieve these goals.

Patients who present with restricted movement but minimal pain frequently benefit from manual manipulation and an exercise program designed to increase mandibular motion. A flat-plane occlusal stabilization appliance to decrease the adverse effects of bruxism on the affected joint is appropriate. Sato and colleagues reported that a combination of a flat-plane stabilization splint and anti-inflammatory drugs was successful in reducing pain and increasing the range of motion in over 75% of patients.[285] The success of this therapy was attributed to decreased inflammation and to the gradual elongation of the posterior attachment, permitting increased translation of the condyle. Patients with severe pain on mandibular movement may benefit from either arthrocentesis or arthroscopy. Flushing the joint and deposition of intra-articular corticosteroids to decrease inflammation or sodium hyaluronate to increase joint lubrication and decrease adhesions have been reported to decrease pain associated with nonreducing disc displacements.[290] A significant reduction in the range of movement was associated with a less favorable treatment outcome.[291]

Kurita and colleagues reported on a 2½-year follow-up on patients with ADD without reduction. Approximately 40% of patients became asymptomatic, 33% continued to have symptoms at a decreased level, and 25% had no improvement. An association was noted between continued TMD symptoms and radiographically detectable degenerative changes.[281] Permanent disc displacement promotes the development of fibrous adhesions in the superior joint compartment.[292] In most cases discs do not reduce but show increased mobility.[293]

Temporomandibular Joint Arthritis

OSTEOARTHRITIS (DEGENERATIVE JOINT DISEASE)

Degenerative joint disease (DJD), also referred to as osteoarthrosis, osteoarthritis, and degenerative arthritis, is primarily a disorder of articular cartilage and subchondral bone, with secondary inflammation of the synovial membrane. It is a localized joint disease without systemic manifestations. The process begins in loaded articular cartilage that thins, clefts (fibrillation), and then fragments. This leads to sclerosis of underlying bone, subchondral cysts, and osteophyte formation.[294] The articular changes are essentially a response of the joint to chronic microtrauma or pressure. Microtrauma may be in the form of continuous abrasion of the articular surfaces as in natural wear associated with age or due to increased loading possibly related to chronic parafunctional activity. The fibrous tissue covering in patients with degenerative disease is preserved.[295] This may be a factor in remodeling and the recovery that is usually expected in osteoarthrosis and osteoarthritis of the TMJs. The relationship between internal derangements and DJD is unclear, but a higher frequency of radiographic signs of DJD was observed in subjects with disc displacement without reduction.[296]

DJD may be categorized as primary or secondary, although both are similar on histopathologic examination. Primary DJD is of unknown origin, but genetic factors play an important role. It is often asymptomatic and is most commonly seen in patients above the age of 50 years, although early arthritic changes can be observed in younger individuals. Secondary DJD results from a known underlying cause, such as trauma, congenital dysplasia, or metabolic disease.

Proposed risk factors include gender, diet, genetics, and psychological stress. Epidemiologic studies suggest a female predisposition to TMDs, including osteoarthritis.[139] How estrogen might contribute to osteoarthritis is unknown, but estrogen receptors have been identified on TMJ articular tissues.[297] The possibility that a diet of excessively hard or chewy foods might cause increased loads on the joints and lead to degenerative changes has been proposed but is speculative. Psychological stress leading to parafunctional activities such as tooth clenching or bruxing has been proposed as a factor. In addition to loading the joint, psychological stress might lead to biologic, biochemical, and hormonal changes that might contribute to changes in the joints, leading to osteoarthritis. A significant association has been observed between ADD and osteoarthritis.[398] The mechanisms and pathogenesis remain unknown.

The present model suggests that excessive mechanical loading on the joints produces a cascade of events leading to the failure of the lubrication system and destruction of the articular surfaces. These events include the generation of free radicals, the release of proinflammatory neuropeptides, signaling by cytokines, and the activation of enzymes capable of matrix degradation.[299]

Clinical Manifestations. DJD of the TMJ begins early and has been observed in over 20% of joints in individuals over the age of 20 years.[300] A study of patients below the age of 30 years presenting to a TMD clinic demonstrated that two-thirds of the patients had degenerative changes detected on tomograms.[301] The incidence of degenerative changes increases with age. Degenerative changes are found in over 40% of patients over 40 years of age. A direct relationship irrespective of age was observed between the rate and extent of dental attrition and degenerative disease of the TMJs in cadavers of aboriginal humans.[302] Many patients with mild to moderate DJD of the TMJ have no symptoms, although arthritic changes are observed on radiographs.

Degenerative changes of the TMJ detected on radiographic examination may be incidental and may not be responsible for facial pain symptoms or TMJ dysfunction; however, some degenerative changes may be underdiagnosed by conventional radiography because the defects are confined to the articular soft tissue. These soft tissues changes are better visualized with MRI.[303]

Patients with symptomatic DJD of the TMJ experience pain directly over the affected condyle, limitation of mandibular opening, crepitus, and a feeling of stiffness after a period of inactivity. Examination reveals tenderness and crepitus on intra-auricular and pretragus palpation. Deviation of the mandible to the painful side may be present. Radiographic findings in DJD may include narrowing of the joint space, irregular joint space, flattening of the articular surfaces, osteophyte formation, anterior lipping of the condyle, and the presence of subchondral cysts. These changes may be seen best on tomograms or CT scans (see Figure 11). The presence of joint effusion is most accurately detected in T2-weighted MRIs.

RHEUMATOID ARTHRITIS (RA)

RA is an inflammatory disease affecting periarticular tissue and secondarily bone. The percentage of RA patients with TMJ involvement ranges from 40 to 80%, depending on the group studied and the imaging technique used.[303–306] Studies using conventional radiography and tomography find fewer abnormalities than detectable on CT.[303] TMJ changes on CT were found in 88% of RA patients, but changes were also detected in more than 50% of controls.[306] CT changes did not correlate with clinical complaints. Avrahami and colleagues detected condylar changes in approximately 80% of RA patients using high-resolution CT.[303] Ackerman and colleagues, using tomography, detected erosive condylar changes in two-thirds of RA patients and stated that symptoms were related to the severity of radiographic changes.[244,307] The disease process starts as a vasculitis of the synovial membrane. It progresses to chronic inflammation marked by an intense round cell infiltrate and subsequent formation of granulation tissue. The cellular infiltrate spreads from the articular surfaces eventually to cause an erosion of the underlying bone.

Clinical Manifestations. The TMJs in RA are usually involved bilaterally. Pain is usually associated with the early acute phase of the disease but is not a common complaint in later stages. Other symptoms often noted include morning stiffness, joint sounds, and tenderness and swelling over the joint area.[308] The symptoms are usually transient in nature, and only a small percentage of patients with RA of the TMJs experience permanent clinically significant disability.

The most consistent clinical findings include pain on joint palpation, limited mouth opening, and crepitus. Micrognathia and an anterior open bite are commonly seen in patients with juvenile idiopathic arthritis. Larheim attributes the micrognathia to a combination of direct injury to the condylar head and altered orofacial muscular activity.[309] Ankylosis of the TMJ related to RA is rare. Radiographic changes in the TMJ associated with RA may include a narrow joint space, destructive lesions of the condyle, and limited condylar movement. There is little evidence of marginal proliferation or other reparative activity in RA in contrast to the radiographic changes often observed in degenerative joint disease. High-resolution CT of the TMJs in RA patients shows erosions of the condyle and glenoid fossa that are not detected on conventional radiography.[303]

Treatment. Involvement of the TMJ in RA is usually treated with anti-inflammatory drugs in conjunction with the therapy for the systemic disease.[310] The patient should be placed on a soft diet during the acute exacerbation. Use of a flat-plane occlusal appliance may be helpful, particularly if parafunctional habits are present. An exercise program to increase mandibular movement should be instituted as soon as possible after the acute symptoms subside. Intra-articular steroids should be considered.[311] Prostheses appear to decrease symptoms in fully or partially edentulous patients.[312]

Surgical treatment of the joints, including placement of prosthetic joints, is indicated in patients who have severe functional impairment or intractable pain not successfully managed by other means. Orthognathic surgery and orthodontics are required for correction of facial deformity resulting from arthritis during growth.

SERONEGATIVE SPONDYLOARTHROPATHIES

Several arthropathies that are distinct from RA are not associated with positive serology (rheumatoid factor). These disorders, characterized by arthritis, are known as the seronegative spondyloarthropathies and include ankylosing spondylitis, psoriatic arthritis, and Reiter's syndrome. The TMJs can be involved in these arthropathies. The clinical manifestations are joint pain with function, limited mouth opening, and erosion of the superior surface of the condyle on radiography. There are no specific findings that are pathognomonic of involvement of the TMJs.

Ankylosing spondylitis (AS) primarily involves the spine, although other joints are often involved. It causes inflammation that can lead to new bone formation, causing the spine to fuse, reducing mobility, and producing a forward, stooped posture. The disease usually involves the sacroiliac joints where the spine joins the pelvis. TMJ involvement has been reported in AS, but the prevalence has not been established. Wenneberg estimated that the TMJ was involved in about 15 to 20% of patients with AS.[313] Significantly decreased mouth opening, TMJ pain, crepitus, and muscle pain are frequent clinical findings.[314]

Psoriatic arthritis (PA) is a chronic disease characterized by psoriasis and inflammation of the joints. Approximately 10% of patients who have psoriasis develop joint inflammation. The skin lesions may precede the joint involvement by several years. PA commonly involves the fingers and spine, and pitting of the nails is common. The cause is unknown, and the disease presents in a variety of forms.[315]

The masticatory system is affected in about 50% of patients.[316,317] The symptoms of PA of the TMJ are similar to those noted in RA, except that the signs and symptoms are likely to be unilateral.[318] TMJ pain with chewing is a common finding.[317] Limitation of mouth opening may occur.[319] The most common radiographic finding is erosion of cortical outline of the mandibular condyle.[320] Coronal CT is particularly useful in showing TMJ changes of PA.[321]

Reiter's syndrome includes polyarthritis, urethritis, and conjunctivitis. It is thought to be triggered by infection, but the arthritis is not septic. Reiter's syndrome occurs more frequently in males in the third decade. The syndrome usually follows venereal infection most often involving *Chlamydia*, *Mycoplasma*, or *Yersinia*. Approximately 25% of male patients with Reiter's syndrome reported recurrent pain, swelling, and/or stiffness of the TMJ.

CONNECTIVE TISSUE DISEASE

Connective tissue diseases that affect the TMJ include systemic lupus, systemic sclerosis (scleroderma), undifferentiated connective tissue disease, and mixed connective tissue disease. When the TMJ is involved, the clinical presentation is similar to other disorders causing inflammation and subsequent degenerative changes. A clinical examination supplemented with diagnostic imaging is usually adequate to confirm involvement of the TMJ.

DISEASES ASSOCIATED WITH CRYSTAL DEPOSITS IN JOINTS

Gout is a disease that includes hyperuricemia, recurrent arthritides, renal disease, and urolithiasis. The disease primarily affects men. Acute pain in a single joint is the characteristic clinical presentation. The TMJ is not commonly involved. Calcium pyrophosphate deposition is also known as pseudogout. Deposits of microcrystals in affected joints are responsible for the clinical manifestations. The TMJ is rarely involved. Examination of aspirated synovial fluid from the involved joint by polarized light and detection of monosodium urate crystals confirms the diagnosis. Treatment includes colchicine, NSAIDs, and intra-articular steroid injection. Pseudogout affecting the TMJ has been treated with colchicine and arthrocentesis.

TREATMENT

Osteoarthritis, the spondyloarthropathies, RA, and other connective tissue diseases that affect the TMJs result in TMJ inflammation. The process eventually leads to the degenerative changes that manifests as joint pain and crepitus, loss of function and range of movement, and, in severe cases, facial deformity. Treatment is directed toward the systemic disease with supportive local therapy consisting of jaw self-care, physiotherapy, oral appliance therapy, topical NSAID, and intra-articular corticosteroid injection.

The DJD of the TMJ can usually be managed by conservative treatment with an emphasis on physical therapy and NSAIDS that control both pain and inflammation. In osteoarthritis, significant improvement is noted in many patients after 9 months, and a "burning out" of many cases occurs after 1 year.[322] Nonsurgical management may consist of jaw self-management, including behavior modification, heat application, soft diet, physical therapy including jaw exercises, NSAID, and oral appliance therapy. When nonsurgical management is not effective, then direct joint therapy; intra-articular corticosteroid injection is indicated.[323] Arthrocentesis is a relatively conservative joint procedure if intra-articular steroid injection is ineffective.[324] Arthroscopy, arthroplasty, and arthrotomy are surgical procedures that may be indicated depending on the response to more conservative treatment and the severity of pain and disability.[325] It seems prudent to manage a patient with conservative treatment for 6 months to 1 year before considering surgery unless severe pain or dysfunction persists after an adequate trial of nonsurgical therapy.

Only when there is intractable TMJ pain or disabling limitation of mandibular movement is surgery indicated. Arthroplasty or condylectomy with placement of costochondral grafts has been performed successfully.[326]

SYNOVIAL CHONDROMATOSIS

Synovial chondromatosis (SC) is an uncommon benign disorder characterized by the presence of multiple cartilaginous nodules of the synovial membrane that break off resulting in clusters of free-floating loose calcified bodies in the joint. It is theorized that SC originates from embryonic mesenchymal remnants of the subintimal layer of the synovium that become metaplastic, calcify, and break off into the joint space.[327,328] SC most commonly involves one joint, but cases of multi-articular SC have been reported.[329] Some cases appear to be triggered by trauma, whereas others are of unknown etiology. The knee and elbow are most commonly involved, and less than 100 cases of SC of the TMJ have been reported in the world medical literature.

More sophisticated imaging techniques, such as CT, and arthroscopy have revealed cases of SC that previously would have received other diagnoses, causing authors of recent publications to suspect that SC is more common than previously believed.[330–333] Extension of SC from the TMJ to surrounding tissues (including the parotid gland, middle ear, or middle cranial fossa) may occur.[333]

Slow progressive swelling in the pretragus region, pain, and limitation of mandibular movement are the most common presenting features. TMJ clicking, locking, crepitus, and occlusal changes may also be present.[328] The extension of the lesion from the joint capsule and involvement of surrounding tissues may make diagnosis difficult, causing SC to be confused with parotid, middle ear, or intracranial tumors. Cases of SC that were mistaken for a chondrosarcoma have been reported. Intracranial extension may lead to neurologic deficits such as facial nerve paralysis. Conventional radiography may not lead to the diagnosis due to superimposition of cranial bones that may obscure the calcified loose bodies.[334] A CT scan should be obtained if SC is suspected after clinical evaluation. The lesion may appear as a single mass or as many small loose bodies.[330] Arthroscopy may be necessary for accurate diagnosis, particularly when the loose bodies are not calcified and cannot be visualized by conventional radiology or CT.[335]

Treatment should be conservative and consist of removal of the mass of loose bodies. This may be done arthroscopically when only a small lesion is present, but arthrotomy is required for larger lesions. The synovium and articular disc should be removed when they are involved. Lesions that extend beyond the joint space may require extensive resection.

SEPTIC ARTHRITIS

Septic arthritis of the TMJ most commonly occurs in patients with previously existing joint disease such as RA or underlying medical disorders (particularly diabetes). Patients receiving immunosuppressive drugs or long-term corticosteroids also have an increased incidence of septic arthritis. The infection of the TMJ may result from bloodborne bacterial infection or by extension of infection from adjacent sites, such as the middle ear, maxillary molars, and parotid gland.[336] Gonococci are the primary bloodborne agents causing septic arthritis in a previously normal TMJ, whereas *Staphylococcus aureus* is the most common organism involved in previously arthritic joints.[337]

Symptoms of septic arthritis of the TMJ include trismus, deviation of the mandible to the affected side, severe pain on movement, and an inability to occlude the teeth, owing to the presence of inflammation in the joint space. Examination reveals redness and swelling over the involved joint. In some cases, the swelling may be fluctuant and extend beyond the region of the joint.[337] Large tender cervical lymph nodes are frequently observed on the side of the infection. Diagnosis is made by detection of bacteria on Gram's stain and culture of aspirated joint fluid.

Serious sequelae of septic arthritis include osteomyelitis of the temporal bone, brain abscess, and ankylosis. Facial asymmetry may accompany septic arthritis of the TMJ, especially in children. Of the 44 cases of ankylosis of the TMJ reviewed by Topazian, 17 resulted from infection.[338] The primary sources of these infections were the middle ear, teeth, and the hematologic spread of gonorrhea.

Evaluation of patients with suspected septic arthritis must include a review of signs and symptoms of gonorrhea, such as purulent urethral discharge or dysuria. The affected TMJ should be aspirated and the fluid obtained tested by Gram's stain and cultured for *Neisseria gonorrhoeae*.

Treatment of septic arthritis of the TMJ consists of surgical drainage, joint irrigation, and 4 to 6 weeks of antibiotics.

Developmental Defects

Developmental disturbances involving the TMJ may result in anomalies in the size and shape of the condyle. Hyperplasia, hypoplasia, agenesis, and the formation of a bifid condyle may be evident on radiographic examination of the joint. Local factors, such as trauma or infection, can initiate condylar growth disturbances.

True condylar hyperplasia usually occurs after puberty and is completed by 18 to 25 years of age. Limitation and deviation of mouth opening and facial asymmetry may be observed.

Facial asymmetry often results from disturbances in condylar growth because the condyle is a site for compensatory growth and adaptive remodeling. The facial deformities associated with condylar hyperplasia involve the formation of a convex ramus on the affected side and a concave shape on the normal side. If the condylar hyperplasia is detected and surgically corrected at an early stage, the facial deformities may be prevented. Bone scintigraphy is recommended as part of a presurgical evaluation to identify activity in the joint.[339]

Deviation of the mandible to the affected side and facial deformities also are associated with unilateral agenesis and hypoplasia of the condyle. Rib grafts have been used to replace the missing condyle to minimize the facial asymmetry in agenesis. In cases of hypoplasia, there is a short wide ramus, shortening of the body of the mandible, and antegonial notching on the affected side, with elongation of the mandibular body and flatness of the face on the opposite side. Early surgical intervention is again emphasized to limit facial deformity.

Hyperplasia of the coronoid process is an uncommon cause of restricted mouth opening but may be missed in the differential diagnosis of restricted mouth opening. One study estimated that 5% of 163 patients had restricted mouth opening due to elongation of the coronoid process.[340]

Fractures

Fractures of the condylar head and neck often result from a blow to the chin (see Figure 15). The patient with a condylar fracture usually presents with pain and edema over the joint area and limitation and deviation of the mandible to the injured side on opening. Bilateral condylar fractures may result in an anterior open bite. The diagnosis of a condylar fracture is confirmed by diagnostic imaging. Intracapsular nondisplaced fractures of the condylar head are usually not treated surgically. Early mobilization of the mandible is emphasized to prevent bony or fibrous ankylosis.

Dislocation

In dislocation of the mandible, the condyle is positioned anterior to the articular eminence and cannot return to its normal position without assistance. This disorder contrasts with subluxation, in which the condyle moves anterior to the eminence during wide opening but is able to return to the resting position without manipulation. It has been

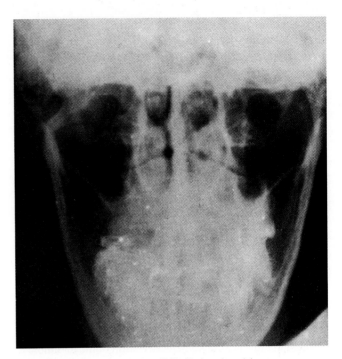

FIGURE 15 Fractured and medially displaced condyle.

demonstrated that subluxation is a variation of normal function and that the normal range of motion of the condyle is not limited to the fossa.

Dislocations of the mandible usually result from muscular incoordination in wide opening during eating or yawning and less commonly from trauma; they may be unilateral or bilateral. The typical complaints of the patient with dislocation are an inability to close the jaws and pain related to muscle spasm. On clinical examination, a deep depression may be observed in the pretragus region corresponding to the condyle being positioned anterior to the eminence.

The condyle can usually be repositioned without the use of muscle relaxants or general anesthetics. If muscle spasms are severe and reduction is difficult, the use of intravenous diazepam (approximately 10 mg) can be beneficial. The practitioner who is repositioning the mandible should stand in front of the seated patient and place his or her thumbs lateral to the mandibular molars on the buccal shelf of bone; the remaining fingers of each hand should be placed under the chin. The condyle is repositioned by a downward and backward movement. This is achieved by simultaneously pressing down on the posterior part of the mandible while raising the chin. As the condyle reaches the height of the eminence, it can usually be guided posteriorly to its normal position.

Postreduction recommendations consist of limiting mandibular movement and the use of NSAIDs to lessen inflammation. The patient should be cautioned not to open wide when eating or yawning because recurrence is common, especially during the period initially after repositioning. Long periods of immobilization are not advised due to the risk of fibrous ankylosis.

Chronic recurring dislocations have been treated with surgical and nonsurgical approaches. Injections of sclerosing solutions have been used but are not used as often now because of difficulty in controlling the extent of fibrosis and condylar limitation. Various surgical procedures have been advocated for treating recurrent dislocations of the mandible; these include bone grafting to the eminence, lateral pterygoid myotomy, eminence reduction, eminence augmentation with implants, shortening the temporalis tendon by intraoral scarification, plication of the joint capsule, and repositioning of the zygomatic arch.

Ankylosis

True bony ankylosis of the TMJ involves fusion of the head of the condyle to the temporal bone. Trauma to the chin is the most common cause of TMJ ankylosis, although infections also may be involved.[338] Children are more prone to ankylosis because of greater osteogenic potential and an incompletely formed disc. Ankylosis frequently results from prolonged immobilization following condylar fracture. Limited mandibular movement, deviation of the mandible to the affected side on opening, and facial asymmetry may be observed in TMJ ankylosis. Osseous deposition may be seen on radiographs. Ankylosis has been treated by several surgical procedures. Gap arthroplasty using interpositional materials between the cut segments is the technique most commonly performed.

Bruxism

Nocturnal bruxing is thought to aggravate or contribute to the persistence of pain symptoms associated with TMD. The etiology is not understood, but the evidence suggests that occlusal abnormalities are not the cause.[341,342] Occlusal appliances may protect the teeth from the effects of bruxism but cannot be expected to prevent or decrease the bruxing activity.[343] When bruxing is considered to be the cause or a factor of TMD symptoms, oral appliance therapy is effective, but symptoms are likely to return when appliance therapy is withdrawn.[344] In one report, nocturnal aversive biofeedback and splint therapy caused a decrease in the frequency and duration of bruxing, but bruxing activity returned after treatment was withdrawn.[345] Occlusal splints worn during sleep have not been found to stop bruxing but do reduce the signs of bruxing.[346]

Recently, reports of bruxism and symptoms of facial pain, earache, and headache associated with the use of selective serotonin reuptake inhibitors (SSRIs) have been published.[347] Symptoms of bruxing resolved when the dosage was decreased or when buspirone was added.[348] Buspirone has a postsynaptic dopaminergic effect and may act to partially restore suppressed dopamine levels associated with the use of SSRIs.

Tang and Jankovic injected severe bruxers in the masseter muscles with botulinum toxin in an open-label prospective trial and reported significant improvement in symptoms and minimal adverse effects.[349] The treatment effect lasted approximately 5 months and had to be repeated. Botulinum toxin exerts a paralytic effect on the muscle by inhibiting the release of acetylcholine at the neuromuscular junction.

Oral Dyskinesia

Oral dyskinesias are abnormal, involuntary movements of the tongue, lips, and jaw. The term *tardive dyskinesia* was introduced in 1964 to describe a dyskinesia associated with antipsychotic medication.[350] The prevalence of tardive dyskinesia in patients treated chronically with conventional antipsychotic medication is estimated to be approximately 20%.[351] Oral dyskinesias may be a factor contributing to muscle stiffness, TMJ degenerative changes, mucosal lesions, damage to teeth, and dental prostheses. Tardive dyskinesia has been reported to cause facial pain.[352]

Complete loss of teeth is considered to be one cause of oral dyskinesia. Ill-fitting dentures or the lack of replacements may initiate dyskinesia.[353]

Oromandibular dystonia produces involuntary and excessive contractions of tongue, lip, and jaw muscles. The etiology and pathophysiology are unknown. The proposed mechanism is related to defective inhibitory control of the basal ganglia of the forebrain, thalamus, and brainstem.

Dyskinesias are characterized clinically by the observation of involuntary mouth movements and the effects of these movements on the jaw muscles, TMJs, oral mucosa, and teeth. Emphasis on management is prevention since no one treatment is predictably effective and safe. A dentist observing dyskinesia in a patient taking conventional antipsychotics should inform the physician managing the medication. Tardive dyskinesia may be persistent even after drug therapy is stopped.

Palliative treatment using tetrabenazine, a central monoamine depleter, clonazepam, and baclofen has been tried.[353] Injection of botulinum toxin has been used in cases of oromandibular dystonia.[354] Severely disabling and refractory conditions have been treated with neurosurgical intervention.[355]

▼ SELECTED READINGS

Clark GT, Minakuchi H. Oral appliances. In: Laskin DM, Greene CS, Hylander WL, editors. TMDs, an evidence-based approach to diagnosis and treatment. Chicago: Quintessence; 2006. p. 377–90.

Clark GT, Seligman DA, Solberg WK, Pullinger AG. Guidelines for the examination and diagnosis of temporomandibular disorders. J Craniomandib Disord 1989;3:7–14.

Dworkin S, LeResche L. Research Diagnostic Criteria for Temporomandibular Disorders: review, criteria, examinations, and specifications, critique. J Craniomandib Disord 1992;6:301–35.

Dworkin SF. Psychological and psychosocial assessment. In: Laskin DM, Greene CS, Hylander WL, editors. TMDs, an evidence-based approach to diagnosis and treatment. Chicago: Quintessence; 2006. p. 203–17.

Fricton J, Kroening R, Hathaway K. TMJ and craniofacial pain: diagnosis and management. St. Louis: Ishiyaku Euroamerica; 1988.

Kreiner M, Betancor E, Clark GT. Occlusal stabilization appliances. Evidence of their efficacy. J Am Dent Assoc 2001;132:770–7.

Kurita K, Westesson PL, Yuasa H, et al. Natural course of untreated symptomatic temporomandibular joint disc displacement without reduction. J Dent Res 1998;77:361–5.

Lund JP. Muscular pain and dysfunction. In: Laskin DM, Greene CS, Hylander WL, editors. Temporomandibular disorders, an evidence-based approach to diagnosis and treatment. Chicago: Quintessence; 2006. p. 99.

Milam SB. TMJ osteoarthritis. In: Laskin DM, Greene CS, Hylander WL, editors. TMDs, an evidence-based approach to diagnosis and treatment. Chicago: Quintessence; 2006. p. 105–23.

National Institutes of Health. Management of temporomandibular disorders: NIH technology assessment statement. 1996.

National Institutes of Health Technology Assessment Conference on Management of Temporomandibular Disorders. Oral Surg Oral Med Oral Pathol Oral Radiol Endod 1997;83:49–183.

Okeson J, editor. Orofacial pain: guidelines for assessment, diagnosis, and management. Chicago: Quintessence; 1996.

Rammelsberg P, Leresche L, Dworkin S, Mancl L. Longitudinal outcome of temporomandibular disorders: a 5-year epidemiologic study of muscle disorders defined by Research Diagnostic Criteria for Temporomandibular Disorders. J Orofac Pain 2003;17:9–20.

Sato S, Takahashi K, Kawamura H, Motegi K. The natural course of nonreducing disc displacement of the temporomandibular joint. Int J Oral Maxillofac Surg 1998;27:173–8.

Wanman A. Longitudinal course of symptoms of craniomandibular disorders in men and women. A 10-year follow-up study of an epidemiologic sample. Acta Odontol Scand 1996;54:337–42.

For the full reference list, please refer to the accompanying CD ROM.

10

OROFACIAL PAIN

BRUCE BLASBERG, DMD, FRCD(C)

ELI ELIAV, DMD, PhD

MARTIN S. GREENBERG, DDS

Orofacial pain (OFP) is the presenting symptom of a broad spectrum of diseases. As a symptom, it may be due to disease of the orofacial structures, generalized musculoskeletal or rheumatic disease, peripheral or central nervous system (CNS) disease, or psychological abnormality; or the pain may be referred from other sources (eg, cervical muscles or intracranial pathology). OFP may also occur in the absence of detectable physical, imaging, or laboratory abnormalities. Some of these disorders are easily recognized and treated, whereas others defy classification and are unresponsive to present treatment methods. The possible causes of orofacial pain are considerable and cross the boundaries of many medical and dental disciplines. An interdisciplinary approach is often required to establish a diagnosis and for treatment.

This chapter discusses new developments that have led to a better understanding of chronic pain and reviews the diagnosis and treatment of OFP disorders. Disorders of the musculoskeletal system that cause OFP are discussed in Chapter 9, "Temporomandibular Disorders."

▼ DEFINING PAIN

The concept of pain has evolved from that of a one-dimensional sensation to that of a multidimensional experience encompassing sensory-discriminative, cognitive, motivational, and affective qualities. The most recent definition of pain, produced by the Task Force on Taxonomy of the International Association for the Study of Pain (IASP) is, "An unpleasant sensory and emotional experience associated with actual or potential tissue damage, or described in terms of such damage."[1] An accompanying explanatory note emphasizes the subjective and emotional nature of pain, as well as the lack of correlation between pain and tissue damage:

Note: Pain is always subjective. Each individual learns the application of the word through experiences related to injury in early life. Biologists recognize that those stimuli which cause pain are liable to damage tissue. Accordingly, pain is that experience we associate with actual or potential tissue damage. It is unquestionably a sensation in a part or parts of the body, but it is also always unpleasant and therefore also an emotional experience. Experiences which resemble pain but are not unpleasant, eg, pricking, should not be called pain. Unpleasant abnormal experiences (dysesthesias) may also be pain but are not necessarily so because, subjectively, they may not have the usual sensory qualities of pain.

Many people report pain in the absence of tissue damage or any likely pathophysiological cause; usually, this happens for psychological reasons. There is usually no way to distinguish their experience from that due to tissue damage if we take the subjective report. If they regard their experience as pain and if they report it in the same ways as pain caused by tissue damage, it should be accepted as pain. This definition avoids tying pain to the stimulus. Activity induced in the nociceptor and nociceptive pathways by a noxious stimulus is not pain, which is always a psychological state, even though we may well appreciate that pain most often has a proximate physical cause.[1]

Pain, in the medical model, is considered a symptom of disease, to be diagnosed and treated. Unfortunately, a cause and a diagnosis cannot always be established. Repeated attempts to identify a physical cause may result in unnecessary and sometimes harmful investigations and treatments. Establishing a precise diagnosis and providing effective treatment have become major challenges in medicine and dentistry. This has led to the development of a biobehavioral or biopsychosocial model to explain the phenomena observed in patients experiencing chronic pain. In this model, pain is not divided into physical versus psychological components. Instead, physical, psychological, and social factors are viewed as mutually influential forces with the potential to create an infinite number of unique pain experiences.[2] The biologic system deals with the anatomic, structural, and molecular substrates of disease. The psychological system deals with the effects of motivation and personality on the experience of illness and on reactions to illness. The social system deals with cultural, environmental, and familial influences on the expression and experience of illness. Each system affects and is affected by all of the others.[3]

The words *pain* and *suffering* have often been used synonymously, but the experience of suffering has been differentiated from pain. Suffering has been defined as including the experience of pain but as also including vulnerability, dehumanization, a lost sense of self, blocked coping efforts, a lack of control over time and space, and an inability to find meaning or purpose in the painful experience.[2] The term *suffering* attempts to convey the experience of pain beyond sensory attributes.

Anatomic Considerations

Cranial nerve V (CN V), the trigeminal nerve, is the dominant nerve that relays sensory impulses from the orofacial area to the CNS. The facial (CN VII), glossopharyngeal (CN IX), and vagus (CN X) nerves and the upper cervical nerves (C2 and C3) also relay sensory information from the face and surrounding area (Table 1). (For a more detailed study of this topic, the reader is referred to the sources listed in the "Suggested Readings" section at the end of this chapter.)

Primary sensory neurons associated with pain (nociceptors) are characterized by small-diameter axons with slow conduction velocities (ie, finely myelinated Aδ fibers and unmyelinated C fibers) (Figure 1). Nociceptors are activated by intense or noxious stimuli. Some are unimodal and respond only to thermal or mechanical stimuli; others are polymodal and respond to mechanical, thermal, and chemical stimuli. Nociceptors encode the intensity, duration, and quality of a noxious stimulus.

Information associated with pain is carried in the three divisions of the trigeminal nerve to the trigeminal sensory ganglion. The central processes of these neurons enter the pons, where they descend in the brainstem as the spinal trigeminal tract. Fibers from the spinal trigeminal tract synapse in the adjacent trigeminal nucleus that extends parallel to the tract in the brainstem. The spinal nucleus of CN V extends from the chief sensory nucleus of CN V to the spinal cord, where it merges with the dorsal gray matter. The spinal nucleus is divided into three nuclei; the most caudal, the nucleus caudalis, is continuous with and resembles the dorsal horn of the cervical spinal cord.[4] Morphologic, clinical, and electrophysiologic observations indicate that the nucleus caudalis is the principal site in the brainstem for nociceptive

TABLE 1 Cranial and Cervical Nerves that Provide Somatic and Visceral Sensation to the Orofacial Area

Nerve	General Area Served
V: Trigeminal	Skin of the face, forehead, and scalp as far as the top of the head; conjunctiva and bulb of the eye; oral and nasal mucosa; part of the external aspect of the tympanic membrane; teeth; anterior two-thirds of the tongue; masticatory muscles; TMJ; meninges of The anterior and middle cranial fossae
VII: Facial	Skin of the hollow of the auricle of the external ear; small area of skin behind the ear
IX: Glossopharyngeal	Mucosa of the pharynx; fauces; palatine tonsils; posterior one-third of the tongue; internal surface of the tympanic membrane; skin of the external ear
X: Vagus	Skin at the back of the ear; posterior wall and floor of external auditory meatus; tympanic membrane; meninges of posterior cranial fossa; pharynx; larynx
Cervical nerve 2	Back of the head extending to the vertex; behind and above the ear; submandibular, anterior neck
Cervical nerve 3	Lateral and posterior neck

TMJ = temporomandibular joint.

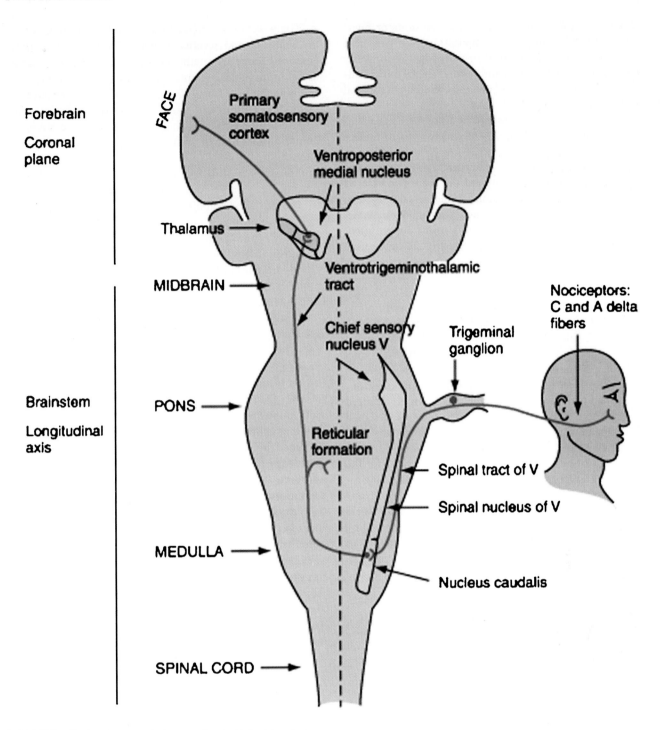

FIGURE 1 Nociceptive transmission associated with the trigeminal nerve.

information.[5–7] Axons from the spinal nucleus of CN V cross to the opposite side and ascend to the ventral posteromedial nucleus of the thalamus and also project to the reticular formation and the medial and intralaminar thalamic nuclei. From the thalamus, neurons course and end at the somatosensory cortex.

Measurement of Pain and Disability

There is no simple method of measuring pain. The intensity of an individual's pain is based on what is verbally or nonverbally communicated about the experience. Patients often express difficulty describing pain, and two people may have very different descriptions for pain that accompanies a similar injury. Within a specific diagnosis, great variability exists regarding the disabling effects of pain on an individual's life. Adding to this complexity is the lack of a direct correlation between the severity of a chronic pain disorder and the magnitude of the anatomic or pathologic change described by the clinical diagnosis.[8] In assessing OFP patients, pain intensity, emotional distress, and associated disability are important and cannot be captured with one scale or questionnaire. This has important implications for treatment because addressing the anatomic or pathologic abnormality alone may not eliminate pain and restore health. Individuals with cognitive impairment, infants, and children pose special challenges to the assessment of pain.

Pain intensity can be measured by using ratings such as a visual analogue scale (VAS). A VAS consists of a 10 cm line on which 0 cm is "no pain" and 10 cm is "pain as bad as it could be." The patient marks the point along the line that best represents his or her pain, and the score is measured from the "no pain" end of the scale. Numeric scales (eg, 1 to 10) and descriptive rating scales (eg, no pain, mild, moderate, severe pain) are also used. VASs are sensitive to treatment effects, can be incorporated into pain diaries, and can be used with children.[9,10]

The multidimensional aspects of pain are not well measured by scales that rate intensity. The McGill Pain Questionnaire (MPQ) (Figure 2) was created to measure the motivational-affective and the cognitive-evaluative qualities of pain, in addition to the sensory experience.[11] The questionnaire was designed to capture the multidimensional nature of pain and to provide quantitative measures of clinical pain that can be treated statistically. The questionnaire enables patients to choose from 78 adjectives (arranged in 20 groups) that describe pain. The form is designed to assess the sensory (groups 1 to 10), affective (groups 11 to 15), and evaluative (group 16) dimensions of pain and to produce a pain-rating index. There are also sections for the location and temporal characteristics of pain and a rating for present pain intensity.

The MPQ is used both by clinicians and researchers and has been helpful in pain research and treatment by providing a common language for assessing and comparing different pain experiences and treatment effects. Verbal descriptors have been shown to discriminate between reversible and irreversible damage of nerve fibers in a tooth and between trigeminal neuralgia (TN) and atypical facial pain (AFP).[12,13] Toothache pain and pain from burning mouth syndrome (BMS) were found to be equal in magnitude but significantly different in pain quality as assessed by the MPQ.[12]

Clinicians should include a rating or scale that can be used initially and during treatment to provide a reference for the course of the disorder and the treatment progress. VASs and numeric scales require no specific forms and are easily administered. The MPQ is available from the IASP and is used in pain clinics and by clinicians focusing on pain management.[14]

Patients experiencing pain may display a broad range of observable behaviors that communicate to others that they are experiencing pain (Table 2). These may be observable during the diagnostic interview or in response to physical examination procedures. An awareness of pain behaviors is valuable, but their presence or absence in any given situation is not necessarily diagnostic. These behaviors are often diminished or absent in patients with chronic pain and cannot be correlated with the presence or absence of pain or pain intensity.

The patient's self-report must be relied on for assessing the character and severity of pain. The scales and ratings described above are attempts to provide a rating that can be useful in diagnosis, treatment planning, treatment progress, and outcome assessment. Pain ratings also give the patient a method for keeping a pain diary to provide insight into what activities and events make the pain better or worse. VASs and numeric scales are relatively easy methods of charting pain intensity.

Assessments of disability related to a pain disorder and psychological status are important parts of any evaluation of chronic pain. Disability is defined as "a lack of the ability to function normally, physically or mentally."[15] The level of disability cannot be predicted on the basis of the anatomic diagnosis. One of the primary goals of chronic pain management (in addition to pain reduction) is the restoration of function. Since complete resolution of pain is often not possible, increasing function is an important measure of treatment success. There is no universally accepted method of assessing pain-related disability, but pain-related interference with activities and psychological impairments associated with pain are important aspects.

Turk and Rudy have developed the Multiaxial Assessment of Pain (MAP) classification and have tested it on several pain populations, including a group of patients with temporomandibular disorders (TMDs).[8,16,17] Their assessment included a 61-item questionnaire, the West Haven-Yale Multidimensional Pain Inventory (WHYMPI), which measures adjustment to pain from a cognitive-behavioral perspective.[18] The following three distinct profiles emerged: (1) "dysfunctional, characterized by patients who perceived the severity of their pain to be high, reported that pain interfered with much of their lives, reported a higher degree of affective distress, and maintained low levels of activity; (2) interpersonally distressed, characterized by a common perception that 'significant others' were not very understanding or supportive of the patient's problems; and (3) adaptive copers, patients with high levels of social support, relatively low levels of pain perceived interference, affective distress, and higher levels of activity and perceived control."[19] Turk and Rudy found that when they used the MAP profiles, psychosocial and behavioral response patterns to pain were similar despite different medical and dental diagnoses. An assessment in this domain can be combined with any classification scheme related to OFP disorders, to provide a more comprehensive profile of the presenting problem. Establishing a specific OFP diagnosis and assessing the psychosocial and behavioral issues are critical in the treatment and prognosis of chronic pain.

Dworkin and LeResche have developed a method for assessing dysfunctional chronic pain as part of a classification system, the Research Diagnostic Criteria.[20] They used the Graded Chronic Pain Severity scale, the depression and vegetative-symptom scales from the Symptom Checklist-90-Revised (SCL-90-R), and a "jaw disability checklist."[21,22] All three of these scales are based on questionnaires that are

Measurement of Pain

McGill Pain Questionnaire

Patient's Name ____________________ Date ____________ Time ______ am/pm

PRI: S ________ A ________ E ________ M ________ PRI(T) ________ PPI ________

(1-10) (11-15) (16) (17-20) (1-20)

1 FLICKERING, QUIVERING, PLUSING, THROBBING, BEATING, POUNDING

2 JUMPING, FLASHING, SHOOTING

3 PRICKING, BORING, DRILLING, STABBING, LANCINATING

4 SHARP, CUTTING, LACERATING

5 PINCHING, PRESSING, GNAWING, CRAMPING, CRUSHING

6 TUGGING, PULLING, WRENCHING

7 HOT, BURNING, SCALDING, SEARING

8 TINGLING, ITCHY, SMARTING, STINGING

9 DULL, SORE, HURTING, ACHING, HEAVY

10 TENDER, TAUT, RASPING, SPLITTING

11 TIRING, EXHAUSTING

12 SICKENING, SUFFOCATING

13 FEARFULL, FRIGHTFUL, TERRIFYING

14 PUNISHING, GRUELLING, CRUEL, VICIOUS, KILLING

15 WRETCHED, BLINDING

16 ANNOYING, TROUBLESOME, MISERABLE, INTENSE, UNBEARABLE

17 SPREADING, RADIATING, PENETRATING, PIERCING

18 TIGHT, NUMB, DRAWING, SQUEEZING, TEARING

19 COOL, COLD, FREEZING

20 NAGGING, NAUSEATING, AGONIZING, DREADFUL, TORTURING

PPI

0 NO PAIN
1 MILD
2 DISCOMFORTING
3 DISTRESSING
4 HORRIBLE
5 EXCRUCIATING

BRIEF	RHYTHMIC	CONTINUOUS
MOMENTARY	PERIODIC	STEADY
TRANSIENT	INTERMETTENT	CONSTANT

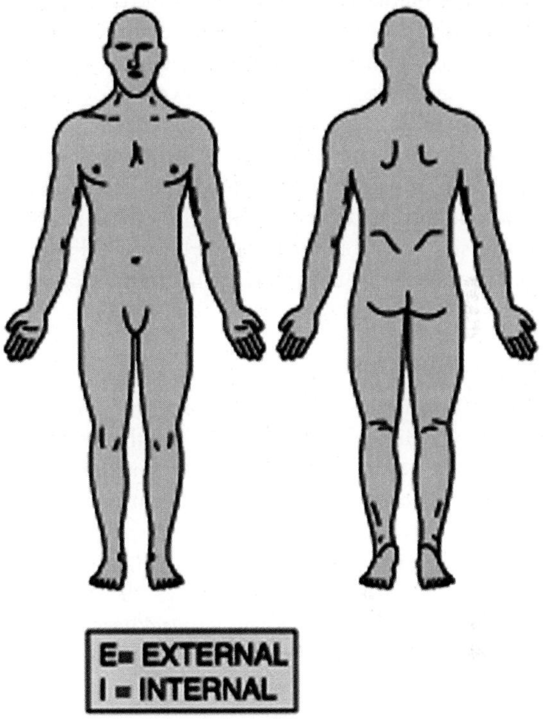

COMMENTS:

FIGURE 2 The McGill Pain Questionnaire.

TABLE 2   Observable Pain Behaviors

Behavior	Observations
Guarding	Abnormally slow, stiff, or interrupted movement
Bracing	Stiff, pain-avoidant posturing while in a static position
Rubbing	Touching, rubbing, or holding of the painful area
Sighing	Pronounced exhalation of air
Grimacing	Obvious facial expression of pain

Adapted from Keefe F et al.[14]

completed by the patient. The criteria were developed to advance the research in TMDs. The criteria require validation, but the design of the classification makes it applicable to clinical practice. The Graded Chronic Pain Severity scale has four grades of disability and pain intensity based on seven questions, of which three are related to pain intensity and four are related to disability. The SCL-90-R depression scales are used to identify patients who may be experiencing significant depression, a problem commonly associated with chronic pain. These issues are discussed further in the section on assessment in this chapter.

Quantitative Sensory Testing

The response to external stimuli has been part of the formal neurologic evaluation since the nineteenth century. Quantitative Sensory Testing (QST) is a set of sensory tests based on normal and non-normal responses to various noninvasive stimuli. QST is an accepted tool for the assessment of diabetic neuropathies and other sensory abnormalities.[23,24] However, it is important to note that, currently, QST cannot stand alone as a diagnostic tool.[23] The major weakness of the method is test accuracy dependent on patient response. Several stimulus randomizing protocols have been developed to overcome this problem.[25–27]

QST modalities (thermal, mechanical, electrical, etc.) selectively activate different sensory nerve fibers. Heat stimuli activate the thin nonmyelinated C fibers (0.3–1.5 μm diameter, conduction velocity 0.4–2 m/s) that comprise 60 to 90% of the cutaneous nerve fibers. In addition to the prevalent heat-activated C fibers, an important subset of C fibers is the polymodal nociceptors that respond to chemical, mechanical, and thermal nociceptive stimuli. Aδ fibers have a thin myelinated sheath (1–5 μm diameter, conduction velocity 4–30 m/s) and are activated mainly by cold stimuli, fast-onset contact, radiant (including laser) heat, and punctuate mechanical stimulation, such as a pin. Aβ fibers have a thicker myelin coat (6–12 μm diameter, conduction velocity 35–70 m/s) and mediate touch and vibratory sensations. Aα fibers are preferentially activated by pulsed electrical stimuli at the threshold for detection.

Three major levels of sensation can describe the response to external sensory stimuli: detection threshold, pain threshold, and pain tolerance.

The threshold value describes the lowest stimulus level that is either detected or produces pain. In the presence of pathology, both the pain and detection thresholds may be altered.

Data gathered from studies employing QST in various orofacial pathologies can provide an important clinical tool.

Joint-related TMDs revealed reduced electrical detection threshold,[28] whereas myogenic TMDs (either clinical or experimental) demonstrated mechanical, electrical, and vibrotactile elevated detection thresholds.[28–30] Sensory assessment of early oral malignant lesions demonstrated reduced electrical detection threshold in the nerve's territory that were exposed to the malignant process.[31] A paranasal sinusitis QST study demonstrated reduced electrical detection threshold in acute sinusitis and elevated heat and electrical detection threshold in chronic sinusitis.[32] Patients studied after mandibular third molar extractions demonstrated reduced mechanical and electrical thresholds of both lingual and mental nerves.[33] This hypersensitivity was reversed by steroid treatment.[34] Not like the detection threshold that returned to normal level 8 days following third molar extraction, pain threshold has been reduced up to 30 days following third molar extraction.[35] BMS studies revealed a normal tongue heat detection threshold but reduced thermal pain tolerance.[36–38] In another BMS study, electrical stimulation was used to differentiate chorda tympani (electrical taste) and lingual nerve function.[39,40] This study documented an elevated taste threshold supporting a theory that chorda tympani nerve hypofunction can contribute to this pathology.[41]

Studies in patients with TN have found increased thresholds to warm and cold that are resolved after neurosurgical decompression of the trigeminal nerve root.[42,43]

Employing QST as part of the routine OFP examination can add to the sensory and pain evaluation. Hyperalgesia, for instance to heat stimulus, suggests thin unmyelinated nerve fiber pathology, whereas tactile hyperalgesia may suggest involvement of myelinated fibers. Severe mechanical nerve damage and total nerve transection are characterized by elevated detection thresholds to heat, electrical, and mechanical stimulation.[44] In contrast to mechanical nerve damage, perineural inflammation produces hypersensitivity of large myelinated nerve fibers.[33,45–50] Moreover, QST methods can distinguish between several allodynia conditions. In addition to the pain threshold reduction that defines allodynia, detection threshold and pain tolerance may or may not be affected as well. The interval between detection and pain thresholds can be used to better describe the conditions. This feature may have a clinical relevance in centrally mediated pain conditions.[51] Evidence-based systematic QST methods can support diagnosis and treatment follow-up. However, routine use of QST in OFP clinics requires further research.

▼ CHRONIC PAIN

Although a precise definition of chronic pain has not been established, a distinction between acute and chronic pain has emerged. The somatosensory system serves the valuable function of warning the individual of actual or potential tissue damage. Nociceptors, specialized receptors that signal tissue damage, terminate in a highly ordered manner in the dorsal horn of the spinal cord and its homologous subnucleus caudalis in the spinal trigeminal nucleus. Information is transferred directly or through relay to the ventrobasal thalamus and then to the cortex. In the spinal cord, other pathways from the dorsal horn pass to the ventral horn and activate flexor motor neurons, generating the withdrawal flexion reflex.

This model draws attention to the protective aspect of the sensation of pain and is consistent with the qualities of acute pain. In other circumstances following peripheral tissue or nerve injury, a pathologic state may develop, resulting in persistent pain long after the injured tissue has healed. In this state, pain no longer represents a warning signal of potential or actual tissue damage; pain itself becomes the disorder.

Chronic pain is now recognized as a complex disorder that is influenced by biologic factors and by a range of psychosocial factors, including emotion, psychological distress, family and work environment, cultural background, the meaning of the pain, and appraisals of the controllability of the pain. Chronic pain has been defined as pain that persists past the normal time of healing, but this may not be an easy determination.[52] Alternatively, chronic pain has been related to duration (ie, pain that lasts longer than 6 months). Recently, pain lasting longer than 3 months has been used to define chronic pain. In the IASP publication on classification, Merskey et al. describes chronic pain as "a persistent pain that is not amenable, as a rule, to treatments based on specific remedies, or to the routine methods of pain control such as non-narcotic analgesics."[1]

As pain persists, psychosocial issues (including depression, maladaptive beliefs about pain, medication abuse, strained interpersonal relationships, and ineffective coping strategies) become prominent aspects of the disorder.[53,54] The term *chronic pain syndrome* has been used to describe a condition that may have started because of an organic cause but is now compounded by psychological and social problems. The term has been criticized since it may obscure more accurate physical and psychiatric diagnoses. It has sometimes been used pejoratively and has been interpreted by some to suggest a pain disorder that is psychological.[1] Originally, this label was used in an attempt to characterize a disorder that (regardless of its original cause) had evolved into a condition in which psychological and social problems were contributing to the persistence or exacerbation of the illness and in which significant disability was present.

In situations in which no ongoing peripheral injury was present to explain the pain, it was assumed that the pain was psychological. Patients need to be educated about the psychological distress and depression that can be a consequence of chronic pain. This is an important issue for clinicians and patients because of the demoralization and doubt patients develop about the condition and about their mental health.

Pathophysiology

The gate-control theory, introduced by Melzak and Wall in 1965, articulated a model that explained the pain experience as a multidimensional process with many modulating influences.[55] The proposed explanation for the persistence of pain after healing relates to changes (neuroplasticity) in the CNS.[56] Neurons are thought to be capable of altering their structure and function in response to stimuli, resulting in new stimulus-response relationships. This sensitization does not require ongoing peripheral input but is a consequence of changes in the sensitivity of neurons in the spinal cord.[57] These changes include the following:

1. A reduction in the stimulation threshold, with the result that the neurons no longer require a noxious stimulus to be activated
2. An alteration in the temporal pattern of the response, so that a transient stimulus evokes a sustained burst of activity
3. An increase in the general responsiveness of the motor neurons, so that a noxious stimulus produces a greater effect
4. The expansion of receptive fields, with the result that responses are evoked over a much wider area

The clinical manifestations of these changes include hyperalgesia (an increased response to a stimulus that is normally painful), allodynia (pain due to a stimulus that does not normally provoke pain), and spontaneous, radiating, and referred pain.

The interaction between the sympathetic and somatosensory nervous systems has been associated with chronic pain and thought to be the cause of many but not all cases of complex regional pain syndrome (CRPS). The relationship may be a coupling mediated by the neurotransmitter noradrenaline, which is released from sympathetic nerve endings acting on α-adrenoreceptors in the membrane of afferent neurons, causing depolarization. The mechanism is thought to be more likely a sensitivity of the somatosensory system than a hyperactivity of the sympathetic efferent system.[58]

Behavioral Issues

The observation that some individuals with high levels of pain continue to work whereas others are completely disabled led to the exploration of behavioral assessment and theories as a possible explanation.[59] Behavioral theories suggest that pain behaviors influence and are influenced by the patient's social environment.[59,60] The behavioral model views the pain behavior and associated disability as being as important as the underlying pathophysiology. A major goal in therapy is to modify pain behavior, thus improving function even when pain itself cannot be treated directly. Behavior therapy focuses on eliminating or reducing maladaptive behavior without theorizing about inner conflicts. It is based on principles of learning theory, particularly operant and classic conditioning.[3]

Pain itself can be viewed as a stress. The consequences of chronic pain (eg, loss of income, marital difficulties) are also significant stressors. Emotional distress is a component of pain, but it is also a consequence of pain, a cause of pain, or a concurrent problem with independent sources. These distinctions have not always been made clear, and there has been debate and confusion concerning whether emotional processes should be conceptualized as causes or consequences of pain.[61] The belief that chronic pain is a psychological disorder arose from two unproven assumptions: (1) chronic pain patients are a homogeneous group whose pain can be explained in terms of a more or less consistent constellation of personality characteristics, and (2) psychosocial disturbances (such as anxiety, depression, and social isolation) in pain patients reflect life events before the pain and are thus significant in explaining its onset.

The prevalence of depression is substantially higher in chronic pain patients compared with individuals without pain, but the majority of chronic pain patients are not depressed.[62] An association between chronic pain and depression exists, but no one hypothesis has emerged or has been proven to explain the relationship. Theories proposed include the following:

1. Depression causes hypersensitivity to pain.
2. Pain is a "masked" form of depression.
3. Depression is caused by the stress of chronic pain.

Depression, anxiety, and anger frequently coexist with chronic illness, but these reactions are not necessarily "psychopathological."[63] The literature suggests that, in general, pain is more likely to cause emotional disturbances than to be precipitated by them.[64] The fourth edition of the *Diagnostic and Statistical Manual of Mental Disorders* (*DSM-IV*) uses the classification "mood disorder due to a general medical condition" to describe this.[65] This classification is not considered to be a mental disorder.

A substantial group of chronic pain patients can be characterized as "dysfunctional" because of a consistent pattern of high levels of pain severity, affective distress, life interference, and lower-than-average levels of life control and activity.[66] The loss of customary roles at work, in the family, and in social settings, accompanied by the realization that neither one's own best efforts nor the interventions of highly respected health care professionals have been effective, is a major stressor. Challenges to the legitimacy of the complaints also represent a major source of stress. Excess use of medical services, hospitalizations for surgery, and abuse of medications are part of the profile of patients with dysfunctional chronic pain.

Chronic Pain: Genetics

In the last two decades, genetics has become central to the science of medicine. Current knowledge of the genetic code has encouraged studies at the molecular level that have increased our knowledge of both prevention and treatment.

It is apparent that genetic factors play a role in pain perception; however, the relative importance of these factors is unclear.

Nerves are often damaged as a result of either orofacial trauma or routine dental procedures, such as third molar extraction or pulpal extirpation during endodontic therapy. These are common nerve injuries that occur a thousand times daily, yet only certain individuals undergoing these procedures develop neuropathic pain.[67] A similar question can be posed regarding postamputation neuropathic pain (phantom limb pain).[68,69]

Since a genome search is expensive, most genetic studies are association studies, aimed at detecting increased frequency of certain alleles compared with controls. The research is even more complicated in pain-related genetic studies since pain pathways contain many molecular components, and dysfunction of any one of them can produce abnormal pain perception. Animal studies provided a list of candidate genes; however, only a few were found to be associated with pain perception in human. Moreover, only one has relevance to pain processing per se: cathechol-O-methyltransferase (COMT). Marbach and Levitt reported that patients with TMD show increased urinary levels of cathecholamine metabolites and express diminished erythrocytic COMT activity, suggesting a role for COMT in chronic orofacial pain conditions.[70] Recently, Maixner's group showed pain perception variability among the three major COMT haplotypes that determined its enzymatic activity.[71] The LPS type is associated with low pain sensitivity, the APS is associated with higher pain sensitivity, and the HPS is associated with highest pain sensitivity. A different study demonstrated a correlation between COMT variance and experimental pain induced by hypertonic saline injection to the masseter muscle, accompanied by differences in μmu-opiod activation in the brain.[72,73] Interestingly, fibromyalgia, a generalized myogenic pain condition that may be related to muscle-oriented OFP, was found to be correlated to the COMT V158M variant.[74,75]

The accumulating evidence suggests an important role for COMT in chronic muscle pain.

Another example of gene correlation to a specific pain condition is familial hemiplegic migraine.[76–78]

Treatment

Treatment that is specific to a particular pain disorder is discussed in a later section. The following is a discussion of general principles of treatment.

Even though it may occur in different locations, chronic pain tends to have certain characteristics regardless of the anatomic diagnosis or site. This tendency has led to the development of treatments to address the effects of chronic pain and to restore activity. These therapies are applied in multidisciplinary pain clinics (MPCs) regardless of whether pain is arising from the jaw, neck, back, or other anatomic site. MPCs have been organized in response to the recognition that pain is a complex physiologic, psychological, and sociologic experience beyond the expertise of any individual or discipline. Interdisciplinary therapy includes education, counseling, medication, pain management techniques (eg, electrical nerve stimulation techniques, nerve-blocking procedures, and acupuncture), psychological therapy (eg, cognitive, behavioral), relaxation training (eg, biofeedback, mental imagery, yoga, and meditation), hypnosis, occupational therapy, physical therapy modalities (eg, thermal and ultrasonic therapies, postural training), and stretching, strengthening, and conditioning programs. Treatment goals usually focus on managing medication misuse or abuse, increasing function, reducing the use of medical resources, decreasing pain intensity, and managing associated depression and anxiety. Behavioral therapy has been shown to be effective at reducing pain and improving function at work and at home.[79]

Pain reduction is a primary goal, but it is not always achieved. Published studies of pain reduction after treatment in pain clinics report pain reduction ranges from 14 to 60%, with an average pain reduction of between 20 and 30%.[80–82] Other treatment outcome criteria include reductions in addictive medication, reductions in the use of health care services, increased activity (including return to work), and closures of disability claims.[83] Providing effective treatment of chronic pain is challenging, and many of the treatments that are effective for acute pain fail to relieve chronic pain. Individuals suffering from chronic pain often seek care from many different practitioners and may be willing to submit to treatments that may complicate the problem or be harmful. This can result in more suffering and disability.

Chronic pain management is often seen as a low priority among health care providers; it is perceived as complicated, time-intensive, and often ineffective.[2] Ineffective medications are often overprescribed, repetitive examinations are conducted in an attempt to find a simple anatomic problem that is causing the pain, and comorbidities are ignored.[66] The failure to understand that chronic pain is a relevant clinical entity with physiologic and psychological consequences has been a barrier to improved care. This is complicated by the reluctance of patients to learn pain management or coping techniques because their energy and attention are usually focused on finding a cure.

COGNITIVE THERAPY

Cognitive therapy is based on the theory that an individual's affect and behavior are largely determined by the manner in which she or he structures the world. A person's structuring of the world is based on ideas and assumptions (developed from previous experiences). For example, "I am stronger if I don't need medicine" is a cognition that contributes to poor adherence to prescribed medication.[3]

In chronic OFP practice, it is not unusual to encounter patients who express ideas that are based on faulty assumptions. Examples include the following:

1. A firm belief that an allergy or an undiscovered or low-grade infection is the cause of pain. Diagnostic testing that fails to find evidence of infection or allergy is not always sufficient to redirect a patient's energy and attention to the pursuit of other factors or treatment. Infection and allergies are possible causes of pain, but when clinical findings are not supportive, the patient's persistent beliefs or attitudes may become a barrier to effective treatment.

2. Acceptance of the possibility that the pain is not a signal of ongoing or increasing tissue damage or life-threatening disease. This often prompts the patient to seek several consultations and to submit to invasive tests or procedures in an attempt to find a cause and (ultimately) a cure.

3. Anxiety about the possibility of further injury when pain increases with activity, resulting in deconditioning, inactivity, and increased emotional distress and limiting the potential for restored function and activity.

4. A focus on an orofacial structure or on a deviation from the ideal with respect to teeth and jaws, even though it is not responsible for the pain. This may complicate the situation and make it more difficult for the patient to accept a more multidisciplinary approach that includes behavioral management.

These are examples of maladaptive thoughts that lead to behaviors that contribute to the disability. Cognitive therapy is an effective method of exploring these thoughts and addressing them as part of the management. Cognitive-behavioral therapy attempts to alter patterns of negative thoughts and dysfunctional attitudes to foster more healthy and adaptive thoughts, emotions, and actions.[85] The cognitive-behavioral model suggests that patients develop negative and distorted convictions regarding their functional capacities, diagnoses, prognoses, and futures. These convictions about illness affect behavior and are reinforced when activity or reconditioning proves to be painful. Cognitive therapy interventions share four basic components: education, skill acquisition, cognitive and behavioral rehearsal, and generalization and maintenance.[84] Treatment is intended to identify and reframe negative cognitions while increasing the patient's range of activity.[63]

RELAXATION THERAPY

Relaxation techniques are used for nondirected calming rather than for achieving a specific therapeutic goal. They do not always reduce pain intensity and are recommended as an adjunctive treatment. The results of relaxation therapy may be more significant in reducing the distress associated with pain. Other benefits may include improved sleep, reduced skeletal-muscle tension, and decreased fatigue. Guided imagery, sometimes considered a relaxation technique, involves the recall of a pleasant or peaceful experience. Patients should be reassured that they are receiving this therapy not because "the pain is imaginary and they just need to relax" but because the therapy addresses an important area of distress that arises from having chronic pain.

Relaxation techniques share two basic components: (1) a repetitive focus on a word, sound, prayer, phrase, body sensation, or muscular activity and (2) the adoption of a passive attitude toward intruding thoughts and a return to focus.[84]

Relaxation training produces physiologic effects that are opposite to those of anxiety (ie, slower heart rate, increased peripheral blood flow, and decreased muscle tension or activity). Relaxing muscle groups in a fixed order (progressive relaxation), imagining oneself in a place associated with pleasant, relaxing memories (guided imagery), and doing yoga are examples. The reader is referred to the references listed in "Suggested Readings" at the end of this chapter for a more detailed discussion and specific exercises that can be applied in management.

DRUG THERAPY

Drug therapy is a significant part of chronic pain management. Analgesics are generally divided into three groups: nonopioids, opioids, and adjuvants. (Adjuvants are drugs that have been approved for use for conditions other than pain; anticonvulsants are an example.) The drugs in these groups have different pharmacologic actions, although their analgesic actions are often not well understood. With the exception of clonazepam, benzodiazepines are not thought to be analgesic and are not recommended for long-term chronic pain management, although they may be helpful for relief of muscle pain due to tension or spasm. Drug therapy for chronic pain often involves the simultaneous use of more than one drug. This takes advantage of the different mechanisms of action of different drugs. It may also allow the use of smaller doses and may reduce adverse effects or risks. The most common example of this in dentistry is the combination of an opioid (such as codeine) with aspirin or acetaminophen, in which each drug acts at different sites.

Choosing the analgesic group (or groups) and the specific drugs is the first step in management. Drug therapy requires the individualizing of regimens for the greatest effect. In chronic pain management, a drug should also be selected to deal with "breakthrough" pain, an episode of increased pain that the regular regimen is not able to control. This drug is usually a mu-receptor agonist with a relatively rapid rate of onset for a brief period. The oral route is preferred for compliance and convenience, and the drug dose requires titration to establish the appropriate regimen. An analgesic is most likely to be effective when given before pain increases and is usually best prescribed with a fixed dose schedule that does not require an increase in pain to signal the need for analgesia.

Nonopioid Analgesics This group consists primarily of acetaminophen and the large group of nonsteroidal anti-inflammatory drugs (NSAIDs). Acetaminophen is dispensed over the counter and is also available in controlled formulations in combination with codeine and other opioids. Acetaminophen generally has fewer adverse effects when compared with NSAIDs. It does not affect platelet function, rarely causes gastrointestinal (GI) disturbances, and can be given to patients who are allergic to aspirin or other NSAIDs. Caffeine has been shown to enhance the effectiveness of nonopioid drugs and is often added to the analgesic.[85] The mechanism of action of acetaminophen is different from that of the NSAIDs but remains unknown; there is some evidence that suggests a central action.[86] Acetaminophen is generally used for mild pain of all types and is also combined with opioids for an additive analgesic effect or to reduce the amount of opioid required. Due to its potential to cause liver damage, it may pose a danger to patients with liver disease, patients who regularly consume moderate to large amounts of alcohol, and patients who are fasting.[87] Acetaminophen has an analgesic "ceiling," and the recommended maximum dose in a 24-hour period is 4 g.[88]

NSAIDs are thought to work primarily at the site of injury by inhibiting the enzyme cyclooxygenase (COX), which is required for the synthesis of prostaglandins (PGs), substances that sensitize peripheral sensory nerves and contribute to the experience of pain. Users of NSAIDs do not exhibit tolerance or physical dependence, but these drugs do have an analgesic ceiling. Patients may vary in their response to NSAIDs, and if appropriate dosage adjustment does not produce an analgesic effect after several days to 1 week, it is appropriate to switch to a different NSAID. It is inadvisable to prescribe two different NSAIDs at the same time; rather, one NSAID should be used and its dose and timing adjusted for maximum analgesic effect. Combinations of NSAIDs increase the risk of side effects. Several NSAIDs (aspirin, ibuprofen, ketoprofen, and naproxen) are available in nonprescription formulations. The usual starting dose for these drugs is the dose recommended by the manufacturer. Titrating doses by starting at a lower dose and assessing incremental effects every 5 to 7 days has been recommended to achieve the greatest effect with the lowest dose.[89]

PGs perform other functions in the body, and this is responsible for many of the side effects. PGs maintain the protective layer of gastric mucosa, and the loss of this layer makes the mucosa more vulnerable to erosion. The longer NSAIDs are administered, the greater the risk of GI bleeding. This effect is a systemic one and is not avoided by administering the drug by other routes (eg, rectal suppository). NSAIDs should be taken with food or at least with a full glass of water. Coadministration of misoprostol (a PG analogue) has resulted in a reduced risk of GI bleeding.[90] Risk factors that are indications for using misoprostol include age of more than 60 years, concurrent steroid therapy, high doses of the NSAID, and a history of ulcer disease. Proton pump inhibitors have also been used concurrently to reduce the risk of gastric erosion. Although all NSAIDs pose a risk of GI bleeding, ibuprofen and diclofenac are considered to pose a lower risk, and ketoprofen and piroxicam are considered to pose a higher risk.[91] Nabumatone is also considered to be less likely to cause GI effects.[50] With any NSAID, the risk increases when high doses are prescribed.

NSAIDs are available that selectively inhibit only one of the isoforms of COX, namely, COX-2. The inhibition of COX-2 seems to be related to the anti-inflammatory and analgesic effects, whereas the inhibition of COX-1 is thought to be responsible for many of the side effects. The COX-2 inhibitors celecoxib and rofecoxib pose less risk of GI bleeding and do not inhibit platelet aggregation.

Recent evidence indicates that patients treated with selective COX-2 inhibitors may be at increased risk of cardiovascular problems.[92–96] The recent concerns led to the removal of rofecoxib and valedocoxib from the market.

Opioids The largest group of opioids that are commonly used for analgesia consists of the morphine-like agonists. Their most important effects are on the CNS and GI system. These drugs bind to m-opioid receptors, resulting in actions that lead to the analgesic effects. Opioids exert a number of effects after binding to receptor sites. Effects at the membrane level include opening potassium channels and inhibiting voltage-gated calcium channels, leading to a decrease in neuronal excitability. Opioids increase activity in some neuronal pathways (such as the descending inhibitory pathways) but may do so by suppressing the firing of inhibitory interneurons. At the spinal level, morphine inhibits the transmission of nociceptive impulses through the dorsal horn.[97] All mu agonists relieve pain by the same mechanism, but patients may vary in their responsiveness to the analgesic and to the adverse effects of specific agents. The use of opioid therapy in moderate to severe acute pain and cancer pain is well established. There has been an increased interest in the use of opioid analgesics for chronic nonmalignant pain. The practice remains controversial, and concern about addiction and behavior is the argument presented against opioid use. The concern relates to the risk of additional disability and antisocial behavior with long-term opioid use. The anecdotal literature suggests that in certain circumstances, opioids are an effective part of management and do not cause the predicted problems of addiction and antisocial behavior.[98] An agreement between the patient and doctor, along with close monitoring, minimizes potential misuse.

Agonist-antagonist drugs, such as buprenorphine, butorphanol, and pentazocine, are used to treat moderate to severe acute pain. As a group, they have a more limited role than the mu agonists. Agonist-antagonist drugs may cause withdrawal symptoms in patients who are taking mu agonists, and they are more likely to cause psychotomimetic effects, such as agitation, dysphoria, and confusion. Butorphanol nasal spray (Stadol, Bristol-Myers Squibb, New York, NY) is used for the treatment of migraine headache.

Adjuvant Drugs This group of drugs has been approved for use in conditions other than pain. Alone or in combination with other analgesics and adjuvants, they have been found to be of value in pain management. Sequential trials are often necessary due to the variability of side effects and treatment responses; this may mean trying different drugs in the same group and in different groups. In controlled clinical trials, carbamazepine (an anticonvulsant) has proven to be effective for the treatment of TN.[99]

Amitriptyline (a tricyclic antidepressant [TCA]), the antidepressant that has been most frequently studied in clinical trials, has been proven to be effective in chronic OFP treatment.[100,101] A patient with chronic pain who is receiving an antidepressant is considered to be better off than 74% of chronic pain patients who are receiving a placebo.[102] The magnitude of the analgesic effect was not different (1) for pain with an organic or psychogenic basis, (2) in the presence or absence of depression (masked or manifest), (3) in the presence or absence of an antidepressant effect, (4) in normal doses and in doses smaller than those that are usually effective in depression, and (5) for sedating and nonsedating drugs.

Information relating to pain from the periphery crosses a common synaptic pathway in the dorsal horn of the spinal cord and its homologue, the spinal trigeminal nucleus in the brainstem. The neurotransmitters serotonin and norepinephrine are thought to play a role in the descending inhibitory transmissions from the brain to the dorsal horn, modulating nociceptive impulses. TCAs block the reuptake of serotonin and norepinephrine, and this is thought to enhance the central inhibitory system in pain processing. These effects occur at doses that are lower than those required for an antidepressant effect, but further evidence is still required to explain the mechanism. TCAs are usually introduced at low doses and are gradually increased in an attempt to reduce the adverse effects, which can be intolerable even at low doses. Side effects such as dry mouth, increased appetite and weight gain, cardiac effects, sedation, and dysphoria may prevent the use of these drugs.

Anticonvulsant drugs are effective in the treatment of TN and diabetic neuropathy and for migraine prophylaxis.[103] There have been no clinical trials for the treatment of other OFP disorders with anticonvulsants. These drugs frequently produce side effects (including sedation, dizziness, ataxia, and mood changes) that can limit their usefulness. Newer anticonvulsants (specifically felbamate, lamotrigine, and gabapentin) are receiving attention as possible therapies for pain.[104–107] Gabapentin has become commonly used in pain management partly because of its relatively few side effects.[108] Movement disorders have been reported with gabapentin. The disorders resolve after administration of the drug is stopped.[109]

A new medication that was designed specifically to relieve neuropathic pain is pregablin,[110] which has a mechanism of action similar to that of gabapentin: binding to calcium channels and modulating calcium influx as well as influencing GABAergic neurotransmission.

A variety of other drugs are used in the treatment of chronic pain, although there is little research involving chronic OFP. These drugs include mexiletine, clonidine, clonazepam, and alprazolam.[111–114]

Topical Medications Topical analgesic therapy on the skin or oral mucosa has the advantage of reduced systemic absorption and thus a reduced risk of side effects. Capsaicin used as a topical cream has been the most researched drug in this field. It is effective in treating postherpetic neuralgia (PHN). Capsaicin is a natural product (extracted from the pungent red chili pepper) that has been used topically to treat a variety of pain conditions.[115] In a single application, neurogenic inflammation occurs and causes a burning sensation, followed by hyperalgesia. After multiple applications, the burning and hyperalgesia resolve. Topical application blocks C-fiber conduction, inactivates the release of neuropeptides from peripheral nerve endings, and subsequently depletes the stores of substance P from sensory neurons.[116,117] The therapeutic effect is thought to be due to the depletion of substance P in C fibers, decreasing their input to the CNS neurons.[118] Topical NSAIDs have been demonstrated to be effective for musculoskeletal pain.[119] Doxepin, clonidine, ketamine, cyclobenzaprine, and carbamazepine have been used topically in a variety of vehicles but have not been subjected to controlled trials.

Drug therapy for chronic pain is complex and often involves multiple drugs with different routes of administration. Patients often express anxiety about dependence on medication and may sometimes feel that drug therapy is used or recommended in place of "getting to the real cause" of the pain. When using drug therapy to treat the pain as the disorder, patients need information and education about the potential value of drug therapy as part of the comprehensive management of chronic pain.

▼ CLASSIFICATION OF OFP

Classification is more than an academic exercise as it provides researchers and practitioners with a way of communicating and understanding groups of individuals who share a set of relevant characteristics. An understanding of the mechanisms of a disorder, the prescription of treatment, and the prognosis are important clinical issues that can be addressed in an effective classification system. Most of the present classifications are based on a consensus of existing knowledge and on unstructured examination findings or assumptions about the consistency of signs and symptoms. This weakness was illustrated in a study of 35 patients who were diagnosed with AFP and whose findings were compared with the criteria established by the International Headache Society (IHS). Bilateral pain, pain-free periods, and paroxysms of pain were common in the patient group but were inconsistent with the criteria.[119]

Current Classification Schemes

Chronic pain classifications that address the physical, psychological, and social aspects of chronic pain provide a more comprehensive view of the disorder. Turk and Rudy proposed the MAP, which integrates physical, psychosocial, and behavioral data.[8] They also developed a classification of chronic pain patients that is based on psychosocial and behavioral data alone.[16] They hypothesized that certain patterns exist in chronic pain patients regardless of the medical diagnosis. Three different response patterns emerged: dysfunctional patients, interpersonally distressed patients, and adaptive copers. The study indicated that despite differences

in medical/dental diagnoses, patients had similar psychosocial and behavioral responses. A classification such as the MAP may be useful when combined with a classification that focuses on biomedical or physical conditions. The TMJ Scale, the computer-based assessment system for psychosocial and behavioral issues (IMPATH), and the Research Diagnostic Criteria (RDC) are assessment systems for OFP that include psychosocial parameters.[120–122]

The IHS, the American Academy of Orofacial Pain (AAOP), and the IASP have all produced classification schemes that include OFP. The IASP classification, originally published in 1986 and revised in 1994, is composed of five axes (Table 3).[1] The IASP has categorized OFP within the section termed "Relatively Localized Syndromes of the Head and Neck" (Table 4); listed within this section are 67 different disorders. The IASP publication includes a comparison between the IASP and IHS diagnostic categories that shows that there are significant differences between these two systems.

Two of 13 categories in the IHS classification specifically relate to OFP disorders: category 11, "headache or facial pain associated with disorders of cranium, neck, eyes, ears, nose, sinuses, teeth, mouth or other facial or cranial structures,"

TABLE 3 Scheme for Coding Chronic Pain Diagnoses*

Axis	Definition
1	Regions (eg, head, face, and mouth)
2	Systems (eg, nervous system)
3	Temporal characteristics of pain (eg, continuous, recurring irregularly, paroxysmal)
4	Patient's statement of intensity: time since onset of pain (eg, mild, medium, severe; 1 mo or less; more than 6 mo)
5	Etiology (eg, genetic, infective, psychological)

Adapted from Merskey H and Bogduk N.[1]
*International Association for the Study of Pain (IASP) classification.

TABLE 4 Classification of Localized Syndromes of the Head and Neck*

Neuralgias of the head and face

Craniofacial pain of musculoskeletal origin

Lesions of the ear, nose, and oral cavity

Primary headache syndromes, vascular disorders, and cerebrospinal fluid syndromes

Pain of psychological origin in the head, face, and neck

Suboccipital and cervical musculoskeletal disorders

Visceral pain in the neck

Adapted from Merskey H and Bogduk N.[1]
*International Association for the Study of Pain (IASP) classfication.

and category 13, "cranial neuralgias, and central causes of facial pain."[76,123] Category 11 includes temporomandibular joint disease and disorders of teeth, jaws, and related structures. Some of the disorders in category 13 are listed in Table 5. The AAOP has used the IHS classification as the basis for a classification on OFP disorders.[124] A separate axis (not included in the publication) is recommended for defining psychosocial factors and diagnosing mental disorders. OFP disorders in this classification are listed in Table 6.

Classification of Idiopathic Facial Pain

ATYPICAL FACIAL PAIN

The use of the term *atypical facial pain* as a diagnostic classification has been recently discouraged.[1,124] Originally, the term was used to describe patients whose response to neurosurgical procedures was not "typical."[125] The term has been applied to various facial pain problems and has been considered to represent a psychological disorder, although no specific diagnostic criteria have ever been established.

AFP is defined more by what it is not than by what it is. Feinmann characterized AFP as a nonmuscular or joint pain that has no a detectable neurologic cause.[100] Truelove and colleagues described AFP as a condition characterized by the absence of other diagnoses and causing continuous, variable-intensity, migrating, nagging, deep, and diffuse pain.[126]

TABLE 6 Differential Diagnosis of Orofacial Pain*

Intracranial pain disorders	Neoplasm, aneurysm, abscess, hemorrhage, hematoma, edema
Primary headache disorders	Migraine, migraine variants, cluster headache, paroxysmal hemicrania, cranial arteritis,
(neurovascular disorders)	carotodynia, tension-type headache
Neurogenic pain disorders	Paroxysmal neuralgias (trigeminal, glossopharyngeal, nervus intermedius, superior laryngeal)
	Continuous pain disorders (deafferentation, neuritis, postherpetic neuralgia, post-traumatic and postsurgical neuralgia)
	Sympathetically maintained pain
Intraoral pain disorders	Dental pulp, periodontium, mucogingival tissues, tongue
Temporomandibular disorders	Masticatory muscle, temporomandibular joint, associated structures
Associated structures	Ears, eyes, nose, paranasal sinuses, throat, lymph nodes, salivary glands, neck

Reproduced with permission from Okeson J.[124]
*American Academy of Orofacial Pain classification.

In the TMD classification of the AAOP, AFP is listed in the glossary of terms and is defined as "a continuous unilateral deep aching pain sometimes with a burning component." AFP was not included as a diagnostic category.[127] The IHS classification (IHS 13.18.4) uses the term "persistent idiopathic facial pain" (Table 7).[123,128] Recent advances in the understanding of chronic pain suggest that at least a portion of patients who have been diagnosed with AFP may be experiencing neuropathic pain.

ATYPICAL ODONTALGIA

Atypical odontalgia (AO), described as a chronic pain disorder characterized by pain localized to teeth or gingiva, has been considered to be a variant of AFP.[1] The condition has also been called "phantom tooth pain" and defined as persistent pain in endodontically treated teeth or edentate areas for which there is no explanation to be found by physical or

TABLE 5 Classification of Cranial Neuralgias, Nerve Trunk Pain, and Deafferentation Pain*

IHS Category	Specific Disorders or Definition
13.1 Trigeminal neuralgia (TN)	Idiopathic TN, symptomatic TN (caused by demonstrable structural lesion)
13.2 Glossopharyngeal neuralgia (GN)	Idiopathic GN, symptomatic GN (caused by demonstrable structural lesion)
13.3 Nervus intermedius neuralgia	Rare disorder characterized by brief paroxysms of pain felt deeply in the auditory canal
13.4 Superior laryngeal neuralgia	Rare disorder characterized by severe pain in the lateral aspect of the throat, submandibular region, and underneath the ear, precipitated by swallowing, shouting, or turning the head
13.8 Occipital neuralgia	Paroxysmal jabbing pain in the distribution of the greater or lesser occipital nerves, accompanied by diminished sensation or dysesthesia in the affected area; commonly associated with tenderness over the nerve concerned
13.18 Central causes of head and facial pain	Anesthesia dolorosa, central post-stroke pain, facial pain attributed to multiple sclerosis, persistent idiopathic facial pain, burning mouth syndrome

Reproduced with permission from Olesen J.[124]
*International Headache Society (IHS) classification.

TABLE 7 Classification of Idiopathic Orofacial Pain*

A. Pain in the face, present daily and persisting for all or most of the day, fulfilling criteria B and C

B. Pain is confined at onset to a limited area on one side of the face1 and is deep and poorly localized

C. Pain is not associated with sensory loss or other physical signs

D. Investigation, including radiography of face and jaws are negative

Reproduced with permission from Committee on Headache Classification, International Headache Society.[128]
*International Headache Society (IHS) classification 13.18.4: persistent idiopathic facial pain.

radiographic examination.[129] In the AAOP classification, AO is listed within the category "facial pain not fulfilling other criteria" and is considered to be a deafferentation pain.[124] AO appears in the IASP classification under "lesions of the ear, nose, and oral cavity" and is defined as a severe throbbing pain in the teeth in the absence of a major pathology.

In an attempt to identify chronic OFP due to neuropathic injury, Lynch and Elgeneidy suggested additional categories to the IASP taxonomy.[130] They also recommended replacing AFP with the term "not otherwise specified." This is the terminology used in the *DSM-IV* for a condition that does not conform to criteria in another category.[65] Although the term *atypical facial pain* has a long history and has been associated with a number of different etiologies, it still is used by clinicians to identify an OFP disorder that does not meet other diagnostic criteria and that is characterized by its chronicity and lack of response to most treatments. The term may fade away as new knowledge identifies causes for these disorders and allows for better classifications and treatment.

NEURALGIA-INDUCING CAVITATIONAL OSTEONECROSIS

The significance and validity of this condition have been discussed extensively in the literature; however, ischemic osteonecrosis of the jaws has been presented as a cause of idiopathic facial pain. The term given to describe this disorder is *neuralgia-inducing cavitational osteonecrosis* (NICO). The pain is described as slowly progressive over time and spreading. It may be intermittent and may vary in extent, location, and character. This disorder has been described as occurring at a wide range of ages but is more frequent in the fourth and fifth decades of life. It is thought to occur most frequently in the mandibular molar area. Most NICO sites are thought to involve edentulous areas or areas associated with radiographically successful endodontic procedures. No specific imaging criteria are diagnostic.[131] Significant debate continues about NICO as a cause of facial pain.[132] Treatment by surgically entering and curretting these cavities raises a concern about the possibility of exacerbating the disorder rather than controlling it. Procedures that risk nerve injury are generally not recommended for patients with persistent neuropathic pain. The lack of clearly defined criteria for the diagnosis of these conditions raises the risk of additional injury and aggravation of the symptoms.

▼ EXAMINATION AND ASSESSMENT OF THE PATIENT WITH CHRONIC OFP

The examination and assessment of patients with chronic OFP is challenging for all clinicians. In most disorders, no specific biologic marker, validated diagnostic criteria, or "gold standard" exists. Biologic markers, including tyramine, oxygen free radicals, and metabolites of neurotransmitters in lumbar cerebrospinal fluid, have been studied in a limited manner in regard to OFP and are not applicable in diagnosis.[133–135] Even test procedures that are considered

objective, such as local anesthetic nerve blocking and the testing of sensation after nerve damage, have yielded inconsistent results.[136,137] A systematic approach for collecting diagnostic information is needed to minimize the risk of missing critical information. A formal and systematic approach increases the probability of identifying disease that occurs from time to time and is life threatening.[138]

History, physical examination, and behavioral assessment usually serve as the basis for diagnosis. Frequent reevaluation, including assessment of the effects of treatment, is an important part of this process. In circumstances in which treatment is ineffective or only partially successful, patients are at risk of seeking additional and alternative treatments that may be inappropriate and potentially dangerous.[139] Even when a diagnosis is uncertain or when previous treatment has failed, the clinician can make a valuable contribution by coordinating the further use of medical and dental services and by being available to advise the patient about possible treatments. Validating patients' feelings and symptoms in these times is critically important and serves to reduce suffering.

History

Evaluation of OFP symptoms must include all of the standard components of a medical interview: chief complaint, history of present illness, past medical history, medications, review of systems, and family and social history. A diagnosis can sometimes be made on the basis of the history, or the possibilities can be significantly narrowed. Since a number of OFP disorders do not produce physical abnormalities, the history and description of pain may serve as the basis for the diagnosis.

HISTORY OF THE PRESENT ILLNESS

A history of the present illness should include a detailed description of the pain and its location (Table 8). The VAS or numeric scale described above can be used to assess intensity, and a questionnaire such as the MPQ can capture the multidimensional experience of the pain. Details of previous injuries, surgeries, and radiation therapy should be obtained.

TABLE 8   Pain Characteristics

Intensity

Quality

Location

Onset

Associated events at onset

Duration and timing of pain

Course of symptoms since onset

Activities or experiences that increase pain

Activities or experiences that decrease pain

Associated symptoms (eg, altered sensation, swelling)

Previous treatments and their effects

Questions about habits such as gum chewing and tooth clenching or grinding may reveal important contributing factors of which the patient is unaware. The effects of eating, opening the mouth wide, rest, exercise, and heat and cold on pain should be explored. Referred pain to the orofacial region is an important clinical consideration. The location of pain, therefore, will not always correspond to its source. A mechanism that has been proposed to explain referred pain is convergence, in which primary afferent fibers from different sites converge on the same second-order neuron in the brainstem nucleus.[140–142] Patients should mark the location and extent of pain on a diagram.

PAST MEDICAL HISTORY AND REVIEW OF SYSTEMS

The past medical history and review of systems should help provide an insight into the general health of the patient and may provide clues regarding the present pain complaint. Pain may be a presenting feature or an ongoing complaint in systemic disease (eg, connective tissue disease, demyelinating disease of the CNS, metastatic disease).

The patient's use of medication (including over-the-counter preparations, naturopathic and homeopathic remedies, and prescription drugs) should be recorded. Prescription medication is often used incorrectly; therefore, the directions, as well as the actual use, should be determined. The medication list may uncover a medical condition that the patient failed to mention in other questioning. Drug effects such as fatigue, dizziness, anxiety, insomnia, or depression may affect the patient's pain complaints. The use of tobacco, alcohol, caffeine, or illicit drugs should be explored.

FAMILY, SOCIAL, AND OCCUPATIONAL HISTORY

Chronic pain can have disastrous effects on one's ability to maintain daily activities and fulfill responsibilities. Pain has profound and often negative effects on family and social relationships, and it is important to assess the level of dysfunction that may have occurred. Traumatic events or emotional distress prior to the onset of pain, a history of other close family members with chronic illness or pain, and changes in work and/or marital status should be explored because these can be significant stressors.

Physical Examination

The physical examination may identify an abnormality that explains the cause of pain. It can also help eliminate from diagnosis the presence of serious disease related to the pain. The examination should include the following:

1. Inspection of the head and neck, skin, topographic anatomy, and swelling or other orofacial asymmetry
2. Palpation of masticatory muscles, tests for strength and provocation
3. Assessment and measurement of the range of mandibular movement
4. Palpation of soft tissue (including lymph nodes)
5. Palpation of the temporomandibular joint
6. Palpation of cervical muscles and assessment of cervical range of motion
7. Cranial nerve examination (Table 9)
8. General inspection of the ears, nose, and oropharyngeal areas
9. Examination and palpation of intraoral soft tissue
10. Examination of the teeth and periodontium (including occlusion)

MUSCLE EXAMINATION

Pain that is reproduced or increases as a result of muscle palpation may point to the source of the pain and to a diagnosis. The degree of finger pressure will influence the result of the palpation examination, and patients' responses to palpation may vary with time. Pressure algometers have been used in research to help standardize examination procedures but are not commonly used in clinical practice.[143] Muscle palpation has been shown to yield reliable scores among examiners, but the diagnostic validity and reliability of muscle palpation have not been established. The masseter and temporalis muscles can be palpated bilaterally to identify differences in size or firmness. The suprahyoid muscles, mylohyoid muscle, and anterior belly of the digastric muscle should be included in the palpation examination. Intraoral techniques have been described for palpating the medial and lateral pterygoids. The ability to perform a meaningful palpation examination of the lateral pterygoid has been questioned.[144] Palpation techniques have been described, but it may be difficult to distinguish tenderness associated with the procedure from an actual muscle abnormality.[145] The temporalis tendon, where it inserts onto the coronoid process, can also be reached intraorally for palpation. Testing muscles against resistance in a static position and having the patient clench on separators to prevent the teeth from coming together may help identify the source of pain.[146]

Palpation of cervical muscles and a general assessment of the cervical range of motion may indicate an abnormality contributing to the pain complaint. Pain localized to the orofacial region can be referred from neck muscles.[140] The cervical muscles to be palpated include the trapezii and the sternocleidomastoid muscle and the muscles that lie deeper between them, including the capitus and scalene muscles and the levator scapulae.

RANGE OF MOTION ASSESSMENT

Mandibular and cervical ranges of motion should be assessed. Movements with and without pain should be noted. Mandibular movements with comfort, with pain, and with examiner assistance should be measured and recorded. Cervical motion can be examined during active, passive, and resisted motions. When restrictions in movement are thought to be caused by muscle guarding, the application of a vapo-coolant spray such as Fluori-Methane Spray (Gebauer Co., Cleveland, OH) followed by stretching may significantly increase range, confirming a muscle cause. Alternatively, injection of a local anesthetic into muscle may block pain and thus identify the source of the pain and the restricted movement.

TABLE 9   Summary of Cranial Nerve Examination

Cranial Nerve	Function	Usual Complaint	Test of Function	Physical Findings
I (olfactory)	Smell	None or loss of "taste" if bilateral	Sense of smell with each nostril; no response to olfactory stimuli	
II (optic)	Vision	Loss of vision	Visual acuity; decreased visual acuity or loss of visual field; visual fields of each eye	
III (oculomotor)	Eye movement Pupillary constriction	Double vision	Pupil and eye movement; failure to move eye in field of motion of muscle Pupillary abnormalities	
IV (trochlear)	Eye movement	Double vision, especially on down- and medial gaze	Ability to move eye down and in may be difficult to detect anything if third nerve intact	
V (trigeminal)	Facial, nasal, and oral sensation Jaw movement	Numbness Paresthesia	Light touch and pinprick; decreased pin and absent corneal reflex sensation on face; weakness of masticatory muscles Corneal reflex Masseter contraction	
VI (abducens)	Eye movement	Double vision on lateral gaze	Move eyes laterally; failure of eye to abduct	
VII (facial)	Facial movement	Lack of facial movement, eye closure Dysarthria	Facial contraction; asymmetry of facial contraction Smiling	
VIII (auditory and vestibular)	Hearing Balance	Hearing loss Tinnitus Vertigo	Hearing test; decreased hearing Nystagmus Balance; ataxia	
IX (glossopharyngeal)	Palatal movement	Trouble with swallowing	Elevation of palate; asymmetric palate	
X (vagus)	Vocal cords	Trouble swallowing	Vocal cords; brassy voice	
XI (spinal accessory)	Turns neck	None	Contraction of sternocleidomastoid muscle; paralysis of sternocleidomastoid muscle and trapezius	
XII (hypoglossal)	Moves tongue	Dysarthria	Protrusion of tongue; wasting and fasciculation or deviation of tongue	

INTRAORAL EXAMINATION

A systematic intraoral inspection looking for changes in form, symmetry, color, and surface texture should be carried out. The examination should include manipulation of the tongue and mandible to clearly visualize all areas. Pooling of saliva on the floor of the mouth should be observed. The palate and tongue should be examined at rest and during function to detect underlying masses that might displace or alter the normal structures. The examiner's finger should palpate the alveolar processes, lateral and posterior parts of the tongue, floor of the mouth, buccal mucosa, and hard and soft palate to identify abnormalities that may not be readily observed. The finger should not meet significant resistance as it moves across a normally lubricated mucosa. The openings of the submandibular and parotid salivary gland ducts should be isolated and dried with cotton; the glands should then be "milked" to verify a clear flow of saliva.

The dentition should be examined for wear, damaged teeth, and evidence of caries. This inspection should be followed by probing, palpation for tooth mobility, and percussion of teeth. If a pulpal problem is suspected, thermal and vitality tests should be included. Applying differential pressure on the teeth by having the patient bite down on cotton rolls, wooden bite sticks, or one of the commercially available instruments designed to apply concentrated pressure on cusps may identify pain associated with a vertical crown or root fracture. Periodontal structures should be examined for color changes suggestive of inflammation, altered gingival architecture that occurs with chronic disease, swelling, or other surface changes. Periodontal probing should be performed to identify bleeding points and pocket depths. Tooth contacts in the maximum intercuspal position, in centric relation, and during excursive movements should be identified. Heavy contacts or interferences in association with tooth mobility or tooth sensitivity may indicate conditions contributing to occlusal trauma.

Pain-Related Disability and Behavioral Assessment

An interview most often serves as the basis for a behavioral assessment. Self-report questionnaires and instruments that include methods of scoring are also in use to assess disability and psychological factors. The assessment should explore the following[147]:

1. Events that precede and follow exacerbation of pain
2. The patient's daily activities:
   - How time is spent during the day and in the evening
   - Activities that have been performed more often or less often since the onset of pain
   - Activities that have been modified or eliminated since the onset of pain

3. Relatives or friends who suffer chronic pain or disabilities of a similar nature
4. The degree of affective disturbance:
   - Change in mood or outlook on life
   - Satisfaction level with friends and family relationships
   - Vegetative signs of depression (sleep disturbance, change in food intake, decreased sexual desire)

Although psychosocial factors are of great importance in pain disorders, studies indicate that physicians and dentists do not always adequately recognize psychological problems.[148–150] One of the problems dentists face is the lack of formal training in psychological assessment. A great deal of study has been focused on the use of questionnaires to assess psychosocial status. Inventories that are completed by the patient, such as the Minnesota Multiphasic Personality Inventory (MMPI), the Beck Depression Inventory, the Zung Self-Rating Depression Scale, the Personality Diagnostic Questionnaire, and the General Health Questionnaire, are examples of self-report questionnaires used for psychological assessment.[151–153] The TMJ Scale, IMPATH, and (more recently) the RDC are instruments designed for evaluating OFP, and they include behavioral assessments.[20,120,121] No one method has gained widespread acceptance for evaluating OFP patients. One strategy for addressing the lack of psychological assessment skills among physicians and dentists is to provide a method of screening that identifies OFP patients who might benefit from a more thorough behavioral assessment. Gale and Dixon found that the following two questions correlated with lengthier questionnaires[154]:

1. How depressed are you?
2. Do you consider yourself more tense than calm or more calm than tense?

Oakley and colleagues used a five-item questionnaire that allows patients to rate levels of depression, anxiety, and recent life stresses that showed moderate to strong association with results from extensive psychological testing.[155] Two of the questions were similar to those used by Gale and Dixon.

Being asked open-ended questions about common areas of life experience provides the patient with an opportunity to express concerns or problems that may not otherwise be communicated, such as what the patient feels may be the cause of pain, activities or problems in the common areas of life (work, love, and play), and complaints of current or previously diagnosed or undiagnosed pain elsewhere in the body. Responses to these questions may be helpful in identifying abnormal thought patterns, external stressors, or other symptoms that are suggestive of a more generalized pain disorder. Recent research indicates that the prevalence of a history of physical and sexual abuse in patients with chronic pain is higher than expected, but how to identify patients who should be referred to experienced therapists remains a challenge.[147]

Self-report instruments are used for clinical and research purposes to assess psychological variables associated with pain. They provide standardized assessments and are sensitive to treatment-related changes. Instruments such as the MMPI and the revised MMPI (MMPI-2) have been used to evaluate psychological distress in chronic pain patients.[156] The use of the MMPI or MMPI-2110 with chronic pain patients has been questioned because the subjects who were used to standardize the inventories were not chronic pain patients.[157–159] In chronic pain patients, elevations on the hypochondriasis, depression, and hysteria scales have been associated with severe pain, affective disturbance, and disability.[160,161] MMPI profiles have been unable to predict treatment outcomes.[147] Other shorter and simpler instruments such as the Beck Depression Inventory are used in place of the MMPI.[162] The shorter inventories are likely to get better patient compliance as well. Questionnaires such as the SCL-90-R, the Millon Behavioral Health Inventory, and the Illness Behavior Questionnaire are examples of shorter inventories that take less time to complete.[22,163,164] A universally accepted assessment instrument for chronic pain patients does not exist.

Dworkin and LeResche published (as part of the RDC) a classification for assessing pain-related disability, identifying depression, and characterizing limitations related to mandibular functioning.[20] The RDC were produced to increase the standardization of assessment and classification applied to clinical research on TMD. Although this assessment/classification requires further validation, it may be of value to clinicians. The pain-related disability assessment is based on the "Graded Chronic Pain Status," a seven-item questionnaire, and specific scoring.[21] An explanation of the scoring and the scale can be found in Von Korff and colleagues' article.[21] The assessment method, scoring, and discussion of the pain-related disability status have been published by Dworkin and LeResche.[20]

From the discussion above, it should be apparent that there is no universal standard that can be relied on to provide a screening assessment of behavioral and pain-related disability. Table 10 lists questions discussed in this section

TABLE 10   Questions to Consider for Screening Assessment
What events precede and follow increased episodes of pain?
How is time spent during the day and the evening?
What activities are performed more often or less often since the onset of pain?
What activities have been modified or eliminated since the onset of pain?
Do relatives or friends suffer chronic pain or disabilities of a similar nature?
Do you characterize yourself as depressed?
Do you have changes in sleep pattern, food habits, sexual desire (vegetative signs of depression)?
Have there been changes in your relationships with friends, family, coworkers?
Do you characterize yourself as being anxious or tense?
Do you think you have experienced a lot of stressful situations over the past year?
What do you think is causing the pain?
Do you presently have any diagnosed or undiagnosed pain complaints elsewhere in the body?

that may be valuable as part of this assessment. These questions may be posed during the interview to explore possible behavioral, psychological, or other systemic problems that may have an impact on the diagnosis and management of an OFP disorder. This is not a scale or instrument with scoring but questions that may provide an opportunity for the patient to communicate issues that may be important to the complaint. The threshold for deciding when the information obtained indicates a more thorough investigation is a clinical judgment. There are no well-defined rules to govern this decision.

When psychosocial issues are thought to be significant and to require assessment and possible management by a psychologist or psychiatrist, the patient should be so advised. This should be done in a conversation that allows the patient to respond and that asks for feedback since the patient may have some insight into the issue. The interviewer's opinion may help validate the patient's own assessment, and the possibility of successfully addressing these issues may be increased. Communicating with the patient's general physician or referring the patient to his or her general physician to explore this further may be an effective method of managing the situation.

When a psychiatric disorder is suspected, a direct referral to a psychiatrist or psychologist may be indicated.[165] The patient may resist this referral for the following reasons:

1. Perception of the referral as a judgment that the problem is only psychological or as a personal rejection
2. Beliefs about the legitimacy of psychiatric therapy and about the kind of people who consult psychologists or psychiatrists
3. Beliefs about the condition that do not include the possibility of a psychological or emotional component

A patient is most likely to accept a recommendation if a trusting relationship is present. The following are suggestions that may facilitate the referral:

1. Make the referral a part of the evaluation. Inform the patient that the consultation is part of your complete evaluation and that it will be part of the other clinical findings for determining the diagnosis and management.
2. Arrange the appointment at the same time that the patient is in the office if the patient agrees. This will facilitate the process.
3. Provide the patient with information about what the consultation will involve.
4. Schedule a follow-up appointment to review the findings and discuss treatment.

Diagnostic Imaging

Imaging can be used to confirm a suspected abnormality, to screen or rule out possible abnormalities that are not detectable by other methods, or to establish the extent of an identified disorder. It is the best method for evaluating a suspected tumor, infection, or ongoing inflammation in sites that are not easily accessible. Many OFP disorders do not produce abnormalities demonstrable with imaging, and its greatest value may be to rule out serious life-threatening disease.

Diagnostic Nerve Blocks

Nerve blocks interrupt the transmission of nociceptive impulses through specific pathways. If pain relief occurs, it is presumed to be due to the interruption of the nerves via the pathways suspected of being involved. Conversely, the absence of pain after a successful block suggests the possibility of a central process.[166] False-positive results may occur due to systemic effects of local anesthetics, blockade of afferent pathways other than those intended, and placebo effects. Conversely, lack of pain relief may be due to technical or anatomic factors.[167] Diagnostic nerve blocks are a valuable part of an assessment, but the results can be equivocal and do not always contribute to an accurate diagnosis. There is a high frequency of placebo response to local anesthetic blocking, even among patients diagnosed with neuropathic pain.[136]

Nerve blocks to diagnose sympathetically maintained pain include local anesthetic block of the sympathetic chain (eg, stellate ganglion), regional guanethedine block (intravenous injection into an arm or leg), and intravenous phentolamine to block the α-adrenoreceptor, preventing the excitation of afferent nociceptors by noradrenaline. The interpretation of these tests has been challenged because of the lack of placebo-controlled procedures and because of a high placebo response, but the weight of evidence supports the hypothesis that the sympathetic nervous system contributes to chronic pain in some circumstances.[168,169]

Local anesthetic blocking should be considered in the context of all of the clinical findings. Topical, intraligament, infiltration, and regional block anesthesia may identify a peripheral site that is responsible for pain. A complete resolution of pain after local anesthetic application or injection should prompt an investigation for a local cause. The injection of local anesthesia may produce ambivalent results when patients report a change in symptoms but not necessarily resolution of pain. In these circumstances, one should consider a more central cause of pain.

Laboratory Tests

Laboratory tests have limited value except in special circumstances. Most OFP disorders do not cause abnormalities that can be identified in laboratory specimens. Exceptions include temporal arteritis, in which the erythrocyte sedimentation rate (ESR) is elevated and temporal artery biopsy is abnormal, and collagen vascular diseases that cause detectable immunologic abnormalities.

Consultation and Referral

Referral and consultation are recommended for a number of reasons, and there are few rigid rules. For a complex pain problem, it may be necessary to include examinations by other dental specialists, otolaryngologists, neurologists, psychologists or psychiatrists, and internists. Referrals may be of value when (1) the referral is for confirming or establishing a suspected or unknown diagnosis, (2) the referral is for the purpose of treatment after a diagnosis has been made, and (3) the referral is for obtaining a second opinion to review an established diagnosis or treatment recommendation.

Suggesting referral to a patient may be met with ambivalence and anxiety. Concerns about the seriousness of the problem, financial issues, time commitments, and having to establish a new relationship with another health care provider may be sources of resistance. The practitioner may feel pressure to do something before a diagnosis is established, and this may lead to ineffective and inappropriate treatment.

Special Circumstances in Assessment of OFP Patients

OFP DISORDERS POSSIBLY CONFUSED WITH TOOTHACHE

Patients who choose to consult a dentist regarding a pain complaint do so because they believe it may be a tooth-related problem. Several OFP disorders have characteristics that may be confused with those of a toothache (Table 11). This confusion may occur because of (1) the location of the pain, (2) the quality of pain that suggests an inflammatory process, or (3) increased pain associated with stimulation of the teeth or surrounding tissues.

OFP SYMPTOMS INDICATING SERIOUS DISEASE

Presenting signs or symptoms may suggest the possibility of a serious or life-threatening disorder and indicate an urgent need to establish a diagnosis. These conditions may warrant referral as part of a thorough and timely evaluation (Table 12).[170]

▼ HEADACHE AND OFP SYMPTOMS ASSOCIATED WITH SYSTEMIC DISEASE

For most of the systemic diseases that manifest in the oral cavity, there is little information on the frequency with which signs and symptoms identified in the oral cavity lead to the

TABLE 12 Orofacial Pain Symptoms that Indicate Serious Disease

Orofacial Pain Symptom	Disease Indicated
Pain at the angle of the mandible, brought on by exertion, relieved by rest	Cardiac ischemia
New-onset; localized progressive headache; superficial temporal artery swelling, tenderness, and lack of pulse; severe throbbing temporal pain; transient visual abnormalities; systemic symptoms of fever, weight loss, anorexia, malaise, myalgia, chills, sweating	Temporal arteritis
New onset of headache in adult life; increasing severe illness or migraine; nocturnal occurrence; precipitated or increased by changes in posture; confusion, seizures, or weakness; any abnormal neurologic sign	Intracranial tumor
Earache, trismus, altered sensation in the mandibular branch distribution	Carcinoma of the infratemporal fossa
Trigeminal neuralgia in a person less than 50 years of age	Multiple sclerosis
Pain associated with altered sensation confirmed by physical examination	Neurogenic disorder; tumor invasion of nerve

recognition and diagnosis of systemic disease. Table 13 lists systemic diseases that have been associated with headache and OFP.[171–179] The literature in this area is primarily case reporting and is a poor guide to the likelihood of finding evidence that implicates a previously undiagnosed systemic disease process as the cause of a patient's unexplained facial OFP. Hyperparathyroidism and metastatic disease will eventually produce radiologic findings that lead to a diagnosis. In other situations, physical signs or laboratory evidence will direct the diagnostic process, but in the early stage of disease, pain (with or without altered sensation) may be the first indication of the disorder.

Diseases such as diabetes mellitus (which occurs with some frequency in the population) will often be found,

TABLE 11 Orofacial Disorders Confused with Toothache

Trigeminal neuralgia

Trigeminal neuropathy (due to trauma or tumor invasion of nerves)

Idiopathic facial pain and atypical odontalgia

Cluster headache

Acute and chronic maxillary sinusitis

Myofascial pain of masticatory muscles

TABLE 13 Systemic Diseases Associated with Headache and Orofacial Pain

Paget's disease

Metastatic disease

Hyperthyroidism

Multiple myeloma

Hyperparathyroidism

Vitamin B deficiencies

Systemic lupus erythematosus

Vincristine therapy for cancer

Folic acid and iron deficiency anemias

but evidence associating the systemic disease and the oral symptoms may be harder to find. Clinical investigation of the majority of patients referred after initial evaluation by dentists and physicians for an unsolved oral complaint only rarely detects undiagnosed systemic disease. More often, abnormal blood values, such as glucose or iron levels, have been noted at earlier examinations. Treating the abnormality does not always eliminate the oral symptoms. Alternatively, both patient and physician are aware of the presence of the systemic disease, but the methods used to control it have been inadequate. Referral consultations for unexplained oral complaints may thus result in recommendations for additional treatment of systemic disease noted at the time of consultation. In many cases, however, these conditions are not specifically related to the oral complaint.

Despite the time and money invested in extensive searches for systemic disease that only rarely find a possible cause of unexplained oral symptoms, such searches are sometimes justified. Unexplained chronic oral symptoms generate considerable anxiety in addition to the discomfort experienced by the patient, and a "leave no stone unturned" approach often seems necessary to allay these anxieties. Patients with problems sometimes demand a continued battery of sophisticated studies. In these circumstances, the clinician's judgment is needed to prevent the unnecessary repetition of tests and to advise the patient on the likelihood of a particular procedure providing additional useful diagnostic information.

ABSENCE OF A CONVINCING PHYSICAL EXPLANATION FOR SYMPTOMS

Patients who have no convincing physical explanation for their symptoms are the most difficult patients for the practitioner. The resultant problems are not restricted to oral medicine, and all who practice medicine and dentistry usually become aware of them early in their careers. Such patients are seen with greater frequency in specialty practices simply because unresolved problems commonly lead to a referral for further diagnostic testing. For residents in specialty training, it is often a discovery that a considerable number of patients will not be concerned with clearly defined pathologic states that are amenable to treatment. Patients with unexplained oral sensory abnormalities still require management and some form of treatment even when a thorough diagnostic search fails to find an explanation.

▼ RESPONSES TO UNEXPLAINED SYMPTOMS

The assumption underlying all diagnostic procedures is that an explanation will be found for the patient's complaint of pain. When extensive and reasonably adequate diagnostic investigations fail to find such an explanation, the initial response by the patient and doctor is that further testing

to probe for more unusual conditions is needed. When this approach fails, the doctor may begin to assume that the symptoms are not real and that they represent exaggeration for some secondary gain or a psychiatric abnormality. Alternatively, the doctor may judge that a borderline abnormality found by palpation or by diagnostic imaging might be more serious than was first considered and might represent evidence of a lesion. Both of these responses on the doctor's part may be exaggerated, and they represent two pitfalls that may complicate the diagnostic and treatment process. First, concluding that symptoms are evidence of a psychiatric abnormality may deny the patient the opportunity for further diagnostic testing that may provide an explanation and solution to the unusual symptoms. Second, performing surgical treatment (even when there are only minimal physical findings) risks complications from the surgical procedure. Although all clinicians are vulnerable to these errors, awareness of these pitfalls does help prevent such extremes of response on the doctor's part.

Patients may respond to the lack of an adequate explanation and treatment by requesting further tests or consultation or by independently seeking further consultation. Considering the wide variety of training and traditions that exist in the health professions, it is not difficult to appreciate that a patient will find a practitioner who will provide some treatment that the patient feels might alleviate the symptoms. Multiple consultation and heavy use of surgical services are characteristic features of patients with chronic disorders, especially among those whose symptoms remain unexplained.[180–184] In three separate studies, OFP patients averaged 5, 6, and 7.5 physician/dentist consultations.[119,185,186]

▼ ORAL SYMPTOMS OUT OF PROPORTION TO RECOGNIZED ORAL LESIONS

Patients with unexplained oral symptoms do not always present completely free of dental, periodontal, and mucosal lesions that might be considered possible causes for the unusual symptoms. The evaluation of these patients commonly involves decisions as to whether a degenerating pulp, a coarsely fissured tongue, or muscle tension, for example, may explain complaints of chronic pain or a burning and painful tongue. When possible, treatment of the abnormality by root canal therapy, increased oral and tongue hygiene, or administration of muscle relaxants (in the situations just described) may resolve the question. However, when symptoms persist in the face of apparently adequate treatment, the clinician must decide whether the patient's symptoms possibly arise from another cause or whether they represent an exaggerated response to the particular oral abnormality that has been found and presumably adequately treated.

Among patients with unexplained oral symptoms, there is a group of patients whose salient features are the atypical or exaggerated response to the pain focus and (perhaps) the length of time their symptoms have persisted. It is important to identify the patient whose problem appears to be an inability to cope with minor oral sensory abnormality and who reacts to chronic low-grade pain in the same manner as he or she reacts to pain of greater intensity. Although this identification must be made cautiously and must be reviewed from time to time as treatment progresses, it does help focus treatment on the behavioral component of the patient's pain problem and help reduce continued and unnecessary diagnostic searches.

PSYCHOLOGICAL AND EMOTIONAL FACTORS

Clues that a patient may be reacting in an unusual fashion to abnormal sensory stimuli of low intensity can come from a variety of inquiries during the diagnostic interview. Patients may reveal evidence of a thought disorder during the interview. Patients may reveal the inability to provide clear and consistent statements about symptoms or events that can be checked with reasonable certainty. Confusion between symptoms and an emotionally charged event or personal relationship; the use of bizarre, mechanical, or animalistic explanations for oral symptoms; and the patient's inability to separate himself or herself from real or imaginary objects or people indicate a need for further psychological evaluation. The dentist also will recognize those who express marked paranoia (eg, the pain that is due to an object purposely left behind by the surgeon, who is acting as the agent of God or an enemy of the patient).

None of these phenomena alone substantiate a diagnosis of mental disease. Specific diagnoses (such as schizophrenia, paranoia, and depression) made by the dentist on this basis are unjustified, but the dentist who becomes aware of compromised mental ability in his or her patient should consider the likelihood that abnormal psychological factors may be complicating the diagnostic situation. Such mental confusion may involve organic or functional mental disease that will require further consultation and assessment.

Mental disease, mental retardation, and the inability to conform to society do not produce oral symptoms, but they may affect the individual's ability to handle sensory abnormality. Conversely, pain and other abnormal oral sensations also are experienced by mentally ill persons in response to physical causes, and the clinician must always be on guard against discounting oral symptoms in mentally ill individuals in favor of a psychological explanation without thorough examination of the patient. Table 14 lists the IASP classification categories of "pain of psychological origin in the head, face, and neck."[1]

The *DSM-IV* includes the classification entitled "pain disorder" within a larger category of "somatoform disorders."[65] Somatoform disorders are characterized by the presence of physical symptoms that suggest a general medical condition but that are not fully explained by the medical condition, the direct effects of a substance, or another mental disorder. A pain disorder is characterized by "pain as the

TABLE 14   Classification of Pain of Psychological Origin*

Classification	Definition
Muscle tension	Virtually continuous pain in any part of the body due to sustained muscle contraction and provoked by persistent overuse of particular muscles
Delusional or hallucinatory	Pain of psychological origin and attributed by the patient to a specific delusional cause
Hysterical, conversion, or hypochondriacal	Pain specifically attributable to the thought process, emotional state, or personality of the patient in the absence of an organic or delusional cause or tension mechanism
Associated with depression	Pain occurring in the course of a depressive illness usually not preceding the depression and not attributable to any other cause (not to be confused with depression that commonly occurs with chronic pain arising from physical reasons)

Reproduced with permission from Merskey H and Bogduk N.[1]
*International Association for the Study of Pain (IASP) classification.

predominant focus of clinical attention where psychological factors are judged to have an important role in its onset, severity, exacerbation, or maintenance."

The majority of patients for whom emotional factors obviously complicate their oral symptoms do not have diagnosable mental disease, although they may often be referred to as "crazy." Periods of increased emotional stress, whether brought about by interpersonal conflicts, external pressure from work or family, or an individual's own physical and personal drives, are normal for everyone, but such episodes also frequently reduce pain tolerance and the ability to handle chronic low-grade sensory abnormality. To the observer, the influence of the patient's emotions on the oral symptoms may at times be quite evident; for the patient, the interaction of emotional distress and physical disease may be impossible to manage, and he or she may be unable to control either aspect without assistance from the clinician. The following factors are clues that may provide insight into complicating emotional factors:

1. The setting of the story. The time of onset of the symptoms may have occurred in a period of increased personal, family, or work stress.
2. A history of extensive medical/dental treatment. Unusually extensive and (perhaps) multiple surgical procedures and the use of many medications despite minimal signs of "disease" that others tolerate as part of life indicate "increased help-seeking behavior" that may be maladaptive.[187]
3. The "naive" or medically inexperienced patient. Patients who have been free of oral disease until adulthood and who then need dental procedures may respond with excessive anxiety.[188] Paradoxically, those who have suffered painful traumatic and surgical

episodes in childhood and have learned excessively apprehensive or other maladaptive responses within their families may also become intolerant of the discomfort associated with dental procedures.[189]

4. The presence of a psychiatric illness or personality disorder. An association exists between chronic pain and psychiatric illness.[190,191] However, this does not confirm an etiologic relationship; rather, it is important to appreciate that psychiatric illness requires concomitant treatment to effectively treat the OFP.

5. Normal oral structures mistakenly identified as physical disease. Under the stress of the death of a friend or family member or the discovery of life-threatening disease in a close relative or friend, normal structures or sensations may be thought of as potential signs of disease.

6. Disrupted oral functions. The mouth serves as a means to obtain food, a modulator for producing speech, and a part of facial expression in interpersonal communication; it also features prominently in sexual encounters. It is not surprising that a limitation of oral function due to oral sensory abnormality can lead to a strong emotional reaction.

7. Imagined or symbolic functions traditionally assigned to the mouth that may be threatened. Unsupported by facts of physiology and anatomy, these functions of the mouth feature prominently in our language and thoughts and may be perceived by the patient as being threatened.

The extent to which these traditional images exist in the thoughts of patients with oral disease is largely undocumented and could probably be revealed only by psychoanalysis. However, comments patients make in regard to their oral symptoms during regular diagnostic interviews suggest that such symbolism is a common accompaniment of oral disease. It is important that the clinician recognize these psychological interactions because it may allow him or her to distinguish complaints that are essentially psychological in nature from those that are more directly related to altered physiologic states; the treatment of one is quite different from the treatment of the other, and simultaneous treatment of both problems may be needed. It is an error to consider the patient who uses symbolic images in relating oral problems to be necessarily psychologically abnormal even when the images appear to be somewhat bizarre and overly graphic.[192] It is likely that oral symbolism is normally well developed in most minds, and concern about oral pain and discomfort simply allows patients to be somewhat less reserved about expressing their thoughts than they might usually be. The following metaphors are examples: the "mouthpiece of the mind" (a source of pleasant, virtuous, complimentary, and encouraging statements, as well as smiles, laughs, and blessings, versus an invective tight-lipped mouth); an "organ of perception" (the ability to distinguish pleasurable from noxious foods and, by extension, pleasurable from unhappy aspects of life); and a "source of pleasure" (the mouth can provide kisses or caresses or can mark an aggressive, hostile personality).

If the clinician suspects a psychological cause for OFP, it is important to keep the following in mind:

1. However sophisticated the diagnostic procedures used, no diagnosis is final, and time may often reveal a previously unrecognized organic problem underlying the patient's symptoms.

2. The diagnostic procedures used should be as exhaustive as possible, even in the presence of major psychological dysfunction.

3. Psychological and psychogenic pains cannot be clearly distinguished from pain that has an obvious organic cause; psychological factors are a component of all painful experiences.

4. Pain associated with overwhelming psychological dysfunction (psychogenic pain) is as real to the patient as is pain from an obvious organic cause and cannot be dismissed as something that is "just in the patient's head."

5. A diagnosis of psychological pain should be confirmed by psychiatric evaluation of the patient.

IMPORTANCE OF FOLLOW-UP AND REPEATED EXAMINATION AND TESTING

Of prime importance in the management of patients with unexplained oral symptoms is the recognition that an identification of the cause of the symptoms may come only with time. Several studies of chronic oral sensory complaints have shown that with time, as many as half of patients with unexplained OFP were found to have specific pathologic diagnoses that explained their symptoms (provided that repeated examinations and diagnostic tests were continued beyond the initial period of consultation).[182,183]

The success of referral clinics in managing problems of this type derives partly from a program of continued surveillance of the patient by a coordinated group of consultants and partly from the availability of sophisticated diagnostic equipment.[183,193] With time, small lesions such as tumors in the nasopharynx, parotid gland, infratemporal fossa, and cranium that can impinge on oral sensory and motor nerves increase in size and become apparent through the development of other abnormalities. Systemic neurologic diseases such as multiple sclerosis develop from a prodromal stage, in which only unusual oral symptoms are present, to a stage in which a variety of tests will reveal the presence of disease and explain the patient's oral symptoms.[194] The literature contains numerous references to patients whose oral symptoms remained unexplained for varied periods of time until further growth of a tumor revealed the focus of the patient's symptoms.[171,195–205] Included among these reports are many descriptions of tumors of the parotid gland, infratemporal space, and cranial cavity that initially mimicked the symptoms of a TMD. Such reports emphasize the need for continuous awareness of such possibilities.[204] Newer imaging techniques may reveal such lesions and are important tools in the management of undiagnosed chronic OFP.[198,206–208]

▼ DIAGNOSIS AND MANAGEMENT OF SPECIFIC OFP DISORDERS

Facial Neuralgias

The classic neuralgias that affect the craniofacial region are a unique group of neurologic disorders involving the cranial nerves and are characterized by (a) brief episodes of shooting, often electric shock–like pain along the course of the affected nerve branch; (b) trigger zones on the skin or mucosa that precipitate painful attacks when touched; and (c) pain-free periods between attacks and refractory periods immediately after an attack, during which a new episode cannot be triggered. These clinical characteristics differ from neuropathic pain, which tends to be constant and has a burning quality without the presence of trigger zones. Neuropathic pain most often results from disorders that involve the spinal nerves, whereas involvement of the cranial nerves may result in either chronic neuropathic pain or the classic brief episodes of shooting pain. Whether a lesion involving a cranial nerve causes constant neuropathic pain or brief episodes of shooting pain depends on both the nature of the underlying disorder and the position of the lesion along the course of the nerve. For example, tumors involving the trigeminal nerve between the pontine angle in the posterior cranial fossa and the ganglion in the middle cranial fossa will usually result in the lancinating pain of TN, whereas more peripheral lesions will usually result in neuropathic pain. The major craniofacial neuralgias include TN, glossopharyngeal neuralgia, and occipital neuralgia. Geniculate neuralgia involving the sensory portion of CN VII is a similar but rare disorder. PHN and post-traumatic neuralgia are common causes of neuropathic pain.

TRIGEMINAL NEURALGIA

TN, also called tic douloureux, is the most common of the cranial neuralgias and chiefly affects individuals older than 50 years of age. TN is classified as either classic TN when it is not associated with an underlying neurologic disease or symptomatic TN when no neurologic disorder can be detected.

Etiology and Pathogenesis. The cause of classic TN remains controversial, but approximately 10% of cases are symptomatic and have detectable underlying pathology, such as a tumor of the cerebellopontine angle, a demyelinating plaque of multiple sclerosis, or a vascular malformation. The most frequent tumor is a meningioma of the posterior cranial fossa.

The most widely accepted theory is that a majority of cases of classic TN are caused by an atherosclerotic blood vessel (usually the superior cerebellar artery) pressing on and grooving the root of the trigeminal nerve. This pressure results in focal demyelinization and hyperexcitability of nerve fibers, which will then fire in response to light touch, resulting in brief episodes of intense pain.[209]

Evidence for this theory includes the observation that neurosurgery that removes the pressure of the vessel from the nerve root by use of a microvascular decompression procedure eliminates the pain in a majority of cases. In a study of 1,185 patients who had microvascular decompression surgery for TN that did not respond to drug therapy, 70% of the patients were pain free 10 years after the surgery.[210] Additional evidence for this theory was obtained from a study using tomographic magnetic resonance imaging (MRI), which showed that contact between a blood vessel and the trigeminal nerve root was much greater on the affected side.[211]

Evidence against this theory includes the finding by neurosurgeons that manipulation of the area of the nerve root may eliminate the painful episodes even when an atherosclerotic vessel is not pressing on the nerve root. Other investigators believe that a major factor in the etiology of TN is a degeneration of the ganglion rather than the nerve root.[212]

Clinical Features. The majority of patients with TN present with characteristic clinical features, which include episodes of intense shooting, stabbing pain that lasts for a few seconds and then completely disappears. The pain characteristically has an electric shock–like quality and is unilateral except in a small percentage of cases. The maxillary branch is the branch that is most commonly affected, followed by the mandibular branch and (rarely) the ophthalmic branch. Involvement of more than one branch occurs in some cases.

Pain in TN is precipitated by a light touch on a "trigger zone" present on the skin or mucosa within the distribution of the involved nerve branch. Common sites for trigger zones include the nasolabial fold and the corner of the lip. Shaving, showering, eating, speaking, or even exposure to wind can trigger a painful episode, and patients often protect the trigger zone with their hand or an article of clothing. Intraoral trigger zones can confuse the diagnosis by suggesting a dental disorder, and TN patients often first consult a dentist for evaluation. The stabbing pain can mimic the pain of a cracked tooth, but the two disorders can be distinguished by determining whether placing food in the mouth without chewing or whether gently touching the soft tissue around the trigger zone will precipitate pain. TN pain will be triggered by touching the soft tissue, whereas pressure on the tooth is required to cause pain from a cracked tooth. Just after an attack, there is a refractory period when touching the trigger zone will not precipitate pain. The number of attacks may vary from one or two per day to several per minute. Patients with severe TN may be severely disabled by attacks that are triggered by speaking or other mouth movements.

Diagnosis. The diagnosis of TN is usually based on the history of shooting pain along a branch of the trigeminal nerve, precipitated by touching a trigger zone, and possibly examination that demonstrates the shooting pain. A routine cranial nerve examination will be normal in patients with idiopathic TN, but sensory and/or motor changes may be evident in patients with underlying tumors or other CNS pathology. A recent study demonstrated that an examination alone was often insufficient to distinguish symptomatic from classic TN and that electrophysiologic testing of trigeminal reflexes was much more accurate.[213] Local anesthetic blocks, which temporarily eliminate the trigger zone, may also be helpful in diagnosis. Since approximately 10% of TN cases are caused by detectable underlying pathology, enhanced MRI of the brain is indicated to rule out tumors, multiple sclerosis, and vascular malformations. Magnetic resonance angiography may also be needed to detect difficult to visualize vascular abnormalities.

Management.   Initial therapy for TN should consist of trials of drugs that are effective in eliminating the painful attacks. Anticonvulsant drugs are most frequently used and are most effective. Carbamazepine is the most commonly used drug and is an effective therapy for greater than 85% of newly diagnosed cases of TN. The drug is administered in slowly increasing doses until pain relief has been achieved. Skin reactions, including generalized erythema multiforme, are serious side effects. Patients receiving carbamazepine must have periodic hematologic laboratory evaluations because serious life-threatening blood dyscrasias occur in rare cases. Monitoring of hepatic and renal function is also recommended. Patients who do not respond to carbamazepine alone may obtain relief from baclofen or by combining carbamazepine with baclofen.[214] Oxcarbamazepine is the 10-ketoanalogue of carbamazepine with a similar mode of action. Its principal advantage over carbamazepine is that the former causes little, if any, induction of hepatic enzyme with a consequent lack of autoinduction and a lower risk of blood dyscrasias. Hyponatremia may be a problem for elderly patients with cardiovascular disease.

Gabapentin, a newer anticonvulsant that also has fewer serious side effects than carbamazepine, is effective in some patients but does not appear to be as reliable as carbamazepine or oxcarbamazepine. Pregablin, a new gabapentin potent synthetic analogue, may be useful treatment; however, trials have not been performed to evaluate pregablin in TN. Use of sumatriptan has also recently shown promise in the management of TN.[215]

Other drugs that are effective for some patients include phenytoin, lamotrigine, baclofen, topiramate, and pimozide.[216] Since TN may have temporary or permanent spontaneous remissions, drug therapy should be slowly withdrawn if a patient remains pain free for 3 months.

Clinicians treating TN must be aware that drug therapy, especially with carbamazepine, may become less effective over time and that progressively higher doses may be required for pain control. In cases in which drug therapy is ineffective or in which the patient is unable to tolerate the side effects of drugs after trials of several agents, surgical therapy is indicated. A number of surgical procedures that result in temporary or permanent remission of the painful attacks have been described. These include procedures performed on the peripheral portion of the nerve, where it exits the jaw; at the gasserian ganglion; and on the brainstem, at the posterior cranial fossa. Peripheral surgery includes cryosurgery on the trigeminal nerve branch that triggers the painful attacks. This procedure is most frequently performed at the mental nerve for cases involving the third division and at the infraorbital nerve for cases involving the second division. The potential effectiveness of this procedure can be evaluated prior to surgery by determining whether a long-acting local anesthetic eliminates the pain during the duration of anesthesia. This procedure is usually effective for 12 to 18 months, at which time it must be repeated or another form of therapy must be instituted.

The most commonly performed procedure at the level of the gasserian ganglion is percutaneous radiofrequency thermocoagulation, although some clinicians continue to advocate glycerol block at the ganglion or compression of the ganglion by balloon microcompression.[217–219] An infrequent but severe surgical complication is anesthesia dolorosa, which is numbness combined with severe intractable pain. The most extensively studied surgical procedure is microvascular decompression of the nerve root at the brainstem. In a report of 1,185 patients who were observed for 1 to 6 years, 70% of the patients experienced long-term relief of symptoms.[220] It should be noted that 30% of the patients experienced a recurrence of symptoms and required a second procedure or alternative therapy. Complications were rare but included stroke, facial numbness, and facial weakness.

Gamma knife stereotactic radiosurgery is a new minimally invasive technique for the treatment of TN. The technique uses multiple beams of radiation, usually in doses of 70 to 90 Gy units, converging in three dimensions to focus precisely on a small volume. The method relies on precise MRI sequencing that helps localization of the beam and allows a higher dose of radiation to be given with more sparing of normal tissue. This technique is particularly helpful for elderly patients with a high surgical risk.[221–224] In summary, therapy for TN presently includes a variety of both medical and surgical approaches, each of which is effective for some patients. Drug therapy, including trials of several drugs or combinations of drugs, should be attempted before surgery is recommended. When surgery is necessary, the patient should be carefully counseled regarding the advantages and disadvantages of the available surgical procedures. Clinicians should also remember that since spontaneous remissions are a feature of TN, procedures resulting in temporary relief might be all that is necessary for some patients.

GLOSSOPHARYNGEAL NEURALGIA

Glossopharyngeal neuralgia is a rare condition that is associated with paroxysmal pain that is similar to, although less intense than, the pain of TN. The location of the trigger zone and pain sensation follows the distribution of the glossopharyngeal nerve, namely, the pharynx, posterior tongue, ear, and infra-auricular retromandibular area. Pain is triggered by stimulating the pharyngeal mucosa during chewing, talking, and swallowing. The pain can be easily confused with that of geniculate neuralgia (because of the common ear symptoms) or with that of TMDs (because of pain following jaw movement).

Glossopharyngeal neuralgia may occur with TN, and when this occurs, a search for a common central lesion is essential. Glossopharyngeal neuralgia also may be associated with a vasovagal reflex, which may cause syncope, asystole, bradycardia, hypotension, and cardiac arrest.[225] Insertion of a pacemaker may be required to prevent syncopal episodes.[226] The application of a topical anesthetic to the pharyngeal mucosa eliminates glossopharyngeal nerve pain and can aid in distinguishing it from the pain of other neuralgias. The most common causes of glossopharyngeal neuralgia are intracranial or extracranial tumors and vascular abnormalities that compress CN IX. Treatment is similar to that for TN, with a good response to carbamazepine and oxcarbazepine[227] Refractory cases are treated surgically by intracranial or extracranial section of CN IX, microvascular decompression in the posterior cranial fossa, or percutaneous radiofrequency thermocoagulation of the nerve at the jugular foramen.[228]

NERVOUS INTERMEDIUS (GENICULATE) NEURALGIA

Nervous intermedius (geniculate) neuralgia is an uncommon paroxysmal neuralgia of CN VII, characterized by pain in the ear and (less frequently) the anterior tongue or soft palate. The location of pain matches the sensory distribution of this nerve (ie, the external auditory canal and a small area on the soft palate and the posterior auricular region). Pain may be provoked by the stimulation of trigger zones within the ipsilateral distribution of the nerve. The pain is not as sharp or intense as in TN, and there is often some degree of facial paralysis, indicating the simultaneous involvement of the motor root. Geniculate neuralgia commonly results from herpes zoster of the geniculate ganglion and nervus intermedius of CN VII, a condition referred to as Ramsay Hunt syndrome. Viral vesicles may be observed in the ear canal or on the tympanic membrane. The symptoms result from inflammatory neural degeneration, and a short course (2 to 3 weeks) of high-dose steroid therapy is beneficial.[229] Acyclovir significantly reduces the duration of the pain.

Patients with geniculate neuralgia can be treated with anticolvusants such as oxcarbazepine, carbamazepine, and gabapentin. Patients who do not respond to these medications may undergo surgery for excision of the nervus intermedius and geniculate ganglion[230] or microvacular decompression.[231]

OCCIPITAL NEURALGIA

Occipital neuralgia presents as a paroxysmal stabbing pain in the distribution of the greater or lesser occipital nerves. It may be caused by trauma, myofascial pain of the neck muscles, neoplasms, infections, and aneurysms. Palpation below the superior nuchal line may reveal an exquisitely tender spot. Treatment has included occipital nerve block,[232] corticosteroids, neurolysis, C2 dorsal root gangionectomy,[233] and peripheral nerve stimulation.[234]

POSTHERPETIC NEURALGIA

Etiology and Pathogenesis. Herpes zoster (shingles), described in detail in Chapter 3, is caused by the reactivation of latent varicella-zoster virus infection that results in both pain and vesicular lesions along the course of the affected nerve. Approximately 15 to 20% of cases of herpes zoster involve the trigeminal nerve, although the majority of these cases affect the ophthalmic division of the fifth nerve, resulting in pain and lesions in the region of the eyes and forehead. Herpes zoster of the maxillary and mandibular divisions is a cause of facial and oral pain as well as of lesions. In a majority of cases, the pain of herpes zoster resolves within a month after the lesions heal. Pain that persists longer than a month is classified as PHN, although some authors do not make the diagnosis of PHN until the pain has persisted for longer than 3 or even 6 months.[235] PHN may occur at any age, but the major risk factor is increasing age. Few individuals younger than 30 years of age experience PHN, whereas more than 25% of individuals older than 55 years of age and two-thirds of patients older than over 70 years of age will suffer from PHN after an episode of herpes zoster.[236] Elderly patients also have an increased risk of experiencing severe pain for an extended period of time,[237] and the incidence of PHN is higher in women.[238] Greater than 25% of patients with herpes zoster will experience PHN for over 1 year.[239] The pain and numbness of PHN results from a combination of both central and peripheral mechanisms. The varicella-zoster virus injures the peripheral nerve by demyelination, wallerian degeneration, and sclerosis, but changes in the CNS, including atrophy of dorsal horn cells in the spinal cord, have also been associated with PHN.[240,241] This combination of peripheral and central injury results in the spontaneous discharge of neurons and an exaggerated painful response to nonpainful stimuli.[240] There is also evidence to support the theory that a low-grade persistent infection of the trigeminal ganglion contributes to PHN pain and that antiviral therapy with intravenous acyclovir or oral valacyclovir or famciclovir reduces the pain.[242]

Clinical Manifestations. Patients with PHN experience persistent pain, paresthesia, hyperesthesia, and allodynia months to years after the zoster lesions have healed. The pain is often accompanied by a sensory deficit, and there is a correlation between the degree of sensory deficit and the severity of pain.[243]

Management. Prevention of PHN is now possible, and use of a live attenuated varicella-zoster vaccine for patients over 60 years of age significantly reduces the incidence of herpes zoster and the sequelae of PHN.[239,244] For patients who develop herpes zoster, use of antiviral drugs early in the course of the disease reduces the risk of PHN.[245] For patients who develop PHN, the method of treatment chosen should depend on the severity of the symptoms and the general medical status of the patient. Treatment includes topical therapy, drug therapy, and surgery.

Topical therapy includes the use of topical anesthetic agents, such as lidocaine, or analgesics, particularly capsaicin. A lidocaine patch is available that was shown to be effective in managing PHN.[246] Combinations of topical anesthetics such as EMLA cream (AstraZeneca) have also been reported as helpful.[247] Capsaicin, an extract of hot chili peppers that depletes the neurotransmitter substance P when used topically, has been shown to be helpful in reducing the pain of PHN, but the side effect of a burning sensation at the site of application limits its usefulness for many patients.

The use of TCAs such as amitriptyline, nortriptyline, doxepin, and desipramine is a well-established method of reducing the chronic burning pain that is characteristic of PHN.[248–251] A recent trial showed that desipramine is superior to both amitriptyline and fluoxetine for management of PHN.[252] Because a significant number of elderly patients cannot tolerate the sedative or cardiovascular side effects associated with TCAs, the use of other drugs, particularly gabapentin, has been advocated. In one controlled clinical trial, the use of gabapentin reduced pain by more than 30% and also improved sleep and overall quality of life.[253] Randomized clinical trials showed that pregablin significantly reduced mean pain scores compared with placebo in patients with PHN.[254,255]

Patients who undergo episodes of shooting pain may experience relief through the use of anticonvulsant drugs, such as carbamazepine or phenytoin.[251] When medical therapy has been ineffective in managing intractable pain, nerve blocks or surgery at the level of the peripheral nerve or dorsal root has been effective for some patients.

POST-TRAUMATIC NEUROPATHIC PAIN

Etiology and Pathogenesis. Trigeminal nerve injuries may result from facial trauma or from surgical procedures, such as the removal of impacted third molars, the placement of dental implants, the removal of cysts or tumors of the jaws, genioplasties, or osteotomies.

Some patients may develop chronic pain following negligible trauma, such as root canal therapy, or even following periodontal treatment.[256] The severity of the injury does not always predict the chronic neuropathic pain intensity.[257,258] Sensory loss following dental implant insertion occurs in 1 to 8% of cases and following orthognathic surgery in up to 30% of the cases.[259–261] However, the incidence of chronic pain and persistent altered sensation following these procedures has never been studied. Chronic pain following endodontic treatment is more common than after any other dental treatment; it was found to occur in 3 to 13% of surgical or nonsurgical endodontic cases.[262] Transient anesthesia and paresthesia in the lingual or inferior alveolar nerves are common following third molar extraction, and altered sensation may persist in 0.3 to 1% of cases.[263–265] However, long-term follow-up of both nerves failed to demonstrate chronic neuropathic pain cases.[266]

The incidence of trigeminal post-traumatic neuropathic pain is extremely low, taking into consideration the number of surgical and interventional procedures performed by dentists. The lack of a consistent classification reduces the ability to study the condition's characteristics and treatment options.[267]

The pain associated with nerve injury often has a burning quality due to spontaneous activity in nociceptor C fibers.[268] Minor nerve injuries (classified as neurapraxia) do not result in axonal degeneration but may cause temporary symptoms of paresthesia for a few hours or days. More serious nerve damage (classified as axonotmesis) results in the degeneration of neural fibers, although the nerve trunk remains intact. These injuries cause symptoms for several months but have a good prognosis for recovery after axonal regeneration is complete. Total nerve section (neurotmesis) frequently causes permanent nerve damage, resulting in anesthesia and/or dysesthesia.[269] Central sensitization probably plays a role in the symptoms of neuropathy.

Clinical Manifestations. The pain associated with peripheral nerve injury may be persistent or may occur only in response to a stimulus, such as a light touch. Patients with nerve damage may experience anesthesia (loss in sensation), paresthesia (a feeling of "pins and needles"), allodynia (pain caused by a stimulus that is normally not painful), or hyperalgesia (an exaggerated response to a mildly painful stimulus).

The pain may be diffuse and spread across dermatomes; the pain intensity is usually moderate to severe.

Management. Treatment of neuropathic pain may be surgical, nonsurgical, or a combination of both, depending on the nature of the injury and the severity of the pain.

However, the microsurgical procedures are complicated and should be performed in selected cases.[270,271] Systemic corticosteroids are considered helpful in decreasing the incidence and severity of traumatic neuropathies when administered within the first week after a nerve injury. Steroids used after this initial period are of little value. The most frequently used medications for the management of neuropathic pain include TCAs and gabapentin.

TCAs such as amitriptyline, doxepin, and nortriptyline have been extensively studied and widely used to treat neuropathic pain, including traumatic neuropathies of the trigeminal nerve.[272] The TCAs can be used alone; in severe intractable cases, they potentiate the effect of narcotic analgesics. The clinician prescribing TCAs must be aware of potentially serious side effects in patients with cardiac arrhythmias or glaucoma and must be able to help the patient manage common side effects, which include drowsiness, weight gain from increased appetite, and dry mouth.

Gabapentin and its synthetic analogue pregabalin, anticonvulsant drugs approved for the treatment of epilepsy, have been used with increasing frequency to treat a variety of neuropathic pain syndromes, including diabetic neuropathy and PHN. The low incidence of serious side effects has encouraged widespread use of this drug. A controlled clinical trial that compared the effectiveness of gabapentin with that of the TCA amitriptyline demonstrated that both were equally effective in controlling neuropathic pain associated with diabetic neuropathy.[273,274]

Topical capsaicin may also be effective in controlling pain and is especially useful for patients who are unable to tolerate the side effects of systemic therapy.

Complex Regional Pain Syndrome I (Reflex Sympathetic Dystrophy)

CRPSs are chronic pain conditions that develop as a result of injury. CRPS I was previously termed reflex sympathetic dystrophy (RSD), and CRPS II was previously termed causalgia. CRPs patients suffer from allodynia, hyperalgesia, and spontaneous pain that extends beyond the affected nerve dermatome. The painful condition is accompanied by motor and sweat abnormalities, trophic changes in muscles and skin, edema, and abnormal blood flow in the skin. CRPS I may develop following relatively minor local trauma, whereas CRPS II follows obvious injury to a major nerve.

ETIOLOGY AND PATHOGENESIS

The constellation of signs and symptoms associated with CRPS is believed to result from changes after trauma that couples sensory nerve fibers with sympathetic stimuli. Evidence for the existence of CRPS includes studies that show that surgical or drug-induced blockades of the sympathetic nervous system relieve the symptoms. In a new taxonomy included in the classification of chronic pain, CRPS I is used in place of RSD, and CRPS II replaces causalgia, which is a pain syndrome resulting from a major nerve injury. RSD has rarely been described as involving the trigeminal nerve distribution, and the role of the sympathetic nervous system in chronic facial pain is unknown. One study of chronic facial pain patients who also had evidence of autonomic dysfunction described a subset of patients who improved after a stellate ganglion block, suggesting a possible role for the sympathetic nervous system.[275] Other reports describe facial pain resolving after cervical sympathectomy, clonidine, guanethidine, and stellate ganglion blockade.[276]

CLINICAL MANIFESTATIONS

The most constant symptom of CRPS is spontaneous chronic burning pain and tenderness, frequently accompanied by motor dysfunction, sweating, and cutaneous atrophy. The involved skin may also be edematous and erythematous as a result of changes in blood flow, and the underlying bone is commonly demineralized. Allodynia and hyperesthesia are common symptoms, and movement exacerbates the pain. This syndrome most commonly involves the extremities distal to an injury. The existence of this disorder in the head and facial region is controversial.

TREATMENT

The recommended therapy for CRPS involves a multidisciplinary approach that includes physical therapy, nerve blocks, and drug therapy. Blockades of regional sympathetic ganglia or regional intravenous blockades with guanethidine, reserpine, or phenoxybenzamine, combined with a local anesthetic, have been reported as successful and are used in anesthesia pain clinics.[277] Bisphosphonates such as alendronate or pamidronate have decreased pain in some RSD patients when used intravenously. It is unclear whether these drugs are helpful because of their effect on bone or because of anti-inflammatory properties.[278]

Atypical Odontalgia (Atypical Facial Pain)

A classification that includes the diagnoses of AO and AFP is controversial, and many workers in the field of facial pain believe that these terms should be discarded because they are often used either as catchalls to denote patients who have not been adequately evaluated or because they imply that the pain is purely psychological in origin. Some classification systems, including the IHS system, use the term "facial pain not fulfilling other criteria" to describe patients in this category. The disputed terms are still commonly used in clinical practice, however, since a group of individuals exists who (1) have a chronic facial pain syndrome with characteristic clinical features, (2) have been thoroughly investigated and have other detectable cause of pain, and (3) do not fall into any other diagnostic categories. The term *atypical odontalgia* is used in this context when the pain is confined to the teeth or gingivae, whereas the term *atypical facial pain* is used when other parts of the face are involved.

ETIOLOGY AND PATHOGENESIS

There are several theories regarding the etiology of AO and AFP. One theory considers AO and AFP to be a form of deafferentation or phantom tooth pain. This theory is supported by the high percentage of patients with these disorders who report that the symptoms began after a dental procedure such as endodontic therapy or an extraction. Others have theorized that AO is a form of vascular, neuropathic, or sympathetically maintained pain. Other studies support the concept that at least some of the patients in this category have a strong psychogenic component to their symptoms and that depressive, somatization, and conversion disorders have been described as major factors in some patients. It is frequently difficult to accurately study the psychological aspects of a chronic pain syndrome since anxiety and depression are part of the clinical picture of all patients with chronic pain.

There is often strong disagreement between facial pain experts who stress the biologic basis of AO and AFP and others who stress the emotional basis, but the etiology remains unknown at this time. It is likely that there are subgroups of patients who fall into the category of AO and AFP, some of whom have a strong component of deafferentation pain, whereas others have a psychological basis for similar symptoms. It is also possible that a combination of both neuropathic and psychological mechanisms is important in the etiology of this presently poorly understood facial pain syndrome.

CLINICAL MANIFESTATIONS

The major manifestation of AO and AFP is a constant dull, aching pain without an apparent cause that can be detected by examination or laboratory studies. AO occurs most frequently in women in the fourth and fifth decades of life, and most studies report that women make up more than 80% of the patients. The pain is described as a constant dull ache, instead of the brief and severe attacks of pain that are characteristic of TN. There are no trigger zones, and lancinating pains are rare. The patient frequently reports that the onset of pain coincided with a dental procedure, such as oral surgery or an endodontic or restorative procedure. Patients also report seeking multiple dental procedures to treat the pain; these procedures may result in temporary relief, but the pain characteristically returns in days or weeks. Other patients will give a history of sinus procedures or of receiving trials of multiple medications, including antibiotics, corticosteroids, decongestants, or anticonvulsant drugs. The pain may remain in one area or may migrate, either spontaneously or after a surgical procedure. Symptoms may remain unilateral, cross the midline in some cases, or involve both the maxilla and mandible.

A thorough history and examination including evaluation of the cranial nerves, oropharynx, and teeth must be performed to rule out dental, neurologic, or nasopharyngeal disease. A thorough examination of the masticatory muscles should also be performed to eliminate myofascial pain as a cause of the symptoms. Laboratory tests should be carried out when indicated by the history and examination. Patients with AO or AFP have completely normal radiographic and clinical laboratory studies.

MANAGEMENT

Once the diagnosis has been made and other pathologies have been eliminated, it is important that the symptoms are taken seriously and are not dismissed as imaginary. Patients should be counseled regarding the nature of AO and reassured that they do not have an undetected life-threatening disease and that they can be helped without invasive procedures. When indicated, consultation with other specialists, such as otolaryngologists, neurologists, or psychiatrists, may be helpful. TCAs such as amitriptyline, nortriptyline, desipramine, and doxepin, given in low to moderate doses, are often effective in reducing or (in some cases) eliminating the pain. Other recommended drugs include gabapentin, pregablin, and clonazepam. Some clinicians report benefit from topical desensitization with capsaicin, topical anesthetics, or topical doxepin.

Burning Mouth Syndrome (Glossodynia)

Burning sensations accompany many inflammatory or ulcerative diseases of the oral mucosa, but the term *burning mouth syndrome* is reserved for describing oral burning that has no detectable cause. The burning symptoms in patients with BMS do not follow anatomic pathways, there are no mucosal lesions or known neurologic or systemic disorders to explain the symptoms, and there are no characteristic laboratory abnormalities.

ETIOLOGY AND PATHOGENESIS

The cause of BMS remains unknown; however, oral and perioral burning can be a symptom of local factors or systemic diseases including hormonal and allergic disorders, salivary gland hypofunction, chronic low-grade trauma, and psychiatric abnormalities. Burning mouth may also be a complication of drug therapy with angiotensin-converting enzyme (ACE) inhibitors such as enalapril or quinapril.[279] The increased incidence of BMS in women after menopause has led investigators to suspect an association with hormonal changes, but there is little evidence that women with BMS have more hormonal abnormalities than matched controls who do not have BMS. Studies of estrogen replacement therapy used to treat BMS have yielded mixed results, and few investigators recommend hormone replacement as a primary therapy for BMS in patients who do not require it for other reasons.

Allergic reactions have also been suspected, but there is no evidence to support the hypothesis that BMS is the result of allergic reactions to food, oral hygiene products, or dental materials. A contact allergy can affect the oral mucosa and result in burning sensations, but inflammatory, lichenoid, or ulcerative lesions are present in cases of contact allergy and absent in BMS patients.

BMS has been associated with psychological disorders in many studies. Depression is frequently associated with BMS, and in some studies, close to one-third of BMS patients have significant depression scores, although, as with any chronic pain disorder, it is unclear if depression is the cause or the effect of the symptoms.[280–282] It is likely that some cases of BMS have a strong psychological component, but other factors, such as chronic low-grade trauma resulting from parafunctional oral habits (eg, rubbing the tongue across the teeth or pressing it on the palate), are also likely to play a role.

Changes in taste have been reported in over 60% of patients with BMS, and BMS patients have been shown to have different thresholds of taste perception than matched controls.[283] Dysgeusia (particularly an abnormally bitter taste) has been reported by 60% of BMS patients.[284] This association has led to a concept that BMS may be a defect in sensory peripheral neural mechanisms.[285] Functional MRI of the brain of BMS patients demonstrated brain activation patterns similar to other neuropathic pain disorders, suggesting that brain hypoactivity may play a role.[286]

CLINICAL MANIFESTATIONS

Women experience symptoms of BMS seven times more frequently than men.[287] When questioned, 10 to 15% of postmenopausal women are found to have a history of oral burning sensations, and these symptoms are most prevalent 3 to 12 years after menopause.[288] The tongue is the most common site of involvement, but the lips and palate are also frequently involved. The burning can be intermittent or constant, but eating, drinking, or placing candy or chewing gum in the mouth characteristically relieves the symptoms. This contrasts with the increased oral burning noted during eating that occurs in patients with lesions or neuralgias affecting the oral mucosa. Patients presenting with BMS are often apprehensive and admit to being generally anxious or "high-strung." They may also have symptoms that suggest depression, such as decreased appetite, insomnia, and a loss of interest in daily activities.

Other causes of burning symptoms of the oral mucosa must be eliminated by examination and laboratory studies before the diagnosis of BMS can be made. Patients with unilateral symptoms should have a thorough evaluation of the trigeminal and other cranial nerves to eliminate a neurologic source of pain. A careful clinical examination for oral lesions resulting from candidiasis, lichen planus, or other mucosal diseases should be performed. Patients complaining of a combination of xerostomia and burning should be evaluated for the possibility of a salivary gland disorder, particularly if the mucosa appears to be dry and the patient has difficulty swallowing dry foods without sipping liquids. When indicated, laboratory tests should be carried out to detect undiagnosed diabetic neuropathy, anemia, or deficiencies of iron, folate, or vitamin B_{12}.

TREATMENT

Once the diagnosis of BMS has been made by eliminating the possibility of detectable lesions or underlying medical disorders, the patient should be reassured of the benign nature of the symptoms. Counseling the patient in regard to the nature of BMS is helpful in management, particularly because many patients will have had multiple clinical evaluations without an explanation for the symptoms. Counseling and reassurance may be adequate management for individuals with mild burning sensations, but patients with symptoms that are more severe often require drug therapy. The drug therapies that have been found to be the most helpful are low doses of TCAs, such as amitriptyline and doxepin, or clonazepam (a benzodiazepine derivative). It should be stressed to the patient that these drugs are being used not to manage psychiatric illness but for their well-documented analgesic effect. Clinicians prescribing these drugs should be familiar with potential serious and annoying side effects.

Topical anesthetics for the treatment of BMS are not as useful as the nonpredictable effect; the pain can either decrease or increase.[289] On the other hand, topical clonazepam applied by sucking (not swallowed) was effective in reducing pain intensity[290]; moreover, in another study, the positive effect was carried over up to 6 months following 2 weeks of treatment.[291] Recently, drugs from a different category have shown a potential to benefit BMS patients. A 2-month course of 600 mg daily of alpha-lipoic acid has been shown to reduce BMS pain,[292,293] and systemic capsaicin (0.25% capsule 3/d for 30 days) demonstrated some positive effects on BMS pain intensity.[294]

Vascular Pain

Pain originating from vascular structures may cause facial pain that can be misdiagnosed and mistaken for other oral disorders, including toothache or TMDs. This section discusses the major pain disorders of vascular etiology that have prominent orofacial signs and symptoms.

CRANIAL ARTERITIS

Cranial arteritis (temporal arteritis, giant cell arteritis) is an inflammatory disorder involving the medium-sized branches of the carotid arteries. The temporal artery is the most commonly involved branch. The blood vessel abnormality may be localized to the head and face or may be part of the generalized disease polymyalgia rheumatica.

Etiology and Pathogenesis. Both cranial arteritis and polymyalgia rheumatica are caused by immune abnormalities that affect cytokines and T lymphocytes, resulting in inflammatory infiltrates in the walls of arteries. This infiltrate is characterized by the formation of multinucleated giant cells. The underlying trigger of the inflammatory response is unknown.

Clinical Manifestations. Cranial arteritis most frequently affects adults above the age of 50 years. Patients have a throbbing headache accompanied by generalized symptoms, including fever, malaise, and loss of appetite. Patients with polymyalgia rheumatica will have accompanying joint and muscle pain. Examination of the involved temporal artery reveals a thickened, pulsating vessel. Since the mandibular and lingual arteries may be involved, a throbbing pain in the jaw or tongue may be an early sign or even a presenting sign. A serious complication in untreated patients is ischemia of the eye, which may lead to progressive loss of vision or sudden blindness. These visual manifestations may be prevented by early diagnosis and prompt therapy.

Laboratory abnormalities include an elevated ESR and anemia. Abnormal C-reactive protein may also be an important early finding. The most definitive diagnostic test is a biopsy specimen (from the involved temporal artery) that demonstrates the characteristic inflammatory infiltrate. Since the entire vessel is not involved, an adequate specimen must be taken to detect the changes. A negative biopsy result does not rule out temporal arteritis, and the diagnosis should continue to be considered in patients over 50 years of age who have chronic pounding head or OFP and an elevated ESR.

Treatment. Individuals with cranial arteritis should be treated with systemic corticosteroids as soon as the diagnosis is made. The initial dose ranges between 40 and 60 mg of prednisone per day, and the steroid is tapered once the signs of the disease are controlled. The ESR may be used to help monitor disease status. Patients are maintained on systemic steroids for 1 to 2 years after symptoms resolve. Steroids may be supplemented by adjuvant therapy with immunosuppressive drugs, such as cyclophosphamide, to reduce the complications of long-term corticosteroid therapy. Immediate steroid therapy should be initiated if visual symptoms are present.

CLUSTER HEADACHE

Cluster headache (CH) is a distinct pain syndrome characterized by episodes of severe unilateral head pain occurring chiefly around the eye and accompanied by a number of autonomic signs. The term *cluster* is used because individuals who are susceptible to CH experience multiple headaches per day for 4 to 6 weeks and then may be without pain for months or even years.

Etiology and Pathogenesis. There are several theories regarding the etiology of CH and its characteristic combination of both severe localized pain and autonomic symptoms. Some investigators postulate that a CH attack originates in the hypothalamus, which stimulates both the trigeminal and vascular systems in the brain.[295] Others believe that the pain originates peripherally in the cavernous sinus since sympathetic, parasympathetic, and sensory fibers from the first division of the trigeminal nerve are present and because organic lesions of the cavernous sinus can result in symptoms that resemble CH.[296]

Clinical Manifestations. Eighty percent of patients with CH are men. The attacks are sudden, unilateral, and stabbing, causing patients to pace, cry out, or even strike objects. Some patients exhibit violent behavior during attacks. This contrasts with the behavior of migraine patients, who lie down in a dark room and try to sleep. Individuals with CH frequently describe the pain as a hot metal rod in or around the eye. The symptoms most commonly affect the area supplied by the first division of the trigeminal nerve, but second-division symptoms may also occur, causing patients to consult a dentist to rule out an odontogenic etiology. Unnecessary extractions of maxillary teeth are often performed before a correct diagnosis is made. The severe painful episodes begin without an aura and become excruciating within a few minutes. Each attack lasts from 15 minutes to 2 hours and recurs several times daily. A majority of the painful episodes occur at night, often waking the patient from sleep. The pain is associated with autonomic symptoms, particularly nasal congestion and tearing. Sweating of the face, ptosis, increased salivation, and edema of the eyelid are also common signs. During a cluster period, ingestion of alcohol or use of nitroglycerin will provoke an attack.

Treatment. An acute attack of CH can be aborted by breathing 100% oxygen, and CH patients may keep an oxygen canister at bedside to use at the first sign of an attack. Injection of sumatriptan or sublingual or inhaled ergotamine may also be effective therapy. Several drug protocols are recommended for preventing CH during active periods. Lithium is effective therapy for those who can tolerate the side effects, and patients who are using long-term lithium must be monitored for renal toxicity. Other drugs that are useful for preventing attacks include ergotamine, prophylactic prednisone, and calcium channel blockers. Methylsergide is also effective therapy, but pulmonary or cardiac fibrosis is a potential side effect, particularly during prolonged use.

CHRONIC PAROXYSMAL HEMICRANIA

Chronic paroxysmal hemicrania (CPH) is believed to be a form of CH that occurs predominantly in women between the ages of 30 and 40 years. The episodes of pain tend be shorter, but attacks of 5 to 20 minutes' duration can occur up to 30 times daily. Initially, episodes of CPH occur with a periodicity similar to that of CH; however, CPH symptoms tend to become chronic over time. CPH responds dramatically to therapy with indomethacin, which stops the attacks within 1 to 2 days. CPH will recur if indomethacin is discontinued.

MIGRAINE

Until recently, headaches were believed to be either vascular or muscular in origin, but studies performed in the past decade have indicated that many patients with frequent or chronic headaches have a mixture of both vascular and muscular pain and that headaches are frequently somewhere on a continuum between being purely vascular and purely muscular. Migraine is the most common of the vascular headaches, which may occasionally also cause pain of the face and jaws. It may be triggered by foods such as nuts, chocolate, and red wine; stress; sleep deprivation; or hunger. Migraine is more common in women.

Etiology and Pathogenesis. The classic theory is that migraine is caused by vasoconstriction of intracranial vessels (which causes the neurologic symptoms), followed by vasodilation (which results in pounding headache). Newer research techniques suggest a series of factors, including the triggering of neurons in the midbrain that activate the trigeminal nerve system in the medulla, resulting in the release of neuropeptides such as substance P. These neurotransmitters activate receptors on the cerebral vessel walls, causing vasodilation and vasoconstriction. There are several major types of migraine: classic, common, basilar, and facial migraine (also referred to as carotidynia).

Clinical Manifestations. Classic migraine starts with a prodromal aura that is usually visual but that may also be sensory or motor. The visual aura that commonly precedes classic migraine includes flashing lights or a localized area of depressed vision (scotoma). Sensitivity to light, hemianesthesia, aphasia, or other neurologic symptoms may also be part of the aura, which commonly lasts from 20 to 30 minutes. The aura is followed by an increasingly severe unilateral throbbing headache that is frequently accompanied by nausea and vomiting. The patient characteristically lies down in a dark room and tries to fall asleep. Headaches characteristically last for hours or up to 2 or 3 days.

Common migraine is not preceded by an aura, but patients may experience irritability or other mood changes. The pain of common migraine resembles the pain of classic migraine and is usually unilateral, pounding, and associated with sensitivity to light and noise. Nausea and vomiting are also common.

Basilar migraine is most common in young women. The symptoms are primarily neurologic and include aphasia, temporary blindness, vertigo, confusion, and ataxia. These symptoms may be accompanied by an occipital headache. Facial migraine (carotidynia) causes a throbbing and/or sticking pain in the neck or jaw. The pain is associated with involvement of branches of the carotid artery rather than the cerebral vessels.[297] The symptoms of facial migraine usually begin in individuals who are 30 to 50 years of age. Patients often seek dental consultation, but unlike the pain of a toothache, facial migraine pain is not continuous but lasts minutes to hours and recurs several times per week. Examination of the neck will reveal tenderness of the carotid artery. Face and jaw pain may be the only manifestation of migraine, or it may be an occasional pain in patients who usually experience classic or common migraine.[298]

Treatment.   Patients with migraine should be carefully assessed to determine common food triggers. Attempts to minimize reactions to the stress of everyday living by using relaxation techniques may also be helpful to some patients. Drug therapy may be used either prophylactically to prevent attacks in patients who experience frequent headaches or acutely at the first sign of an attack. Drugs that are useful in aborting migraine include ergotamine and sumatriptan, which can be given orally, nasally, rectally, or parenterally. These drugs must be used cautiously since they may cause hypertension and other cardiovascular complications. Drugs that are used to prevent migraine include propranolol, verapimil, and TCAs.[299] Methylsergide or monoamine oxidase inhibitors such as phenelzine can be used to manage difficult cases that do not respond to safer drugs.

▼ SELECTED READINGS

Assessment and Management of Orofacial Pain. Eds. JM Zakrzewska & SD Harrison Elsevier, 2002, Amsterdam Orofacial Pain From Basic Science to Clinical Management Eds. JP Lund, GJ Lavigne, R Dubner, BJ Sessle. Quintessence Chicago 2001

Bergdahl J, Anneroth G, Perris H. Personality characteristics of subjects with resistant burning mouth syndrome. Acta Odontol Scand 1995;53:7–11.

Caudill MA. Managing pain before it manages you. New York: The Guildford Press; 1995.

Cheung LK, Lo J. The long-term clinical morbidity of mandibular step osteotomy. Int J Adult Orthodon Orthognath Surg 2002;17:283–90.

Davis M, Robbins E, Eshelman M. The relaxation and stress reduction workbook. 4th ed. Oakland (CA): New Harbinger Publications; 1995.

Gilman S, Newman S. Essentials of clinical neuroanatomy and neurophysiology. 9th ed. Philadelphia: C.A. Davis; 1996.

Gilron I, Flatters SJ. Gabapentin and pregabalin for the treatment of neuropathic pain: a review of laboratory and clinical evidence. Pain Res Manag 2006;11 Suppl A:16A–29A.

Jung BF, Johnson RW, Griffin DRJ, Dworkin RH. Risk factors for postherpetic neuralgia in patients with herpes zoster. Neurology 2004;62:1545–51.

Kost RG, Straus SE. Drug therapy: postherpetic neuralgia — pathogenesis, treatment, and prevention. N Engl J Med 1996;335:32–42.

McCaffery M, Pasero C. Pain, a clinical manual. 2nd ed. St. Louis: Mosby; 1999.

Reskin A. Imaging aspects of new approaches to the differential diagnosis of chronic orofacial pain. In: Lipton JA, Bryant PS, editors. New approaches to the differential diagnosis of chronic orofacial pain. Proceedings of the Research Workshop on Chronic Orofacial Pain sponsored by National Institute of Dental Research, April 1989. Anesth Prog 1990;37:127.

The International Classification of Headache Disorders: 2nd edition. Cephalalgia 2004;24 Suppl 1:9–160.

Vickers ER, Cousins MJ, Walker S, Chisholm K. Analysis of 50 patients with atypical odontalgia. Oral Surg Oral Med Oral Pathol Oral Radiol Endod 1998;85:24–32.

Wilson-Pauwels L, Akesson E, Stewart P. Cranial nerves: anatomy and clinical comments. Toronto: BC Decker; 1988.

For the full reference list, please refer to the accompanying CD ROM.

11

▼

HEADACHE

SCOTT S. DEROSSI, DMD
JOHN A. DETRE, MD

Headache is one of the most common complaints in both adolescents and adults. Estimates of headache prevalence vary, but most surveys report that as many as 90% of all individuals experience at least one headache annually, with severe, disabling migraine headache affecting over 35% of the population.[1–3] Headaches are relatively rare in children but increase with age. Headache in general and migraine specifically increase in frequency during adolescence, particularly in women due to hormonal modulation. Since there is significant anatomic proximity of structures of the head and face and because dentists are often consulted to evaluate orofacial pain, it is imperative that dentists be familiar with the clinical manifestations of headache disorders. This chapter reviews the pain-sensitive structures of the head and discusses the etiology and pathophysiology, diagnostic considerations, and treatment recommendations of headache appropriate for dental professionals.

▼ PAIN-SENSITIVE STRUCTURES OF THE HEAD

Somatic pain occurs when peripheral nociceptors are stimulated in response to tissue injury or inflammation. Visceral pain often arises from distention and may be referred to external locations. In such cases, pain is a normal physiologic response mediated by a healthy nervous system. However, pain can also be as a result of damaged or inappropriately activated pain-sensitive pathways of the central or peripheral nervous system. Headache pain may result from both mechanisms. Very few of the cranial structures are pain sensitive, with intracranial pain arising primarily from blood vessels and meninges. Sensory stimuli from these intracranial tissues are conveyed to the central nervous system via trigeminal nerves for areas above the tentorium in the anterior and middle cranial fossae and may be referred to trigeminal distributions in the face and head. Causes of headache are multifactorial but can occur as the result of distention or dilation of intracranial and extracranial arteries; displacement of large intracranial vessels or their dural envelope; compression or inflammation of cranial or spinal nerves; inflammation, spasm, or trauma to cranial, facial, and cervical muscles; or meningeal irritation and increased intracranial pressure.[4]

▼ CLASSIFICATION OF HEADACHE

A useful classification of the numerous causes of headache has been established by the International Headache Society (IHS) to be highly specific based on reliable signs and symptoms as well as stable inclusion and exclusion criteria (Table 1).[5] Since there are no specific diagnostic tests to allow a guaranteed diagnosis, the clinical diagnosis of headache relies heavily on the ability of the examiner to elicit the relevant history and the reliability of patients to report accurately their symptoms and the absence of other etiologic factors.

▼ GENERAL CLINICAL CONSIDERATIONS

The first and most important consideration in evaluating patients with complaints of orofacial or headache is to rule out an underlying progressive structural lesion or systemic diseases, such as intracranial tumors, severe infection, aneurysms, hypertension, and stroke. Headache is generally a benign symptom, but it is estimated that 5% of patients with headache in emergency settings are found to have a serious underlying disorder, emphasizing the need for rapid and accurate diagnosis of headache.[6,7]

The history of present illness, including the quality, location, duration, and timing of headache, along with the modifying factors that produce, worsen, or relieve headache, needs to be carefully reviewed in each patient. Ascertaining

characteristic pain qualities is often helpful for diagnosis. For instance, most tension-type headaches (TTHs) are described as tight "band-like" pain or deep, aching pain. The location of pain might be important in diagnosing a temporal arteritis since pain is localized to the site of the vessel. Pain duration and time intensity are often diagnostically useful since ruptured aneurysm, migraine, and cluster headache all have unique pain peaks and duration. In general, progressive headaches that are associated with neurologic deficits are the most concerning as being secondary to a serious underlying disorder.

Patients who present with their first severe headache raise different diagnostic possibilities compared with those who have recurring headache. Features or "diagnostic alarms" of acute, new-onset headache caused by underlying disorders are reviewed in Table 2. A complete neurologic examination is a vital first step in patient evaluation. Diagnostic imaging, such as computed tomography (CT) or magnetic resonance imaging (MRI), is useful in screening for intracranial pathology. Whereas CT is typically more readily available than MRI, MRI provides much greater sensitivity, particularly for vascular lesions and lesions in the posterior fossa. AN MRI and magnetic resonance angiography of the brain with contrast is the most sensitive noninvasive diagnostic study for headache and should be the diagnostic modality of choice in nonemergent cases. In addition, the psychological state of the patient needs to be assessed given the well-demonstrated relationship between head pain and depression.

▼ MIGRAINE

Epidemiology

Migraine typically presents as an episodic "sick" headache that interferes with normal daily activities. The migraine headache is frequently accompanied by nausea, vomiting, photophobia (aversion to light), phonophobia (aversion to sound), and osmophobia (aversion to odors). It may be preceded by an aura of neurologic dysfunction, such as visual disturbances, vertigo, numbness, weakness, or even alterations of consciousness. The pain may be moderate or incapacitating. Migraine frequency varies considerably. In many patients, migraine is triggered by specific factors, such as

---

TABLE 1 International Headache Society Classification of Headache

1.	Migraine
2.	Tension-type headache
3.	Cluster headache and trigeminal autonomic cephalgias
4.	Other primary headaches
5.	Headache associated with head and/or neck trauma
6.	Headache attributed to cranial or cervical vascular disorders
7.	Headache associated with nonvascular intracranial disorders
8.	Headache associated with substances or their withdrawal
9.	Headache attributed to infection
10.	Headache attributed to disorders of hemostasis
11.	Headache or facial pain attributed to disorders of the cranium, neck, eyes, ears, nose, sinuses, teeth, mouth, or other facial or cranial structures
12.	Headache attributed to psychiatric disorders
13.	Cranial neuralgias and central causes of face pain
14.	Other headache, cranial neuralgia, central or primary facial pain

---

TABLE 2 Headache Symptoms Suggesting a Serious Underlying Disorder

First severe headache

"Worst" headache ever

Headache worsening over days or weeks

Abnormal neurologic examination

Fever or other unexplained systemic signs/symptoms

Vomiting precedes headaches

Headache induced by bending, lifting, or coughing

Disturbing sleep or present immediately upon waking

Onset after age 55

menses, weather changes, irregular sleep, alcohol, or certain foods. Migraine is also often relieved by sleep. The lifetime prevalence of migraine is estimated to be near 35%, and it affects greater than 17% of women and 6% of men.[8] Migraine headache has a staggering economic impact, including absenteeism and loss productivity totaling $13 billion dollars in the United States.[9] The direct medical cost of caring for migraineurs is estimated at $1 billion.[9,10]

Pathophysiology

There appears to be a genetic and familial risk as more than half of all migraineurs report having other family members who suffer from migraine. In addition, specific mutations leading to rare causes of vascular headache have been identified.[11–13] The pathogenesis of migraine is only now becoming more clearly understood but involves the role of serotonin and dopamine in both vascular and neuronal dysfunction.

Vascular Theory

The aura of migraine was thought to be caused by cerebral vasoconstriction and the headache by reactive vasodilation, which explained the throbbing quality of migraine and relief by ergots. It is now believed that the aura is caused by neuronal dysfunction rather than ischemia. Migrainous fortification spectrum (an aura consisting of scintillating zigzag figures of bright luminous geometric lines and shapes) experienced by many patients corresponds to cortical hypoperfusion that begins in the visual cortex and spreads forward at 2 to 3 mm/min, and frontal spread continues as the headache phase begins.[14] It is unlikely that these changes fully explain the symptoms of migraine. Specifically, the decreased vascular perfusion seen is not significant enough to cause focal neurologic symptoms.[15] In addition, the increase in blood flow and vasodilation do not account for the local edema and tenderness observed in migraine patients.[16] Although some cerebral blood flow changes do occur in aura, migraine without aura demonstrates no flow abnormalities; thus, it is unlikely that simple vasoconstriction and vasodilation are the fundamental pathophysiologic feature.

Neuronal Theory and the Trigeminovascular System

Migraine aura is believed to result from a slow-moving, spreading depression of cortical activity that liberates potassium and is preceded by a wavefront of increased metabolic activity, suggesting that dysregulation of normal neuronal function is a cause of migrainous attacks. Migraine probably results from pathologic activation of meningeal and vessel nociceptors combined with a change in central pain modulation.[16] Both headache and the associated neurovascular changes are served by the trigeminal system; activation of the trigeminovascular system results in vasoactive polypeptide release, including substance P and calcitonin gene–related peptide (CGRP).[17] These neuropeptides interact with the blood vessel wall to produce dilation, plasma protein extravasation, and platelet activation, producing a sterile inflammation that activates trigeminal nociceptive afferents

originating on the vessel wall, leading to further pain production.[18,19] Inhibiting this trigeminovascular activation is at the core of attempts to link headache with temporomandibular disorders (TMDs) and to treat headache with occlusal appliance therapy.[20,21] The pathophysiology of migraine and the potential role of TMD as a mechanical trigger is summarized in Figure 1.

Role of Serotonin and Dopamine

Pharmacologic data point to a strong role of the neurotransmitter serotonin in migraine dating back to 40 years ago, when methysergide was found to antagonize certain peripheral actions of serotonin and was introduced as the first drug capable of preventing migraines.[22] More recently, the triptan class of drugs has renewed interest in the role of 5-hydroxytryptamine (5-HT) in migraine because of their ability to stimulate selectively a crucial subtype of 5-HT receptors (ie, 5-HT$_{1D}$).[23]

A growing body of data supports a role of dopamine in the pathophysiology of certain types of migraine. Biologic, genetic, and pharmacologic evidence includes the following: (1) most migraine symptoms can be induced by dopamine, (2) there is dopamine receptor hypersensitivity in migraineurs, and (3) dopamine receptor antagonists are effective agents in migraine.[24]

Clinical Findings

The clinical features of migraine are separated into two types of headache: migraine without aura (common migraine) and migraine with aura (classic migraine). In migraine without aura, there is an absence of focal neurologic symptoms preceding headache. Clinically, patients have moderate to severe pulsating, unilateral head pain aggravated by walking stairs or similar routine activity. In addition, nausea and vomiting, photophobia, and phonophobia are usually associated with these multiple attacks, each lasting 4 to 72 hours.

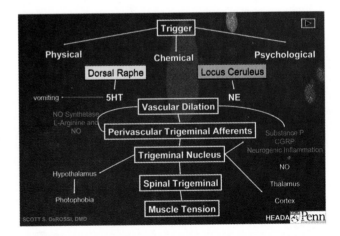

FIGURE 1 Pathogenesis of migraine. CGRP = calcitonin gene–related peptide; 5HT = 5-hydroxytryptamine; NE = ; NO = nitric oxide.

In migraine with aura, the headache is preceded by stereotyped sensory, motor, and visual symptoms. The most common premonitory symptoms in migraine include visual scotomas and hallucinations, and one-third of all migraineurs are affected.[25] Paresthesias involving the face, lips, and tongue; allodynia; and muscle weakness may occur. The median frequency of migraine attacks is 1.5 per month, and the typical headache is a unilateral, gradual-onset, throbbing, moderate to severe pain aggravated with movement. After the headache, there may be a resolution phase in which the patient feels tired, irritable, and listless.

Management

Treatment of migraine begins with making an accurate diagnosis, appropriate patient explanation and education, and a treatment plan including nonpharmacologic and pharmacologic therapies. Generally, migraine management is divided into three specific strategies: (1) prophylactic or preventive therapy, (2) abortive therapy, and (3) palliative or rescue therapy.

The mainstay of pharmacologic therapy is the judicious use of one or more migraine-effective drugs. The selection of the most optimal drug regimen is dependent on several factors, including individual patient response, but primarily on the frequency and severity of the attacks. Patients experiencing more than four to six migraines per month or a fewer number of protracted migraines are candidates for prophylactic therapy. Less frequent headaches can be managed with abortive therapy alone. Patients with severe and refractory headaches may require rescue therapy to avoid frequent visits to the emergency room. A staged approach to the medical management of migraine is summarized in Table 3.

Mild migraine can often be successfully managed by oral agents, whereas fulminant attacks with accompanying nausea may require parenteral drugs. Most abortive agents for migraine fall into one of three classes: (1) anti-inflammatory agents, (2) 5-HT$_1$ agonists, and (3) dopamine antagonists. The response to migraine treatment is highly variable and must be individualized for each patient.

Preventive protocols for migraine include a substantial number of drugs now available that have been shown to stabilize migraine. β-Adrenergic agents, anticonvulsants, tricyclic antidepressants, monoamine oxidase inhibitors, serotoninergic drugs, and calcium channel antagonists have all been used with varied success, although not all of them have received a specific indication for migraine by the Food and Drug Administration (FDA). These drugs must be taken daily and usually have a 2- to 6-week lag before an effect is observed. As none of the agents currently used for migraine prevention are specifically intended for this purpose and may have side effects, a period of trial and error is usually required to arrive at an effective and tolerable regimen. Preventive agents are ultimately effective in at least 50 to 75% of cases. A reasonable goal for preventive therapy is at least a 50% reduction in headache frequency and/or severity. To assess this, some idea of the baseline headache frequency and severity is essential prior to initiating therapy. Once effective stabilization is achieved, the drug should be continued for at least 6 months and then tapered to assess continued need.[26,27]

The mainstay of abortive therapy for migraine centers on the use of ergotamine derivatives and the "triptan" drugs, although both the severity and duration of migraine can be reduced by anti-inflammatory agents, especially when taken early in a migraine attack.[28] Specifically, the combination of acetaminophen, aspirin, and caffeine has been approved by the FDA for the treatment of mild to moderate migraine. Stimulation of 5-HT$_1$ receptors can stop a migraine attack. Ergotamine derivatives are nonselective receptor agonists, whereas the triptan drugs are selective 5-HT$_1$ receptor agonists. Each of the triptans has similar pharmacologic properties, but they vary in clinical effectiveness. Available in oral, nasal, and parenteral formulations, triptan drugs unfortunately do not result in rapid, consistent, and complete relief in all migraine patients. The drugs often used for treatment of acute migraine are reviewed in Table 4.

Dopamine antagonists may be used as an adjunctive therapy in the treatment of migraine. Gastrointestinal

TABLE 3 Staged Approach to Treating Migraine

Stage	Diagnosis	Therapy
Mild migraine	Occasional throbbing HA No major impairment of daily function	NSAIDs Combination analgesics Oral serotonin agonists
Moderate migraine	Moderate to severe headache Nausea Some impairment of functioning	Oral, nasal, or subcutaneous serotonin agonists Oral dopamine antagonists
Severe migraine	Severe headaches (> 3 times/mo) Marked nausea and/or vomiting Significant functional impairment	Intramuscular or intravenous dopamine antagonists Prophylactic medications

HA = headache; NSAIDs = nonsteroidal anti-inflammatory drugs.

TABLE 4 Medications/Treatments Effective for Acute Migraine

Trade Name	Drug	Dose
Amerge	Naratriptan	2.5 mg tablet at onset; repeat once after 4h prn
Axert	Almotriptan	12.5 mg tablet at onset; repeat once after 2h prn
Ergomar	Ergotamine	One 2 mg sublingual tablet at onset and q30min
Excedrine Migraine	Acetaminophen, aspirin, caffeine	Two q6h
Frova	Frovatriptan	2.5 mg tablet at onset; repeat once after 2h prn
Imitrex	Sumatriptan	50–100 mg tablet at onset; repeat once after 2h prn 5–20 mg intranasal spray (4 sprays)
Maxalt	Rizatriptan	5–10 mg tablet at onset; repeat once after 2h prn
Migranal Nasal Spray	Dihydroergotamine	One spray (0.5 mg); repeat in 15 min
Zomig	Zolmitriptan	2.5 mg tablet at onset; repeat once after 2h prn One spray (2.5 mg); repeat after 2h prn

drug absorption can be impaired during attacks because of decreased motility limiting the effectiveness of nonsteroidal anti-inflammatory drugs (NSAIDs) or oral triptans. Dopamine antagonists can decrease nausea/vomiting and restore gastric motility.[28]

▼ TENSION-TYPE HEADACHE

Epidemiology

The most common cause of headache is TTH. Over 80% of adults experience TTH, characterized by bilateral, tight, band-like discomfort periodically, and it is common in both adolescents and children. Women tend to be affected more than men, and in some patients, anxiety and depression are coexisting diagnoses. TTH may be episodic or chronic (ie, present for > 15 days per month). Indeed, musculoskeletal or tension-type headache is the most common cause of chronic daily headache. Patients often describe a slow-building pain that fluctuates in severity. Most patients who experience TTH rely on over-the-counter remedies rather than seek medical attention for their symptoms.[29] A well-recognized "analgesic rebound syndrome" due to analgesic overuse is a major contributing factor to the transformation from episodic TTH to chronic daily headache. Most patients are not aware that they can develop a tolerance and even a dependence on over-the-counter analgesics and that more than occasional use of these drugs can be counterproductive. Determining the frequency and dosing of over-the-counter analgesics is an important part of the headache history. In many cases, dramatic improvements can be achieved simply by stopping daily analgesics, albeit with increased discomfort for the first few days.

Pathophysiology

The pathophysiologic basis for TTH is not fully known. Many investigators believe that periodic TTH is biologically indistinguishable from migraine, whereas others believe that TTH and migraine are, in fact, two distinct clinical entities. It is generally agreed that TTH is triggered by psychophysiologic changes related to stress, anxiety, and depression.[30]

Abnormalities of cervical and masticatory muscle contraction are likely to exist, but the exact nature of any dysfunction has yet to be elucidated. Tender pericranial muscles during headache are not a universal finding in TTH, leading some investigators to postulate a central mechanism leading to peripheral pain in some patients.[31] There appears to be a central disinhibitory phenomenon, probably with neurotransmitter changes underlying personality traits, defective pain control, and sensitivity to myofascial and vascular input.[32]

Clinical Findings

The clinical presenting symptoms and signs of TTH include bilateral, holocephalic, band-like tightness and pressure with a pounding character beginning usually in late morning and persisting throughout the day. Unlike migraine, nausea and vomiting are rare, occurring only in cases of severe pain in a minority of patients, and those patients are most likely manifesting a mixed headache syndrome with triggering of secondary migrainous headache by intense musculoskeletal pain.

Management

Treatment of TTH includes psychological, physiologic, and pharmacologic therapies. Psychological management includes simple counseling and hypnosis, whereas relaxation and biofeedback measures, including acupuncture, are helpful physiologic treatments. TTH is most often effectively treated with over-the-counter analgesics, including $NSAID_S$, acetaminophen or aspirin, and tricyclic antidepressants. Medications to treat TTH are reviewed in Table 5.

TABLE 5 Medications Effective in Tension-Type Headache

Nonsteroidal anti-inflammatory agents

    Acetaminophen

    Aspirin

    Diclofenac

    Ibuprofen

    Etodolac

    Naproxen sodium

Combination analgesics

    Acetaminophen plus butalbital

    Acetaminophen plus butalbital plus caffeine

    Aspirin plus butalbital

    Aspirin plus butalbital plus caffeine

Prophylactic medications

    Amitryptiline

    Doxepin

    Nortriptyline

▼ CLUSTER HEADACHE

Cluster headache is a distinctive vascular headache disorder that is less prevalent but often confused with migraine because of the extreme severity of pain. There are both episodic and chronic types. The episodic form is characterized by one or several short-lived attacks of periorbital pain per day over a 1- to 2-month span. The chronic form is characterized by the absence of sustained periods of remission and can transform from the episodic type.

Epidemiology

Cluster is more common in males over the age of 25, and men are affected seven to eight times more than women. Alcohol provokes the attacks in 70% of cases initially but ceases to be provocative when the bout remits.

Pathophysiology

The etiology of cluster, although not fully understood, is classified as a vascular headache disorder with features of both migraine and neuralgias. Although no consistent cerebral blood flow changes have been demonstrated with cluster attacks, the strongest evidence for a central mechanism includes the periodicity of attacks and the association with autonomic symptoms.[33] Although dysfunction of the trigeminovascular system appears to be central to the pathophysiology of cluster, the hypothalamus is probably the site of activation in this disorder, which would explain the symptoms of cluster headache.[34] Oxygen desaturation may lead to abnormal serotoninergic neurotransmission combined with hypersensitive chemoreceptors in the carotid body and neurogenic inflammation with elevations of CGRP, substance P, and other neuropeptides during attacks.

Clinical Features

Cluster headache is unilateral and among the most painful of all headache disorders. Attacks last from 30 minutes to 2 hours and have a nocturnal onset in half of cases, waking patients several hours after falling asleep. Periorbital pain is commonly associated with autonomic symptoms, including homolateral lacrimation, reddening of the eye, nasal stuffiness, ptosis, and nausea. In addition, 10 to 20% of patients report superimposed paroxysms of stabbing, ice pick–like pains in the periorbital region that last for a few seconds and may occur once or several times in rapid succession; this paroxysmal pain usually heralds the end of an attack. The symptoms often resolve in 1 to 2 minutes. The pain usually begins in, around, or above the eye or the temple; occasionally, the face, neck, ear, or hemicranium may be affected, and the pain can be confused with pain of odontogenic origin.

Management

Management of cluster headache includes use of medications to prevent cluster attacks until the bout is over as well as abortive therapies. Individual headaches are difficult to treat because they are short-lived. Abortive medications, including the use of 100% oxygen at the outset of an episode, are often useful in confirming a diagnosis of cluster. Oxygen inhalation (9 L/min) results in rapid resolution of symptoms in over 70% of cases. Intranasal sprayed lidocaine 4% is also effective in nearly half of cases.[35] Triptan therapy can be effective, although, typically, parenteral forms are required due to their more rapid absorption. Most cluster headaches occur repeatedly and require more than just abortive therapy. Short courses of oral glucocorticoids are typically effective in aborting repeated clusters of headaches. For more chronic cluster, effective prophylactic medications include lithium, methysergide, ergotamine, sodium valproate, and verapamil. Since cluster occurs as a series of episodes with a period of remission, preventive measures should be discontinued to see if remission has occurred.

▼ TEMPORAL ARTERITIS

Epidemiology

Temporal (or giant cell) arteritis is a systemic inflammatory disorder that often involves the extracranial carotid circulation. This is commonly a disorder of elderly individuals, with an annual incidence of 77:100,000 individuals, usually over age 50. The average age at onset is 70 years, and women account for 65% of cases. This is a rare form of chronic daily headache with clinical importance because it is treatable. Failure to treat giant cell arteritis may lead to serious ischemic complications, including blindness, stroke, and myocardial infarction.

Pathophysiology

Inflammation of the temporal artery on biopsy is seen in over half of cases and can spread to arteries other than the temporal artery and extracranial vessels. The inflammatory process appears to be similar to both an acute immune-mediated vasculitis and chronic noncaseating granulomatous inflammation similar to that seen in sarcoid. Blindness occurs when the posterior ciliary artery is affected, which supplies the optic disk, leading to ischemic papillopathy and atrophy.

Clinical Features

Symptoms include diffuse unilateral headache, polymyalgia rheumatica, chest pain, jaw pain and claudication, fever, and weight loss. Symptoms initially are low grade; progress in severity and duration, increasing in the evening when the patient reclines; and are reported as a bitemporal constant dull ache. Most patients are able to recognize that their pain is superficial and extracranial and associated with scalp tenderness that interferes with hair brushing or resting the head on a pillow. Pain in the temporal and masseter muscles on chewing is virtually pathognomonic of temporal arteritis, making it easily confused with other causes of facial pain (eg, myofascial pain and TMDs) in a clinical setting. Erythrocyte sedimentation rate and C-reactive protein are frequently, although not always, elevated, and patients may be anemic. A temporal artery biopsy should be performed to confirm the diagnosis.

Management

Approximately half of patients with untreated temporal arteritis develop blindness due to involvement of the ophthalmic artery.[36] This significant complication can be prevented by immediate initiation of glucocorticoid therapy (75 mg daily), underscoring the importance of prompt recognition. Steroid doses are reduced by 5 mg per week to a maintenance dose of 10 mg daily and then continued for 3 months.

▼ CHRONIC PAROXYSMAL HEMICRANIA

Chronic paroxysmal hemicrania (CPH) is a vascular headache disorder that is frequently confused with odontogenic pain, TMD, or regional pathology of structures of the face and head. It has features similar to migraine headache and may share some etiology and pathophysiology.

Epidemiology

Paroxysmal hemicrania is a rare syndrome. Although the precise prevalence of CPH is unknown, it is estimated to be 1 in 50,000. In contrast to cluster headache, CPH has a distinct female predominance, with a gender ratio of 2:1. The condition usually begins in adulthood during the midthirties and can last several years to decades.

Clinical Features

CPH has a rapid onset and is associated with severe, consistently unilateral head pain lasting a few minutes to an hour. It differs from cluster in its high frequency and shorter duration of attacks, but they have numerous overlapping characteristics. Most often, the temporal and orbital regions are the site of pain, with the jaw and face also affected. Episodic attacks are more frequent than cluster and can number greater than five per day during acute periods of recurrence. Like cluster, there are associated symptoms, including conjunctival injection, lacrimation, rhinorrhea or nasal stuffiness, and swelling of the painful areas.[37] Since no confirmatory diagnostic test exists, diagnosis is made via the patient history and confirmation of symptoms and signs during attacks. Indomethacin in doses of 25 to 150 mg daily is effective in nearly all cases of CPH, in contrast to cluster.[38]

Over the past 30 years, there have emerged several rare headache disorders that respond selectively to indomethacin, including CPH, cough or exertional headache, and the ice-pick headache syndrome. Other headaches also may be sensitive to indomethacin, and a trial of this drug should be considered in patients in whom these headache syndromes are suspected.[39]

▼ OTHER CAUSES OF HEADACHES

Brain Tumor

Headache associated with intracranial masses is usually nondescript. Approximately 30% of patients with brain tumors consider headache to be their chief complaint or first presenting symptom.[40] Intermittent deep, dull, and aching pain of moderate intensity that worsens with physical exertion or position change and is associated with nausea and vomiting is the symptom most commonly described in migraine but is also seen in brain tumor headaches. Sleep disturbances occur in 10% of patients, and vomiting preceding headaches by weeks is highly characteristic of tumors of the posterior cranial fossa.[41] Tumors should be suspected in patients with progressively severe new "migraine" headaches that are unilateral.

Intracranial Hemorrhage

Most vascular disorders associated with headache require immediate medical or surgical intervention. Severe, acute headaches associated with a stiff neck in the absence of fever are highly suggestive of subarachnoid hemorrhage (SAH). Sudden onset of the "worst headache of life" is a medical emergency, and aneurysmal SAH must be excluded by a CT scan, which is approximately 90% sensitive for SAH, and a lumbar puncture if the CT scan is negative.[42] Other causes of headache can include ruptured aneurysm, arteriovenous malformation, or intraparenchymal hemorrhage, but these often present as headache alone without nausea, vomiting, and mental and emotional changes.

Lumbar Puncture

Headache following lumbar puncture usually begins 48 hours to 2 weeks following the procedure. It is relatively common, with an incidence of 10 to 30%, and is associated with head pain that worsens with positional changes. Nausea, stiff neck, vertigo, photophobia, tinnitus, and blurred vision are frequent complaints. Loss of cerebrospinal fluid (CSF) decreases the brain's supportive cushion, resulting in dilation and tension on pain-sensitive dural structures when patients are upright. Intracranial hypotension often occurs, but severe lumbar puncture headache can be present in patients with normal CSF pressure.[43] Spontaneous CSF leaks can also occur due to exertion or following surgical procedures near the dura and are also characterized by positional modulation.

Idiopathic Intracranial Hypertension

Headache resembling that of brain tumor is a common presenting symptom of raised intracranial pressure, usually resulting from impaired CSF absorption by arachnoid villi.[44] This disorder, called pseudotumor cerebri, is most commonly seen in young, obese adult females and is associated with morning headaches that worsen with coughing or straining. The pain is usually retro-ocular and worsened by eye movements, which are often restricted by sixth cranial nerve dysfunction. Patients may have a history of exposure to precipitating agents such as tetracycline, vitamin A, or glucocorticoids. Intracranial hypertension is diagnosed by lumbar puncture, which can also provide temporary relief. Chronic management includes diuretics or surgical implantation of a shunt.[45] Ophthalmologic evaluation for visual field testing is required in patients with intracranial hypertension as it can enlarge the blind spot due to pressure transduced along the optic nerve. Patients with enlarging blind spots can be treated surgically with an optic nerve sheath fenestration.

Postconcussion

Many patients following relatively trivial head injuries, such as extension-flexion injuries (ie, whiplash), report symptoms such as headache, dizziness, vertigo, and impaired memory. Symptoms may resolve after a few weeks or can persist months to years after injury. In nearly all cases, clinical neurologic examination and radiographic and imaging studies are normal.[46] Although the etiology of this headache is poorly understood, it does not appear to be entirely psychogenic, and symptoms usually persist after a pending legal settlement.[47] These headaches may be part of a TMD also related to direct or indirect trauma to the temporomandibular complex.[48–50]

▼ SUGGESTED READINGS

Bendtsen L, Jensen T. Tension-type headache: the most common, but also the most neglected, headache disorder. Curr Opin Neurol 2006;19:305–9.

Boes CJ, Swanson JW. Paroxysmal hemicrania, SUNCT, and hemicrania continua. Semin Neurol 2006;26:260–70.

Capobianco DJ, Dodick DW. Diagnosis and treatment of cluster headache. Semin Neurol 2006;26:242–59.

Ebell MH. Diagnosis of migraine headache. Am Fam Physician 2006;74:2087–8.

Evans RW. Post-traumatic headaches. Neurol Clin 2004;22:237–49, viii.

May A, Jurgens TP. Trigeminal-autonomic headaches in daily clinical practice. Expert Rev Neurother 2006;6:1531–43.

Olesen J. Are headache disorders caused by neurobiological mechanisms? Curr Opin Neurol 2006;19:277–80.

Silberstein SB. Chronic daily headache. J Am Osteopath Assoc 2005;105(4 Suppl 2):23S–9S.

Wright EF, Clark EG, Paunovich ED, Hart RG. Headache improvement through TMD stabilization appliance and self-management therapies. Cranio 2006;24:104–11.

For the full reference list, please refer to the accompanying CD ROM.

12

DISEASES OF THE RESPIRATORY TRACT

SANDHYA DESAI, MD

FRANK A. SCANNAPIECO, DMD, PhD

MARK LEPORE, MD

ROBERT ANOLIK, MD

MICHAEL GLICK, DMD

Given the fact that the oral cavity is contiguous with the trachea and lower airway, it would not be surprising to learn that conditions within the oral cavity might influence lung function. Respiratory infections are commonly encountered among dental patients. Commonalities between chemotherapeutic options and the anatomic proximity with the oral cavity lead to much interplay between oral and respiratory infections. Recent studies have reported on oral bacteria as causative pathogens in respiratory diseases and conditions associated with significant morbidity and mortality. Furthermore, some respiratory illnesses (such as asthma) may have an effect on orofacial morphology or even on the dentition. This chapter discusses the more common respiratory illnesses and explores the relationship between these conditions and oral health.

▼ UPPER AIRWAY DISEASES

There are several major oral health concerns for patients with upper respiratory infections. These concerns are about infectious matters, such as the possible transmission of pathogens from patients to health care workers and reinfection with causative pathogens through fomites such as toothbrushes and removable oral acrylic appliances. Furthermore, antibiotic resistance may develop because of the use of similar types of medications for upper respiratory infections and odontogenic infections. Lastly, oral mucosal changes (such as dryness due to decongestants and mouth breathing) and increased susceptibility to oral candidiasis in patients using long-term glucocorticosteroid inhalers may be noticed.

Viral Upper Respiratory Infections

The most common cause of acute respiratory illness is viral infection, which occurs more commonly in children than in adults. Rhinoviruses account for the majority of upper respiratory infections in adults.[1] These are ribonucleic acid (RNA) viruses, which preferentially infect the respiratory tree. At least 100 antigenically distinct subtypes have been isolated. Rhinoviruses are most commonly transmitted by close person-to-person contact and by respiratory droplets. Shedding can occur from nasopharyngeal secretions for up to 3 weeks, but 7 days or less is more typical. In addition to rhinoviruses, several other viruses, including coronavirus, influenza virus, parainfluenza virus, adenovirus, enterovirus, coxsackievirus, and respiratory syncytial virus (RSV), have also been implicated as causative agents. Infection by these viruses occurs more commonly during the winter months in temperate climates.

PATHOPHYSIOLOGY

Viral particles can lodge in either the upper or lower respiratory tract. The particles invade the respiratory epithelium, and viral replication ensues shortly thereafter. The typical incubation period for rhinovirus is 2 to 5 days.[2] During this time, active and specific immune responses are triggered, and mechanisms for viral clearance are enhanced. The period of communicability tends to correlate with the duration of clinical symptoms.

CLINICAL AND LABORATORY FINDINGS

Signs and symptoms of upper respiratory tract infections are somewhat variable and are dependent on the sites of inoculation.[3] Common symptoms include rhinorrhea, nasal congestion, and oropharyngeal irritation. Nasal secretions can be serous or purulent. Other symptoms that may be present include cough, fever, malaise, fatigue, headache, and myalgia.[4] A complete blood count (CBC) with differential may demonstrate an increase in mononuclear cells, lymphocytes, and monocytes ("right shift").

Laboratory tests are typically not required in the diagnosis of upper respiratory infections. Viruses can be isolated by culture or determined by rapid diagnostic assays. However, these tests are rarely clinically warranted.

DIAGNOSIS

The diagnosis is made on the basis of medical history as well as confirmatory physical findings. Diagnoses that should be excluded include acute bacterial rhinosinusitis, allergic rhinitis, and group A streptococcal pharyngitis.

MANAGEMENT

The treatment of upper respiratory infections is symptomatic as most are self-limited. Analgesics can be used for sore throat and myalgias. Antipyretics can be used in febrile patients, and anticholinergic agents may be helpful in reducing rhinorrhea. Oral or topical decongestants, such as the sympathomimetic amines, are an effective means of decreasing nasal congestion. Adequate hydration is also important in homeostasis, especially during febrile illnesses.

Antimicrobial agents have no role in the treatment of acute viral upper respiratory infections.[5] Presumptive treatment with antibiotics to prevent bacterial superinfection is not recommended.[6] The excessive use of antibiotics can result in the development of drug-resistant bacteria.[7]

PROGNOSIS

As most patients recover in 5 to 10 days, the prognosis is excellent. However, upper respiratory infections can put patients at risk for exacerbations of asthma, acute bacterial sinusitis, and otitis media; this is especially so in predisposed patients, such as children and patients with an incompetent immune system.

ORAL HEALTH CONSIDERATIONS

The most common oral manifestation of upper respiratory viral infections is the presence of small round erythematous macular lesions on the soft palate. These lesions may be caused directly by the viral infection, or they may represent a response of lymphoid tissue. Individuals with excessive lingual tonsillar tissue also experience enlargement of these foci of lymphoid tissue, particularly at the lateral borders at the base of the tongue.

Treatment of upper respiratory infections with decongestants may cause decreased salivary flow, and patients may experience oral dryness (see Chapter 9 for a discussion of the treatment of oral dryness).

Although there has been some discussion in the dental literature in regard to a relationship between dentofacial morphology and mouth breathing, this association has not been verified in prospective longitudinal studies.[8]

Allergic Rhinitis and Conjunctivitis

Allergic rhinitis is a chronic recurrent inflammatory disorder of the nasal mucosa. Similarly, allergic conjunctivitis is an inflammatory disorder involving the conjunctiva. When both conditions occur, the term *allergic rhinoconjunctivitis* is used. The basis of the inflammation is an allergic hypersensitivity (type I hypersensitivity) to environmental triggers. Allergic rhinoconjunctivitis can be seasonal or perennial. Typical seasonal triggers include grass, tree, and weed pollens. Common perennial triggers include dust mites, animal dander, and mold spores.

Allergic rhinitis is the most prevalent chronic medical disorder. More than 35 million Americans are affected. Allergic rhinitis is associated with a significant health care cost burden, and more than $2 billion (US) are spent annually in the United States on medication for this condition alone. In addition, allergic rhinitis accounts for more than

2 million lost school days per year and more than 3 million lost workdays per year.[9]

PATHOPHYSIOLOGY

Patients with allergic rhinoconjunctivitis have a genetically predetermined susceptibility to allergic hypersensitivity reactions (atopy). Prior to the allergic response, an initial phase of sensitization is required. This sensitization phase is dependent on exposure to a specific allergen and on recognition of the allergen by the immune system. The end result of the sensitization phase is the production of specific immunoglobulin E (IgE) antibody and the binding of this specific IgE to the surface of tissue mast cells and blood basophils. Upon reexposure to the allergen, an interaction between surface IgE and the allergen takes place, which results in IgE cross-linking. The cross-linking of surface IgE triggers degranulation of the mast cell and the release of mast cell mediators. This is the early-phase allergic reaction. Histamine is the primary preformed mediator released by mast cells, and it contributes to the clinical symptoms of sneezing, pruritus, and rhinorrhea. Mast cells also release cytokines that permit amplification and feedback of the allergic response. These cytokines cause an influx of other inflammatory cells, including eosinophils, resulting in the late-phase allergic reaction. Eosinophils produce many proinflammatory mediators that contribute to chronic allergic inflammation and to the symptom of nasal congestion.

CLINICAL AND LABORATORY FINDINGS

The symptoms of allergic rhinoconjunctivitis can vary from patient to patient and depend on the specific allergens to which the patient is sensitized. Conjunctival symptoms may include pruritus, lacrimation, crusting, and burning. Nasal symptoms may include sneezing, pruritus, clear rhinorrhea, and nasal congestion. Other symptoms can occur, such as postnasal drainage with throat irritation, pruritus of the palate and ear canals, and fatigue.

The clinical signs of allergic rhinoconjunctivitis include injection of the conjunctiva with or without "cobblestoning"; prominent infraorbital creases (Dennie-Morgan folds/pleats), swelling, and darkening ("allergic shiners"); a transverse nasal crease; and frequent upward rubbing of the tip of the nose (the allergic "salute"). Direct examination of the nasal mucosa reveals significant edema and a pale blue coloration of the turbinates. A copious clear rhinorrhea is often present. Nasal polyps may also be visible. Postnasal drainage or oropharyngeal cobblestoning might be identified upon examination of the oropharynx. A high-arched palate, protrusion of the tongue, and overbite may be seen.

Laboratory investigations are usually kept to a minimum. Patients with allergic rhinitis might have elevated levels of serum IgE and an elevated total eosinophil count. These findings are not, however, sensitive or specific indicators of atopy. Microscopic examination of nasal secretions often demonstrates significant numbers of eosinophils. The radioallergosorbent test (RAST) is a method of testing for specific allergic sensitivities that is based on circulating levels of specific IgE. Specific IgE levels are determined by using serum samples and are quantified by using radioactive markers. Although the RAST is somewhat less reliable than skin testing (see below), it is a useful test in certain situations (such as pregnancy or severe chronic skin disorders, including atopic dermatitis).

CLASSIFICATION

There is no universal classification system for allergic rhinoconjunctivitis. Many authors make the distinction between perennial and seasonal illness, with the former being caused mainly by indoor allergens (eg, house dust mites, cockroaches, pets) and the latter being triggered primarily by outdoor allergens (eg, trees, grasses, weeds). Perennial allergic rhinitis sufferers might benefit more from specific environmental control measures than would seasonal allergic rhinitis sufferers.

DIAGNOSIS

The diagnosis of allergic rhinoconjunctivitis is usually apparent, based on history and physical examination. Patients present with a history suggestive of allergic sensitivity, recurrent symptoms with specific exposures, or predictable exacerbations during certain times of the year. Symptoms that have recurred for 2 or more years during the same season are very suggestive of seasonal allergic disease. Alternatively, the history might indicate a pattern of worsening symptoms while the patient is at home, with improvement while the patient is at work or on vacation; this pattern is highly suggestive of perennial allergic disease with indoor triggers. The presence of the characteristic physical findings described above would confirm the presence of allergic rhinoconjunctivitis.

The preferred method of testing for allergic sensitivities is skin testing, which is performed with epicutaneous (prick/scratch) tests, often followed by intradermal testing. Prick skin testing is the type most widely used. With prick testing, a small amount of purified allergen is inoculated through the epidermis only (ie, epicutaneously) with a pricking device. Positive (histamine) and negative (albumin-saline) controls are used for comparison. Reactions are measured at 15 minutes, and positive reactions indicate prior allergen sensitization. Tests that yield negative results may be repeated intradermally to increase the sensitivity of the testing. All tests with positive results need to be interpreted carefully, with attention to each patient's history and physical findings.

MANAGEMENT

Three general treatment modalities are used in the treatment of allergic rhinoconjunctivitis: allergen avoidance, pharmacotherapy (medication), and immunotherapy (allergy injections).[10] The best treatment is avoidance of the offending allergen. This requires the accurate identification of the allergens implicated and a thorough knowledge of effective interventions that can minimize or eliminate the exposure. Complete avoidance is rarely possible.

Pharmacotherapy is often recommended for patients with incomplete responses to allergen avoidance and for patients who are unable to avoid allergen exposures. Many treatment options are available. For patients with prominent sneezing, pruritus, or rhinorrhea, antihistamines are an excellent treatment option. Second-generation nonsedating antihistamines such as loratadine and fexofenadine are now widely available. These medications deliver excellent antihistaminic activity with few side effects.[11] Oral decongestants (sympathomimetic amines) can be added to oral antihistamines to relieve nasal congestion and obstruction. Combination medications are available in once-daily and twice-daily dosage forms for ease of administration. CysLT1-receptor antagonists may have additional benefit as well. Some studies have demonstrated that therapy with a cysLT$_1$-receptor antagonist plus antihistamine may have a greater effect than either agent administered alone.[11,12] For patients with daily nasal symptoms or severe symptoms that are not relieved with antihistamine-decongestants, topical anti-inflammatory agents for the nasal mucosa are available. These medications include cromolyn sodium and topical corticosteroid sprays. The benefits of topical corticosteroids include once-daily dosing, superior efficacy (when compared with cromolyn sodium), and relief of the total symptom complex.

Immunotherapy is an effective means of treatment for patients with allergic rhinoconjunctivitis. Numerous studies have shown the efficacy of long-term allergen immunotherapy in inducing prolonged clinical and immunologic tolerance.[13] Immunotherapy is available for a variety of airborne allergens, including grass, tree, and weed pollens; dust mites; animal dander; and mold spores. Excellent candidates for immunotherapy include those patients who are unable to avoid exposures, patients with suboptimal responses to pharmacotherapy, patients who prefer to avoid the long-term use of medications, and women who are contemplating pregnancy.

PROGNOSIS

Although allergic rhinoconjunctivitis is not a life-threatening disorder, it does have a significant impact on the patient's quality of life. With proper allergy care, most patients can lead normal lives, with an excellent quality of life.

ORAL HEALTH CONSIDERATIONS

The use of decongestants and first-generation antihistamines may be associated with oral dryness. There may also be an increased incidence of oral candidiasis in long-term users of topical corticosteroid-containing sprays.

It has been reported that dental personal are at risk for allergic respiratory hypersensitivity from exposure to dental materials such as methacrylates and natural rubber latex.[14] It is thus important for dental health care workers to minimize exposure to allergenic materials in the workplace.

Otitis Media

Otitis media is inflammation of the middle-ear space and tissues. It is the most common illness that occurs in children who are 8 years of age or younger. Approximately 70% of children experience at least one episode of otitis media by age 3 years; of these, approximately one-third experience three or more episodes in this same time interval.[15]

Otitis media can be subdivided into acute otitis media, recurrent otitis media, otitis media with effusion, and chronic suppurative otitis media. The underlying problem in all types of otitis media is dysfunction of the eustachian tube. A poorly functioning eustachian tube does not ventilate the middle-ear space sufficiently. This lack of proper ventilation results in pressure changes in the middle ear and subsequent fluid accumulation. The fluid frequently becomes infected, resulting in acute otitis media. The most common infectious causes are viruses, *Streptococcus pneumoniae*, *Haemophilus influenzae*, and *Moraxella catarrhalis*.[1] In infants younger than 6 weeks of age, other bacteria, including *Staphylococcus aureus*, *Escherichia coli*, *Klebsiella*, and *Enterobacter*, have also been implicated.

PATHOPHYSIOLOGY

There are several factors that influence the pathogenesis of otitis media. Nasopharyngeal colonization with large numbers of pathogenic viruses and bacteria such as *S. pneumoniae*, *H. influenzae*, or *M. catarrhalis* can increase the risk of otitis media. The likelihood of aspiration of these nasopharyngeal pathogens can be increased by nasal congestion or obstruction, negative pressure in the middle-ear space, acute viral upper respiratory infections, and exposure to tobacco smoke.[16] For infants, breast-feeding can decrease the risk of otitis media, whereas impaired immune responsiveness can increase this risk.

Under normal circumstances, the eustachian tube acts to ventilate the tympanomastoid air cell system during the act of swallowing. Any process that impairs normal eustachian tube function can lead to negative pressure in the middle-ear space. Transient impairments of eustachian tube function are seen in conditions that cause nasopharyngeal mucosal edema and obstruction of the eustachian tube orifice, such as allergic rhinitis and viral upper respiratory infections. Chronic eustachian tube obstruction can be seen with several conditions, including cleft palate and nasopharyngeal masses. Aspiration of nasopharyngeal pathogens can then occur due to negative pressure in the middle-ear space, with subsequent infection by these pathogens. This leads to the clinical manifestations of otitis media.

CLINICAL AND LABORATORY FINDINGS

The most common symptoms in acute otitis media are fever and otalgia. Other symptoms include irritability, anorexia, and vomiting. Parents may note their child pulling or tugging at one or both ears. Symptoms of a viral upper respiratory infection might also be present, preceding the development of otitis media. On physical examination, the tympanic membrane may appear erythematous and bulging, suggesting inflammation of the middle ear. Other otoscopic findings include a loss of landmarks and decreased mobility of the tympanic membrane as seen by pneumatic otoscopy.

In otitis media with effusion, patients often complain of "clogged" ears and "popping." Otoscopic examination reveals serous middle-ear fluid, and air-fluid levels may be present. The mobility of the tympanic membrane is usually diminished, and mild to moderate conductive hearing loss may be demonstrated. In chronic suppurative otitis media, otorrhea is present and can be visualized either from a tympanic membrane perforation or from surgically placed tympanostomy tubes.

Investigations that can aid in the diagnosis or management of otitis media include tympanometry and myringotomy with aspiration. Tympanometry is a technique that measures the compliance of the tympanic membrane by using an electroacoustic impedance bridge. Decreased compliance of the tympanic membrane indicates a middle-ear effusion. Myringotomy with aspiration can be useful in situations when culture of the middle ear fluid is needed, such as with immunocompromised hosts or with patients who have persistent effusions despite medical management.

CLASSIFICATION

Acute otitis media is defined as middle-ear inflammation with an infectious etiology and a rapid onset of signs and symptoms. Otitis media with effusion is defined as a middle-ear effusion (often asymptomatic) that can be either residual (3 to 16 weeks following acute otitis media) or persistent (lasting more than 16 weeks). Recurrent otitis media is defined as three new episodes of acute otitis media in 6 months' time or four new episodes in a 12-month period. Chronic suppurative otitis media is defined as persistent otorrhea lasting longer than 6 weeks.

DIAGNOSIS

The diagnosis of otitis media is made on the basis of the history and physical examination. The most useful tool for diagnosing otitis media is pneumatic otoscopy, which allows the clinician not only to visualize the tympanic membrane but also to assess its mobility. As stated above, an immobile tympanic membrane probably represents the presence of middle-ear fluid, and (in the context of a confirmatory medical history) the diagnosis of otitis media is made in such a case.

MANAGEMENT

In recent years, meta-analyses of acute otitis media have demonstrated that close observation in most children with mild disease is often justified.[17] There is evidence that suggests that antibiotics may be more beneficial in certain children, specifically those aged less than 2 years with bilateral acute otitis media and in those with both acute otitis media and otorrhea.[18,19] If antibiotics are indicated, initial antibiotic therapy is directed toward the most common middle-ear pathogens. Common choices include amoxicillin,

azithromycin, and trimethoprim-sulfamethoxazole. In recalcitrant cases, treatment is directed toward (β-lactamase-producing organisms and antibiotic-resistant strains of *S. pneumoniae*. Common choices include high-dose amoxicillin or amoxicillin-clavulanate, the second- and third-generation cephalosporins, and clindamycin. The duration of therapy varies from 3 to 14 days.[20]

Multiple surgical modalities currently are used for the management of otitis media, including myringotomy with or without tympanostomy tube insertion, tympanocentesis, and adenoidectomy. Insertion of tympanostomy tubes is indicated when a patient experiences more than six acute otitis media episodes during a 6-month period or has recurrent otitis media in addition to otitis media with effusion or persistent bilateral effusions for longer than 3 months.[21] A trial of antibiotic prophylaxis is commonly carried out prior to surgical consultation.[22]

Antihistamines and decongestants are ineffective for otitis media with effusion and are not recommended for treatment.[23] The management of chronic suppurative otitis media often includes parenteral antibiotics to cover infection by *Pseudomonas* species and anaerobic bacteria.

PROGNOSIS

The prognosis for acute otitis media is excellent. Recent studies show that over 80% of children in the United States who were treated symptomatically for acute otitis media without antibiotics had complete resolution of otitis without suppurative complications.[24] However, complications can occur, more commonly in patients younger than 1 year of age. The most common complication is conductive hearing loss related to persistent effusions. Serious complications, including mastoiditis, cholesteatoma, labyrinthitis, extradural or subdural abscesses, meningitis, brain abscess, and lateral sinus thrombosis, are uncommon.[25]

ORAL HEALTH CONSIDERATIONS

Many children with recurrent otitis media are treated frequently (and sometimes for extensive periods) with various antibiotics. Included in the antibiotic armamentarium are medications that are also used for odontogenic infections. Oral health care providers need to be aware of what type of antibiotics the patient has taken within the previous 4 to 6 months, to avoid giving the patient an antibiotic to which resistance has already developed. It has been demonstrated that antibiotic regimens used for the treatment of otitis media promote the emergence of antibiotic-resistant bacteria.[26] Furthermore, the extended use of antibiotics may result in the development of oral candidiasis.

Sinusitis

Sinusitis is defined as an inflammation of the epithelial lining of the paranasal sinuses. The inflammation of these tissues causes mucosal edema and an increase in mucosal secretions. The most common trigger is an acute upper respiratory infection, although other causes (such as exacerbations of allergic rhinitis, dental infections or manipulations, and direct trauma) can be implicated. If blockage of sinus drainage occurs, retained secretions can promote bacterial growth and subsequent acute bacterial sinusitis.

Acute sinusitis is a very common disorder, affecting more than 31 million Americans per year. This accounts for more than 18 million office visits to primary care physicians per year and for 124 million lost days from work each year. Chronic sinusitis is also very common.[27]

PATHOPHYSIOLOGY

The paranasal sinuses are air-filled cavities that are lined with pseudostratified columnar respiratory epithelium. The epithelium is ciliated, which facilitates the clearance of mucosal secretions. The frontal, maxillary, and ethmoid sinuses drain into an area known as the ostiomeatal complex. Rhythmic ciliary movement and the clearance of secretions can be impaired by several factors, including viral upper respiratory infections, allergic inflammation, and exposure to tobacco smoke and other irritants. In addition, foreign bodies (accidental or surgical) or a severely deviated nasal septum can cause obstruction. If blockage of the sinus ostia or obstruction of the ostiomeatal complex occurs, stasis of sinus secretions will allow pooling in the sinus cavities, which facilitates bacterial growth.

The most common organisms found in acute sinusitis are *S. pneumoniae*, *H. influenzae*, and *M. catarrhalis*. In approximately 8 to 10% of cases of acute sinusitis, *Bacteroides* spp and *S. aureus* are causative. Organisms that are commonly associated with chronic sinusitis are anaerobic bacteria such as *Bacteroides* spp, *Fusobacterium* spp, *Streptococcus*, *Veillonella*, and *Corynebacterium* spp. Sinusitis due to a fungal infection rarely occurs, usually in immunocompromised patients and in patients who are unresponsive to antibiotics.[28]

CLINICAL AND LABORATORY FINDINGS

The symptoms of acute sinusitis include facial pain, tenderness, and headache localized to the affected region. Sinusitis affecting the sphenoid sinuses or posterior ethmoid sinuses can cause headache or pain in the occipital region. Other symptoms that are commonly described include purulent nasal discharge, fever, malaise, and postnasal drainage with fetid breath. Occasionally, there may be toothache or pain with mastication. Patients with chronic sinusitis often present with other symptoms that are often vague and poorly localized. Chronic rhinorrhea, postnasal drainage, nasal congestion, sore throat, facial "fullness," and anosmia are common complaints.

Physical examination reveals sinus tenderness and purulent nasal drainage. On occasion, erythema and swelling of the overlying skin may be evident. The nasal mucosa will appear edematous and erythematous, and nasal polyps might be visible.

In routine cases of suspected acute bacterial sinusitis, imaging studies are not required.[29] Then there are more persistent symptoms as in chronic sinusitis or an incomplete response to initial management; imaging studies become appropriate. Plain-film radiography is not helpful for establishing osteomeatal complex disease.[30] Computed tomography (CT) is the study of choice for documenting chronic sinusitis with underlying disease of the osteomeatal complex and is superior to magnetic resonance imaging (MRI) for the identification of bony abnormalities. CT can also accurately assess polyps, reactive osteitis, mucosal thickening, and fungal sinusitis.[31]

CLASSIFICATION

Sinusitis is classified as either acute, subacute, or chronic, based on the duration of the inflammation and underlying infection. Acute sinusitis is defined as inflammation of less than 4 weeks, subacute as 4 to 12 weeks, and chronic as longer than 12 weeks in duration.[32]

DIAGNOSIS

The diagnosis of acute sinusitis is made on the basis of history and physical examination. As previously noted, radiologic evaluations may be helpful in certain situations. Patients with recurrent disease need to be evaluated for underlying factors that can predispose patients to sinusitis. Allergy evaluation for allergic rhinitis is often helpful. Other predisposing factors, such as tobacco smoke exposure, immunodeficiency, and septal deviation, should be considered.[33]

CT usually aids the diagnosis of chronic sinusitis. Evaluation of the osteomeatal complex is crucial in the management of these patients. In addition, rhinoscopy may be helpful for direct visualization of sinus ostia.

MANAGEMENT

Initial medical treatment consists of antibiotics to cover the suspected pathogens, along with topical or oral decongestants to facilitate sinus drainage. First-line antibiotics such as amoxicillin are often effective, although second-generation cephalosporins, azithromycin, and amoxicillin-clavulanate can be helpful in resistant cases. Comprehensive treatment of bacterial sinusitis may also include adequate hydration, steam inhalation, and pharmacologic measures intended to treat underlying disease, such as rhinitis, and to restore ostial patency. Nasal glucocorticosteroids are thought to be potentially effective adjuncts to antibiotic therapy, but available objective data have not unequivocally demonstrated effectiveness.[32] Acute frontal or sphenoid sinusitis is very serious because of the potential for intracranial complications. Intravenous antibiotics are indicated, and surgical intervention is considered, based on the condition's response to medical management.[34]

The management of chronic sinusitis involves antibiotics of a broader spectrum, and a prolonged treatment course may be required.[35] Topical corticosteroids or short courses of oral corticosteroids may help reduce the swelling and/or obstruction of the osteomeatal complex.[36] Avoidance of exacerbating factors such as allergens or tobacco smoke should be emphasized. Patients with histories suggestive of allergy should undergo a thorough allergy evaluation.

Patients who have chronic sinusitis with evidence of disease of the osteomeatal complex who fail medical management often require surgical intervention. Functional endoscopic sinus surgery involves the removal of the osteomeatal obstruction through an intranasal approach. This procedure can be performed with either local or general anesthesia and without an external incision. The recovery time from this procedure is short, and morbidity is generally low.

PROGNOSIS

Patients treated for acute sinusitis usually recover without sequelae. Children with sinusitis, particularly ethmoid and maxillary sinusitis, are at risk for periorbital or orbital cellulitis. Periorbital cellulitis is most often treated on an outpatient basis with broad-spectrum antibiotics and rarely leads to complications. Orbital cellulitis, on the other hand, requires hospital admission with broad-spectrum intravenous antibiotics. Further treatment is tailored on a case-by-case basis and may entail surgical or endoscopic drainage of the infection.[37]

Frontal sinusitis can extend through the anterior wall and present as Pott's puffy tumor. Sinusitis can also spread intracranially and result in abscess or meningitis. These complications, although uncommon, are more likely to occur in male adolescent patients.

Patients with chronic sinusitis are more likely to require a prolonged recovery period, with a resultant decrease in quality of life. Chronic medication use can lead to side effects or other complications, such as rhinitis medicamentosa from prolonged use of topical decongestants. Surgical intervention and underlying-factor assessment will often reverse the chronic process, leading to an improvement in quality of life.

ORAL HEALTH CONSIDERATIONS

Patients with sinus infections who present with a complaint of a toothache are commonly encountered in a dental office. The oral health care professional evaluating the patient must be able to differentiate between an odontogenic infection and sinus pain. On history, sinus infections usually present with pain involving more than one tooth in the same maxillary quadrant, whereas a toothache usually involves only a single tooth. Ruling out odontogenic infections by a dental examination and appropriate periapical radiography strengthens a diagnosis.

Chronic sinus infections are often accompanied by mouth breathing. This condition is associated with oral dryness and (in long-time sufferers) increased susceptibility to oral conditions such as gingivitis.[38]

As with other conditions for which the prolonged use of antibiotics is prescribed, the potential development of bacterial resistance needs to be considered. Switching to a different class of antibiotics to treat an odontogenic infection is preferable to increasing the dosage of an antibiotic that the patient has recently taken for another condition.

The use of decongestants may be associated with oral dryness, which may need to be addressed.

Laryngitis and Laryngotracheobronchitis

The upper airway is the site of infection and inflammation during the course of a common cold, but respiratory viruses can attack any portion of the respiratory tree. Laryngitis is defined as an inflammation of the larynx, usually because of a viral infection. Laryngotracheobronchitis (also termed viral croup) is an inflammation (also due to a viral illness) involving the larynx, trachea, and large bronchi. Although these illnesses have distinct presenting features, both result from a similar infectious process and the reactive inflammation that follows. Laryngitis can present at any age, although it is more common among the adult population.[39] In contrast, laryngotracheobronchitis is an illness seen primarily in young children and has a peak incidence in the second and third years of life. These infections are most common during the fall and winter months, when respiratory viruses are more prevalent.

The viruses most commonly implicated in laryngitis are parainfluenza virus, coxsackieviruses, adenoviruses, and herpes simplex virus. The viruses most commonly associated with laryngotracheobronchitis are parainfluenza virus, RSV, influenza virus, and adenovirus.[40]

Acute laryngitis can also result from excessive or unusual use of the vocal cords, gastroesophageal reflux, or irritation due to tobacco smoking.

PATHOPHYSIOLOGY

The underlying infectious process is quite similar to that seen in viral infections of the upper respiratory tract (see above). After infection of the respiratory epithelium occurs, an inflammatory response consisting of mononuclear cells and polymorphonuclear leukocytes is mounted. As a result, vascular congestion and edema develop. Denudation of areas of respiratory epithelium can result. In addition to edema, spasm of laryngeal muscles can occur. Because the inflammatory process is triggered by viral infection, the disease processes are usually self-limited.

CLINICAL AND LABORATORY FINDINGS

Patients with laryngitis usually have an antecedent viral upper respiratory infection. Complaints of fever and sore throat are common. The most common manifestation of laryngitis is hoarseness, with weak or faint speech.[41] Cough is somewhat variable in presentation and is more likely when the lower respiratory tract is involved.

Children presenting with viral croup commonly have an antecedent upper respiratory infection, which may include fever. Shortly thereafter, a barking cough and intermittent stridor develop. Stridor at rest, retractions, and cyanosis can occur in children with severe inflammation. Neck radiography will demonstrate subglottic narrowing (a finding termed "steeple sign") on an anteroposterior view.

CLASSIFICATION

There is no universal classification system for these illnesses. The anatomic site most affected describes these diseases.

DIAGNOSIS

The diagnosis of laryngitis is based on the suggestive history. There are no specific findings on physical examination or laboratory tests, although the presence of hoarseness is suggestive. The differential diagnosis includes other causes of laryngeal edema, including obstruction of venous or lymphatic drainage from masses or other lesions, decreased plasma oncotic pressure from protein loss or malnutrition, increased capillary permeability, myxedema of hypothyroidism, and hereditary angioedema. Carcinoma of the larynx can also present with hoarseness.

The diagnosis of laryngotracheobronchitis is usually apparent and is based on a suggestive history. Radiologic evaluation may or may not aid physicians in the diagnosis. Only 50% of patients with laryngotracheobronchitis show the classic steeple sign on plain neck radiography (Figure 1).[42] With children, it is important to rule out other causes of

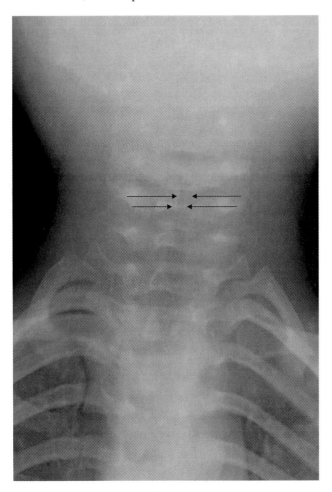

FIGURE 1 Anteroposterior radiograph of the neck show narrowing of the upper trachea that is most evident on the anteroposterior view (black arrows). This type of narrowing is typically present in croup and is known as the steeple sign on the anteroposterior radiograph given its similarity to a church steeple.

stridor, including foreign-body aspiration, acute bacterial epiglottitis, and retropharyngeal abscess.[43]

MANAGEMENT

Most cases of laryngitis are mild and self-limited, so only supportive care need be prescribed. The use of oral corticosteroids in severe or prolonged cases can be considered, although their routine use is controversial.[44]

The most important aspect in the management of laryngotracheobronchitis is airway maintenance. The standard therapy includes mist therapy, corticosteroids, and racemic epinephrine. Any child with evidence of respiratory distress should be considered a candidate for steroid treatment. Less frequently, hospitalization and intubation or tracheotomy are necessary.[42]

PROGNOSIS

As with viral upper respiratory infections, most cases of laryngitis and laryngotracheobronchitis are self-limited and require minimal medical intervention. Recovery within a few days to a week is the rule. In some cases, laryngotracheobronchitis can recur, although the factors influencing this are not well understood.

Pharyngitis and Tonsillitis

Inflammation of the tonsils and pharynx is almost always associated with infection, either viral or bacterial. More than 90% of cases of sore throat are related to viral infections. These infections can be associated with fever, rhinorrhea, and cough. The major viral etiologies are Epstein-Barr virus, coxsackievirus A, adenovirus, rhinovirus, and measles virus.[45]

The most common bacterial cause of acute tonsillopharyngitis is group A β-hemolytic *Streptococcus* (GABHS) infection, specifically *Streptococcus pyogenes* infection. Proper diagnosis and treatment of this infection are extremely important in order to prevent disease sequelae, namely, acute rheumatic fever and glomerulonephritis. Less common bacterial causes include *Corynebacterium diphtheriae*, *Neisseria gonorrhoeae*, *Chlamydia*, and *Mycoplasma pneumoniae*.

Chronic mouth breathing, chronic postnasal drainage, and inflammation due to irritant exposure can also cause pharyngitis and tonsillitis.

PATHOPHYSIOLOGY

Streptococcal infections are spread through direct contact with respiratory secretions. Transmission is often facilitated in areas where close contact occurs, such as schools and day-care centers. The incubation period is 2 to 5 days.

CLINICAL AND LABORATORY FINDINGS

Sore throat is the predominant symptom. Associated clinical findings are based on the infectious etiology. Patients with Epstein-Barr virus infections develop infectious mononucleosis, a disease characterized by exudative tonsillopharyngitis, lymphadenopathy, fever, and fatigue. Physical examination can reveal hepatosplenomegaly. Common laboratory findings include leukocytosis, with more than 20% atypical lymphocytes on blood smear. Blood chemistries may reveal elevated liver enzymes.

Infection with coxsackievirus can cause several distinct illnesses, each associated with tonsillopharyngitis. Herpangina is a disease that is characterized by ulcers that are 2 to 3 mm in size and located on the anterior tonsillar pillars and possibly the uvula and soft palate. Hand-foot-and-mouth disease is characterized by ulcers on the tongue and oral mucosa, in association with vesicles found on the palms and/or soles. Small yellow-white nodules on the anterior tonsillar pillars characterize lymphonodular pharyngitis; these nodules do not ulcerate.

Pharyngoconjunctival fever is a disorder characterized by exudative tonsillopharyngitis, conjunctivitis, and fever. Infection is due to an adenovirus.

Measles is a disease with a prodromal phase that is characterized by symptoms of upper respiratory infection, tonsillopharyngitis, and small white lesions with erythematous bases on the buccal mucosa and inner aspect of the lower lip (Koplik's spots). These lesions are pathognomonic of early measles infection.

Streptococcal pharyngitis is characterized by exudative tonsillitis and fever. Physical examination often reveals a beefy red uvula, cervical adenitis, and oral petechiae. Laboratory evaluation should include a throat culture for group A *Streptococcus*.[46]

CLASSIFICATION

Pharyngotonsillitis is classified on the basis of etiology and clinical presentation (see above).

DIAGNOSIS

Diagnosis is based on a history of sore throat and is established by appropriate physical findings and results of a throat culture (see above). A rapid antigen detection test is available for diagnosing streptococcal pharyngitis. The test has a high specificity (95+%) and slightly lower sensitivity (80 to 90%).[47] The importance of confirmatory cultures is still controversial, with some studies concluding that culture confirmation of negative rapid antigen detection tests may not be necessary in all circumstances.[48]

Antistreptococcal antibody titers reflect past and not present immunologic events and are of no value in the diagnosis of acute GABHS pharyngitis. They are valuable for confirmation of prior GABHS infections in patients suspected of having acute rheumatic fever or poststreptococcal acute glomerulonephritis.

MANAGEMENT

The viral causes of tonsillopharyngitis are treated symptomatically. Gargle solutions, analgesics, and antipyretics are often helpful. The course is always self-limited.[5]

Acute streptococcal pharyngitis is treated with oral penicillin V, cephalosporins, macrolides, clindamycin, or an intramuscular injection of benzathine penicillin G. Failure

rates for penicillin vary from 6 to 23%, so an additional antibiotic course may be necessary.[46]

PROGNOSIS

The prognosis for viral tonsillopharyngitis is very good as the infections are self-limited. Late sequelae from group A streptococcal tonsillitis can be avoided by prompt diagnosis and treatment.[49] Other complications due to streptococcal tonsillitis are uncommon but include cervical adenitis, peritonsillar abscesses, otitis media, cellulitis, and septicemia.

Oral Health Considerations

The association between GABHS infection and the development of severe complications, such as rheumatic fever and its associated heart condition, is well known. Although failure to successfully treat GABHS infections was more common in the prepenicillin era, there are some concerns today regarding reinfection in cases in which penicillin is unable to eradicate the organism. One study found a significant association between the persistence of GABHS on toothbrushes and removable orthodontic appliances and the recovery of GABHS in the oropharynx of symptomatic patients after 10 days of treatment with penicillin.[50] Interestingly, when toothbrushes were rinsed with sterile water, organisms could not be cultured beyond 3 days, whereas nonrinsed toothbrushes harbored GABHS for up to 15 days. Thus, patients with GABHS infections should be instructed to thoroughly clean their toothbrushes and removable acrylic appliances daily. It is also advisable to change to a new toothbrush after the acute stage of any oropharyngeal infection.

▼ LOWER AIRWAY DISEASES

The association between oral health and respiratory diseases has recently received renewed attention. Several articles have suggested that dental plaque may be a reservoir for respiratory pathogens involved in pneumonia and chronic obstructive pulmonary disease (COPD).[51–56] Although this may not be a critical problem for ambulatory healthy individuals, deteriorating oral health may be a major factor for both morbidity and mortality among institutionalized elderly persons, as well as for patients in critical care units.

Acute Bronchitis

Acute bronchitis is an acute respiratory infection involving the large airways (trachea and bronchi) that is manifested predominantly by cough with or without phlegm production that lasts up to 3 weeks. In patients who are otherwise healthy and without underlying pulmonary disease, bronchitis is most commonly caused by a viral infection.[57] The viruses most commonly implicated are influenza B, influenza A, parainfluenza, and RSV. Viruses that are predominantly associated with upper respiratory tract infection, including coronavirus, rhinovirus, and adenovirus, have also been implicated as causes of acute bronchitis.[58] Acute bronchitis due to bacterial infection is less common and is seen more commonly in patients who have chronic lung disease.[59] The bacteria that have been causally linked to acute bronchitis in otherwise healthy individuals include only *Mycoplasma pneumoniae*, *Chlamydia pneumoniae*, *Bordetella pertussis*, and *Bordetella parapertussis*.[60] *Staphylococcus* and gram-negative bacteria are common causes of bronchitis among hospitalized individuals.

PATHOPHYSIOLOGY

The pathophysiology of acute bronchitis is similar to that of other respiratory tract infections. Following infection of the mucosal cells, congestion of the respiratory mucosa develops. Inflammation causes an increase in secretory activity, resulting in increased sputum production. Polymorphonuclear leukocytes infiltrate the bronchial walls and lumen. Desquamation of the ciliated epithelium may occur, and spasm of bronchial smooth muscle is common.

CLINICAL AND LABORATORY FINDINGS

Acute viral bronchitis usually presents with sudden onset of cough, with or without sputum expectoration and without evidence of pneumonia, the common cold, acute asthma, or an acute exacerbation of chronic bronchitis.[58] Chest discomfort may occur; this usually worsens with persistent coughing bouts.[61] Other symptoms, such as dyspnea and respiratory distress, are variably present. Physical examination may reveal wheezing. The presentation may closely resemble an acute asthma exacerbation. Symptoms gradually resolve over a period of 1 to 2 weeks. Patients with underlying chronic lung disease might also experience respiratory compromise, with a significant impairment in pulmonary function.

The presentation of acute bacterial bronchitis is very similar to that of bacterial pneumonia (see below). Symptoms may include fever, dyspnea, productive cough with purulent sputum, and chest pain. Bacterial bronchitis can be differentiated from pneumonia by the lack of significant findings on chest radiography.

CLASSIFICATION

Although there is no universal classification scheme, acute bronchitis can be differentiated on the basis of etiology. Viral bronchitis presents differently from bacterial bronchitis, as described above.

DIAGNOSIS

Diagnosis of acute bronchitis is based on a suggestive history and a physical examination. Neither blood cell counts nor sputum analyses are particularly diagnostic in otherwise healthy patients. Chest radiography may be helpful in distinguishing bacterial bronchitis from pneumonia. Patients with recurrent bouts of acute bronchitis should be evaluated for possible asthma. This evaluation would include pulmonary function testing.

Patients with persistent symptoms in the course of presumed viral bronchitis should be evaluated to determine possible underlying etiologies. Sputum cultures might prove useful in these circumstances but are not performed routinely.[62]

MANAGEMENT

Viral bronchitis can be managed with supportive care only as most individuals who are otherwise healthy recover without specific treatment.[7] If significant airway obstruction or hyperreactivity is present, inhaled bronchodilators, such as albuterol, can be useful. Cough suppressants, such as codeine, can also be used for patients whose coughing interferes with sleep.

The treatment of bacterial bronchitis includes amoxicillin, amoxicillin-clavulanate, macrolides, and cephalosporins. For suspected or confirmed pertussis infection, treatment with a macrolide or trimethoprim-sulfamethoxazole is appropriate. Inhaled β_2-agonist bronchodilators were commonly used in the past but are no longer recommended to alleviate cough.[58]

PROGNOSIS

Acute bronchitis carries an excellent prognosis for patients who are without underlying pulmonary disease, and recovery without sequelae is the norm. However, for patients with chronic lung disease and respiratory compromise, bronchitis can be quite serious and may often lead to hospitalization and respiratory failure. In other high-risk individuals, such as those with human immunodeficiency virus (HIV) infection or other immunodeficiencies, acute bronchitis may lead to the development of bronchiectasis.

ORAL HEALTH CONSIDERATIONS

Resistance to antibiotics may develop rapidly and last for 10 to 14 days.[63] Thus, patients who are taking amoxicillin for acute bronchitis should be prescribed another type of antibiotic, (such as clindamycin or a cephalosporin) when an antibiotic is needed for an odontogenic infection.

Pneumonia

Pneumonia is defined pathologically as an infection and a subsequent inflammation involving the lung parenchyma. Both viruses and bacteria are causes, and the presentation is dependent on the causative organism. There are an estimated 5.6 million cases of pneumonia each year.[64] Pneumonias can be broadly classified as either community acquired or nosocomial. Nosocomial infections are infections that are acquired in a hospital or health care facility and often affect debilitated or chronically ill individuals. Community-acquired infections can affect all persons but are more commonly seen in otherwise healthy individuals.

The most common bacterial cause of community-acquired pneumonia is *S. pneumoniae*, followed by *H. influenzae*. The organisms responsible for nosocomial pneumonia include aerobic gram-negative bacilli, such as *P. aeruginosa*, *Escherichia coli*, *Klebsiella pneumoniae*, and *Acinetobacter* species. Infections due to gram-positive cocci, such as *S. aureus*, particularly methicillin-resistant *S. aureus* (MRSA), have been rapidly emerging in the United States as well.[65] A related condition is aspiration pneumonia, which is typically caused by anaerobic organisms, often with their source from the gingival crevice.[66] Aspiration pneumonia often occurs in patients with dysphagia, depressed consciousness, or other risks for aspiration of oral contents into the lung. Aspiration pneumonia occurs both in the community and in institutional settings.

Atypical organisms commonly associated with pneumonia include *M. pneumoniae*, *Legionella*, and *Chlamydia*.[67] The atypical organisms may cause a pneumonia that differs in clinical presentation from that caused by the aforementioned bacteria (see below). Pneumonia can also be caused by viruses (such as influenza, pararinfluenza, adenovirus, and RSV); by fungi such as *Candida*, *Histoplasma*, *Cryptococcus*, and *Aspergillus*; and by protozoa such as *Pneumocystis carinii* (seen in immunocompromised hosts), *Nocardia*, and *Mycobacterium tuberculosis*. Infection with these organisms can often be differentiated by chest radiography.

PATHOPHYSIOLOGY

The pathophysiology of pneumonia is dependent on the causative infectious organism. In bacterial pneumonia caused by *S. pneumoniae*, for example, the bacteria first enter the alveolar spaces after inhalation. Once inside the alveoli, the bacteria rapidly multiply, and extensive edema develops. The bacteria cause a vigorous inflammatory response, which includes an influx of polymorphonuclear leukocytes. In addition, capillary leakage is pronounced. As the inflammatory process continues, the polymorphonuclear leukocytes are replaced by macrophages. Subsequent deposition of fibrin ensues as the infection is controlled, and the inflammatory response resolves.[68]

Atypical infections of the lung (ie, viral, mycoplasmal, etc.) are interstitial processes. The organisms are first inhaled into the alveolar spaces. The organisms then infect the type I pneumocytes directly. As these pneumocytes lose their structural integrity and necrosis ensues, alveolar edema begins. Type II pneumocytes proliferate and line the alveoli, and an exudative cellular debris accumulates. An interstitial inflammatory response is mounted, primarily by mononuclear leukocytes. This process can occasionally progress to interstitial fibrosis, although resolution is the norm.

CLINICAL AND LABORATORY FINDINGS

Pneumonia due to community-acquired bacterial infection typically presents acutely, with a rapid onset of symptoms. A prodrome similar to that seen with acute infections of the upper respiratory tract is unusual. Common symptoms include fever, pleuritic chest pain, and coughing that produces purulent sputum.[61] Chills and rigors are also common. Pneumonia due to *H. influenzae*, which is seen more commonly in patients with COPD or alcoholism, presents with fever, cough, and malaise. Chest pain and rigors are less common.

Nosocomial pneumonia with *Staphylococcus* secondary to aspiration presents with fever, dyspnea, cough, and purulent sputum. In cases acquired hematogenously, signs and symptoms related to the underlying endovascular infection predominate. Otherwise, respiratory tract symptoms are mild or absent despite radiographic evidence of multiple pulmonary infiltrates. The classic clinical features of nonbacteremic Enterobacteriaceae or *Pseudomonas* pneumonia are abrupt onset of dyspnea, fever, chills, and cough in an older patient who is either hospitalized or chronically ill.[69]

Physical examination demonstrates crackles (rales) in the affected lung fields. Decreased breath sounds and dullness to percussion might also be noted. Signs of respiratory distress may be present in severely affected individuals.

As many as 37% of all outpatient cases of community-acquired pneumonia are considered atypical.[69] Symptoms usually develop over 3 to 4 days and initially consist of low-grade fever, malaise, a nonproductive cough, and headache. Sputum production, if present, is usually minimal. Findings on physical examination of the chest are usually unremarkable, with only scattered rhonchi. Infection due to *Mycoplasma* is common among younger patients. Pneumonias due to viral causes have a similar presentation but can have a more rapid onset.

Infection with *Legionella* spp (legionnaires' disease) begins with a prodrome consisting of fever and malaise and progresses rapidly to an acute phase of high fever, rigors, pleuritic chest pain, gastrointestinal complaints, and confusion. The cough is typically nonproductive and is only variably present. Elevated liver enzymes and proteinuria indicate renal and hepatic involvement. Hypoxia can also develop and can rapidly progress. Legionnaires' disease was first described at an American Legion convention in Philadelphia in 1976. The causative organisms have a predilection for moist areas such as air-conditioning ducts and cooling towers. The infection tends to occur more commonly among middle-aged men with a history of tobacco smoking.

CLASSIFICATION

Pneumonia is initially classified on clinical presentation as either viral, bacterial, or atypical. Different classifications based on radiologic or pathologic manifestations are less commonly used.

DIAGNOSIS

When a patient with probable pneumonia is being evaluated, the possible causative organism will be suggested by (1) the clinical presentation and course of the illness, (2) the degree of immunocompetency of the patient, (3) the presence or absence of underlying lung disease, and (4) the place of acquisition (hospital or community). Ultimately, the goal is rapid diagnosis to establish an etiology so that appropriate antimicrobial therapy can be initiated. With community-acquired pneumonia, the diagnosis should be based on a clinical history and physical examination findings. Chest radiography, laboratory studies, and blood cultures may be considered.[70]

In nosocomial infection, the presence of pneumonia is defined by new lung infiltrate on radiography plus clinical evidence that the infiltrate is of an infectious origin. The presence of a new or progressive radiographic infiltrate plus at least two of three clinical features (fever greater than 38°C, leukocytosis or leukopenia, and purulent secretions) represents the most accurate combination of criteria for starting empiric antibiotic therapy.[65]

Sputum analysis is the traditional tool used for diagnosis and management. Spontaneously coughed or induced sputum is analyzed by Gram stain and allows for the identification of a select group of pathogens and thus a more directed antibiotic therapy. For example, gram-positive cocci in pairs (diplococci) are suggestive of pneumococcal infection. Gram-positive cocci in grape-like clusters suggest infection with S. aureus. Gram-negative pleomorphic rods are typical of H. influenzae, whereas Klebsiella is identified by its short plump gram-negative-rod appearance. Numerous polymorphonuclear leukocytes are also often seen. This method, however, is limited since very often sputum contains bacteria of the normal flora that may be confused with pathogens.

Quantitative cultures for hospital-acquired infections can be performed on endotracheal aspirates or samples collected either bronchoscopically or nonbronchoscopically. These techniques may aid in diagnosis and management as well. Routine culture can identify S. pneumoniae, H. influenzae, S. aureus, and gram-negative rods. Specialized culturing techniques are needed to identify Legionella, Mycobacterium, Nocardia, Mycoplasma, and fungi. Tissue cultures are used to identify viruses and Chlamydia. In patients with hospital-acquired pneumonia, a lower respiratory tract culture should be collected before antibiotic therapy, but collection of cultures should not delay the initiation of therapy in critically ill patients.[65]

Chest radiography can be a valuable tool in the evaluation of the patient with pneumonia. The radiologic presentation is dependent on the infectious etiology and the underlying medical condition of the patient. A pattern of lobar consolidation and air bronchograms is seen most commonly in cases of pneumococcal pneumonia (Figure 2). The lower lobes and

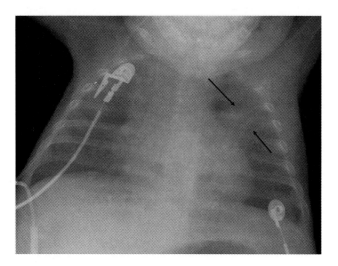

FIGURE 2   Anteroposterior radiograph of the chest in an infant shows an infiltrate in the left upper lobe (black arrows). Blood cultures obtained on this infant were positive for pneumoccous.

right middle lobe are most commonly involved. A pattern of patchy nonhomogeneous infiltrates, pleural effusion, and cavitary lesions is common with staphylococcal pneumonia. Klebsiella pneumonia typically involves multiple lobes and can also be associated with effusion and cavitation. Viral or atypical organisms usually present with an interstitial infiltrative pattern or patchy segmental infiltrates. Organisms such as Nocardia, Mycobacterium, and fungi often cause nodular or cavitary lesions, which are demonstrable on chest radiography. Rapid accumulation of pleural fluid or empyema is seen most often with bacterial infection.

The presence of cold agglutinins is suggestive of Mycoplasma infection. Cold agglutinins are antibodies (produced in response to Mycoplasma infection) that agglutinate red blood cells upon cold exposure. Titers reach maximal levels in 3 to 4 weeks but can be detected 1 week after the onset of disease. These antibodies can be found in 60 to 70% of patients with Mycoplasma pneumonia but are not specific to this disease.

Legionella pneumonia is diagnosed either by culture of the organisms, using specialized media, or by direct fluorescent antibody staining of sputum.

MANAGEMENT

Empiric treatment is started immediately upon diagnosis of pneumonia. Treatment options for outpatients with community-acquired pneumonia include β-lactams (eg, amoxicillin-clavulanate), macrolides, and fluoroquinolones. Patients who have received antimicrobial therapy within the previous 3 months are at increased risk for infection with antimicrobial-resistant S. pneumoniae and may require newer agents, including extended-release amoxicillin-clavulanate, the ketolide telithromycin, and the oxazolidinone linezolid.[71]

In the case of nosocomial pneumonia, patients with low risk of infection by an antibiotic-resistant organism should be treated with empiric therapy such as a third-generation cephalosporin or fluoroquinolone. However, more aggressive broad-spectrum therapy (such as an antipseudomonal cephalosporin, carbepenem, or fluoroquinolone, along with linezolid or vancomycin for MRSA), is required for high-risk patients, such as those with a prolonged duration of hospitalization (5 days or more), admission from a health care–related facility, or recent prolonged antibiotic therapy.[65]

Nonspecific treatment for patients with pneumonia includes aggressive hydration to aid in sputum clearance. Chest physiotherapy is advocated by many clinicians, although evidence of efficacy is lacking. If hypoxia is present, supplemental oxygen is given.[72]

A pneumococcal vaccine is available for active immunization against pneumococcal disease. The vaccine is effective for preventing disease from 85% of pneumococcal serotypes. It is effective for adults and for children older than 2 years of age and is recommended for high-risk individuals, such as those with asplenia and all individuals over the age of 65 years.

PROGNOSIS

Mortality due to community-acquired pneumonia is low. The risk of mortality is higher for older patients, patients with underlying pulmonary disease, patients with immuno-deficiency (ie, asplenia), and patients with positive blood cultures. Most deaths occur within 5 days of the onset of disease.

Mortality due to staphylococcal pneumonia is high, and patients who do recover often have residual pulmonary abnormalities. Mortality due to atypical pneumonia is low, with the exception of *Legionella* pneumonia, which has a 15% mortality rate if left untreated.

ORAL HEALTH CONSIDERATIONS

The aspiration of salivary secretions containing oral bacteria into the lower respiratory tract can cause pneumonia. Numerous periodontally associated oral anaerobes and facultative species have been isolated from infected pulmonary fluids.[73] Although most reports suggest increased susceptibility to the development of nosocomial pneumonia from periodontal pathogens, other oral bacteria (such as *Streptococcus viridans*) have been implicated in community-acquired pneumonia.[74]

The connection of oral health to pneumonia involves aspiration of a pathogen from a proximal site, for example, the oral-pharyngeal cavity, into the lower airway. The teeth or dentures have nonshedding surfaces upon which oral bio-films, that is, dental plaque, form, which are susceptible to colonization by respiratory pathogens. Indeed, intensive care subjects were found to harbor greater levels of dental plaque than nonhospitalized control patients, and bacterial pathogens known to cause pneumonia were found to be prevalent in the dental plaque from the intensive care subjects.[53] In some cases, up to 100% of the aerobic flora was found to be *S. aureus, P, aeruginosa*, or several enteric species. In contrast, the control dental patients were only rarely colonized by respiratory pathogens. Poor oral hygiene therefore may predispose high-risk patients to oral colonization by respiratory pathogens and therefore increase the risk for lung infection. In addition, the host response to oral biofilms results in inflammation of the periodontal tissues.[75] Thus, inflammatory products from the gingival tissues as well as pathogenic bacteria shed from oral biofilms into the secretions can be aspirated into the lower airway to promote lung infection.[73]

Elderly individuals residing in nursing homes also have an increased prevalence of poor oral health, including increased plaque retention.[76] Studies have evaluated the occurrence of pneumonia in cohorts of elderly individuals who were receiving and not receiving oral care. In one such study, the relative risk of developing pneumonia increased 67% in the group without access to oral health interventions compared with individuals who had access to oral care.[77] These data support the benefit of increased awareness and increased oral health interventions in hospitalized and institutionalized individuals. More intervention studies are needed to assess the impact of oral pathogens on the incidence of pneumonia, but at present, there is ample evidence that poor oral health status is a risk indicator for the development of pneumonia.

These and other studies support the notion that institutionalized subjects, especially those in hospital intensive care and nursing home settings, have a greater risk for dental plaque colonization by respiratory pathogens than do community-dwelling subjects. This suggests that oral intervention to reduce or control dental plaque may serve as a simple, cost-effective method to reduce pathogen colonization in high-risk populations. A recent systematic review of the literature that examined the association between poor oral hygiene and the risk for nosocomial pneumonia and chronic lung disease showed that interventions aimed at improving oral hygiene can significantly reduce the incidence of pulmonary disease.[78] The studies included in this analysis, together with several subsequent studies, suggest that improved oral hygiene prevents pneumonia (Table 1). Interventions tested to date include topical disinfections using chlorhexidine[79–81] and supervised mechanical plaque control augmented with topical agents.[82] Most studies have found a reduction in the incidence of pneumonia in the intervention group to be reduced up to 60% compared with the control group. Taken together, the available evidence suggests that there is a relationship between poor oral hygiene and bacterial pneumonia in special care populations, including those in hospital and nursing home settings. Interventions designed to improve oral hygiene may reduce the risk of pneumonia in these populations.

Bronchiolitis

Bronchiolitis is a disease that affects children under the age of 2 years; it is most common among infants aged 2 to 12 months. It is characterized by infection of the lower respiratory tract, with the bronchioles being most affected. The inflammatory response can be caused by various pathogens, including RSV, human metapneumovirus, parainfluenza virus, influenza virus, adenovirus, and *M. pneumoniae*.[83–85]

PATHOPHYSIOLOGY

Infection of the bronchioles leads to a marked inflammatory response with a prominent mononuclear cell infiltrate. This inflammatory response results in edema and necrosis of epithelial cells lining small airways, mucosal thickening and mucus hypersecretion, plugging, and bronchospasm.[85] Bronchiolar spasm is an occasional feature. Due to these changes, the lumina of the bronchioles are critically narrowed, leading to areas of microatelectasis and emphysema. Respiratory compromise is common, with decreased blood oxygen saturation, hypercarbia, respiratory acidosis, and, in severe cases, respiratory failure.

CLINICAL AND LABORATORY FINDINGS

Infants first develop signs and symptoms of an infection of the upper respiratory tract, with low-grade fever, profuse clear rhinorrhea, and cough. Signs of infection in the lower respiratory tract soon follow, including tachypnea, retractions, wheezing, and (on occasion) cyanosis. Crackles can be audible, and thoracic hyperresonance can be noted on percussion. Associated findings can include conjunctivitis, otitis media, and pharyngitis.

TABLE 1   Recent Intervention Studies of Oral Hygiene and Pneumonia

Study	Number of Subjects (Study/Placebo/Control)	Outcome Variables	Result (Placebo vs Control)	Comments
DeRiso et al, 1996[79]	Randomized study of cardiovascular ICU subjects undergoing heart surgery. Experimental group ($n = 173$) received 0.12% CHX oral rinse (with 11.6% EtOH), 0.5 oz for 30 s $2 \times$ /d. Control group ($n = 180$) received placebo (with EtOH 3.2%) 0.5 oz for 30 s $2 \times$ /d.	Overall nosocomial infection rate, upper and lower respiratory infection rates, in-hospital mortality rate. Pneumonia diagnosis: progressing pulmonary infiltrate, fever, leukocytosis, purulent tracheobronchial secretions.	69% reduction in the incidence of total respiratory tract infections in the CHX group ($p < .05$). A reduction in mortality in the CHX group (1.16% vs 5.56%).	CHX oral rinse reduces the total nosocomial respiratory infection rate and the use of nonprophylactic systemic antibiotics in patients under going heart surgery
Fourrier et al, 2000[80]	60 ICU patients requiring mechanical ventilation. Test group ($n = 30$) received 0.2% CHX gel $3 \times$ /d. Controls ($n = 30$) received oral rinsing with bicarbonate isotonic serum and oropharyngeal aspiration $4 \times$ /d.	Pneumonia diagnosis: temperature $> 38°C$ or $< 36°C$, presence of infiltrates in chest radiographs, leukocytosis or leukopenia, positive culture from tracheal aspirate and/or of BAL	8/30 test patients and 17/30 control patients had nosocomial infections. Number of VAP for 1,000 days of mechanical ventilation was significantly lower in the treated group (10.7 vs 32.3 d, respectively; $p < .05$). Trend, but not statistical difference, in a shorter length of stay in the ICU, a shorter duration of mechanical ventilation, and a lower mortality rate in the treated group.	Antiseptic decontamination of dental plaque with 0.2% CHX gel may reduce the incidence of nosocomial infections. The correlation between oral intervention and the incidence of nosocomial pneumonia was, however, not clearly stated.
Koeman et al, 2006[81]	Randomized, prospective study comparing oral decontamination with either CHX (2%) ($n = 127$) or 2% CHX + 2% colistin (COL) ($n = 128$) or control (no intervention) ($n = 130$)	VAP and oropharyngeal colonization by respiratory pathogens	The daily risk of VAP was reduced in both treatment groups compared with control: 65% (HR = 0.352; 95% CI [0.160–0. 791]; $p = .012$) for CHX and 55% (HR = 0.454; 95% CI [0.224–0.925]; $p = .030$) for CHX/COL. CHX/COL provided significant reduction in oropharyngeal colonization by both gram-negative and gram-positive microorganisms, whereas CHX mostly affected gram-positive microorganisms.	No differences noted in duration of mechanical ventilation, ICU stay, or ICU survival between groups
Yoneyama et al, 2002[82]	Randomized prospective study of elderly residents from 11 nursing homes. Test group ($n = 184$) received toothbrushing after each meal plus in some cases swabbing with povidone-iodine 1%. Controls ($n = 182$) received unsupervised care.	New pulmonary infiltrate in chest radiograph and cough or temperature $> 37.8°C$ or subjective dyspnea	RR 1.67 of developing pneumonia on no active oral care compared with oral care ($p = .04$)	Oral care may be useful in preventing pneumonia in older patients in nursing homes

BAL = bronchoalveolar lavage; CHX = chlorhexidine; CI = confidence interval; COL = colistin; EtOH = ethyl alcohol; HR = hazard ratio; ICU = intensive care unit; RR = relative risk; VAP = ventilator-associated pneumonia.

Chest radiography shows peribronchial cuffing, flattening of the diaphragms, hyperinflation, and increased lung markings.

Laboratory studies reveal a mild leukocytosis with a prominence of polymorphonuclear leukocytes ("left shift").

CLASSIFICATION

Bronchiolitis can be classified by the causative agent, as is the case with acute bronchitis.

DIAGNOSIS

The diagnosis is clinical, based on the history and physical examination. Laboratory and radiologic studies for diagnosis are not generally required. The etiology can be determined (and the diagnosis confirmed) by performing a nasopharyngeal culture for RSV and other respiratory viruses. Rapid viral diagnostic assays are also available.

The differential diagnosis includes many other causes of wheezing and respiratory distress in this age group, such as asthma, congenital heart disease, and cystic fibrosis (CF).

MANAGEMENT

Clinical treatment of these infants is generally limited to supportive care. Infants may be placed in cool-mist oxygen tents, where continuous oxygen administration can be given. Due to an increase in insensible water losses, hydration must be ensured. Aerosolized bronchodilators should not be used routinely in the management of bronchiolitis, although a carefully monitored trial may be attempted if there is a documented positive clinical response. Corticosteroid medications are generally not indicated.[86]

Antiviral therapy with ribavirin is rarely used, although it may be considered for use in highly selected situations involving documented RSV bronchiolitis with severe disease or in those who are at risk for severe disease (eg, immunocompromised and/or hemodynamically significant cardiopulmonary disease).[85] Ribavirin is delivered by aerosol on a semicontinuous basis for up to 1 week.[87]

Mechanical ventilation is required in the infant with respiratory failure. Very young infants (less than 1 month of age) are at risk for apnea due to RSV infection, so close observation is required.

An intramuscular monoclonal antibody to the RSV F protein, palivizumab, is effective in preventing severe RSV disease in high-risk infants when given before and during the RSV season. This prophylaxis is currently recommended only for high-risk patient populations such as those with chronic lung disease, a history of prematurity, or congenital heart disease.[88]

PROGNOSIS

Although mortality due to bronchiolitis is not uncommon, most patients recover without sequelae. Epidemiologic studies with a several-year follow-up of index and control children show a higher incidence of wheezing and asthma in children with a history of bronchiolitis, unexplained by family history or other atopic syndromes. It is unclear whether bronchiolitis incites an immune response that manifests as asthma later or whether those infants have an inherent predilection for asthma that is merely unmasked by their episode of RSV.[88]

Asthma

Asthma is a chronic inflammatory disorder of the airways. It is characterized by recurrent and often reversible airflow limitation due to an underlying inflammatory process. The etiology of asthma is unknown, but allergic sensitivity is seen in most patients with asthma.[4] There is a significant hereditary contribution, but no single gene or combination of genes has yet been identified as causative. Multiple risk factors for the development of asthma have been indentified, including family history of asthma, atopy, respiratory infections, inhaled pollutants in indoor and outdoor air and in the workplace, allergens, food sensitivities, and other exposures (such as tobacco smoke).[89]

In the United States, asthma affects more than 14 million people. Its onset is most commonly during childhood, and almost 5 million children are affected. Asthma mortality numbers 5,000 people per year.[90] In addition, the care of asthmatic persons represents a significant economic and social burden, accounting for numerous hospitalization days and days missed from school and work. These trends do not appear to be declining despite advances in our understanding of asthma and despite new pharmacologic modalities.

PATHOPHYSIOLOGY

The clinical features of asthma are due to the underlying chronic inflammatory process. Although the etiology is not known, certain histopathologic features provide insights into the chronic process. Infiltration of the airway by inflammatory cells such as activated lymphocytes and eosinophils, denudation of the epithelium, deposition of collagen in the subbasement membrane area, and mast cell degranulation are often features of mild or moderate persistent asthma. In fatal disease and severe persistent asthma, other features are also seen, including occlusion of the bronchial lumen by mucus, hyperplasia and hypertrophy of the bronchial smooth muscle, and goblet cell hyperplasia.[91]

Airway inflammation contributes significantly to many of the hallmark features of asthma, including airflow obstruction, bronchial hyperresponsiveness, and the initiation of the injury-repair process (remodeling) found in some patients. Bronchial smooth muscle spasm is instrumental in the excessive airway reactivity. Resident airway cells, including mast cells, alveolar macrophages, and airway epithelium, as well as immigrating inflammatory cells, secrete a variety of mediators that directly contract the bronchial smooth muscle. These same mediators, such as histamine, cysteinyl leukotrienes, and bradykinin, increase capillary membrane permeability to cause mucosal edema of the airways.[92]

Atopy is the strongest risk factor associated with the development of asthma. Persistent exposure to relevant allergens in a sensitized individual can lead to chronic allergic inflammation of the airways. Although atopy is seen more commonly in childhood-onset asthma, it can also play an important role in asthma in adults.

CLINICAL AND LABORATORY FINDINGS

The hallmark clinical features of asthma are recurrent reversible airflow limitation and airway hyperresponsiveness. These factors lead to the development of the signs and symptoms of asthma, which include intermittent wheezing, coughing, dyspnea, and chest tightness. Symptoms of asthma tend to worsen at night and in the early morning hours. In addition, well-defined triggers may precipitate asthma symptoms. These triggers include allergens, exercise, cold air, respiratory irritants, emotional extremes, and infections (especially viral infections). Symptoms can progress slowly over time, or they may develop abruptly.[2,93,94]

Historical points that suggest asthma are chronic coughing with nocturnal awakenings, dyspnea or chest tightness with exertion, recurrent "bronchitis" associated with infections of the upper respiratory tract, and wheezing that occurs on a seasonal basis. Physical examination of patients with mild disease often shows no abnormalities. However, common findings in patients with more severe disease include an increased anteroposterior chest diameter, a prolonged expiratory phase, wheezing, and diminished breath sounds.

Digital clubbing is rarely seen. Concurrent allergic disease such as allergic rhinitis may be present. During acute exacerbations, patients may show signs of respiratory distress, with tachypnea, intercostal retractions, nasal flaring, and cyanosis.

Pulmonary function testing or spirometry is recommended in the initial assessment of most patients with suspected asthma. These tools can often be useful to monitor the course of asthma and a patient's response to therapy. The technique involves a maximal forced expiration following a maximal inspiration. The key measurements are the forced vital capacity (FVC), which is the amount of air expired during the forced expiration, and the forced expiratory volume in 1 second (FEV_1), which is the volume of air expired during the first second of expiration; FEV_1 is a measure of the rate at which air can be exhaled. Given the FEV_1 and the FEV_1/FVC ratio, an objective determination of airflow limitation is possible. Reversibility can be demonstrated after administration of a short-acting bronchodilator (such as albuterol) and a repeat spirometric measurement. In patients with normal baseline spirometry values, a demonstration of bronchial hyperresponsiveness is useful. This is performed by bronchoprovocation, using nonspecific triggers such as histamine or methacholine. When delivered by aerosol, these agents allow the determination of bronchial hyperreactivity by triggering a decrease in the FEV_1 immediately following inhalation. Subsequent measurements of peak expiratory flow rate (PEFR) at home may also be helpful to assess symptoms, to alert to worsening of airflow obstruction, and to monitor therapeutic responses.[92] The PEFR is easy to determine, and durable metering devices are available at little cost.

Allergen skin testing is another valuable tool. This testing allows the accurate identification of allergic triggers, which can translate into more specific therapies, such as allergen avoidance and immunotherapy (see "Allergic Rhinitis and Conjunctivitis," above). Chest radiography may be useful, especially as a means of excluding other diseases from the diagnosis.

CLASSIFICATION

Asthma is classified according to its severity. Although there is no universal classification scheme, the guidelines set forth by the National Asthma Education and Prevention Program (NAEPP) are the most widely used in the United States.[91,95] Asthma patients are classified as having mild-intermittent, mild-persistent, moderate-persistent, or severe-persistent disease. The categories are defined by both subjective (historical) and objective (spirometric) points. Treatment guidelines are based on the level of severity of the patient's disease, and the classification can therefore change over time.[96] Asthma may also be classified by the underlying trigger (eg, exercise-induced asthma and occupational asthma).

DIAGNOSIS

The diagnosis of asthma is made on the basis of a suggestive history, confirmatory physical findings, and the demonstration of reversible airflow limitation. This can be documented during hospitalization, by outpatient use of spirometry or PEFR determinations, or by clinical assessment after therapeutic trials.

The differential diagnosis of asthma includes other causes of chronic coughing and wheezing. The diseases that are usually considered are chronic rhinitis or sinusitis, CF, gastroesophageal reflux disease, airway narrowing due to compression (ie, masses), and COPD (chronic bronchitis). Factors favoring the diagnosis of asthma include intermittent symptoms with asymptomatic periods, complete or nearly complete reversibility with bronchodilators, the absence of digital clubbing, and a history of atopy.

MANAGEMENT

The goals of asthma management include the patient having little or no chronic symptoms, few or no exacerbations, no hospitalizations, and minimal or no activity limitation. Ideal control would include no need for short-acting bronchodilators, normal PEFRs, no PEFR variability, and no adverse effects from controller medications. All patients with asthma, regardless of its severity, should have an asthma control plan to aid in understanding the underlying process and treatment options and to effectively treat asthma exacerbations. Regular monitoring of asthma is important; spirometry, PEFR measurement, exhaled nitric oxide levels,[97] and questionnaires may be useful tools for this purpose. Avoidance control measures are regularly emphasized, focusing on allergen and irritant triggers. Treatment for concomitant diseases that may exacerbate asthma (such as allergic rhinitis, gastroesophageal reflux disease, and chronic sinusitis) should be instituted.[98]

Pharmacotherapy of asthma is based on the severity of disease. NAEPP guidelines provide written algorithms to aid in treatment plan development (Figure 3). Patients with mild-intermittent disease usually require short-acting bronchodilators on an as-needed basis. These medications (such as albuterol) are preferably administered by inhalation. In addition to relaxing airway smooth muscle, β-agonists enhance mucociliary clearance and decrease vascular permeability.[99]

Patients with mild-persistent asthma usually require routine therapy for control of underlying airway inflammation. Inhaled corticosteroids are the most widely used and most effective asthma anti-inflammatory agents.[100] Strong evidence establishes that inhaled corticosteroids improve long-term outcomes for children of all ages with mild or moderate persistent asthma, compared with as-needed β_2-agonists, as measured by prebronchodilator FEV_1, reduced hyperresponsiveness, improvements in symptom scores, fewer courses of oral corticosteroids, and fewer urgent care visits or hospitalizations.[91] They have an excellent safety profile at conventional doses, although high-dose therapy can put patients at risk for corticosteroid side effects. These medications have been used for decades in both children and adults without significant long-term side effects in most patients. Although there is the potential for but small risk of delayed

Stepwise Approach for Managing Asthma in Adults and Children Older Than 5 Years of Age: Treatment

Classify Severity: Clinical Features Before Treatment or Adequate Control			Medications Required To Maintain Long-Term Control
	Symptoms/Day Symptoms/Night	PEF or FEV₁ PEF Variability	Daily Medications
Step 4 Severe Persistent	Continual Frequent	≤ 60% > 30%	■ **Preferred treatment:** – **High-dose inhaled corticosteroids** AND – **Long-acting inhaled beta₂-agonists** AND, if needed, – Corticosteroid tablets or syrup long term (2 mg/kg/day, generally do not exceed 60 mg per day). (Make repeat attempts to reduce systemic corticosteroids and maintain control with high-dose inhaled corticosteroids.)
Step 3 Moderate Persistent	Daily > 1 night/week	> 60% – < 80% > 30%	■ **Preferred treatment:** – **Low-to-medium dose inhaled corticosteroids and long-acting inhaled beta₂-agonists.** ■ Alternative treatment (listed alphabetically): – Increase inhaled corticosteroids within medium-dose range OR – Low-to-medium dose inhaled corticosteroids and either leukotriene modifier or theophylline. If needed (particularly in patients with recurring severe exacerbations): ■ **Preferred treatment:** – **Increase inhaled corticosteroids within medium-dose range and add long-acting inhaled beta₂-agonists.** ■ Alternative treatment (listed alphabetically): – Increase inhaled corticosteroids within medium-dose range and add either leukotriene modifier or theophylline.
Step 2 Mild Persistent	> 2/week but < 1x/day > 2 nights/month	≥ 80% 20–30%	■ **Preferred treatment:** – **Low-dose inhaled corticosteroids.** ■ Alternative treatment (listed alphabetically): cromolyn, leukotriene modifier, nedocromil, OR sustained-release theophylline to serum concentration of 5–15 mcg/mL.
Step 1 Mild Intermittent	≤ 2 days/week ≤ 2 nights/month	≥ 80% < 20%	■ No daily medication needed. ■ Severe exacerbations may occur, separated by long periods of normal lung function and no symptoms. A course of systemic corticosteroids is recommended.

Quick Relief All Patients	■ Short-acting bronchodilator: 2–4 puffs **short-acting inhaled beta₂-agonists** as needed for symptoms. ■ Intensity of treatment will depend on severity of exacerbation; up to 3 treatments at 20-minute intervals or a single nebulizer treatment as needed. Course of systemic corticosteroids may be needed. ■ Use of short-acting beta₂-agonists >2 times a week in intermittent asthma (daily, or increasing use in persistent asthma) may indicate the need to initiate (increase) long-term-control therapy.

 Step down
Review treatment every 1 to 6 months; a gradual stepwise reduction in treatment may be possible.

 Step up
If control is not maintained, consider step up. First, review patient medication technique, adherence, and environmental control.

Note
- The stepwise approach is meant to assist, not replace, the clinical decisionmaking required to meet individual patient needs.
- Classify severity: assign patient to most severe step in which any feature occurs (PEF is % of personal best; FEV₁ is % predicted).
- Gain control as quickly as possible (consider a short course of systemic corticosteroids); then step down to the least medication necessary to maintain control.
- Minimize use of short-acting inhaled beta₂-agonists. Overreliance on short-acting inhaled beta₂-agonists (e.g., use of approximately one canister a month even if not using it every day) indicates inadequate control of asthma and the need to initiate or intensify long-term-control therapy.
- Provide education on self-management and controlling environmental factors that make asthma worse (e.g., allergens and irritants).
- Refer to an asthma specialist if there are difficulties controlling asthma or if step 4 care is required. Referral may be considered if step 3 care is required.

Goals of Therapy: Asthma Control
- Minimal or no chronic symptoms day or night
- Minimal or no exacerbations
- No limitations on activities; no school/work missed
- Maintain (near) normal pulmonary function
- Minimal use of short-acting inhaled beta₂-agonist
- Minimal or no adverse effects from medications

FIGURE 3 Stepwise approach for treating asthma in adults and children older than 5 years of age. Reproduced with permission from <http://www.nhlbi.nih.gov/guidelines/asthma/asthsumm.htm>.

growth, strong evidence from clinical trials following children for up to 6 years suggests that the use of inhaled corticosteroids at recommended doses does not have long-term, clinically significant, or irreversible effects.[91] Alternative medications include the nonsteroidal anti-inflammatory agents nedocromil and cromolyn, leukotriene receptor antagonists (LTRAs), or sustained-release theophylline.

Patients with moderate and severe persistent disease require more intensive therapy. Long-acting bronchodilators such as salmeterol and formoterol have been shown to have an additive effect when used with inhaled corticosteroids and are useful additions to inhaled corticosteroid therapy.[101] LTRAs also are often a helpful addition to inhaled corticosteroids. A minority of patients might require long-term corticosteroids; these patients are difficult to manage, but adequate symptom control while minimizing the dose is of paramount importance.[102] Omalizumab, a recombinant humanized monoclonal anti-IgE antibody, currently indicated for moderate to severe asthma, has been shown to improve asthma symptom scores, decrease exacerbations, and decrease inhaled corticosteroid dosese.[103] Newer promising agents that are also currently under investigation include PDE4 inhibitors[104] and anti–tumor necrosis factor (TNF) biologic agents. In recent studies, anti-TNF biologic agents have been shown to result in a marked improvement in asthma symptoms, lung function, and bronchial hyper-responsiveness.[105,106] Patients with allergic triggers may benefit from allergen immunotherapy. Many studies have now documented improvement from following a 3- to 5-year course of specific immunotherapy.[107] This is an excellent means of minimizing medications while maintaining control for many patients.

PROGNOSIS

Although asthma is not a curable disease, it is a controllable disease. Asthma education programs are extremely important in making early diagnosis and interventions possible. Despite an increase in our knowledge of the underlying pathophysiology, asthma mortality rates have not declined. With early diagnosis and a comprehensive management plan, patients with asthma can experience a normal life expectancy with good quality of life.

ORAL HEALTH CONSIDERATIONS

The main concern when treating any medically complex patient is to avoid exacerbation of the underlying condition. Several protocols suggesting appropriate procedures for dental treatment of asthmatic patients have been put forth.[108–111] However, few studies assessing the respiratory response of patients to dental care have been performed. One recent study indicated that although 15% of asthmatic pediatric patients will have a clinically significant decrease in lung function, no clinical parameter or historical data pertaining to asthma can predict this phenomenon.[112]

However, numerous dental products and materials, including toothpaste, fissure sealants, tooth enamel dust,

and methylmethacrylate, have been associated with the exacerbation of asthma, whereas other items (such as fluoride trays and cotton rolls) have been suggested as being so associated.[108, 113–117]

There is still no consensus regarding the association between asthma and dentofacial morphology.[118,119] Although nasal respiratory obstruction resulting in mouth breathing has been implicated in the development of a long and tapered facial form, an increased lower facial height, and a narrow maxillary arch, this relationship has never been substantiated with unequivocal evidence.

Oral manifestations include candidiasis, decreased salivary flow, increased calculus, increased gingivitis, increased periodontal disease, increased incidence of caries, and adverse effects of orthodontic therapy.[120–124]

It is possible that prolonged use of β_2-agonists may cause reduced salivary flow, with a resulting increase in cariogenic bacteria and caries and an increased incidence of candidiasis.[125] The increased incidence of caries is further accelerated by the use of cariogenic carbohydrates and sugar-containing antiasthmatic medications.[126]

Dental treatment for asthmatic patients needs to address the oral manifestations of this condition, as well as its potential underlying systemic complications. Elective dental procedures should be avoided in all but those whose asthma is well controlled. The type and frequency of asthmatic attacks, as well as the type of medications used by the patient, indicate the severity of the disease.

The following are considerations and recommendations for administering dental care to patients who have asthma:

1. Fluoride supplements should be instituted for all asthmatic patients, particular those taking R$_2$-agonists.
2. The patient should be instructed to rinse his or her mouth with water after using inhalers.
3. Oral hygiene should be reinforced to reduce the incidence of gingivitis and periodontitis.
4. Antifungal medications should be administered as needed, particularly in patients who are taking inhaled corticosteroids.
5. Steroid prophylaxis needs to be used with patients who are taking long-term systemic corticosteroids (see Chapter 10).
6. Use stress-reducing techniques. Conscious sedation should be performed with agents that are not associated with bronchoconstriction, such as hydroxyzine. Barbiturates and narcotics should be avoided due to their potential to cause bronchospasm and reduce respiratory functions. Nitrous oxide can be used for all but patients with severe asthma as it may irritate the airways.[127]
7. Avoid dental materials that may precipitate an attack. Acrylic appliances should be cured prior to insertion. Dental materials without methylmethacrylate should be considered.
8. Schedule these patients' appointments for late morning or later in the day to minimize the risk of an asthmatic attack.[128]

9. Have oxygen and bronchodilators available in case of an exacerbation of asthma.

10. There are no contraindications to the use of local anesthetics containing epinephrine, but preservatives such as sodium metabisulfite may contribute to asthma exacerbation in susceptible patients.[129] Nevertheless, interactions between epinephrine and R$_2$-agonists may result in a synergistic effect, producing increased blood pressure and arrhythmias.

11. Judicious use of rubber dams will prevent reduced breathing capability.

12. Care should be used in the positioning of suction tips as they may elicit a cough reflex.

13. Up to 10% of adult asthmatic patients have an allergy to aspirin and other nonsteroidal anti-inflammatory agents.[130] A careful history concerning the use of these types of drugs needs to be elicited. Although the use of acetaminophen has been proposed as an alternative to the use of aspirin, recent data suggest caution because these types of drugs have also been associated with more severe asthma.[131]

14. Drug interactions with theophylline are common. Macrolide antibiotics may increase the level of theophylline, whereas phenobarbitals may reduce the level. Furthermore, drugs such as tetracycline have been associated with more accentuated side effects when given together with theophylline.

15. During an acute asthmatic attack, discontinue the dental procedure, remove all intraoral devices, place the patient in a comfortable position, make sure the airway is opened, and administer a R$_2$-agonist and oxygen. If no improvement is noted, administer epinephrine subcutaneously (1:1,000 concentration, 0.01 mg/kg of body weight, up to a maximum of 0.3 mg) and alert emergency medical assistance.

Chronic Obstructive Pulmonary Disease

COPD is a disease state characterized by airflow limitation. The airflow is usually both progressive and associated with an abnormal inflammatory response of the lungs to noxious particles or gases.[132] COPD includes emphysema, an anatomically defined condition characterized by destruction and enlargement of the lung alveoli; chronic bronchitis, a clinically defined condition with chronic cough and phlegm; and small airways disease, a condition in which small bronchioles are narrowed. COPD is present only if chronic airflow obstruction occurs; chronic bronchitis without chronic airflow obstruction is not included within COPD.[133]

COPD is the fourth leading cause of chronic morbidity and mortality in the United States.[132] The diagnosis should be considered in any patient with symptoms of cough, sputum production or dyspnea, and/or a history of exposure to risk factors for the disease.

Risk factors for the disease can include environmental exposures and host factors, such as a rare hereditary deficiency in the enzyme α_1-antitrypsin. This enzyme is responsible for inhibiting the activity of trypsin and other proteases in the serum and tissues. The characteristic panlobular emphysematous changes that are seen in α_1-antitrypsin deficiency are related to the loss of alveolar walls. More commonly, risk factors for the disease include environmental exposure to tobacco smoke, heavy exposure to occupational dusts and chemicals (vapors, irritants, fumes), and indoor/outdoor pollution.[132]

The clinical course of patients with COPD is quite varied. Most patients display some degree of progressive dyspnea, exercise intolerance, and fatigue. In addition, patients are susceptible to frequent exacerbations, usually caused by infections of the upper or lower respiratory tract. Most patients with COPD have little respiratory reserve. Therefore, any process that causes airway inflammation can lead to clinical deterioration.

PATHOPHYSIOLOGY

Three processes are thought to be important in the pathogenesis of COPD: chronic inflammation throughout the airways, parenchyma, and pulmonary vasculature; oxidative stress; and an imbalance of proteases and antiproteases in the lung. These pathologic changes lead to the physiologic changes characteristic of the disease, including mucus hypersecretion, ciliary dysfunction, airflow limitation, pulmonary hyperinflation, gas exchange abnormalities, pulmonary hypertension, and cor pulmonale.[132]

Expiratory airflow limitation is the primary physiologic change in COPD. Airflow limitation results from fixed airway obstruction mainly. Patients with COPD may also have smooth muscle hypertrophy and bronchial hyperreactivity, although these features are not as prominent as in asthma.[133] Mucus hypersecretion and ciliary dysfunction lead to chronic cough and sputum production. In advanced COPD, peripheral airway obstruction, parenchymal destruction, and pulmonary vascular abnormalities reduce the lung's capacity for gas exchange, producing hypoxemia and, later, hypercapnia.[132]

Many toxins in tobacco smoke can cause a vigorous inflammatory response. In humans, chronic exposure to tobacco smoke results in an increase in the number of goblet cells because of hyperplasia and metaplasia. Acrolein, for example, causes both impairment of both ciliary and macrophage activities, as well as increases mucin hypersecretion.[134] Nitrogen dioxide causes direct toxic damage to the respiratory epithelium. Hydrogen cyanide is responsible for the functional impairment of enzymes that are required for respiratory metabolism. Carbon monoxide causes a decrease in the oxygen-carrying capacity of red blood cells by associating with hemoglobin to form carboxyhemoglobin. Lastly, polycyclic hydrocarbons have been implicated as carcinogens.

Hypoxemia is the result of the ventilation-perfusion mismatch that accompanies airway obstruction and emphysema. Portions of the lung that are not aerated due to obstruction cannot oxygenate the blood. This causes a decrease in overall oxygen concentrations. In addition, emphysema causes a decreased diffusion capacity because of a loss of air-space capillary units. Hypercarbia also develops and is often progressive and asymptomatic. Pulmonary hypertension can result from chronic hypoxia due to vasoconstriction of pulmonary vessels.

Patients with emphysema alone have less ventilation-perfusion mismatching early in the course of the disease; this is due to the loss of both air space and supplying blood vessels. Severe hypoxia, pulmonary hypertension, and cor pulmonale are generally not seen until late in the disease process. Emphysema manifests as loss of the elastic recoil of the lungs, making the lungs more compliant. The work of breathing is therefore not significantly increased. However, the decrease in recoil allows the easy collapse of the peripheral airways, leading to further airway obstruction and airflow limitation.[135]

CLINICAL AND LABORATORY FINDINGS

Patients with COPD have symptoms of dyspnea, cough, and sputum production. An increase in the production of purulent sputum is a sign of exacerbation due to respiratory infection. Physical findings include diffuse wheezing, possibly associated with signs of respiratory distress, including the use of accessory muscles of respiration (retractions) and tachypnea.[136] Liver enlargement due to congestion, ascites, and peripheral edema can develop as the disease progresses to pulmonary hypertension and cor pulmonale. This leads to the characteristic clinical patient presentation termed the "blue bloater."

Patients with emphysema present primarily with dyspnea. Patients can be adequately oxygenated in the early stages of the disease and thus can have fewer signs of hypoxia; the term *pink puffer* has been used to describe these patients. Physical findings include an increase in chest wall size. Wheezing is present to varying degrees.

Chest radiography may show evidence of an increase in lung compliance, with flattened diaphragms, hyperexpansion, and an increase in anteroposterior diameter (Figure 4). Spirometry will show evidence of airflow limitation, with decreases in the FEV_1 and the FEV_1/FVC ratio. Complete pulmonary function studies will also indicate an increase in residual volume and total lung capacity.[136] Pulmonary diffusion capacity will be decreased due to a loss of gas-exchanging units.

CLASSIFICATION

COPD is now classified into five stages: at risk, mild, moderate, severe, and very severe. The at-risk stage is defined by normal spirometry, but patients have chronic symptoms of cough and sputum production. Mild, moderate, and severe COPD has evidence of increasing airway obstruction on spirometry in each progressive stage. Finally, very severe COPD is defined by severe airway obstruction with chronic respiratory failure. At this stage, quality of life is significantly impaired and exacerbations may be life-threatening.[132]

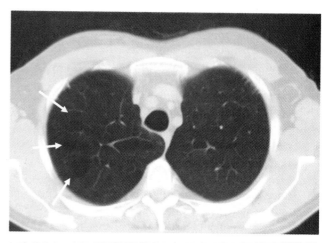

FIGURE 4 Axial computed tomography image of the upper chest demonstrates decreased attenuation of the lung tissue bilaterally, especially on the right (white arrows) where there is evidence of centrilobular emphysema.

DIAGNOSIS

The diagnosis is suggested by the history and physical findings. Patients often have cough, dyspnea, and sputum production and/or a history of exposure to risk factors. Alternative diagnoses, such as asthma, CF, and congestive heart failure, should be considered. Complete pulmonary function tests are a valuable means of assessing airflow limitation and the reversibility of airway obstruction. For patients with more severe disease, assessment of oxygen status with pulse oximetry is a valuable office procedure. A determination of arterial blood gases is important for patients who are clinically deteriorating and for the management of hospitalized patients.[137] Chest radiography can be helpful to exclude alternative diagnoses but is rarely diagnostic in COPD.

MANAGEMENT

There are no curative treatments for chronic bronchitis and emphysema. Smoking cessation is the single most important intervention to stop the progression of COPD. Reduction of exposures to occupational dusts and chemicals and indoor/outdoor pollution can also decrease the progression of disease.[132]

Management focuses on maintaining quality of life and preventing exacerbations. Maintenance therapy includes trials of inhaled bronchodilators such as β-agonists and ipratropium bromide. Long-acting bronchodilators, such as formoterol or salmeterol, may be added also according to the guidelines provided by the Global Initiative for Obstructive Lung Disease (Figure 5). Theophylline products have also been used with some efficacy. Inhaled corticosteroids are appropriate in patients with severe and very severe COPD staging.[132] Although they have not been shown to alter the decline in lung function in COPD patients, inhaled corticosteroids result in fewer exacerbations,[134] a decrease in pulmonary symptoms, and improved sensitivity of the lungs to external stimuli.[105] Long-term treatment with oral corticosteroids is not recommended.[132]

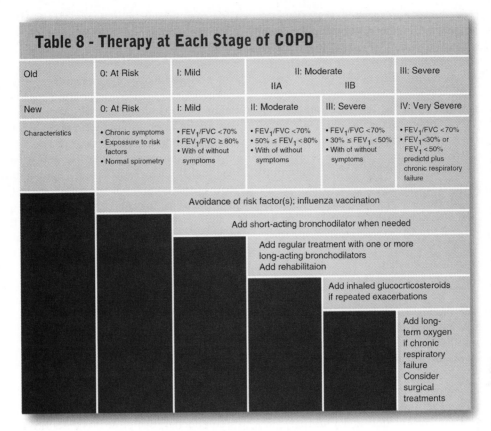

Table 8 - Therapy at Each Stage of COPD

Old	0: At Risk	I: Mild	II: Moderate		III: Severe
			IIA	IIB	
New	0: At Risk	I: Mild	II: Moderate	III: Severe	IV: Very Severe
Characteristics	• Chronic symptoms • Exposure to risk factors • Normal spirometry	• FEV_1/FVC <70% • FEV_1/FVC ≥80% • With of without symptoms	• FEV_1/FVC <70% • 50% ≤ FEV_1 <80% • With of without symptoms	• FEV_1/FVC <70% • 30% ≤ FEV_1 <50% • With of without symptoms	• FEV_1/FVC <70% • FEV_1 <30% or FEV_1 <50% predictd plus chronic respiratory failure

Avoidance of risk factor(s); influenza vaccination

Add short-acting bronchodilator when needed

Add regular treatment with one or more long-acting bronchodilators
Add rehabilitaion

Add inhaled glucocrticosteroids if repeated exacerbations

Add long-term oxygen if chronic respiratory failure Consider surgical treatments

FIGURE 5 Therapy at each stage of chronic obstructive pulmonary disease (COPD). Reproduced with permission from the Global Initiative for Obstructive Lung Disease. Global strategy for the diagnosis, management, and prevention of chronic obstructive pulmonary disease – executive summary. Updated 2005. Available at: http://www.goldcopd.com/Guidelineitem.asp?l1=2&l2=1&intId=996.

Chest physiotherapy has not been proven to be of value in the management of COPD.

The long-term administration of oxygen therapy to patients with chronic respiratory failure increases survival. Additionally, during exacerbations, oxygen therapy is often required. Caution must be used when administering oxygen to patients with COPD as their ventilatory drive will often be diminished. This is the result of chronic retention of carbon dioxide and subsequent insensitivity to hypercarbia. As a result, patients with COPD are sensitive to increases in oxygen tension, which provides the major stimulus for respiratory drive. Oxygen therapy during sleep can also be a useful means of limiting hypoxemia and subsequent pulmonary hypertension.

Antibiotics are often used during exacerbations of COPD. The presence of purulent sputum during an exacerbation of symptoms generally requires treatment with 7 to 10 days of an oral broad-spectrum antibiotic such as a second- or third-generation cephalosporin. The primary pathogens in COPD exacerbations include *S. pneumoniae*, *H. influenzae*, and *M. catarrhalis*. If an infectious exacerbation does not clinically respond to initial antibiotic treatment, a sputum culture should be obtained.[132]

PROGNOSIS

The prognosis is poor for patients who are frequently symptomatic due to COPD. The need for hospital admission for an exacerbation, especially if intensive care is required, is an ominous prognostic sign in COPD; at least half of such patients do not survive a year after admission.[138]

ORAL HEALTH CONSIDERATIONS

The association, if any, between oral disease and lung disease was analyzed by the National Health and Nutrition Examination Survey I (NHANES I).[139] Of 23,808 individuals, 386 reported a suspected respiratory condition (as assessed by a physician) categorized as a confirmed chronic respiratory disease (chronic bronchitis or emphysema) or acute respiratory disease (influenza, pneumonia, acute bronchitis), or not to have a respiratory disease.

Significant differences were noted between subjects having no disease and those having a chronic respiratory disease confirmed by a physician. Individuals with a confirmed chronic respiratory disease had a significantly greater oral hygiene index than subjects without a respiratory disease. Logistic regression analysis was performed to simultaneously control for multiple variables, including gender, age, race, oral hygiene index (OHI), and smoking status. The results of this analysis suggest that for patients having the highest OHI values, the odds ratio for chronic respiratory disease was 4.5.

Another study of elderly subjects (aged 70 to 79) found that, after controlling for smoking status, age, race, and gender, there was a significant association between periodontal health and airway obstruction in former smokers.[140]

A more recent study, however, suggested that cigarette smoking may be a cofactor in the relationship between periodontal disease and COPD.[141] Further longitudinal epidemiologic studies and clinical trials are necessary to determine the role of oral health status in COPD.

Apart from the periodontal pathogens mentioned above, *S. viridans* has been shown to be the causative pathogen of exacerbation in 4% of individuals with COPD.[142] One prospective study suggested that oral colonization with respiratory pathogens in patients residing in a chronic care facility was significantly associated with COPD.[51] The relationship between oral pathogens and exacerbations of COPD clearly deserves serious consideration. It is essential that elderly individuals (particularly institutionalized patients) receive adequate oral hygiene in order to minimize respiratory complications.

Drug interactions with theophylline may arise (see above), and a change of medications by the oral health care provider may be appropriate.

As mentioned above, increased oxygen tension may diminish respiratory function in patients with COPD. Extreme caution must be exercised when administering supplemental oxygen in emergencies.

Cystic Fibrosis

CF is a multisystem genetic disorder that is characterized chiefly by chronic airways obstruction and infection and by exocrine pancreatic insufficiency, with its effects on gastrointestinal function, nutrition, growth, and maturation.[143]

The disorder is caused by numerous mutations in the gene that encodes the cystic fibrosis transmembrane conductance regulator (CFTR) that helps regulate ion flux at epithelial surfaces. The disease is characterized by hyperviscous secretions in multiple organ systems. Thickened secretions affect the pancreas and intestinal tract, causing malabsorption and intestinal obstruction. In the lungs, viscid mucus causes airway obstruction, infection, and bronchiectasis. Pulmonary complications are the major factors affecting life expectancy in patients with CF. This section focuses on the pulmonary manifestations of CF.

CF is an autosomal recessive trait resulting from mutations at a single gene locus on the long arm of chromosome 7. The incidence of CF among whites is approximately 1 in 2,000 to 3,000 births; the incidence is lower among those of other races.[144]

PATHOPHYSIOLOGY

The primary defect in the *CFTR* gene results in a defective chloride transport system in exocrine glands. As a result, mucus production occurs without sufficient water transport into the lumen. The resultant mucus is dry, thick, and tenacious and leads to inspissation in the affected glands and organs. In the airways, the viscid secretions impair mucociliary clearance and promote airway obstruction and bacterial colonization. Most airway injury in CF is believed to be mediated by neutrophil products, including proteases and oxidants, liberated by the abundance of neutrophils in the

CF airway at almost all ages.[145] Bacterial superinfection is common and can lead to respiratory compromise.

CLINICAL AND LABORATORY FINDINGS

Patients with CF may present in infancy with extrapulmonary manifestations such as meconium ileus or failure to thrive. Pulmonary manifestations include cough, recurrent infections of the lower respiratory tract, refractory lung infiltrates, and bronchospasm. Tachypnea and crackles can be found on physical examination. As the disease progresses, digital clubbing and bronchiectasis (Figure 6) may become apparent. Most of the nonpulmonary pathology in CF occurs in the gastrointestinal tract and related organs.

Spirometry and pulmonary function testing are useful tools for documenting and monitoring airflow limitation. Airway obstruction tends to worsen with disease progression, although some patients with CF have mild pulmonary disease. CT analysis of the remarkable lung structural changes may be another potential outcome measure to monitor disease progression.[145]

CLASSIFICATION

There is no universally accepted classification system for CF.

DIAGNOSIS

The diagnosis of CF is based on the presence of pulmonary or extrapulmonary symptoms, as described above. A sweat test can be performed to confirm the diagnosis. The procedure involves the collection of sweat after stimulation with pilocarpine. Samples containing > 60 mEq/L chloride are considered positive. Patients with indeterminate values (40 to 60 mEq/L) can be further assessed by using deoxyribonucleic acid (DNA) analysis. Characteristic nasal epithelial bioelectric abnormalities can also serve as laboratory evidence of CFTR dysfunction and be used to diagnose CF when phenotypic clinical features are present.[143] Due to the importance of

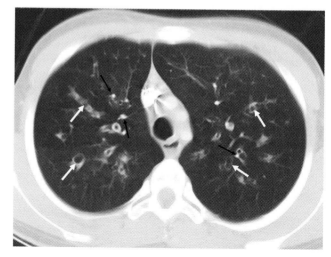

FIGURE 6 Axial computed tomography scan shows thickening of the bronchial walls in the upper lobes and bronchiectasis (dilation of the bronchi) bilaterally (white arrows). The bronchi should be approximately the same size as its associated pulmonary artery (black arrows).

early diagnosis, many states have implemented newborn screening programs in all infants as well.

MANAGEMENT

Treatment of CF includes antibiotics, bronchodilators, anti-inflammatory agents, chest physiotherapy with postural drainage, and mucolytic agents. In addition to oral and parenteral antibiotics, inhaled antibiotics such as tobramycin are used to help minimize systemic effects.[146,147] Long-term macrolide antibiotics have been used to effectively treat diffuse panbronchiolitis as well.[143] The use of anti-inflammatory agents in young patients with mild disease may help slow the decline of lung function.[148] Recombinant enzyme deoxyribonuclease therapy has also been shown to offer benefit to some patients with purulent airway secretions.[149,150] Finally, proper nutrition and exercise are essential. Approximately 90% of patients with CF require mealtime pancreatic enzymes,[143] and vitamin and caloric supplementation is essential as well. Exercise is generally considered beneficial for patients with CF and should be encouraged, except for those with the most severe lung disease and hypoxemia.[151]

PROGNOSIS

Although the mortality rate is high, the most recent statistics from the Cystic Fibrosis Foundation indicate that 50% of patients can now be expected to survive beyond age 30 years.[143] The severity of lung disease often determines long-term survival. Lung transplantation has become an accepted treatment for respiratory failure secondary to CF.[152] New treatment modalities that are being investigated to help prolong survival include pharmacologic interventions targeted to epithelial cell pathophysiology and gene transfer to airway epithelium.

ORAL HEALTH CONSIDERATIONS

It has been suggested that patients with CF may have the same type of dentofacial morphology as other mouth-breathing patients.[153] However, larger prospective studies are need to confirm this.

Several studies have reported that the number of decayed, missing, and filled teeth and plaque, calculus, and gingival bleeding of CF patients is lower than that of non-CF control subjects and those heterozygous for CF.[154,155] This finding may be due to more antibiotic use by CF patients.

It has also been reported that the tongue, buccal mucosa, dental plaque, and saliva serve as a reservoir of colonization by both mucoid and nonmucoid strains of *P. aeruginosa*, an important bacterial pathogen for CF patients.[156,157] This suggests that oral hygiene strategies may help reduce the level of these pathogens in the mouth and thus reduce potential lung infection.

As with other patients with chronic lower respiratory infections, improved oral hygiene may minimize exacerbation of the underlying condition.

Pulmonary Embolism

Pulmonary embolism (PE) is a result of an exogenous or endogenous material traveling to the lung and causing blockage of a pulmonary arterial vessel. The embolus may originate anywhere, but it is usually due to a thrombosis in the lower extremities.[158] Other substances, such as neoplastic cells, air bubbles, carbon dioxide, intravenous catheters, and fat droplets, are also potential sources of emboli.[159] Risk factors for PE include prolonged immobilization (such as in a postoperative state), lower extremity trauma, a history of deep venous thromboses, and the use of estrogen-containing oral contraceptives (especially in association with tobacco smoking).[160]

Pathophysiology

PE causes occlusion of pulmonary arterial vessels, which results in a ventilation-perfusion mismatch. Massive PE causes right-sided heart failure and is rapidly progressive. Local bronchoconstriction may occur due to factors released by platelets and mast cells at the sites of occlusion. Pulmonary hypertension due to vessel occlusion and arterial vasospasm is a common finding.

CLINICAL AND LABORATORY FINDINGS

Patients usually present with dyspnea. Other features that are variably present include chest pain, fever, diaphoresis, cough, hemoptysis, and syncope. Physical findings can include evidence of a lower extremity deep venous thrombosis, tachypnea, crackles or rub on lung auscultation, and heart murmur.

Hypoxemia is common in acute PE. Measurements of arterial blood gases are helpful as patients may demonstrate a decrease in partial pressure of arterial oxygen (PaO_2) and partial pressure of arterial carbon dioxide ($PaCO_2$), with an increase in hydrogen ion concentration (pH). However, normal arterial blood gases do not rule out the possibility of PE.

CLASSIFICATION

Four separate PE syndromes have been described: (1) massive PE, (2) PE with pulmonary infarction, (3) PE without infarction or cor pulmonale, and (4) organized emboli in central arteries. There is significant overlap among these syndromes.[161]

DIAGNOSIS

The diagnosis is made on the basis of history and physical findings. The diagnostic utility of plasma measurements of circulating D-dimer (a specific derivative of cross-linked fibrin) has been found to have a high negative predictive value of 99.5%.[162] Although a negative D-dimer may strongly suggest that venous thromboembolism is absent, a high clinical suspicion should not be ignored.[159]

Chest radiography is often unhelpful but may reveal suggestive signs such as elevated hemidiaphragm, pleural effusions, and pulmonary artery dilatation. Troponin levels may be elevated, the echocardiogram may be abnormal with increased right ventricular volume, and electrocardiography may help establish or exclude alternative diagnoses, such as acute myocardial infarction.

Although the ventilation-perfusion scan has historically been the most common diagnostic test used when PE is suspected, spiral (helical) CT scanning has essentially replaced it at many centers.[159] Pulmonary arteriography is the "gold standard" study and is usually performed when the results of other studies are inconclusive.[163]

MANAGEMENT

Heparin, both unfractionated and low molecular weight, remains the mainstay of therapy. For most patients with PE, systemic thrombolytic therapy (such as streptokinase, urokinase, and tissue-type plasminogen activator) is not required unless the patient is hemodynamically unstable. Pulmonary embolectomy may be indicated in select patients who are unable to receive thrombolytic therapy or whose critical status does not allow sufficient time to infuse thrombolytic therapy.[164] Oxygen is administered as necessary, and the need for intubation and mechanical ventilation in massive PE is considered. Patients with recurrent disease may be candidates for vena caval interruption by placement of an inferior vena cava filter.

PROGNOSIS

Although many patients with PE die before medical attention is received, the rate of mortality due to PE once adequate anticoagulation therapy is initiated is less than 5%.

ORAL HEALTH CONSIDERATIONS

The main concern in the provision of dental care for individuals with PE is the patient who is being managed with oral anticoagulants. As a general rule, dental care (including simple extractions) can safely be provided for patients with prothrombin times of up to 20 seconds or an international normalized ratio of 2.5. However, it is recommended that any dental care for these patients be coordinated with their primary medical care provider.

Pulmonary Neoplasm

Lung cancer is the leading cause of cancer deaths in both men and women. More than 100,000 people in the United States die each year due to lung cancer. Men and women who are over the age of 45 years and who have a long history of tobacco smoking are at highest risk.[165]

Squamous cell carcinomas account for one-third of all lung cancers. The neoplasm derives from bronchial epithelial cells that have undergone squamous metaplasia. This is a slow-growing neoplasm that invades the bronchi and leads to airway obstruction.

Small cell carcinomas account for approximately one-fourth of all lung cancers. This type of lung cancer has the highest association with smoking, almost never arising in the absence of a smoking history. These derive from neuroendocrine cells in the airways and metastasize rapidly. Most small cell tumors have metastasized prior to diagnosis.

Adenocarcinomas account for approximately one-third of all lung cancers. These neoplasms are of glandular origin and develop in a peripheral distribution. They grow more rapidly than squamous cell carcinomas and tend to invade the pleura. The bronchoalveolar tumor (a type of adenocarcinoma) is derived from bronchiolar or alveolar epithelium. This cancer is not associated with exposure to tobacco smoke.[166]

Large cell carcinomas, which account for most of the remaining lung cancers, include anaplastic and giant cell tumors. They are poorly differentiated tumors that resemble neither squamous cell carcinomas nor adenocarcinomas.

PATHOPHYSIOLOGY

Metaplasia of the respiratory epithelium occurs in response to injury, such as that induced by tobacco smoking. With continued injury, the cells become dysplastic, with the loss of differentiating features. Neoplastic change first occurs locally; invasive carcinoma usually follows shortly thereafter.[167]

CLINICAL AND LABORATORY FINDINGS

A chronic nonproductive cough is the most common symptom. Sputum production may occur, usually associated with obstructive lesions. Hemoptysis is present in up to 30% of patients.[168] Dyspnea is variably present. Facial edema, cyanosis, and orthopnea indicate the possibility of superior vena cava syndrome, caused by compression of the superior vena cava by tumor. The acute onset of hoarseness may signal tumor compression of the recurrent laryngeal nerve. Shoulder and forearm pain might suggest the presence of Pancoast's tumor, which is found in the apical region of the lungs below the pleura.

Metastatic and paraneoplastic effects are also common. The symptoms of metastasis depend on the sites involved and on the size of the tumor. The bones, the brain, and the liver are common sites of metastasis. Paraneoplastic effects include endocrine abnormalities that are due to tumors that secrete hormones such as antidiuretic hormone, adrenocorticotropic hormone, and parathyroid hormone–related peptides.[169]

CLASSIFICATION

The World Health Organization has differentiated pulmonary neoplasms into 12 distinct histologic types. The major clinical distinction is between small cell types and non–small cell types; each type has different therapeutic implications. The four major pathologic categories are squamous cell carcinoma, small cell carcinoma, adenocarcinoma, and large cell carcinoma.

DIAGNOSIS

Diagnosis is suggested by the history and physical examination. The method of diagnosis of suspected lung cancer depends on the type of lung cancer (ie, small cell lung cancer or non–small cell lung cancer), the size and location of the primary tumor, the presence of metastasis, and the overall clinical status of the patient. CT scanning is the anatomic imaging modality of choice and is performed in virtually all

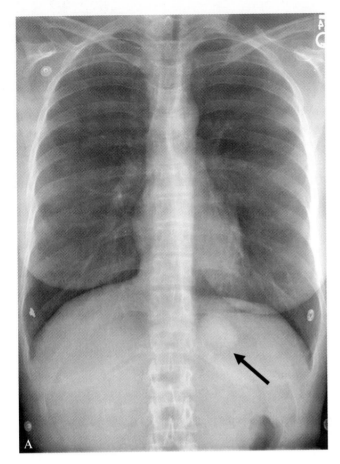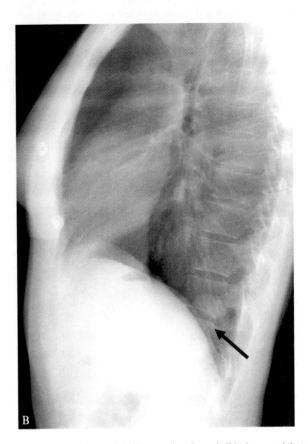

FIGURE 7 Anteroposterior (A) and lateral (B) chest radiographs demonstrate a rounded mass in the medial left costophrenic angle (black arrows) that is seen to be located in the posterior portion of the left lower lobe. This is best seen on the lateral view.

patients with suspected or known lung cancer (Figure 7). Other diagnostic modalities include sputum or pleural fluid cytology, excisional biopsy, transthoracic needle aspiration, and bronchoscopy.[170]

MANAGEMENT

Complete surgical resection of localized lung cancer offers patients the best chance for cure. However, treatment is based on the stage of the disease and the patient's clinical status. In general, early-stage disease is surgically managed, locally advanced disease is managed with chemotherapy and radiotherapy, and advanced disease is managed with chemotherapy with supportive care or supportive care alone. Radiation therapy is an important palliative measure, especially for patients with superior vena cava syndrome, brain metastases, or bone lesions.

PROGNOSIS

Despite the presence of developed modalities for treatment, the prognosis for patients with lung cancer has remained poor, with the overall 5-year survival being approximately 10 to 14%. Unfortunately, most pulmonary cancers are found too late for a cure; only about 20% of patients undergo a radical surgical procedure, which is the only curative treatment.[171,172]

▼ ACKNOWLEDGMENT

Douglas P. Beall, MD, chief of radiology, Clinical Radiology of Oklahoma, LLC. and associate professor of orthopedics, University of Oklahoma.

▼ SELECTED READINGS

Fourrier F, Duvivier B, Boutigny H, et al. Colonization of dental plaque: a source of nosocomial infections in intensive care unit patients. Crit Care Med 1998;26:301–8.

Katancik JA, Kritchevsky S, Weyant RJ, et al. Periodontitis and airway obstruction. J Periodontol 2005;76(11 Suppl):2161–7.

Marik PE. Aspiration pneumonitis and aspiration pneumonia. N Engl J Med 2001;344:665–71.

Ramsey BW, Pepe MS, Quan JM, et al. Intermittent administration of inhaled tobramycin in patients with cystic fibrosis; The Cystic Fibrosis Inhaled Tobramycin Study Group. N Engl J Med 1999;340:23–30.

Reilly JJ, Silverman EK, Shapiro SD. Chronic obstructive pulmonary disease. In: Braunwald E, Fauci AS, Kasper DL, et al, editors. Harrison's internal medicine. 16th ed. New York: McGraw-Hill Professional; 2004.

Sandler NA, Johns FR, Braun TW. Advances in the management of acute and chronic sinusitis. J Oral Maxillofac Surg 1996;54: 1005–13.

Scannapieco FA. Role of oral bacteria in respiratory infection. J Periodontol 1999;70:793–802.

Scannapieco FA, Bush RB, Paju S. Associations between periodontal disease and risk for nosocomial bacterial pneumonia and chronic obstructive pulmonary disease. A systematic review. Ann Periodontol 2003;8:54–69.

Simons D, Kidd EAM, Beighton D. Oral health of elderly occupants in residential homes. Lancet 1999;353:1761.

Spurlock BW, Dailey TM. Shortness of (fresh) breath: toothpaste-induced bronchospasm. N Engl J Med 1990;323:1845–6.

Yoneyama T, Yoshida M, Ohrui T, et al. Oral care reduces pneumonia in older patients in nursing homes. J Am Geriatr Soc 2002;50:430–3.

Zhu JF, Hidalgo HA, Holmgreen WC, et al. Dental management of children with asthma. Pediatr Dent 1996;18:363–70.

For the full reference list, please refer to the accompanying CD ROM.

13

▼

Diseases of the Cardiovascular System

Peter B. Lockhart, DDS

Laszlo Littmann, MD

Michael Glick, DMD

With 16.7 million deaths worldwide in 2003, cardiovascular disease (CVD) is the leading cause of mortality in the world, representing over 29% of all global deaths.[1] There are approximately 71 million American adults with CVD, and of the more than 2,440,000 deaths in the United States in 2003, CVD was listed as the primary cause in 37% of cases.[1] According to the Centers for Disease Control and Prevention (CDC) and the National Health and Nutrition Examination Survey (NHANES) III, the probability at birth of dying from CVD is 47%, compared with 22% from cancer, 2% from diabetes, and less than 1% from human immunodeficiency virus (HIV) disease. The largest proportion of this high mortality is attributed to coronary artery disease (CAD) or coronary heart disease (CHD), which was the primary contributing cause of death in 479,305 Americans in 2003.[1] During the past decades, the age-adjusted death rate in the United States has declined overall. However, racial and ethnic disparities exist, with African Americans exceeding that of whites, with 32%.[2]

CVD includes hypertension, CAD, congestive heart failure (CHF), congenital cardiovascular defects, and stroke (Table 1).[1] Although these diseases are associated with a high mortality, the associated morbidity affects all walks of life and has a great impact on the quality of life of affected individuals. This chapter presents a brief overview of common cardiovascular conditions and their implications for the practice of dental medicine.

▼ HYPERTENSION

General Description and Incidence

About 29% of the entire US population has hypertension at any one time, and many will develop it as they age (Table 2). This sobering statistic translates into more than 65,000,000 Americans, and over 1 billion worldwide, with high blood pressure (BP).[1] However, although the majority of individuals are aware of their elevated BP, only an estimated 23 to 49% of hypertensive patients are being treated and may have achieved normotensive control.[1–3]

TABLE 1 Prevalence of Cardiovascular Disease in the United States

Type of Cardiovascular Disease	No. of Patients
High blood pressure	65,000,000
Coronary artery disease	13,200,000
Myocardial infarction	7,200,000
Angina pectoris	6,500,000
Stroke	5,500,000
Congenital cardiovascular disease	1,000,000
Congestive heart failure	5,500,000
Total	71,300,000*

Adapted from Thom T et al.[1]
*Due to overlap among patients, the added numbers will exceed the total.

TABLE 2 Hypertension among Persons over 20 Years of Age and Over, United States, 2001–2004

Age Category (yr)	Male	Female
20–34	6.4	*
35–44	16.8	14.0
45–54	30.2	32.6
55–64	45.8	54.6
65–74	58.5	74.3
75 and over	68.8	81.7

Adapted from National Center for Health Statistics.[2]
*Unreliable estimate.

Hypertension is defined as having systolic blood pressure (SBP) ≥ 140 mm Hg or diastolic blood pressure (DBP) ≥ 90 mm Hg or as having to use antihypertensive medications. Approximately every 5 years, the National Heart, Lung, and Blood Institute (NHLBI), through its Joint National Committee on Prevention, Detection, Evaluation, and Treatment of High Blood Pressure, puts forth recommendations for the treatment of high BP. Its seventh and latest recommendations (JNC 7) was initially published in 2003 and in its entirety in a National Institutes of Health publication in 2004.[3] This document defines cardiovascular risk stratification and treatment strategies and BP classifications for adults (Tables 3 through 5). The purpose of these guidelines is to reduce the morbidity and mortality associated with hypertension as several clinical trials have suggested that the lowering of BP reduces the risk of end-organ disease.[4,5]

Hypertension is classified as primary (or essential) and secondary. Ninety-five percent of all hypertension is of unknown cause. The use of new molecular biologic tools will likely serve to better delineate some of the basic mechanisms of primary hypertension. There are many secondary causes, including renal disorders such as renal parenchymal disease, renovascular disease, renin-producing tumors, and primary sodium retention. Endocrinologic disturbances that may result in hypertension include thyroid disease, adrenal disorders, carcinoid, and exogenous hormones. Remaining causes include aortic coarctation, complications of pregnancy (such as preeclampsia), neurologic causes, acute stress, alcohol

TABLE 3 Classification of Blood Pressure for Adults

Blood Pressure Classification	SBP (mm Hg)		DBP (mm Hg)
Normal	< 120	and	< 90
Prehypertension	120–139	or	80–89
Stage 1 hypertension	140–159	or	90–99
Stage 2 hypertension	≥ 160	or	≥ 100

Adapted from US Department of Health and Human Services, National Institutes of Health, National Heart, Lung, and Blood Institute, National High Blood Pressure Eduction Program.[3]
DBP = diastolic blood pressure; SBP = systolic blood pressure.

TABLE 4 Cardiovascular Risk Factors

Major risk factors
  Hypertension
  Age (older than 55 yr for men, 65 yr for women)
  Diabetes mellitus
  Elevated LDL (or total) cholesterol or low HDL cholesterol
  Estimated GFR <60 mL/min
  Family history of premature CVD (men < 55 yr of age or women < 65 yr of age)
  Microalbuminuria
  Obesity (BMI > 30 kg/mm^2)
  Physical inactivity
  Tobacco use, particularly cigarettes

Target organ damage
  Heart
    LVH
    Angina/prior MI
    Prior coronary revascularization
    Heart failure
  Brain
    Stroke or transient ischemic attack
    Dementia
  Chronic kidney disease
  Peripheral arterial disease
  Retinopathy

Adapted from US Department of Health and Human Services, National Institutes of Health, National Heart, Lung, and Blood Institute, National High Blood Pressure Eduction Program.[3]

BMI = body mass index; CVD = cardiovascular disease; GFR = glomerular filtration rate; HDL = high-density lipoprotein; LDL = low-density lipoprotein; LVH = left ventricular hypertrophy; MI = myocardial infarction.

ingestion, nicotine use, increased intravascular volume, and the use of drugs such as cyclosporine or tacrolimus.

Risk Factor Modification

Hypertension is a well-recognized risk factor for CAD. With improved control of BP, there has been a steady decrease in mortality from CHD and an even greater decrease in mortality from stroke. It is important to realize that hypertension is a chronic disease with long-term sequelae. Therefore, treatment focuses on prevention to reduce complications that eventually affect target organs such as the brain, heart, kidneys, eyes, and peripheral arteries (see Table 4). Complications of hypertension include cerebral hemorrhage, left ventricular hypertrophy, CHF, renal insufficiency, aortic dissection, and atherosclerotic disease of various vascular beds.

Diagnosis

Because hypertension usually has a long, asymptomatic course, many patients are undiagnosed and/or have only a mild elevation in BP. The diagnosis is made only after an elevated BP has been recorded on multiple occasions. Stage 1 hypertension refers to an SBP of 140 to 159 mm Hg or a DBP of 90 to 99 mm Hg. Stage 2 hypertension is defined as an SBP of ≥ 160 mm Hg or a DBP of ≥ 100 mm Hg (see Table 3). The BP level, as well as other clinical factors, determines the severity of hypertension. These other factors include certain demographic features (age, sex, race), the extent of the vascular damage induced by the high BP (ie, target organ involvement), and the presence of other risk factors for premature CVD, especially diabetes (see Table 4).

The three main goals of the medical evaluation of patients with hypertension are to identify treatable (secondary) or curable causes, to assess the impact of persistently elevated BP on target organs, and to estimate the patient's overall risk profile for the development of premature CVD. A routine history and physical examination should be performed. The history should focus on the duration of the hypertension and any prior treatment. Asking the patient about the duration of their high BP may be misleading as in many cases, the patient often will not have had a BP measurement for many years prior to the discovery of hypertension. Symptoms of organ dysfunction, lifestyle habits, diet, and psychosocial factors should be included.

TABLE 5 Lifestyle Modifications to Prevent and Manage Hypertension

Modification	Recommendation	Approximate SBP Reduction
Weight reduction	Maintain normal body weight (BMI 18.5–24.9 kg/mm^2)	5–20 mm Hg/10 kg
Adopt DASH eating plan	Consume a diet rich in fruits, vegetables, and low-fat dairy products with a reduced content of saturated and total fat	8–14 mm Hg
Dietary sodium reduction	Reduce dietary sodium intake to no more than 100 mmol/d (2.4 g sodium or 6 g sodium chloride)	2–8 mm Hg
Physical activity	Engage in regular aerobic physical activity such as brisk walking (at least 30 min/d, most days of the week)	4–9 mm Hg
Moderation of alcohol consumption	Limit consumption to no more than 2 drinks (eg, 24 oz beer, 10 oz wine, or 3 oz 80-proof whiskey) per day in most men and to no more than 1 drink/d in women and lighter persons	2–4 mm Hg

Adapted from US Department of Health and Human Services, National Institutes of Health, National Heart, Lung, and Blood Institute, National High Blood Pressure Eduction Program.[3]

BMI = body mass index; DASH = Dietary Approaches to Stop Hypertension; SBP = systolic blood pressure.

Physical Examination

The main goals of the physical examination are to identify signs of end-organ damage (see Table 14) and a cause of secondary hypertension. Thus, the peripheral pulses should be palpated, and the abdomen should be auscultated for renal artery bruit that would indicate renovascular hypertension. The physical examination should include a funduscopic assessment.

Laboratory and Additional Testing

Routine laboratory procedures include hemoglobin, urinalysis, routine blood chemistries (glucose, creatinine, electrolytes), and a fasting lipid profile consisting of total and high-density lipoprotein (HDL) cholesterol and triglycerides. Twelve-lead electrocardiography (ECG) should also be performed. Additional tests, outlined below, may be indicated in certain clinical settings.

ELECTROCARDIOGRAPHY

Echocardiography can reveal signs suggestive of left atrial enlargement, left ventricular hypertrophy (LVH) with or without associated repolarization abnormality, abnormal Q waves suggestive of a previous myocardial infarction (MI), and signs of myocardial ischemia or injury. This procedure is a more sensitive method of detecting LVH than is routine ECG, and limited echocardiography offers a less expensive alternative to a complete echocardiographic examination when the sole question is whether the patient has LVH. LVH is an independent predictor of mortality in patients with hypertension. This hypertrophy of the ventricle initially results in the impairment of left ventricular (LV) diastolic function and, if progressive, may impair systolic function as well, thus diminishing the normal function of pumping blood out of the heart through the aortic valve and into the aorta. This increase in LV mass may result in increased myocardial oxygen demand, which can result in myocardial ischemia and, ultimately, myocardial fibrosis with CHF. Thus, the main indication for echocardiography is possible end-organ damage to the heart in a patient with borderline elevated BP values. Echocardiography may also identify patients who would not be treated on the basis of clinical criteria alone (Figures 1 to 4).

AMBULATORY BP MONITORING

Ambulatory BP monitoring may identify patients with "white-coat hypertension" and also ensures the adequacy of therapy in the outpatient setting. However, at the present, many insurers do not reimburse for this procedure. As a result, the main indication for ambulatory BP monitoring is persistent hypertension in the office setting but normal BP readings in the ambulatory setting.

The term *white-coat hypertension* is used to describe a phenomenon in which individuals present with persistent elevated BP in a clinical setting but present with nonelevated BP in an ambulatory setting. The relationship between white-coat hypertension and the development of essential hypertension has not been thoroughly elucidated, but it is estimated that about 20% of mild hypertensive individuals may present with white-coat hypertension. Since BP readings in the ambulatory BP setting reflect BP throughout the day, an accurate ambulatory measure would theoretically better predict end-organ damage than would occasional clinical or office BP readings, yet it is not clear if white-coat hypertension is associated with end-organ damage.[6]

PLASMA RENIN ACTIVITY TESTING

Although plasma renin activity testing may provide prognostic information, it is usually performed only in patients with possible low-renin forms of hypertension, such as primary hyperaldosteronism. Unexplained hypokalemia is the primary clinical clue to this disorder, and its presence should prompt further diagnostic testing.

RADIOLOGIC TESTING

Radiographic testing for renovascular disease is indicated only for patients whose history is suggestive and in whom a corrective procedure will be performed if significant renal artery stenosis is detected. Intra-arterial digital subtraction angiography has historically been the initial test when the history is highly suggestive; however, spiral computed tomography and magnetic resonance angiography are becoming the standard screening tests when renovascular hypertension is strongly suspected.[7] Renal ultrasonography is often used in a hypertensive patient with a family history of polycystic kidney disease.

Assessment of Cardiovascular Risk

Numerous aspects contribute to the detrimental association between hypertension and CVD.[8] Most studies have shown a strong correlation between long-term sustained elevated BP and the subsequent development of CVD. Recent prospective longitudinal studies suggest that BP that is even slightly elevated above normal is associated with increased mortality.[9] The underlying causes include the promotion of atherosclerosis and thrombogenesis, reduced coronary vasodilatory reserve, and LVH.[10–15]

The incidence of CVD increases stepwise with increasing BP. Studies have indicated that the risk of a cardiac event increases by 1.6 times in men and 2.5 times in women when BP increases from an optimal level (< 120/80 mm Hg) to a high normal level (130 to 139/85 to 89 mm Hg).[16] As is well defined by data from the Framingham Heart Study, a number of other risk factors interact with hypertension to affect the overall risk status of the individual patient.[11,17] These include hypercholesterolemia, diabetes mellitus, and smoking. Increased age of the patient may suggest a more detrimental effect conferred by an elevated systolic rather than diastolic pressure.[18] The presence or absence of other risk factors can influence the decision of whether to institute antihypertensive medications in a patient with borderline values.

Management

The treatment of hypertension is among the leading indications for the use of drugs in the United States. A large

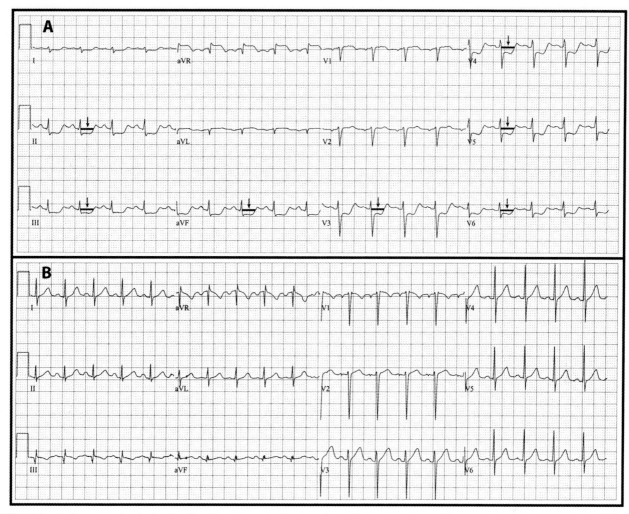

FIGURE 1   Left ventricular ischemia. ***Top:*** Note the marked horizontal and slightly downsloping ST-segment depression seen in leads II, III, aVF, and in chest leads V3-V6 (arrows). ***Bottom:*** The ischemic ST-segment depression resolved. In the setting of chest pain, dynamic ST-segment depression is a high-risk condition associated with elevated early and late mortality. These patients require intensive monitoring and aggressive medical and/or interventional management.

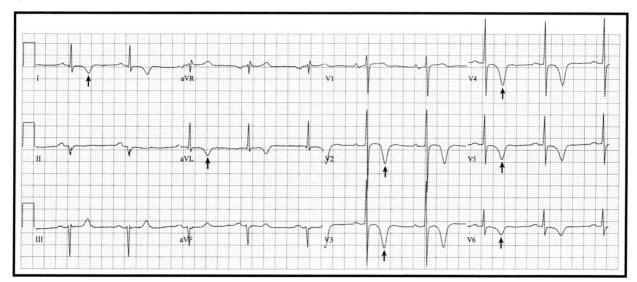

FIGURE 2   Acute coronary syndrome. Note the deep, symmetrical T wave inversion in the anterolateral leads (arrows). This ECG pattern is frequently seen in patients who have tight occlusion of the proximal portion of the left anterior descending coronary artery that supplies the anterior wall of the left ventricle. The most commonly applied treatment is balloon angioplasty with stenting after which the patients are typically treated with the combined anti-platelet regimen of aspirin + clopidogrel (Plavix), a beta-blocker, and statin.

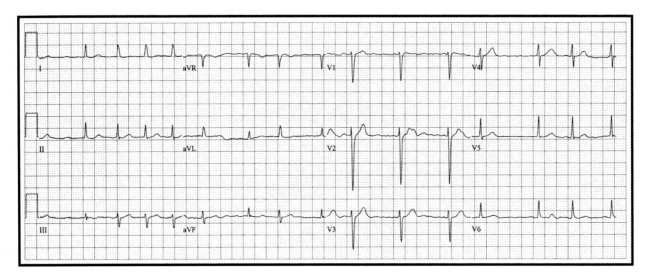

FIGURE 3 **Atrial fibrillation.** Note the irregularly irregular rhythm, the fine baseline undulation, and the absence of distinct P waves in front of the QRS complexes. Patients with atrial fibrillation are usually treated with a beta-blocker for ventricular rate control, and with warfarin (Coumadin) anticoagulation for stroke prevention. The risk of stroke without anticoagulation is significant; the degree of risk depends on a number of clinical factors including age, hypertension, diabetes, heart failure, and most importantly, a previous history of TIA or stroke.

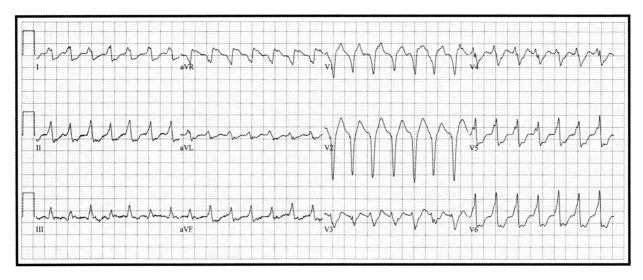

FIGURE 4 **Ventricular tachycardia.** Note the rapid (rate, 170/min), regular wide-complex tachycardia without distinct P waves in front of the QRS complexes. Ventricular tachycardia is most commonly seen in patients with a history of myocardial infarction. This is a potentially life-threatening arrhythmia that requires emergent treatment, usually electrical cardioversion.

number of agents exist, including diuretics, β-blockers, calcium channel blockers, angiotensin-converting enzyme inhibitors (ACEIs), angiotensin II receptor blockers, direct vasodilators, and centrally acting agents. Each of the antihypertensive agents is roughly equally effective, producing a good antihypertensive response in 40 to 60% of cases. Thus, the choice among the different antihypertensive drugs is not generally made on the basis of efficacy. There is, however, wide interpatient variability as many patients will respond well to one drug but not to another. The identification of the particular drug class to which a patient is more likely to respond is therefore one major criterion used in the choice of an antihypertensive agent.

The results of an increasing number of trials suggest that at the same level of BP control, most antihypertensive drugs provide similar degrees of cardiovascular protection. As an example, several major antihypertension drug trials found little overall difference in outcome between older (eg, diuretics and β-blockers) and newer (eg, ACEIs and calcium channel blockers) antihypertensive drugs.[19,20] However, there is some evidence that the use of particular agents may be associated with specific positive outcomes in specific clinical settings. For example, in the Heart Outcomes Prevention Evaluation (HOPE) study, a cardiovascular benefit from angiotensin-converting enzyme inhibition with ramipril was demonstrated in patients who were at high risk for CVD.[21]

High risk was defined as either evidence of vascular disease (including CHD, stroke, peripheral vascular disease) or diabetes and at least one other coronary risk factor. In this trial, the primary end point was any cardiovascular event (cardiovascular death, MI, or stroke). Most of the patients were on other cardioprotective medications, including aspirin, β-blockers, and lipid-lowering agents. Younger patients with high-renin hypertension may benefit more from β-blockers, whereas there is some suggestion that in elderly individuals, β-blockers confer less survival benefit compared with other similarly effective antihypertensive agents, such as calcium channel blockers, diuretics, or ACEIs.[22]

Patient compliance is another important aspect of choosing an antihypertensive agent. Inexpensive once-a-day preparations with few side effects are often desired. The specific antihypertensive agent chosen for a patient may also depend on comorbid diseases. For example, β-blocker therapy is an excellent choice for patients who have CAD and hypertension. An ACEI is usually first-line therapy for a diabetic patient with microalbuminuria since ACEIs retard the progression of diabetic nephropathy. Although the use of diuretics has been decreasing over the past 10 years, diuretics are still among the most frequently prescribed medications for treating hypertension, probably because they are effective, well tolerated, and inexpensive.

The role of education and the importance of patient contact are paramount in successfully treating hypertension. Self-recorded measurements and ambulatory BP monitoring aid in the physician's titration of medications and monitoring of the 24-hour duration of action of antihypertensive agents. The monitoring of BP by oral health care providers will therefore support the overall medical care of their hypertensive patients.

At present, there is no consensus on optimal initial drug therapy for hypertension as four of the major classes of antihypertensive drugs (diuretics, (β-blockers, calcium channel blockers, and ACEIs) appear to provide equal benefit at the same degree of BP control.[23] Many physicians recommend either low-dose therapy (to maximize efficacy in relation to side effects) or "sequential monotherapy." A patient who is relatively unresponsive to one drug has almost a 50% likelihood of becoming normotensive on a second drug. This regimen of trying to find the one drug to which the patient is most responsive should minimize side effects and maximize patient compliance while being as effective as combination therapy.

The Systolic Hypertension in the Elderly Program (SHEP) trial showed that in older patients with systolic hypertension, low-dose thiazide therapy effectively lowered BP and led to a reduction in cardiovascular events as compared with placebo treatment.[24] In a more recent study, therapy based on a long-acting dihydropyridine calcium channel blocker provided protection almost identical to that previously noted with diuretic-based therapy.[25]

In those with uncomplicated hypertension, beginning with a low dose of a thiazide diuretic (eg, 12.5 to 25 mg of hydrochlorothiazide) has the advantages of very low cost and low risk of metabolic complications such as hypokalemia,

lipid abnormalities, and hyperuricemia. If low-dose thiazide monotherapy is ineffective, an ACEI, a β-blocker, or a calcium channel blocker can be sequentially substituted. A calcium channel blocker is likely to be most effective in African American patients. A report suggesting that calcium channel blockers may increase the risk of MI in hypertensive patients has not been confirmed in studies with long-acting dihydropyridines; the appropriate use of these drugs should therefore not be curtailed.[26] However, given the preliminary evidence that the patient who is unresponsive to a diuretic may also have a similar response to a calcium channel blocker, an ACEI or a β-blocker may be the preferred second-line agent.

Managing hypertensive patients who are undergoing surgery poses unique problems because they have an increased risk of perioperative mortality. However, the administration of antihypertensive therapy reduces this risk, and patients taking medications prior to surgery should thus be continued on therapy until surgery. Intravenous preparations are used during surgery and during the postoperative period, while the patient is on a nothing-by-mouth (NPO) order.

Treatment of hypertension is important because it reduces overall mortality. An analysis of the Framingham Heart Study cohort showed that improved control of hypertension contributed to the decline in mortality from CVD over the past 30 years.[27] In randomized controlled trials, antihypertensive pharmacotherapy appears to have its predominant effect on stroke mortality.[28]

Oral Health Considerations

It is clear that patients with high BP are at increased risk for adverse advents in a dental setting when target organ disease is present. However, the absence of target organ disease does not mitigate a careful evaluation and treatment of patients within safe and appropriate parameters of care. Based on the medical model for assessment, risk stratification, and treatment of patients with hypertension, dental guidelines can be proposed (Table 6).[29] These guidelines do not release the dental practitioner from good clinical judgment, and they should be used in accordance with the dental provider's knowledge, training, and experience.

Oral health care providers also need to be aware of medications that (1) may have systemic side effects that are of importance to the provision of care, (2) interact with medications used during dental care, and (3) cause intraoral changes, such as oral dryness, gingival overgrowth, or ulcerations. The use of epinephrine for dental procedures in this patient population is controversial. Some authorities feel that the benefit of epinephrine in attaining a profound and more prolonged anesthesia outweighs the risk of systemic effects. Concentrations of epinephrine greater than 1:100,000 are unnecessary and carry a higher risk.

▼ CORONARY ARTERY DISEASE

General Description and Incidence

CAD accounts for approximately 30 to 50% of all cases of CVD.[1] Approximately 12,400,000 Americans alive today have

TABLE 6   Blood Pressure Measurement in the Dental Setting

Routine BP measurements
　Measure and record BP at initial visit
　Recheck
　　Every two years for patients with BP <120/80 mm Hg
　　Every year for patients with BP 120-139/80-89 mm Hg
　　Every visit for patients with BP > 140-90 mm Hg
　　Every visit for patients with established coronary artery disease, diabetes
　　　mellitus or chronic renal disease with BP > 135-85 mm Hg
　　Every visit for patient with established hypertension

Before initiating dental care
　Assess presence of hypertension
　Determine presence of target organ disease
　Determine dental treatment modifications

Dental treatment modifications for patients with elevated BP
　Asymptomatic, BP <159/99 mm Hg, no history of target organ disease
　　No modifications needed
　　Can safely be treated in a dental outpatient setting
　Asymptomatic, BP 160-179/100-109 mm Hg, no history of target organ disease
　　Assessment on an individual basis with regard to type of dental procedure
　BP > 180/110 mm Hg, no history of target organ disease
　　No elective dental care
　Presence of target organ disease or poorly controlled diabetes mellitus
　　No elective dental care until BP is controlled, preferable below
　　　140–90 mm Hg

already suffered an MI or experienced angina pectoris (chest pain).[1] It is also estimated that in 2006, 700,000 Americans will have a new coronary attack, and 500,000 will have a recurrent attack. The estimated incidence for MI is 565,000 new attacks and 300,000 recurrent attacks annually.[1] Atherosclerosis, the most common cause of CAD, results from a wide variety of pathologic processes that interact with and disrupt the vascular endothelium. The result is plaque formation, with compromise of effective arterial luminal area. In the coronary circulation, this process may cause a chronic reduction in coronary blood flow and ensuing myocardial ischemia or it may cause acute plaque rupture, with intracoronary thrombus formation and subsequent MI. Atherosclerosis may affect any vascular bed, including the coronary, cerebral, renal, mesenteric, and peripheral vascular systems. When end-organ blood flow is compromised, the resulting ischemia can cause subsequent organ dysfunction.

Etiology

Atherosclerosis is responsible for almost all cases of CAD. This insidious process begins with a fatty streak, first seen in early adolescence; these lesions progress into plaques in early adulthood and may result in thrombotic occlusions and coronary events in middle age and later life. Other lipid metabolism abnormalities, systemic hypertension, diabetes mellitus, and cigarette smoking contribute to the total atherosclerotic plaque burden, although these factors differ in their impact on CAD in clinical subgroups. For example, diabetes and a

low HDL cholesterol to total cholesterol ratio have a greater impact in women, cigarette smoking has more of an impact in men, and SBP and isolated systolic hypertension are major risk factors at all ages and in either sex.

Risk Factors

Risk factor assessment is useful as a guide to therapy for dyslipidemia, hypertension, and diabetes; multivariable prediction rules can be used to help estimate risks for subsequent coronary disease events. An emerging model uses the risk of cardiovascular events over a 10- to 20-year period as a basis for initiating risk factor–modifying therapy for lipid abnormalities.[30]

Based on the increased risk conferred by the various CAD risk factors, concepts of "normal" have continued to evolve from "usual" or "average" to more biologically optimal values associated with long-term freedom from disease. As a result, acceptable BP, blood sugar, and lipid values have been continually revised downward in the past 20 years.[4,31,32]

Lipids

The total cholesterol concentration in serum is a major and clear-cut risk factor for CHD. In the Multiple Risk Factor Intervention Trial of more than 350,000 middle-aged American men, the risk of CHD progressively increased with higher values of serum total cholesterol.[33] More recent data emphasize the advantages in knowing the concentrations of lipid subfractions, such as low-density lipoprotein (LDL) and HDL, in addition to total cholesterol.[31] Conversely, the concentration of serum HDL cholesterol is inversely associated with CHD incidence, consistent with its suggested role in reverse cholesterol transport.[34] Data from the Framingham Heart Study suggest that the risk for MI increases by about 25% for every 5 mg/dL decrement below median values for men and women.[35]

The HDL cholesterol to total cholesterol ratio represents a simple and efficient way to estimate coronary disease risk. Data from the Lipid Research Clinics and the Framingham Heart Study show that among men, a ratio of ≥ 6.4 identified a group that was at a 2 to 14% greater risk than that predicted from serum total or LDL cholesterol; among women, a ratio of ≥ 5.6 or more identified a group at a 25 to 45% greater risk than that predicted from serum total or LDL cholesterol.[36] In contrast, serum total or LDL cholesterol did not add an independent predictive value to the ratio.

Recommendations for lipid evaluation and therapy in adults were formulated by an expert committee of the National Cholesterol Education Program (NCEP) and were revised in 2001 as the ATP III. Stepped care for abnormal lipid levels considers individuals' overall risk factor burden and their 20-year risk of cardiovascular events. Treatment includes the dietary restriction of fat and cholesterol and recommends medications when certain LDL cholesterol levels are exceeded despite dietary interventions and other lifestyle modifications (Table 7).

TABLE 7   Common Cholesterol-Lowering Medications

Drug	Trade Name	Side Effects
HMG CoA reductase inhibitors (statins)*		Myopathy; increased liver transaminases
Atorvastatin	Lipitor	
Fluvastatin	Leschol	
Lovastatin	Mevacor	
Pravastatin	Pravachol	
Simvastatin	Zocor	
Bile acid sequestrants		Decreased absorption of other drugs
Cholestyramine	—	
Colestipol	—	
Colesevelam	Welchol	
Nicotinic acid		Flushing; hyperglycemia; upper GI distress; hepatotoxicity
Crystalline nicotinic acid	—	
Sustained-release nicotinic acid	—	
Extended-release nicotinic acid	Niaspan	
Fibric acid derivatives		Dyspepsia; upper GI distress; myopathy
Gemfibrozil	Lopid	
Fenofibrate	Tricor	
Clofibrate	—	

GI = gastrointestinal; HMG CoA = 3-hydroxy-3-methylglutaryl coenzyme A.
*Avoid use with macrolide antibiotics.

A number of clinical trials, including the Scandinavian Simvastatin Survival Study, the Cholesterol and Recurrent Events (CARE) trial, and the West of Scotland Coronary Prevention Study, have shown that reductions in total and LDL cholesterol levels through the use of 3-hydroxy-3-methylglutaryl coenzyme A (HMG CoA) reductase enzyme inhibitors reduce coronary events and mortality when given for primary and secondary prevention.[37–40] A number of recent trials have demonstrated that high-dose statin therapy resulting in LDL cholesterol levels of ≤ 70 mg/dL can further decrease the incidence of major cardiovascular events compared with conventional doses and LDL cholesterol targets of 100 mg/dL.[22,40a–42]

Hypertension

Hypertension and LVH are well-established risk factors for adverse cardiovascular outcomes, including CHD morbidity and mortality, stroke, CHF, and sudden death. SBP is as powerful a coronary risk factor as DBP, and isolated systolic hypertension is now established as a major hazard for CHD and stroke, especially in the elderly population.[18,43]

However, although controlled trials have demonstrated clear benefits with BP reduction in terms of stroke and heart failure risk, they have not consistently demonstrated a benefit in coronary events, particularly in patients with mild degrees of hypertension. The increased coronary risk associated with hypertension is primarily seen in subgroups that have other risk factors or underlying target organ damage, and individuals in these subgroups derive the greatest benefit from antihypertensive therapy. The recommendations of the Seventh Joint National Committee on Prevention, Detection, Evaluation, and Treatment of High Blood Pressure provide guidelines for therapy according to stratification based on BP level and the presence or absence of underlying target organ disease.[3]

Glucose Intolerance and Diabetes Mellitus

Insulin resistance, hyperinsulinemia, and glucose intolerance all appear to promote atherosclerosis. As diabetic individuals have a greater number of additional atherogenic risk factors (including hypertension, hypertriglyceridemia, increased cholesterol to HDL ratio, and elevated levels of plasma fibrinogen) than do nondiabetic individuals, the CHD risk for diabetic persons varies greatly with the severity of these risk factors. Thus, aggressive treatment of these additional risk factors may help reduce cardiovascular events in diabetic patients. For example, there is increasing evidence of the value of aggressive BP control in diabetic patients.[44] JNC 6 and recent guidelines published by the NCEP help provide goals for aggressive risk factor modification in diabetic patients.[3,32]

Cigarette Smoking

Cigarette smoking is an important and potentially reversible risk factor for CHD and CHD events such as MI. For both men and women, the risk increases with increasing tobacco consumption.[45] For example, in one study, the risk of MI was sixfold increased for women and threefold increased for men who smoked at least 20 cigarettes per day compared with nonsmoking control patients.[46]

Lifestyle and Dietary Factors

Dietary factors such as a high-calorie, high-fat, and high-cholesterol diet contribute to the development of other risk factors, such as obesity, hyperlipidemia, and diabetes, which predispose patients to CHD. Conversely, a diet that emphasizes fruits and vegetables and the increased intake of dietary fiber and the so-called Mediterranean-style diet rich in olive oil and nuts are associated with a decreased risk of CAD.[47,48] Weight gain and obesity directly worsen the major cardiovascular risk factors, whereas weight loss appears to improve them.[49] Epidemiologic data indicate that the moderate intake of alcohol has a cardioprotective effect.[50–52] Elevation of serum HDL levels appears to be the primary mechanism by which alcohol imparts this benefit. It should be stressed that the benefits of alcohol apply only to moderate consumption and are not seen in those who "abuse" alcohol. Furthermore, the protective effects of alcohol are not seen in regard to the risks of hemorrhagic stroke, death due to trauma, or cancer, all of which may be increased in individuals who consume greater amounts of alcohol.

Exercise

Even a moderate degree of exercise appears to have a protective effect against CHD.[53] In one study of middle-aged men, participation in moderately vigorous physical activity was associated with a 23% lower risk of death than that associated with a less active lifestyle, and this improvement in survival was equivalent and additive to other lifestyle measures, such as smoking cessation, hypertension control, and weight control.[54] Mechanisms that could account for the benefits of exercise include elevated serum HDL cholesterol levels, reduced BP, weight loss, and a lower incidence of insulin resistance.

Obesity

As stated above, obesity is associated with the development of a number of risk factors for CHD, including systemic hypertension, impaired glucose metabolism, insulin resistance, hypertriglyceridemia, reduced HDL cholesterol, and elevated fibrinogen. Data from the Framingham Heart Study, the Nurses' Health Study, and other studies have shown the risk of developing CHD that is associated with obesity.[55–57] The distribution of body fat appears to be an important determinant as patients with abdominal (central) obesity are at greatest risk for subsequent CHD.[58] Patients with central obesity, elevated levels of serum triglycerides and (to a lesser degree) LDL cholesterol, low HDL cholesterol, insulin resistance, and hypertension are classified as having atherogenic dyslipidemia (metabolic syndrome).[59] This syndrome is more difficult to treat and is associated with a worse prognosis than is an isolated increased LDL level.[60]

Vitamins and Homocysteine

Multiple studies have now linked elevated serum levels of homocysteine with increased risk of CHD. For example, in the Physicians' Health Study of almost 15,000 male physicians who were without prior CHD events, those with homocysteine levels that were above the 95th percentile had a threefold increase in the risk of MI when compared with those in the lower 90th percentile.[61] Elevated homocysteine may be associated with reduced levels and intake of folate and vitamin B_{12}, as was shown in older subjects from the Framingham Heart Study.[62] Dietary supplementation with high levels of vitamins such as folate, vitamin B_{12}, and pyridoxine has been demonstrated to reduce serum homocysteine levels, but whether this translates into improved CHD end points is an active area of investigation.[63,64]

Plasma Fibrinogen

Plasma fibrinogen levels have recently been shown to be predictors of CVD, and there is a linear relationship between fibrinogen and other cardiovascular risk factors, including age, smoking, diabetes, body mass index, total and LDL cholesterol, and triglycerides.[65] Data from the Framingham Offspring Study suggest that the measurement of fibrinogen is a useful screening tool for identifying individuals who are at increased thrombotic risk and therefore at increased risk of CVD.[66]

Antioxidants

The oxidation of LDL particles is an integral part of the atherosclerotic process; this suggests that antioxidant therapy may reduce the incidence of CVD. Antioxidant vitamins such as vitamin E, vitamin C, and β-carotene have been studied in smaller clinical trials, with earlier studies demonstrating benefit only for vitamin E.[67] Despite these early data, the HOPE trial demonstrated that vitamin E use was associated with no protective effect on cardiovascular end points; therefore, its routine administration cannot be recommended at this time.[68]

Endothelial Dysfunction

Endothelial dysfunction appears to be an early step in the atherosclerotic process and may result from dyslipidemia, hypertension, and diabetes. Recent studies have suggested that coronary artery endothelial dysfunction predicts the long-term progression of atherosclerosis and an increased incidence of cardiovascular events.[69]

Risk Factor Modification

When atherosclerosis is identified, the immediate goals are to relieve symptoms and to improve organ perfusion. Aggressive risk factor modification to retard or prevent ongoing atherosclerosis is among the most important parts of long-term management. Smoking cessation, meticulous control of hypertension and diabetes, weight management, and aggressive lipid-lowering therapy should all be advised. Lipid-lowering therapy with HMG CoA reductase inhibitors has been shown to reduce mortality in patients with CAD, even when total cholesterol and LDL are only modestly elevated.[38,70] A low-fat, low-calorie diet may result in improved serum lipid levels as well as improved weight management, and a cardiovascular exercise program may result in reduced morbidity and mortality from CHD.[71]

Diagnosis

The diagnosis of chronic CAD is usually suspected from the clinical presentation. A history of exertional or resting symptoms including (but not limited to) chest tightness, jaw discomfort, left arm pain, dyspnea, or epigastric distress should raise the suspicion of CAD. Many patients deny "chest pain" per se, but the clinician should recognize subtle symptoms (such as dyspnea, diaphoresis, or epigastric distress) that may limit activity. Some patients with CAD have no symptoms that are identified during careful questioning but have "silent ischemia" that is demonstrated by noninvasive testing, such as exercise testing or ambulatory ECG.[72] Careful attention should be directed to the risk factor profile for CAD since the probability of atherosclerosis is increased in these individuals.[8,73] A statistical extrapolation of the most recent NHANES data suggested that oral health care professionals can effectively screen and identify patients who are unaware of their risk for developing CHD.[74]

Diagnostic testing begins with baseline 12-lead ECG. Unfortunately, this is neither sensitive nor specific for the presence of CAD or prior MI. The presence of Q waves on the ECG may suggest prior MI, although these are not invariably present, and often only nonspecific changes of the ST segments are observed in patients with chronic CAD. Even a normal ECG does not exclude the presence of severe or even life-threatening CAD. Exercise stress testing, often combined with nuclear or echocardiographic imaging modalities, remains the mainstay of a noninvasive diagnosis.[75] Exercise testing with ECG monitoring is associated with a relatively low sensitivity and specificity for the detection of CAD and should be performed only if the resting ECG is normal. Myocardial perfusion imaging with agents such as thallium 201 and technetium 99m sestamibi is used to assess coronary perfusion at rest and with physical stress. Since the uptake of these agents into the myocardium is an active process, ischemic or infarcted cells exhibit a reduced or absent uptake. A 70 to 90% stenosis of a coronary artery typically is associated with decreased myocardial perfusion on the stress images but with normal myocardial perfusion at rest. This reversible defect is the perfusion pattern associated with stress-induced myocardial ischemia. A fixed defect demonstrates reduced myocardial perfusion both at rest and on exercise. This abnormality usually implies (1) prior MI without viable tissue or (2) severe resting ischemia due to high-grade coronary stenosis with inadequate collateral blood flow. Stress echocardiography detects myocardial ischemia by demonstrating regional differences in LV contractile function during stress. If there is an isolated lesion in the coronary arterial bed, the segmental wall motion abnormality will typically correlate to the distribution of a coronary artery. Ischemic myocardial tissue exhibits both diastolic and systolic dysfunction; the latter is more easily identified on two-dimensional echocardiographic images following exercise or pharmacologic stress with agents such as dobutamine. Both myocardial perfusion imaging and stress echocardiography offer greater sensitivity and specificity than does exercise ECG alone, and they provide important prognostic information as well. The sensitivity of either modality has been reported as between 85 and 90%, and specificity has been reported to be as high as 90%, but each modality has distinct advantages and disadvantages. Stress echocardiography may offer higher specificity, allows concomitant evaluation of cardiac anatomy and function, and is less expensive than perfusion imaging. Up to 5 to 10% of referred patients will have technically inadequate resting images and will require a perfusion imaging study for diagnostic accuracy. Stress perfusion imaging offers a higher technical success rate, higher sensitivity for the detection of single-vessel CAD, and better accuracy when multiple resting LV wall motion abnormalities are present.[76,77] The role of exercise testing in asymptomatic individuals is highly controversial.[78,79] Coronary angiography is often needed to define the anatomy and to assist in planning an appropriate management strategy for selected intermediate- to high-risk patients.

Management

The management of chronic, stable CAD depends on a number of clinical factors, including the extent and severity of ischemia, exercise capacity, prognosis based on exercise testing, overall LV function, and associated comorbidities,

such as diabetes mellitus. Patients with a small ischemic burden, normal exercise tolerance, and normal LV function may be safely treated with pharmacologic therapy. The front line of modern medical therapy includes the selected use of aspirin, β-blockers, ACEIs, and HMG CoA reductase inhibitors. These agents have been shown to reduce the incidence of subsequent MI and death.[77,80] Nitrates and calcium channel blockers may be added to the primary agents to relieve angina in selected patients. Percutaneous coronary intervention (PCI) with percutaneous transluminal coronary angioplasty (PTCA) and intracoronary stenting relieves symptoms of chronic ischemia, improves mortality when used acutely in patients with MI, and may improve regional or global LV function.[81,82] There is no evidence that in patients with chronic stable angina, PCI is superior to medical management in the prevention of heart attack and death.[83,84] Patients with complex multivessel CAD may not be completely revascularized with PCI because of the technical limitations of the procedure and commonly require PCI with adjunct medical therapy or surgical revascularization. Early randomized trials in the 1970s, comparing then-current medical therapy with bypass surgery, demonstrated that patients with reduced LV function and severe ischemia, often associated with left main or multivessel CAD, are often best served by coronary artery bypass graft surgery.[85–88] More recently, certain subgroups of patients, such as those with multivessel disease or patients with diabetes mellitus, have been shown to have improved survival when treated with surgery as compared with treatment by PCI.[89,90]

Prognosis

Recent improvements in pharmacologic therapy, PCI, and surgical technique have resulted in significant improvements in morbidity and mortality in patients with CAD. Risk factor modification is a critical element of the therapy and may result in improved prognosis as well. Despite these improvements, over 1 million Americans die each year of CAD.

▼ ACUTE CORONARY SYNDROMES

The sudden rupture of an atherosclerotic plaque, with ensuing intracoronary thrombus formation that acutely reduces coronary blood flow, causes the acute coronary syndromes (ACSs).[91,92] This results in myocardial ischemia and subsequent infarction if there is a prolonged and severe reduction in blood flow. ACSs represent a continuous spectrum of disease ranging from unstable angina to non-ST-elevation MI to acute ST-elevation myocardial infarction (STEMI).

If the intraluminal thrombus following acute plaque rupture is not completely occlusive, the corresponding clinical presentation is that of unstable angina.[93] There is a sudden change in anginal pattern relating to the frequency or duration of the symptoms. In some cases, the patient may present with symptoms at rest. With a greater degree of obstruction of the epicardial coronary arterial lumen, a non-Q-wave myocardial infarction (NQWMI) may develop. This presents with prolonged symptoms of resting ischemia, typically without ST-segment elevation or the development of pathologic Q waves. ECG in an NQWMI patient may show resting ST-segment depression or deep symmetric T-wave inversions, consistent with severe ischemia. If a large epicardial coronary artery becomes obstructed for a relatively long duration of time, a larger MI results, and the ECG findings will be STEMI and, without prompt restoration of blood flow, the subsequent development of pathologic Q waves.

Diagnosis of Acute Unstable Coronary Syndromes

The diagnosis of an ACS is usually made on the basis of clinical data. The patient's history suggests a change in anginal pattern or ischemic symptoms at rest. Acutely, the ECG is important to risk-stratify the patient and to make decisions regarding treatment. A normal ECG does not exclude the presence of acute myocardial infarction (AMI). If the MI is located in the posterior wall of the LV, it will typically not be well represented on the standard 12-lead ECG. Resting ST-segment depression or T-wave inversions in the distribution of an epicardial coronary artery often accompany unstable angina or NQWMI; however, ST-segment elevation is the hallmark of an acute STEMI. Patients presenting with a history suggestive of an AMI who have a left bundle branch block pattern on the 12-lead ECG are usually treated as if they had STEMI, given the difficulty of interpreting the ECG when this conduction delay is present.

Levels of serum cardiac enzymes, such as creatine phosphokinase (CPK) and the more cardiac-specific CPK MB fraction, can be used to establish myocardial injury and infarction. It is important to remember that these levels do not rise significantly until 8 to 12 hours following an MI. Newer, more sensitive and specific cardiac serum markers such as troponin T and troponin I can be used to risk-stratify patients with cardiac injury or infarction.[94] The serum levels become elevated approximately 4 to 8 hours after the acute insult and persist for 5 to 7 days following the event. As both markers can be normal in the early phases of unstable angina or AMI, neither CPK nor troponin is significantly useful in the acute management of patients who may be at the highest risk because of STEMI. Patients with ACS and positive troponin T or I have been shown to have an increased risk of recurrent cardiac events.[95,96] These patients are typically treated more aggressively and are referred for diagnostic and therapeutic cardiac catheterization.

Therapy for Unstable Coronary Syndromes

The treatment of the unstable coronary syndromes is the relief of myocardial ischemia and the institution of pharmacologic therapy targeting the underlying thrombotic mechanism.[97] Aspirin should be promptly administered to inhibit platelet function. The selective use of β-blockers may relieve ischemia by lowering heart rate and BP, which subsequently decreases myocardial oxygen demand (MVO_2). β-Blockers are also antiarrhythmic agents and reduce the risk of malignant ventricular arrhythmias. β-Blockers should not be administered to those with heart failure, bradycardia, heart block, or severe bronchospasm. Sublingual or intravenous nitroglycerin results in venodilation with a resultant decrease in LV preload and MVO_2, thereby reducing myocardial ischemia. They may also contribute to reducing ischemia by their action as epicardial coronary vasodilators.

Antithrombotic therapy with intravenous unfractionated or low molecular weight heparin and newer agents such as the platelet IIb/IIIa inhibitors (ie, tirofiban and abciximab) results in improved coronary blood flow and reduced MI size. Procedural outcomes are improved when these agents are used during angioplasty and stenting.

In patients with STEMI, thrombolytic therapy with agents such as streptokinase, tissue plasminogen activator, and reteplase have all been shown to improve coronary blood flow and to reduce mortality.[98,99] This benefit has not been demonstrated in patients with unstable angina or NQWMI. As an alternative to thrombolytic therapy, percutaneous revascularization with balloon angioplasty and stenting may be performed acutely to improve coronary blood flow and reduce MI size. Prospective randomized trials have shown that primary angioplasty with or without stenting in patients with STEMI is superior to thrombolytic therapy when it is completed within 1 to 2 hours of clinical presentation. If a patient with STEMI presents to a center that lacks the ability to perform primary angioplasty, thrombolytic therapy is then the treatment of choice if immediate transfer to such a center cannot be arranged. Certain subgroups of patients, including those in cardiogenic shock due to massive AMI, may not derive as great a benefit from thrombolytic therapy.[100–102] Transfer to a facility capable of PTCA and bypass surgery may be preferred for this selected patient population. Support with inotropic agents such as dobutamine or milrinone or with an intra-aortic balloon pump may be necessary in hemodynamically compromised patients while awaiting more definitive therapy.[103–105]

Oral Health Considerations

Several considerations need to be addressed when treating dental patients with CAD. The primary concern is to prevent ischemia or infarction. The risk for such an event is determined by numerous factors, including the degree and type of CAD (ie, stable vs unstable angina or history of MI). In rare situations, impaired hemostasis due to one or more medications may also require dental modifications.[106] In addition, side effects from cardiac drugs may cause oral changes, and drug interactions with medications used for dental care may occur. The current cardiac status and medications should be discussed with the patient's physicians prior to stressful or invasive procedures.

▼ GENERAL PRECAUTIONS REGARDING DENTAL PROCEDURES

It is beneficial, but not necessary, for oral health care professionals treating patients with a history of ischemic heart disease to be versed in advanced cardiac life support. The use of a pulse oximeter to determine the level of oxygenation and the availability of an automatic external defibrillator are also advantageous. The determination of vital signs prior to dental care is an important preventive measure, to include blood pressure and pulse rate and rhythm, and any abnormal findings should be noted and taken into consideration before dental treatment.[107]

Patients with CAD are at increased risk of demand-related ischemia with increased heart rate and BP, as well as for plaque rupture and acute unstable coronary syndromes. Anxiety can increase the heart rate and BP and can provoke angina or ischemia,[108] but this risk is low during outpatient dental procedures. Protocols to reduce the anxiety of the patient should be considered according to the level of anticipated stress. Premedication with antianxiety medications and inhalation nitrous oxide are commonly used for this purpose.

Numerous studies have indicated the influence of circadian variation on the triggering of acute coronary events.[109] Most such events occur between 6:00 am and noon. It has been proposed that sympathetic nervous system activation and an increased coagulative state may be precipitating factors.[110] Medications designed to prevent these events, such as β-blockers, aspirin, and antihypertensives, should be continued. Therefore, dental care for high-risk patients might ideally be provided in the late morning or the early afternoon.

Elective procedures, especially those requiring general anesthesia, should be avoided for at least 4 weeks following an MI as there is a small increased risk of reinfarction.[111] Limited data indicate that the acute risk of administering local anesthesia for dental procedures 3 weeks after an uncomplicated AMI is very low; however, consultation with the patient's primary physician or cardiologist prior to dental therapy is recommended.

Anticoagulation Therapy and Dental Care

Patients with CAD may require the use of aspirin or other antiplatelet drug, such as clopidogrel or ticlopidine, which are frequently used in patients with a history of ACS and in all patients after coronary artery stenting (Table 8). The combination of acetylsalicylic acid and clopidogrel is usually continued for a minimum of 4 weeks after stent placement and for a minimum of 3 to 6 months following the use of the newer drug-eluting stents, to prevent subacute thrombosis. Daily aspirin is typically continued lifelong. These agents may increase the risk of bleeding when used alone or in combination. Data that address the risks of bleeding from dental extractions in patients who use antiplatelet agents are limited. Although a bleeding time test is often recommended to evaluate the qualitative defect in platelets, this test has not been shown to have a good correlation with impaired intraoral hemostasis unless bleeding time is significantly longer than 15 to 20 minutes.[112,113]

Anticoagulant therapy is used both to treat and to prevent thromboembolism, and different types of medications are

TABLE 8 Common Antiplatelet and Antithrombin Medications	
Drug	Trade Name
Antiplatelet medications	
Aspirin	—
Ticlopidine	Ticlid
Clopidogrel	Plavix
Glycoprotein IIb/IIIa receptor antagonists	
Abciximab	ReoPro
Eptifibatide	Integrilin
Tirofiban	Aggrastat
Antithrombin medications	
Indirect thrombin inhibitors	
Unfractionated heparin	Heparin
Low-molecular-weight heparin	Enoxaparin
Direct thrombin inhibitors	
Lepirudin	Hirudin
Dicumarols	
Warfarin	Coumadin

used to achieve anticoagulation, based on the patient's underlying medical condition. Dental providers treating ambulatory patients in an outpatient setting will almost exclusively treat patients who are using anticoagulation therapy for prophylactic purposes. Medical conditions for which prophylactic anticoagulation therapy is instituted include (but are not limited to) atrial fibrillation (AF) (with and without concomitant systemic embolism), valvular heart disease, the presence of prosthetic heart valves, ischemic heart disease, cerebrovascular accidents, pulmonary embolism, and deep venous thrombosis.

Two major types of medications are used for anticoagulation: drugs with antiplatelet activity and drugs with antithrombin activity.

The most common antiplatelet drug is aspirin, which is used chronically in low doses to prevent cardiovascular and cerebrovascular events. Aspirin irreversibly decreases platelet aggregation, and patients will take between 81 and 325 mg of aspirin once per day.[114] The dose and duration of aspirin use may be irrelevant as it appears that one aspirin tablet essentially blocks platelet aggregation for their lifetime. If the patient has other underlying medical conditions that predispose patients to impaired hemostasis (such as uremia or liver disease) or takes other anticoagulants (including nonaspirin, nonsteroidal anti-inflammatory drugs [NSAIDs]), the possibility of oral bleeding following oral surgical procedures increases greatly.[106,115]

If emergency surgery needs to be performed and there is concern about aspirin therapy, 1-desamino-8-D-arginine vasopressin (DDAVP) can be instituted to improve hemostasis.[116] DDAVP is administered parenterally at 0.3 μg/kg of body weight, with a maximum dose of 20 to 24 μg within 1 hour of surgery. A nasal spray containing 1.5 mg of DDAVP per milliliter can be given in a dose of 300 mg/kg body weight. In routine clinical practice, the need for DDAVP is extremely uncommon. There have been no studies indicating the need to discontinue or alter anticoagulation therapy prior to routine oral surgical procedures for patients taking antiplatelet medications other than aspirin, and there seems to be a consensus that the risk to the patient (eg, thromboembolism) if these drugs are discontinued far exceeds the problem of prolonged bleeding (see Table 8 for a list of antiplatelet medications).

The most commonly used antithrombin medications are the dicumarols (eg, warfarin), which inhibit the biosynthesis of vitamin K–dependent coagulation proteins (factors II [prothrombin (PT)], VII, IX, and X). The full therapeutic effect of warfarin is reached after 48 to 72 hours and lasts for 36 to 72 hours if the drug is discontinued. The efficacy of warfarin therapy is monitored by the international normalized ratio (INR) as PT has been shown to vary depending on the source and brand of thromboplastin as well as the type of instrumentation used to perform the test. The INR is calculated on the basis of the international sensitivity index of the specific thromboplastin used in the test (see Chapter 17, "Bleeding and Clotting Disorders," for more information on PT, INR, and normal hemostatic values). The therapeutic level of the INR is dependent on the underlying condition but is usually kept in the range of 2.0 to 3.5. For an accurate assessment of an individual's anticoagulation status, an INR measurement should be performed within several hours of surgery. There is little indication that anticoagulation therapy should be discontinued before minor oral surgical procedures when the patient's INR is <3.5.[106,117] This conclusion is based on the minimal increase of intraoral bleeding tendency at this level of anticoagulation, the ease with which most intraoral bleeding can be stopped with local measures, and the potentially devastating consequences of thromboembolic events if warfarin is held, especially those of an embolic stroke.

Three different protocols can be used to treat patients with markedly elevated INR. In the first protocol, warfarin is continued without a change in the dose. This minimizes adverse thromboembolic events but may increase the risk of prolonged oral bleeding after surgery. If localized antihemostatic measures are inadequate to stop bleeding after surgery, antifibrinolytic mouthrinses can be instituted and vitamin K injections used with physician approval.[118] With the second protocol, warfarin therapy is discontinued for 2 to 3 days prior to surgery, and the patient is not placed on any alternative anticoagulation therapy. It takes an additional 2 to 3 days after surgery to regain the therapeutic effect of the medication. During this period, the patient may be in a hypercoagulable state and therefore at an increased risk for developing a thromboembolic event. In patients who are at the highest risk of thromboembolism, such as those with mechanical prosthetic heart valves, AF with a history of stroke, or recent deep venous thrombosis and/or pulmonary embolism, this second approach of holding warfarin without "bridging" heparin (see below) may be too risky. In the third protocol, warfarin therapy is discontinued, and the patient is placed on an alternative anticoagulation therapy. This protocol has both advantages and disadvantages. The greatest advantage is that

the patient's risk for developing thromboembolic events is minimized by comparison with the second protocol above. When unfractionated heparin is used for bridging the warfarin-free period, the patient is typically admitted to a hospital, has his or her oral anticoagulation (warfarin) therapy discontinued, and is administered vitamin K and started on parenteral (heparin) therapy. Heparin is continued until approximately 6 hours before surgery and is reinstituted after surgery in combination with oral anticoagulation therapy until a desirable INR has been reached. This is both a time-consuming and costly course of action. The advantages of using heparin are its short half-life of 4 to 6 hours and the availability of an antidote, protamine sulfate, that has an immediate effect. An alternative to using standard unfractionated heparin is to have the patient self-administer a subcutaneous injection of low molecular weight heparin on an outpatient basis.[119] This is becoming the treatment of choice in most clinical practices.

There are also limited data addressing the risk from dental procedures performed following coronary stenting.[120] It is prudent to wait approximately 1 month after this procedure, to allow endothelialization of the stent to decrease the risk of subacute thrombosis. Reendothelialization is considered to be complete approximately 4 weeks after bare metal stent placement and at 3 to 6 months following the use of a drug-eluting ("coated") stent. There is some new concern that patients who receive drug-eluting stents continue to be at a slightly increased risk of stent thrombosis even when Plavix is discontinued as late as 6 to 12 months following stent placement. Premature discontinuation of antiplatelet therapy has been significantly associated with adverse cardiac events, such as MI and death.[121] As the risk of bleeding from anything but highly invasive dental procedures is small, and bleeding is relatively easy to manage, antiplatelet therapy should never be discontinued for elective dental procedures. The patient's cardiologist should be contacted prior to carrying out invasive dental procedures.[121]

Recent guidelines from the American Heart Association (AHA) suggest not using antibiotic prophylaxis for dental procedures in patients after coronary stent placement unless the patient presents with an acute odontogenic infection.[122]

Considerations for dental patients who have undergone coronary artery bypass grafting are similar to those who have had a stent procedure. In addition, due to the cardiac surgical procedure involved, such patients may be in significant pain when sitting in a dental chair, even several weeks after their surgery. Elective dental care should therefore be postponed until the patient can sit comfortably for the required time period.

Dental care for patients who are on anticoagulation therapy has been discussed in numerous dental and medical publications, and various protocols have been suggested.[123] The debate surrounding the dental management of patients with anticoagulation therapy, when invasive dental procedures are to be performed, centers on the potential risk for excessive bleeding after the procedures if anticoagulation therapy is not reduced or stopped versus the risk of the patient experiencing a thromboembolic event if the anticoagulation therapy is altered.[124] Various authors have suggested a wide range of alternatives, including discontinuing all anticoagulation therapy before invasive procedures, altering the anticoagulation regimen, and making no changes. Ultimately, the core of the problem of developing a uniform protocol for anticoagulated patients is the ability to quantify risk, using parameters that can be applied to the majority of patients. Several relevant issues need to be considered, including the underlying medical condition requiring anticoagulation therapy, the type of medications used to achieve anticoagulation, the level of anticoagulation, the timing of dental care, and the cost and convenience to the patient.

▼ VALVULAR HEART DISEASE

Mitral Valve Disease

The most common types of mitral valve disease include mitral valve prolapse (MVP), mitral regurgitation (MR), and mitral stenosis. In addition to the hemodynamic alterations that are present in patients with these conditions, there are additional issues with regard to the prevention of bacterial endocarditis.

Definition and Incidence

MVP typically occurs as a result of myxomatous degeneration of the mitral leaflets and their supporting apparatus. This results in abnormal movement or prolapse of the mitral leaflets posteriorly toward the left atrium during mechanical systole. Thus, there is abnormal coaptation of the valve with varying degrees of MR. MVP has been reported in 2.4% of the Framingham Heart Study population and in up to 4 to 5% of the general population.[125] A small percentage of those with MVP have significant MR and ensuing LV volume overload. Acute chordal rupture within the subvalvular apparatus can occur, and this leads to the rapid development of a flail mitral leaflet with acute severe MR. Rarely, MVP can be accompanied by malignant dysrhythmias such as ventricular tachycardia or fibrillation. Typically, more benign atrial dysrhythmias are seen and manifest clinically as palpitations. Cardiac auscultation frequently reveals a midsystolic click, late systolic murmur, or the combination of click and murmur. The gold standard for diagnosing and risk-stratifying MVP is echocardiography. Patients with MVP may exhibit increased sympathetic autonomic activity and an enhanced sense of cardiac perception. Patients often complain of atypical chest pain or palpitations, and this generates a sense of anxiety regarding their cardiac situation. Often patients are diagnosed as having MVP with a similar symptom complex, but the rigorous clinical and echocardiographic criteria for its diagnosis are not strictly applied.[126]

MR occurs as a result of a wide variety of abnormalities of the mitral leaflets.[127] These abnormalities have various causes, including myxomatous degeneration and leaflet prolapse, rheumatic heart disease, endocarditis, and use of anorectic agents such as fenfluramine and phentermine (fen-phen).[128–130] Another mechanism of MR is secondary to

dilation of the base of the LV in patients with dilated cardiomyopathy. Regardless of the mechanism, if MR is left untreated, the final common end point is significant LV volume overload, with subsequent eccentric hypertrophy of the LV and resultant progressive heart failure.

Mitral stenosis most often occurs as a result of rheumatic heart disease. In rheumatic heart disease, there is characteristic thickening and fusion of the mitral commissures as well as thickening and calcification of the leaflets and subvalvular apparatus. This results in a restriction to LV inflow, subsequent left atrial hypertension and enlargement, atrial arrhythmias, and secondary pulmonary hypertension.

The clinical diagnosis of mitral disease requires a careful history suggesting a previously heard heart murmur, exertional or resting dyspnea, or symptoms of heart failure, such as orthopnea, paroxysmal nocturnal dyspnea, or peripheral edema. Auscultatory findings include a midsystolic click in MVP, a holosystolic murmur in rheumatic MR, and an opening snap and diastolic rumble in mitral stenosis. Ancillary findings such as pulmonary or peripheral edema may be present as well.

Transthoracic echocardiography (TTE) remains the mainstay of noninvasive diagnosis in the vast majority of patients with mitral valve disease, and Doppler techniques are extremely useful in establishing the severity of stenosis or regurgitation.[131] Transesophageal echocardiography (TEE) is occasionally needed to further define the mechanism of MR or mitral stenosis and to better assess the severity of the hemodynamic lesion[132]; this is instrumental in planning appropriate surgical therapy. TEE offers improved image quality due to the proximity of the transducer to the mitral valve and left atrium, which allows much greater anatomic definition of the mitral apparatus than can be attained with TTE. It is also widely used to help guide intraoperative management in patients who are referred for valve repair or replacement. Recently, exercise stress echocardiography has been used to evaluate the LV contractile reserve in patients with MR, allowing better timing of operative intervention.[133] Cardiac catheterization has a limited role in the diagnosis of mitral valve disease and is primarily reserved for those patients who are referred for cardiac surgery.[134]

Treatment of Mitral Valvular Disease

The American College of Cardiology and the AHA have published guidelines for treating valvular heart disease that are based on the strength of the currently available evidence in the medical literature.[135] MVP with relatively minor degrees of MR can be observed with serial clinical and echocardiographic examinations to screen for worsening degrees of regurgitation. Symptomatic patients with significant degrees of MR or mitral stenosis are typically referred for operative or other mechanical intervention. Asymptomatic patients with MR can be observed with serial clinical and echocardiographic examinations. The development of symptoms or, in the asymptomatic patient, an increase in LV dimension or a decrease in the LV ejection fraction are important factors in determining the timing of surgical intervention. Unfortunately, ideal criteria for proceeding to intervention prior to irreversible LV enlargement and contractile decompensation do not exist. MR can be treated by either repair of the mitral valve or replacement with a mechanical or biologic prosthesis. Mitral repair is usually accomplished with the resection of the prolapsing or flail segment of the mitral leaflets and the placement of an annuloplasty ring to decrease mitral annular dimension in order to improve mitral coaptation. More complicated mitral repair is possible and includes the resection and transposition of the chordal structures. If significant fibrosis or calcification of the mitral valve is present, replacement with either a biologic or mechanical prosthesis may be necessary. Mitral stenosis can be treated with percutaneous balloon valvuloplasty (PBV) or mitral valve replacement. PBV may be the initial treatment of choice in carefully selected patients, although many will require repeat PBV or valve replacement over time. Patients with highly calcified valves or those with significant degrees of MR that accompanies mitral stenosis are typically referred for valve replacement.

Aortic Valve Disease

The three major causes of aortic stenosis (AS) are congenital, rheumatic, and senile calcific valve disease. The leaflet excursion is restricted, and a pressure gradient develops from the LV to the aorta, causing subsequent LV pressure overload. This leads to concentric hypertrophy of the LV. The natural history of untreated AS is eventual LV failure due to afterload mismatch.

Aortic regurgitation (AR) results from a wide variety of processes that directly affect the aortic leaflets, including congenital abnormalities, rheumatic disease, infective endocarditis, senile calcific valve degeneration, and the use of anorexigens.[136] Additionally, abnormalities of the aortic root, such as aneurysm or aortic dissection, may dilate or disrupt the aortic annulus, resulting in malcoaptation and regurgitation. AR imposes an acute or chronic volume load to the LV, with subsequent eccentric hypertrophy, LV enlargement, and eventual LV contractile failure if the regurgitation is not corrected.

Diagnosis

The clinical diagnosis of aortic valve disease requires a careful history suggesting a previously heard heart murmur, exertional or resting dyspnea, or symptoms of heart failure, such as orthopnea, paroxysmal nocturnal dyspnea, or peripheral edema. Severe AR may produce angina due to impaired coronary filling, which results from a decrease in aortic diastolic pressure and an increase in LV diastolic pressure.

The auscultatory findings of AS include a harsh systolic crescendo-decrescendo murmur and a diminished or absent aortic component of the second heart sound. Congenital AS may be accompanied by an ejection click in the early stages because the valve remains relatively pliable. AR is manifest on physical examination by a diastolic murmur heard best at the left sternal border when the patient is sitting upright with

breath held after exhalation. Pulmonary or peripheral edema may also be clinically evident. Chronic AR often yields findings of a hyperdynamic circulation with bounding or "water hammer" pulses, head bobbing (titubation), "to-and-fro" murmurs heard in the femoral arteries, and Quincke's pulse (visible in the nail beds). Acute AR may present with heart failure and acute pulmonary edema, without the characteristic murmur of AR. Because of early closure of the mitral valve with acute severe AR, the only auscultatory finding may be a soft or absent first heart sound (S1).

TTE remains the mainstay of noninvasive diagnosis in the vast majority of patients with aortic valve disease. Doppler techniques are useful in establishing the severity of stenosis or regurgitation.[137] TEE may be needed to define the mechanism of AR or AS, to evaluate the aortic root and ascending aorta, and to investigate the possibility of endocarditis. It is also used to guide intraoperative management in patients who are referred for valve replacement.[138,139] As in cases of MR, exercise stress echocardiography can be used to evaluate the LV contractile reserve in patients with AR.[133] The ability to predict the LV contractile decompensation earlier allows optimal timing of operative intervention. A role exists for cardiac catheterization in the diagnosis of aortic valve disease as well; it is primarily reserved for both evaluating the possibility of coexisting CAD and determining the need for surgical revascularization in patients who are being considered for cardiac surgery. Hemodynamic data obtained by cardiac catheterization are used to corroborate Doppler-derived measures of aortic valve area and pressure gradients.

Treatment of Aortic Valvular Disease

Aortic disease with relatively minor degrees of stenosis or regurgitation can be observed clinically, with serial clinical and echocardiographic examinations to monitor progression. In cases of AS, the development of symptoms and, to a lesser degree, the severity of AS determine the timing of surgery.[140] Both retrospective and prospective studies have demonstrated that the risk of sudden death is low in asymptomatic patients with even a severe degree of stenosis.[141] Although largely unproved, some have suggested that asymptomatic patients should undergo operative intervention if they have critical AS (aortic valve area < 0.6 cm^2 and a mean gradient > 50 mm Hg on Doppler echocardiography) or if they have severe AS and are found to have significant ventricular arrhythmia or myocardial ischemia, progressive decline in systolic function, or a rapid increase in the aortic jet velocity (> 0.3 m/s), as measured by Doppler echocardiography, over 1 year.[142]

In patients with AR, the key factors to observe are the development of symptoms and a worsening of LV enlargement.[135] Heart failure symptoms typically develop in the late or decompensated stages of LV volume overload. Symptomatic patients with significant degrees of AR or AS are typically referred for surgery. Unfortunately, as with MR, ideal criteria for proceeding to operative intervention prior to irreversible LV enlargement and contractile decompensation do not exist. Severe AR or AS is usually treated with aortic valve replacement with either a mechanical or biologic valve prosthesis. AS can be treated with PBV; however, minimal hemodynamic improvements postprocedure and rapid restenosis rates limit the usefulness of this procedure in AS. It is usually reserved for patients who are not operative candidates but who require end-stage symptomatic palliation or temporary hemodynamic improvements to tolerate additional noncardiac surgery or to overcome acute illness.

Prosthetic Heart Valves

There are numerous types and models of prosthetic heart valves, each with its own unique characteristics. These valves are either mechanical or bioprosthetic. The mechanical valves, which are classified according to their structure, include the oldest type caged-ball (Starr-Edwards) valve, the single tilting-disk (Bjork-Shiley) valve, and the currently most widely used bileaflet tilting-disk valves (ie, St. Jude, Edwards-MIRA). Bioprosthetic valves are either (1) heterografts made from porcine or bovine tissue or (2) homografts from preserved human aortic valves. Patients with mechanical valves require chronic anticoagulation therapy (typically with warfarin) to prevent thromboembolism. The degree of anticoagulation varies according to the type of the mechanical heart valve. The thrombogenic potential is the highest for caged-ball valves, moderate for single tilting-disk valves, and the lowest for bileaflet tilting-disk valves. In patients with mechanical valves, the risk of systemic embolization is approximately 4% per patient per year without anticoagulation, 2.2% with aspirin therapy, and 0.7 to 1.0% with warfarin therapy.[143] Patients with mitral valve prostheses are at approximately twice the risk of those with aortic valve prostheses.[144] The risk of thromboembolism is highest in the period following placement of the valve and decreases over time as the valve becomes endothelialized. Bioprosthetic valves have a lower thrombogenic potential and do not require long-term anticoagulation except for the early postoperative period. The recommended anticoagulation therapy for each type of prosthetic valve is summarized in Table 9. It is important that although these recommendations serve as broad guidelines, the level of chronic anticoagulation should be individualized and based on the location, type, and number of prosthetic valves, as well as the patient's age, comorbidities, and additional thromboembolic risk factors, such as a history of AF or stroke. Thus, the intensity of anticoagulation is determined by weighing the patient's risk of thromboembolic events against the risk of adverse anticoagulation consequences (bleeding risks).[145]

Prosthetic heart valves increase the risk for infectious endocarditis, which typically manifests as fever and as other systemic symptoms.[146] Although endocarditis within 60 days of surgery typically is caused by nonoral bacteria, the cause of endocarditis that occurs 60 days after valve surgery is similar to that of native-valve endocarditis.

Oral Health Considerations

The AHA issues recommendations based on analysis of the relevant literature regarding the risk of infective endocarditis, results of animal studies, and results of retrospective analyses

TABLE 9 Anticoagulation Therapy for Patients with Prosthetic Heart Valves

Risk of Thromboembolism	Type of Valve	Recommended INR	Antiplatelet Therapy
Low	Mechanical		
	More than one prosthesis	4.0–4.9	Not indicated
	Caged ball	4.0–4.9	Not indicated
	Single tilted disk	3.0–3.9	Not indicated
	Bileaflet tilted disk	2.5–2.9	Not indicated
	Bioprosthetic		
	Heterograft	2.0–3.0 (1st 3 mo)	ASA, 325 mg/d
	Homograft	Not indicated	Not indicated
High*	Mechanical	3.0–4.5	ASA, 80–160 mg/d
	Bioprosthetic		
	Heterograft	2.0–3.0	Not indicated
	Homograft	2.0–3.0	Not indicated

Adapted from Salem DN et al.[146]

ASA = acetylsalicylic acid; INR = international normalized ratio.

*High-risk patients are those with a history of atrial fibrillation, previous systemic embolism, left ventricular thrombus, or severe left ventricular dysfunction.

in humans (Tables 10 and 11).[147] According the 2007 AHA recommendations, prophylaxis is no longer recommend for the group of people defined in the previous (1997) recommendations as being at moderate risk. This is a significant departure from previous guidelines since prophylaxis is now recommended only for people defined as being in higher risk for a poor outcome should they acquire IE. The 2007 recommendations are significant also for the definition of dental procedures recommended for coverage (Table 12). It is important to note that although the AHA recommendations for antibiotic prophylaxis have been adopted for use in well over 20 patient populations, there is little or no scientific

TABLE 10 Cardiac Conditions Associated with the Highest Risk of Adverse Outcome from Endocarditis for Which Prophylaxis with Dental Procedures Is Recommended

- Prosthetic cardiac valve
- Previous infective endocarditis
- Congenital heart disease (CHD)
  - Unrepaired cyanotic congenital heart disease, including those with palliative shunts and conduits
  - Completely repaired CHD with prosthetic material or device either by surgery or catheter intervention during the first six months after the procedure*
  - Repaired CHD with residual defects at the site or adjacent to the site of a prosthetic patch or prosthetic device (which inhibit endothelialization)
  - Except for the conditions listed above, antibiotic prophylaxis is no longer recommended for any other form of congenital heart disease
- Cardiac transplantation recipients who develop cardiac valvulopathy

*Prophylaxis is recommended because endothelialization of prosthetic material occurs within 6 months after the procedure

TABLE 11 Regimens for a Dental Procedure

Situation	Agent	Regimen—Single Dose 30–60 minutes before procedure	
		Adults	**Children**
Oral	Amoxicillin	2 gm	50 mg/kg
Unable to take oral medication	Ampicillin or	2 g IM or IV*	50 mg/kg IM or IV
	Cefazolin or ceftriaxone	1 g IM or IV	50 mg/kg IM or IV
Allergic to penicillins or ampicillin	Cephalexin**† or	2 g	50 m/kg
	Clindamycin	600 mg	20 mg/kg
Oral	Azithromycin or clarithromycin	500 mg	15 mg/kg
Allergic to penicillins or ampicillin and unable to take oral medication	Cefazolin or ceftriaxone†	1 g IM or IV	50 mg/kg IM or IV
	Clindamycin phosphate	600 mg IM or IV	20 mg/kg IM or IV

*IM – intramuscular; IV – intravenous.
**or other first or second generation oral cephalosporin in equivalent adult or pediatric dosage.
†Cephalosporins should not be used in an individual with a history of anaphylaxis, angioedema, or urticaria with penicillins or ampicillin

TABLE 12 Dental Procedures for which Endocarditis Prophylaxis is Recommended for Patients in Table 10

All dental procedures that involve manipulation of gingival tissue or the periapical region of teeth or perforation of the oral mucosa*

* The following procedures and events do not need prophylaxis: routine anesthetic injections through noninfected tissue, taking dental radiographs, placement of removable prosthodontic or orthodontic appliances, adjustment of orthodontic appliances, placement of orthodontic brackets, shedding of deciduous teeth and bleeding from trauma to the lips or oral mucosa.

TABLE 13 Diseases and Conditions Associated with Different Types of Heart Murmurs

Type of Murmur	Associated Abnormality	Possible Associated Diseases or Conditions
Early systolic	MR	A fib, LVH, SLE, CTD
	TR	A fib, JVD, CTD
	VSD	A fib, L-to-R shunt, CHF
	AS	A fib, LVH
Midsystolic	AS	A fib, LVH
	PS	R-sided CHF
Late systolic	MVP	CTD, Stickler's disease, trisomy 21
Holosystolic	MR	A fib, LVH, SLE, CTD
	TR	A fib, JVD, CTD
	VSD	A fib, L-to-R shunt, CHF
Early diastolic	AI	CHF
	PI	CHF
Mid-diastolic	Rheumatic MS	A fib
Late diastolic	Rheumatic MS	A fib
Continuous	Aortopulmonary and arteriovenous connection	CHF, LVH
Early diastolic	AI	CHF

Adapted from Lessard E et al.[149]
A fib = atrial fibrillation; AS = aortic stenosis; CHF = congestive heart failure; CTD = connective tissue disease; JVD = jugular vein distention; LVH = left ventricular hypertrophy; MR = mitral regurgitation; MS = mitral stenosis; MVP = mitral valve prolapse; SLE = systemic lupus erythematosus.

evidence to support this practice in any of these populations of people.[147a]

Antibiotic prophylaxis is indicated for patients with specific types of heart murmurs, and it is important to be aware that murmurs are sometimes associated with underlying non-cardiac medical conditions that may also require modification in the dental management of these patients.[148] When patients present with specific types of heart murmurs, a consultation with the patient's cardiologist may be warranted (Table 13).

Although patients with prosthetic heart valves are generally maintained at higher INR levels (3.0-4.0), only in rare situations should the INR be lowered for dental procedures.[106] It is therefore prudent to continue anticoagulation therapy in patients who require intensive high INR levels (see Table 9 and the above discussion on anticoagulation therapy and dental care).

▼ HEART FAILURE

Definition and Incidence

Heart failure represents a clinical syndrome that is broadly defined as the inability of the cardiovascular system to meet the demands of the end-organs.[149,150] Heart failure may be due to pericardial disease, valvular heart disease, and, most commonly, myocardial disease resulting in abnormal contractile function (systolic dysfunction) or impaired relaxation (diastolic dysfunction). Diastolic dysfunction is characterized by clinical heart failure syndrome with normal LV systolic function on cardiac testing.[151,152] In many series, it represents one of the most common types of heart failure encountered in the general population.[153] Common causes of diastolic dysfunction include hypertension, CAD, long-standing diabetes, and advanced age. In addition, diastolic dysfunction is almost always present in patients with any type of advanced systolic heart failure (Table 14).

Diagnosis

Dyspnea, orthopnea, and paroxysmal nocturnal dyspnea are classic symptoms, but nonspecific complaints, such as chest discomfort, fatigue, palpitations, dizziness, and syncope, are not uncommon. The onset of symptoms may be insidious, and symptoms may present for medical attention only when an acute decompensation occurs. For example, a patient with asymptomatic LV dysfunction develops rapid AF, resulting in decompensated heart failure. Asymptomatic patients are sometimes diagnosed when routine testing is performed for other reasons that reveal abnormalities on ECGs, chest radiographs, or echocardiograms.

The physical examination findings in heart failure are numerous. A relative decrease in SBP (due to reduced cardiac output) and an increase in DPB (due to peripheral vasoconstriction) may result in a decrease in pulse pressure. Cardiac

TABLE 14 Heart Failure Etiologies

Coronary artery disease (ischemic cardiomyopathy)

Hypertension

Idiopathic dilated cardiomyopathy

Hypertrophic cardiomyopathy

Alcohol

Diabetes

Viruses (coxsackievirus, enterovirus, HIV)

Infiltrative disorders (amyloidosis, hemochromatosis, sarcoidosis)

Toxins (chemotherapeutic agents)

Metabolic disorders (hypothyroidism)

Valvular heart disease

Pericardial disease

Incessant tachyarrhythmia

High-output states (thyrotoxicosis, AV fistula, thiamine deficiency)

AV = atrioventricular; HIV = human immunodeficiency virus.

percussion and palpation reveal an enlarged heart with a laterally displaced and diffuse apical impulse. Auscultation may reveal an apical systolic murmur of MR and the lower parasternal murmur of tricuspid regurgitation. Third and fourth heart sounds can be heard, signifying evidence of systolic and diastolic dysfunction. Rales suggest pulmonary congestion secondary to elevated left atrial and LV end-diastolic pressures. Jugular venous distention, peripheral edema, and hepatomegaly are markers of elevated right-heart pressures and right ventricular dysfunction. In advanced heart failure, additional findings may include cool extremities with decreased pulses, generalized cachexia, muscle atrophy, and profound weakness.

Chest radiography may demonstrate cardiac enlargement, pulmonary congestion, and pleural effusions. The ECG is frequently abnormal in a nonspecific manner and may be the only indication of heart disease in asymptomatic individuals.

ECG may reveal prolonged repolarization (ie, Q–T interval), and nonspecific ST and T-wave abnormalities. Conduction disturbances such as atrioventricular (AV) block, bundle branch block, and hemiblocks are also seen. Criteria for LVH with a repolarization abnormality may suggest hypertension as an etiology. ECG may also reveal evidence of arrhythmias such as AF and atrial flutter, as well as premature atrial or ventricular contractions. Supraventricular tachyarrhythmias and nonsustained ventricular tachycardia are also associated with heart failure, as is the development of ventricular fibrillation leading to sudden cardiac death.

TTE is the most useful noninvasive diagnostic tool for the initial evaluation of a patient with heart failure.[154] TTE provides information not only on overall heart size and function but also on valvular structure and function, wall motion and thickness, LV mass, and the presence of pericardial disease. Doppler-derived hemodynamic measurements accurately predict the severity of valvular regurgitation seen in heart failure and give a noninvasive estimation of pulmonary artery pressures. Doppler techniques may also be used to evaluate LV diastolic abnormalities, which are frequently present in those with heart failure.

Nuclear imaging techniques such as perfusion heart scans with thallium 201 and technetium 99m sestamibi, radionuclide ventriculography with multiple gated acquisition scanning, and positron emission tomography may be useful in evaluating cardiac size and function and in screening for coronary disease as a cause of heart failure. However, because of the inability of these tests to answer important etiologic questions with absolute certainty and their inherent use of radiation, these tests are often unnecessary in the routine evaluation of patients with a known cause of heart failure.

Cardiac catheterization (with measurement of intracardiac pressures and cardiac output), along with coronary angiography, is useful in evaluating the etiology of heart failure when ischemic cardiomyopathy is suspected. In middle-aged and elderly patients, the most common cause of heart failure and cardiomyopathy is CAD. In patients with heart failure, typical findings at catheterization include elevated LV end-diastolic, wedge, pulmonary artery, and right-heart pressures; increased LV size with decreased overall systolic function; and MR. Regional wall motion abnormalities may be seen in either ischemic or dilated cardiomyopathy but are usually less prominent in patients who do not have ischemic heart disease.

Therapy

The treatment of heart failure must be individualized to the etiology of the heart failure and to the patient. Patients with CAD and heart failure should be evaluated for ischemia as well as viable but hibernating myocardium that would improve systolic and diastolic performance with revascularization.[155–157] Patients with alcoholic cardiomyopathy should be advised to abstain from alcohol, in addition to the usual therapeutic options, as this often leads to an improvement in LV performance.[158] Hypertension should be aggressively treated with pharmacologic intervention and dietary measures.

The initial treatment in decompensated heart failure is with intravenous or oral diuretics. Intravenous vasodilators such as nitroglycerin may also be used. The majority of patients with symptomatic heart failure will need to stay on oral diuretic therapy. The dose of the diuretic must always be individualized. For patients with systolic heart failure, ACEIs are one of the mainstays of chronic drug therapy. These agents have clearly been shown to decrease mortality and to prolong survival. They also delay onset and reduce the symptoms of heart failure in patients with LV systolic dysfunction. When ACEIs cannot be tolerated, angiotensin receptor antagonists or the combination of hydralazine and nitrate derivatives may be substituted. Digoxin is effective in reducing morbidity and hospitalizations but has little effect on overall mortality. Loop diuretics control symptoms but have not been shown to affect mortality. Conversely, the RALES trial found that spironolactone improves survival in patients with advanced CHF.[159] Additionally, data exist to support the use of "triple therapy" with ACEIs, digoxin, and diuretics in preference to ACEIs used alone.[160] Over the last 10 years, β-blockers, which were previously contraindicated in patients with heart failure, became the most important component of therapy in patients with clinically stable heart failure regardless of severity. β-Blockers improve symptoms, reduce hospitalizations, and markedly prolong survival. They are the only class of medications that can significantly improve LV systolic function. This is not a class effect. Only those β-blockers should be used that have been shown in clinical studies to improve outcome. In the United States, the most widely used β-blockers in patients with heart failure include carvedilol and Toprol-XL. Doses should be initiated at low levels and gradually titrated up over weeks to months. Symptoms of heart failure may initially worsen, and other medication doses may need to be adjusted during the initial stages of β-blocker therapy.[161] The long-term benefits, however, are robust.[162,163]

Anticoagulation with warfarin (Coumadin) in patients with LV dysfunction may reduce morbidity and mortality from cardioembolic events that develop secondary to chamber enlargement and stasis of blood; however, the risks of bleeding need to be considered.[164] Anticoagulation therapy is likely to be most beneficial for patients with AF or atrial flutter or for patients in sinus rhythm with a LV ejection fraction of less than 20%.

For those patients who remain highly symptomatic, despite optimum medical management, intravenous therapy with diuretics and inotropes may need to be initiated. Some patients respond well to this treatment, and oral therapy can subsequently be resumed rapidly; other patients require long-term intravenous therapy. For the subset of patients who cannot be successfully weaned from intravenous treatment and who do not have other significant morbidities, cardiac transplantation is another therapeutic option.

Cardiac resynchronization therapy with implanted biventricular pacemakers has been recently shown to have a significant beneficial effect on morbidity and mortality in a subgroup of patients with heart failure who have wide QRS complexes in the ECG, mostly due to left bundle branch block.[165] Implantation cardioverter-defibrillators (ICDs) are also increasingly used for primary prevention of sudden death in patients with chronic heart failure whose LV ejection fraction remains below 30 to 35% despite optimum medical management.[166]

Oral Health Considerations

For well-compensated patients with heart failure, no special dental modifications are necessary unless the underlying causes for the heart failure require modifications. However, when patients suffer from uncompensated CHF, it is prudent to inquire about the patient's ability to be placed in a supine position as this may cause severe dyspnea.

▼ ARRHYTHMIA

Definition and Incidence

Abnormalities of cardiac rhythm can be broadly defined as any deviation from the normal cardiac pacemaker and conduction mechanism. Tachyarrhythmias, when the heart rate is > 100 bpm, occur as a result of increased automaticity of cardiac pacemaker cells or due to a reentrant mechanism where the electrical impulse circulates rapidly in certain areas of the heart. Bradyarrhythmias occur as a result of sinoatrial node dysfunction or conduction block at any level of the conduction system, including the AV node, His-Purkinje system, or distal branches of the left and right bundles. Bradyarrhythmias are associated with heart rates of < 60 bpm. Both tachyarrhythmias and bradyarrhythmias may be hemodynamically well tolerated in patients with normal cardiac function, or they may result in cardiovascular collapse if cardiac output is significantly compromised.

Supraventricular Tachycardia

Reentrant supraventricular tachycardias such as atrioventricular nodal reentrant tachycardia (AVNRT) occur commonly in the absence of structural heart disease and are usually well tolerated from a hemodynamic standpoint. AVNRT is the most common form where the AV node is functionally dissociated into two discrete electrical pathways.[167,168] These pathways have different refractory periods and conduction velocities, which are both prerequisites for reentry. AVNRT is usually triggered by a fortuitously timed premature atrial or ventricular impulse and therefore may be observed in settings where there is increased atrial ectopy due to anxiety or other types of sympathetic stimulation.[169] Interrupting conduction within the reentrant circuit in the AV node can terminate AVNRT. Therefore, vagal maneuvers (such as Valsalva's maneuver) or drugs that act on the AV node (such as adenosine, β-blockers, and diltiazem or verapamil) are particularly effective in terminating AVNRT. Recently, radiofrequency ablation with modification of the normally quiescent slow pathway in the AV node has been used to interrupt the reentrant circuit, thereby preventing the recurrence of the tachycardia.[170] Patients with frequent symptomatic episodes, who experience presyncope or frank syncope, or who do not wish or cannot tolerate medication therapy may be referred for this procedure.

Wolff-Parkinson-White (WPW) syndrome is characterized by the presence of an accessory pathway that enables conduction from atria to ventricles outside the normal conduction system.[171] This produces AV reentrant tachycardia, a narrow complex tachycardia with retrograde P waves on the surface ECG following each QRS complex. The surface ECG of a patient with WPW syndrome is characterized by a short P–R interval and the slurred onset of the QRS complex (called a delta wave), representing atrial-to-ventricular conduction via the accessory pathway. This may result in either orthodromic or antidromic AV reentrant tachycardia, depending on whether the reentrant rhythm conducts antegrade or retrograde through the AV node, or rapidly conducted AF with an increased ventricular response due to the rapid conduction of the accessory pathway. This may precipitate ventricular fibrillation if not promptly terminated with electrical cardioversion or intravenous procainamide.

Atrial Fibrillation

AF is the most common sustained dysrhythmia that occurs both with and without structural heart disease.[172] It represents rapid and chaotic atrial activity with an irregular and rapid ventricular response. AF can be classified as valvular as it frequently accompanies mitral stenosis or regurgitation. Nonvalvular AF may accompany a structurally normal heart (lone AF), hypertensive heart disease, cardiomyopathy, and a wide variety of other clinical conditions (Table 15). In AF, the chaotic atrial activity results in ineffective atrial contraction and in stasis of blood within the left atrium and left atrial appendage. This stasis may lead to thrombus formation and may increase the risk of embolic events, including cerebral and peripheral embolization. Embolic stroke occurs in 1.6 to about 18% of patients per year, and the risk increases with increasing age, comorbidities, and CVD.[173] The highest risk of embolic stroke is that of patients with valvular AF. In nonvalvular AF, a history of previous transient ischemic attack or stroke, age above 75, significant hypertension, systolic heart failure, and diabetes are major clinical risk factors. Frequently, younger patients with brief episodes of paroxysmal AF are treated with antiplatelet drugs such as acetylsalicylic acid because the risk of stroke is low; however, anticoagulation with warfarin is typically used in older patients and in those who have one or more of the listed high-risk characteristics.[173] A number of trials have shown that warfarin use is associated with a 45 to 82% reduction in the risk of stroke in patients with chronic AF.[174,175]

TABLE 15   Etiologies of Atrial Fibrillation

Hypertension
Rheumatic valvular disease
Coronary artery disease (including acute MI and ischemic cardiomyopathy)
Atrial septal defects
Hypertrophic cardiomyopathy
Congenital heart disease (Ebstein's disease, patent ductus arteriosus, tetralogy of Fallot)
Dilated cardiomyopathy
Alcoholic cardiomyopathy
Holiday heart syndrome
Pulmonary embolism
Pericardial disease
Chronic obstructive lung disease, cor pulmonale
Peripartum cardiomyopathy
Sleep apnea
Thyrotoxicosis
Autonomic dysfunction
Post–cardiac surgery and transplantation
Noncardiac surgery (thoracic and esophageal)
Medications (theophylline, caffeine, digitalis)
Familial
Pheochromocytoma
MI = myocardial infarction.

A wide variety of strategies have been used in the attempt to restore and maintain normal sinus rhythm, including β-blocker drugs, antiarrhythmic therapy, and electrical cardioversion.[176] Historically, chemical or electrical cardioversion has been performed after at least 3 to 4 weeks of anticoagulation with warfarin as this has been shown to reduce the risk of thromboembolism. TEE can be used to facilitate earlier cardioversion by evaluating the LA and LAA for thrombus.[177]

Whether antiarrhythmic drugs should be used to maintain sinus rhythm is controversial. Earlier studies revealed an increased risk of death due to proarrhythmia with quinidine therapy. More limited data exist on the use of newer agents, such as amiodarone, sotalol, and propafenone. However, even the newer agents are not always effective and are associated with side effects, including the risk of proarrhythmia. A newer investigational approach is the percutaneous catheter ablation of focal AF. The long-term safety and efficacy of this procedure have not been determined. It is now thought that in elderly patients with recurrent AF, a simple rate-control and anticoagulation approach (leaving the patients in AF) is at least as effective clinically as an attempt to restore and maintain sinus rhythm at all costs.[178]

Dental protocols for patients with AF have been proposed. These protocols specifically address the underlying cause of AF and the subsequent need for antibiotic prophylaxis, the need to alter dental care on the basis of the patient's anticoagulation therapy, and the use of anxiety-reducing strategies.[179]

Ventricular Tachycardia and Fibrillation

Ventricular tachycardia (VT) and ventricular fibrillation (VF) typically occur in patients with structural heart disease of the LV, such as those with CAD, various forms of dilated cardiomyopathy, and hypertrophic cardiomyopathy. Rarely, VT may occur as an idiopathic event in an individual with a structurally normal heart or may originate in the right ventricle as in the case of arrhythmogenic right ventricular dysplasia. VF may occur in the setting of acute ischemia and infarction, in dilated and hypertrophic cardiomyopathy, and as a result of a variety of drug and electrolyte effects. VF causes sudden death. The percentage of patients successfully resuscitated is very low.

Patients with sustained VT and resuscitated VF typically require a thorough evaluation for the underlying structural or functional abnormality. Prevention of subsequent episodes may be achieved by treating the underlying cause. If such a treatable cause is found, patients with a structurally normal heart and a history of clinically stable VT may undergo antiarrhythmic drug therapy trials. β-Blockers appear to be the safest and most effective class of medications for this indication.[180] Patients who had a hemodynamically unstable VT or resuscitated VF, on the other hand, typically undergo implantation of a cardioverter-defibrillator (ICD). ICDs are also frequently implanted for primary prevention in patients who never had a VT or VF event but who are at a high risk for sudden arrhythmic death. Patient populations who may be candidates for an ICD for primary prevention include those with a remote history of MI and an LV ejection fraction of 30% or less and patients with either ischemic or nonischemic cardiomyopathy and an ejection fraction of 30 to 35% despite optimum medical therapy.[181,182]

▼ PERMANENT PACEMAKERS

Permanent cardiac pacing is used in a wide variety of cardiac conditions, including symptomatic heart block and brady-cardia, brady-tachy syndrome, carotid hypersensitivity, neurocardiogenic syncope, heart failure, and hypertrophic cardiomyopathy. Single- (typically ventricular) or dual-chamber (atrial and ventricular) models are typically employed. Guidelines for the implantation of cardiac pace-makers have been established by the American College of Cardiology and the AHA joint task force on the basis of available evidence in the medical literature.[183]

Oral Health Considerations

The severity and type of a patient's arrhythmia will govern dental care considerations. In particular, patients with severe supraventricular tachycardia should only be treated after consultation with the patient's cardiologist. Patients with AF may have an associated heart murmur and be taking anticoagulant medications to prevent thromboembolic events.

Dental treatment modifications for patients with defibril-lators or pacemakers are today of little concern. According to the AHA, no antibiotic prophylaxis is indicated for patients with pacemakers or defibrillators, unless the patient presents with an acute odontogenic infection.[122] Furthermore, a most recent in vivo study suggested that modern pacemakers are not influenced by any type of dental equipment, including high-speed rotary instruments or even the proximity of ultrasonic baths.[184]

▼ SELECTED READING

Aframian DJ, Lalla RV, Peterson DE. Management of dental patients taking common hemostasis-altering medications. Oral Surg Oral Med Oral Pathol Oral Radiol Endod 2007;103 Suppl:41–5.

Baddour LM, Bettman MA, Bolger AF, et al. Nonvalvular cardiovascular device-related infections. Circulation 2003;108:2015–31.

Bardy GH, Lee KL, Mark DB, et al. Amiodarone or an implantable cardioverter-defibrillator for congestive heart failure. N Engl J Med 2005;352:225–37.

Bonow RO, Carabello BA, Chatterjee K, et al. ACC/AHA 2006 guidelines for the management of patients with valvular heart disease. J Am Coll Cardiol 2006;48:e1–148.

Brennan MT, Shariff G, Kent ML, et al. Relationship between bleeding time test and postextraction bleeding in a healthy control population. Oral Surg Oral Med Oral Pathol Oral Radiol Endod 2002;94:439–43.

Estruch R, Martínez-González MA, Corella D, et al. Effects of a Mediterranean-style diet on cardiovascular risk factors. Ann Intern Med 2006;145:1–11.

Glick M, Greenberg BL. The potential role of dentists in identifying patients' risk of experiencing coronary heart disease. J Am Dent Assoc 2005;136:1541–6.

Heart Outcomes Prevention Evaluation (HOPE) 2 Investigators. Homocysteine lowering with folic acid and B vitamins in vascular disease. N Engl J Med 2006;354:1567–77.

Lessard E, Glick M, Ahmed S, Saric M. The patient with a heart murmur: evaluation, assessment and dental considerations. J Am Dent Assoc 2005;136:347–56.

Lindholm LH, Carlberg B, Samuelsson O. Should β-blockers remain first choice in the treatment of primary hypertension? A meta-analysis. Lancet 2005;366:1545–53.

Miller TD, Redberg RF, Wackers FJT. Screening asymptomatic diabetic patients for coronary artery disease: why not? J Am Coll Cardiol 2006;48:761–4.

Owan TE, Hodge DO, Herges RM, et al. Trends in prevalence and outcome of heart failure with preserved ejection fraction. N Engl J Med 2006;355:251–9.

Ray KK, Cannon CP, McCabe CH, et al. Early and late benefits of high-dose atorvastatin in patients with acute coronary syndromes: results from the PROVE-IT – TIMI 22 trial. J Am Coll Cardiol 2005;46:1405–10.

The third report of the National Cholesterol Education Program (NCEP) Expert Panel on Detection, Evaluation, and Treatment of High Blood Cholesterol in Adults (Adult Treatment Panel III). Bethesda (MD): NCEP/National Heart, Lung, and Blood Institute/National Institutes of Health; 2002.

Thom T, Haase N, Rosamond W, et al. Heart disease and stroke statistics—2006 update: a report from the American Heart Association Statistics Committee and Stroke Statistics Subcommittee. Circulation 2006;113:e85–151.

Vasbinder CBC, Nelemans PJ, Kessels AGH, et al. Accuracy of computed tomographic angiography and magnetic resonance angiography for diagnosing renal artery stenosis. Ann Intern Med 2004;141:674–82.

Wilson W, Taubert KA, Gewitz M, et al. Prevention of infective endocarditis: guidelines from the American Heart Association‹a guideline from the American Heart Association Rheumatic Fever, Endocarditis and Kawasaki Disease Committee, Council on Cardiovascular Disease in the Young, and the Council on Clinical Cardiology, Council on Cardiovascular Surgery and Anesthesia, and the Quality of Care and Outcomes Research Interdisciplinary Working Group. JADA 2007;138(6):739–60.

For the full reference list, please refer to the accompanying CD ROM.

14

DISEASES OF THE GASTROINTESTINAL TRACT

MICHAEL A. SIEGEL, DDS, MS

This chapter is intended to review diseases affecting the gastrointestinal tract, with an emphasis on the medical aspects, the dentist's role as a primary health care professional in screening for undiagnosed conditions, and the dentist's role in monitoring patient compliance with recommended medical therapy for gastrointestinal conditions that are likely to be encountered in the general practice of dentistry. Oral health care professionals (OHCPs) are expected to recognize, diagnose, and treat oral conditions associated with gastrointestinal diseases, as well as provide dental care for afflicted individuals. To provide safe and appropriate dental care, dentists are typically concerned with the proper diagnosis of oral manifestations of gastrointestinal disorders, homeostasis, risk of infection, drug actions and interactions, the patient's ability to withstand the stress and trauma of dental procedures, and, when necessary, proper medical referral. These dental management issues are discussed, where appropriate, for each gastrointestinal disorder.

Both OHCPs and gastroenterologists have their primary focus within the alimentary canal. The common embryogenesis of the oral cavity and gastrointestinal tract is occasionally reinforced for the clinician when he or she finds heterotopic gastric mucosal cysts in the oral mucous membranes or on the tongue.[1,2] However, in addition to these relatively rare anomalies, the paths of gastroenterologists and dentists cross quite frequently in clinical practice. The digestive tract is a long muscular tube that moves food and accumulated secretions from the mouth to the anus. As ingested food is slowly propelled through this tract, the gut assimilates calories and nutrients that are essential for the establishment and maintenance of normal bodily functions. Protein, fats, carbohydrates, vitamins, minerals, water, and orally ingested drugs (prescription and nonprescription) are digested in this tract. This digestive process depends on the hydrolysis of large nonabsorbable molecules into smaller absorbable molecules through secreted enzymes and the absorption of substances through the epithelial lining of the digestive tract. From there, digested substances are transported by blood vessels and lymphatic channels through the body. The remaining contents of undigested food, typically cellulose fiber, are excreted out of the digestive tract through the rectum and anus. The digestion and absorption of nutrient materials depend on (1) an optimal hydrogen ion concentration (pH) in the gut; (2) the presence of conjugated bile salts; (3) adequate concentrations of enzymes to split fats, proteins, and carbohydrates; and (4) adequate intestinal mobility.

Some of the foods entering the blood from the digestive tract can be used by cells without being altered. However, the majority of the absorbed food passes to special organs, where it is changed into new substances that are needed by cells. One such special organ is the liver, where this intermediate metabolism takes place. Additionally, the gastrointestinal tract is a primary route for drug administration, absorption, biotransformation, detoxification, and excretion. Many dental patients require drug therapy in which pharmacokinetic parameters may be altered by gastrointestinal and hepatobiliary dysfunction. Consequently, OHCPs must have a comprehensive understanding of the gastrointestinal system and of how normal and abnormal function may affect the oral health care of patients.

The digestive system is composed of the esophagus, stomach, small intestine, and large intestine. Each of these components performs specific functions as ingested substances move through the different anatomic areas. Additionally, the exocrine functions of the pancreas, liver, and gallbladder combine to complete the assimilation of dietary calories and nutrients.

This chapter is organized such that disorders are presented under the following anatomic divisions: esophagus, stomach, small intestine, large intestine, and hepatobiliary tree. A final section on gastrointestinal syndromes introduces disorders that affect both the oral cavity and the gastrointestinal tract but that are not primarily of oral or gastrointestinal etiology.

▼ DISEASES OF THE UPPER DIGESTIVE TRACT

Gastroesophageal Reflux Disease

MEDICAL ASPECTS

Gastroesophageal reflux disease (GERD) is one of the most commonly occurring diseases affecting the upper gastrointestinal tract. The incidence of GERD is increasing in the developed world; upwards of 10% of the population experience heartburn daily. Symptoms can range from mild to severe. There is no difference between the percentage of men and the percentage of women who are affected by GERD. GERD is a disease that has a significant effect on activities of daily living as well as an economic effect on individuals and society.

During gastroesophageal reflux, gastric contents (chyme) passively move up from the stomach into the esophagus.

Although this can occur normally, it may be attributed to GERD if it is associated with symptoms. GERD is often considered a syndrome because it can present with a wide variety of symptoms. Patients may experience mild symptoms with an esophagus that appears to be clinically normal, or they may have severe symptoms with surface abnormalities that can be detected with an endoscope. A presumptive diagnosis of GERD may be made for any symptomatic condition that is the result of gastric contents moving into the esophagus. Functional bowel disease is a syndrome with similar symptoms and may mimic GERD; it is often misdiagnosed as GERD.

Heartburn is the cardinal symptom of GERD and is defined as a sensation of burning or heat that spreads upward from the epigastrium to the neck.[3] Although symptoms of GERD can be quite varied, they are primarily symptoms that are associated with the sequelae of mucosal injury. These resultant injuries include esophagitis, esophageal ulceration, stricture, and dysplasia. Chest pain is another important symptom that is related to disorders of the esophagus. Chest pain can mimic the symptoms of an acute cardiovascular disorder and is often the impetus for patients seeking medical care. Dysphagia is also a common presenting complaint that may serve to prompt the dentist to refer the patient to the patient's physician. Several studies have shown that a number of airway problems that were previously thought to be idiopathic, such as laryngitis, chronic cough, hoarseness, and asthma, are, in fact, the result of microaspiration of refluxate into the airway.[4,5] Alternatively, these symptoms may also arise from disorders of the upper or lower respiratory tracts. GERD complications include premalignant and malignant conditions of the esophagus.

Barrett's esophagus is a variant of GERD in which normal squamous epithelium is replaced by columnar epithelium.[6] Patients with this phenomenon show an increased incidence of adenocarcinoma. This condition may increase the incidence of carcinoma by as much as 10%.[7] However, it has become clear that the majority of patients with Barrett's esophagus die from causes not related to adenocarcinoma of the esophagus.[8] The major reason to evaluate patients with chronic symptoms of GERD is to recognize Barrett's esophagus. The factors of gender, race, and age can be used to determine the threshold for endoscopy in patients with GERD to screen for the presence of Barrett's esophagus. The highest yield of Barrett's esophagus would be expected in white men with chronic symptoms of GERD. However, the specific criteria to select patients to screen for Barrett's esophagus are not yet defined.[9]

The relaxation of the lower esophageal sphincter for the purpose of relieving pressure in the stomach (from gas and the ingestion of food) is called the "burp" mechanism. This phenomenon is a normal process and occurs only when a person is in an erect posture; gastric contents are thereby prevented from flowing into the esophagus and possibly being aspirated. The gastroesophageal junction, which prevents the regurgitation (retrograde or upward flow) of gastric contents, is composed of an internal lower esophageal sphincter. External pressure on the junction by the diaphragm also assists in this function. When this barrier fails, gastric contents may make their way into the esophagus and cause symptoms. The cause of lower esophageal sphincter incompetence is unknown; however, it does not appear to be mechanical. Hiatal hernia was historically recognized as a cause of GERD, but there is no correlation between sphincter pressure and the presence of a hiatal hernia, which leads to the widely accepted position that GERD is not caused by hiatal hernia. Surgery, scleroderma, and drugs such as anticholinergics, cardiac vasoconstrictors, and nicotine can also cause an incompetent sphincter. Estrogen-progesterone combinations used in contraceptives and during pregnancy also have been shown to decrease sphincter pressures.

Symptoms occur when refluxate proceeds through the junction. The severity of the symptoms depends on the amount of acid in the refluxate, the speed with which the esophagus can clear the refluxate, and the presence of buffering agents, such as swallowed saliva. An insufficient amount of alkaline fluid prohibits the esophagus from properly buffering the acid that has moved up from the stomach. Patients who smoke, take certain drugs, have had head and neck radiation, or suffer from diseases such a Sjögren's syndrome often do not produce enough saliva to protect the esophagus from the acid in the refluxate. Increased abdominal pressure as a result of obesity, pregnancy, or a large meal may predispose patients to gastric content reflux. Moving into or out of various positions (eg, lying down too soon after eating) will also promote reflux.

MEDICAL MANAGEMENT

Significant success in preventing or reducing the symptoms of GERD is seen with lifestyle modification. Weight loss reduces the pressure difference between the abdomen and the thorax, thereby reducing reflux. Smoking cessation will increase the production of saliva and therefore counteract the symptoms of GERD. Fatty meals slow down gastric emptying and produce distention and reflux. An increase in the fat content of meals may be an important factor in explaining the increase of reflux in the Western world in recent years. Eating large meals and reclining too soon after meals also predispose individuals to reflux disease. Sleeping with the head of the bed elevated may help empty the esophagus of any refluxate and may prevent symptoms.

Since the mid-1970s, H_2 receptor antagonists have been used to treat GERD and ulcer disease. In patients with GERD, H_2 receptor antagonists improve the symptoms of heartburn and regurgitation and heal mild to moderate esophagitis. Symptoms have been eliminated in up to 50% of patients by twice-a-day prescription dosages of H_2 receptor antagonists. Approximately 50% of patients require higher or more frequent doses to promote the healing of esophagitis. Only about 25% of patients will remain in remission while taking these agents only.

Proton pump inhibitors (PPIs) such as omeprazole and (more recently) lansoprazole have been found to heal erosive esophagitis more efficaciously than do H_2 receptor antagonists. PPIs provide not only symptomatic relief but also resolution of signs, including those that involve significant ulcers and/or esophageal damage.[10] Studies have shown that PPI therapy can provide complete endoscopic mucosal healing of esophagitis at 6 to 8 weeks in 75 to 100% of cases. Daily PPI treatment provides the best long-term reduction of symptoms for patients with moderate to severe esophagitis. Remission for as long as 5 years has been seen.

Promotility drugs are effective in the treatment of mild to moderately symptomatic GERD. These drugs increase lower esophageal sphincter pressure (which helps decrease acid reflux) and improve the movement of food from the stomach. They decrease heartburn symptoms, especially at night, by improving the clearance of acid from the esophagus. Cisapride is the most effective of the promotility agents.[10]

During the last decade, a significant change has been seen in the role of surgery for the treatment of GERD. Once relatively rare and reserved for patients who had failed every form of medical treatment, antireflux operations are now common and are considered part of the regular armamentarium by those who treat this disease.[11] Patients with a good initial response to medical therapy but who have severe functional and anatomic abnormalities of the gastroesophageal junction are the ones who are most commonly treated with surgery.

ORAL HEALTH CONSIDERATIONS

Patients who experience GERD complain of dysgeusia (foul taste), dental sensitivity related to hot or cold stimuli, dental erosion, and/or pulpitis. Dental thermal sensitivity is generally due to erosion of enamel by gastric acid. Study of esophageal sphincter pressure, sphincter length, and esophageal motility in patients with dental erosion suggests that poor esophageal motility may be a risk factor in regurgitation erosion.[12] Erosion of enamel leads to exposed dentin and thermal sensitivity. On occasion, if the erosion is severe, irreversible pulpal (nerve) damage may result that requires root canal therapy. No relationship between GERD and changes in the oral cavity can be established through the use of saliva tests. However, histopathologic morphometric analysis of the palatal mucosa in patients with GERD may disclose an association with microscopic alteration manifesting as epithelial atrophy and increased fibroblast number.[13] Mild baking soda mouthrinses may be swished and expectorated to minimize dysgeusia due to acid reflux. Dental management should provide topical fluoride applications using custom-made occlusive tray delivery in order to ensure optimal dental mineralization and reduction of thermal sensitivity. The dentist can restore tooth structure destroyed by gastric acid erosion in order to provide comfort and esthetics and to minimize further hard tissue damage. It is preferable to institute oral preventive measures at the earliest possible time in order to minimize the need for extensive dental restoration.

Medical therapy can affect the dental management of patients with GERD in a number of ways. Patients taking cimetidine (Tagament) or other H_2 receptor antagonists may experience a toxic reaction to lidocaine (or other amide local anesthetics) if the anesthetic is injected intravascularly.[14] Cimetidine also has been shown to inhibit the absorption and, therefore, the blood concentration of azole antifungal drugs such as ketaconazole via the potent inhibition of the cytochrome P-450 3A4 enzyme system. Soft tissue changes such as esophageal stricture and fibrosis may complicate intubation if the patient requires general anesthesia for an oral maxillofacial procedure. Oral mucosal changes are minimal; however, erythema and mucosal atrophy may be present as a result of chronic exposure of tissues to acid. Mild sodium bicarbonate rinses may again be useful if mild signs of stomatitis are present.

H$_2$ receptor antagonists may also cause central nervous system effects in a continuum from fatigue and lethargy to confusion, delirium, and seizures. These effects are dose dependent; thus, they may be seen more commonly in elderly persons or in those with impaired kidney or liver function.

Hiatal Hernia

MEDICAL ASPECTS

The esophagus passes through the diaphragmatic hiatus and into the stomach just inferior to the diaphragm. The hiatus causes an anatomic narrowing of the opening into the stomach and thus helps prevent reflux of stomach contents into the esophagus. Some patients have a weakened or enlarged hiatus, perhaps due to hereditary factors. It may also be caused by obesity, exercising (eg, weight lifting), or chronic straining when passing stools. When a weakened or enlarged hiatus occurs, a portion of the stomach herniates into the chest cavity through this enlarged hole, resulting in a hiatal hernia. Hiatal hernias are quite common; occurrence rates of between 20 and 60% have been reported in the medical literature.[3] The incidence of hiatal hernia increases with age, although the condition is also seen in infants and children. Because the diaphragm separates the thorax from the abdomen, symptoms of hiatal hernia often include chest pain, which may radiate in patterns similar to those of myocardial infarction pain. If the hiatal hernia is small, there may be no symptoms. On the other hand, if the area of the hiatus is very weak, the function of preventing reflux may be compromised, resulting in the entry of acidic digestive juices into the esophagus.

Hiatal hernias are classified into three major types.[3] The sliding type is the most common. In this type, the herniated portion of the stomach slides back and forth through the diaphragm into the chest. These hernias are normally small and often present with minimal (if any) symptoms. In the fixed type of hiatal hernia, the upper part of the stomach is fixed through the diaphragm into the chest. There may be few symptoms with this type as well. However, the potential for problems in the esophagus increases. The complicated type is the most serious and least common form of hiatal hernia. This form includes a variety of herniation patterns of the stomach, including those in which the entire stomach moves into the chest. The likelihood of significant medical problems with this type is high; its treatment requires surgery.

Infants with hiatal hernia usually regurgitate bloodstained food and may also have difficulty in breathing and swallowing. Adult patients with hiatal hernia may experience chronic acid reflux into the esophagus. Chronic gastrointestinal reflux can erode the esophageal lining, causing bleeding, which may lead to anemia. Additionally, chronic esophageal inflammation may produce scarring, resulting in esophageal narrowing. This narrowing causes dysphagia, and because food does not pass easily into the stomach, patients experience an uncomfortable feeling of fullness or "bloating." Adults typically present with heartburn that is exacerbated when bending forward or lying down. The pain may spread to the jaw and down the arms, similar to an attack of angina pectoris. Other symptoms include hiccups, a dry cough, and an increase in the contractile force of the heart. In contrast to abdominal hernias, hiatal hernias have no outward physical signs. Diagnosis is made through a combination of endoscopy and contrast radiography.

MEDICAL MANAGEMENT

Defects present at birth may sometimes correct themselves. Until this occurs, however, the infant should sleep in a crib with the head raised and be given an altered diet consisting of food that has a thicker-than-normal consistency. With adults, anything that will increase abdominal pressure and cause reflux, such as bending, abdominal exercises, and tight belts and girdles, should be avoided. Because obesity increases intra-abdominal pressure, weight loss may be recommended to relieve symptoms. Sleeping with the head elevated will also prevent the symptoms of hiatal hernia. Antacids help relieve heartburn by neutralizing stomach acids. H$_2$ receptor antagonists are effective in inhibiting the action of histamine on parietal cells, which reduces the production of gastric acids.[10] Patients should also eat smaller and more frequent meals and should have their main meal at lunchtime. This should be followed by a light supper, with nothing being consumed within 2 to 3 hours of bedtime. Foods and habits that increase the reflux of acid should be avoided or significantly reduced. These foods or habits include nicotine (tobacco products), alcohol, caffeine, chocolate, fatty foods, and peppermint or spearmint oil flavorings.

Drug therapy usually allows patients to avoid all symptoms of hiatal hernia without significant inconvenience. The disadvantage to this approach is that many patients object to taking daily medications for the rest of their lives or find the process too onerous to carry out. When conservative medical measures fail to control the condition, the hernia is surgically corrected. However, surgical correction is complex, and nonsurgical remedies are preferable.[15,16] Surgery is currently considered to be a treatment of last resort, and some authors argue that surgery is never indicated for a hiatal hernia. Surgical access is gained either through the chest or through the abdomen. These approaches carry high risks of operative and perioperative morbidity. Recent surgical advances have made it possible to do the repair laparoscopically.[15]

ORAL HEALTH CONSIDERATIONS

If a hiatal hernia is treated with medications that cause xerostomia (dry mouth), the dose or drug type may need to be altered by the patient's physician. Various treatment modalities for dry mouth, such as artificial saliva, alcohol-free mouthwashes, or increased fluid intake, may need to be prescribed. Class V caries, or root caries, are sequelae of dry mouth, even in patients who have been relatively free of caries prior to developing the disease. If reflux into the oral cavity is present, oral manifestations that are the same as those of GERD may be present.

▼ DISEASES OF THE LOWER DIGESTIVE TRACT

Disorders of the Stomach

The stomach serves primarily as a secretory organ and as a reservoir. The stomach secretes acid, mucus, pepsinogen, and intrinsic factor. The secreted hydrochloric acid is essential for killing swallowed bacteria while the mucus helps coat and lubricate the stomach's lining epithelium in order to propel the ingested contents through the digestive system. Pepsinogen is a proteolytic enzyme that helps digest protein and intrinsic factor, a glycoprotein that permits the adequate absorption of dietary vitamin B_{12}. The stomach collects food that is often ingested in bursts and then slowly empties the chyme—the semifluid mass of partly digested food—into the duodenum over time.

Peptic Ulcer Disease

Peptic ulcer disease is a common benign (nonmalignant) ulceration of the epithelial lining of the stomach (gastric ulcer) or duodenum (duodenal ulcer). When patients or physicians refer to ulcers or ulcer disease, they are usually referring to a duodenal or gastric ulcer. About 6% of patients attending a dentist office will have peptic ulcer disease.[17,18] Since peptic ulcer disease includes both gastric (stomach) ulcers and duodenal ulcers, a general discussion of peptic ulcer disease is presented first, followed by specific information on gastric and duodenal ulcers, under the corresponding anatomic region.

Peptic ulcer disease represents a serious medical problem largely because of its frequency; there are approximately 500,000 new cases and 4,000,000 recurrences each year in the United States. The estimated annual direct cost for treatment of patients with ulcer disease is approximately $8 billion to $10 billion (US). It is likely that the growing geriatric population in the United States, coupled with the increasing use of nonsteroidal anti-inflammatory drugs (NSAIDs) that have inherent damaging effects on the gastroduodenal mucosa, will contribute to the costs of this disease.[19,20]

Data indicate that the lifetime prevalence of peptic ulcers ranges from 11 to 14% for men and 8 to 11% for women. The 1-year point prevalence of active gastric and duodenal ulcers in the United States is about 1.8%.[17–20] Genetic factors appear to play a role in the pathogenesis of ulcers. The concordance for peptic ulcers among identical twins is approximately 50%. In first-degree relatives of ulcer patients, the lifetime prevalence of developing ulcers is about threefold greater than that in the general population.[17–20]

Within the last decade, it has become accepted that gastric ulcers primarily result from altered mucosal defenses, whereas duodenal ulcers are associated with increased acid production. It has become clear that *Helicobacter pylori* plays a vital role in peptic ulcer development at both sites. A complex relationship exits between host defense mechanisms, the presence of elevated acid, pepsin levels, and *H. pylori*. The incidence of duodenal ulcers also increases in cigarette smokers, patients with chronic renal disease, and alcoholics. *H. pylori* is observed in the gastric mucosa in 90 to 100% of patients with duodenal ulcers and 70 to 90% of patients with gastric ulcers. Consequently, it has been proposed that the bacteria may be the cause of both the gastritis and the reduced mucosal resistance that leads to ulcer formation in the stomach.[18] It is noteworthy that healing of peptic ulcers of either the stomach or duodenum is usually facilitated by specific antimicrobial treatment and by the elimination of this bacterium.[19]

Many patients with duodenal ulcers have demonstrable hyperacidity, and it is thought that this is the dominant factor in the development of ulcer disease. Concomitant inflammation and infection with *H. pylori* are noted in the gastric antrum in more than 80% of cases of duodenal ulcers. In gastric ulcers, however, the relative importance of the two major factors of acid amounts and mucosal resistance is reversed. Typically, the concentration of gastric acid is normal or reduced, and prior injury (mucosal) from other causes appears to be a prerequisite for the development of gastric ulcers. Most patients with the disease have recurrent pain and consult their physician periodically for relief of symptoms and to prevent recurrence. About 10 to 20% of these patients have a life-threatening complication (ie, hemorrhage, perforation, or obstruction).[17,18,20] Failure to recognize and manage these patients properly on these occasions can have grave consequences. Since about 6% of the patients attending a dental office will have a peptic ulcer, it is essential that dentists (1) recognize the morbidity associated with peptic ulcers and the symptoms associated with undiagnosed or poorly managed peptic ulcer disease and (2) make a referral to the primary care physician or gastroenterologist when these symptoms are recognized.

It is important to discuss gastric and duodenal ulcers separately because each has implications for dentists and the patients they treat.

MEDICAL ASPECTS

Gastric ulcers are only one-tenth to one-fourth as frequent as duodenal ulcers. They are also more common in lower socioeconomic groups. Gastric ulcers occur more often after 50 years of age and are seen at a male to female ratio of 3:1. Gastric ulcers are generally of more concern because approximately 3 to 8% of gastric ulcers represent malignant ulceration of the gastric mucosa.[17–21] Therefore, accurate diagnosis requires multiple biopsies and brush specimens for cytologic examination. These additional diagnostic tests are often performed by a gastroenterologist. In general, the diagnostic procedures are the same as those performed in cases of duodenal ulcers, except that the diagnosis is more urgent and additional diagnostic studies other than gastroscopy are warranted. It is essential to ascertain gastric acidity levels with ulcers of the stomach because a stomach ulcer in the presence of histamine-fast achlorhydria has a very high chance of being a malignant ulcer rather than a peptic ulcer.

Patients with gastric ulcers often present with epigastric pain radiating to the back. In contrast to the symptoms of duodenal ulcers, the pain is aggravated by food. The management and the treatment of gastric ulcers are similar to those of duodenal ulcers, except that gastric ulcers are usually diagnosed and treated more vigorously. Follow-up studies to document the healing process are essential for gastric ulcers. Nevertheless, the standard medical treatment of gastric ulcers involves antacid compounds, antibiotics to eradicate *H. pylori*, H_2 blocking agents, and other protective drugs. Additional information about peptic ulcer disease and management in the dental office is presented in the following section on duodenal ulcers.

Disorders of the Intestines

The small intestine comprises the duodenum, jejunum, and ileum. The duodenum is the principal site of digestion and absorption. When chyme enters the duodenum, it stimulates the pancreas to secrete sodium bicarbonate (to neutralize the gastric acid) and to secrete digestive enzymes for normal digestion of food. Additionally, chyme in the duodenum stimulates the gallbladder to discharge stored bile through the common bile duct. Vitamin B_{12} in the presence of intrinsic factor is absorbed in the distal small intestine (ileum). The bile acids that promote fat absorption in the duodenum are themselves also reabsorbed in the small bowel, returned to the liver, and resecreted into the bile. The motor activity of the small intestine propels the chyme forward to the large intestine. The major role of the large intestine is to receive the ileal effluent, absorb most of the water and salt, and thus produce solid feces.

Duodenal Ulcer Disease
MEDICAL ASPECTS

A duodenal ulcer represents a break through the mucosa into the submucosa or deeper. The base of the ulcer is necrotic tissue consisting of pus and fibrin. When the ulcer erodes into an adjacent blood vessel, there is hemorrhage. If erosion continues through the serous outer layer of the duodenum, adjacent organs or perforation into the peritoneal cavity occurs. When conditions are favorable, the ulcer heals, with granulation tissue and new epithelium. If the ulcer is present for prolonged periods, it becomes associated with scar tissue and possible deformity.

The incidence of duodenal ulcer is thought to be declining, but it is still a common disorder developing in about 10% of the US population. Of all peptic ulcers, 80 to 85% are duodenal, and duodenal ulcers occur at a male to female ratio of 4:1. The most common primary cause is *H. pylori* infection, but NSAID use can also be an associated etiologic factor. Less commonly, factors such as stress, exogenous glucocorticosteroids, parathyroid disease, malignant carcinoid, cirrhosis, gastrinoma of the pancreas (Zollinger-Ellison disease), polycythema vera, and chronic lung disease have been associated with duodenal ulcers.[17–21] The ulceration is usually located in the first part of the duodenum because the acidic chyme ordinarily becomes alkaline after pancreatic secretions enter the intestines in the second part of the duodenum.

The most common symptom of an uncomplicated ulcer is epigastric pain. The pain is often perceived as a burning or gnawing sensation sometimes associated with nausea and vomiting and usually occurs when the stomach is empty or when not enough of a meal remains in the stomach to adequately buffer the acid stimulated by the meal. Therefore, the pain often begins 1 or more hours after eating and when the patient is asleep. The pain is characteristically relieved within a few minutes by buffering or diluting the gastric acid with ingestion of an antacid, milk, food, or even water. Once an individual has had a duodenal ulcer, the chance of recurrence is high. Frequently, these attacks will occur with a change of season, especially in spring or autumn. When an ulcer perforates and hemorrhages, the patient often vomits gross blood. When the blood interacts with acid, it can appear as coffee grounds. Also, the stools can appear black or tar-like or may sometimes contain gross blood. The blood loss can lead to iron deficiency anemia, and if the blood loss is acute, the patient may be weak, lightheaded, and short of breath.

Physical examination is usually of little use in the diagnosis of duodenal ulcers. The early diagnostic cues are based on the history of a periodic pain pattern. Duodenal ulcers usually feel better postprandially, and the pain of gastric ulcers is frequently exacerbated by meals. The mainstay of the diagnosis of a duodenal ulcer is an upper gastrointestinal radiologic examination, which will demonstrate the presence of an ulcer in up to 85% of patients. In this procedure, the patient swallows a barium salt that outlines the lumen and mucosal surface of the gastrointestinal tract and thereby demonstrates any disruption of the mucosal surface. Endoscopy is an acceptable and sometimes preferable means of diagnosis. If the ulceration is too superficial to be detected by a gastrointestinal radiologic examination or if a gastric ulcer with the possibility of malignancy is suspected, endoscopy is recommended.[21] The presence of *H. pylori* can be demonstrated by biopsy if endoscopy is used. Serologic tests and tests that detect the presence of labeled carbon dioxide in the breath after oral administration of labeled urea are available.[18]

In cases of Zollinger-Ellison syndrome caused by a gastrinoma of the pancreas, specific determination of the etiology is necessary because this disease is treatable and is particularly severe, causing multiple ulcers and debilitating diarrhea. The tumor of Zollinger-Ellison syndrome secretes gastrin, a potent acid producer, and the diagnosis is made on the basis of extremely high levels of gastric acid and elevated levels of serum gastrin.[20] The usual laboratory tests include a complete blood count for detecting anemia and leukocytosis, an examination of the stool for occult blood, and a serum calcium test for detecting an occasional elevation from an associated hyperparathyroidism or endocrine tumors with Zollinger-Ellison syndrome.

MEDICAL MANAGEMENT

In the absence of complications such as massive bleeding, obstruction due to scarring, and perforation, medical rather than surgical treatment is preferred. Obviously, foods that cause discomfort to the patient should be avoided. Substances or drugs that have potent acidogenic properties with little ability to neutralize acid should be avoided; among these are alcohol, tobacco, aspirin, and NSAIDs. If NSAIDs cannot be avoided, the patient should also be treated with misoprostol. Attempts to eradicate *H. pylori* are necessary in all patients with a peptic ulcer in which the organism can be demonstrated. Bismuth, metronidazole, amoxicillin, and tetracycline have been shown to be effective.[17–21] In addition to the drugs used to eliminate *H. pylori*, medical treatment involves the following six other classes of drugs: (1) sedatives to reduce mental stress if anxiety is thought to be etiologic; (2) antacids to neutralize acid; (3) drugs that act by covering and protecting the ulcer; (4) anticholinergic drugs to decrease the production of acid by the gastric mucosa; (5) histamine H_2 receptor antagonists (cimetidine, famotidine, nizatidine, or ranitidine), which block the action of histamine on the gastric parietal cells, thus reducing food-stimulated acid secretion up to 75%; and (6) omeprazole, which also suppresses gastric acid secretion but which has a different mechanism of action from that of anticholinergics or H_2 receptor antagonists. Antacids and dietary changes are the mainstays of therapy. Anticholinergics are sometimes prescribed, particularly for reducing acid production at night. However, limited effectiveness and side effects such as mouth dryness make anticholinergics less attractive than histamine H_2 receptor antagonists. In most patients, the pain is controlled within 1 week, and most ulcers heal by the sixth week. Intractable symptoms or complicated duodenal ulcers may require surgery.[17,20]

ORAL HEALTH CONSIDERATIONS

If a patient presents with symptoms of epigastric pain, as described previously, the dentist should refer this person to the primary care physician for diagnostic workup. Oral manifestations of peptic ulcer disease are rare unless there is severe anemia from gastrointestinal bleeding or persistent regurgitation of gastric acid as a result of pyloric stenosis that leads to dental erosion, typically of the palatal aspect of the maxillary teeth. Vascular malformations of the lip have been reported and range from a very small macule to a large venous pool.[22,23] *H. pylori* has been islolated from dental plaque implicating the oral cavity as a potential source of this organism which is responsible for both peptic ulcer disease and gastric cancer.[24] Oral health status may play a role in peptic ulcer disease of the stomach as low salivary secretion may contribute to the decrease in efficacy of *H. pylori* eradication from the stomach in some patients treated with certain drug regimens.[25]

Aggravation of the peptic ulcer disease might be minimized by avoidance of actions that increase the production of acid. Thus, lengthy dental procedures should be avoided or spread out over shorter appointments to minimize stress. To avoid aspirations, patients should not be left in a supine or subsupine position for lengthy periods during dental appointments. Dentists should avoid administering drugs that exacerbate ulceration and cause gastrointestinal distress such as aspirin and other NSAIDs. Instead, acetaminophen products should be recommended. Additionally, because many of the antacids contain calcium, magnesium, and aluminum salts that bind antibiotics, such as erythromycin and tetracycline, dentists should remember that administering one of these drugs within 1 hour of antacid therapy may decrease the absorption of the antibiotic as much as 75 to 85%. Consequently, erythromycin and tetracycline should be taken 1 hour before or 2 hours after ingestion of antacids. Exogenous steroid administration is likely to exacerbate the ulcer because of the increased production of acid caused by the steroid and should be avoided. Although it is generally good policy to prescribe penicillin V instead of penicillin G (because of the destruction of penicillin G by gastric acid), it is essential with patients who have peptic ulcers.[26]

Hyposalivation and dry mouth (xerostomia) are common complaints in patients taking anticholinergic drugs. Patients who wear either complete or partial dentures are particularly troubled by oral dryness. Denture adhesives and artificial saliva may aid in the retention of their dental prostheses. Dentate patients are at an increased risk of dental caries if the hyposalivation is prolonged or if the patient places sugar-containing candies or antacids into the mouth in an effort to stimulate saliva flow. In these cases, dental management is prudent to ensure that appropriate preventive measures are instituted. Medical management of peptic ulcer disease often includes the use of medications that may cause xerostomia. If the patient specifically complains of dry mouth, it may be possible to alter the specific drug type or dosage in consultation with the patient's physician. Various therapeutic modalities for dry mouth are available, such as artificial saliva, alcohol-free mouthrinses, or increased fluid intake. Class V (root) caries are sequelae of dry mouth, even in patients who have been relatively caries free prior to the disease. Commonly used sialogogues, such as pilocarpine or cevimeline, may be contraindicated due to their parasympathomimetic action. If reflux into the oral cavity is present, referral to the dentist for restorative dental therapy is indicated. [14,27]

Prior to extensive oral surgical or periodontal procedures, physicians should be consulted in order to ascertain the patient's serology, especially if the patient has had a history of ulcer perforation and subsequent hemorrhage resulting in anemia. Delayed healing and risk of bacterial infection, particularly anaerobic bacterial infection due to tissue hypoxia, and the potentially grave side effects of respiratory depression induced by narcotic analgesics are examples of such associated oral surgical risks in the chronically anemic gastrointestinal patient. Cimetidine and rantidine, drugs commonly prescribed for duodenal ulcer patients, have occasionally been associated with thrombocytopenia and may compete with antibiotics or antifungal medications.[14]

Inflammatory Bowel Disease

Inflammatory bowel disease (IBD) is a general classification of inflammatory processes that affect the large and small intestines. Ulcerative colitis and Crohn's disease together make up IBD. Since many other intestinal diseases with known etiologies also have an inflammatory basis, it has been suggested that Crohn's disease and ulcerative colitis should more appropriately be designated as idiopathic IBD. Ulcerative colitis involves the mucosa and submucosa of the colon. Crohn's disease or regional enteritis is an inflammatory condition involving all layers of the gut. The precise etiology and pathogenesis of ulcerative colitis and Crohn's disease are unknown, and the two diseases share many features. Accordingly, the diagnostic separation of these two disorders often depends on the results of the radiographic, endoscopic, and histologic examinations. The two conditions are presented separately in this chapter since the management and prognosis of each may be different.

The medical and dental literature is replete with articles describing extra-abdominal and oral signs of IBDs, including pyostomatitis vegetans, chronic stomatitis, aphthous ulcerations, cobblestone appearance of the oral mucosa, oral epithelial tags and folds, gingivitis, persistent lip swelling, lichenoid mucosal reactions, granulomatous inflammation of minor salivary gland ducts, candidiasis, and angular cheilitis.[28–39] Current dental literature focuses on the oral status of IBD patients with regard to the potential use of thalidomide against antitumor necrosis factor α for the treatment of recalcitrant oral granulomatous lesions, caries rate, salivary antimicrobial proteins, and infections of bacterial and fungal origins.[40–46] In fact, it is accepted that oral manifestations of IBD may precede the onset of intestinal radiographic lesions by as much as 1 year or more.[33,47] Both diseases are of interest to the dentist because of their associated oral findings and the impact of their medical management, particularly the use of glucocorticosteroids on dental management.

Once IBD is established, patients may suffer episodic acute attacks during the chronic disease progression. As a result, the patient is likely to suffer from disabling disease for decades. The annual incidence of IBD in the United States ranges from 3.9 to 10 new cases per 100,000 persons. Incidence rates for both diseases are higher in urban areas than in rural areas. Crohn's disease occurs less frequently than ulcerative colitis, but both are slightly on the rise.[17–21,48] Overall, both diseases show three peak prevalence rates. The first and highest peak occurs between the ages of 20 and 24 years, the second at ages 40 to 44 years, and the third at ages 60 to 64 years. By the age 60 years, the incidence of ulcerative colitis far exceeds that of Crohn's disease. Northern European and English women appear to have a 30% increased risk of developing ulcerative colitis or Crohn's disease. IBD more frequently affects Caucasians, and Ashkenazi Jews, especially those originating in Middle Europe, Poland, or Russia, exhibit a particularly high IBD risk.[17–21]

Ulcerative Colitis

MEDICAL ASPECTS

The inflammation in ulcerative colitis may affect all or part of the large intestine. Macroscopically, the mucosa may have a granular appearance if the disease is mild. When fulminant, the disease may include stripping of the mucosa, with areas of sloughing, ulceration, and bleeding. Ulcerative colitis remains a disease of unknown etiology. Despite intense interest in possible bacterial, viral, immunologic, and psychological factors, there has been no firm etiology established. Although much has been written about psychological factors associated with IBD, most gastroenterologists no longer accept the idea that the disease is primarily a psychiatric disorder. Rather, the frequent psychiatric problems experienced by patients are a result of the disease, not the cause of it. The most likely explanation of the evidence involves an autoimmune reaction, with sensitization and destruction of the colonic mucosa in the setting of abnormal immunologic regulation. As the superficial mucosal lesions enlarge, they may be perpetuated by secondary bacterial invasion.[17–21]

The hallmark of ulcerative colitis is rectal bleeding and diarrhea. The frequency of bowel movements and the amount of blood present reflect the activity of the disease. Typically, the diarrhea is severe, possibly five to eight bowel movements in 24 hours. Patients usually complain of pain that is in both abdominal quadrants and that is crampy in nature and exacerbated prior to bowel movement. Along with the change in the pattern of bowel movements, the patient may have nocturnal diarrhea. Extraintestinal manifestations may be prominent. Erythema nodosum, characterized by red swollen nodules that are usually on the thighs and legs, may be present. Eye changes such as episcleritis, uveitis, corneal ulcers, and retinitis may cause pain and photophobia. Joint symptoms occur in up to 20% of patients with the disease, usually affecting the ankles, knees, and wrists. Perhaps the most pernicious complication of ulcerative colitis is liver disease. Although other extraintestinal manifestations usually undergo remission with control of the colon inflammation, liver disease may continue, and the dentist must recognize this risk.[17–21] Anemia is commonly associated with ulcerative colitis. It is most likely caused by blood loss and is typically a microcytic hypochromic anemia of iron deficiency. Leukocytosis occurs in active disease and is usually associated with intra-abdominal abscess. Electrolyte imbalances, hypoalbuminemia, and low serum magnesium and potassium levels may occur because of the severe diarrhea.[17–21]

MEDICAL MANAGEMENT

Diagnosis of ulcerative colitis is made on the basis of careful history, physical examination, gastrointestinal radiography, and endoscopy, which involves direct visualization of the intestinal mucosa. Most important is the sigmoidoscopic examination, which usually reveals the characteristic picture of multiple tiny mucosal ulcers covered by blood and pus. Lacking any specific markers, the diagnosis of ulcerative colitis is essentially one of exclusion.[20]

The therapy for ulcerative colitis is aimed at reducing the inflammation and correcting the effects of the disease. Sulfasalazine is used to initiate and maintain a remission in ulcerative colitis. Its active moiety, 5-aminosalicylate, has a direct anti-inflammatory effect on intestinal tissues without altering the colon flora. Corticosteroids and corticotropin (adrenocorticotropic hormone [ACTH]) are used in patients who have not responded satisfactorily to sulfasalazine. They are administered in high doses (eg, 40 to 60 mg of oral prednisone daily initially and then maintenance doses of 10 to 20 mg of prednisone daily). Immunosuppressive agents such as azathioprine, cyclosporine, and mercaptopurine are being used, with varying results. Because of the risk of hematologic suppression and superinfection in patients taking these medications, they are reserved for patients who have not responded to traditional medical therapy. Approximately 15 to 20% of patients will receive surgery for intractable disease. Proctocolectomy combined with ileostomy is a curative procedure for ulcerative colitis. With the new disposable ileostomy equipment available today, most patients can look forward to an active lifestyle and normal life expectancy.[17,20]

ORAL HEALTH CONSIDERATIONS

Due to the symptoms of severe frequent diarrhea and abdominal pain or cramping, it is unlikely that a patient will be seeking routine dental care with undiagnosed ulcerative colitis. Nonetheless, should an undiagnosed patient attend a dental office for care, then the risks associated with anemia, such as delayed healing, an increased risk of infection, the side effects of narcotic analgesics, and depression of respiration, may collectively contraindicate surgical treatment until the disease is under control. Obviously, following a history and a thorough examination, signs and symptoms of ulcerative colitis and/or anemia would warrant a referral to the patient's primary care physician. More likely is the situation of a diagnosed and medically managed patient attending a dental office for routine or episodic oral health care. The following section addresses those issues a OHCP should be knowledgeable about when treating patients with ulcerative colitis.

The oral changes that occur in ulcerative colitis cases are nonspecific and uncommon, with an incidence of less than 8%. Aphthous stomatitis of the major and minor variety has been reported in patients with active ulcerative colitis. There is nothing unique about these lesions, and it has been suggested that their appearance is coincidental.[23] However, they may result from nutritional deficiencies of iron, folic acid, and vitamin B_{12} due to poor absorption in the gut and/or blood loss directly related to the ulcerative colitis. In addition, anti-inflammatory medications such as the 5-aminosalicylates, which often represent the mainstay of therapy for IBD patients and which are excreted in saliva,

are known to cause recurrent aphthous ulcers in some patients.[49–51] In patients who are prone to develop aphthous ulcers, the appearance of a new crop of oral ulcers often heralds a flare-up of the bowel disease. Other nonspecific forms of ulceration associated with skin lesions have been reported. Pyoderma gangrenosum may occur in the form of deep ulcers that sometimes ulcerate through the tonsillar pillar.[23]

Pyostomatitis vegetans, a purulent inflammation of the mouth, may also occur. These oral lesions are characterized by deep tissue vegetating or proliferative lesions that undergo ulceration and then suppuration. As the lesions disappear with a total colectomy, it is speculated that these manifestations are due to the effects of circulating immunocomplexes induced by antigens that are derived from the gut lumen or the damaged colonic mucosa.[22] Lastly, ulcerative colitis patients also can develop hairy leukoplakia, a lesion more commonly associated with human immunodeficiency virus (HIV) disease.[52] This lesion probably serves as a marker of severe immunosuppression and may result from the use of corticosteroids or other immunosuppressive agents. Medical management for ulcerative colitis may necessitate alterations of dental therapy or special precautions. Sulfasalazine interferes with folate metabolism, and supplemental folic acid may be needed, especially if a macrocytic anemia is revealed in a complete blood count.

Medical management of ulcerative colitis may necessitate alterations of dental therapy. A number of oral health care considerations are related to the therapeutic use of glucocorticosteroids. These are the many side effects associated with the use of corticosteroids and ACTH, including hypertension and hyperglycemia. Obtaining a blood pressure reading and a blood glucose measurement by finger prick in the office and/or consultation with the treating physician to understand the patient's current medical status is highly recommended. Long-term glucocorticosteroid therapy may also cause osteoporosis and vertebral compression fractures; thus, carefully positioning the patient in the dental chair and encouraging the patient to take dietary calcium supplements may help prevent fractures.

Chronic use of glucocorticosteroids can also result in adrenal suppression. Major operative or surgical procedures can precipitate adrenal insufficiency if the glucocorticosteroid dosing is not adjusted properly. Patients undergoing surgery may require supplemental glucocorticosteroids before and after the procedure because their own adrenal response to stress is blunted. Patients who were formerly on glucocorticosteroid therapy may also experience adrenal suppression. Routine maintenance dental therapy such as cleanings or simple restorations should be unaffected by steroid or immunosuppressive therapy.[14] Consultation with the patient's physician is warranted prior to surgical procedures. The details of steroid dosage adjustment for various dental procedures are described on pages XX to XX.

Ulcerative colitis can be associated with chronic bleeding. Prior to dental procedures, blood studies that include hemoglobin, hematocrit, and a red blood cell count should be undertaken to rule out the presence of anemia. Patients taking the immunosuppressive agent azathioprine may suffer from additional side effects that impact dental management. Patients on azathioprine might be expected to have changes in white and red blood cell counts, and total and differential white blood cell counts should be ascertained before embarking on surgical procedures. Suppression of the liver can be expected, and liver function tests should be completed in those patients who will receive dentist-prescribed medications that are metabolized in the liver. Abnormal liver function tests should be discussed with the attending dentist who might need to prescribe analgesic or antibiotic medications that are metabolized in the liver. Typically, patients taking an immunosuppressive agent such as azathioprine are monitored by their primary care physician with liver function tests. Consequently, consultation with the patient's physician will help the dentist determine the patient's liver function. Obviously, toxic doses of the same drugs may be reached if reduced drug metabolism is not taken into consideration. Patients who have extensive bowel surgery may suffer from malabsorption of vitamin K, vitamin B_{12}, and folic acid. Before any surgical procedures are completed, these patients should be evaluated for both macrocytic and microcytic anemia and bleeding disorders from insufficient levels of vitamin K (fibrin clot formation). Clotting factors II, VII, IX, and X are all dependent on vitamin K. A prothrombin time/international normalized ratio (INR) and a partial thromboplastin time will provide information about the patient's ability to form a blood clot.

Crohn's Disease

MEDICAL ASPECTS

Crohn's disease is an inflammatory disease of the small or large intestine. The inflammation involves all the layers of the gut. Gross examination may reveal mucosal ulceration (aphthous ulcers within the mucosa that appear normal, deep ulcers within areas of swollen mucosa, or long linear serpiginous ulcers). Recent epidemiologic evidence suggests that there are two forms of Crohn's disease: a nonperforating form that tends to recur slowly and a perforating or aggressive form that evolves more rapidly. Patients with the aggressive perforating type are more prone to develop fistulae and abscesses, whereas the more indolent nonperforating type tends to lead to stenotic obstruction.[17–21] With the involvement of either the colon or small intestine, microscopic examination reveals inflammatory infiltrate in all layers of affected bowel, with plasma cells and lymphocytes predominating in the lamina propria.

Crohn's disease shares many epidemiologic features with ulcerative colitis. There has been a steady rise in the incidence and prevalence of Crohn's disease, but no clear correlation exists between the increased incidence and environmental or lifestyle changes. Crohn's disease affects all ages and both sexes and occurs most frequently in urban women aged 20 to 39 years. The prevalence of Crohn's disease among first-degree relatives is 21 times higher than that among non-relatives. Evidence for familial association in Crohn's disease

includes increased incidence in Jewish populations, strong familial aggregation, and increased concordance among monozygotic twins or triplets.[17–21]

The cause and evolution of Crohn's disease are unknown. The single strongest risk factor for Crohn's disease, overpowering any influences of diet, smoking, stress, or hygiene, is having a relative with the disease. The fact that first-degree relatives of Crohn's disease patients exhibit increased intestinal permeability supports the theory of an inheritable permeability defect in Crohn's disease. This abnormal intestinal barrier could result in the increased uptake of injurious materials and/or enhanced immune reaction to intestinal antigens. Other theories have included vascular disease, lymphatic obstruction, and emotional stress. Whatever the process, tiny erosions of the overlying normal mucosal lymphoid tissues eventually coalesce to form small aphthous ulcers or more diffuse ulceration of the mucosa. With progression, there is marked hyperplasia of the lymphoid tissue extending through the wall, fibrosis and muscular hypertrophy leading to constrictures, and inflammatory tracts. Granulomas are present in about 50% of patients.[17–21]

The clinical presentation of Crohn's disease depends on the extent of inflammation and on the site of intestinal involvement. The usual presentation is that of a young person in the late teens or twenties who has been ill for an indefinite period and whose disease suddenly worsens. The history often reveals intermittent episodes of abdominal distress, fever, and crampy abdominal pain accompanied by loose stools. Although bleeding is a prominent feature of ulcerative colitis, it is rare in cases of small bowel Crohn's disease.[20]

Inflammation of the small intestine may impair its absorption of vital nutrients. Calcium, iron, and folate are absorbed in the duodenum, and their decreased absorption due to inflammation can lead to deficiencies. Disease in the terminal ileum may interfere with the absorption of bile salts and vitamin B_{12}. Inflammation of the small or large intestines may impair the absorption of fat, fat-soluble vitamins, salt, water, protein, and iron.

The absorptive function of the small bowel is more likely to be altered in patients with Crohn's disease than in those with ulcerative colitis. Electrolyte abnormalities and low albumin levels commonly occur in cases of severe diarrhea. Anemia, usually resulting from an iron or folate deficiency, may also be present. Leukocytosis, cell counts of $>15,000/cm^3$, is suggestive of abscess or perforation.

The signs and symptoms of Crohn's disease are often more subtle than those associated with ulcerative colitis, frequently delaying the diagnosis. However, the diagnosis can usually be made on the basis of a careful history, physical examination, and diagnostic testing. The most reliable and sensitive method for differentiating between ulcerative colitis and Crohn's disease is a colonoscopy with endoscopically directed colonic biopsies. The following features distinguish Crohn's disease from ulcerative colitis: (1) involvement of the small intestine or the upper part of the alimentary canal; (2) segmental disease of the colon, with "skip" areas of normal rectum; (3) the appearance of fissures or sinus tracts; and (4) the presence of well-formed sarcoid-type granulomas.[17–21]

In the case of ulcerative colitis, the signs and symptoms of disease are rather dramatic, and it is unlikely that a patient would attend a dentist's office with undiagnosed disease. The probabilities are greater that someone with undiagnosed Crohn's disease could visit the dentist. Consequently, a thorough history and examination may uncover signs and symptoms of this inflammatory bowel disease, in which case, a referral to the primary care physician is warranted. The associated risks of proceeding with dental care in a patient with undiagnosed Crohn's disease are essentially the same as those described for patients with ulcerative colitis. Anemias, vitamin K–dependent blood clotting disorders, and general nutritional deficiencies may occur if the diagnosis and treatment of Crohn's disease are delayed.

ORAL HEALTH CONSIDERATIONS

Oral lesions, both symptomatic and asymptomatic, affect 6 to 20% of Crohn's disease patients. Most oral manifestations of Crohn's disease occur in patients with active intestinal disease, and their presence frequently correlates with disease activity. Recurrent aphthous ulcers are the most common oral manifestation of Crohn's disease.[23,34] It is not clear whether these oral manifestations are true expressions of Crohn's disease, preexisting and/or coincidental findings, direct results of medical treatment, or manifestations of an associated problem, such as anemia. Certainly, pyostomatitis vegetans, cobblestone mucosal architecture, and minor salivary gland duct pathology represent granulomatous changes that constitute the hallmark of Crohn's disease. Biopsy specimens of these multiple small nonhealing aphthous ulcers reveal granulomatous inflammation. Less often, Crohn's disease patients develop diffuse swelling of the lips and face, inflammatory hyperplasias of the oral mucosa with a cobblestone pattern, indurated polypoid tag-like lesions in the vestibule and retromolar pad area, and persistent deep linear ulcerations with hyperplastic margins. Granulomatous lesions have also been observed in the salivary glands, where they may cause rupture of the ducts and localized mucocele formation.

Numerous medications, including anti-inflammatory and sulfa-containing preparations that are commonly used to manage IBD patients, have been reported to cause oral lichenoid drug reactions.[53,54] Superinfection with *Candida albicans* is often associated with IBD and may represent a primary manifestation of the disorder, a reaction to the bacteriostatic effect of sulfasalazine, or an impaired ability of neutrophils to kill this granuloma-provoking organism.[55] Of interest is the possibility that oral lesions may precede the radiologic changes of the disease by up to 1 year. This underscores the sometimes subtle signs and symptoms of Crohn's disease and the possibility that a dentist may encounter a patient with undiagnosed Crohn's disease. Frequently, patients will complain of pain associated with ulcerative lesions in the oral cavity. Palliative rinses, ointment, and topical steroids may be helpful. There appears to be an increased risk of dental caries that is probably related to dietary changes in patients with IBD.[41] The causes of the dental caries and increased incidence of bacterial and fungal infections are multifactorial but appear to be related to either the patient's altered immune status or diet.[40–45]

Oral effects of malabsorption may also be seen. Pallor, angular cheilitis, and glossitis, all oral manifestations of anemia, may occur, particularly in undiagnosed or poorly controlled disease. Nutritional deficiencies that are directly related to the section of the bowel affected by the disease can occur. Malnutrition is often a problem, and monitoring the patient's compliance with dietary supplementation is essential.[23,34]

As with ulcerative colitis, the medical management of a patient with Crohn's disease may require modifications to standard oral health care routines The underlying assumption of this management change is that patients with IBD are at increased risk for the development of oral infections, including dental caries. Consequently, dental management of patients with IBD should include frequent preventive and routine dental care to monitor oral health and to prevent the destruction of hard and soft tissue. If the patient is taking a systemic glucocorticosteroid, monitoring of blood pressure and evaluation of blood glucose are necessary. A determination needs to be made regarding the need for glucocorticosteroid replacement therapy. This is based on the dosages and length of time taking glucocorticosteroids and the type of planned dental procedure. Screen, diagnose, and treat any oral inflammatory, infectious, or granulomatous lesions as necessary. Palliative rinses and topical steroid therapy, such as fluocinonide 0.05% gel, may be helpful. Topical steroid therapy should be short term and monitored because of the side effect of mucosal atrophy and systemic absorption. To completely comprehend the medical management of the patient, knowledge of the effects, side effects, and drug interactions of any medications the patient is taking is important and may necessitate a consultation with the patient's physician.

Depending on the results of the consultation with the patient's physician, the following laboratory studies may be indicated before surgical procedures are performed: (1) complete blood count; (2) hematocrit level; (3) hemoglobin level; (4) platelet count; (5) coagulation studies (prothrombin time/INR, and partial thromboplastin time); (6) liver function test; and (7) blood glucose level. Coordination and collaboration with the patient's primary care physician will enhance the overall outcome for the patient.

OHCPs are responsible for treatment of oral manifestations of IBD, particularly if the lesions are symptomatic. Palliative sodium bicarbonate mouthrinses (one-half teaspoon of baking soda in 8 ounces of water) may be used as swish and expectorate. Moderate-potency topical steroid preparations, such as 0.05% fluocinonide, desoximetasone, and triamcinolone, or ultrapotency preparations, such as clobetasol and halobetasol, can be topically applied to the lesions, four times daily (not to exceed 2 continuous weeks).[14,27] Ointments and creams are useful when the lesions are localized and direct topical application is possible. In cases when lesions are disseminated or oropharyngeal in distribution, dexamethasone elixir 0.5 mg/5 mL can be used as a rinse or gargle for 1 minute, four times daily, and expectorated. The patient must be advised that prolonged use of topical steroids will result in mucosal atrophy, systemic glucocorticosteroid absorption (especially with the ultrapotency preparations), and an increased incidence of mucosal candidiasis.

IBD patients appear to be at an increased risk of dental caries as well as bacterial and fungal infections. These are multifactorial in etiology but appear to be related to either the patient's altered immune status or diet.[40–45] Oral manifestations of anemia may be noted in patients with ulcerative colitis, especially in undiagnosed or poorly controlled disease. The oral manifestations include pallor, angular cheilitis and glossitis.

Antibiotic-Induced Diarrhea and Pseudomembranous Enterocolitis

MEDICAL ASPECTS

In patients who are receiving antibiotic therapy, diarrhea may occur as a result of an alteration of the colonic flora. Often, this condition is mild and subsides when antibiotic therapy is discontinued. Occasionally, a severe disease results, with the development of a thick mucosal exudate that has the appearance of a membrane and is termed pseudomembranous enterocolitis. This condition is extremely serious and demands aggressive treatment. Practically all antibiotics can be associated with this condition. Patients who are debilitated or who have renal failure seem to be at a higher risk of contracting the disease. Recent studies have shown a major role for *Clostridium difficile* in the pathogenesis of antibiotic-produced pseudomembranous enterocolitis. Infections with *C. difficile* account for 10 to 25% of cases of antibiotic-associated diarrhea and virtually all cases of antibiotic-associated pseudomembranous colitis.[56]

The type of antibiotic and the route of its administration influence disease incidence. More cases occur when the drug is given orally than when it is administered parenterally. Clindamycin, ampicillin, and the cephalosporins are most commonly associated with antibiotic-associated pseudomembranous colitis, but virtually any antibiotic may produce this disorder. Symptoms typically occur during antibiotic treatment, with the majority occurring within 14 days of antibiotic administration. However, cases have been documented to occur up to 3 months after antibiotic exposure.[57] Pseudomembranous colitis is known to follow the administration of clindamycin, amoxicillin, or the cephalosporins, all of which are now recommended for antibiotic prophylaxis of infective endocarditis and late prosthetic joint infections. Presumably, the normal colonic flora is inhibited when antibiotics are administered, allowing *C. difficile* to proliferate and produce a cytopathic toxin. The precise mechanism is not known but probably involves both the cytotoxic and vasoconstrictive effects of toxins. The timing is highly variable, with some cases appearing after a single dose and

about one-third of cases occurring after the medicine is stopped. About 1 to 3 of 100,000 individuals who take antimicrobial agents develop *C. difficile* colitis.[20,56] Diarrhea is present in all cases and is associated with colitis and hemorrhage in 20% of cases. Bowel movements may occur every 15 to 20 minutes. The patient may be febrile and may have lost considerable fluid, electrolytes, and protein. Sigmoidoscopy may reveal mild or severe inflammation, along with yellow raised membranous plaques of exudate. Stool cultures may demonstrate *C. difficile* or may be tested for the enterotoxin.[17–21]

Pseudomembranous colitis is a life-threatening disease, and individuals must be treated aggressively with fluids and electrolyte replacement. Vancomycin, given orally in dosages of 125 to 500 mg four times daily for 10 to 14 days, is effective in eliminating *C. difficile* infection. Metronidazole, in doses of 250 to 500 mg three times daily, is also effective and is less expensive.[17–21]

ORAL HEALTH CONSIDERATIONS

The primary role of the dentist is to recognize the signs and symptoms of antibiotic-associated diarrhea and pseudomembranous colitis in patients who either are taking an antibiotic or have a recent history of an antibiotic regimen. Cessation of the antibiotic and prompt referral to the patient's physician are necessary for definitive diagnosis.

Diseases of the Hepatobiliary System

In this section, the liver, biliary tract, and pancreas are considered together due to their interrelated functions with regard to the digestive system. The liver dominates this group of structures in size and multiplicity of roles. Consequently, the majority of this section focuses on liver disease and dental management in patients with disease or dysfunction.

The liver serves as the major locus of synthetic, catabolic, and detoxifying activities in the body. The intermediary metabolism of all foodstuffs occurs here. The liver is essential in the excretion of heme pigments, and it participates in the immune response. Impairment of the hepatocyte will interfere with the liver's ability to synthesize and store glycogen, a major source of glucose. Should glycogen stores be depleted, liver gluconeogenesis from amino acids is initiated to maintain glucose levels. Lipids are metabolized in the liver to form cholesterol and triglycerides. Cholesterol is the major building block of cell membranes, steroids, and bile salts. Bile salts are essential in the absorption of fat in the small intestine. Proteins, albumin, and clotting factors are synthesized and stored in the liver; specifically, clotting factors I, II, V, VII, IX, and X are synthesized in the liver. Since some of the clotting factors are also dependent on vitamin K (eg, II, VII, IX, and X), coagulopathy can occur from hepatocyte dysfunction and/or vitamin K malabsorption due to biliary problems. The metabolism of drugs is principally performed by the cytochrome P-450 microsomal enzyme system in the hepatocyte. Local anesthetics, analgesics, sedatives, antibiotics, and antifungals are all metabolized in the liver. Consequently, cautious use of these drugs in a person with liver dysfunction is essential. Lastly, the liver inactivates or metabolizes hormones such as insulin, aldosterone, antidiuretic hormone, estrogens, and androgens. Clearly, liver dysfunction can express itself through multiple signs and symptoms. Liver disease commonly manifests itself through jaundice, and the disease process can lead to liver failure and cirrhosis.[58–61] Accordingly, jaundice and cirrhosis are considered separately below.

Jaundice

Jaundice (or icterus), which is a sign rather than a disease, results from excess bilirubin in the circulation and the accumulation of bilirubin in the tissues. Jaundice is a yellow discoloration most often seen in the skin, in mucous membranes, and in the sclera of the eye. This excess bile pigment may be caused by (1) excess production of bilirubin by hemolysis of red blood cells (hemolytic jaundice); (2) obstruction in the biliary tree, preventing the excretion of bilirubin (obstructive jaundice); or (3) liver parenchymal disease (hepatocellular jaundice). Each of these three processes is briefly reviewed in this section, and the role of the dentist is discussed with regard to dental management.

Hemolytic Jaundice

Hemolytic jaundice is not a gastrointestinal disease. Hemolytic anemias are the most common cause of this disorder, so it is critical to understand the implications of hemolytic jaundice. Excessive destruction of erythrocytes will lead to mild hyperbilirubinemia. This excess destruction is often due to an inherent abnormality in the cells (eg, sickle cell disease, hereditary sphenocytosis, thalassemia, and glucose-6-phosphate dehydrogenase deficiency). Additionally, drugs and poisonous agents (eg, nitrobenzene, toluene, and phenacetin), as well as acquired immune disease (eg, systemic lupus erythematosus), can lead to hemolytic jaundice. Even with a thorough history and examination, it would be difficult for a dentist to make a diagnosis of hemolytic jaundice with only a presenting sign of jaundice. Referral to the patient's primary care physician is necessary to elucidate the source of the excess pigmentation of the tissues. Medical diagnosis of jaundice by a hemolytic process is based on laboratory studies demonstrating the presence of anemia with a high reticulocyte count, a decreased level of serum haptoglobins, and elevated serum bilirubin. The specific cause of the increased hemolysis of red blood cells is determined by studies such as hemoglobin electrophoresis, erythrocyte fragility studies, and Coombs' test for antibodies to red cells. Typically, once a proper diagnosis is made and the underlying disorder (excessive hemolysis) is controlled, the jaundice resolves as the liver functions normally to remove bilirubin. Since the liver has enormous reserve capacity, the dentist should anticipate little to no residual damage to the liver unless liver function tests indicate otherwise.

Obstructive Jaundice (Cholestasis)

As its name implies, this form of jaundice is caused by a partial or complete stoppage in bile flow. The causes of this disorder are obstructions of the extrahepatic biliary tree and those associated with intrahepatic abnormalities. In either case, the flow of bile through the liver and out of the common bile duct can be impeded, resulting in an increase in bilirubin in the tissues. Gallstones and malignancies are the causes of most cases of extrahepatic cholestasis. Tumors of the pancreatic head are the most common malignant cause of extrahepatic cholestasis, and adenocarcinoma is the most frequent. The causes of intrahepatic cholestasis include neoplasms (eg, metastatic carcinomas, lymphomas), toxic drugs and chemicals (eg, phalloidin, the toxic component of mushrooms), hepatitis, IBD, and metabolic derangements.[59]

The OHCP's primary function is recognition of the clinical signs of jaundice and timely referral to a primary care physician for appropriate diagnosis and treatment. Once successful disease management is achieved, routine dental care can continue. Consultation with the patient's physician to ascertain the patient's liver function and ability to undergo dental treatment is necessary. Oral surgical procedures in the jaundiced patient should be deferred whenever possible. The main danger in surgery on the patient with obstructive jaundice is excessive bleeding resulting from vitamin K malabsorption. If surgery is essential, vitamin K should be given parenterally at a dose of 10 mg daily for several days. General anesthesia in a severely jaundiced patient can lead to renal failure.

Hepatocellular Jaundice

Hepatocellular jaundice can be caused by hepatitis and cirrhosis. Alcoholic hepatitis and drug-induced hepatotoxicity are discussed in this section, along with cirrhosis.

Alcoholic Hepatitis
MEDICAL ASPECTS

Alcoholic hepatitis is a term used to describe the clinical presentation of alcoholic patients with jaundice. Alcoholic hepatitis is a form of toxin-induced liver disease that runs a wide clinical spectrum from subclinical disease to cirrhosis and fulminant hepatic failure. Excessive use of alcohol remains the most important cause of cirrhosis in the Western world and a leading cause of death and mortality during midlife. Although alcoholic hepatitis is somewhat dose related, the variability and extent of injury are remarkable. Clearly, it is a matter not only of how much alcohol is ingested but by whom. Ingestion of at least 40 to 60 g of ethanol per day for more than 15 years is necessary for development of alcoholic cirrhosis; this is equal to about six 12-ounce beers per day, four glasses of wine, or three 2-ounce shots of whisky. Hepatocyte injury from alcohol develops predominantly as a consequence of the direct cellular toxicity of acetaldehyde, the major metabolite of alcohol. However, there are important contributions from the associated nutritional deficiencies that often accompany alcoholism. There is compelling evidence that the tendency to alcoholism is inherited. Only 1 in 12 alcoholics develops evidence of severe liver injury. Genetic variation in the metabolism of ethanol may explain the higher prevalence of alcoholic liver injury in some populations. Clinicians from around the world are generally convinced that females are at greater risk of developing alcohol-induced liver disease than are males. The reasons for this observation remain obscure. However, women have lower levels of alcohol dehydrogenase (essential for metabolizing alcohol into acetaldehyde) in the gut; consequently, more alcohol reaches the liver.[61]

Due to the large number of individuals who have only mild symptoms, the true incidence of alcoholic hepatitis can only be estimated. In a US study involving veterans with liver disease who underwent liver biopsy, approximately 35% of subjects had changes consistent with alcoholic hepatitis. There have been numerous efforts to identify cofactors that may affect the progression of alcohol-induced injury. Nutrition, genetics, cytokines, hepatitis B and C, and therapeutic drugs all have been implicated. However, the evidence to date is only suggestive.[61]

There is a broad spectrum of clinical manifestations of alcoholic liver disease. Often there is little correlation and sometimes considerable disassociation between the apparent severities of injury as based on clinical findings and as based on evidence found on liver biopsy. Alcoholic hepatitis is often found superimposed on cirrhosis that is already established. Alcoholic hepatitis is considered to be at least partially reversible. The earliest indication of alcoholic liver disease is an enlarged liver. The patient may also exhibit signs of both acute hepatitis (jaundice, fever, anorexia, and malaise) and more chronic liver disease, which may include spider angiomas, gynecomastia, jaundice, ascites, and ethanol intoxication.[59,61]

The clinical problems associated with alcoholic hepatitis reflect the disordered metabolism and circulation in the liver. Jaundice reflects the inability of the hepatocyte to conjugate and excrete bilirubin, and bleeding is secondary to decreased synthesis of clotting factors by the hepatocytes. Also, there can be an associated thrombocytopenia in cases of alcoholic jaundice. Mental confusion results from failure of the liver cells to metabolize and excrete toxins such as ammonia. Spider angiomas and gynecomastia result from elevated levels of estrogen, which is normally metabolized by hepatocytes.[59,61]

MEDICAL MANAGEMENT

Alcoholic hepatitis requires consideration in the case of any patient who has a history of regular alcohol use. Confirmation of the diagnosis and assessment of the extent of injury is best done by performing a liver biopsy. There are no biochemical tests that have proven to be sufficiently helpful in establishing a diagnosis of alcohol-induced injury. Even with a liver biopsy, one can only guess the extent of reversible injury. However, the severity of alcoholic hepatitis can be objectively measured by using the laboratory criteria of prothrombin time and bilirubin. This measure is called a Maddrey discriminate function or Child-Pugh classification. Values of > 32 in this measure indicate severe disease and poor prognosis with significant mortality.[61]

Abstinence is the mainstay of the treatment of alcoholic hepatitis. However, this is difficult to achieve. Nutritional support for the malnourished patient is also important. Although medications such as corticosteroids, anabolic steroids, propylthiouracil, colchicine, and insulin/glucagon show promise, there is insufficient evidence to support their general use. In those patients with alcoholic hepatitis without liver cirrhosis, the disease is reversible.[61]

ORAL HEALTH CONSIDERATIONS

The oral lesions that may be seen in patients with alcoholic hepatitis are primarily related to dysfunction of the hepatocyte. Jaundice (yellow pigmentation) may be observed on the mucosa and may be accompanied by cutaneous and scleral jaundice. Jaundice usually occurs when total serum bilirubin reaches levels ≥ 3 mg/dL. There may be extraoral and/or intraoral petechiae and ecchymoses, gingival crevicular hemorrhage due to the deficient clotting factors associated with dysfunctioning hepatocytes, and thrombocytopenia associated with alcohol. Additional oral findings can include manifestations of malnutrition, such as vitamin deficiencies and anemia. Consequently, pallor, angular cheilitis, and glossitis may be exhibited as expressions of related problems. Additionally, the sweet ketone breath, indicative of liver gluconeogenesis, should raise the suspicion of hepatotoxicity. The presentation of the above clinical signs, as well as a history or symptoms suggestive of alcohol abuse, should warrant a referral to the patient's primary care physician for evaluation. Liver impairment would necessitate specific dental management procedures before proceeding with dental treatment.[58] Adverse interactions between alcohol or resultant alcoholic liver disease and medications used in dentistry include but are not limited to acetaminophen, aspirin, ibuprofen, some cephalosporins, erythromycin, metronidazole, tetracycline, ketoconazole, pentobarbital, secobarbital, diazepam, lorazepam, chloral hydrate, and opiod analgesics.[62]

The prevalence of dental disease is usually extensive because of disinterest in performing appropriate oral hygiene techniques and a decrease in salivary flow.[62] Obviously, elective dental treatment should not be carried out in a patient who has ingested a large amount of alcohol. Conversely, routine dental treatment of a patient with a history of alcoholic liver disease is not contraindicated unless there is significant cirrhosis. Cirrhotic changes due to alcoholism are not reversible, whereas noncirrhotic changes generally are. Consequently, the dentist must determine the functioning level of the liver through consultation with the patient's physician and through appropriate liver function tests. To obtain the appropriate information from the physician, the dentist must be familiar with the laboratory tests used in evaluating the patient's status.[58,61,63]

Drug-Induced Hepatotoxicity
MEDICAL ASPECTS

Drug-induced liver disease can mimic any acute or chronic liver disease. Patients may present with fulminant hepatic failure from an intrinsic hepatotoxin such as acetaminophen or may simply have had an abnormal liver function test result on a laboratory screening panel. Ingested drugs are absorbed into the portal circulation and pass through the liver en route to distant sites of action. The liver is responsible for the conversion of lipid-soluble drugs, which are difficult to excrete, into polar-soluble metabolites that are easily excreted through the kidneys. This solubilization and detoxification may paradoxically produce toxic intermediates. Fortunately, death from drug-induced hepatic injury is uncommon. Nevertheless, the dentist's role in recognizing the potential for drug-induced hepatotoxicity from drugs prescribed by the dentist, other medications (either prescribed or over the counter) being taken by the patient, and drug interactions are critical. Herbal and other alternative (nontraditional) drugs, which are increasing in popularity, have been reported to elicit hepatocellular toxicity as well.[59]

Drugs may be conjugated, oxidized, or reduced through the cytochrome P-450 system. This system can be induced by the long-term use of alcohol, barbiturates, or other drugs. With some hepatotoxic drugs, the relative activity of the cytochrome P-450 system is crucial; a drug that exerts its toxic actions through the generation of cytochrome P-450 metabolites may be relatively more toxic in a patient who uses alcohol or other agents that are capable of inducing cytochrome P-450. An example is the enhanced toxicity of acetaminophen in chronic alcoholics.[59,61]

Most drug reactions occur in one of two general patterns: dose-dependent drug toxicity and idiosyncratic drug reaction. In dose-dependent drug toxicity, a particular agent may be expected to produce hepatic injury in virtually all persons who take a large enough dose. A classic example of this type of toxicity is associated with acetaminophen. Toxicity usually occurs with weeks or months of use, is usually reversible, and recurs at approximately the same dose if stopped and then reintroduced.[59]

Idiosyncratic drug reactions occur at an unpredictable dose, recur at lower doses if stopped and reintroduced, and are occasionally associated with features suggesting involvement of the immune system. Sulfonomides and phenytoin are examples of drugs associated with this type of drug-induced hepatotoxicity. Because of the nature of the reaction, a small dose is as likely to produce a serious reaction as is a full therapeutic dose. Consequently, death may occur upon rechallenge, even at low doses. Idiosyncratic hypersensitivity reactions make up the most common type of drug-induced hepatotoxicity.[59]

Regardless of the mechanism involved, drug-induced hepatotoxicity can result in hepatocellular injury, cholestatic drug reactions, abnormal lipid storage, cirrhosis, and vascular injury. Hepatocellular injury and cholestatic drug reactions account for the majority of drug reactions encountered in dentistry. Hepatocellular injury is the most commonly recognized drug-induced injury, with acetaminophen toxicity probably being the most frequent risk in the practice of dentistry. Nonetheless, there are many categories of drugs that are known to have demonstrated hepatotoxicity that are not covered in this chapter.

ORAL HEALTH CONSIDERATIONS

As stated previously, drug-induced liver disease can present as any acute or chronic disorder. Also, since idiosyncratic reactions often have an immunoallergic basis, the patient can present not only with jaundice and other features of chronic liver disease but also with fever, dermatitis, arthralgias, and eosinophilia. Regardless of clinical presentation, referral to the patient's primary care physician is necessary should the dentist suspect drug-induced hepatotoxicity. It is simplistic to recommend that, since any drug may produce hepatotoxicity, the drug in question should be stopped. Rather, consultation with the physician is necessary to weigh the relative risks of stopping or changing therapy. Fortunately, most of the drugs that dentists might use or prescribe that are known to be hepatotoxic have safe and effective alternatives, and stopping the most likely offending drug is a prudent course of action. Nonetheless, coordination of dental therapy and medical therapy is critical. For example, the alternative agent in the case of NSAID toxicity would be a drug from a different subclass. However, after starting the alternative agent, the patient should be followed for at least 4 to 8 weeks with biochemical tests in order to ensure that the original drug reaction has resolved.

Since many drugs produce idiosyncratic drug toxicity, there is no way to predict or prevent such reactions. A patient who experiences an abrupt episode of hepatocellular injury should be considered to have an idiosyncratic drug reaction and should not be challenged again. For patients who take drugs associated with dose-dependent drug reactions, the obvious precaution is to keep the dose to a minimum. Since it is possible to take a toxic dose of acetaminophen without greatly exceeding the recommended doses, patients with chronic pain should be warned of the potential toxicity of acetaminophen. Also, patients who are taking large doses of acetaminophen should be advised to avoid alcohol and to ensure adequate nutrition.

Because most drug reactions are hepatocellular and may lead to hepatocyte failure and death, patients with a history of drug-induced hepatotoxicity should be evaluated with serial liver function tests. There may be cell death to the extent that drug metabolism and homeostasis are affected and that the patient's ability to undergo dental care is significantly affected.

Liver Cirrhosis

MEDICAL ASPECTS

Cirrhosis is neither a single process nor a single disease; rather, it is the end result of a variety of conditions, primarily alcoholism, that produce chronic inflammatory change and liver cell injury. The progressive scarring leads to abnormal fibrosis and nodular regeneration. Alcohol-induced liver disease is either the first or second commonest specific indication for liver transplant throughout Europe and the United States.[60] Symptoms are the result of hepatocellular dysfunction, portal hypertension, or a combination of the two conditions. The most common symptoms include malaise, weakness, dyspepsia, anorexia, and nausea. One-third of the patients complain of abdominal pain, and 30 to 78% of patients present with ascites. Approximately 65% of cirrhotic individuals are jaundiced at presentation. Increased pigmentation, particularly on overexposed surfaces, is seen in hemochromatosis, whereas xanthomas are suggestive of biliary cirrhosis. Less frequently seen are nonspecific findings of clubbing, cyanosis, and spider angiomas.[59,61]

MEDICAL MANAGEMENT

The medical management of liver cirrhosis is dependent on the underlying etiology. The main objective is to prevent further injury to the liver. Discontinuation of alcohol and other toxins is essential. Some patients may benefit from taking corticosteroids and other immunosuppressive agents, such as methotrexate. Phlebotomy to deplete iron stores and deferoxamine is used as an iron-chelating agent in patients with hemochromatosis. Liver transplantation is reserved for irreversible progressive liver disease.[59,61]

ORAL HEALTH CONSIDERATIONS

Oral findings may be associated with vitamin deficiencies and anemia; these findings include angular cheilitis, glossitis, and mucosal pallor. Yellow pigmentation may be observed on the oral mucosa and may be accompanied by scleral and cutaneous jaundice. Salivary gland dysfunction secondary to Sjögren's syndrome may be associated with primary biliary cirrhosis. Pigmentation of the oral mucosa is only rarely observed in cases of hemochromatosis.

The dental patient who presents with a history of liver cirrhosis deserves special attention. First, patients with cirrhosis may have significant hemostatic defects, both because of an inability to synthesize clotting factors and because of secondary thrombocytopenia. These deficits can be overcome with replacement with fresh frozen plasma and platelets. Therefore, laboratory evaluation prior to any surgical or periodontal procedures should be directed at bleeding parameters; specifically, complete blood count, prothrombin time or INR, partial thromboplastin time, and platelet count should be obtained.[58]

Second, the ability to detoxify substances is also compromised in patients with hepatic insufficiency, and drugs and toxins may accumulate. Patients may become encephalopathic due to an ammonia buildup from the incomplete detoxification of nitrogenous wastes. Patients with encephalopathy are likely to be taking neomycin or lactulose. The use of sedatives and tranquilizers should be avoided in patients with a history of taking encephalopathy narcotics. Additionally, there may be an induction of liver enzymes, leading to a need for increased or decreased dosages of certain medications. Consequently, consultation with the patient's physician is essential to the proper management of the dental patient with liver cirrhosis. The patient with ascites may not be able to fully recline in the dental chair because of increased pressure on abdominal vessels. Lastly, liver transplantation patients who are on immunosuppressive therapy should be monitored for systemic infection of oropharyngeal origin, oral viral infection (herpes simplex virus, cytomegalovirus), and oral ulcers of unknown origin. Oral manifestations of acute graft-versus-host disease in the post-transplant patient can present as a mucositis, whereas chronic graft-versus-host disease may resemble oral lichen planus.[14]

▼ GASTROINTESTINAL SYNDROMES

Eating Disorders: Anorexia and Bulimia
MEDICAL ASPECTS

The two most common eating disorders are anorexia nervosa and bulimia.[64] A variety of specialists, including psychiatrists, psychologists, dentists, internists, clinical social workers, nurses, and dietitians, must provide the treatment of eating disorders.[65] Anorexia involves individuals who intentionally starve themselves when they are already underweight. People suffering from this disorder have an intense fear of becoming fat, even when they are extremely underweight (defined as body weight that is 15% or more below the recommended levels). Those who suffer from anorexia are unable to perceive their physical appearance accurately.

In contrast to those with anorexia, persons with bulimia nervosa consume large amounts of food during "binge" episodes in which they feel out of control of their eating. Bulimic individuals are also not as successful in dieting as are those with anorexia. They may successfully diet for a short time, but they often again lose the ability to restrict food intake, often as a result of some emotional trauma. They then try to prevent weight gain after such episodes by vomiting, using laxatives or diuretics, dieting, and/or exercising aggressively. Persons with bulimia, like those with anorexia, are very dissatisfied with their body shape and weight, and their self-esteem is unduly influenced by their appearance. To be diagnosed with bulimia nervosa, an individual must engage in bingeing and purging at least twice a week for 3 months; exhibit a feeling of lack of control over eating; regularly use self-induced vomiting, laxatives, or diuretics to prevent weight gain; and exhibit a persistent excessive concern with body shape and weight.

The diagnosis of anorexia or bulimia is not always clear. For example, some anorexic persons may binge and purge, whereas some bulimic persons may restrict food intake and overcompensate for overeating by exercising. If an individual eats through bingeing but is 15% or more below recommended weight, then anorexia nervosa is the appropriate diagnosis.

Both of these disorders seem to be most prevalent in industrialized societies, particularly where thinness is espoused as the ideal. Anorexia usually develops in adolescence, between the ages of 14 and 18 years, whereas bulimia is more likely to develop in the late teens or early twenties. It is estimated that anorexia occurs in about 0.5% of adolescent girls and that bulimia occurs in about 1 to 2% of adolescent girls. However, 5 to 10% of young women may exhibit less severe signs and symptoms of these diseases. Anorexia affects 0.3 to 0.7%, whereas bulimia affects 1.7 to 2.5% of women.[66] Studies indicate that by their first year of college, 4.5 to 18% of women and 0.4% of men have a history of bulimia and that as many as 1 in 100 females between the ages of 12 and 18 years have anorexia.

Anorexia and bulimia are both considered psychiatric disorders with physical complications.[67] Before diagnosing either of these eating disorders, other possible causes of significant changes in weight or appetite (eg, tumors, immunodeficiency, malabsorption, and alcohol) must be ruled out. Symptoms of eating disorders can also be primary signs of depression and schizophrenia. Eating disorders can be differentiated from these other disorders by the presence of a distorted body image and preoccupation with losing weight. Because patients may develop a good rapport with their dentists, dentists may be the first health care providers to sense that a diagnosis of an eating disorder is appropriate.

Although many people with an eating disorder recover fully, relapse is common and may occur months or even years after treatment. An estimated 5 to 10% of anorexic patients will die from the disorder; their deaths most commonly result from starvation, suicide, or electrolyte imbalance.

ORAL HEALTH CONSIDERATIONS

The cardinal oral manifestation of eating disorders is severe erosion of the enamel on the lingual surfaces of the maxillary teeth. Acids from chronic vomiting are the cause.[68,69] Examination of the patient's fingernails may disclose abnormalities related to the use of fingers to initiate purging. Mandibular teeth may be affected but not as severely as the maxillary teeth. Parotid enlargement may develop as a sequela of starvation. Rarely does one observe soft tissue changes of the oral mucosa because of trauma from gastric acids.

The dentist should be aware of a possible eating disorder when these symptoms are encountered and should take steps to arrange for referral to other practitioners.[70] Support of the patient both physically, by treatment of tooth desensitization and esthetics, and psychologically, by demonstrating a caring and compassionate attitude, is a part of the dental practitioner's treatment responsibility to these patients.

Gardner's Syndrome

Gardner's syndrome consists of intestinal polyposis (which represents premalignant lesions) and multiple impacted supernumerary (extra) teeth. This disorder is inherited as an autosomal dominant trait, and few patients afflicted with this syndrome reach the age of 50 years without surgical intervention.[71] In a young patient with a family history of Gardner's syndrome, dental radiography (such as a panoramic radiograph) can provide the earliest indication of the presence of this disease process.[72]

Plummer-Vinson Syndrome

Plummer-Vinson syndrome, originally described as "hysterical dysphagia," is noted primarily in women in the fourth and fifth decades of life. The hallmark of this disorder is dysphagia resulting from esophageal stricture, causing many patients to have a fear of choking.[73] Patients may present with a lemon-tinted pallor and with dryness of the skin, spoon-shaped fingernails, koilonychia, and splenomegaly. The oral manifestations are the result of an iron deficiency anemia. Oral findings include atrophic glossitis with erythema or fissuring, angular cheilitis, thinning of the vermilion borders of the lips, and leukoplakia of the tongue. Inspection of the oral mucous membranes will disclose atrophy and hyperkeratinization. These oral changes are similar to those encountered in the pharynx and esophagus. Carcinoma of the upper alimentary tract has been reported in 10 to 30% of patients.[74] Thorough oral, pharyngeal, and esophageal examinations are mandatory to ensure that carcinoma is not present. Artificial saliva may reduce the sensation (and thereby the fear) of choking.

PEUTZ-JEGHERS SYNDROME

Peutz-Jeghers syndrome is characterized by multiple intestinal polyps throughout the gastrointestinal tract but primarily in the small intestine. Malignancies in the gastrointestinal tract and elsewhere in the body have been reported in approximately 10% of patients with this syndrome. Pigmentation (present from birth) of the face, lips, and oral cavity is a hallmark of this syndrome.[75] Interestingly, the facial pigmentation fades later in life, although the intraoral mucosal pigmentation persists. No specific oral treatment is necessary.

Cowden's Syndrome

Cowden's syndrome (multiple hamartoma and neoplasia syndrome) is an autosomal dominant disease characterized chiefly by facial trichilemmomas, gastrointestinal polyps, breast and thyroid neoplasms, and oral abnormalities. Cowden's syndrome is considered to be a cutaneous marker of internal malignancies.[76] Pebbly papilloma-like lesions and multiple fibromas may be found widely distributed throughout the oral cavity.[77]

▼ SELECTED READINGS

Bartlett DW, Evans DF, Anggiansah A, Smith BGN. The role of the esophagus in dental erosion. Oral Surg Oral Med Oral Pathol Oral Radiol Endod 2000;89:312–5.

Calobrisi SD, Mutasim DF, McDonald JS. Pyostomatitis vegetans associated with ulcerative colitis: temporary clearance with fluocinonide gel and complete remission after colectomy. Oral Surg Oral Med Oral Pathol Oral Radiol Endod 1995;79:452–4.

Glick M. Medical considerations for dental care of patients with alcohol-related liver disease. J Am Dent Assoc 1997;128:61–70.

Golla K, Epstein JB, Cabay RJ. Liver disease: current perspectives on medical and dental management. Oral Surg Oral Med Oral Pathol Oral Radiol Endod 2005;98:516–21.

Hegarty A, Hodgson T, Porter S. Thalidomide for the treatment of recalcitrant oral Crohn's disease and orofacial granulomatosis. Oral Surg Oral Med Oral Pathol 2003;95:576–85.

Namiot Z, Namiot DB, Kemona A, Stasiewicz J. Effect of antibacterial therapy and salivary secretion on the efficacy of *Helicobacter pylori* eradication in duodenal ulcer patients. Oral Surg Oral Med Oral Pathol Oral Radiol Endod 2004;97:714–7.

National Institutes of Health Consensus Development Panel statement. *Helicobacter pylori* in peptic ulcer disease. JAMA 1994; 272:65–9.

Sampliner RE. Practice Parameters Committee of the American College of Gastroenterology. Updated guidelines for the diagnosis, surveillance, and therapy of Barrett's esophagus. Am J Gastroenterol 2002;97:1888–95.

Siegel MA, Silverman SS, Sollecito TP, editors. Clinician's guide to the treatment of common oral lesions. 6th ed. Hamilton (ON): BC Decker; 2006.

Siegel MA, Hupp WS. Oral considerations in patients with gastrointestinal disorders. In: Bayless TM, Diehl AM, editors. Advanced therapy in gastroenterology and liver disease. 5th ed. Burlington (ON): BC Decker; 2005. p. 43–8.

Siegel MA, Jacobson JJ. Inflammatory bowel diseases and the oral cavity. Oral Surg Oral Med Oral Pathol Oral Radiol Endod 1999;87:12–4.

Silva MA, Damante JH, Stipp AC, et al. Gastroesophageal reflux disease: new oral findings. Oral Surg Oral Med Oral Pathol Oral Radiol Endod 2001;91:301–10.

For the full reference list, please refer to the accompanying CD ROM.

15

RENAL DISEASE

SCOTT S. DeROSSI, DMD
DEBBIE L. COHEN, MD

Diseases of the kidney are a major cause of morbidity and mortality in the United States, affecting close to 20 million Americans.[1] The kidneys are vital organs for maintaining a stable internal environment (homeostasis). The kidneys have many functions, including regulating the acid-base and fluid-electrolyte balances of the body by filtering blood, selectively reabsorbing water and electrolytes, and excreting urine. In addition, the kidneys excrete metabolic waste products, including urea, creatinine, and uric acid, as well as foreign chemicals. Apart from these regulatory and excretory functions, the kidneys have a vital endocrine function, secreting renin, the active form of vitamin D, and erythropoietin. These hormones are important in maintaining blood pressure, calcium metabolism, and the synthesis of erythrocytes, respectively.

Disorders of the kidneys can be classified into the following diseases or stages: disorders of hydrogen ion concentration (pH) and electrolytes, acute renal failure (ARF), chronic renal failure (CRF), and end-stage renal failure or uremic syndrome. Approximately 1 of 20 hospitalized patients develops ARF, most often related to the trauma of surgery. Death from ARF occurs in 30 to 80% of patients, depending on their underlying medical conditions. Almost 1 in 10,000 persons develops end-stage renal failure annually. whereas mortality related to CRF accounts for more than 50,000 deaths each year in the United States. Oral health care professionals are frequently challenged to meet the dental needs of medically complex patients. This chapter reviews the etiology and pathophysiology of renal disorders and reviews considerations for the provision of dental care.

▼ KIDNEY STRUCTURE AND FUNCTION

The human kidneys are bean-shaped organs located in the retroperitoneum at the level of the waist. Each adult kidney weighs approximately 160 g and measures 10 to 15 cm in length. Coronal sectioning of the kidney reveals two distinct regions: an outer region, or cortex, and an inner region known as the medulla (Figure 1A). Structures that are located at the corticomedullary junction extend into the kidney hilum and are called papillae. Each papilla is enclosed by a minor calyx that collectively communicates with the major calyces to form the renal pelvis. The renal pelvis collects urine flowing from the papillae and passes it to the bladder via the ureters. Vascular flow to the kidneys is provided by the renal artery, which branches directly from the aorta. This artery subdivides into segmental branches to perfuse the upper, middle, and lower regions of the kidney. Further subdivisions account for the arteriole-capillary-venous network or vas recta. The venous drainage of the kidney is provided by a series of veins leading to the renal vein and ultimately to the inferior vena cava.

The kidney's functional unit is the nephron (Figure 1B), and each kidney is made up of approximately one million nephrons. Each nephron consists of Bowman's capsule, which surrounds the glomerular capillary bed; the proximal convoluted tubule; the loop of Henle; and the distal convoluted tubule, which empties into the collecting ducts. The glomerulus is a unique network of capillaries that is suspended between afferent and efferent arterioles enclosed within Bowman's capsule and that serves as a filtering funnel for waste. The filtrate drains from the glomerulus into the tubule, which alters the concentration along its length by various processes to form urine. The glomerulus funnels ultrafiltrate to the remaining portion of the nephron, or renal tubule. Following filtration, the second step of urine formation is the selective reabsorption of filtered substances, which occurs along the length of the tubule via active and passive transport processes.

TABLE 1 Major Functions of the Kidneys

Nonexcretory functions

Degradation of polypeptide hormones

Insulin

Glucagon

Parahormone

Prolactin

Growth hormone

Antidiuretic hormone

Gastrin

Vasoactive intestinal polypeptide

Synthesis and activation of hormones

Erythropoietin (stimulates erythrocyte production by bone marrow)

Prostaglandins (vasodilators that act locally to prevent renal ischemia)

Renin (important in regulation of blood pressure)

1,25-Dihydroxyvitamin D_3 (final hydroxylation of vitamin D to its most potent form)

Excretory functions

Excretion of nitrogenous end products of protein metabolism (eg, creatinine, uric acid, urea)

Maintenance of ECF volume and blood pressure by altering Na^+ excretion

Maintenance of plasma electrolyte concentration within normal range

Maintenance of plasma osmolality by altering water excretion

Maintenance of plasma pH by eliminating excess H^+ and regenerating HCO_3^-

Provision of route of excretion for most drugs

ECF = extracellular fluid; H^+ = hydrogen; HCO_3^- = bicarbonate; Na^+ = sodium; pH = hydrogen ion concentration.

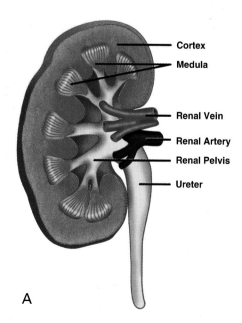

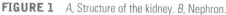

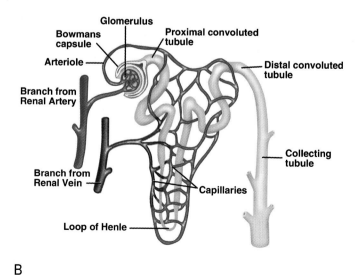

FIGURE 1 *A*, Structure of the kidney. *B*, Nephron.

Each day, the kidneys excrete approximately 1.5 to 2.5 L of urine; although the removal of toxic and waste products from the blood remains their major role, the kidneys are also essential for the production of hormones such as vitamin D and erythropoietin and for the modulation of salt and water excretion. The major functions of the kidney are summarized in Table 1.

Once destroyed, nephrons do not regenerate. However, the kidney compensates for the loss of nephrons by hypertrophy of the remaining functioning units. This theory, often referred to as the intact nephron hypothesis, maintains that diseased nephrons are totally destroyed. Normal renal function can be maintained until approximately 50% of the nephrons per kidney are destroyed, at which point abnormal laboratory values and changes in the clinical course occur. This hypothesis is most useful in explaining the orderly pattern of functional adaptation in progressive renal failure.

▼ FLUIDS, ELECTROLYTES, AND PH HOMEOSTASIS

With advancing nephron destruction, water and electrolyte regulation becomes increasingly more difficult. Adaptations to sudden shifts in intake occur slowly, resulting in wide swings in water and solute concentrations. The first clinical sign of diminished renal function is a decreased ability to concentrate the urine (isosthenuria). As a result of this inability to conserve water, dehydration ensues. With early renal insufficiency, sodium is also lost in the urine. This loss is often independent of the amount of water lost. As renal disease progresses, volume overload leading to hypertension and congestive heart failure can be serious sequelae. When glomerular filtration becomes markedly diminished, the distal tubule can no longer secrete sufficient potassium, leading to hyperkalemia.

In a healthy body, the acid-base balance is maintained via buffers, breathing, and the amounts of acid or alkaline wastes in the urine; this is because the daily load of endogenous acid is excreted into the urine with buffering compounds such as phosphates. As the glomerular filtration rate (GFR) progressively decreases, the tubular excretory capacity for positive hydrogen (H^+) ions is overwhelmed because renal ammonia production becomes inadequate. In its early phases, the resultant acidosis usually has a normal anion gap. As the kidney deteriorates, metabolically derived acids accumulate, leading to an increase in the anion gap. Clinically, this metabolic acidosis is manifested as anorexia, nausea, fatigue, weakness, and Kussmaul's respiration (a deep gasping respiration similar to that observed in patients with diabetic ketoacidosis).

▼ DIAGNOSTIC PROCEDURES IN RENAL DISEASE

Serum Chemistry

In the presence of renal dysfunction, changes in homeostasis are reflected in serum chemistry. Sodium, chloride, blood urea nitrogen (BUN), glucose, creatinine, carbon dioxide, potassium, phosphate, and calcium levels provide a useful tool to evaluate the degree of renal impairment and disease progression. Serum creatinine and BUN are often important markers to the GFR. Both of these products are nitrogenous waste products of protein metabolism that are normally excreted in the urine, but they may increase to toxic levels in the presence of renal dysfunction. A characteristic profile of changes occurs with advancing renal dysfunction, including elevations in serum creatinine, BUN, and phosphate, compared with low levels of serum calcium. Laboratory findings commonly seen in renal disease are summarized in Table 2.

Urinalysis

The most important aspects of urine examination in patients with renal disease include the detection of protein or blood in the urine, determination of the specific gravity or osmolality, and microscopic examination. The hallmarks of renal dysfunction detected by urinalysis are hematuria and proteinuria. Hematuria (the presence of blood in the urine) can result from bleeding anywhere in the urinary tract. Rarely is hematuria a sign of clinically significant renal disease. Microscopic hematuria in patients less than 40 years of age is almost always benign, and further workup is rarely indicated. Occasionally, significant underlying disease, such as a neoplasm or proliferative glomerulonephritis, can cause hematuria. However, the accompanying active sediment of proteins and red blood cell casts makes the diagnosis relatively straightforward. In older people, hematuria warrants further evaluation, including urologic studies to rule out prostatic hypertrophy and neoplasia, urine cultures to rule out infection, urine cytology, and advanced renal studies (such as an intravenous pyelography [IVP]) to rule out intrinsic abnormalities.

Proteinuria is probably the most sensitive sign of renal dysfunction. However, many benign conditions (including exercise, stress, and fever) can produce elevated protein in the urine, or the proteinuria may be idiopathic. A 24-hour urine

TABLE 2 Laboratory Changes in Progressive Renal Disease		
Laboratory Test	Normal Range	Level in Symptomatic Renal Failure
Glomerular filtration rate	100–150 mL/min	< 6–10 mL/min
Creatinine clearance	85–125 mL/min (female)	10–50 mL/min (moderate failure)
	97–140 mL/min (male)	< 10 mL/min (severe failure)
Serum creatinine	0.6–1.20 mg/dL	> 5 mg/dL
Blood urea nitrogen	8–18 mg/dL	> 50 mg/dL
Serum calcium	8.5–10.5 mg/dL	Depressed
Serum phosphate	2.5–4.5 mg/dL	Elevated
Serum potassium	3.8–5.0 mEq/L	Elevated

collection should be done in the presence of persistent proteinuria. The upper limit of normal urinary protein is 150 mg per day; patients who excrete > 3 g of protein per day carry a diagnosis of nephrotic syndrome (discussed below). Specific gravity is measured to determine the concentration of urine. In chronic renal disease, the kidney initially loses its ability to concentrate the urine and then loses its ability to dilute the urine, resulting in a relatively fixed osmolality near the specific gravity of plasma. This occurs when 80% of the nephron mass has been destroyed.

Creatinine Clearance Test

The GFR assesses the amount of functioning renal tissue and can be calculated indirectly by the endogenous creatinine clearance test. Creatinine is a breakdown product of muscle, liberated from muscle tissue and excreted from the urine at a constant rate. This results in a steady plasma concentration of 0.7 to 1.5 mg/dL (often slightly higher in men because of increased muscle mass). Creatinine is 100% filtered by the glomerulus and is not reabsorbed by the tubule. Although a very small portion is secreted by the tubule, this test is an effective way to estimate the GFR. The creatinine clearance test is performed by collecting a 24-hour urine specimen and a blood sample in the same 24-hour period. In CRF and in some forms of acute disease, the GFR is decreased below the normal range of 100 to 150 mL/min. Advancing age also diminishes the GFR, by approximately 1 mL/min every year after age 30 years. The most accurate way to measure the GFR is by the inulin clearance test. However, this clinical test is infrequently used because it requires intravenous (IV) infusion at a constant rate and timed urine collection by catheterization.

Intravenous Pyelography

IVP is the most commonly used and relied upon radiologic examination of the kidneys. Following the IV injection of a contrast medium, a plain-film abdominal radiograph is taken. Further films are exposed every minute for the first 5 minutes, followed by a film exposed at 15 minutes and a final film exposed at 45 minutes. Since various diseases of the kidney alter its ability to concentrate and excrete the dye, the extent of renal damage can be assessed. The location and distribution of the dye itself give information regarding the position, size, and shape of the kidneys. This examination has limited application, particularly since in severely azotemic patients (whose BUN > 70 mg/dL), this test is deferred because there is sufficiently low glomerular filtration to prevent the excretion of the dye, rendering information about the kidney nondiagnostic.

Renal Ultrasonography

Ultrasonography of the kidneys finds its usefulness in the enhanced ability to distinguish solid tumors from fluid-filled cysts.[1] This diagnostic procedure uses high-frequency sound waves (ultrasound) directed at the kidneys to produce reflected waves or echoes from tissues of varying densities, thereby forming images (sonograms). Renal ultrasonography is particularly useful for patients with severe renal failure who are not candidates for IVP. It is most often indicated to determine kidney size, to view an obstruction, to evaluate renal transplants for abscesses or hematomas, and to localize the organ during percutaneous renal biopsy.

Computed Tomography and Magnetic Resonance Imaging

Computed tomography (CT) and magnetic resonance imaging (MRI) have limited application for imaging the kidney and associated areas of interest. Because CT is more expensive than conventional radiographic studies, its clinical application has been limited to the detection of retroperitoneal masses that are difficult to detect with other modalities. MRI gives the same information as renal CT but does not use ionizing radiation or require IV contrast media.

Biopsy

The development and growing use of renal biopsy have considerably advanced the knowledge of the natural history of kidney diseases. Percutaneous needle biopsy guided by ultrasonographic or radiographic reference is usually performed by nephrologists, with the patient in the supine position. Intrarenal and perirenal bleeding may be common sequelae, with serious postprocedural bleeding and hematuria occurring in 5% of cases. Patients are placed on bed rest for 24 hours following the procedure while vital signs and abdominal changes are monitored.

▼ RENAL FAILURE

The classification of renal failure is based on two criteria: the onset (acute versus chronic failure) and the location that precipitates nephron destruction (prerenal, renal or instrinsic, and postrenal failure). CRF or chronic kidney disease (CKD) is a slow, irreversible, and progressive process that occurs over a period of years, whereas ARF develops over a period of days or weeks. The distinction between acute and chronic disease is important; acute disease is usually reversible if managed appropriately, whereas CRF is a progressive and irreversible process that leads to death in the absence of medical intervention. In both cases, the kidneys lose their normal ability to maintain the normal composition and volume of bodily fluids. Although the terminal functional disabilities of the acute and chronic diseases are similar, ARF has some unique aspects that warrant its separate discussion.

▼ ACUTE RENAL FAILURE

ARF is a clinical syndrome characterized by a rapid decline in kidney function over a period of days to weeks, leading to severe azotemia (the building up of nitrogenous waste products in the blood). It is very common in hospitalized patients; ARF occurs in up to 5% of all admitted patients and in as many as 30% of patients admitted to intensive care units. Medications, surgery, pregnancy-related complications, and trauma are the most common causes of ARF. Unlike patients who develop CRF, patients with ARF usually have normal baseline renal function, yet mortality from ARF (even with medical intervention including dialysis) can reach 80%, demonstrating the critical illness of these patients.[2] The clinical course of ARF most often progresses through three stages: oliguria (urine volume <400 mL per day), diuresis (high urine volume output >400 mL per day), and, ultimately, recovery.[3] The causes of ARF are often divided into three diagnostic categories: prerenal failure, postrenal failure, and acute intrinsic renal failure.

Prerenal Failure

Prerenal failure, defined as any condition that compromises renal function without permanent physical injury to the kidney, is the most common cause of hospital-acquired renal failure. This condition, often referred to as prerenal azotemia, results from reversible changes in renal blood flow and is the most common cause of ARF, accounting for more than 50% of cases.[4] Some etiologic factors commonly associated with prerenal failure include volume depletion, cardiovascular diseases that result in diminished cardiac output, and changes in fluid volume distribution that are associated with sepsis and burns.[5]

Postrenal Failure

Postrenal causes of failure are less common (<5% of patients) than prerenal causes. Postrenal failure refers to conditions that obstruct the flow of urine from the kidneys at any level of the urinary tract and that subsequently decrease the GFR. Postrenal failure can cause almost total anuria, with complete obstruction or polyuria. Renal ultrasonography often shows a dilated collecting system (hydronephrosis). Most commonly, obstruction results from prostatic enlargement (benign hypertrophy or malignant neoplasia) or cervical cancer. It is usually seen in older men as a result of the enlargement of the prostate gland. Although postrenal failure is the least common cause of ARF, it remains the most treatable.

Acute Intrinsic Renal Failure

Glomerular disease, vascular disease, and tubulointerstitial disease comprise the three major causes of acute intrinsic renal failure and describe the sites of pathology. Glomerulonephritis is an uncommon cause of ARF and usually follows a more subacute or chronic course. However, when fulminant enough to cause ARF, it is associated with active urinary sediment. Prominent clinical and laboratory findings include hypertension, proteinuria, hematuria, and red blood cell casts. Postinfectious, membranoproliferative, and rapidly progressive glomerulonephritis, as well as glomerulonephritis associated with endocarditis and infections of the vascular access, are the most common glomerular diseases to cause a sudden renal deterioration. The pathogenesis of glomerulonephritis appears to be related to the immunocomplex and complement-mediated damage of the kidney.[6]

Vascular occlusive processes such as renal arterial or venous thromboses are also causes of acute intrinsic renal failure. The clinical presentation is archetypal, consisting of a triad of severe and sudden lower back pain, severe oliguria, and macroscopic hematuria. By far, the most common causes of acute intrinsic failure are tubulointerstitial disorders (>75% of cases), including interstitial nephritis and acute tubular necrosis (ATN). Infiltrative diseases (such as lymphoma or sarcoidosis), infections (such as syphilis and toxoplasmosis), and medications are the leading causes of interstitial nephritis. With drug-induced interstitial nephritis, there are accompanying systemic signs of a hypersensitivity reaction, and the presence of eosinophils is a common finding in the urine. Although renal function usually returns to normal with the discontinuation of the offending drug, recovery may be hastened with corticosteroid therapy.[7] ATN is a renal lesion that forms in response to prolonged ischemia or exposure to a nephrotoxin.[8] ATN remains more of a clinical diagnosis of exclusion than a pathologic diagnosis. The period of renal failure associated with ATN can range from weeks to months, and the major complications of this transient failure are imbalances in fluid and electrolytes, as well as uremia. Serum levels of BUN and creatinine peak, plateau, and slowly fall, accompanied by a return of renal function over 10 to 14 days in most cases.[9]

Sudden renal failure in hospitalized patients is often very apparent from either oliguria or a rise in BUN and creatinine levels. However, renal dysfunction in the outpatient population is often more subtle. A patient can present to the dental office with vague complaints of lethargy and fatigue or entirely without symptoms. These patients can often go undiagnosed but for abnormal results on routine urinalysis, the most common test for screening for renal disease.[10,11]

▼ CHRONIC RENAL FAILURE

CRF is now termed chronic kidney disease or CKD. CKD is defined by the National Kidney Foundation Kidney Disease Outcomes Quality Initiative as either of the following: (1) the presence of markers of kidney damage for >3 months, as defined by structural or functional abnormalities of the kidney with or without a decrease in GFR manifest either by pathologic abnormalities or other markers of kidney damage, including abnormalities in the composition of blood or urine, or abnormalities in imaging tests; (2) the presence of GFR <600 cc/min/1.73 m^2 for >3 months, with or without other signs of kidney damage.[12]

CRF can be caused by many diseases that devastate the nephron mass of the kidneys. Most of these conditions involve diffuse bilateral destruction of the renal parenchyma. Some renal conditions affect the glomerulus (glomerulonephritis), others involve the renal tubules (polycystic kidney disease or pyelonephritis), whereas others interfere with blood perfusion to the renal parenchyma (nephrosclerosis). Ultimately, nephron destruction ensues in all cases unless this process is interrupted.

The United States Renal Data System has generated statistics showing that the most common primary diagnosis for CRF or end-stage renal disease (ESRD) patients is diabetes

TABLE 3 Etiology of End-Stage Renal Disease

Disorder	Percentage of New Dialysis Patients
Diabetes mellitus	44.4
Hypertension	26.6
Glomerulonephritis	12.2
Interstitial nephritis, pyelonephritis, and polycystic kidney disease	7.2
Other disorders	9.6

Adapted from United States Renal Data System report. Available at: http://www.usrds.org.

mellitus (DM), followed by hypertension, glomerulonephritis, and others (Table 3). Despite the varying causes, the clinical features of CRF are always remarkably similar because the common denominator remains nephron destruction.

The prognosis of the patient with renal disease has improved significantly during the last two decades. The improvement of antimicrobial therapy to combat increased susceptibility to infection, along with advances in dialysis and transplantation techniques, has provided patients with the opportunity for survival in the face of a complete loss of renal function. However, despite these advances, the current annual mortality rate for patients with ESRD in the United States is approximately 24%.[1]

Clinical Progression

CKD is divided into stages according to the level of renal function present or the GFR. CKD is classified from stage 1 to stage 5 as shown in Table 4. In stage 1 CKD, patients have normal renal function (GFR > 90 cc/min) but may have proteinuria or hematuria. In stage 2 CKD, patients have reduced renal function with GFR between 60 and 90 cc/min. Stage 3 CKD reflects a GFR between 30 and 60 cc/min. During stage 3 CKD, patients often start developing manifestations related to CKD, such as anemia and secondary hyperparathyroidism (HPTH). In the United States, most patients with CKD have stage 3 CKD (see Table 4). These patients are more likely to die from other comorbidities than before they progress to advanced CKD or ESRD. Stage 4 CKD reflects

TABLE 4 Stages of Chronic Kidney Disease

Stage	GFR cc/min	Manifestation
1	> 90 n	Asymptomatic; may have hematuria or proteinuria
2	60–90	Asymptomatic; may have hematuria or proteinuria
3	30–60	May develop anemia, SHPT
4	15–30	Start to prepare for dialysis or transplantation
5	< 15	Initiate dialysis (< 15 cc/min in diabetic and < 10 cc/min in nondiabetic patients)

GFR = glomerular filtration rate; SHPT = secondary hyperparathyroidism.

a GFR of 15 to 30 cc/min, and during this stage of CKD, patients are medically prepared for dialysis. Stage 5 CKD, or GFR of < 15 cc/min, reflects significantly reduced renal function, and this is the stage when patents will require long-term chronic dialysis treatments. Stages of CKD can be calculated by the modified Modification of Diet in Renal Disease (MDRD) equation, which can be found at the following Web site: <www.nephron.com>. The GFR varies depending on the gender, age, and race of the patient. It is important to estimate this accurately as the treatment varies according to the different stages of CKD. A 70-year-old white female with a serum creatinine of 1.2 mg/dL has an estimated creatinine clearance or GFR of 47 cc/min or stage 3 CKD, whereas a 35-year-old black male with a serum creatinine of 1.2 has an estimated GFR of 90 cc/min or stage 1 CKD. In stage 1 and 2 CKD, patients have diminished renal reserve, which is characterized by normal or minimal elevations in serum creatinine and BUN levels. Patients have no symptoms or prominent biochemical disturbances aside from an abnormal serum creatinine level. As nephron destruction progresses, the GFR falls, and the BUN and creatinine levels rise. Patients may develop mild azotemia, nocturia, polyuria, and an impaired ability to concentrate urine. As renal function deteriorates, patients become more symptomatic and progress to ESRD. Patients usually require chronic dialysis when the GFR level is 15 cc/min or less in diabetic patients and 10 cc/min or less in patients without diabetes. During late stage 4 disease or early stage 5 disease, patients often become symptomatic and may develop uremic symptoms, which include nausea, vomiting, weight loss, decreased appetite, metallic taste in the mouth, and fluid gains, including leg swelling or edema and shortness of breath due to pulmonary edema. Patients may also develop severe biochemical abnormalities, including severe anemia, hyperkalemia, metabolic acidosis, hyperphosphatemia, hypocalcemia, and raised parathyroid hormone levels. The complex biochemical changes, including anemia, hypocalcemia, hyperphosphatemia, and metabolic acidosis, together with systemic symptoms patients experience, are termed the "uremic syndrome." At this point in the disease process, renal replacement therapy or dialysis is a necessity or death is a certain consequence.[13]

Etiology and Pathogenesis

The progression of the varied renal diseases, culminating in CRF, ranges from a few months to 30 to 40 years. The most common causes of renal failure are summarized in Table 3. Currently, diabetes and hypertension account for 44.4% and 26.6%, respectively, of the total cases of ESRD. Glomerulonephritis is the third most common cause of ESRD (12.2% of cases). Interstitial nephritis, pyelonephritis, and polycystic kidney disease account for 7.2% of cases. The remaining 9.6% of the causes of ESRD include systemic lupus erythematosus (SLE) and relatively uncommon conditions such as obstructive uropathy.[1–3,7]

Age, race, gender, and family history have been identified as risk factors for the development of ESRD. The average age of a newly diagnosed patient with ESRD is 61.1 years, and 53.1% of ESRD patients are male. White people, including Hispanics, account for 63.5% of ESRD patients; black people account for 28.7% of ESRD patients, and people of Asian ancestry make up 2.9%.[1–3,7,11–13] Family history is a risk factor for diabetes and hypertension, both of which adversely affect the kidneys and therefore constitute a risk for developing ESRD. Recent evidence suggests that smoking is a major renal risk factor, increasing the risk of nephropathy and doubling the rate of progression to end-stage disease.[14]

GLOMERULONEPHRITIS

Glomerulonephritis represents a heterogeneous group of diseases of varying etiology and pathogenesis that produce irreversible impairment of renal function. This is often initiated by an attack of acute glomerulonephritis of streptococcal or nonstreptococcal origin. Glomerulonephritis also may enter the chronic stage from a nephritic syndrome. The most typical examples of this are focal segmental glomurulosclerosis, idiopathic membranous glomerulonephritis, and membranoproliferative glomerulonephritis.[15] In most cases, the patients present with the features of CRF and hypertension or with a chance proteinuria that has progressed to chronic nephritis over a period of years.

Chronic glomerulonephritis is usually insidious in onset. The course is very slow but is steadily progressive, leading to renal failure and uremia in up to 30 years. It is thought to be a disorder of immunologic origin. The continuous nature of the immunologic injury is shown by the recurrence of disease in kidneys that have been transplanted to patients with some type of glomerulonephritis, even after their own kidneys had been removed.[16]

NEPHROTIC SYNDROME

Nephrotic syndrome is the clinical manifestation of any glomerular lesion that causes an excess of more than 3.5 g of protein excretion in the urine per day. Nephrotic syndrome is caused by multiple diseases, all of which enhance the permeability of the glomerulus to plasma proteins. Excessive protein excretion leads to a decline of plasma osmotic pressure, with consequent edema and serosal effusions. The differential diagnosis of nephrotic syndrome is vast but includes sickle cell anemia, DM, multiple myeloma, SLE, and membranous glomerulonephritis. Bacterial infections secondary to hypogammaglobulinemia have been described as a cause of death in children with nephrotic syndrome.

PYELONEPHRITIS

Pyelonephritis refers to the effects of bacterial infection in the kidney, with *Escherichia coli* being the most frequent cause of infection.[17] Pyelonephritis may present in an acute form with active pyogenic infection or in a chronic form in which the principal manifestations are caused by an injury sustained during a preceding infection. The chronic form of bacterial pyelonephritis can be further subdivided into reactive and inactive forms, and one or both kidneys may be affected.

Any lesion that produces an obstruction of the urinary tract can predispose a patient to active pyelonephritis. Pyelonephritis also may occur as part of a generalized sepsis, as seen in patients with bacterial endocarditis or staphylococcal septicemia.

The clinical picture of acute pyelonephritis is often characteristic, consisting of a sudden rise in body temperature (to 38.9–40.6°C), shaking chills, aching pain in one or both costovertebral areas or flanks, and symptoms of bladder inflammation. Microscopic evaluation of the urine reveals large numbers of bacteria and a polymorphonuclear leukocytosis. There are no signs of impaired renal function or acute hypertension as is sometimes seen in patients with acute glomerulonephritis. Patients with chronic active pyelonephritis often suffer from recurrent episodes of acute pyelonephritis or may have persistent smoldering infections that gradually result in end-stage renal failure secondary to destruction from the scarring of renal parenchyma. This process may continue for many years. The inability to conserve sodium (a feature in any patient with impaired renal function) is more pronounced in patients with pyelonephritis than in those with glomerulonephritis. This "salt-losing" defect may be pronounced and may dominate the clinical picture.

POLYCYSTIC RENAL DISEASE

Polycystic kidney disease exhibits autosomal dominant inheritance.[18] Most patients present with microscopic or gross hematuria, abdominal or flank pain, and recurrent urinary tract infections. The disease causes renal insufficiency in 50% of individuals by age 70 years.[19] Clinically, these patients have large palpable kidneys, and the diagnosis is confirmed via renal ultrasonography, CT, or IVP. Most patients develop hypertension during the course of their disease, and more than one-half of patients are hypertensive at the time of presentation. Although no preventive therapies have proven to be effective, treating the hypertension with angiotensin-converting enzyme inhibitors may help slow the progression of polycystic disease. Another form of polycystic kidney disease is an acquired reactive process that is seen in over 50% of patients treated by hemodialysis or peritoneal dialysis for longer than 3 years. The development of adenocarcinomas is seen in approximately 5% of these multiple cysts throughout the remnant kidneys.

HYPERTENSIVE NEPHROSCLEROSIS

The association between the kidneys and hypertension is recognized, yet the primary disease often is not. Hypertension may be the primary disorder damaging the kidneys, but, conversely, severe CRF may lead to hypertension or perpetuate it through changes in sodium and water excretion and/or in the renin-angiotensin system.[20] Hypertension remains one of the leading causes of CRF, especially in nonwhite populations (see Chapter 13, "Diseases of the Cardiovascular System," for detailed discussion of hypertension). The heart, brain, eyes, and kidneys comprise the four major target organs of hypertension. Long-standing hypertension leads to fibrosis and sclerosis of the arterioles in these organs and throughout the body. Benign nephrosclerosis results from arteriosclerotic changes due to long-standing hypertension. It is the direct result of ischemia caused by narrowing of the lumina of the intrarenal vascular supply. The progressive closing of the arteries and arterioles leads to atrophy of the tubules and destruction of the glomerulus. "Malignant nephrosclerosis" refers to the structural changes that are associated with the malignant phase of essential hypertension.

CONNECTIVE TISSUE DISORDERS

Renal diseases are very prevalent among patients with connective tissue disorders, commonly referred to as collagen vascular diseases. Approximately two-thirds of patients with SLE and scleroderma or progressive systemic sclerosis (PSS) have clinical evidence of renal involvement. In rheumatoid arthritis, the prevalence of renal involvement is considerably less and is often related to complications of treatment with gold salts or D-penicillamine.

End-stage renal failure occurs in 25% of patients with SLE. Lupus nephritis, caused by circulating immune complexes that become trapped in the glomerular basement membrane, produces a clinical picture similar to that of acute glomerulonephritis or nephrotic syndrome.[21] PSS is characterized by the progressive sclerosis of the skin and viscera, including the kidneys and their vasculature, leading to changes resembling the nephrosclerosis seen in patients with long-standing hypertension.

METABOLIC DISORDERS

The most common metabolic disorders that may lead to CRF include DM, amyloidosis, gout, and primary HPTH. By far, DM is one of the most important causes of CRF and accounts for nearly one-half of new ESRD patients (data from US Renal Data System, 2005). The type of diabetes the patient has affects the probability that the patient will develop ESRD. It has been estimated that about 50% of patients with type 1 DM develop ESRD within 15 to 25 years after the onset of diabetes compared with 6% for patients with type 2 DM. The term *diabetic nephropathy* refers to the various changes that affect the structure and function of the kidneys in the presence of diabetes. Glomerulosclerosis is the most characteristic lesion of diabetic nephropathy. Other lesions include chronic tubulointerstitial nephritis, papillary necrosis, and ischemia. The natural progression of diabetic nephropathy follows five stages, beginning with early functional changes (stage 1) and progressing through early structural changes (stage 2), incipient nephropathy (stage 3), clinical diabetic nephropathy (stage 4), and, finally, progressive renal insufficiency or failure (stage 5). The final stage is characterized by azotemia (elevated BUN and serum creatinine) resulting from a rapid decline in the GFR and leading to ESRD.

TOXIC NEPHROPATHY

The kidney is particularly exposed to the toxic effects of chemicals and drugs because it is an obligatory route of excretion for most drugs and because of its large vascular perfusion.[22] There are medications and other agents (referred to as "classic" nephrotoxins) whose use leads directly to renal failure. However, abuse of nonsteroidal anti-inflammatory drugs (NSAIDs) can also result in CRF. The renal protective effects of prostaglandins are inhibited by NSAIDs. Currently, abuse of analgesics accounts for 1 to 2% of all ESRD cases in the United States.[1,11]

▼ MANIFESTATIONS OF RENAL DISEASE: UREMIC SYNDROME

Two groups of symptoms are present in patients with uremic syndrome: symptoms related to altered regulatory and excretory functions (fluid volume, electrolyte abnormalities, acid-base imbalance, accumulation of nitrogenous waste, and anemia) and a group of clinical symptoms affecting the cardiovascular, gastrointestinal, hematologic, and other systems (Table 5).

Biochemical Disturbances

Metabolic acidosis is a common biochemical disturbance experienced by patients with renal failure. As kidney function fails, excretion of hydrogen (H^+) ions diminishes, leading to systemic acidosis that results in a lower plasma pH and bicarbonate (HCO_3^-) concentration. Ammonium (NH_4^+) excretion, decreased because of reduced nephron mass, is the most important factor in the kidney's ability to eliminate H^+ and regenerate HCO_3^-. These patients often suffer from a moderate acidosis (serum bicarbonate level stabilized at 18 to 20 mEq/L). The symptoms of anorexia, lethargy, and nausea frequently observed in patients with uremia may be due partly to this metabolic acidosis. Kussmaul's breathing, a symptom

TABLE 5 Systemic Disturbances in Renal Disease (Uremic Syndrome)	
Body System	**Manifestations**
Gastrointestinal	Nausea, vomiting, anorexia, ammoniacal taste and smell, stomatitis, parotitis, esophagitis, gastritis, gastrointestinal bleeding
Neuromuscular	Headache, peripheral neuropathy, paralysis, myoclonic jerks, seizures, asterixis
Hematologic-immunologic	Normocytic and normochromic anemia, coagulation defect, increased susceptibility to infection, decreased erythropoietin production, lymphocytopenia
Endocrine-metabolic	Renal osteodystrophy (osteomalacia, osteoporosis, osteosclerosis), secondary hyperparathyroidism, impaired growth and development, loss of libido and sexual function, amenorrhea
Cardiovascular	Arterial hypertension, congestive heart failure, cardiomyopathy, pericarditis, arrhythmias
Dermatologic	Pallor, hyperpigmentation, ecchymosis, uremic frost, pruritus, reddish brown distal nail beds

caused by acidosis, is a deep sighing respiration aimed at increasing carbon dioxide excretion and reducing the metabolic acidosis. Disturbances in potassium balance are serious sequelae of renal dysfunction since only a narrow plasma concentration (normal = 3.5 to 5.5 mEq/L) is compatible with life. As kidney function deteriorates, hyperkalemia ensues. Fatal dysrhythmias or cardiac standstill will occur when the potassium level reaches 7 to 8 mEq/L. The normally functioning kidney allows great flexibility, excreting and conserving sodium in response to changing intake. Patients with CKD lose this adaptability, and small fluctuations often have serious consequences. Initially, patients experience osmotic diuresis and excess sodium excretion because of the polyuria. Sodium loss is more common in those conditions that are likely to affect the tubules (polycystic kidney disease and pyelonephritis). When oliguria develops in end-stage renal failure, sodium retention invariably occurs, resulting in edema, hypertension, and congestive heart failure.

Gastrointestinal Symptoms

The gastrointestinal system, particularly the esophagus, stomach, duodenum, and pancreas, shows a myriad of symptoms in cases of uremic syndrome. The more common symptoms are often the first signs of the disease and include nausea, vomiting, and anorexia. Gastrointestinal inflammations such as gastritis, duodenitis, and esophagitis are common in late renal failure and can affect the entire gastrointestinal tract. Mucosal ulceration in the stomach, small intestine, and large intestine may hemorrhage, resulting in lowered blood pressure and a resultant lowered GFR. Digestion of hemorrhagic blood may lead to a rapid increase in BUN.[23]

Neurologic Signs and Symptoms

Some of the early signs and symptoms of advanced CKD are related to changes in the neurologic system.[24] Both central and peripheral nervous systems are involved, with diverse consequences. The degree of cerebral disturbance roughly parallels the degree of azotemia. The patient's electroencephalogram becomes abnormal, with changes that are commensurate with metabolic encephalopathy. As the disease progresses, asterixis and myoclonic jerks may become evident; central nervous system irritability and eventual seizures may occur. Seizures also can occur secondary to hypertensive encephalopathy, electrolyte disturbances (such as hyponatremia), and alkalosis, which induces hypocalcemia.

Along with neurologic hyperirritability, peripheral neuropathy is commonly present as a result of a disturbance of the conduction mechanism rather than a quantitative loss of nerve fiber. The clinical picture is dominated by sensory symptoms and signs. Impairment of vibratory sense and loss of deep tendon reflexes are the earliest, most frequent, and most constant findings. The predominant patient complaint is paresthesia or "burning feet," which may progress to eventual muscle weakness, atrophy, and, finally, paralysis; there is a tendency toward increasing incidence with decreasing renal function. This predominantly affects the lower extremities

but can affect the upper extremities as well. Rarely, facial, oral, and perioral regions also can be affected. Severe uremic neuropathy is less commonly seen today because dialysis or transplantation is usually performed before uremic symptoms become prolonged or severe. Renal replacement therapy may halt the progress of peripheral neuropathy, but once these changes occur, sensory changes are poorly reversible, whereas motor changes are considered irreversible.

The treatment of renal failure also may lead to the development of neurologic abnormalities in the form of dialysis disequilibrium, which may be seen during the first or second dialysis treatments and is characterized by headache, nausea, and irritability that can progress to seizures, coma, and death. This is uncommon as precautions are taken in the first few treatments not to reduce the uremic toxins from the blood too rapidly.

Hematologic Problems

Patients with CKD will often have hematologic problems, most commonly anemia and increased bleeding. The anemia associated with renal disease is a function of decreased erythropoiesis in the bone marrow and is usually normocytic and normochromic. It is not uncommon for these patients to have hematocrit levels in the 20 to 35% range (normal levels are 42 to 54% in males and 37 to 47% in females). The pathogenesis of the anemia is multifactorial, with nutritional deficiencies, iron metabolism abnormalities, and circulating uremic toxins that inhibit erythropoiesis all playing a role.[25] The major factor, however, is the inability of the diseased kidney to produce erythropoietin, which stimulates (through a feedback mechanism) the bone marrow to produce red blood cells. Hypertension, retention of waste products, and altered body fluid pH and electrolyte composition create a suboptimal environment for living cells; therefore, an accelerated destruction of red blood cells contributes to the anemia. Another cause of anemia in many dialysis patients is the frequent blood sampling and loss of blood in hemodialysis tubing and coils.

These patients may also have a microcytic hypochromic anemia that may be caused by deficiencies in iron stores. Previously, patients were given aluminum-containing medications, often given as phosphate-binding agents to control hyperphosphatemia, which could also contribute to the anemia. Aluminum also can be found in domestic tap water supplies or in nondealuminized dialysis water. This form of anemia is treated by chelation with deferoxamine.[25] This form of anemia is extremely rare in this modern era, and aluminum-containing medications are not used anymore in chronic dialysis patients.

Interestingly, these patients tolerate their anemia quite well. Whole-blood transfusions are usually unnecessary, with the exception of cases of significant surgical blood loss or when the patient exhibits severe symptoms of anemia. These symptoms and signs of anemia may include pallor, tachycardia, systolic ejection murmur, a widened pulse pressure, and angina pectoris (in patients with underlying coronary artery disease). Transfusions may further suppress the production of red blood cells. The risk of hepatitis B and C, human immunodeficiency virus (HIV) infection, and other bloodborne infections is increased with the number of transfusions, although blood screening techniques continue to minimize these risks.

Recombinant human erythropoietin (epoetin alfa) (Epogen Amgen, Procrit Ortho Biotech Products; Aranesp, Amgen) corrects the anemia of ESRD and eliminates the need for transfusions in virtually all patients.[26] A dosage of 50 to 150 U/kg of body weight IV three times a week produces an increase in hematocrit of approximately 0.01 to 0.02 per day.[27–29] During early therapy, iron deficiency will develop in most patients. It is therefore initially essential to monitor the body's iron stores monthly.[30] With all patients, except those with transfusion-related iron overloads, prophylactic supplementation with ferrous sulfate (325 mg up to three times daily) or IV iron is recommended.[25,31,32] Onset or exacerbation of hypertension has been observed as a possible complication of recombinant human erythropoietin therapy for the anemia of ESRD.[33] This effect is attributed to an overly rapid rise in the hematocrit level in the accompanying increased hemoglobin, blood viscosity, and renal cell mass.[34]

Bleeding may be a significant problem in patients with end-stage renal failure, and it has been attributed to increased prostacyclin activity, increased capillary fragility, and a deficiency in platelet factor 3. The bleeding risk in renal failure results from an acquired qualitative platelet defect secondary to uremic toxins that decrease platelet adhesiveness. In addition, the low hematocrit levels commonly found in uremic patients negatively influence the rheologic component of platelet–vessel wall interactions. Platelet defects secondary to uremia are best remedied by dialysis but are also treated successfully by cryoprecipitate or l-deamino-8-D-arginine vasopressin (DDAVP).[35] Platelet numbers affect bleeding, and mechanical trauma to the platelets during dialysis can cause a decrease of up to 17% in the platelet count. In addition to lowered platelet counts (which are usually not clinically significant) and qualitative platelet defects, the effects of medications on platelets contribute to bleeding episodes.

During dialysis, patients are given heparin to facilitate blood exchange and to maintain access patency. However, since the effects of heparinization during dialysis last only approximately 3 to 4 hours after infusion, the risk of excessive clinical bleeding because of anticoagulation is minimal in dentistry.[36] Some patients have a tendency to be hypercoagulable; for these patients, a regimen of warfarin sodium (Coumadin) therapy may be instituted to maintain a continuous anticoagulated state and to ensure shunt patency.

Calcium and Skeletal Disorders (Renal Osteodystrophy)

"Renal osteodystrophy" (RO) refers to the skeletal changes that result from chronic renal disease and that are caused by disorders in calcium and phosphorus metabolism,

abnormal vitamin D metabolism, and increased parathyroid activity. In early renal failure, intestinal absorption of calcium is reduced because the kidneys are unable to convert vitamin D into its active form. Upon exposure to sunlight, 7-dehydroxycholesterol in the skin is converted to cholecalciferol (vitamin D_3) and is subsequently metabolized in the liver to a more biologically active form, 25-hydroxycholecalciferol (25-HCC). Further conversion to either 1,25-dihydroxycholecalciferol (1,25-DHCC) or 21,25-dihydroxycholecalciferol (21,25-DHCC) then occurs in the kidney parenchyma.

When the serum calcium level is high, 25-HCC is metabolized to 21,25-DHCC; conversely, a hypocalcemic state initiates the conversion of 25-HCC to 1,25-DHCC. This form is the most biologically active for absorbing calcium from the digestive tract. Impaired absorption of calcium because of defective kidney function and the corresponding retention of phosphate cause a decrease in the serum calcium level. This hypocalcemia is associated with a compensatory hyperactivity of the parathyroid glands (parathyroid hormone production) that increases the urinary excretion of phosphates, decreases urinary calcium excretion, and augments the release of calcium from bone.

The most frequently observed changes associated with compensatory HPTH are those that involve the skeletal system. These changes can appear before and during treatment with hemodialysis. Although it is a lifesaving therapy, hemodialysis unfortunately fails to perform vital metabolic or endocrine functions and does not correct the crucial calcium-phosphate imbalance. In some cases, RO becomes worse during hemodialysis. Some of the changes that are accelerated are bone remodeling, osteomalacia, osteitis fibrosa cystica (a rarefying osteitis with fibrous degeneration and cystic spaces that result from hyperfunction of the parathyroid glands), and osteosclerosis.[37]

The bone lesions are usually in the digits, the clavicle, and the acromioclavicular joint. Other lesions that can be seen are mottling of the skull erosion of the distal clavicle and margins of the symphysis pubis, rib fractures, and necrosis of the femoral head.[37] The manifestations of metabolic RO of the jaws include bone demineralization, decreased trabeculation, a "ground-glass" appearance, loss of lamina dura, radiolucent giant cell lesions, and metastatic soft tissue calcifications.

In children, the predominant lesion is osteomalacia (a deficiency or absence of osteoid mineralization), which is associated with bone softening that leads to deformities of the ribs, pelvis, and femoral neck (renal rickets). Early stages of RO may be detected histologically or biochemically without the presence of definitive radiographic changes because dependable radiographic evidence of bone disease appears only after 30% of bone mineral contents have been lost.

Osteodystrophy patients are placed on protein-restricted diets and phosphate binders (calcium carbonate or calcium acetate) to keep the serum phosphorus within the normal range (between 3.5 and 5.0 mg/dL). They also are given vitamin D supplements (such as 1,25-DHCC) and medications to target the calcium receptor (Sensipar).[38] If these measures fail, a parathyroidectomy may be performed, whereby two or more of the four glands are removed, leaving residual parathyroid hormone–secreting tissue.[39]

Most recently, a new form of renal bone disease termed adynamic bone disease has emerged as the most frequent finding on bone biopsy of patients who are on dialysis. The etiology of this new condition is not fully understood, but relatively low levels of intact serum parathyroid hormone are often associated with this disorder and may play a role in its pathogenesis.[40]

Cardiovascular Manifestations

Hypertension and congestive heart failure are common manifestations of uremic syndrome. Alterations in sodium and water retention account for 90% of cases of hypertension in CRF patients.[41] The association of circulatory overload and hypertension caused by disturbances in sodium and water balance contributes to an increased prevalence of congestive heart failure. In addition, retinopathy and encephalopathy can result from severe hypertension. Because of the early initiation of dialysis, the once frequent complication of pericarditis resulting from metabolic cardiotoxins is rarely seen.[42] Accelerated coronary artery disease is also seen in patients with ESRD and accounts for the largest cause of mortality in dialysis patients.[43]

Respiratory Symptoms

Kussmaul's respirations (the deep sighing breathing seen in response to metabolic acidosis) is seen with uremia. Initially, however, dyspnea on exertion is a more frequent and often overlooked complaint in patients with progressing disease. The other respiratory complications, pneumonitis and "uremic lung," result from pulmonary edema associated with fluid and sodium retention and/or congestive heart failure.

Immunologic Changes

The significant morbidity experienced by patients with renal failure can be attributed to their altered host defenses. Uremic patients appear to be in a state of reduced immunocapacity, the cause of which is thought to be a combination of uremic toxemia and ensuing protein and caloric malnutrition compounded by protein-restricted diets. Uremic plasma contains nondialyzable factors that suppress lymphocyte responses that are manifested at the cellular and humoral levels, such as granulocyte dysfunction, suppressed cell-mediated immunity, and diminished ability to produce antibodies.[44] In addition, impaired or disrupted mucocutaneous barriers decrease protection from environmental pathogens. Together, these impairments place uremic patients at a high risk of infection, which is a common cause of morbidity and mortality.

Oral Manifestations

With impaired renal function, a decreased GFR, and the accumulation and retention of various products of renal failure, the oral cavity may show a variety of changes as the body progresses through an azotemic to a uremic state (Table 6). The oral health care professional should be able

TABLE 6 Oral and Radiographic Manifestations of Renal Disease and Dialysis
Oral manifestations
Enlarged (asymptomatic) salivary glands
Decreased salivary flow
Dry mouth
Odor of urea on breath
Metallic taste
Increased calculus formation
Low caries rate
Enamel hypoplasia
Dark brown stains on crowns
Extrinsic (secondary to liquid ferrous sulfate therapy)
Intrinsic (secondary to tetracycline staining)
Dental malocclusions
Pale mucosa with diminished color demarcation between attached gingiva and alveolar mucosa
Low-grade gingival inflammation
Petechiae and ecchymosis
Bleeding from gingiva
Prolonged bleeding
Candidal infections
Burning and tenderness of mucosa
Erosive glossitis
Tooth erosion (secondary to regurgitation associated with dialysis)
Dehiscence of wounds
Radiographic manifestations
Demineralization of bone
Loss of bony trabeculation
Ground-glass appearance
Loss of lamina dura
Giant cell lesions, "brown tumors"
Socket sclerosis
Pulpal narrowing and calcification
Tooth mobility
Arterial and oral calcifications

to recognize these oral symptoms as part of the patient's systemic disease and not as an isolated occurrence. In studies of renal patients, up to 90% were found to have oral symptoms of uremia. Some of the presenting signs were an ammonia-like taste and smell, stomatitis, gingivitis, decreased salivary flow, xerostomia, and parotitis.

As renal failure develops, one of the early symptoms may be a bad taste and odor in the mouth, particularly in the morning. This uremic fetor, an ammoniacal odor, is typical of any uremic patient and is caused by the high concentration of urea in the saliva and its subsequent breakdown to ammonia. Salivary urea levels correlate well with the BUN levels, but no fixed linear relationship exists. An acute rise in the BUN level may result in uremic stomatitis, which may appear as an erythemopultaceous form characterized by red mucosa covered with a thick exudate and a pseudomembrane or as an ulcerative form characterized by frank ulcerations with redness and a pultaceous coat. In all reported cases, intraoral changes have been related to BUN levels > 150 mg/dL and disappear spontaneously when medical treatment results in a lowered BUN level. Although its exact cause is uncertain, uremic stomatitis can be regarded as a chemical burn or as a general loss of tissue resistance and inability to withstand normal and traumatic influences. White plaques called "uremic frost" and occasionally found on the skin can be found intraorally, although rarely. This uremic frost results from residual urea crystals left on the epithelial surfaces after perspiration evaporates or as a result of decreased salivary flow. A more common oral finding is significant xerostomia, probably caused by a combination of direct involvement of the salivary glands, chemical inflammation, dehydration, and mouth breathing (Kussmaul's respiration). Salivary swelling can occasionally be seen. Another finding associated with increased salivary urea nitrogen, particularly in children, is a low caries activity. This is observed despite a high sugar intake and poor oral hygiene, suggesting an increased neutralizing capacity of the urea arising from urea hydrolysis. With the increased availability and improved techniques of dialysis and transplantation, many of the oral manifestations of uremia and renal failure are less commonly observed.

Other oral manifestations of renal disease are related to RO or secondary HPTH. These manifestations usually become evident late in the course of the disease. The classic signs of RO in the mandible and maxilla are bone demineralization, loss of trabeculation, ground-glass appearance, total or partial loss of lamina dura, giant cell lesions or brown tumors, and metastatic calcifications (Figure 2). These changes appear most frequently in the mandibular molar region superior to the mandibular canal. The rarefaction in the mandible and maxilla is secondary to generalized osteoporosis. The finer trabeculae disappear later, leaving a coarser pattern. Small lytic lesions that histologically prove to be giant cell or brown tumors may occur.

The compact bone of the jaws may become thinned and eventually disappear. This may be evident as loss of the lower border of the mandible, the cortical margins of the inferior dental canal and floor of the antrum, and lamina dura. Studies have shown that the finding of decreasing thickness of cortical bone at the angle of the mandible correlates well with the degree of RO. Spontaneous and pathologic fractures may occur with the thinning of these areas of compact bone and may complicate dental extractions.

Although the skeleton may undergo decalcification, fully developed teeth are not directly affected; however, in the presence of significant skeletal decalcification, the teeth will appear more radiopaque. The loss of lamina dura is neither pathognomonic for nor a consistent sign of HPTH. A similar loss of lamina dura also may be seen in Paget's disease, osteomalacia, fibrous dysplasia, sprue, and Cushing's and Addison's diseases. Various studies indicate changes in lamina dura in only 40 to 50% of known HPTH patients.

The radiolucent lesions of HPTH are called "brown tumors" because they contain areas of old hemorrhage and appear brown on clinical inspection. As these tumors increase in size, the resultant expansion may involve the cortex. Although the tumor rarely breaks through the periosteum, gingival swelling may occur. The brown tumor lesion contains an abundance of multinucleated giant cells, fibroblasts, and hemosiderin. This histologic appearance is also consis-

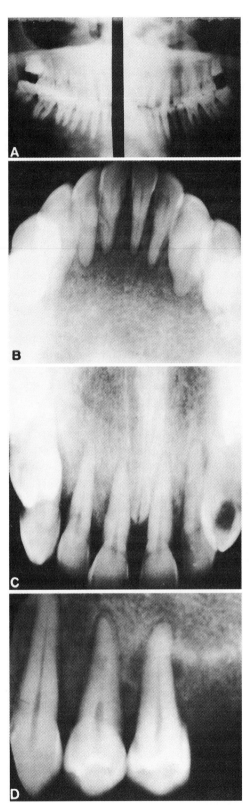

FIGURE 2 *A,* Panoramic image showing trabecular changes. Also note erupted lower third molars without fully developed root formations. *B,* Mandibular anterior loss of trabeculation. *C,* Maxillary anterior loss of trabeculation. *D,* Loss of lamina dura.

tent with central giant cell tumor and giant cell reparative granuloma. Associated bone changes consist of a generalized osteitis fibrosa, with patches of osteoclastic resorption on all bone surfaces. This is replaced by a vascular connective tissue that represents an abortive formation of coarse-fibered woven bone. This histologic picture also may be seen in fibrous dysplasia, giant cell reparative granuloma, osteomalacia, and Paget's disease.

Other clinical manifestations of RO include tooth mobility, malocclusion, and metastatic soft tissue calcifications. Increasing mobility and drifting of teeth with no apparent pathologic periodontal pocket formation may be seen. Periapical radiolucencies and root resorption also may be associated with this gradual loosening of the dentition. The teeth may be painful to percussion and mastication, and positive thermal and electric pulp test responses often will be elicited. Splinting is a useful adjunct to prevent pain and further drifting, and the splint should be maintained until adequate treatment of the HPTH results in bone remineralization. Malocclusion may result from the advanced mobility and drifting of the dentition. Extreme demineralization and collapse of the temporomandibular and paratemporomandibular bones may also produce a malocclusion.

Metastatic calcification can occur particularly when the calcium-phosphate multiplication sign (Ca x P) is >70. In normal subjects, a relationship exists between plasma calcium and inorganic phosphate. When expressed in terms of total calcium and inorganic phosphate (both as milligrams per deciliter), the ion product or calcium-phosphate solubility product (Ca x P) is normally an average of 35. A rise in the calcium-phosphate ion product in the extracellular fluid may cause metastatic calcifications because of the precipitation of calcium-phosphate crystals into the soft tissues, such as the sclera, corner of the eye, subcutaneous tissue, skeletal and cardiac muscle, and blood vessels. This also may occur in the oral and associated perioral soft tissues. These calcifications are often visible radiographically.

Abnormal bone repair after extraction, termed "socket sclerosis" and radiographically characterized by a lack of lamina dura resorption and by the deposition of sclerotic bone in the confines of the lamina dura, has been reported in patients with renal disease, although it is not unique to them (Figure 3).

Enamel hypoplasia (a white or brownish discoloration) is frequently seen in patients whose renal disease started at a young age. The location of the hypoplastic enamel on the permanent teeth corresponds to the age at onset of advanced renal failure. Prolonged corticosteroid administration also may contribute to this deficiency (Figure 4). Another frequent dental finding is pulpal narrowing and calcifications. In some patients who are on dialysis, severe tooth erosion as a result of the nausea and extensive vomiting that often follows dialysis treatment may be seen. Because of the platelet changes with renal disease itself and with dialysis therapy, gingival bleeding may be a common patient complaint.

▼ MEDICAL MANAGEMENT OF CRF

The treatment of CRF is often divided into (1) conservative therapy aimed at delaying progressive renal dysfunction and (2) renal replacement therapy, instituted when conservative measures are no longer effective in sustaining life.

Conservative Therapy

Once the extent of renal impairment is established and reversible causes are excluded, medical management is devoted to the elimination of symptoms and the prevention of further deterioration.[45] Conservative measures are initiated when the patient becomes azotemic. Initial conservative therapy is directed toward managing diet, fluid, electrolytes, and calcium-phosphate balance and toward the prevention and treatment of complications.[45] Dietary modifications are initiated with the onset of uremic symptoms. Dietary regulation of protein (20 to 40 g per day) may improve acidosis, azotemia, and nausea. The restriction of protein reduces not only BUN levels but also potassium and phosphate intake and hydrogen ion production. Also, a low-protein intake reduces the excretory load of the kidney, thereby reducing glomerular hyperfiltration, intraglomerular pressure, and secondary injury of nephrons.[46,47] This restricted diet is often supplemented with multivitamins specific to the needs of the renal patient. Despite difficulties with hypertension, edema, and weight gain, salt and fluid excess and depletion must be avoided. For patients with early renal insufficiency, prevention of hyperphosphatemia by limiting the intake of phosphate-containing foods and by supplementing the diet

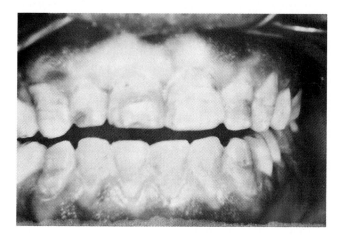

FIGURE 3. Enamel hypoplasia and tetracycline stains in a young patient with end-stage renal disease.

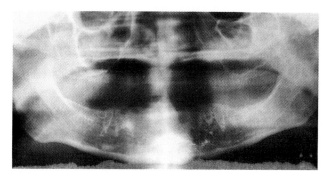

FIGURE 4 Panoramic radiograph of extraction sites representative of socket sclerosis. Teeth were extracted 6 years before the radiograph and 2 years before diagnosis of end-stage renal disease

with calcium carbonate (which prevents intestinal absorption) may potentially minimize the sequelae of uremic osteodystrophy.[48]

Recently, a practical clinical approach to the management of patients with CRF, using the acronym BEANS, has gained popularity. To temper renal dysfunction, attenuate uremic complications, and prepare patients for renal replacement therapy, medical care providers should "take care of the BEANS," as follows.[49] Blood pressure should be maintained in a target range lower than 130/80 mm Hg. (Toward this end, the use of angiotensin-converting enzyme inhibitors or angiotensin receptor blockers, because of their renal protective effects, has gained favor with many clinicians.[50]) Hemoglobin levels should be maintained at 10 to 12 g/dL with erythropoietin-stimulating agents. Hyperlipidemia should be treated with a "statin" lipid-lowering medication.[51] Smoking cessation should also be encouraged.[52] Access for dialysis should be created when the serum creatinine reaches >4.0 mg/dL or the GFR falls to <20 mL/min. This is also the appropriate time to refer patients for renal transplant evaluation. Close monitoring of nutritional status is important to avoid protein malnutrition, correct metabolic acidosis, prevent and treat hyperphosphatemia, administer vitamin supplements, and guide the initiation of dialysis therapy. Specialty evaluation by a nephrologist should be instituted when serum creatinine is >1.2 mg/dL in a female and >1.5 mg/dL in a male or patients with stage 3 kidney disease or an estimated GFR <60 cc/min.[53]

Renal Replacement Therapy

For patients with ESRD, dialysis has significantly decreased the mortality of this once invariably fatal disease. Long-term maintenance dialysis therapy has been a reality since 1961. In 1964, there were fewer than 300 patients in the United States receiving dialysis. Because of amendments to the Social Security Act in 1972 and the extension of Medicare benefits in 1973, dialysis therapy was made available to virtually everybody who developed ESRD. Although access to treatment is of less concern today, discrepancies between the morbidity and mortality rates of for-profit and not-for-profit dialysis centers remain a source of controversy.[54,55] Today, approximately 450,000 people are given treatments in more than 3,000 dialysis facilities in the United States. The total cost of the ESRD program in the United States was approximately $27 billion dollars in 2003. The projected number of ESRD patients by 2010 has been estimated to be 660,000 and the total Medicare ESRD program in excess of 28 billion dollars.[1]

There are no clear guidelines for determining when renal replacement therapy should begin. Most nephrologists base their decisions on the individual patient's ability to work full time, the presence of peripheral neuropathy, and the presence of other signs of clinical deterioration or uremic symptoms. Most nephrologists will initiate dialysis when the GFR is <15 cc/min in a diabetic patient and <10 cc/min in a nondiabetic patient. There are a number of absolute clinical indications to initiate maintenance dialysis. These include pericarditis, fluid overload or pulmonary edema refractory to diuretics, accelerated hypertension poorly responsive to antihypertensive medications, progressive uremic encephalopathy or neuropathy (confusion, asterixis, myoclonus, wrist or foot drop, seizures), clinically significant bleeding attributable to uremia, and persistent nausea and vomiting.[56] There are two major techniques of dialysis: hemodialysis and peritoneal dialysis. Each follows the same basic principle of diffusion of solutes and water from the plasma to the dialysis solution in response to a concentration or pressure gradient.

▼ HEMODIALYSIS

Hemodialysis is the removal of nitrogenous and toxic products of metabolism from the blood by means of a hemodialyzer system. Exchange occurs between the patient's plasma and dialysate (the electrolyte composition of which mimics that of extracellular fluid) across a semipermeable membrane that allows uremic toxins to diffuse out of the plasma while retaining the formed elements and protein composition of blood (Figure 5). Dialysis does not provide the same degree of health as normal renal function provides because there is no resorptive capability in the dialysis membrane; therefore, valuable nutrients are lost, and potentially toxic molecules are retained. The usual dialysis system consists of a dialyzer, dialysate production unit, roller blood pump, heparin infusion pump, and various devices to monitor the conductivity, temperature, flow rate, and pressure of dialysate and to detect blood leaks and arterial and venous pressures.[57]

Dialysis therapy can be delivered to the patient in outpatient dialysis centers, where trained personnel administer therapy on a regular basis, or in the home, where family members trained in dialysis techniques assist the patient in dialysis therapy. It has been shown that patients who undergo dialysis at home fare better psychologically, have a better quality of life, and have lower rates of morbidity and mortality than hospital dialysis patients.[58,59] Unfortunately, home dialysis may not be applicable for all patients because it is more difficult and requires a high degree of motivation.

The frequency and duration of dialysis treatments are related to body size, residual renal function, protein intake, and tolerance to fluid removal. The typical patient undergoes hemodialysis three times per week, with each treatment lasting approximately 3 to 4 hours on standard dialysis units and slightly less time on high-efficiency or high-flux dialysis units. Nocturnal dialysis and daily dialysis are newer forms of hemodialysis that are gaining acceptance due to improved control of both biochemical abnormalities and blood pressure and volume status. During treatments and for varying amounts of time afterward, anticoagulants are administered by regional or systemic methods.

There are three major types of vascular access for maintenance hemodialysis: primary arteriovenous (AV) fistula, synthetic AV graft, and double-lumen, cuffed tunneled

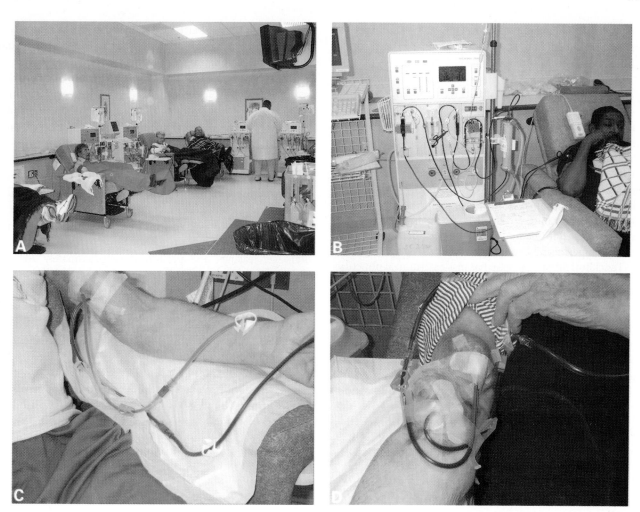

FIGURE 5 *A*, Dialysis Unit replacing of picture of Dialysate. *B*, Dialysis unit. *C*, Patient receiving dialysis. *D*, Close-up of access.

catheters.[60] Vascular accesses for hemodialysis can be created by a shunt or external cannula system or by an AV fistula; the fistula is preferred for long-term treatment. The classic construction is a side-to-side anastomosis between the radial artery and the cephalic vein at the forearm. In patients with very thin veins, it can be technically impossible to create a direct AV fistula, and in some patients, fistulae have clotted in both arms, resulting in a demand for other forms of vascular access (sometimes the thigh is used as a site). A great advance in access capability was the introduction of subcutaneous artificial AV grafts, beginning with Gore-Tex heterografts (W.L. Gore, Flagstaff, AZ). Fistulae are now constructed between arteries and veins by means of saphenous vein, autografts, polytetrafluoroethylene (PTFE) grafts, Dacron, and other prosthetic conduits. Hemodialysis is performed by direct cannulation of these grafts or vascular anastomoses (Figure 6).[61,62] There is an increasing trend toward the use of indwelling central venous catheters for maintenance hemodialysis.[63]

Despite optimal dialysis, these patients remain chronically ill with hematologic, metabolic, neurologic, and cardiovascular problems that are more or less permanent. Growth alterations may be seen in very young renal disease patients,

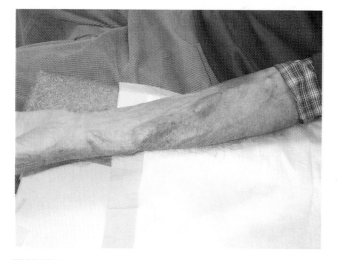

FIGURE 6 Vascular access site in the arm.

particularly if they are maintained on hemodialysis. This growth deficiency has been attributed to the poor caloric intake of these patients and to the uremic state.[64] Dietary supplements have produced accelerated growth spurts, and successful kidney transplantation may restore a normal growth rate.[65] The major determining factor is the bone age. For patients older than 12 years of age, it is doubtful that significant growth would be attained.

▼ PERITONEAL DIALYSIS

Peritoneal dialysis accounts for only 10% of dialysis treatments. During peritoneal dialysis, access to the body is achieved via a catheter through the abdominal wall into the peritoneum. One to two liters of dialysate is placed in the peritoneal cavity and is allowed to remain for varying intervals of time. Substances diffuse across the semipermeable peritoneal membrane into the dialysate. Compared with the membranes used for hemodialysis, the peritoneal membrane has greater permeability for high molecular weight species. The Tenckhoff Silastic catheter has made peritoneal puncture for each dialysis unnecessary. The Tenckhoff catheter is a permanent intraperitoneal catheter that has two polyester felt cuffs into which tissue growth occurs. If used with a sterile technique, it permits virtually infection-free long-term access to the peritoneum (Figure 7).

Several regimens can be used with peritoneal dialysis. In one, chronic ambulatory peritoneal dialysis, 2 L of dialysis fluid is instilled into the peritoneal cavity, allowed to remain for 30 minutes, and then drained out. This is repeated every 8 to 12 hours, 5 to 7 days per week. A popular variation of this is continuous cyclic peritoneal dialysis, in which 2 to 3 L of dialysate is exchanged every hour over a 6- to 8-hour period overnight, 7 days per week.[66]

Two of the benefits of peritoneal dialysis are that heparinization is unnecessary and that there is no risk of air embolism and blood leaks. It also allows a great deal of personal freedom; for this reason, it is often used as the primary therapy or as a temporary measure. These features, along with its simplicity, make peritoneal dialysis safe for patients who are at risk when hemodialysis is used (eg, the young, elderly patients, those with high-risk coronary and cerebral vascular disease, and those with vascular access problems).[67] Some of the problems encountered with peritoneal dialysis are pain, intra-abdominal hemorrhage, bowel infarction, inadequate drainage, leakage, and peritonitis (approximately 70% of which is caused by a single gram-positive microorganism that is indigenous to the patient's skin or upper respiratory tract and that infects the peritoneal cavity).[68] Recent studies have shown inferior mortality data in peritoneal dialysis versus hemodialysis patients, especially in patients with diabetes and coronary artery disease.[69]

Today, renal transplantation is the treatment of choice for patients with irreversible kidney failure. However, the use of transplantation is limited by organ availability. Renal transplantation and its specific dental management

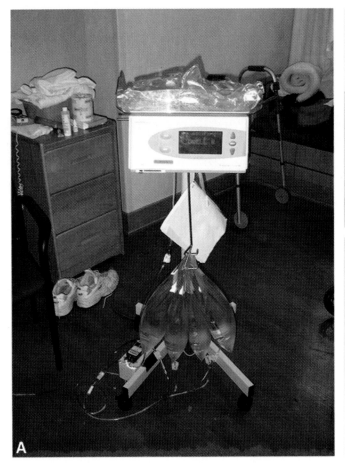
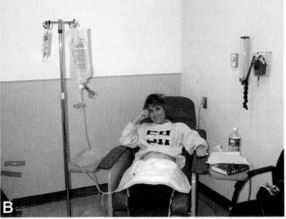
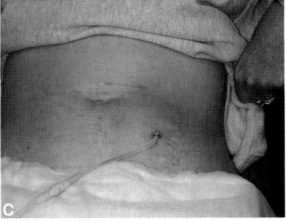

FIGURE 7   *A,* Dialysate for chronic ambulatory peritoneal dialysis. *B,* Close-up of patient receiving dialysis. *C,* Close-up of peritoneal access.

considerations are discussed in Chapter 19, "Transplantation Medicine."

▼ OTHER APPROACHES TO SOLUTE REMOVAL

Many patients continue to have various disturbances in metabolic functions despite optimal dialysis, maintaining uremic metabolites (eg, urea, creatinine, and phosphate) at nearly normal levels. These observations have led investigators to postulate that uremic toxins of a molecular weight between that of urea (<500 Da) and that of plasma proteins (>50,000 Da), effectively unfiltered by dialysis, account for these clinical abnormalities. This theory, termed the middle molecular hypothesis, has led to the development of two techniques: hemofiltration (HF) and absorbent therapy. Hemofiltration is based on the principle of convection instead of diffusion and is based on the physiologic function of the glomerulus.[70] In HF, the standard dialysis technique is modified by sequentially prediluting the blood with an electrolyte solution that is similar to plasma and subsequently "ultrafiltering" it under high hydraulic pressures. This technique is more efficient than dialysis in removing solutes in the middle molecular range and results in patients who feel well and have little hemodynamic instability. Adjunctive techniques used with maintenance dialysis or for patients with significant residual renal function (a GFR of 5 to 10 mL/min) include the use of absorbent materials for solute removal. These absorbents may be used through direct action on the bloodstream (hemoperfusion), through regeneration of dialysate (REDY sorbent hemodialysis), or indirectly, through introduction into the gut. The REcirculating DialYsis System (REDY 2000, REDY Sorbent system), which was manufactured initially by Organon Teknika and now by Gambro Healthcare, Inc., differs from regular single-pass dialysis in that after passing through the dialyzer, the REDY dialysate fluid is regenerated, rather than discarded, by passing through a sorbent cartridge.

▼ ORAL HEALTH CONSIDERATIONS

For the purposes of dental management, patients with renal disease can be categorized into two groups: patients with ARF and patients with chronic progressing renal failure or end-stage renal failure who are undergoing dialysis. The dental management considerations for patients with renal disease is summarized in Table 9.

ARF Patients

ARF is most commonly observed in young healthy adults after injury to the renal tubules as a result of toxic agents, severe necrotizing glomerular disease, or complications of surgery, including hemorrhage and transfusion. Patients with ARF are not candidates for elective dental care, and some patients with ARF require the institution of dialysis therapy. In such cases, elective dental care should be deferred until the patient makes a complete renal recovery. Peritoneal dialysis generally poses no contraindications to dental treatment. The exceptions are in times of acute peritoneal infections, when elective care should be postponed.

CRF and ESRD Patients

Many patients with chronic renal disease have poor oral health. The results of a study assessing the dental needs of hemodialysis patients showed that 64% of these patients needed dental treatment and that the majority of these patients were not aware of the possible complications of dental neglect while on hemodialysis.[71] In addition to the more common reasons for not receiving routine dental treatment, these patients have limited access to dental care because many general dentists are reluctant to treat patients with severe systemic diseases. Because most dialysis centers refer their patients to general practitioners for most forms of treatment, it is important that more general dentists become familiar with the management problems associated with patients with ESRD who are undergoing dialysis.

Excessive bleeding and anemia are the two major hematologic conditions that most commonly affect patients with uremia and renal failure. Bleeding tendencies in these patients are attributed to a combination of qualitative and quantitative platelet defects, increased prostacyclin activity, intrinsic coagulation defects, and capillary fragility. This hemorrhagic tendency can be magnified in the presence of uremia. Hemorrhagic episodes in the gingiva are not uncommon. Ulcerations and purpural or petechial lesions may be noted throughout the oral mucosa. Bruising after trauma is common, and hematoma formation should be expected after alveolectomy or periodontal surgery. Adjunctive hemostatic measures should be considered for patients who are at risk. DDAVP (1-deamino-8-D-arginine vasopressin), the synthetic analogue of the antidiuretic hormone vasopressin, has been shown to be effective in the short-term management of bleeding in patients with renal failure. The effects of conjugated estrogen, used for longer-term hemostasis, commonly last for up to 2 weeks, compared with a few hours for DDAVP. Tranexamic acid (an antifibrinolytic agent) administered in the form of a mouthrinse or soaked gauze significantly reduces operative and postoperative bleeding. Meticulous surgical technique, primary closure, and local hemostatic aids such as microfibrillar collagen and oxidized regenerated cellulose should be used as the standards of care. Although rare, hemorrhagic effusions into the temporomandibular joint space presenting as pain and swelling have been reported in a patient who was on dialysis and systemic anticoagulant therapy.

The timing of dental care for the patient who is undergoing dialysis has long been a source of discussion in the literature. Since dialysis will return hydration, serum electrolytes, urea nitrogen, and creatinine toward normal levels, arguments have been made for treating patients in a dental setting on the day of dialysis treatment. This argument is countered by the facts that patients often do not feel well immediately after undergoing dialysis and that they are heparinized. Ideally, elective dental procedures, as well as extractions and other surgery, should be done on nondialysis days as early as possible from the next dialysis treatment. At this point, the blood is free of uremic toxins, and the patient is far enough removed from dialysis to allow sufficient time after surgery for clotting before the next cycle and reheparinization. Also, it is less likely that the patient will have a clotting defect that is due to uremia-related platelet dysfunction, which develops because of retained urea metabolites. A platelet count and complete blood count are important guides for the dental practitioner with regard to the management of bleeding tendencies and anemic conditions. However, since patients are physically and emotionally exhausted and do not feel well following dialysis treatments, elective dental procedures should be scheduled on nondialysis days, when patients are more likely to tolerate care.

Apart from serving as a potential site for infection, the AV site should never be jeopardized. The arm with the vascular access should be identified and noted on the patient's chart with instructions to avoid both intramuscular and IV injection of medication into this arm, and the access site should not be used as an injection site. The blood flow through the arm should not be impeded by requiring the patient to assume a cramped position or by using that arm to measure blood pressure. When the access site is located in a leg, the patient should avoid sitting for long periods. Obstructing venous drainage by compression at the groin or behind the knee must be avoided, especially because it tends to occur normally when the patient is in the sitting position. Such patients should be permitted to walk about for a few minutes every hour during a lengthy dental procedure.

Susceptibility to infection is a serious concern for patients with uremia or ESRD who are undergoing hemodialysis.[72] These patients have an increased susceptibility to bacterial infections that results from altered cellular immunity secondary to the effects of uremic toxins combined with malnutrition from protein-restricted diets. Oral diseases and dental manipulation create bacteremias that may lead to significant morbidity and potential mortality in patients with renal failure who are undergoing hemodialysis. A majority of septicemic infections have been attributed to the vascular access site, but oral diseases such as periodontal disease, pulpal infection, and oral ulcerations, along with dental treatment, may provide microorganisms with a convenient portal of entry into the circulatory system. Therefore, every effort should be made to eliminate potential sources of infection. Meticulous oral hygiene, including good home care, frequent oral health maintenance, and routine use of antifungal and antimicrobial oral rinses, may reduce the risk of dentally induced infections.

Infective endocarditis is a serious concern in hemodialysis patients. Sepsis and bacterial endarteritis occur from infections at the access site by organisms seeded through punctures. Infective endocarditis has been reported in patients with access-site grafts on hemodialysis after receiving dental treatment. The incidence of infective endocarditis in patients undergoing hemodialysis is 2.7%. In those patients with a history of vascular access-site infection, the incidence increases to 9.0%. *Streptococcus viridans* accounts for almost one-third of the cases of infective endocarditis, whereas staphylococcal organisms such as *Staphylococcus epidermidis* and *Staphylococcus aureus* account for the majority of cases. The cause of endocarditis in these patients is debatable but seems to be related to a combination of vascular access and intrinsic cardiovalvular pathology. The presence of an AV shunt or synthetic graft (fistula) sutured in place increases the risk for infective colonization at the suture lines or at the surface discrepancies between normal arterial intima and the so-called prosthetic pseudointima. These sites may provide a nidus for intravascular lodgment of bacteria, leading to the persistence of an otherwise transient bacteremia (such as one resulting from dental manipulation), with subsequent endarteritis, embolization, and possible endocardial infection.[73] A period of high susceptibility to infection is usually seen within the first 3 months after implantation (the risk is highest in the first 3 weeks), after which there is a gradual decline in risk. This reduced risk is possibly caused by an "insulating effect" of the developing pseudointima and endothelialization.

Endocarditis infection is more likely to affect previously abnormal cardiac valves, yet there is a high incidence of endocarditis in hemodialysis patients with no previously demonstrated valvulopathy. A possible explanation may lie in the theory that changes in fluid volume with uremia and hemodialysis may affect blood flow through the heart and cardiac function, creating mechanical stresses on the valves that play a role in the development of infective endocarditis. Therefore, according to the American Heart Association's protocol for prevention of infective endocarditis, antimicrobial premedication should be used routinely prior to appropriate dental procedures in those patients with a risk of developing endocarditis or a prior history and those with patent and active vascular access sites for dialysis.

The choice of antibiotic depends on many variables but is primarily based on the type of microorganisms that have been cultured at the site of manipulation. In patients who were reported to have acquired infective endocarditis after dental treatment, either viridans streptococci or *Enterococcus* spp were the causative agents. This indicates a prophylactic regimen of either (1) amoxicillin or clindamycin or (2) a broad-spectrum antibiotic such as oral clarithromycin (as recommended by the American Heart Association) or IV vancomycin given at the time of dialysis in patients with hypersensitivity to penicillin or clindamycin. Limited insurance reimbursement for vancomycin infusion historically has limited many patients' access to this therapy.

Because these patients are exposed to a large number of blood transfusions and exchanges and also because of their renal failure–related immune dysfunction, they are at greater risk of hepatotropic viral infections (such as hepatitis B and C), HIV infection, and tuberculosis. Many patients with renal disease may have viral hepatitis without clinical manifestations. In these patients, the disease tends to run a chronic and persistently active (although subclinical) course. With the

TABLE 7 Drug Therapy for Renal Disease

		Adjustments for Renal Failure	
Drug	Normal	Moderate (GFR = 10–50 mL/min)	Severe (GFR <10 mL/min)
Antifungal agents			
Amphotericin	q24h	Unchanged	Unchanged
Fluconazole	q24h	Unchanged	Unchanged
Miconazole	q8h	Unchanged	Unchanged
Aminoglycosides			
Gentamicin	q8h	q12–24h	Avoid if possible
Tobramycin	q8h	q8–24h	Avoid if possible
Streptomycin	q12h	Avoid if possible	Avoid if possible
Other antimicrobials			
Penicillin G	q6–8h	q8–12h	q12–18h
Penicillin V	q6h	q6h	q6h
Erythromycin	q6h	Unchanged	Unchanged
Ampicillin	q6h	q6–12h	q12–16h
Amoxicillin	q8h	q8–12h	q12–16h
Cephalothin	q6h	Unchanged	q8–12h
Carbenicillin	q4h	q8–12h	Avoid if possible
Clindamycin	q8h	q8h	q8h
Metronidazole	q8h	q8h	q12–16h
Vancomycin	q6h	q72–240h	q240h
Tetracycline	q6h	q6h	q6h
Doxycycline	q12–24h	q12–24h	q12–24h
Analgesics			
Acetaminophen	q4h	q6h	q8h
Acetylsalicylic acid	q4h	q4–6h	Avoid
Ketorolac	q6h	Avoid	Avoid
Phenacetin	q6h	Avoid	Avoid
Ibuprofen	q6h	Avoid	Avoid
Local anesthetics	Unchanged	Unchanged	Unchanged
Narcotics			
Codeine	q4h	Unchanged	Unchanged
Meperidine (Demerol)	q4h	Unchanged	Unchanged
Morphine	q4h	Unchanged	Unchanged
Pentazocine (Talwin)	q4–6h	Unchanged	Unchanged
Propoxyphene (Darvon)	q4h	Unchanged	Unchanged
Naloxone (Narcan)	Bolus	Unchanged	Unchanged
Sedatives, hypnotics, barbiturates, and tranquilizers			
Chlordiazepoxide (Librium)	q6–8h	Unchanged	Unchanged
Diazepam (Valium)	q8h	Unchanged	Unchanged
Flurazepam (Dalmane)	q24h	Unchanged	Unchanged
Meprobamate (Miltown)	q6h	q9–12h	q12–18h
Methaqualone (Quaalude)	q8h	Unchanged	Unchanged
Amitriptyline (Elavil)	q8h	Unchanged	Unchanged
Secobarbital	q8h	Unchanged	Unchanged
Phenobarbital	q8h	Unchanged	Unchanged
Pentobarbital	q8h	Unchanged	Unchanged
Antihistamines			
Chlorpheniramine (Chlortrimeton)	q4–6h	Unchanged	Unchanged
Diphenhydramine (Benadryl)	q6h	q6–9h	q9–12h
Corticosteroids			
Cortisone	q8h	Unchanged	Unchanged
Hydrocortisone	q8h	Unchanged	Unchanged
Prednisone	q8h	Unchanged	Unchanged
Neurologic agents			
Phenytoin (Dilantin)	q8h	Unchanged	Unchanged
Lidocaine	—	Unchanged	Unchanged

GFR = glomerular filtration rate.

advent of prophylactic immunoglobulin and the hepatitis B vaccine, the number of dialysis unit outbreaks of hepatitis has decreased; however, the dialysis patient should still be considered to be in a high-risk group. The prevalence of hepatitis C virus infection in dialysis patients ranges from 3.9 to 71%.[74,75] Patients undergoing dialysis should be encouraged to undergo periodic testing for hepatitis infectivity. Hemodialysis patients with accompanying conditions such as HIV disease, viral hepatitis (and associated liver dysfunction), and tuberculosis have complicating issues that affect the provision of dental care. CRF patients who are on hemodialysis have been reported to be at increased risk of developing tuberculosis.[76] (The dental management of patients with infectious diseases is discussed in Chapter 20, "Infectious Diseases.")

As a result of changes in fluid volume, sodium retention, and the presence of vascular access, these patients are commonly affected by a host of cardiovascular conditions. Often, hypertension, postdialysis hypotension, congestive heart failure, and pulmonary hypertension can be seen in patients who are undergoing hemodialysis.[77] Hypertension in the presence of ESRD can lead to accelerated atherosclerosis. Although the medical management of these patients includes the aggressive use of antihypertensive agents, the dental practitioner should obtain blood pressure readings at every visit, prior to and during procedures. Avoiding excessive stress in the dental chair is important to minimize intraoperative elevations of systolic pressure. The use of sedative premedication should be considered for patients who are to undergo stressful procedures. Hypotension resulting from fluid depletion is a common complication of hemodialysis and occurs in up to 30% of dialysis sessions. Cerebrovascular accidents, angina, fatal dysrhythmias, and myocardial infarction are less common but serious sequelae of hemodialysis and most commonly present during or immediately following dialysis. Therefore, elective dental care should be performed on nondialysis days, when the patients are best able to tolerate treatment.

Pharmacotherapeutics are a serious concern for dentists treating patients who have renal disease. Most drugs are excreted at least partially by the kidney, and renal function affects drug bioavailability, the volume of drug distribution, drug metabolism, and the rate of drug elimination. The dentist can obviate problems of drug reactions and further renal damage by following simple principles related to drug administration and by altering dosage schedules according to the amount of residual renal function. Many ordinarily safe drugs must not be administered to the uremic patient, and many others must be prescribed over longer intervals (Table 7). The plasma half-lives of medications that are normally eliminated in the urine are often prolonged in renal failure and are effectively reduced by dialysis. Even drugs that are metabolized by the liver can lead to increased toxicity because the diseased kidneys fail to excrete them effectively. Theoretically, a 50% decrease in creatinine clearance

corresponds to a twofold increase in the elimination half-life of any medication excreted fully by the kidneys. For drugs that are partially excreted by the kidneys, the change in plasma half-life is proportionally less. For most drugs, it is proper to give a loading dose similar to that given to patients without renal disease; this provides a clinically desirable blood concentration that can be sustained by the necessary dosage adjustments. Whenever reliable blood drug level measurements are available, they can be used to monitor therapy. In the absence of precise blood levels, the best guide to therapy is carefully obtained data on biologic half-lives of drugs in humans with varying degrees of renal failure.

Certain drugs are themselves nephrotoxic and should be avoided. Particular medications may be metabolized to acid and nitrogenous waste or may stimulate tissue catabolism. NSAIDs may induce sodium retention, impair the action of diuretics, prevent aldosterone production, affect renal artery perfusion, and cause acidosis. Tetracyclines and steroids are antianabolic, increasing urea nitrogen to approximately twice the baseline levels. Other drugs, such as phenacetin, are nephrotoxic and put added strain on an already damaged kidney (Table 8). The challenge for dentists in prescribing medications is to maintain a therapeutic regimen within a narrow range, avoiding subtherapeutic dosing and toxicity.

The safety of a fluoridated community water supply for patients undergoing hemodialysis has been questioned in regard to whether such water is a contributing factor to the incidence of renal osteodystrophy, fluoride toxicity, and fluorosis. There is no satisfactory evidence that the fluoride content of fluoridated drinking water is harmful to patients with severe renal disease. Dialysis patients, however, should receive dialysates that are water-purified and deionized. No studies have reported on the dental use of topical fluoride in

TABLE 8   Drugs to Limit or Avoid When Treating Dialysis Patients

Indication	Drug
Magnesium content	Antacids (Maalox, Milk of Magnesia), laxatives
Potassium content	IV fluids Salt substitutes Massive penicillin therapy (1.7 mEq/million U)
Sodium content	Carbenicillin (4.7 mEq/g) Alka Seltzer (23 mEq tablet), IV fluid
Acidifying effects	Ascorbic acid, ammonium chloride (in cough syrup), nonsteroidal anti-inflammatory agents
Catabolic effects	Tetracyclines, steroids
Nephrotoxicity	Phenacetin, ketorolac Cephalosporins*
Alkalosis effect	Absorbed antacids Carbenicillin (large doses), penicillin (large doses)

*Long term, especially when combined with gentamicin.

TABLE 9 Summary of Dental Considerations and Management of the Patient with Renal Disease

Before treatment
  Determine dialysis schedule and treat on day after dialysis.
  Consult with the patient's nephrologist for recent laboratory tests and discussion of antibiotic prophylaxis.
  Identify arm with vascular access and type; notate in chart and avoid taking blood pressure measurement/injection of medication on this arm.
  Evaluate patient for hypertension/hypotension.
  Institute preoperative hemostatic aids (DDAVP, conjugated estrogen) when appropriate.
  Determine underlying cause of renal failure (underlying disease may affect provision of care).
  Obtain routine annual dental radiographs to establish presence and follow manifestations of renal osteodystrophy.
  Consider routine serology for HBV, HCV, and HIV antibody.
  Consider antibiotic prophylaxis when appropriate.
  Consider sedative premedication for patients with hypertension.

During treatment
  Perform a thorough history and physical examination for the presence of oral manifestations.
  Aggressively eliminate potential sources of infection/bacteremia.
  Use adjunctive hemostatic aids during oral/periodontal surgical procedures.
  Maintain the patient in a comfortable uncramped position in the dental chair.
  Allow the patient to walk or stand intermittently during long procedures.

After treatment
  Use postsurgical hemostatic agents.
  Encourage meticulous home care.
  Institute therapy for xerostomia when appropriate.
  Consider use of postoperative antibiotics for traumatic procedures.
  Avoid use of respiratory-depressant drugs in the presence of severe anemia.
  Adjust dosages of postoperative medications according to the extent of renal failure.
  Ensure routine recall maintenance.

DDAVP = 1-deamino-8-D-arginine vasopressin; HBV = hepatitis B virus; HCV = hepatitis C virus; HIV = human immunodeficiency virus.

Adapted from De Rossi SS, Glick M. Dental considerations for patients with renal disease receiving hemodialysis. JADA 1996;127:211–9

patients with renal disease or on any related problems. If a patient with renal disease needs fluoride supplements for caries control (particularly because of diminished salivary flow), the preferred route should be fluoride rinses until more definitive studies are carried out.

▼ SELECTED READINGS

Chonchol M. Neutrophil dysfunction and infection risk in end-stage renal disease. Semin Dial 2006;19:291–6.

Collins AJ, Kasiske B, Herzog C, et al. Excerpts from the United States Renal Data System 2004 annual data report: atlas of end-stage renal disease in the United States. Am J Kidney Dis 2005;45(1 Suppl 1):A5–7.

de Francisco AL. Medical therapy of secondary hyperparathyroidism in chronic kidney disease: old and new drugs. Expert Opin Pharmacother 2006;7:2215–24.

De Rossi SS, Glick M. Dental considerations for patients with renal disease receiving hemodialysis. JADA 1996;127:211–9.

El-Kishawi AM, El-Nahas AM. Renal osteodystrophy: review of the disease and its treatment. Saudi J Kidney Dis Transpl 2006;17:373–82.

Fishbane S. Iron supplementation in renal anemia. Semin Nephrol 2006;26:319–24.

Liu J, Kalantarinia K, Rosner MH. Management of lipid abnormalities associated with end-stage renal disease. Semin Dial 2006;19:391–401.

Ganesh Sk, Hulbert-Shearon TE, Port FK, et al. Mortality differences by dialysis modality among incident ESRD patients with and without coronary artery disease. J Am Soc Nephrol 2003;14:415–28.

Ledebo I, Lamiere N, Charra B, et al. Improving the outcome of dialysis—opinion vs scientific evidence. Nephrol Dial Transplant 2000;15:1310–6.

Maggiore Q, Pizzarelli F, Dattolo P, et al. Cardiovascular stability during hemodialysis, hemofiltration, and hemodialfiltration. Nephrol Dial Transplant 2000;15 Suppl 1:68–73.

Orth SR. Effects of smoking on systemic and intrarenal hemodynamics: influence on renal function. J Am Soc Nephrol 2004;15 Suppl 1:S58–63.

Pereira BJ. Optimization of pre-ESRD care; the key to improved dialysis outcomes. Kidney Int 2000;57:351–65.

St Peter WL, Obrador GT, Roberts TL, Collins AJ. Trends in intravenous iron use among dialysis patients in the United States (1994-2002). Am J Kidney Dis. 2005;46:650–60.

For the full reference list, please refer to the accompanying CD ROM.

16

HEMATOLOGIC DISEASES

LAUREN L. PATTON, DDS

▼ PROCESS OF HEMATOPOIESIS

The production of all types of blood cells occurs in the bone marrow as a result of differentiation from pluripotential precursor or primitive stem cells. This is a self-regulating process, with normal target distribution of cell types and maintenance of a steady state of production balanced with natural senescence and removal from the system. The hematopoietic system can respond to demands placed upon it by triggers such as infection, immune challenges, hemorrhage, or hypoxia by altering the distribution of cell types, through increasing or decreasing production of certain cell types. Feedback signals are provided by cytokines to the stem cells to produce more mature cells of the certain type in the quantity needed by the body. For example, thrombopoietin is the primary cytokine known to trigger the megakaryocyte to differentiate and proliferate into additional platelets, erythropoietin for erythrocytes, and granulocyte colony-stimulating factor (G-CSF) for the granulocyte line, although cross-stimulation is also possible.[1] An exception occurs for lymphocytes, which can be produced in larger numbers each day than needed by the body, of which many are destroyed during production.

The pluripotent stem cell matures into two common precursor lines, lymphopoietic and hematopoietic. The lymphopoietic common precursor cell becomes committed to either the B-cell or T-cell lines, which undergo cellular differentiation and maturation into the B memory and B plasma cells and T memory helper suppressor and large granular lymphocyte, respectively. The hematopoietic common precursor cell becomes committed to megakaryocytic cells that mature to platelets, erythroid cells that mature to erythrocytes, or the myelomonocytic cell line, which undergoes cellular differentiation and maturation to the following cell types: monocytes, eosinophils, neutrophils, and basophils.

Examination of the peripheral blood complete blood count (CBC) and differential of the white blood cells and peripheral blood smear to detect erythrocyte morphology, the presence of abnormal or immature white blood cells, and platelet size, combined with bone marrow examination by biopsy, can reveal much about homeostasis and is important in the diagnosis and management of a variety of clinical disorders. Disorders are both neoplastic and non-neoplastic. Morphologic and biochemical identification may be required to distinguish primitive cell types that have become disordered in acute leukemias. Subtypes of leukemias and lymphomas can also be distinguished by the use of labeled monoclonal antibodies directed against cell surface antigens or by the use of immunohistochemical techniques to demonstrate cytoplasmic antigens in tissue sections. Electron microscopy, cytogenetics, and demonstration of genetic defects and gene rearrangements may also be of diagnostic value.

Once formed, different cell types have different normal life spans (eg, 120 days for erythrocytes, 5–10 days for platelets, 6 hours to 3 days for neutrophils) before they become senescent. Senescent or otherwise damaged erythrocytes are recognized and destroyed by the reticuloendothelial system. At least half of senescent erythrocytes are destroyed in the spleen by splenic macrophages and the remaining red cells are destroyed in the liver, bone marrow, or other sites of the mononuclear phagocyte system. Neutrophils undergo death by apoptosis; however, the trigger is unknown. Aging platelets are also sequestered in the spleen and are subject to phagocytosis by macrophages.

▼ RED BLOOD CELL DISORDERS

Erythrocyte levels may be increased or decreased in various disease states. Table 1 shows the key laboratory tests for red cell disorders.

Erythrocytoses

Erythrocytosis describes conditions with an increase in circulating red blood cells (RBCs), characterized by a consistently raised hematocrit (HCT). Conditions of increased circulating RBCs include apparent erythrocytosis, relative erythrocytosis and absolute erythrocytoses (both primary and secondary causes), and idiopathic erythrocytosis (IE).

Measurement of the RBC mass should be done to evaluate patients with a persistently raised venous HCT (> 52% males, > 48% females for over 2 months).[2] Apparent erythrocytosis is diagnosed when individuals have an elevated venous HCT but whose RBC mass falls within the reference range. Relative erythrocytosis generally only exists with the state of significant dehydration, use of diuretics, diarrhea, or burns, where hemoconcentration occurs, such that the RBC mass is in the normal reference range, whereas the plasma volume is below the reference range. Absolute erythrocytosis is diagnosed when an individual's measured RBC mass is more than 25% above the mean predicted value. Once an absolute erythrocytosis has been confirmed, it is desirable to identify the underlying etiology.[2]

Absolute erythrocytoses are usually subdivided into primary and secondary forms. Primary erythrocytosis is a condition in which the erythropoietic compartment is expanding independently of extrinsic influences or by responding inadequately to them. Primary erythrocytoses include primary familial and congenital polycythemia due to mutations of the erythropoietin (Epo) receptor gene and the myeloproliferative disorder polycythemia vera (PV).[3]

Secondary erythrocytoses are driven by hormonal factors (predominantly by Epo) extrinsic to the erythroid compartment. The increased Epo secretion may represent either a physiologic response to tissue hypoxia, an abnormal autonomous Epo production, or a dysregulation of the

TABLE 1 Key Laboratory Tests for Red Cell Disorders

Test Name	Normal Range (SI units)	Increased	Decreased	Oral Findings
Red blood cell (RBC)	Adult male: $4.5–9.0 \times 10^6/\mu$ Adult female: $4.5–5.1 \times 10^6/\mu$	Polycythemia; erythrocytosis; fluid loss due to dehydration, diuretics, diarrhea, burns	Anemia	Pale, atrophic oral mucosa; in chronic anemia, possible large trabecular pattern on dental radiographs from hypertrophic marrow
RBC indices Mean corpuscular volume	Adult: $80–93 \ \mu m^2$	Macrocytosis Vitamin B_{12} and folate deficiency	Microcytosis Iron deficiency anemia; thalassemia	
Mean corpuscular hemoglobin	27.5–33.2 pg	Hyperchromia	Hypochromic anemia	
Mean corpuscular hemoglobin concentration	33.4–35.5% (concentration fraction 0.334–0.355)	Hyperchromia	Hypochromic anemia	
Hemoglobin	Adult male: 14.0–17.5 g/dL Adult female: 12.3–15.3 g/dL	Same as RBC results	Same as RBC results	Same as RBC results
Hematocrit	Adult male: 41.5–50.4% Adult female: 35.9–44.6%	Same as RBC results	Same as RBC results	Same as RBC results

oxygen-dependent Epo synthesis.[3] Secondary erythrocytoses may also result from congenital high–oxygen affinity hemoglobin, hypoxia because of smoking and chronic lung disease, congenital cyanotic heart disease with intracardiac shunts, hypoventilation syndromes, chronic high altitude, and post–renal transplantation.[4]

IE is also characterized by an increase in RBC mass of unknown cause. Its diagnosis is based on the exclusion of PV and various congenital primary and secondary acquired erythrocytoses. The frequency of IE has been estimated to be 110 per 100,000 subjects, which is higher than that observed in PV.[5] Heterogeneous mechanisms underlying IE have been suggested, including 'early' PV and unrecognized secondary or congenital polycythemia. IE is a stable disease with a low thrombotic risk and rare spontaneous progression to acute leukemia or myelofibrosis. Phlebotomy is controversial, and myelosuppressive drugs should be avoided.

Polycythemia Vera

PV is a chronic myeloproliferative disease characterized by a predominant proliferation of the erythroid cell line and primary bone marrow dysfunction that results in hemorrhage, thrombosis, and increased RBC mass. Both erythrocytes and megakaryocytes play essential roles in causing complications of the disease. PV represents a histopathologic spectrum of two recognized stages, the polycythemic and the postpolycythemic phase.[6] Diagnosis of PV is based mainly on clinical criteria.

First described in 1892 by Vasquez as an autonomous erythrocytosis, the cause of PV remains unknown. PV is a rare disorder, with a minimum incidence of 2.6 per 100,000, and is particularly prevalent in persons of Ashkenazi Jewish ancestry.[7] Peak incidence occurs in the sixth decade, with approximately equal gender distribution. Characteristic features of PV are Epo-independent in vitro erythroid colony formation and hypersensitivity to many other hematopoietic growth factors.[7] Recently, a specific point mutation (V617F) in the Janus tyrosine kinase 2 (JAK2) gene was described in a majority of PV patients.[6,7]

DIAGNOSIS

Diagnosis is made using criteria developed by the Polycythemia Vera Study Group. Major criteria include elevated RBC mass, normal oxygen saturation, and palpable splenomegaly.[8] Screening for JAK2 V617F can now be added to both diagnostic algorithms.

CLINICAL MANIFESTATIONS

PV is usually asymptomatic. When symptoms occur, they may include pruritis, vertigo, gastrointestinal pain, headache, paresthesias, fatigue, weakness, visual disturbances, tinnitus, plethora, and bleeding gums. PV should be suspected in patients with elevated hemoglobin or HCT levels, splenomegaly, or portal venous thrombosis.

ORAL MANIFESTATIONS

PV can manifest intraorally with erythema (red-purple color) of mucosa, glossitis, and erythematous, edematous gingiva.[9]

Spontaneous gingival bleeding can occur because the principal sites for hemorrhage, although rare, are reported to be the skin, mucous membranes, and gastrointestinal tract.

TREATMENT

Prognosis is strongly associated with thrombosis risk and disease progression; thus, treatment is directed toward minimizing coagulopathic complications and preventing myeloid metaplasia with myelofibrosis or transformation to acute myeloid leukemia. Untreated patients may survive for 6 to 18 months, whereas adequate treatment may extend life expectancy to more than 10 years.[8] Cytoreductive treatment of blood hyperviscosity by phlebotomy (to remove RBCs) or chemotherapy is the treatment of choice. The general target levels for the HCT have been accepted as $\leq 45\%$ for men and $\leq 42\%$ for women.[10] Low-dose aspirin therapy (80–100 mg/d) is successful in the primary prophylaxis of vascular complications. These techniques used together have dramatically reduced the number of thrombotic complications and substantially improved survival.[11]

Most patients require myelosuppressive therapy during the course of their disease due to progressive myeloproliferation. Hydroxyurea is the primary drug used across the age span, and α-interferon is an alternative in younger patients. Both agents have potential side effects even when used properly. Radioactive phosphorus (^{32}P) has been used in the past, with a success rate of 80 to 90%; however, its association with an increased incidence of acute leukemic transformation severely restricts its usefulness. With the exception of the rare bone marrow transplantation, there is no known curative treatment for PV.[12]

ORAL HEALTH CONSIDERATIONS

Control of hemorrhage after dental surgery should be considered. Hemorrhage in patients with PV may be associated with high platelet counts, acquired von Willebrand's disease, and high doses of antiplatelet drug therapy. Low-dose aspirin is rarely associated with hemorrhagic complications from dental extractions.[13] Although not predictive of bleeding, a wide variety of platelet function defects are reported in PV. Clinically significant bleeding may paradoxically require platelet transfusion[14] and a role for ε-aminocaproic acid and tranexamic acid has been suggested by some.[15] Other measures to consider in preparing the patient with PV for routine dental surgery include obtaining better control of blood counts by phlebotomy or drug therapy and adjustment of any concomitant antiplatelet and/or anticoagulant therapy.[16]

Anemia

Anemia is a disordered process in which the rate of red cell production fails to match the rate of destruction, which results in a reduction in hemoglobin concentration. This can occur as a result of an acute hemorrhagic diathesis or chronic disease. Red cell transfusion can elevate hemoglobin concentration in the short term for acute anemias but does nothing to address the underlying disorder associated with chronic anemias. The aim of chronic anemia management is to restore patient functionality and quality of life by restoring effective red cell production. Patients with anemia of chronic disease may benefit from intravenous or oral iron therapy and/or erythropoiesis-stimulating agents.[17]

Anemia Owing to Blood Loss: Iron Deficiency Anemia

Iron deficiency is defined as a reduction in total body iron to an extent that iron stores are fully exhausted and some degree of tissue iron deficiency is present. In epidemiologic studies, it has been common practice to determine the prevalence of both mild iron deficiency without anemia and more advanced iron deficiency anemia.[18] Globally, iron deficiency is a serious health threat. Iron deficiency contributes annually to 841,000 deaths and 35,057,000 disability-adjusted life-years lost as a risk factor for maternal and perinatal mortality and through its direct contributions to cognitive impairment, decreased work productivity, and death from severe anemia.[19]

DIAGNOSIS

Diagnosis of iron deficiency anemia, which is a microcytic hypochromic anemia due to inadequate supply of iron for normal hemoglobin synthesis in developing erythroid cells in the bone marrow, involves a battery of tests. Anemia as manifest by reduced hemoglobin and HCT on a CBC is typically the first clue to iron deficiency. In addition, measures of iron-deficient erythropoiesis, such as transferrin iron saturation, mean corpuscular hemoglobin concentration, erythrocyte zinc protoporphyrin, percentage of hypochromic erythrocytes, or reticulocyte hemoglobin concentration, are needed to assist in diagnosis, which is difficult to distinguish from anemia of chronic disease.[18] Screening measurements identify iron-deficient erythropoiesis by demonstrating either a reduced supply of plasma iron or poor hemoglobinization of circulating RBCs. These include hemoglobin, transferrin saturation, mean corpuscular hemoglobin, zinc protoporphyrin, and reticulocyte hemoglobin.[18] A peripheral blood smear and examination of the erythrocytes show microcytic and hypochromic RBCs in chronic iron deficiency anemia.

Definitive tests identify iron deficiency anemia by measuring iron-related proteins derived from either the iron storage compartment in macrophages or the iron utilization compartment in red cell precursors. These include serum ferritin, serum transferrin receptor, and bone marrow iron. Definitive diagnosis of iron deficiency requires evidence that iron stores are fully depleted and demonstration of tissue iron deficiency. The optimal diagnostic approach is to measure the serum ferritin as an index of iron stores and the serum transferrin receptor as an index of tissue iron deficiency. In those at increased risk of iron deficiency because of high physiologic requirements for iron, a serum ferritin level < 30 µg/L in an individual with anemia is diagnostic of iron deficiency anemia, but a higher value does not exclude it.[18]

The diagnosis of iron deficiency must always be followed by a carefully reasoned assessment of the underlying cause or etiology. The various causes of iron deficiency anemia are conveniently classified into two major categories: physiologic and pathologic. The most common cause is physiologic and relates to nutritional deficiency. The prevalence of iron deficiency rises in females during their teenage years when menstrual iron losses become superimposed on growth requirements and among pregnant women with added iron demands of the fetus. Other less common causes of iron deficiency anemia are increased gastrointestinal blood loss from gastritis due to chronic use of aspirin or other nonsteroidal anti-inflammatory drugs and regular blood donations in premenopausal women. Pathologic iron deficiency anemia is invariably due to excessive blood loss. In the vast majority of patients, the source of bleeding is the gastrointestinal tract from hemorrhoids, peptic ulcers, esophageal varices, or carcinoma or from excess uterine bleeding in women.

CLINICAL MANIFESTATIONS

The most important clinical symptom is chronic fatigue. This symptom may be accompanied by certain clinical findings, such as pallor of the conjunctivae, lips, and oral mucosa; brittle nails with spooning, cracking, and splitting of nail beds; and palmar creases that have traditionally been used by physicians in the diagnosis of anemia. Among 50 prospectively examined patients, a statistically significant correlation was noted between hemoglobin concentration and the following: color tint of the lower eyelid conjunctiva, nail-bed rubor, nail-bed blanching, and palmar crease rubor. Results from this study support the contention that the presence and degree of anemia can be estimated clinically by careful physical examination.[20] Other findings may include palpitations, shortness of breath, numbness and tingling in fingers and toes, and bone pain.

ORAL MANIFESTATIONS

Glossitis and stomatitis are recognized oral manifestations of anemia. Oral manifestations of iron deficiency anemia in a study of 12 patients included angular cheilitis (58%), glossitis with different degrees of atrophy of fungiform and filliform papillae (42%), pale oral mucosa (33%), oral candidiasis (25%), recurrent aphthous stomatitis (8%), erythematous mucositis (8%), and burning mouth (8%) for several months to 1 year's duration.[21] Dietary iron deficiency anemia or anemia of chronic disease should be suspected in every case of glossitis, glossodynia, angular cheilitis, erythematous mucositis, oral candidiasis, recurrent oral ulcers, and burning mouth when no other obvious causes are identified.[22–24] The high prevalence of these oral findings in iron deficiency anemia results from impaired cellular immunity, deficient bactericidal activity of polymorphonuclear leukocytes, inadequate antibody response, and epithelial abnormalities.[25] Clinically evident atrophic changes of the tongue, giving a smooth red tongue appearance, in patients with iron deficiency anemia have been associated with a significant reduction in the mean epithelial thickness of the buccal mucosa as determined histologically.[26]

TREATMENT

The treatment of iron deficiency should always be initiated with oral iron supplementation. Ferrous sulfate is the preferred form of oral iron because of low cost and high bioavailability, typically administered at 325 mg (60 mg iron) orally three times daily. Side effects of nausea and epigastric pain are reduced with food consumption. A therapeutic response should occur in 4 to 8 weeks.

When this fails because of large blood losses (eg, from defects in hemostasis, long-term anticoagulant therapy, chronic hemodialysis), iron malabsorption (eg, from coeliac disease, atrophic gastritis, partial gastrectomy, or antacid therapy), or intolerance to oral iron, parenteral iron can be given.[18] The most common preparation is iron dextran, the only formulation marketed in the United States until recently, when iron gluconate and iron sucrose were approved. Iron dextran is no longer first line due to the potential for serious anaphylactic reaction to administration.

ORAL HEALTH CONSIDERATIONS

For dental patients with extremely low hemoglobin levels, physician consultation prior to surgical treatment is recommended. When the hemoglobin is less than 8 g/dL, general anesthesia should be avoided and the potential for clinical bleeding and faulty wound healing should be recognized. Narcotic use should be limited for those with severe anemia, and dentists should be aware that anemia places a patient at increased risk for ischemic heart disease.

PLUMMER-VINSON SYNDROME

Plummer-Vinson syndrome, also called Paterson-Kelly syndrome or sideropenic dysphagia, is a rare syndrome with the classic triad of dysphagia, iron deficiency anemia, and upper esophageal webs or strictures.[27,28] It usually affects middle-aged white women in the fourth to seventh decade of life but has also been described in children and adolescents.

The dysphagia may be intermittent or progressive over years, is usually painless and limited to solids, and sometimes is associated with weight loss. Symptoms resulting from anemia (weakness, pallor, fatigue, tachycardia) predominate the clinical picture, although splenomegaly and enlargement of the thyroid and upper alimentary tract cancers may also be found. Additional features are glossitis, angular cheilitis, and koilonychia. Radiologic examination of the pharynx shows the presence of webs.[28] Etiopathogenesis of Plummer-Vinson syndrome is unknown; however, the most important possible etiologic factor is iron deficiency. Other possible factors include malnutrition, genetic predisposition, or autoimmune processes.

Plummer-Vinson syndrome can often be treated effectively with iron supplementation.[28,29] In cases of significant obstruction of the esophageal lumen by esophageal webs/strictures with persistent dysphagia despite iron supplementation, rupture and mechanical dilation of the web may be required. Since Plummer-Vinson syndrome is associated with an increased risk of squamous cell carcinoma of the pharynx and the esophagus, the patients should be followed closely.[30]

Anemia Owing to Hemolysis

The normal RBC life span is 90 to 120 days in the circulation. Hemolytic diseases result in anemia if the bone marrow is not able to replenish adequately the prematurely destroyed RBCs. The hemolytic anemias can be either inherited or acquired. Accelerated destruction of RBCs can be caused by one of these three basic mechanisms: (1) a molecular defect (hemoglobinopathy or enzymopathy) inside the red cell, (2) an abnormality in membrane structure and function, or (3) an environmental factor, such as mechanical trauma or an autoantibody.

DIAGNOSIS

A careful history and physical examination provide important clues to the diagnosis of hemolytic anemias. Once a patient presents with clinical signs and symptoms of anemia, laboratory testing should be supported by a complete drug and toxin exposure history and the family history. Laboratory tests in the anemic patient may be used initially to demonstrate the presence of hemolysis and define its cause. An elevated reticulocyte count is the most useful indicator of hemolysis, reflecting erythroid hyperplasia of the bone marrow. Assessment of RBC morphology, findings on the peripheral blood smear, and, rarely, bone marrow biopsy may provide additional clues to support the specific diagnosis.

CLINICAL MANIFESTATIONS

With acute hemolytic disease, the signs and symptoms depend on the mechanism that leads to red cell destruction. The release of free hemoglobin occurring in intravascular hemolysis may present as acute back pain, free hemoglobin in the plasma and urine, and renal failure. In patients with chronic or progressive anemias, symptoms depend on the patients' age and adequacy of blood supply to critical organs. With moderate anemia, symptoms may include fatigue, loss of stamina, breathlessness, tachycardia, and, less commonly, jaundice and hemoglobinuria. Physical findings include jaundice of skin and mucosae, splenomegaly, and other findings associated with specific hemolytic anemias.

ORAL MANIFESTATIONS

Oral signs indicating possible hemolytic anemia may include pallor or jaundice of oral mucosa, paresthesia of mucosa, and, for those with chronic conditions, hyperplastic marrow spaces in the mandible, maxilla, and facial bones.

PAROXYSMAL NOCTURNAL HEMOGLOBINURIA

Paroxysmal nocturnal hemoglobinuria (PNH) is an uncommon complement-mediated intravascular hemolytic anemia that results from the clonal expansion of hematopoietic stem cells harboring somatic mutations in an X-linked gene, termed PIG-A.[31] Intravascular hemolysis leads to release of free hemoglobin, which leads to many of the clinical manifestations of PNH, including fatigue, pain, esophageal spasm, erectile dysfunction, and, possibly, thrombosis. Patients with classic PNH are at increased risk for thrombosis and other complications of intravascular hemolysis. Allogeneic bone marrow transplantation was the only effective therapy for these patients until the development of eculizumab. Eculizumab (Soliris, Alexion Pharmaceuticals, Inc., Cheshire, CT) is a humanized monoclonal antibody against C5 that inhibits terminal complement activation and has been shown to reduce hemolysis and greatly improve symptoms and quality of life for PNH patients.[32]

GLUCOSE-6-PHOSPHATE DEHYDROGENASE DEFICIENCY

Glucose-6-phosphate dehydrogenase (G6PD) deficiency is inherited as an X-linked hemolytic anemia that affects 400 million people worldwide, primarily men.[33] It is a prototype hemolytic anemia due to enzymopathy, that is, to a primary abnormality of a red cell enzyme. The majority of cases of hemolysis are triggered by exogenous agents.[34] The disease is highly polymorphic, with more than 300 reported variants. The *G6PD* enzyme acts via the hexose monophosphate shunt to catalyze the oxidation of glucose-6-phosphate to 6-phosphogluconate while concomitantly reducing the oxidized form of nicotinamide adenine dinucleotide phosphate ($NADP^+$) to nicotinamide adenine dinucleotide phosphate (NADPH). NADPH, a required cofactor in many biosynthetic reactions, maintains glutathione in its reduced form. Reduced glutathione acts as a scavenger for dangerous oxidative metabolites in the cell.

RBCs rely heavily upon G6PD activity because it is the only source of NADPH that protects the cells against oxidative stresses. People with G6PD deficiency have blockage of the hexose monophosphate shunt pathway that allows accumulation of oxidants in the RBCs. These produce methemoglobin and denatured hemoglobin that precipitates to form Heinz bodies that attach to cell membranes. Alteration of cell membranes leads to hemolysis.

The five classes of G6PD deficiency include low, normal, or increased levels of the enzyme. G6PD deficiency affects all races; however, because it confers partial protection against malaria, the highest prevalence is among persons of African, Asian, or Mediterranean descent. Severe deficiency variants primarily occur in the Mediterranean population.

Diagnosis   Diagnosis is made by measuring RBC enzyme activity by quantitative assay. The normal RBC G6PD activity level measured at 30°C is 7 to 10 IU/g hemoglobin. In G6PD-deficient males or homozygous females, the level of G6PD in the steady state is, by definition, less than 50% of normal; however, with most variants, it is less than 20% and is practically undetectable in some.[34]

Clinical Manifestations   The vast majority of affected people remain clinically asymptomatic throughout their lives.

They are more likely to manifest neonatal jaundice for incompletely understood reasons and are at risk of developing acute hemolytic anemia in response to three types of triggers: fava beans, viral or bacterial infections, and drugs. Today, consumption of fava beans, common in the Middle Eastern and southern European diet, is the most common trigger or hemolysis.[34] A hemolytic attack often begins with malaise, weakness, and abdominal or lumbar pain. Peripheral vascular collapse is possible. Within several hours to days, jaundice and dark urine appear due to hemoglobinuria. Anemia, largely due to intravascular hemolysis, is moderately to extremely severe, usually normochromic and normocytic. The most serious threat of acute anemia is acute renal failure; however, full recovery is the rule in the absence of comorbidity.[34] A rare variant of this disease, often found among those presenting with neonatal jaundice, may result in a chronic nonspherocytic hemolytic anemia, with associated extravascular hemolysis and hypersplenism.

Treatment   The key to management is prevention of acute hemolysis triggering exposures. Drugs and chemicals to be avoided for patients with G6PD deficiency are shown in Table 2. Neonatal jaundice is usually treated with phototherapy and, when severe, with exchange blood transfusion. Acute hemolysis can be managed with blood transfusion and regular folic acid supplements, and hematologic surveillance is warranted for those rater patients with chronic nonspherocytic hemolytic anemia variant. Infection can also trigger hemolysis, so infection must be promptly treated and immunizations kept up to date.

Oral Health Considerations   Patients should maintain excellent oral hygiene and comply with routine recall visits so as to prevent oral and periodontal infection. Prompt and aggressive treatment of oral infections once diagnosed is important. Patients should avoid the use of aspirin or other drugs known to trigger hemolysis.

Hemoglobinopathies

Hemoglobin is made up of heme (the iron-containing portion of hemoglobin) and globin (amino acid chains that

TABLE 2   Drugs and Chemicals Causing Hemolysis in Glucose-6-Phosphate Dehydrogenase-Deficient Patients

Category	Drug
Analgesics	Acetanilid, aspirin
Antimalarials	Primaquine, pamaquine, dapsone, chloroquine, pentaquine
Antibiotics	Sulfonamides: sulfanilamide, sulfamethoxypyridazine, sulfacetamide, sulfadimidine, sulfapyridine, sulfamerazine, sulfamethoxazole Others: nitrofurantoin, ciprofloxacin, niridazole, norfloxacin, chloramphenicol, nalidixic acid, furazolidone
Miscellaneous	Vitamin K (water-soluble form), vitamin C, doxorubicin, methylene blue, phenazopyridine, isobutyl nitrite, naphthalene (moth balls), phenylhydrazine, pyridium

form a protein). Normal hemoglobin types include adult hemoglobin A (HgbA; about 95–98%); HgbA contains two alpha chains and two beta chains; HgbA$_2$ (2–3%) has two alpha and two delta chains and fetal hemoglobin (HgbF; up to 2%). HgbF has two alpha and two gamma chains. HgbF is the primary hemoglobin produced by the fetus during gestation. Its production usually falls to a low level shortly after birth.

Hemoglobinopathies occur when point mutations or deletions in the globin genes cause changes in the amino acids that make up the globin protein, resulting in abnormal forms of hemoglobin. The structure of the hemoglobin may be abnormal in its behavior, production rate, and/or stability. Several hundred hemoglobin variants have been documented; however, only a few are common and clinically significant. The majority of these are β chain variants that are inherited in an autosomal recessive fashion. Because a person inherits one copy of each β globin gene from each parent, if one normal β gene and one abnormal β gene are inherited, the person is said to be a carrier or heterozygous for the abnormal hemoglobin. The abnormal gene can be passed on to any offspring but does not cause symptoms or disease in the carrier. If two abnormal β genes of the same type are inherited, the person is considered to have the disease and is homozygous for the abnormal hemoglobin. A copy of the abnormal β gene will be passed on to any offspring. If two abnormal genes of different types are inherited, the person is doubly or compound heterozygous and one of the abnormal β genes will be passed on to each offspring.

SICKLE CELL DISEASE/SICKLE CELL ANEMIA

Sickle cell disease, or sickle cell anemia (SCA), is the most prevalent genetic hematologic disorder in the United States. Although autosomal recessive in inheritance, it affects approximately 1 in 350 African American infants each year and approximately 72,000 people.[35] Much progress has been made during the past several decades in gaining understanding about the natural history of SCA and management approaches aimed at treating or even preventing certain disease complications.[36]

SCA is characterized by a hemoglobin gene mutation, consisting of replacement of the amino acid glutamic acid so that valine is encoded instead in the sixth position on the β-hemoglobin chain. As a result, the erythrocytes have their normal biconcave discoid shape distorted, generally presenting a sickle-like shape, which reduces both their plasticity and lifetime from the normal 120 days average down to 14 days. This results in the underlying anemia and hypertrophic bone marrow.

The homozygous disease SCA is characterized by vascular occlusive events. An underlying grasp of sickle cell pathophysiology, which has rapidly accrued new knowledge in areas related to erythrocyte and extraerythrocyte events, is crucial to an understanding of the complexity of this molecular disease with countless clinical manifestations.[37] The vaso-occlusion model has evolved to a complex, wide-ranging schema that involves multistep, heterogeneous, and interdependent interactions among sickle erythrocytes, adherent leukocytes, endothelial cells, plasma proteins, and other factors. Endothelial activation, induced directly or indirectly by the proinflammatory behavior of sickle erythrocytes, is the most likely initiating step toward vaso-occlusion.[38] Stressors that can lead to vaso-occlusion typically include viral and bacterial infection, hypoxia, dehydration, iron overload, and cell and fluid phase–related causes. Microvascular occlusion arises predominantly in localized areas of marrow, leading to necrosis. Inflammatory mediators activate nociceptive afferent nerve fibers, evoking the pain response. Affected areas are the long bones, ribs, sternum, spine, and pelvis, often with multiple-site involvement.

Diagnosis Newborn screening is an important starting point for simple public health strategies such as parental education, immunization, and penicillin prophylaxis, although utilization of prenatal testing has varied by factors such as geographic location.[39] The HbS solubility test (Sickledex) can be performed in 5 minutes for screening of adults for hemoglobinopathies. Prenatal screening by deoxyribonucleic acid (DNA) analysis of amniotic fluid at 14 to 16 weeks can be ordered to investigate alterations and mutations in the genes that produce hemoglobin components. For diagnosis of specific hemoglobinopathies, hemoglobin type determination is usually performed by electorphoresis using cellulose acetate or acid citrate agar, by isoelectric focusing, or by hemoglobin fractionation by high-performance liquid chromatography. Newborn screening is accomplished with the latter technique.

Clinical Manifestations This disease is characterized by periods of latency interrupted by periods of actue crisis. Known sequelae of SCA include invasive infections, painful episodes, acute chest syndrome, cerebrovascular accidents/strokes, aplastic crises leading to severe anemia, chronic leg ulcers, hematuria, aseptic osteonecrosis, retinitis leading to blindness, priapism, pregnancy-associated problems, hyposplenism when young and then hyperspenism due to splenic sequestration, renal failure, and chronic pulmonary hypertension. A major cause of morbidity and mortality is acute chest syndrome.[37] Acute chest syndrome can be defined as a *new* infiltrate on chest radiography and one or more new symptoms of fever, cough, sputum production, dyspnea, or hypoxia.

The femoral head is the most common area of bone destruction in sickle cell patients, although other disease-related problems include avascular necrosis of the humeral head leading to hip joint dysfunction, changes in the thoracic and lumbar spine, infection with encapsulated organisms, particularly *Salmonella* and *Staphylococcus aureus*, and bone and marrow disturbances.[40] One of the precipitating events for a sickle cell crisis is infection, and cases of periodontal infection[41] and mandibular osteomyelitis[42] precipitating sickle cell crises have been reported.

Oral Manifestations Radiographic findings in patients with SCA include a "stepladder" trabeculae pattern (70%), enamel hypomineralization (24%), calcified canals (5%), increased overbite (30–80%), and increased overjet (56%).[43] Patients may also have pallor of the oral mucosa and delayed eruption of the teeth. Figure 1 (A and B) illustrates gnathopathy and Figure 2 illustrates radiographic stepladder appearance. Involvement of the maxillofacial skeleton leading to radiopaque lesions that correspond to bone infarcts in the course of a known vessel or in the apical region of the teeth has been reported in the literature. Such lesions combined with facial pain or sensory changes in the distribution of the inferior alveolar nerve during sickle cell crisis and absence of dental pathology should be considered to be of possible vaso-occlusive origin.[44] Interruption of the blood supply can result in an anesthesia of the inferior alveolar nerve and pulpal

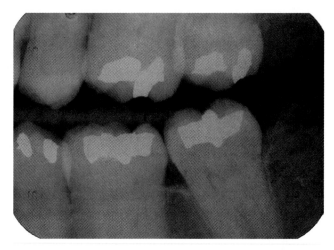

FIGURE 2 Left molar bitewing radiograph in a 32-year-old African American with sickle cell anemia with radiographic stepladder appearance and dense lamina dura, resulting from hyperplastic marrow, evident posterior to the second molar.

necrosis of otherwise sound premolar and molar teeth. A radionuclide scan of the mandible may demonstrate the position and extent of the infarcted area.[45]

In a case-control study, orofacial and dental pain with no obvious cause was detected in 83% of patients with SCA, 67% had deteriorated quality of the bone tissue, 22% of the patients had cortical thinning and irregularity in the mandible as examined radiologically, and 6% of the teeth with no restorations or a history of trauma were determined as being nonvital.[46]

Long-term penicillin prophylaxis in SCA patients under age 6 years likely prevents the acquisition of *Streptococcus mutans*, resulting in significantly lower caries rates in these children. This benefit occurs only during active administration of the twice-daily penicillin, however, and only delays the acquisition of the bacteria and related decay process.[47] In case-control studies involving adults, untreated decay was 24% higher in the patients with SCA, and they were less likely to receive treatment with a restoration than matched controls.[48,49] SCA is not associated with increased levels of gingivitis or periodontitis.[50]

Treatment The mainstay of successful treatment remains high-quality supportive care and judicious use of transfusion therapy to prevent mortality.[51] Management of pain continues to be primarily palliative, including supportive, symptomatic, and preventive approaches to therapy. Most vaso-occlusive episodes resulting in acute pain are managed at home with a combination of anti-inflammatory and analgesic drugs, often with opioids. Episodes of severe pain may require hospitalization for intravenous morphine, hydration, and supplemental oxygen therapy. Chronic sickle cell pain may be due to certain complications of the disease, such as leg ulcers and avascular necrosis; intractable chronic pain may be due to central sensitization. Management of chronic pain should take a multidisciplinary approach.[52] Infection is a

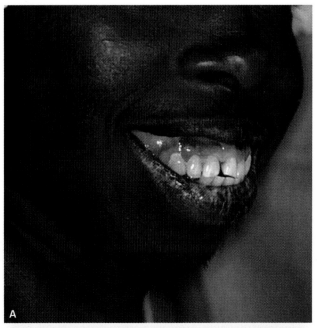

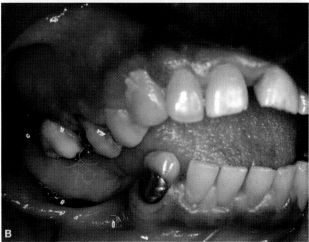

FIGURE 1 Gnathopathy (maxillary excess) of a 28-year-old African American with sickle cell anemia. *A*, Facial image. *B*, Intraoral image.

significant precipitating event for acute crisis. Preventive strategies that decrease the risk of infection are the routine use of daily antibiotics until 5 to 6 years of age, immunization of children with pneumococcal vaccine, annual influenza vaccination after 6 months of age, and meningococcal vaccination after 2 years of age.[53] Nutrition and hydration are important, and folic acid dietary supplements may be needed. Patients are educated to avoid crisis-precipitating events.

Patients with chest pain, fever, or respiratory symptoms and new pulmonary infiltrates on chest radiography require aggressive medical management for acute chest syndrome.[53] This typically necessitates transfusion therapy. Chronic transfusion therapy for primary or secondary stroke prevention requires careful surveillance for iron overload and chelation therapy, as needed.[53]

Existing and emerging therapies to treat the underlying disease process include induction of HbF, modulation of erythrocyte hydration, augmentation of nitric oxide, chronic transfusion, stem cell transplantation, and gene therapy.[54] Hydroxyurea therapy to convert HbF to HbA is used to decrease the frequency of painful episodes and associated comorbidities. To achieve higher levels of HbF that might be necessary for complete amelioration of the clinical manifestations of these disorders, other drugs, including 5-azacytidine, decitabine (an analogue of 5-azacytidine), and butyrate, have been investigated.[55] Hematopoietic stem cell transplantation (HSCT) is curative for a limited subset of patients and the first proof of principle that globin gene transfer into hematopoietic stem cells inhibits in vivo sickling and ameliorates the severity of the disease has been demonstrated.[55]

Persons with SCA are more likely to undergo surgery, for example, cholecystectomy and hip arthroplasty, than are the general population during their lifetime.[56] Because surgery exposes patients to many of the factors, for example, stress, hypoxia, dehydration, infection, and lactic acidosis, that are known to precipitate RBC sickling, persons with SCA undergoing surgery require meticulous clinical care to prevent perioperative sickle cell–related complications. Even with meticulous care, approximately 25 to 30% of patients will have a postoperative complication.[56]

Oral Health Considerations The need for antibiotic prophylaxis is controversial. At least 50% of pediatric dentist and hematologist respondents to a survey recommended antibiotic prophylaxis of children with SCA for the following clinical situations: dental extractions, treatment under general anesthesia, and status postsplenectomy.[57] Amoxicillin was the most commonly chosen antibiotic, and the perceived risk of infectious complication was highest for extractions, followed by restorative treatment and tooth polishing.[57] Other management considerations for patients with SCA include maintaining good oral hygiene, routine care during noncrisis periods, aggressive treatment of oral infection, avoidance of use of aspirin, caution with respiratory-depressing conscious sedation, and avoidance of long, stressful dental visits. Use of nitrous oxide–oxygen for anxiolysis is safe, with maintenance of adequate flow rates.

Preoperative transfusion of SCA patients prior to general anesthesia may be needed to ensure adequate levels of normal HbA to prevent a sickle cell crisis, although delayed hemolytic reaction has been reported as a risk, so individual assessment of the need for preanesthetic transfusion should be done by the patient's hematologist.[58] Because a complete blood supply is so important during application of both intraoral and extraoral forces, such patients who seek orthodontic treatment require multidisciplinary management.[59]

THALASSEMIAS

Thalassemia is a group of genetic disorders of hemoglobin synthesis characterized by a disturbance of either alpha (β) or beta (β) hemoglobin chain production. Worldwide, β-thalassemia is one of the most frequent hemoglobinopathies. An estimated 900,000 births are expected to occur in the next 20 years with clinically significant thalassemia disorders.[60] Many more people are carriers (they have the thalassemia trait with only one β gene affected or one to two α genes affected), and they usually have no symptoms and need no treatment.

The severity of β-thalassemia ranges from a complete lack of symptoms to transfusion dependence. Cooley's anemia, or thalassemia major (both β genes are affected), is the name for the severe form of β-thalassemia. α-Thalassemia diseases, often considered benign, are now recognized to be more severe than originally reported, with hemoglobin H disease being among the more severe.[60] Homozygous α-thalassemia (all four α genes are affected), usually fatal, is also being more commonly detected. Several regions have initiated universal prenatal screening programs to address homozygous α-thalassemia.[60]

Diagnosis Clinically, anemia of variable severity becomes apparent in the first year, accompanied by occasionally massive expansion of erythropoiesis. Thalassemia is diagnosed using blood tests, including a CBC and special hemoglobin studies. People with thalassemia have reduced RBCs, lowered hemoglobin, and defects in α or β chains of hemoglobin. Anemia in children of Mediterranean origin or ancestry (Greek, Italian, Middle Eastern) and people of Asian and African descent is suggestive of β-thalassemia, and anemia in children of Southeast Asian, Indian, Chinese, or Filipino origin or ancestry may indicate α-thalassemia.

Individuals with moderate forms of thalassemia (eg, thalassemia intermedia) may need blood transfusions occasionally, such as when they are experiencing stress due to an infection. If a person with thalassemia intermedia worsens and needs regular transfusions, he or she is then considered to have thalassemia major.

Clinical Manifestations In more severe types of thalassemia, such as Cooley's anemia, signs of severe anemia are seen in early childhood and may include fatigue and weakness, pale skin or jaundice, protruding abdomen with enlarged spleen and liver, dark urine, abnormal facial bones, and poor growth. Ineffective erythropoiesis and expansion of the bone marrow in every part of the skeleton of individuals with untreated thalassaemia result in skeletal changes, including osteoporosis, growth retardation, platyspondyly, and kyphosis.[61]

Oral Manifestations   Radiographic features of jaws and teeth among people with thalassemia major include the appearance of spiky-shaped and short roots, taurodontism, attenuated lamina dura, enlarged bone marrow spaces, small maxillary sinuses, absence of inferior alveolar canal, and thin cortex of the mandible.[62] Craniofacial deformities include universal Class II skeletal base relationship with a short mandible, a reduced posterior facial height, increased anterior facial proportions, and 17% with severe facial disfigurements (grade 3 or "chipmunk faces").[63] Dental arch morphologic changes include a narrower maxilla and smaller incisor widths for the maxillary and mandibular arches.[64] Consistent with general growth retardation, dental development of patients with β-thalassemia major was found to be delayed by a mean of 1.01 years, increased with age, and was higher for boys than girls compared with unaffected children.[65]

Thalassemia is not associated with increased levels of gingivitis or periodontitis but is associated with higher dental caries experience.[66,67] Parotid saliva flow rates in children with thalassemia major are not significantly different from those in the healthy controls; however, median saliva concentrations of phosphorus and IgA are significantly lower in the patients than in the controls, possibly providing an explanation for the higher dental caries experience observed in the thalassemia major group.[68]

Treatment   The rates of survival and complication-free survival of patients with thalassemia major continue to improve due to better treatment strategies. A mainstay of treatment for the most anemic patients is regular RBC transfusions to avoid death from cardiac failure. Today, most patients with a major form of thalassemia receive RBC transfusions every 2 to 3 weeks, amounting to as many as 52 pints of blood a year. Regularly transfused patients require iron chelation to resolve the inevitable iron accumulation that leads to dysfunction, primarily involving the heart, liver, and endocrine system.[69] Deferoxamine mesylate USP (Desferal, Novartis Pharmaceuticals, East Hanover, NJ) is a commonly used chelator and must be delivered by a battery-operated infusion pump worn under the skin of the stomach or legs five to seven times a week for up to 12 hours. Chelated iron is later eliminated, reducing the amount of stored iron. Compliance is difficult, and complications, such as heart disease caused by iron overload, hypothyroidism, hypogonadism, osteoporosis and osteopenia, hepatitis C, and hepatocellular carcinoma, are still frequent and affect the patients' quality of life.[70]

Allogeneic HSCT can result in cure in severely affected subjects with both α- and β-thalassemia.[69] Recent advances in genetic engineering with lentiviral vectors bode well for the continued clinical investigation of stem cell–based gene therapy in the future management of severe hemoglobinopathies.[71]

Infections are major complications and constitute the second most common cause of mortality and a main cause of morbidity in patients with thalassemia. Predisposing factors for infections in thalassemic patients include severe anemia, iron overload, splenectomy, and a range of immune abnormalities.[72] Although major causative organisms of bacterial infections in thalassemic patients are *Klebsiella* spp in Asia and *Yersinia enterocolitica* in Western countries, not common oral microorganisms, it is mandatory to reduce mortality by recognizing and presumptively treating infections in these patients as quickly as possible.[72]

Oral Health Considerations   The primary concern is the level of anemia; however, it is rarely of clinical significance. Hemoglobin levels of 10.0 g/dL or less were found in 3% of 1,000 children needing minor dental surgery who underwent hematologic investigation prior to general anesthesia in a dental outpatient hospital in London, England. The planned general anesthesias were undertaken without transfusion, allowing the authors to conclude that preanesthetic hematologic assessment is rarely of any significant clinical value.[73]

Anemia Owing to Decreased Production of RBCs

Anemia due to ineffective erythropoiesis may be characterized by macrocytosis associated with a megaloblastic marrow. The bone marrow may be hypercellular, showing evidence of abnormal proliferation and maturation of multiple myeloid cell lines. The term *macrocytosis* refers to a blood condition in which RBCs are larger than normal and is reported in terms of mean corpuscular volume (MCV). MCV, the average volume of RBCs, is calculated as HCT × 1,000 divided by RBC (millions/μL). Normal MCV values range from 80 to 100 femtoliters depending on gender, age, and reference laboratory. Macrocytosis can be identified by reviewing peripheral blood smears and/or by automated RBC indices.[74]

There are a large number of causes of macrocytic anemia, with the most frequent being disorders resulting in vitamin B_{12} or folate deficiency.[75] The diagnostic process begins by establishing the presence of vitamin B_{12} or folate deficiency and then determining the cause of deficiency. The primary laboratory investigations include a CBC, peripheral blood smear, serum vitamin B_{12} assay, and RBC and serum folate assays.[75]

MEGALOBLASTIC (PERNICIOUS) ANEMIA AND VITAMIN B12 (COBALAMIN) DEFICIENCY

Vitamin B_{12} (cobalamin) deficiency is a common cause of macrocytic anemia.[76] Vitamin B_{12} deficiency occurs frequently (>20%) among the elderly, but it is often unrecognized because the clinical manifestations are subtle; they are also potentially serious, particularly from a neuropsychiatric and hematologic perspective. Causes of the deficiency most frequently include food-cobalamin malabsorption syndrome (>60% of all cases), pernicious anemia (15–20% of all cases), insufficient dietary intake, and malabsorption.[77]

Megaloblastic or pernicious anemia is an autoimmune disease resulting from autoantibodies directed against intrinsic factor (a substance needed to absorb vitamin B_{12} from the gastrointestinal tract) and gastric parietal cells. Vitamin B_{12} is necessary for the formation of RBCs. Pernicious anemia is more common among people of Celtic and Scandinavian descent and has an average age at diagnosis of 60 years. Deficiency in production of intrinsic factor may result from chronic gastritis or surgical removal of the stomach.

Diagnosis   Diagnosis of vitamin B_{12} deficiency is typically based on measurement of serum vitamin B_{12} levels; however, about 50% of patients with subclinical disease have normal B_{12} levels. A more sensitive method of screening for vitamin B_{12} deficiency is measurement of serum methylmalonic acid and homocysteine levels, which are increased early in vitamin B_{12} deficiency. Use of the Schilling test (which measures cyanocobalamin absorption by increasing urine radioactivity after an oral dose of radioactive cyanocobalamin) for detection of pernicious anemia has been supplanted for the most part by serologic testing for parietal cell and intrinsic factor antibodies.[76]

Clinical Manifestations   Clinical manifestations of vitamin B_{12} deficiency are shown in Table 3.

Oral Manifestations   Patients with pernicious anemia may have complaints of a burning sensation in the tongue, lips, buccal mucosa, and other mucosal sites. The tongue and mucosa may be smooth or patchy areas of erythema. Dysphagia and taste alterations have been reported.[78]

Treatment   Treatment has traditionally been weekly intramuscular injections of 1,000 µg of vitamin B_{12} for the initial 4 to 6 weeks, followed by 1,000 µg per week indefinitely. Contrary to prevailing medical practice, studies show that supplementation with oral vitamin B_{12} is a safe and effective treatment for the B_{12} deficiency state. A recent evidence-based review suggests that 2,000 µg doses of oral vitamin B_{12} daily and 1,000 µg doses initially daily and thereafter weekly and then monthly may be as effective as intramuscular administration in obtaining short-term hematologic and neurologic responses in vitamin B_{12}–deficient patients.[79] Even when intrinsic factor is not present to aid in the absorption of vitamin B_{12} as in pernicious anemia or in other diseases that affect the usual absorption sites in the terminal ileum, oral therapy remains effective.[76]

APLASTIC ANEMIA

Aplastic anemia (AA) is a rare blood dyscrasia in which peripheral blood pancytopenia results from reduced or absent blood cell production in the bone marrow and normal hematopoietic tissue in the bone marrow has been replaced by fatty marrow.[80] The estimated incidence of AA is 2 new cases per 1 million persons per year.[81] The disease is rare in children, and the peak age at occurrence is between 3 and 5 years for children, but in large series of adults with AA, the mean age at presentation is about 25 years.[81]

The disorder can be inherited, idiopathic, or acquired. Environmental exposures, such as to drugs, viruses, and toxins, are thought to trigger the aberrant immune response in some patients, but most cases are classified as idiopathic.[82] Most cases of idiopathic and acquired AA are immune-mediated, with activated type 1 cytotoxic T cells implicated. The molecular basis of the aberrant immune response and deficiencies in hematopoietic cells is now being defined genetically; examples are telomere repair gene mutations in the target cells and dysregulated T-cell activation pathways.[83]

Clinical Manifestations   Like other autoimmune diseases, AA has a varied clinical course. Some patients have mild symptoms and need no therapy, whereas others present with life-threatening pancytopenia representing a medical emergency. The pathophysiologically linked disorders myelodysplastic syndrome and PNH commonly arise in patients with AA.[82] Patients with AA usually present with complaints caused by anemia, such as fatigue and malaise, chest pain, or shortness of breath. There may be a more sudden onset of bleeding caused by thrombocytopenia, manifest as increased bruising, evident by purpura and petechiae, and epistaxis or gingival bleeding. Leukopenia, particularly neutropenia, can result in fever and infection. Occasionally, the diagnosis is established in the absence of symptoms directly related to the low blood counts.

TABLE 3   Clinical Manifestations of Vitamin B_{12} Deficiency

Organ System	Condition
Hematologic	Megaloblastic (macrocytic) anemia Pancytopenia (leukopenia, thrombocytopenia)
Neurologic	Paresthesias, tingling and numbness of hands and feet Peripheral neuropathy Combined systems disease (demyelination of dorsal columns and corticospinal tract) with uncoordination and muscle weakness Impaired sense of smell Syncope
Psychiatric	Fatigue Irritability, personality changes Mild memory impairment, dementia Depression Psychosis
Cardiovascular	Possible increased risk of myocardial infarction and stroke

Oral Manifestations   The most common oral manifestation of AA is hemorrhage, which develops most often in patients with platelet counts less than 25×10^9 cells/L. The second and third most common oral manifestations are candidiasis and viral infection, respectively.[84] In a case-control study, 79 patients with AA were significantly more likely than controls to present with petechiae, spontaneous gingival bleeding, gingival hyperplasia from prior cyclosporine use, and herpetic lesions.[85]

Treatment   The course, treatment, and outcome are related to the severity of the quantitative reduction in peripheral blood cell counts, particularly the neutrophil number. Supportive therapy with blood transfusions to correct anemia and thrombocytopenia can be beneficial for many. Immunosuppression with antithymocyte globulins and cyclosporine is effective at restoring blood cell production in the majority of patients, but relapse and especially evolution of clonal hematologic diseases remain problematic.[83] Ultimately, patients with histocompatible sibling donors can be cured by replacement of the hematopoiesis through allogeneic HSCT.[86] The most serious complication of AA is the high risk of infection secondary to the absence of neutrophils; overwhelming bacterial sepsis and especially fungal infections are the most frequent causes of death.

Oral Health Considerations   Neutropenia, caused by the disorder itself and its treatment, leads to an increased susceptibility to infection, and thrombocytopenia leads to bruising and mucosal bleeding. Neutropenic fevers must be treated aggressively with parenteral, broad-spectrum antibiotics. Antifungal therapy should be added when patients are persistently febrile because aspergillosis infections can be difficult to diagnose early. Attention to details of oral hygiene and hand washing and avoidance of minor injuries or casual exposure to infectious agents can reduce the risk of serious complications.

▼ WHITE BLOOD CELL DISORDERS

White blood cell (WBC) disorders primarily involve one or both of the principal components, the lymphocytes or neutrophilic granulocytes. Table 4 outlines alterations in the WBC and differential cell count that occur clinically in various disorders. Leukocyte defects are also discussed in Chapter 18, "Immunologic Disorders."

Quantitative Leukocyte Disorders
GRANULOCYTOSIS

There are three types of granulocytes, distinguished by their appearance under Wright's stain: neutrophil granulocytes, eosinophil granulocytes, and basophil granulocytes. Their names are derived from their staining characteristics; for example, the most abundant granulocyte is the neutrophil granulocyte, which has neutrally staining cytoplasmic granules. Other WBCs that are not granulocytes ("agranulocytes") are mainly lymphocytes and monocytes.

Granulocytosis is an abnormally large number of granulocytes in the blood. Basophilia and eosinophilia are an excess number of basophils and eosinophils, respectively. Table 4 shows several conditions that are associated with basophilia and eosinophilia. Neutrophilia, an excess of neutrophils, is more common. Causes of neutrophilia are varied and include acute infections caused by cocci, bacilli, certain fungi, spirochetes, viruses, rickettsia, and parasites. Infections may present as furuncles, abscesses, tonsillitis, appendicitis, otitis media, osteomyelitis, cholecystitis, salpingitis, meningitis, diphtheria, plague, and peritonitis. In acute infections, leukocyte counts typically are 15 to 25×10^9/L. Noninfectious causes of neutrophilia include burns, postoperative states, acute myocardial infarction, acute attacks of gout, acute glomerulonephritis, rheumatic fever, collagen vascular diseases, and hypersensitivity reactions. Neutrophilia can also accompany metabolic conditions (diabetic ketoacidosis, preeclampsia, uremia), poisoning (with lead, mercury, digitalis, camphor, antipyrine, phenacetin, quinidine, pyrogallol, turpentine, arsphenamine, and insect venoms), rapidly growing neoplasms, and strenuous exercise.

AGRANULOCYTOSIS (NEUTROPENIA/GRANULOCYTOPENIA)

The terms *agranulocytosis, neutropenia,* and *granulocytopenia* are commonly used interchangeably for a reduced quantity of leukocytes. Clinical symptoms of agranulocytosis include sudden onset of fever, rigors, and sore throat. Neutropenic fevers often reflect an absolute neutrophil count (ANC) of <500 cells/mm³ of blood. The differential diagnosis of agranulocytosis depends upon the severity and duration of neutropenia, leukocyte and bone marrow morphology, and associated hematologic or congenital abnormalities (Table 5).[87] Acquired neutropenias are far more common than congenital forms, often accompany viral infection, or may be drug induced, either due to myelosuppression or antibody-mediated destruction. Many drugs, including antineoplastics, antibiotics, anticonvulsants, anti-inflammatories, antithyroid agents, diuretics, and phenothiazines, have neutropenia as a reported potential side effect. Infection-mediated neutropenias require only monitoring of blood counts until recovery. For potential drug-induced neutropenias, discontinuation of the suspected offending drug provides both the diagnosis and the cure. Neutropenia resulting from myelosuppression in patients on cytotoxic chemotherapy typically reaches a nadir between 7 and 14 days after chemotherapy has been delivered. Congenital forms of neutropenia need to be considered in children and occasionally in adults presenting with low neutrophil counts. Antineutrophil antibodies may be detected by flow cytometry or agglutination assays to support the diagnosis of immune-mediated neutropenia. Bone marrow examination is indicated in cases of severe or persistent neutropenia or when other hematologic lineages are affected.

TABLE 4   Key Laboratory Tests for White Cell Disorders

Test Name	Normal Range (SI units)	Increased	Decreased	Oral Findings
White blood cell (WBC)	4,400–11,000/μL	Infections, inflammation, cancer, leukemia	Hematologic neoplastic disease (early leukemia), drug-induced neutropenia, cyclic neutropenia, viral infection, severe bacterial infections, bone marrow failure, and congenital marrow aplasia	Enlarged gingival, oral ulcers, oral infection due to immune suppression from disease or therapy
Differential WBC				
Polymorphonuclear neutrophils (Segs)*	41–78%	Infections, inflammation, toxic states, tissue destruction, stress, certain drugs (adrenal acute hemorrhage)	Agranulocytosis, drug-induced neutropenia, viral infection, infectious diseases, chemical induced, hypersplenism, collagen-vascular disease	
Band neutrophils*	0–6%	Immature neutrophils; indicates rapid production of cell line often seen in infection		
Lymphocytes	23–44%	Viral infections, mononucleosis, infectious lymphocytosis, hypoadrenalism, hypothyroidism	Immunodeficiencies, adrenal-corticosteroid exposure, severe debilitating illness, defects in lymphatic circulation	
Monocytes	0–7%	Chronic infections (tuberculosis), bacterial endocarditis, granulomatous disease		
Eosinophils*	0–4%	Parasitic diseases, certain allergic diseases, chronic skin diseases, various miscellaneous diseases (sarcoidosis, Hodgkin's disease, metastatic cancer)		
Basophils*	0–2%	Chronic hypersensitivity states, no specific allergen, myeloproliferative disorders		

*Granulocytes.

TABLE 5   Classification of Primary and Secondary Neutropenias

Acquired	Congenital	Complex Syndromes Including Neutropenia
Antibody-mediated (aminopyrine, other drugs)	Cyclic neutropenia	Cartilage-hair hypoplasia
Bone marrow aplasia, dysplasia, or replacement	Familial benign neutropenia	Chédiak-Higashi syndrome
Drug induced (cytotoxic chemotherapy, phenothiazines, other drugs)	Myelokathexis	Dyskeratosis congenital
Hypersplenism	Severe chronic neutropenia	Fanconi's anemia; Diamond-Blackfan anemia
Immune-mediated (alloimmune and autoimmune)		Metabolic disorders (eg, glycogen storage disease type 1b, organic acidurias)
Nutritional (folate, vitamin B$_{12}$)		Primary immunodeficiencies (eg, X-linked hyper-IgM syndrome)
Sepsis with exhaustion of bone marrow storage pool		Reticular dysgenesis
Viral bone marrow suppression		Shwachman-Diamond syndrome

Oral Health Considerations   Prophylactic antibiotics have historically been recommended by some for patients with a hematologic malignancy–caused ANC <1,000 cells/mm³ prior to dental extractions.[88] Typically in the dental setting, the drugs and regimens supported by the most recent American Heart Association guidelines for infective endocarditis prevention are used prior to invasive dental procedures.[89] New evidence from a Cochrane Review shows that antibiotic prophylaxis in afebrile neutropenic patients reduces mortality, febrile episodes, and bacterial infections, without apparent development of antibiotic resistance.[90] Analysis for patients with acute leukemia or HSCT demonstrated that prophylaxis with fluoroquinolones (ciprofloxacin or levofloxacin) reduced infections caused by gram-positive bacteria and diminished the risk of death from any cause by 33%.[91] Hence, prophylaxis with fluoroquinolones is now being recommended as a routine practice for patients with acute leukemia, lymphoma, and solid organ tumors who are anticipated to receive regimens that cause severe neutropenia.[91] Physician consultation is recommended for guidance on management of the severely neutropenic patient.

CYCLIC NEUTROPENIA

Cyclic neutropenia is a rare hematologic disorder, characterized by repetitive episodes of fever, mouth ulcers, and infections attributable to recurrent severe neutropenia. These patients manifest a distinctly cyclical pattern to episodes of neutropenia ($<0.2 \times 10^9$/L). Neutropenia recurs with a regular periodicity of 21 days, persists for 3 to 5 days, and is characterized by infectious events that are usually less severe than in severe chronic neutropenia.[92–94] Autosomal dominant cyclic neutropenia is caused by a mutation of the gene for neutrophil elastase, *ELA2, located at 19p13.3.*[95] This enzyme is synthesized in neutrophil precursors early in the process of primary granule formation. It has been proposed that cyclic hematopoiesis results from the mutant neutrophil elastase functioning aberrantly within the cells to accelerate apoptosis of the precursors, oscillatory production, and loss of a regulatory feedback loop.[93]

Clinical and Oral Manifestations　Periodic oscillations of neutrophil counts associated with fever and mouth ulcers are the key clinical hallmark of this disease. Serial blood counts may be needed to establish the diagnosis. A wide spectrum of symptom severity, ranging from asymptomatic to life-threatening illness, is seen in autosomal dominant cyclic neutropenia.[94] The phenotype changes with age, where children display typical neutrophil cycles with symptoms of mucosal ulceration, lymphadenopathy, and infections. Adults often have fewer episodes and milder chronic neutropenia without distinct cycles. Although commonly described as "benign," four children in nine families who underwent pedigree analysis died of *Clostridium* or *Escherichia coli* colitis, supporting the need for urgent evaluation of abdominal pain.[94] Stomatitis and gingivitis frequently are seen in patients with neutropenia, and a differential WBC count may be essential in the diagnosis of unusual periodontal destruction or severe oral pathoses of obscure origin.[96]

Treatment　Hematopoietic growth factors, such as G-CSF, have reduced the number and severity of infectious episodes, prolonging the survival and the extent of time during which neutropenic patients remained free of life-threatening infections. Clinical trials and reports from international registries suggest that the vast majority of neutropenic patients (>90%) respond within 1 to 2 weeks to treatment with G-CSF at dosages lower than 30 μg/kg (2.4–2.6 μg/kg for patients with cyclic neutropenia) with a mean ANC increase of more than 1.5 to 2.0×10^9 cells/L.[92] Long-term, daily, or alternate-day administration reduces fever, mouth ulcers, and other inflammatory events associated with this disorder.[95]

CHRONIC NEUTROPENIAS

Neutrophils are important for first-line defense and innate immunity. Chronic neutropenia is defined as a low ANC for more than 6 months. Chronic neutropenia can be congenital, acquired, or idiopathic. Neutropenia is an absolute decrease in the number of circulating neutrophils in the blood that results in susceptibility to severe pyogenic infections. Like cyclic neutropenia, severe congenital neutropenia, also known as Kostmann's syndrome, has recently been shown to derive largely from heterozygous germline mutations in a common gene, *ELA2*, encoding neutrophil elastase.[87] Chronic benign idiopathic neutropenia is characterized by a prolonged noncyclic neutropenia as the sole abnormality, with no underlying disease to which the neutropenia can be attributed.[97]

Clinical Manifestations　Manifestations include life-threatening bacterial infections, recurrent gingivitis, and even severe periodontitis, often starting in early childhood.[98] In light of an otherwise unremarkable medical history, periodontitis of the primary dentition and early tooth loss may have been the sole manifestation of a juvenile patient leading to the diagnosis of chronic benign neutropenia.[97]

Treatment　Most patients with severe chronic neutropenia respond to therapy with G-CSF (Neupogen [filgastrim], Amgen, Thousand Oaks, CA), often at higher doses than required for cyclic neutropenia.[87] Prior to the G-CSF era, approximately half of severe chronic neutropenia patients died of bacterial sepsis in the first year of life and the remainder in early childhood. Currently, these survivors are at increased risk for development of acute myeloid leukemia or myelodysplastic syndrome and death from bacterial sepsis.

Oral Manifestations　Various oral findings, such as recurrent gingivitis, severe periodontitis, alveolar bone loss, and ulceration, may be seen in neutropenic patients. G-CSF together with a dental care regimen resulted in resolution of neutropenic ulceration and periodontal breakdown within 2 weeks of treatment initiation in a patient with severe chronic neutropenia,[99] whereas normalized ANC levels were not sufficient to resolve chronic periodontal disease in other severe chronic neutropenia patients, possibly due to continued deficiency of the antibacterial peptide LL-37, normally produced by peripheral blood neutrophils and important to the destruction of periodontal disease–associated bacteria.[99,100]

Qualitative Leukocyte Disorders

CHÉDIAK-HIGASHI SYNDROME

Chediak-Higashi syndrome (CHS) is a rare autosomal recessive immunodeficiency disorder characterized by partial oculoalbinism, easy bruisability and bleeding as a result of deficient platelet-dense bodies, neutropenia and defective neutrophil function with abnormal lysosomal inclusions, impaired chemotaxis and bactericidal activity, and abnormal natural killer cell function contributing to recurrent infections, most commonly involving the skin and respiratory systems.[101,102] The only laboratory diagnostic test is examination of bone marrow aspirate, myeloid precursor cells, granulocytes, and eosinophils for the atypical large cytoplasmic granules that are characteristic of this disorder.[103] The abnormal, large granules in neutrophils lead to an increased susceptibility to infection. These granules are peroxidase positive and contain lysosomal enzymes, suggesting that they are giant lysosomes or, in the case of melanocytes, giant melanosomes. The underlying defect in CHS remains elusive, but the disorder can be considered a model for defects in vesicle formation, fusion, or trafficking.[101]

Clinical Manifestations   The complete syndrome includes oculocutaneous albinism with photophobia, neurologic features, recurrent infections, and enterocolitis. Neurologic involvement is variable but often includes peripheral neuropathy. Abnormalities can be found in the hematopoietic tissues, hair, ocular pigment, skin, adrenal and pituitary glands, gastrointestinal organs, peripheral nerves, and elsewhere. The effects of the abnormality in different tissues depend on granule function in that tissue. Thus, the large but fewer melanin granules produce pigment dilution, which explains the peculiar silver hair color, partial albinism with milky-white to slate gray skin, photophobia, light-colored eyes, and nystagmus. Most patients also undergo an accelerated phase, which is a nonmalignant lymphohistiocytic infiltration of multiple organs resembling lymphoma. Death often occurs in the first decade from infection, bleeding, or development of the accelerated phase.[101]

Oral Manifestations   Patients with CHS may present with serious periodontal destruction with acute inflamed gingiva and ulcers. Patients are particularly susceptible to sinus and oral infections caused by β-hemolytic *Streptococcus*, *S. aureus*, gram-negative organisms, *Candida*, and *Aspergillus*.[101] Early-onset periodontitis seems to be the expression of CHS granulocyte deficiency.[104] Oral radiographic status showed extensive loss of alveolar bone leading, in most cases, to tooth exfoliation. Light and electronic microscopic examinations of periodontal tissue reveal massive bacterial invasion of the epithelial tissue, epithelial cells, and connective tissue. Ultrastructural observations of periodontal polymorphonuclear leukocytes show defective granulation, with abnormal granules not discharging their lysosomal content against engulfed bacteria, and viable dividing bacteria can be found in the cytoplasm.[104] Periodontal treatment of these patients is often unsuccessful.

Treatment   Most of the therapy available in CHS is symptomatic, such as childhood immunizations and antibiotics for infections.[101] Bleeding can be managed with avoidance of aspirin and use of desmopressin, ε-aminocaproic acid, or platelet transfusions for severe bleeding. Chemotherapy, corticosteroids, intravenous immunoglobulin, and splenectomy have been tried for management of the accelerated phase. Current curative treatment for the disorder is HSCT, which alleviates the immune problems and the accelerated phase but does not inhibit the development of neurologic disorders that grow increasingly worse with age.[105]

Oral Health Considerations   When oral surgical procedures are planned, excessive operative blood loss should be anticipated secondary to qualitive defects in platelet function. Intramuscular injections should be avoided. Patients often have photophobia and may be sensitive to the bright operatory lights.[106] Patients can be encouraged to bring sunglasses to dental appointments.

LYMPHOCYTOSIS

Asymptomatic lymphocytosis is not always due to chronic lymphocytic leukemia (CLL) or malignant disease. Evaluation of lymphocytosis begins with a search for a reactive cause, such as infection of postsplenectomy.[107] Flow cytometry and a peripheral blood smear can help distinguish between clonal disorders and a nonclonal process (reactive lymphocytosis). Infectious disease causes include viral (human immunodeficiency virus [HIV], human T-lymphotrophic virus 1 [HTLV-1], cytomegalovirus, hepatitis, Epstein-Barr virus [EBV], and influenza) or other infections (tuberculosis, rickettsia, brucellosis, toxoplasmosis, syphilis) or other causes (drug induced, hyperthyroidism, autoimmune disease, and thymoma). Clonal disorders can be T-cell disorders, such as large granular lymphocyte leukemia, T-cell non-Hodgkin's lymphoma (NHL), T-cell prolymphocytic leukemia, HTLV-1 and T-cell leukemia or lymphoma, or Sézary syndrome, and may require bone marrow or lymph node biopsy to clarify diagnosis.[107] Clonal B-cell disorders can by diagnosed with immunophenotyping and possibly bone marrow or lymph node biopsy as CLL or other B-cell malignancies, such as mantle cell lymphoma, follicular NHL, hair cell leukemia, nodal or splenic marginal zone lymphoma, lymphoplasmacytoid lymphoma, and B-cell prolymphocytic leukemia.[107]

In one retrospective series of 280 consecutive patients in the Central Arkansas Veterans Healthcare System with an absolute lymphocyte count greater than 5×10^9 cells/L on at least two occasions, 51% had spontaneous resolution of lymphocytosis, 30% had CLL, 7% had a malignant lymphoid disease other than CLL, 1% had hepatitis C, <1% had a monoclonal gammopathy of undetermined significance, and 9% had no specific diagnosis.[108]

Leukemia

Leukemia results from the proliferation of a clone of abnormal hematopoietic cells with impaired differentiation, regulation, and programmed cell death (apoptosis). Leukemia is classified based on clinical behavior (acute or chronic) and the primary hematopoietic cell line affected (myeloid or lymphoid). The four principal diagnostic categories are the following: (1) acute myelogenous leukemia (AML), (2) acute lymphocytic leukemia (ALL), (3) chronic myelogenous leukemia (CML), and (4) CLL. Leukemic cells multiply at the expense of normal hematopoietic cell lines, resulting in marrow failure, altered blood cell counts, and, when untreated, death from infection, bleeding, or both.

The expected leukemia incidence in the United States for 2007 is 44,240 cases, distributed equally between acute and chronic forms (ALL, 5,200; AML, 13,410; CLL, 15,340; CML, 4,570; others/unspecified, 5,720), with an anticipated death of 21,790 individuals from leukemia.[109] Annually, leukemias account for 3% of new cancer cases in US adults and 4% of cancer deaths.[109] Leukemia is more common in adults than in children, with most chronic leukemias occurring in adults. Of acute leukemias, ALL is more common in children, whereas AML is more common in adults.

The peripheral granulocyte count is markedly elevated in chronic leukemia but may be increased (with numerous blast forms), decreased, or normal in acute leukemia. The laboratory diagnosis of leukemia is made from the identification of abnormal hematopoietic cells in the peripheral blood and bone marrow. Further characterization is by cytochemical staining (myeloperoxidase, Sudan black B), immunophenotyping (cell surface markers, cytoplasmic immunoglobulin, terminal deoxynucleotide transferase detection), and cytogenetic analysis of chromosomal abnormalities.[110]

ACUTE LEUKEMIA

Acute Lymphocytic/Lymphoblastic Leukemia ALL is the clonal proliferation of lymphoid cells that have undergone maturational arrest in early differentiation. The general mechanisms underlying the induction of ALL include the aberrant expression of proto-oncogenes, chromosomal translocations that create fusion genes encoding active kinases and altered transcription factors, and hyperdiploidy involving more than 50 chromosomes.[111] Philadelphia chromosome–positive ALL is the most common subtype of ALL in adults.

Approximately 5,000 cases are diagnosed annually, with two-thirds occurring in children. ALL accounts for 10 to 15% of adult acute leukemia and 75% of childhood acute leukemia. Acute leukemia presents with flu-like symptoms and bone pain, joint pain, or both, caused by malignant marrow expansion. Marrow failure results in thrombocytopenia, manifested by petechial skin and posterior palate hemorrhages and gingival bleeding, gingival infiltration by leukemic cells, and gingival ulcerations as a result of infection by normal oral flora in the setting of neutropenia. Untreated, acute leukemia has an aggressive course, with death occurring in 6 months or less. Clinical manifestations of ALL are similar to those of AML but with a high incidence of central nervous system disease.

Treatment Factors associated with a poor prognosis in adults are age greater than 30 years, blast count greater than 50,000/mL, and t(9;22)- or t(4;11)-type chromosome translocations. Improved treatment has abolished the prognostic strength of many other clinical and biologic variables that previously were related to outcome. When treated, the 5-year event-free survival rates for childhood ALL generally range from 70 to 83% in developed countries, with an overall cure rate of approximately 80%.[112] Adult ALL cure rates seldom exceed 40%, despite the use of HSCT in many cases.

The recognition that ALL is a heterogeneous disease has led to treatment directed according to phenotype, genotype, and risk. Varying clinical outcomes associated with the subtypes of ALL can be attributed primarily to drug sensitivity or resistance of leukemic blasts harboring specific genetic abnormalities.[111]

The goal of remission-induction therapy is to eradicate more than 99% of the initial burden of leukemia cells and to restore normal hematopoiesis and a normal performance status. This induction treatment phase almost always includes the administration of a glucocorticoid (prednisone, prednisolone, or dexamethasone), vincristine, and at least one other agent (usually L-asparaginase, an anthracycline, or daunorubicin). Complete remission occurs in 80% of patients. Once remission is achieved, intensification therapy is given with high-dose methotrexate, 6-mercaptopurine, high-dose asparaginase C, central nervous system prophylaxis with radiation therapy, and intrathecal methotrexate following induction.

After intensification therapy, consolidation chemotherapy or HSCT is necessary.[112] Reinduction treatment, a repetition of the initial induction therapy administered during the first few months of remission, has become an integral component of successful ALL treatment protocols. Repeat induction will lead to a second complete remission lasting 3 to 6 months in 50 to 60% of patients. Although optimal timing is unclear, HSCT is recommended for high-risk patients in the first complete remission and low-risk patients in the second complete remission.

Acute Myelogenous (Nonlymphocytic) Leukemia AML is a heterogeneous clonal disorder of hematopoietic progenitor cells ("blasts") that lose the ability to differentiate normally and to respond to normal regulators of proliferation.[113] In the absence of treatment, bone marrow failure and fatal infection, bleeding, or organ infiltration (brain and lung) may occur within 1 year of diagnosis. The median age at presentation for patients with AML is 70 years, and three men are affected for every two women. Treatment for patients younger than 60 years consists of cytotoxic chemotherapy with 20 to 75% cure rates, depending primarily on leukemia cell cytogenetics. Cure rates from chemotherapy in the elderly are less than 10% because of their inability to survive treatment and the association of old age with cytogenetic abnormalities involving chromosomes 5 and 7.

Risk factors for acquiring AML include exposure to ionizing radiation, benzene, and cytotoxic chemotherapy.[113] Development of AML after exposure may reflect genetic variation in enzymes that detoxify benzene and other carcinogens. AML has typically been categorized with the French-American-British (FAB) system, which is based on cytomorphology and cytochemistry.[114] In this system, AML is diagnosed when the marrow contains more than 30% blasts. AML is subclassified into seven myeloid cell types that are important from a therapeutic and prognostic standpoint.

Treatment   Treatment of AML generally begins with rapid-induction combination of an anthracycline, such as daunorubicin or idarubicin, and cytarabine.[115] Initial therapy attempts to produce complete response, defined as a marrow with less than 5% blasts, an ANC >1,000, and a platelet count >100,000. Other regimens may add 6-thioguanine or etoposide (VP-16). Remission is achieved in 65 to 75% of all patients and in approximately 80% of patients younger than 40 years.[116] Induction chemotherapy produces severe marrow failure and cytopenia lasting 3 to 4 weeks. This requires maintenance of platelet count above 10,000 to 20,000/mL with platelet transfusions and institution of empiric antimicrobial therapy on the basis of neutropenia and fever. Consolidation high-dose chemotherapy is needed to prolong survival. Allogeneic HSCT, generally reserved for those under the age of 45 years with a suitable sibling donor, will affect a cure at the cost of a 30% mortality rate from complications of transplantation.

Clinical and Oral Manifestations   Symptoms include fever, weight loss, muscle or joint pain, fatigue/malaise, anemia/pallor, mucosal bleeding, petechiae, and local infections. Fever and fatigue/malaise are the most common presenting symptoms in patients with all types of leukemia. The most common manifestations or clinical signs of acute leukemia at initial presentation are lymphadenopathy (71.4% in ALL; 45% in AML), laryngeal pain (52.7% in ALL; 37.3% in AML), gingival bleeding (28.6% in ALL; 43.2% in AML), oral ulceration, and gingival enlargement.[117] Oral problems are more common in patients with acute leukemia than chronic leukemia, and complaints related to oral bleeding were the most common among those seeking a diagnosis for their leukemia because of oral problems.[118]

Gingival hyperplasia secondary to leukemia cell infiltration may be a first sign, heralding the presence of acute leukemia.[119] Figure 3 shows gingival hyperplasia in AML. In addition, extensive leukemic tumor infiltration in the gingiva or oral mucosa can be seen in some patients with acute leukemias. Histologically, these may have inflammatory cell infiltration, epithelium hyperplasia, and an increase in the keratinization of epithelium.[120] Herpes simplex virus–related ulcerations of oral mucosa in patients undergoing oncologic therapy, particularly for AML, may show atypical clinical patterns, leading to misdiagnosis.[121]

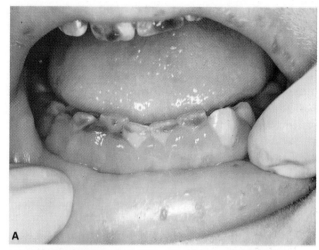
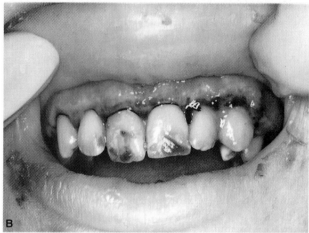

FIGURE 3   Gingival enlargement in a 16-year-old white female with undiagnosed acute myelogenous leukemia (AML) who presented to the dentist with gingival swelling, low-grade fever, and fatigue. *A*, Lower gingiva with leukemic gingival overgrowth. *B*, Upper gingiva 1 week post-gingivectomy with failure to heal and prolonged hemorrhage that led to the AML diagnosis.

Chemotherapy-induced mucositis and infection, including herpes simplex ulcers and oral candidiasis, are commonly observed complications of leukemia in the oral cavity. Primary oral manifestations of leukemia patients under treatment include mucosal pallor secondary to anemia, odontalgia, ulceration of the palate, gingival bleeding, gingivitis, petechiae, and ecchymoses of the hard and soft palate, tongue, and tonsils.[122–124] Among patients with leukemia, fluconazole has the potential to reduce oropharyngeal colonization by *Candida albicans*.[126]

Oral mucositis, beginning with erythema and progressing to ulceration, often begins within 7 to 10 days of the onset of chemotherapy and usually resolves within 2 weeks of cessation of cytotoxic drugs. Mucositis occurs in ≥98% of patients undergoing HSCT for hematologic malignancies and is associated with significant morbidity and mortality. Oral mucosal lesions may also be a manifestation of graft-versus-host disease in patients who have undergone allogeneic HSCT. Mucosal lesions can result in debilitating pain, compromised oral function, difficulty with daily activities such as talking and eating, and the breakdown of the oral mucosal barrier that is important for prevention of systemic bacterial, viral, and fungal infection in the neutropenic patient.

No therapy can predictably prevent or treat mucositis. Management is primarily palliative.[126] A recent Cochrane Review of interventions for preventing oral mucositis among patients receiving treatment for cancer found the following: interventions where there was more than one trial in the meta-analysis finding a significant difference when compared with a placebo or no treatment were amifostine, which provided minimal benefit in preventing moderate and severe mucositis; antibiotic paste or pastille demonstrated a moderate benefit in preventing mucositis; hydrolytic enzymes reduced moderate and severe mucositis; and ice chips prevented mucositis at all levels; other interventions showing some benefit with only one study were benzydamine, calcium phosphate, honey, oral care protocols, povidone, and zinc sulfate.[127]

Meticulous oral hygiene is critically important in the patient with neutropenia. Oral care is facilitated by frequent mechanical cleaning and alternating rinses of sodium bicarbonate with saline solution and 0.12% chlorhexidine gluconate and nystatin. These topical antimicrobials may reduce the risk of systemic infection of oral origin. Topical anesthetics (diphenhydramine, 2% lidocaine, or 0.5–1.0% dyclonine hydrochloride) and systemic analgesics may be required.[126] Novel cytoprotective agents, such as palifermin (Kepivance, Amgen, Thousand Oaks, CA), are currently being used. Palifermin is a keratinocyte growth factor that has been shown to decrease the severity and duration of mucositis, with a concurrent decrease in patient-reported symptoms and use of narcotics and total parenteral nutrition.[128]

A study of dental status of long-term survivors after HSCT at a median age of 9 years for leukemia demonstrated soft deposits in 78%, serious gingivitis in 59%, dentofacial abnormalities in 55%, root hypoplasia in 33%, and tooth abnormalities or agenesis in 63%.[129]

Oral Health Considerations Prechemotherapy dental assessment, maintenance of oral hygiene, and management of periodontal infection that may exacerbate in neutropenic patients have been shown to be effective in preventing oral and systemic complications during treatment.[130] In a study of acute leukemia patients, randomized to receive an intensive dental care protocol (dental treatment and plaque and calculus removal prior to chemotherapy and supervised oral hygiene measures during chemotherapy) or not, those in the intensive dental care group of patients developed less severe and less painful oral complications compared with the limited dental care group of patients.[131]

In a prospective, 13-month, controlled study of 96 children from 1 to 16 years old receiving antineoplastic treatment for ALL, those who received a daily preventive protocol consisting of (1) elimination of bacterial plaque, (2) application

of a mouthwash with a nonalcoholic solution of chlorhexidine 0.12%, and (3) topical application of iodopovidone followed by "swish and swallow" with nystatin 500,000 units had a significant improvement in oral hygiene and a significant decrease in the incidence of mucositis grade 2 and oral candidiasis compared with the control.[132]

Cytopenia is common in patients with acute leukemia and may require management prior to invasive dental treatment. At initial presentation with leukemia, screening laboratory assessment may show platelet counts from 25,000 to 60,000/mm^3, sufficiently low levels to result in spontaneous bleeding, and WBC counts > 10,000/mm^3 in most patients.[117] In a retrospective study to evaluate sequelae and complications after dental extractions among 388 patients with hematologic malignancies, 69 underwent dental extractions and 9 had sequelae and complications after the intervention, giving a complication rate of 13%.[133] Nonetheless, the authors concluded that dental extraction intervention provided in the prechemotherapy and pre-HSCT time frame did not have a negative bearing on medical outcome. In a patient who is on a myelosuppressive chemotherapy regimen, the optimum time to provide invasive dental therapy is often in the week prior to the start of the next cycle, when the platelets and neutrophils have been restored to normal or near-normal levels. Physician consultation should be made to assist in dental treatment planning and sequencing with the delivery of the chemotherapy.

CHRONIC LEUKEMIA

Chronic Myelogenous Leukemia Chronic leukemias with less pronounced marrow failure than acute leukemias have an indolent course that usually lasts several years. CML affects all ages, with a median age of 53 years at diagnosis. CML is a clonal disorder resulting in myeloid marrow hyperplasia and myeloid cells in the blood displaying the t(9;22) chromosome translocation.[134] Risk factors include older age, male gender, and exposure to ionizing radiation and benzene and benzene-containing products.[135] Most patients with CML have an acquired mutation called the Philadelphia chromosome that results from a translocation between chromosomes 9 and 22, producing the *Bcr-Abl* abnormal gene. This abnormal gene produces Bcr-Abl tyrosine kinase, an abnormal protein that causes the excess WBCs typical of CML.

Clinical Manifestations CML is typically chronic and indolent for 3 to 5 years in which patients have no symptoms, followed by an accelerated phase and blast crisis, resembling acute leukemia. In the acute or blast phase, the most common presentations are fever, weakness, fatigue, anorexia, weight loss, splenomegaly, anemia, and infection.[134] In the blast phase, there are mostly immature WBCs (more than 30%) in the blood and bone marrow. CML rarely has oral presentations.

CML Treatment Pre–blast phase treatment is palliative. There are four drugs used in the treatment of chronic phase

CML. First-line therapy involves the newest drug, imatinib mesylate (Gleevec, Novartis, East Hanover, NJ), an oral therapy that is believed to interfere with the action of the abnormal Bcr-Abl tyrosine kinase in CML WBCs.[136] Oral hydroxurea or bisulfan can be used to control granulocytosis. An intravenous treatment, cytarabine, is sometimes used in combination with immune therapy with α-interferon. A 50 to 70% cure rate can be achieved during the chronic phase with bisulfan and cyclophosphamide or cyclophosphamide combined with whole-body radiation therapy followed by allogeneic HSCT.[134] Only 15 to 20% are suitable candidates for allogeneic HSCT. The overall 5-year survival rate is 50%, largely because of HSCT and α-interferon.[137]

Chronic Lymphocytic Leukemia CLL results from the slow accumulation of clonal B lymphocytes in 95% of patients. The median age at diagnosis of CLL is 65 years, but 20 to 30% of patients are age 60 years or younger and 5 to 10% are age 50 years or younger. The etiology of CLL is unknown, although an abnormality of chromosome 12 is noted in leukemic cells in 40% of patients. Lymphocytosis >5,000/mL for a month, with at least 30% of nucleated marrow granulocytes being well-differentiated lymphocytes, in an adult is diagnostic for CLL. Staging is based on the extent of lymph node, liver, or spleen involvement and anemia, thrombocytopenia, or both. The clinical staging systems of Rai and colleagues[138] and Binet and colleagues[139] are commonly used in the United States and Europe, respectively (Table 6).

Median survival after diagnosis of CLL ranges from 2 to 10 years or more, depending on stage at diagnosis.[140] Most patients with CLL, including approximately 50% of those with early-stage disease, will eventually die of disease progression or disease-related complications, including infection or a second malignant condition.[107]

Clinical Manifestations Historically, CLL was frequently recognized when patients presented for evaluation of constitutional symptoms (fever, night sweats, weight loss, fatigue), lymphadenopathy, anemia, or thrombocytopenia.[107] With the widespread use of automated blood counters, 70 to 80% of patients with CLL now have early-stage disease (Rai stage 0 or I or Binet stage A) at diagnosis that is incidentally discovered when lymphocytosis is found on a CBC.[107] Of these,10 to 20% will be symptomatic and require prompt evaluation by a hematologist and initiation of therapy.

Oral Manifestations Oral manifestations at presentation of CLL are infrequent and generally related to bleeding.[118] The oral lesion incidence rate increases once chemotherapy is initiated for treatment. In a prospective study of 50 inpatients with leukemia or NHL under chemotherapy, the oral lesion incidence was 45 in 100 patients/week.[141] The most common oral lesions were exfoliative cheilitis and infections with herpes and *Candida*, followed by hemorrhagic lesions and mucositis. In logistic regression analysis, hemorrhagic lesions correlated with thrombocytopenia and mucositis was associated with etoposide administration, alkylating agents, a prior course of chemotherapy, and neutropenia. Use of the chemotherapeutic agent methotrexate also commonly results in mucositis.[142]

Treatment Treatment decisions are guided by clinical staging using the systems of Rai and colleagues[138] and Binet and colleagues,[139] the presence of symptoms, and disease activity. Early-stage (Rai 0–II; Binet A or B) patients may be monitored until constitutional signs and symptoms of the disease, such as constitutional symptoms, decreased performance status, or symptoms of complications from hepatomegaly, splenomegaly, and lympadenopathy, occur. These individuals should be seen every 6 to 12 months for review of symptoms, physical examination, and CBC.

High disease activity with rapidly growing lymph nodes or lymphocyte doubling in <12 months is an indication to treat. Advanced-stage (Rai III–IV; Binet C) patients with absence of disease progression may justify watchful waiting. In approximately 5 to 10% of patients, CLL transforms to an aggressive NHL or Hodgkin's lymphoma (HL) (the Richter transformation), usually heralded by the development of fever, night sweats, weight loss, or rapid enlargement of a single lymph node region. In addition to the risk for second malignant disease and transformation, patients with untreated early-stage CLL are at higher risk for infection due to defects in humoral and cell-mediated immunity. When anemia or thrombocytopenia develops, the patient is reclassified as having Rai stage III or IV disease and considered for initiation of chemotherapy.

First-line therapy is typically monotherapy with purine analogues (fludarabine, pentostatin, and cladribine) or chlorambucil.[140] Combination chemotherapy or chemo-immunotherapy with rituximab, an anti-CD20 monoclonal antibody, or with alemtuzumab, a recombinant human monoclonal antibody against CD52 antigen, may also be

TABLE 6 Prognostic Stages of Chronic Lymphocytic Leukemia

CLL Stage	Characteristic*	Frequency (%)	Median Survival (yr)
Binet			
A		63	>10
B		30	5
C		7	1.53
Rai			
Low/early			
0	Lymphocytosis only	30	>10
Intermediate			
I	Lymphadenopathy	60	7
II	Organomegaly (liver or spleen)		
High/late			
III	Anemia (hemoglobin <110 g/L)	10	1.5
IV	Thrombocytopenia (platelet <100 × 10⁹cells/L)		

Adapted from Shanafelt TD et al,[107] Rai KR et al,[138] and Hallek M et al.[140]
CLL = chronic lymphocytic leukemia.
*Patients are categorized according to the worst characteristic present.

used. With limited success with HSCT, currently, no treatment is curative, and most patients succumb to bacterial infection from drug-induced neutropenia and disease-associated hypogammaglobulinemia.

Oral Health Considerations CLL is a relatively indolent chronic hematologic malignant disease that often has a prognosis compatible with relatively normal dental treatment planning.[143] Patients in late-stage disease, with severe thrombocytopenia (< 50,000 cells/mm³), might require platelet transfusions prior to dental surgery.

LYMPHOMA

Hodgkin's Lymphoma/Disease The World Health Organization (WHO) classification of lymphoid neoplasms distinguishes between two major subtypes of HL, classic and nodular lymphocyte predominant HL, and has replaced the Rye classification.[144] Approximately 95% of patients with HL will have the classic HL histology, which is characterized by the presence of rare malignant Hodgkin's Reed-Sternberg cells among an overwhelming number of benign reactive cells.[145] Classic HL is further subdivided into four types: nodular sclerosing classic HL (accounts for 70–80% of North American cases), lymphocyte-rich classic HL (5%), mixed cellularity HL (10–15%), and lymphocyte-depleted classic HL (rare).[144]

In 2007 in the United States, there are projected to be 8,190 new HL cases diagnosed (4,470 males, 3,720 females) and 1,070 deaths (770 males, 300 females).[109] HL has a bimodal age distribution at diagnosis, with the first peak in the third decade in life and a second smaller peak after the age of 50 years. The 5-year relative survival rates have improved significantly over the past decades due to the increasing treatment success, to reach 85% in 1995–2001.

The etiology of HL is unknown; however, both genetic and environmental factors, including EBV, play a role in the pathogenesis of HL. The pathognomic morphologic features used to establish the diagnosis of HL include an effacement of the involved lymph node with destruction of its normal architecture; an inflammatory cellular infiltrate consisting of lymphocytes, histiocytes, plasma cells, and fibroblasts; and the presence of the malignant cell, the Reed-Sternberg cell.[146]

Clinical Manifestations The first sign of HL is typically an asymptomatic enlargement of a supradiaphragmatic lymph node, often in the neck, which may wax and wane over a period of a few months. Mediastinal lymph node involvement is common, occurring in 80% of cases. When mediastinal disease is bulky, patients may complain of chest pain, cough, and dyspnea. Systemic symptoms of night sweats, fever, and weight loss are reported in approximately 30% of patients. Less common symptoms are generalized pruritus and alcohol-induced pain localized over the involved lymph node. Infradiaphragmatic sites such as the inguinal, pelvic, or retroperitoneal lymph node regions are rare. Physical examination may reveal involvement of the Waldeyer's ring

structures. The location and size of lymph node masses should be documented. Imaging tests are the key to defining the anatomic extent of disease, with computed tomography of the head and neck, thorax, abdomen, and pelvis being the standard staging procedure, along with increased use of total body positron emission tomography scans.[146]

The Ann Arbor Staging classification (Table 7) is currently used along with pathology and other prognostic factors to guide treatment choice.[147] Approximately 70% of patients present with stage I or II disease.

Treatment Treatment approaches can involve radiation alone and chemotherapy with ABVD (Adriamycin [doxorubicin], bleomycin, vinblastine, dacarbazine) followed by involved-field radiation therapy (IFRT) in doses to 35 Gy.[146] Local control of HL is expected in the majority of patients treated with radiation therapy alone. Cure is being achieved in the majority of HL patients. Management recommendations vary by stage and are shown in Table 8.

TABLE 7 Ann Arbor Staging Classification for Hodgkin's and Non-Hodgkin's Lymphomas

Clinical Stage Hodgkin's Lymphoma and Non Hodgkin's Lymphoma	
I	Involvement of a single lymph node region or lymph node structure (eg, spleen, thymus, or Waldeyer's ring)
II	Involvement of two or more lymph node regions on the same side of the diaphragm
III	Involvement of lymph node regions on both sides of the diaphragm
IV	Disseminated (multifocal) involvement of one or more extralymphatic organs, with or without associated lymph node involvement; or isolated extralymphatic organ involvement with distant (nonregional) nodal involvement

For stages I–III: suffix E = involvement of single extranodal site contiguous or proximal to known nodal site; suffix S = involvement of spleen.
All stages divided into A, without symptoms, or B, with fever (> 38°C), drenching sweats, weight loss (10% body weight over 6 months).

TABLE 8 Management Recommendations for Hodgkin's Lymphoma

Stage IA nodular lymphocyte-predominant Hodgkin's lymphoma	Involved-field RT (35 Gy)
Stages I and II (asymptomatic)	Chemotherapy (ABVDx2–3 cycles) followed by involved-field RT (30 Gy)
Stages I and II (unfavorable*)	Chemotherapy (ABVD, x4–6 cycles) followed by involved-field RT (30–35 Gy)
Stages III and IV	Chemotherapy (ABVDx6–8 cycles) Involved-field RT (30–35 Gy) for initial sites of bulky disease (maximum tumor diameter g10 cm)

ABVD = Adriamycin (doxorubicin), bleomycin, vinblastine, dacarbazine; RT = radiation therapy.
*For stage I and II disease, the presence of one or more of the following adverse factors will place the patient in the group "unfavorable": systemic symptoms (stage IB or IIB); bulky mediastinal disease or peripheral site with bulk g10 cm; extranodal extension (stage IE or IIE); unexplained anemia (< 105 g/L).

The radiation fields for HL that involve bilateral cervical nodes have the potential to result in damage to the salivary glands. These include (1) IFRT when lymphoma involves the oral structures or Waldeyer's ring, (2) mantle, and (3) mini or modified mantle. Of these, the mantle field is largest and involves radiation therapy to all supradiaphragmatic lymph node regions, including the following groups: bilateral cervical, supraclavicular, bilateral axillae, mediastinal, and bilateral lung hilar, treated in contiguity. Mini or modified mantle typically refers to radiation therapy covering bilateral cervical, supraclavicular, and axillary lymph nodes. Autologous HSCT represents the standard of care for patients with relapsed or refractory HL.

Oral Manifestations   Unlike NHLs, HL rarely presents as an extranodal mass in the head and neck region. Waldeyer's ring involvement by HL tumors is uncommon, with < 200 cases reported in the English literature, most involving the tonsil or nasopharynx, and only 6 cases of tongue involvement have been reported.[148,149]

Oral Health Considerations   Patients who receive radiation in fields involving the cervical nodes will invariably have their submandibular and sublingual salivary glands in the field and are at risk for temporary, and occasionally permanent, xerostomia. Because the parotid glands are usually not in the field of radiation for these patients, the risk of radiation-induced caries is minimal; however, topical fluoride varnish, gel, or 1,000 parts per million fluoride toothpaste can be used for caries prevention if the patient's mouth appears to be dry or the caries rate appears elevated. The risk of osteoradionecrosis is very low due to low radiation doses delivered (30–40 Gy) and often exclusion of maxilla and mandible from the fields, with the exception of the inferior border and angle of the mandible.

HL survivors who received mediastinal radiation 10 to 20 years earlier may suffer from late-onset heart disease with heart valve pathology and accelerated atherosclerosis. Physician consultation is warranted for assessment of radiation-induced valvular disease risk and the need for prophylactic antibiotics and ischemic risk and benefit of sedative agents and limitation of epinephrine in local anesthetics.[150]

Non-Hodgkin's Lymphoma   NHLs are a heterogeneous group of malignancies of the lymphoid system. In 2007 in the United States, there are projected to be 63,190 new NHL cases diagnosed (34,200 males, 28,990 females) and 18,660 deaths (9,600 males, 9,060 females).[109] NHL incidence has risen steadily over the past four decades, and 5-year survival rates have also improved. Incidence increases with age.

NHL is known to be associated with chronic inflammatory diseases such as Sjögren's syndrome, celiac disease, and rheumatoid arthritis and immune suppression from HIV and medications to manage patients who have received solid organ transplantation. The risk remains substantially higher for patients with HIV (approximately 100-fold) than in the HIV-noninfected population, with a larger proportion being Burkitt-type lymphomas.[151] Chronic infection is associated with lymphoma, with an association between *Helicobacter pylori* infection and mucosa-associated lymphoid tissue (MALT) lymphoma; HTLV-1 and adult T-cell lymphoma; EBV and Burkitt's lymphoma; *Clamydia psittaci* and ocular adenexal lymphomas; and hepatitis C and splenic or large cell lymphomas.[152]

Histology of biopsied lymph nodes is essential to determine the specific type of lymphoma. Lymphomas are classified based on cytology, immunophenotype, and genetic and clinical features with the use of the WHO classification system.[153] The WHO recognizes three major categories of lymphoid neoplasms: (1) B-cell neoplasms, (2) T- and natural killer cell neoplasms, and (3) HL. B-cell lymphomas represent approximately 90% of NHLs, whereas T-cell lymphomas represent approximately 10%.[154] Expression of cell surface antigens and immunoglobulin proteins (immunoglobulin-heavy and -light chains, CD79a, CD19, CD20, and CD22) is dependent on the type of lymphocyte and its stage of differentiation or maturation. Additional antibodies (CD5, CD10, CD23, cyclin D1) are used to further delineate the subtype of lymphoma and tumor histogenesis. Chromosomal translocations and molecular rearrangements, such as translocation of t(14;18)(q32;q21) that is found in 85% of follicular lymphomas and 28% of diffuse large B-cell lymphomas, are commonly used to confirm the diagnosis.[154]

The initial evaluation of the individual diagnosed with NHL includes a history and physical examination, laboratory studies, a bone marrow aspirate and biopsy, nodal biopsy, computed tomography, positron emission tomography, and lactate dehydrogenase levels to measure tumor proliferation.

Clinical Manifestations   Clinical manifestations on presentation usually include lymphadenopathy and sometimes extranodal involvement of the gastrointestinal tract, skin, bone marrow, sinuses, thyroid, or central nervous system.[152] Slowly progressive, usually painless peripheral lymphadenopathy, sometimes waxing and waning, is characteristic of indolent lymphomas (such as follicular lymphomas). Bone marrow involvement in indolent lymphomas is common and is sometimes associated with cytopenias. More aggressive B-cell lymphomas present with large abdominal or mediastinal masses. Systemic constitutional symptoms such as fever, chills, night sweats, and weight loss occur in approximately one-third of patients with aggressive lymphomas. Splenomegaly is seen in approximately 30 to 40%, but the spleen is rarely the only site of disease involvement at initial presentation.[154]

Treatment   The Ann Arbor Staging Classification of lymphomas is used routinely to classify the extent of disease, and the International Prognostic Index has been used since 1993 to define prognostic subgroups.[155] International Prognostic Index prognostic factors include age > 60 years, performance status > 2, lactate dehydrogenase 1 × normal, extranodal sites > 2, and stage III or IV.[155]

NHLs are divided into indolent (eg, grade I and II follicular lymphoma, chronic lymphocytic leukemia/small lymphocytic lymphoma, marginal zone lymphoma [B cell], and mycosis fungoides) or aggressive lymphomas based on their historical growth. Most patients diagnosed with indolent tumors are elderly and present with an advanced stage of disease. These tumors have a relatively slow growth rate and a median survival of 8 to 10 years with palliation. Patients with follicular lymphomas with early-stage disease generally are treated with radiation therapy, whereas those with stage III and IV disease requiring treatment usually are treated with chemotherapy, immunotherapy, or radioimmunotherapy. Indolent lymphomas can transform into high-grade malignancies in approximately 30% of patients, for which treatment is similar to that of aggressive lymphomas.[152]

Aggressive lymphomas include mantle cell lymphoma, diffuse large B-cell lymphoma, follicular grade III lymphoma, primary effusion lymphoma, adult T-cell leukemia/lymphoma, extranodal natural killer/T-cell lymphoma nasal type, angioimmunoblastic T-cell lymphoma, peripheral T-cell lymphoma, and anaplastic large cell lymphomas.[153] T-cell lymphomas tend to have a poorer survival rate than aggressive B-cell lymphomas. Highly aggressive B-cell lymphomas include precursor B-lymphoblastic lymphoma/leukemia and Burkitt's lymphoma. Aggressive NHLs of intermediate and high grade are potentially curable in 40 to 50% with aggressive combination chemotherapy. For years, the standard regimen has been cyclophosphamide, doxorubicin, Oncovin (vincristine), and prednisone (CHOP) chemotherapy. Randomized controlled trials have shown that the addition of rituximab to the CHOP regimen increases the complete response rate and prolongs event-free and overall survival in elderly patients with diffuse large B-cell lymphoma, without a clinically significant increase in toxicity.[156,157] Patients with limited-stage disease may receive chemotherapy followed by IFRT. For chemosensitive relapsed aggressive lymphomas, high-dose therapy with stem cell support is the treatment of choice when relapse occurs.[151]

Radioimmunotherapy, combining the targeting advantage of a monoclonal antibody with the radiosensitivity of NHL cells, is a novel therapy for relapse. Yttrium 90 ibritumomab tiuxetan and iodine 131 tositumomab are the first two radioimmunoconjugates currently available for clinical use after failure following chemotherapy and/or rituximab.[158] Single doses of radioimmunotherapy, with either agent, on an outpatient basis over 1 week produce an 80% overall response rate, with approximately 20% of patients achieving durable responses, with the risk of reversible myelosuppression.[159]

Oral Manifestations Diagnosis of NHL in the oral cavity may result from gingival or mucosal tissue swelling or masses,[160] whereas intrabony presentation can mimic toothache. This latter presentation can result in dental extraction and then rapid growth of the tumor from the nonhealing extraction site. Figure 4 shows NHL in a nonhealing lower left molar extraction site. Often evidence of rarefaction can

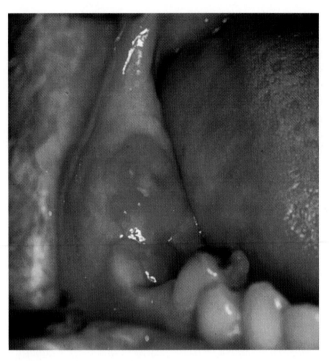

FIGURE 4 Non-Hodgkin's lymphoma in a nonhealing extraction site of teeth 30 and 31 that appeared within 1 week of dental extraction in a 31-year-old HIV-infected man.

be seen around the roots of the symptomatic teeth.[161] Nerve invasion can lead to paresthesia or anesthesia of related oral mucosal tissue. Symptoms may include anesthesia or paresthesia. Presentation can also include nonhealing ulceration with ill-defined borders in the surrounding mucosa, benign-appearing gingival lesions, and erosive mucosal lesions resembling a vesiculobullous disease.[162–164] Involvement of the oral mucosa in cutaneous T-cell lymphoma (mycosis fungoides) is uncommon and is usually associated with a poor prognosis.[165]

A record review in Canada of 88 consecutive patients with extranodal maxillofacial NHL, with age at diagnosis ranging from 22 to 94 years (median 60 years), revealed the affected anatomic site distribution to be the maxillary sinus (22), nasal cavity (8), maxilla (13), mandible (8), salivary glands (14), and other sites (23). Although most presented as nonpainful masses, 72 patients had associated dental symptoms, including intraoral swelling, pain, and loose teeth.[166]

Oral Health Considerations Acute complications of chemotherapy include mucositis, viral and bacterial infections, and hemorrhagic lesions related to bone marrow suppression. Long-term survivors of NHL treated with chemotherapy have limited chronic orodental consequences, including enamel discolorations and root malformations.[167] If radiation therapy is delivered to the mandible/maxilla during tooth formation, the consequences for development include short, blunted, tapered, and V-shaped root malformations, as well as delayed and ectopic eruptions.

Burkitt's Lymphoma Burkitt's lymphoma (BL) is a highly aggressive, small, non–cleaved cell lymphoma that commonly presents as jaw swellings first described in the last century by Denis Burkitt, a surgeon working in Africa.[168] This l ymphoma was initially described in children with grossly distorted faces resulting from tumors on one or both sides of the upper and lower jaws, sometimes accompanied by proptosis and huge abdominal masses, although there was usually no lymph node involvement.[169] Within these lymphomas was found EBV, the first virus identified as involved in the pathogenesis of a tumor in humans.

In the WHO classification, three clinical variants of BL are described: endemic (African), sporadic (American), and immunodeficiency-associated types. In present-day Africa, endemic BL continues to account for most childhood malignancies, whereas HIV-associated BL is now found in African adults.[170] The differential diagnosis of BL is broad, and precise diagnosis based on histologic, immunophenotypic, and genetic features remains the critical first step in planning appropriate therapy. On histopathology, uniform large neoplastic cells with abundant cytoplasm, a high mitotic rate, and numerous macrophages scattered about create a characteristic "starry-sky" pattern. A defining feature of BL is the presence of a translocation between the c-*myc* gene (the first oncogene described in lymphoma) and the *IgH* gene (found in 80% of cases [t(8;14)]) or between c-*myc* and the gene for either the kappa or lambda light chain (*IgL*) in the remaining 20% [t(2;8) or t(8;22)], respectively.[168]

Clinical Manifestations Endemic (African) BL refers to cases occurring in African children, usually 4 to 7 years old, with a male to female ratio of 2:1, nearly all EBV associated, involving primarily the bones of the jaw and other facial bones, as well as the kidneys, gastrointestinal tract, ovaries, breast, and other extranodal sites. Endemic BL is rare in the United States.

Sporadic (American) BL, 15 to 30% of which is EBV associated, occurs worldwide and accounts for 1 to 2% of lymphomas in adults and up to 40% of lymphomas in children in the United States and western Europe.[171] The abdomen, especially the ileocecal area, is the most common site of involvement. Patients may have malignant pleural effusions or ascites and involvement of the lymph nodes, jaws, ovaries, kidneys, breasts, omentum, Waldeyer's ring, and other sites.

Immunodeficiency-associated BL, often EBV associated, occurs mainly in patients infected with HIV but also occurs in organ transplant recipients after a relatively long interval post-transplantation and individuals with congenital immunodeficiency. BL accounts for nearly 30 to 40% of NHLs in HIV-infected patients.[172] Compared with other HIV-infected patients with diffuse large B-cell–type NHLs, those with BL are younger, less often carry a prior diagnosis of acquired immune deficiency syndrome (AIDS), and have higher mean CD4 counts, usually >200 cells/μL.[172]

Treatment Approximately 30% of patients present with limited-stage disease (Ann Arbor stage I or II), whereas 70% present with widespread disease (stage III or IV). Chemotherapy is the mainstay of treatment, with agents including cyclophosphamide, vincristine, methotrexate, and corticosteroids; however, surgical debulking and palliative low-dose radiation therapy to local tumor sites are also considered in treatment planning. Endemic BL is very sensitive to short-duration, high-intensity chemotherapy, sometimes combined with central nervous system prophylaxis. Children with localized disease have a >90% 5-year survival rate, and those with widespread disease (including leukemic presentation) may achieve a >90% complete response rate, with an event-free survival rate at 4 years of 65 to 75%. Adults with sporadic and immunodeficiency-associated BL treated with similar aggressive chemotherapeutic regimens have achieved good outcomes, with complete response rates of 65 to 100% and overall survival rates of 50 to 70%. A recent Cochrane Review was unable to provide any strong evidence on the relative effectiveness of various interventions to treat BL.[173]

Oral Manifestations In a Kenyan study that documented 961 children and 44 adults with rapidly growing BL, the main complaint was swelling.[174] The major sites involved in children were the jaw (52%), abdomen (25%), combined jaw and abdomen (14%), and other sites (10%). In adults, the involved sites were the jaw (4%), abdomen (43%), combined jaw and abdomen (25%), and other sites (27%). For those with jaw involvement, most were male and younger.[174]

In an assessment of cases submitted to the American Burkitt's Lymphoma Registry, American cases resembled African BL's time-space clustering, male predominance, and excellent response to chemotherapy. American BL appears to be a more heterogeneous disease than African BL, with more patients having involvement of cervical lymph nodes and bone marrow at an early stage of disease.[175] An examination of 17 cases of BL diagnosed in North Carolina, over a 10-year period, aged 3 to 23 years with male predominance, demonstrated maxillary or mandibular tumors in nearly 30%.[176] Sixty-three Turkish children with BL diagnosed over a 10-year period in a single institution, aged 3 to 14 years, with male predominance, had an incidence of jaw involvement of 16%.[177]

Clinically evident jaw tumors may result in tooth mobility and pain, intraoral swelling of the mandible and maxilla, and anterior open bite.[178] Mobile teeth may be present even in the absence of clinically detectable jaw tumors.[179] Radiographic features on panoramic images include resorption of alveolar bone, loss of teeth lamina dura, enlargement of tooth follicles, destruction of the cortex around tooth crypts, displacement of teeth and tooth buds by the enlarging tumor, resulting in the impression of "teeth floating in air," and sun-ray spicules as bone forms perpendicular to the mandible from subperiosteal growth.[176,179,180]

MULTIPLE MYELOMA

Multiple myeloma (MM) is a plasma cell neoplasm that is characterized by a bone marrow plasmacytosis, abnormal paraprotein, and complications of bone disease with skeletal destruction, renal insufficiency or failure, anemia, and hypercalcemia.[181] It is the third most common hematologic malignancy after leukemia and lymphoma, with an estimated incidence in 2007 of 19,900 cases in the United States.[109] The median age at diagnosis is 65 to 70 years.

Diagnosis Diagnostic criteria require end-organ damage, the presence of at least 10% plasma cells on examination of the bone marrow (or biopsy of a tissue with monoclonal plasma cells), and monoclonal protein in the serum or urine.[181,182] The diagnosis of MM often results from the workup of unexplained renal disease.

Clinical Manifestations Symptoms include fatigue, weakness, weight loss, bone pain, and recurrent infections. This disease is characterized by a high capacity to induce focal osteolytic bone lesions, diffuse osteopenia, and pathologic fractures. Osteolytic bone lesions in MM result from increased osteoclast formation, osteoblast inhibition induced by MM cells, and activity that occurs in close proximity to myeloma cells.[183]

Oral Manifestations Patients with MM can manifest soft tissue masses that are extramedullary plasmablastic tumors of the jaws.[184,185] Figure 5 shows a plasmablastic tumor of the upper right jaw. Consistent with plasma cell tumor growth in the mandible, initial oral signs of MM may involve pain, paresthesia of the inferior alveolar and mental nerves, swelling, tooth mobility, and radiolucency.[186] Radiographic changes in patients with MM include typical "punched-out" lesions in the skull from the focal proliferation of plasma cells inside the bone marrow and mandibular (more so than maxillary) involvement, ranging from asymptomatic osteolytic lesions to pathologic fracture.[187,188] Figure 6 illustrates the radiographic appearance of MM.

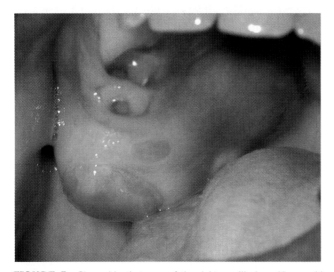

FIGURE 5 Plasmablastic tumor of the right maxilla in a 46-year-old African American woman with multiple myeloma.

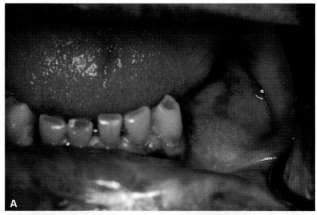
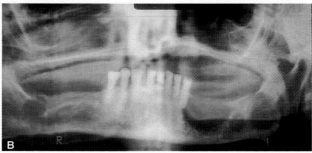

FIGURE 6 Multiple myeloma of the left mandible of a 58-year-old African American woman. *A*, Clinical image of a left mandible plasmablastic tumor. *B*, Panoramic radiographic image with punched-out lesions of the right and left mandible.

Treatment Although treatable, MM remains incurable in virtually all cases, with a median survival of 3 to 4 years after diagnosis. Although not curative, induction chemotherapy with vincristine, doxorubicin, and dexamethasone, or thalidomide plus dexamethasone, followed by HSCT (usually autologous) improves the likelihood of a complete response and prolongs disease-free survival and overall survival.[181] A number of new biologic therapies for management of MM targeted at cellular mechanisms and interactions, that is, with the bone marrow microenvironment, are expected to improve survival and include the use of thalidomide (Thalidomide Pharmion, Pharmion/Celgene, Boulder, CO), lenalidomide (Revlimid, Celgene Corporation, Summit, NJ), and bortezomib (Velcade, Janssen Pharmaceutica N.V., Belgium).[189,190]

To manage focal bone lytic lesions, patients with MM frequently require radiation therapy, surgery, and analgesic medications. Bisphosphonates are specific inhibitors of osteoclastic activity, and monthly intravenous infusions of either zoledronic acid (Zometa, Novartis Oncology, East Hanover, NJ) or pamidronate (Aredia, Novartis Oncology) have reduced the skeletal complications among patients with MM and are now a mainstay of myeloma therapy.[191]

Oral Health Considerations Osteonecrosis of the jaw (ONJ), resulting in symptomatic exposed nonhealing areas of the maxilla and mandible, is increasingly recognized as a serious complication of long-term intravenous bisphosphonate therapy, primarily with zoledronic acid and pamidronate. Figure 7 shows osteonecrosis of the maxilla resulting from

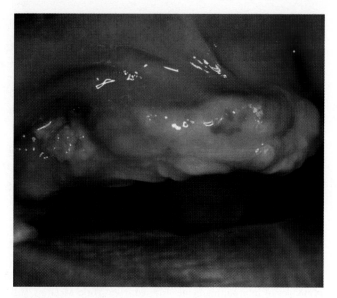

FIGURE 7 Osteonecrosis of the jaw. A 58-year-old African American male with a 2-year history of zoledronic acid use for multiple myeloma who had maxillary tooth extractions 2 months prior to bone necrosis and infection of the bilateral mandible in the molar region.

TABLE 9 Management Recommendations for Prevention of Osteonecrosis of the Jaws among Patients Taking Intravenous Bisphosphonates

Dental Procedure	Modifications/Management Recommendations
Dental examination	Dental examination and radiographs before patients are placed on intravenous bisphosphonates
Scaling and prophylaxis	Scaling and prophylaxis accomplished as atraumatically as possible, with gentle soft tissue management
Restorative procedures	Routine restorative care may be provided, with use of local anesthetics as necessary
Dental extractions	Dental extractions avoided unless the teeth have a mobility score of g3. Extractions performed as atraumatically as possible. Patients followed up weekly for the first 4 weeks and then monthly until the sockets are completely closed and healed.
Endodontic therapy	Endodontic therapy, crown amputation, and overdenture fabrication should be considered for severely decayed teeth
Removable prostheses	Existing prosthetic appliances should be reevaluated to ensure that they fit well. Relining a denture with a soft liner to promote a better fit and to minimize soft tissue trauma and pressure points is recommended.

Adapted from Migliorati CA et al.[194]

intravenous bisphosphonate use. Through case reporting and clinical experience, the incidence of ONJ in patients with cancer receiving intravenous bisphosphonates appears to range between 1 and 10% and is often associated with a recent dental surgical procedure, although spontaneous ONJ can also occur.[192] A multidisciplinary panel consisting of hematologists, dental specialists, and nurses specializing in the treatment of MM at the Mayo Clinic in Minnesota developed guidelines for the use of bisphosphonates, concluding effectiveness in reducing skeletal complications, pamidronate is favored over zoledronic acid; recommending discontinuing bisphosphonates after 2 years of therapy for patients who achieve complete response and/or plateau phase versus for patients whose disease is active, who have not achieved a response, or who have threatening bone disease beyond 2 years, decreasing therapy to every 3 months.[193]

TABLE 10 Recommendations for Management of Bisphosphonate-Associated Osteonecrosis of the Jaws

Evaluation and Management	
Goals	Area of ONJ should be treated only with the objective of eliminating sharp edges of bone that may traumatize soft tissues
Palliation	Superficial débridement may be performed if necessary to eliminate areas that may further traumatize adjacent tissues
	Clinicians should follow up with these patients every 2–3 weeks to reevaluate the areas and to ensure that they have not become suppurative
	Soft vinyl appliances or obturators, not designed for use during mastication, may help cover exposed necrotic bone to prevent further trauma to soft tissues. The interior portion of the appliance flanges must be relieved so as not to deliver pressure to the diseased tissues but rather to serve as a protective barrier.
Medical therapeutic approach	If the area around the exposed bone exhibits tender erythema and suppuration and/or sinus tracts, the patient should be treated with antibiotics until the areas resolve
	Microbiologic culture and sensitivity tests may be helpful
	Use of chlorhexidine mouthrinse 3–4 times a day is recommended to reduce bacterial load and colonization
Surgical therapeutic approach	A surgical approach with the aim of removing the necrotic bone and closing the site with healthy mucosa may be considered for patients with multiple myeloma who will be undergoing high-dose conditioning chemotherapy in preparation for hematopoietic stem cell transplantation
	Surgical manipulation may not lead to the closure of the necrotic site but may result in further increase of the osseous breakdown and dehiscence. If a surgical procedure is needed, patients should be informed of the possible risks and benefits.
	The role of hyperbaric oxygen therapy for the treatment of ONJ is unknown

Adapted from Migliorati CA et al.[194]
ONJ = osteonecrosis of the jaw.

Management of ONJ focuses on maximizing oral health to prevent its occurrence, conservative management with antiseptic mouthrinses and antibiotics, and avoidance of unnecessary invasive dental procedures.[194] Recommendations are listed in Tables 9 and 10. Odontogenic infections should be treated aggressively with systemic antibiotics, such as amoxicillin and/or clindamycin, with adequate bone penetration and a wide spectrum of coverage.

Another consideration for MM patients requiring dental surgery is the risk of hemorrhage.[195] Patients with MM and other disorders associated with high-titer serum paraproteins can manifest unique hemostatic disorders, predisposing the patient to hemorrhage, especially following surgical procedures.[196] Mechanisms can include acquired von Willebrand's syndrome, paraprotein-induced platelet function defects, factor VIII or X deficiency, and local tissue fragility associated with amyloidosis, abnormalities of the function of fibrin, circulating anticoagulants, and thrombocytopenia. Predental surgery assessment should include radiographic assessment for plasma cell tumors of the jaw and CBC and coagulation studies. Prevention of hemorrhage should be managed by consultation with the patient's hematologist regarding the status of treatment of the underlying disease and, depending on clinical circumstances, the need for additional therapies that might include plasmapheresis with appropriate factor replacement, desmopressin acetate (Stimate, Aventis Behring, King of Prussia, PA), fibrinolysis inhibitors ε-aminocaproic acid (Amicar 25% syrup, Xanodyne Pharmacal Inc, Florence, KY) and tranexamic acid (Cyclokapron; Pharmacia Corp, Peapack, NJ), and splenectomy.[196]

▼ SELECTED READINGS

Abbott BL. Diagnosis and management of lymphoma. Clin Lymphoma Myeloma 2006;7:30–2.

Dhaliwal G, Cornett PA, Tierney LM Jr. Hemolytic anemia. Am Fam Physician 2004;69:2599–606.

Duggal MS, Bedi R, Kinsey SE, et al. The dental management of children with sickle cell disease and beta-thalassaemia: a review. Int J Paediatr Dent 1996;6:227–34.

Farber JL, Rubin E, editors. Pathology. 3rd ed. Philadelphia: Lippincott, Williams, and Wilkins; 1999.

Kasper DL, Braunwald E, Fauci AS, et al, editors. Harrison's principles of internal medicine. 16th ed. New York: McGraw-Hill; 2005.

Lockhart PB, Meechan JG, Nunn J, editors. Laboratory tests. In: Dental care of the medically complex patient. 5th ed. Edinburgh: Wright/Elsevier Science; 2004. p. 370–72.

Rund D, Rachmilewitz E. Beta-thalassemia. N Engl J Med 2005; 353:1135–46.

Smith HB, McDonald DK, Miller RI. Dental management of patients with sickle cell disorders. J Am Dent Assoc 1987;114:85–7.

For the full reference list, please refer to the accompanying CD ROM.

17
▼

BLEEDING AND CLOTTING DISORDERS

LAUREN L. PATTON, DDS

▼ OVERVIEW AND EPIDEMIOLOGY

Dental health care professionals are increasingly called upon to provide dental care to individuals whose bleeding and clotting mechanisms have been altered by inherited or acquired diseases. This provides an opportunity for the dentist who is trained in the recognition of oral and systemic signs of altered hemostasis to assist in the screening and monitoring of the underlying condition. Dental procedures resulting in bleeding can have serious consequences for the patient with a bleeding disorder, including severe hemorrhage or even death. Safe dental care may require consultation with the patient's medical provider, institution of systemic management, and dental treatment modifications.

Of the inherited coagulopathies, von Willebrand's disease (vWD) is the most common. It results from quantitative deficiencies or qualitative defects of von Willebrand's factor (vWF) and affects about 0.8 to 1% of the population.[1] Hemophilia A, caused by coagulation factor (F) VIII deficiency, is the next most common, followed by hemophilia B, a F IX deficiency. The age-adjusted prevalence of hemophilia in six surveillance states in 1994 was 13.4 cases in 100,000 males (10.5 for hemophilia A and 2.9 for hemophilia B).[2] Application to the US population resulted in an estimated national prevalence of 13,320 cases of hemophilia A and 3,640 cases of hemophilia B, with an incidence rate of 1 per 5,032 live male births. Hemophilia A accounted for 79% of all hemophiliacs. Forty-three percent of hemophiliacs have a severe factor deficiency (<1% F VIII), whereas 26% have a moderate deficiency (1–5% F VIII) and 31% present with a mild deficiency (6–30% F VIII).[2]

Acquired coagulation disorders can result from drug actions or side effects or underlying systemic disease. A stratified household sample of 4,163 community residents aged 65 years or older living in a five-county area of North Carolina revealed 51.7% to be taking one or more medications (aspirin, warfarin, dipyridamole, nonsteroidal anti-inflammatory drugs [NSAIDs], or heparin) with the potential to alter hemostasis.[3] The use of coumarin anticoagulants is increasing as a result of their demonstrated effectiveness in the treatment of atrial fibrillation and venous thromboembolism and control of thrombosis in the presence of a mechanical heart valve.[4]

▼ PATHOPHYSIOLOGY

Basic Mechanisms of Hemostasis and Their Interactions

Interaction of several basic mechanisms produces normal hemostasis. For clarity and understanding, these are presented separately. Hemostasis can be divided into four general phases: the vascular phase; the platelet phase; the coagulation cascade phase, consisting of intrinsic, extrinsic, and common pathways; and the fibrinolytic phase. The first three phases are the principal mechanisms that prevent or diminish the loss of blood following vascular injury. Briefly,

when vessel integrity is disrupted, platelets are activated, adhere to the site of injury, and form a platelet plug that reduces or temporarily arrests blood loss.[5] The exposure of collagen and activation of platelets also initiates the coagulation cascade, which leads to fibrin formation and the generation of an insoluble fibrin clot that strengthens the platelet plug.[5] Fibrinolysis is the major means of disposing of fibrin after its hemostatic function has been fulfilled, and it can be considered the rate-limiting step in clotting. It leads to fibrin degradation by the proteolytic enzyme plasmin. As seen in Figure 1, multiple processes occur either simultaneously or in rapid sequence, such that, following almost immediate vascular contraction, platelets begin to aggregate at the wound site. The coagulation cascade is under way within 10 to 20 seconds of injury, an initial hemostatic plug is formed in 1 to 3 minutes, and fibrin has been generated and added to stabilize the clot by 5 to 10 minutes.

Vascular Phase

After tissue injury, there is an immediate reflex vasoconstriction that may alone be hemostatic in small vessels. Reactants such as serotonin, histamine, prostaglandins, and other products are vasoactive and produce vasoconstriction of the microvascular bed in the area of the injury.

Platelet Phase

When circulating platelets are exposed to damaged vascular surfaces (in the presence of functionally normal vWF, endothelial cells, collagen or collagen-like materials, basement membrane, elastin, microfibrils, and other cellular debris),

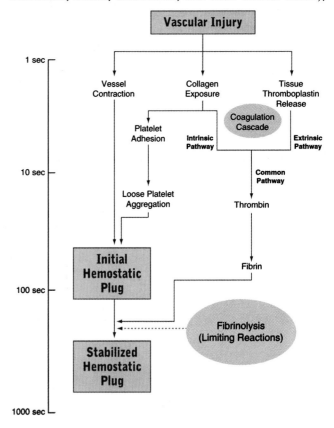

FIGURE 1 Mechanisms of hemostasis following vascular injury.

platelets are activated to experience physical and chemical changes.[5] These changes produce an environment that causes the platelets to undergo the aggregation and release phenomenon and form the primary vascular plug that reduces blood loss from small blood vessels and capillaries. These platelet plugs adhere to exposed basement membranes. As this reaction is occurring, the release reaction is under way, involving the intracellular release of active components for further platelet aggregation as well as promotion of the clotting mechanism. Adenosine diphosphate (ADP) is a potent nucleotide that activates and recruits other platelets in the area, immensely adding to the size of the plug. Platelet factor 3 is the intracellular phospholipid that activates F X and subsequently results in the conversion of prothrombin to thrombin. Additionally, the platelet plug, intermixed with fibrin and cellular components such as red and white cells, contracts to further reduce blood loss and to seal the vascular bed.

Coagulation Phase

The generation of thrombin and fibrin is the end product of the third phase of hemostasis, the coagulation phase. This process involves multiple proteins, many of which are synthesized by the liver (fibrinogen; prothrombin; Fs V, VII, IX, X, XI, XII, and XIII) and are vitamin K dependent (Fs II, VII, IX, and X). The process of coagulation essentially involves three separate pathways. It initially proceeds by two separate pathways (intrinsic and extrinsic) that converge by activating a third (common) pathway.

The blood clotting mechanism is the most studied unit; it was originally outlined in 1903 by Markowitz as the prothrombin-to-thrombin and fibrinogen-to-fibrin conversion system. In 1964, the "cascade" or "waterfall" theory was proposed.[6,7] It offered a useful device for understanding this complex system and its control, as well as the clinically important associated laboratory tests.

Figure 2 depicts the sequence of interactions between the various clotting factors following injury of tissue. The scheme of reaction is a bioamplification, in which a precursor is altered to an active form, which, in turn, activates the next precursor in the sequence. Beginning with an undetectable biochemical reaction, the coagulation mechanism results in a final explosive change of a liquid to a gel. The major steps involve the conversion of a precursor protein to an "activated" form, which activates another precursor protein, and so on down the cascade. The coagulation of blood also requires the presence of both calcium ions and phospholipid (or a phospholipid-containing membrane fragment derived from blood platelets).

The intrinsic pathway is initiated when F XII is activated by surface contact (eg, with collagen or subendothelium), and it involves the interaction of F XII and F XI. The next step of intrinsic coagulation, the activation of F IX to F XIa, requires a divalent cation.[8] Once activated, F IXa forms a complex with F VIII, in a reaction that requires the presence of both calcium ions and phospholipid, which, in turn, converts F X to an activated form—F Xa.

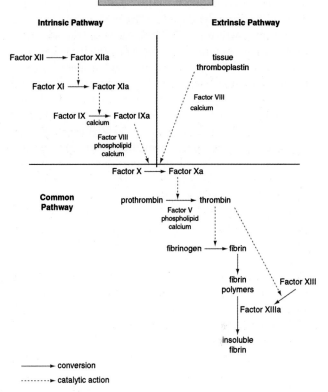

Coagulation Cascade

FIGURE 2   The coagulation cascade.

The extrinsic pathway is initiated by the release of tissue thromboplastin, also called tissue factor, and does not require contact activation. Tissue thromboplastin binds to F VII in the presence of calcium, and this complex is capable of activating Fs IX and X, linking the intrinsic and extrinsic pathways.

It is the activation of FX that begins the common pathway. Once activated, F Xa converts prothrombin to thrombin in a reaction similar to the activation of F X by F IXa. The activation of prothrombin by F Xa requires the presence of calcium ions and phospholipid as well as F V, a plasma protein cofactor.[9] Once formed, thrombin converts fibrinogen, a soluble plasma protein, to insoluble fibrin. Fibrin polymerizes to form a gel, stabilizing the platelet plug. Finally, F XIII, which has been converted to an activated form by thrombin,[10] produces covalent cross-links between the fibrin molecules that strengthen the clot and make it more resistant to lysis by plasmin. Individuals deficient in this clotting factor experience poor wound healing.[11]

FIBRINOLYTIC PHASE

The fourth phase of hemostasis is fibrinolysis; this is considered the major means of disposing of fibrin after its hemostatic function has been fulfilled. Once the microvascular bed is sealed and primary hemostasis is complete, the secondary hemostasis pathway has already commenced in parallel. As the monomeric fibrin is cross-linked with the aid of F XIII (fibrin stabilizing factor), the propagation of the formed clot is limited by several interactions.[12] One of these limiting systems is the fibrinolytic system (Figure 3). Kallikrein, which is an intrinsic activator of plasminogen, is generated when prekallikrein is bound to kininogen, thereby becoming a substrate for F XIIa. Tissue plasminogen activator (tPA) is released from the endothelial cells and converts plasminogen to plasmin that degrades fibrinogen and fibrin into fibrin degradation products (FDPs). tPA is a proteolytic enzyme that is nonspecific and also degrades Fs VIII and V. tPA has been used with great success in therapeutic doses to lyse thrombi in individuals with thromboembolic disorders associated with myocardial infarction.[12] The effectiveness of this drug is limited to the first 6 hours postinfarction. Activation of the fibrinolytic system can be turned off by inhibition of plasmin activity (eg, by α_2-antiplasmin) or inhibition of plasminogen activators (eg, plasminogen activator inhibitor [PAI]-1 and PAI-2).

Extended function of the fibrinolytic system is realized during wound healing. As the wound is revascularized and the capillary beds extend into the fibrin clot, the way for plasmin to remove the cross-linked fibrin is paved by the release of tPA. Without this unique system, wound healing would be impossible. Whereas the fibrinolytic system limits the coagulation process as described above, other systems function to limit the extent of the microvascular thrombosis in the area of injury. Antithrombin III is a potent inhibitor directed at thrombin.

▼ CLINICAL AND LABORATORY FINDINGS

Clinical Manifestations

Clinical manifestations of bleeding disorders can involve various systems, depending on the extent and type of disease.

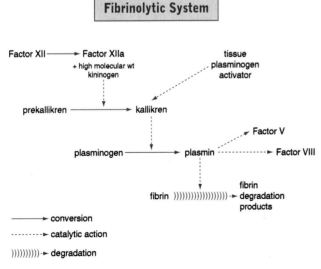

Fibrinolytic System

Factor XII ⟶ Factor XIIa
+ high molecular wt kininogen

tissue plasminogen activator

prekallikren ⟶ kallikren

plasminogen ⟶ plasmin

Factor V

Factor VIII

fibrin))))))))))))))))) ⟶ fibrin degradation products

⟶ conversion
-------- ⟶ catalytic action
)))))))))) ⟶ degradation

FIGURE 3 The fibrinolytic system.

Individuals with mild disease may present with no clinical signs, whereas individuals with severe coagulopathies may have definite stigmata. When skin and mucosa are involved, individuals may present with petechiae, ecchymoses, spider angiomas, hematomas, or jaundice. Deep dissecting hematomas and hemarthroses of major joints may affect severe hemophiliacs and result in disability or death. Disorders of platelet quantity may result in hepatosplenomegaly, spontaneous gingival bleeding, and risk of hemorrhagic stroke. Table 1 illustrates clinical features that distinguish coagulation disorders from platelet or vascular disorders.

Clinical Laboratory Tests

There are a variety of common and less common laboratory tests that help identify deficiency of required elements or dysfunction of the phases of coagulation (Tables 2 and 3). The two clinical tests used to evaluate primary hemostasis are the platelet count and platelet function tests such as bleeding time (BT). Tests to evaluate the status of other aspects of hemostasis include prothrombin time (PT)/international normalized ratio (INR), activated partial thromboplastin time (aPTT), thrombin time (TT), FDPs, specific coagulation factor assays (especially Fs VII, VIII, and IX and fibrinogen), and coagulation factor inhibitor screening tests (blocking antibodies).

PLATELET COUNT

Normal platelet counts are 150,000 to 450,000/mm³. Spontaneous clinical hemorrhage is usually not observed with platelet counts above 10,000 to 20,000/mm³. Many hospitals have established a critical value of 10,000/mm³ platelets, below which platelets are transfused to prevent serious bleeding sequelae, such as hemorrhagic stroke. Surgical or traumatic hemorrhage is more likely with platelet counts below 50,000/mm³.

TESTS OF PLATELET FUNCTION

BT is determined from a standardized incision on the forearm. BT is usually considered to be normal between 1 and 6 minutes (by modified Ivy's test) and is prolonged when greater than 15 minutes. The skin BT test, thought to identify qualitative or functional platelet defects, is a poor indicator of clinically significant bleeding at other sites, and its use as a predictive screening test for oral surgical procedures has been discouraged.[13,14]

A new in vitro system for the detection of platelet dysfunction, Platelet Function Analyzer (PFA-100; Dade-Behring, Deerfield, IL), has been developed.[15] Closure time (CT), measured by the PFA-100 device, is now reportable by many clinical laboratories as a possible alternative or supplement to the BT test.[16] The high sensitivity of the PFA-100 to vWD and its simplicity of use are its greatest strengths. However, because it is a global test system and also sensitive to low hematocrit, low platelet counts, and platelet dysfunction (both congenital and acquired; eg, secondary to medication such as aspirin), it must be recognized that the PFA-100 is neither specific for, nor predictive of, any particular disorder (inclusive of vWD).[17]

TABLE 1 Clinical Features of Bleeding Disorders

Feature	Vascular or Platelet Disorders	Coagulation Disorders
Bleeding from superficial cuts and scratches	Persistent, often perfuse	Minimal
Delayed bleeding	Rare	Common
Spontaneous gingival bleeding	Characteristic	Rare
Petechiae	Characteristic	Rare
Ecchymoses	Characteristic, usually small and multiple	Characteristic, usually large and solitary
Epistaxis	Common	Common
Deep dissecting hematomas	Rare	Characteristic
Hemarthroses	Rare	Characteristic

TABLE 2 Laboratory Tests for Assessing Hemostasis

Test	Normal Range
Platelet count	150,000 to 450,000/mm³
Bleeding time	<7 min (by simplate); 1–6 min (modified Ivy's test)
PFA-100 closure time	CEPI <164 s; CADP <116 s (Ketesztes and Tazbir, 2005)
PT/INR	Control ± 1 s (eg, PT: 11–13 s/INR 1.0)
Activated partial thromboplastin time	Comparable to control (eg, 15–35 s)
Thrombin time	Control ± 3 s (eg, 9–13 s)
Fibrin degradation products	<10 µg/dL
Fibrinogen assay	200–400 mg/dL
von Willebrand's antigen	60–150% vWF activity
Coagulation factor assays (eg, F VIII assay)	60–100% F VIII activity
Coagulation factor inhibitor assays (eg, Bethesda inhibitor assay for F VIII)	0.0 Bethesda inhibitor units

CADP = time it takes blood to block a membrane coated with collagen and adenosine diphosphate; CEPI = time it takes blood to block a membrane coated with collagen and epinephrine; F = factor; INR = international normalized ratio; PT = prothrombin time; vWF = von Willebrand's factor.

TABLE 3 Results of Hemostatic Screening Tests for Selected Bleeding Disorders

Bleeding Disorder	Screening Laboratory Tests			
	Platelet Count	PT/INR	aPTT	BT
Thrombocytopenia Leukemia	↓	N	N	↑
F VIII, IX, XI deficiency Heparin anticoagulation	N	N	↑	N
F II, V, X deficiency Vitamin K deficiency Intestinal malabsorption	N	↑	↑	N
F VII deficiency Coumarin anticoagulation Liver disease	N	↑	N	N
von Willebrand's disease	N, ↓	N	N, ↑	↑
DIC Severe liver disease	↓	↑	↑	↑
F XIII deficiency	N	N	N	N
Vascular wall defect	N	N	N	↑

aPTT = activated partial thromboplastin time; BT = bleeding time; DIC = disseminated intravascular coagulation; INR = international normalized ratio; N = normal; PT = prothrombin time; ↑ = increased; ↓ = decreased.

International consensus opinion is that although the PFA-100 CT is abnormal in some forms of platelet disorders, the test does not have sufficient sensitivity or specificity to be used as a screening tool for disorders of platelet function and is currently best restricted to research studies and prospective clinical trials.[16] A role of the PFA-100 CT in therapeutic monitoring of platelet function remains to be established.

In a comparison of the matched results among 113 hospital patients, the results of BT and PFA-100 CT agreed in 74.3% of patients. Of the 29 patients in whom the BT and PFA-100 results were discordant, whole-blood platelet aggregation studies supported the PFA-100 result in 86.2%.

The PFA-100 was more sensitive to aspirin-induced platelet dysfunction and was more rapidly and cheaply performed than the BT.[18]

PT AND INR

The normal range of PT is approximately 11 to 13 seconds. Because of individual laboratory reagent variability and the desire to be able to reliably compare the PT from one laboratory with that from another, the PT test is now commonly reported with its INR.[19,20] The INR, introduced by the World Health Organization in 1983, is the ratio of PT that adjusts for the sensitivity of the thromboplastin reagents, such that a normal coagulation profile is reported as an INR of 1.0.[21]

This test evaluates the extrinsic coagulation system and measures the presence or absence of clotting Fs I, II, V, VII, and X. Its most common use is to measure the effects of coumarin anticoagulants and reduction of the vitamin K–dependent Fs II, VII, IX, and X. Since the extrinsic system uses only Fs I, II, VII, and X, it does not measure the reduction of Fs VIII or IX, which characterizes hemophilias A and B. Additionally, the PT is used to measure the metabolic aspects of protein synthesis in the liver. Although most patients on coumarin anticoagulants are monitored by monthly venous blood draws and laboratory analysis, the CoaguChek system (Roche Diagnostics, Indianapolis, IN) allows Clinical Laboratory Improvements Amendments (CLIA)-waived point-of-care PT/INR testing of fingerstick blood in physicians' and dentists' offices.

ACTIVATED PARTIAL THROMBOPLASTIN TIME

The aPTT is considered normal if the control aPTT and the test aPTT are within 10 seconds of each other. Control aPTT times are usually 15 to 35 seconds. Normal ranges depend on the manufacturer's limits; each supplier varies slightly. The unactivated partial thromboplastin time (PTT) was originally described by Langdell and colleagues in 1953 as a simple one-stage assay for measuring F VIII.[22] Now it is used to evaluate the intrinsic cascade and measure the functional levels of Fs VIII, IX, XI, and XII. Since the addition of the activator (a rare earth), the test no longer measures Fs XI and XII. As a screening test, the aPTT is prolonged only when the factor levels in the intrinsic and common pathways are less than approximately 30%. It is altered in hemophilias A and B and with the use of the anticoagulant heparin.

THROMBIN TIME

The TT is used specifically to test the ability to form the initial clot from fibrinogen and is considered normal in the range of 9 to 13 seconds. Additionally, it is used to measure the activity of heparin, FDPs, or other paraproteins that inhibit conversion of fibrinogen to fibrin. Fibrinogen can also be specifically assayed and should be present at a level of 200 to 400 mg/dL.

FIBRIN DEGRADATION PRODUCTS

The FDPs are measured using a specific latex agglutination system to evaluate the presence of the D-dimer of fibrinogen and/or fibrin above normal levels. Such presence indicates that intravascular lysis has taken place or is occurring. This state can result from primary fibrinolytic disorders or disseminated intravascular coagulation (DIC). DIC is a catastrophic state that may result from massive trauma, extensive and terminal metastatic cancer, or fulminant viral or bacterial infections. DIC is rarely seen in the practice of dentistry, but it can occur.

FACTOR ASSAYS

To further identify factor deficiencies and their level of severity, specific activity levels of factors can be measured.

Normal factor activity is usually in the 60 to 150% range. Inhibitor screening tests are essential when sufficient factor concentrate to correct the factor deficiency under normal conditions fails to control bleeding. To identify the specific type of vWD (types I–III and platelet type), additional studies, such as the ristocetin cofactor, ristocetin-induced platelet aggregation studies, and monomer studies, are helpful.

TESTS OF CAPILLARY FRAGILITY

The tourniquet test for capillary fragility, which assesses the Rumpel-Leede phenomenon, is useful for identifying disorders of vascular wall integrity or platelet disorders. Stasis is produced by inflating a sphygmomanometer cuff around the arm in the usual manner to a pressure halfway between systolic and diastolic levels. This moderate degree of stasis is maintained for 5 minutes. At 2 minutes following cuff deflation and removal, a 2.5 cm diameter region (size of a quarter) of skin on the volar surface of the arm at 4 cm distal to the antecubital fossa is observed for petechial hemorrhages. Normally, petechiae in men do not exceed 5 in number, and in women and children, they do not exceed 10 in number in the skin region examined.

Vessel wall disorders can result in hemorrhagic features. Bleeding is usually mild and confined to the skin, mucosa, and gingiva. Vascular purpura can result from damage to capillary endothelium, from abnormalities in the vascular subendothelial matrix or extravascular connective tissue bed, or from abnormal vessel formation. The pathogenesis of bleeding is not well defined in many conditions, and the capillary fragility test is the only test to demonstrate abnormal results.

▼ CLASSIFICATION OF BLEEDING DISORDERS

Vessel Wall Disorders

Scurvy, resulting from dietary deficiency of water-soluble vitamin C, is found primarily in regions of urban poverty, among either infants on nonsupplemented processed milk formulas, elderly who cook for themselves, or adults with alcohol or drug dependencies or mental retardation.[23–25] Many of the hemorrhagic features of scurvy result from defects in collagen synthesis. Vitamin C is necessary for the synthesis of hydroxyproline, an essential constituent of collagen. One of the first clinical signs is petechial hemorrhages at the hair follicles and purpura on the back of the lower extremities that coalesce to form ecchymoses. Hemorrhage can occur in the muscles, joints, nail beds, and gingival tissues. Gingival involvement may include swelling, friability, bleeding, secondary infection, and loosening of teeth.[24] Scurvy results when dietary vitamin C falls below 10 mg/d. Implementation of a diet rich in vitamin C and administration of 1 g/d of vitamin C supplements provide rapid resolution.

Cushing's syndrome, resulting from excessive exogenous or endogenous corticosteroid intake or production, leads to general protein wasting and atrophy of supporting connective tissue around blood vessels. Patients may show skin bleeding or easy bruising. Aging causes similar perivascular connective tissue atrophy and lack of skin mobility. Tears in small blood vessels can result in irregularly shaped purpuric areas on arms and hands, called purpura senilis. Other metabolic or inflammatory disorders resulting in purpura include Schönlein-Henoch or anaphylactoid purpura, hyperglobulinemic purpura, Waldenström's macroglobulinemia, multiple myeloma, amyloidosis, and cryoglobulinemia.

Ehlers-Danlos syndrome is an autosomal dominant inherited disorder of connective tissue matrix, generally resulting in fragile skin blood vessels and easy bruising. It is characterized by hyperelasticity of the skin and hypermobile joints. Eleven subtypes have been identified with unique biochemical defects and varying clinical features.[26] Type I is the classic form, with soft, velvety, hyperextensible skin; easy bruising and scarring; hypermobile joints; varicose veins; and prematurity. Type VIII, which was recently mapped to chromosome 12q13,[27] has skin findings similar to those in type I, with easy bruising following minor trauma due mainly to the resulting fragility of the oral mucosa and blood vessels, and is characterized by early-onset periodontal disease with severe loss of alveolar bone and permanent dentition.[28,29] Children with type VII syndrome may present with microdontia and collagen-related dentinal structural defects in primary teeth, in addition to bleeding after tooth brushing.[30] Other oral findings include fragility of the oral mucosa, gingiva, and teeth, as well as hypermobility of the temporomandibular joint and stunted teeth and pulp stones on dental radiographs.[31–33] Oral health may be severely compromised as a result of specific alterations of collagen in orofacial structures. A number of tissue responses (mucosa, periodontium, pulp) and precautions (temporomandibular joint [TMJ] dislocation) should be considered when planning dental treatment.[34]

Rendu-Osler-Weber syndrome, also called hereditary hemorrhagic telangiectasia (HHT), is a group of autosomal dominant disorders with abnormal telangiectatic capillaries, frequent episodes of nasal and gastrointestinal bleeding, and associated brain and pulmonary lesions.[35–37] Perioral and intraoral angiomatous nodules or telangiectases are common with progressive disease, involving areas of the lips, tongue, and palate that may bleed upon manipulation during dental procedures.[38] Diagnosis is facilitated by the history of nosebleeds[37] and the observation of multiple nonpulsating vascular lesions, where arterioles connect to venules representing small arteriovenous malformations. These lesions blanch in response to applied pressure, unlike petechiae or ecchymoses. Mucocutaneous lesions may bleed profusely with minor trauma or, occasionally, spontaneously.[39] Persistently bleeding lesions may be treated with cryotherapy, laser ablation, electrocoagulation, or resection.[40] Blood replacement and iron therapy may be necessary following dental extractions in involved areas.[39] It has been suggested that antibiotic prophylaxis should be considered before dental care for patients with HHT and concomitant pulmonary arteriovenous malformation.[35]

Platelet Disorders

Platelet disorders may be divided into two categories by etiology—congenital and acquired—and into two additional categories by type—thrombocytopenias and thrombocytopathies (Table 4). Thrombocytopenias occur when platelet quantity is reduced and are caused by one of three mechanisms: decreased production in the bone marrow, increased sequestration in the spleen, or accelerated destruction. Thrombocytopathies, or qualitative platelet disorders, may result from defects in any of the three critical platelet reactions: adhesion, aggregation, or granule release. Dysfunctional platelet mechanisms may occur in isolated disorders or in conjunction with dysfunctional coagulation mechanisms.

CONGENITAL PLATELET DEFECTS

Congenital abnormalities of platelet function or production are rare and the causes are quite diverse, ranging from defects in receptors critical to platelet adhesion and aggregation, to defects in signaling molecules or in transcription factors important for production of functional platelets.[41] Glanzmann's thrombasthenia is a qualitative disorder characterized by a deficiency in the platelet membrane glycoproteins IIb and IIIa.[42–44] Clinical signs include bruising,

TABLE 4 Classification of Platelet Disorders

Congenital
  Thrombocytopenic—quantitative platelet deficiency
    May-Hegglin anomaly
    Wiskott-Aldrich syndrome
    Neonatal alloimmune thrombocytopenia
  Nonthrombocytopenic—qualitative or functional platelet defect
    Glanzmann's thrombasthenia
    Platelet-type von Willebrand's disease
    Bernard-Soulier syndrome

Acquired
  Thrombocytopenic—quantitative platelet deficiency
    Autoimmune or idiopathic thrombocytopenia purpura
    Thrombotic thrombocytopenic purpura
    Cytotoxic chemotherapy
    Drug induced (eg, quinine, quinidine, gold salts, trimethoprim-sulfamethoxazole, rifampin)
    Leukemia
    Aplastic anemia
    Myelodysplasia
    Systemic lupus erythematosus
    Associated with infection: HIV, mononucleosis, malaria
    Disseminated intravascular coagulation
  Nonthrombocytopenic—qualitative or functional platelet defect
    Drug induced (eg, by aspirin, NSAIDs, penicillin, cephalosporins)
    Uremia
    Alcohol dependency
    Liver disease
    Myeloma, myeloproliferative disorders, macroglobulinemia
    Acquired platelet-type von Willebrand's disease

HIV = human immunodeficiency virus; NSAIDs = nonsteroidal anti-inflammatory drugs.

epistaxis, gingival hemorrhage, and menorrhagia. Treatment of oral surgical bleeding involves platelet transfusion and use of antifibrinolytics and local hemostatic agents. Wiskott-Aldrich syndrome is characterized by cutaneous eczema (usually beginning on the face), thrombocytopenic purpura, and an increased susceptibility to infection due to an immunologic defect.[45] Oral manifestations include gingival bleeding and palatal petechiae. May-Hegglin anomaly is a rare hereditary condition characterized by the triad of thrombocytopenia, giant platelets, and inclusion bodies in leukocytes. Clinical features and the pathogenesis of bleeding in this disease are poorly defined.[46] Bernard-Soulier syndrome and platelet-type vWD also result from identified defects in platelet membrane glycoproteins.[47] Unlike the other types of vWD, the platelet type is rare and presents with less severe clinical bleeding.

ACQUIRED PLATELET DEFECTS

Two of the most commonly encountered platelet disorders, idiopathic or immune thrombocytopenic purpura (ITP) and thrombotic thrombocytopenic purpura (TTP), have clinical symptoms, including petechiae and purpura over the chest, neck, and limbs—usually more severe on the lower extremities. Mucosal bleeding may occur in the oral cavity and gastrointestinal and genitourinary tracts.

The age-adjusted prevalence of ITP in Maryland was 9.5 per 100,000 persons, with an overall female to male ratio of 1.9.[48] ITP may be acute and self-limiting (2 to 6 weeks) in children. In adults, ITP is typically more indolent in its onset, and the course is persistent, often lasting many years, and may be characterized by recurrent exacerbations of disease. In severe cases of ITP, oral hematomas and hemorrhagic bullae may be the presenting clinical sign.[49,50] Most patients with chronic ITP are young women. Intracerebral hemorrhage, although rare, is the most common cause of death. ITP is assumed to be caused by accelerated antibody-mediated platelet consumption. The natural history and long-term prognosis of adults with chronic ITP remain incompletely defined.[51] ITP may be a component of other systemic diseases. Autoimmune thrombocytopenia associated with systemic lupus erythematosus is often of little consequence but may occasionally be severe and serious, requiring aggressive treatment.[52] Immune-mediated thrombocytopenia may occur in conjunction with HIV disease in approximately 15% of adults, being more common with advanced clinical disease and immune suppression, although less than 0.5% of patients have severe thrombocytopenia with platelet counts below 50,000/mm³.[53] Although there are numerous therapeutic options, neither consensus among experts nor clear algorithms to treat this complex disease exist. In addition to conventional agents such as corticosteroids and intravenous immune globulin and splenectomy, there is a role of newer therapies with diverse mechanisms of action, such as rituximab, anti-D, and thrombopoietin-like agents.[54]

TTP is an acute catastrophic disease that, until recently, was uniformly fatal. Causes include metastatic malignancy, pregnancy, mitomycin C, and high-dose chemotherapy. If untreated, it still carries a high mortality rate. In addition to thrombocytopenia, clinical presentation of TTP includes microangiopathic hemolytic anemia, fluctuating neurologic abnormalities, renal dysfunction, and occasional fever. Microvascular infarcts occurring in gingival and other mucosal tissues are present in about 60% of the cases. These appear as platelet-rich thrombi. Serial studies of plasma samples from patients during episodes of TTP have often shown vWF multimer abnormalities.[55]

Thrombocytopenia may be a component of other hematologic disease, such as myelodysplastic disorders,[56] aplastic anemia,[57] and leukemia.[58] Bone marrow suppression from cytotoxic chemotherapy can result in severe thrombocytopenia, requiring platelet transfusions for prevention of spontaneous hemorrhage. Thrombocytopenia and thrombocytopathy in liver disease are complicated by coagulation defects, as discussed below. Alcohol can, itself, induce thrombocytopenia.[59] The coagulopathy of renal disease consists of an acquired qualitative platelet defect resulting from uremia.[60]

Medications can also reduce absolute numbers of platelets or interfere with their function, resulting in postsurgical hemorrhage.[61–63] Aspirin induces a functional defect in platelets detectable as prolongation of BT and altered PFA-100 CTs. It inactivates an enzyme called prostaglandin synthetase, resulting in inactivation of cyclooxygenase catalytic activity and decreasing biosynthesis of prostaglandin and thromboxanes that are needed to regulate interactions between platelets and the endothelium.[64] A single 100 mg dose of aspirin provides rapid complete inhibition of platelet cyclooxygenase activity and thromboxane production. This type of drug-related platelet disorder is compensated for within 7 to 10 days. Aspirin is commonly used as an inexpensive and effective antiplatelet therapy for thromboembolic protection. Antiplatelet therapy reduces the risk of death from cardiovascular causes by about one-sixth and the risk of nonfatal myocardial infarction and stroke by about one-third for patients with unstable angina or a history of myocardial infarction, transient ischemia, or stroke.[64] Most NSAIDs have a similar but less significant antiplatelet effect. Reversal of this type of platelet dysfunction takes place within 6 to 8 hours after discontinuation of the drug and may be completely reversed within 3 days. A relatively new antiplatelet agent, clopidogrel bisulfate (Plavix, Bristol-Meyers Squibb-Sanofi Pharmaceuticals Partnership, New York, NY), that acts as an inhibitor of ADP-induced platelet aggregation is often prescribed after coronary stent placement and carries less risk of prolonged bleeding than aspirin.[65] The cyclooxygenase-2 inhibitors, such as celecoxib (Celebrex, Pfizer, New York, NY), generally do not inhibit platelet aggregation at indicated doses.

Coagulation Disorders

Coagulation disorders may be either congenital or acquired secondary to drugs or disease processes.

▼ CONGENITAL COAGULOPATHIES

Inherited disorders of coagulation can result from deficiency of a number of factors (Table 5) that are essential in the coagulation cascade or deficiency of vWF. Clinical bleeding can vary from mild to severe, depending on the specific clotting factor affected and the level of factor deficiency.

Hemophilia A

A deficiency of F VIII, the antihemophilic factor, is inherited as an X-linked recessive trait that affects males (hemizygous). The trait is carried in the female (heterozygous) without clinical evidence of the disease, although a few do manifest mild bleeding symptoms. Males with hemophilia transmit the affected gene to all their female offspring, yet their sons are normal, and the effects skip a generation unless their wives were carriers and their daughters received the maternal affected X chromosome as well. Only 60 to 70% of families with newly diagnosed hemophiliacs report a family history of the disease, suggesting a high mutation rate. There is no racial predilection. Clinical symptoms and F VIII levels vary from pedigree to pedigree. Severe clinical bleeding is seen when the F VIII level is less than 1% of normal. In contrast to the more superficial signs of bleeding observed in individuals with platelet-associated disorders, individuals with hemophilia exhibit bleeds into more deep-seated spaces. The more common signs include hematomas, hemarthroses, hematuria, gastrointestinal bleeding, and bleeding from lacerations or head trauma or spontaneous intracranial bleeding that require factor replacement therapy.[66] Retroperitoneal and central nervous system bleeds, occurring spontaneously or induced by minor trauma, can be life threatening. Severe hemorrhage leads to joint synovitis and hemophilic arthropathies, intramuscular bleeds, and pseudotumors (encapsulated hemorrhagic cyst). Since 1965, replacement therapy, prophylaxis, and home treatment have been used with intensification of clotting factor consumption that has led to decreases in the risk of hemophilic arthropathy.[67] Moderate clinical bleeding is found when F VIII levels are 1 to 5% of normal. Only mild symptoms, such as prolonged bleeding following tooth extraction, surgical procedures, or severe trauma, occur if levels are between 6 and 50% of normal.

Hemophilia B

F IX (Christmas factor) deficiency is found in hemophilia B. The genetic background, factor levels, and clinical symptoms are similar to those in hemophilia A. The distinction was made only in the late 1940s between these two X-linked diseases. Concentrates used to treat F VIII and F IX deficiencies are specific for each state; therefore, a correct diagnosis must be made to ensure effective replacement therapy. Further discussion of the clinical management is presented later in this chapter. Circulating blocking antibodies or inhibitors to Fs VIII and IX may be seen in patients with these disorders. These inhibitors are specific for F VIII or F IX and render the patient refractory to the normal mode of treatment with concentrates. Catastrophic bleeding can occur, and only with supportive transfusions can the patient survive.

F XI Deficiency

Plasma thromboplastin antecedent deficiency is clinically a mild disorder seen in pedigrees of Jewish descent; it is transmitted as an autosomal dominant trait. Bleeding symptoms do occur but are usually mild. In the event of major surgery or trauma, hemorrhage can be controlled with infusions of fresh frozen plasma (FFP).

F XII Deficiency

Hageman factor deficiency is another rare disease that presents in the laboratory with prolonged PT and PTT. Clinical symptoms are nonexistent. Treatment is therefore contraindicated.

F X Deficiency

Stuart factor deficiency, also a rare bleeding diathesis, is inherited as an autosomal recessive trait. Clinical bleeding symptoms in the patient with levels less than 1% are similar to those seen in hemophilias A and B.

F V Deficiency

Proaccelerin deficiency, like F XI and F X deficiencies, is a rare autosomal recessive trait that presents with moderate to severe clinical symptoms. When compared with hemophilias A and B, this hemorrhagic diathesis is moderate, only occasionally resulting in soft tissue hemorrhage and only rarely presenting with hemarthrosis; it does not involve the devastating degenerative joint disease seen in severe hemophilias A and B.

TABLE 5 Coagulation Factors			
	Coagulation Factor Affected		
Factor (Name)	Intrinsic	Extrinsic	t1/2 (h)
XIII (fibrin-stabilizing factor)	*	*	336
XII (Hageman factor)	*		60
XI (plasma thromboplastin antecedent)	*		60
X (Stuart factor)	*	*	48
IX (Christmas factor)	*		18–24
VIII (antihemophilic factor)	*		8–12
VII (proconvertin)		*	4–6
V (proaccelerin)	*	*	32
IV (calcium)	*	*	—
III (tissue thromboplastin)		*	—
II (prothrombin)	*	*	72
I (fibrinogen)	*	*	96

t1/2 = half-life.

Fs XIII and I Deficiencies

Fibrin-stabilizing deficiency and fibrinogen deficiency are very rare, and these diagnoses can be made only with extensive laboratory tests usually available only in tertiary care medical centers. Both are autosomal recessive traits. Most dysfibrinogenemias result in no symptoms, others lead to moderate bleeding, and a few induce a hypercoagulable state. F XIII deficiency appears to have different forms of penetrance and in some families appears only in the males.

von Willebrand's Disease

vWD, a unique disorder that was described originally by Erik von Willebrand in 1926,[68] can result from inherited defects in the concentration, structure, or function of von Willebrand's factor (vWF), a multimeric high molecular weight glycoprotein.[69] It promotes its function in two ways: (1) by supporting platelet adhesion to the injured vessel wall under conditions of high shear forces and (2) by its carrier function for factor VIIIc in plasma.[70] Because of the complexity of the disease, diagnosis of vWD is one of the most challenging of any coagulation disorder.

This disorder is usually transmitted as an autosomal dominant trait with varying penetrance. The clinical features of the disease are usually mild and include mucosal bleeding, soft tissue hemorrhage, menorrhagia in women, and rare hemarthrosis.[71] The common genetic profile suggests a heterozygous state, with both males and females affected. Normal plasma vWF level is 10 mg/L, with a half-life of 6 to 15 hours.

vWD is classified into three primary categories.[69] Type 1 (85% of all vWD) includes partial quantitative deficiency, type 2 (10–15% of all vWD) includes qualitative defects, and type 3 (rare) includes virtually complete deficiency of vWF. vWD type 2 is divided into four secondary categories. Type 2A includes variants with decreased platelet adhesion caused by selective deficiency of high molecular weight vWF multimers. Type 2B includes variants with increased affinity for platelet glycoprotein Ib. Type 2M includes variants with markedly defective platelet adhesion despite a relatively normal size distribution of vWF multimers. Type 2N includes variants with markedly decreased affinity for F VIII. These six categories of vWD correlate with important clinical features and therapeutic requirements.[69]

A rare fourth type is called pseudo- or platelet-type vWD, and it is a primary platelet disorder that mimics vWD. The increased platelet affinity for large multimers of vWF results primarily in mucocutaneous bleeding. Due to familial genetic variants, wide variations occur in the patient's laboratory profile over time; therefore, diagnosis may be difficult.[72] The uncovering of all of the biochemical, physiologic, and clinical manifestations of vWD has held experts at bay for many years. As early as 1968, acquired vWD was noted to occur as a rare complication of autoimmune or neoplastic disease, associated mostly with lymphoid or plasma cell proliferative disorders and having clinical manifestations that are similar to congenital vWD.[73]

▼ ANTICOAGULANT-RELATED COAGULOPATHIES

Heparin

Intentional anticoagulation is induced acutely with heparin or as chronic oral therapy with coumarin drugs. Indications for heparin therapy include prophylaxis or treatment for venous thromboembolism, including prophylaxis in medical and surgical patients.[74] Heparin is a potent anticoagulant that binds with antithrombin III to significantly inhibit activation of Fs IX, X, and XI, thereby reducing thrombin generation and fibrin formation. The major bleeding complications from heparin therapy are bleeding at surgical sites and bleeding into the retroperitoneum.

Heparin has a relatively short duration of action of 3 to 4 hours and so is typically used for acute anticoagulation, whereas chronic therapy is initiated with coumarin drugs. For acute anticoagulation, intravenous infusion of 1,000 units unfractionated heparin per hour, sometimes following a 5,000-unit bolus, is given to raise the aPTT to 1.5 to 2 times the preheparin aPTT. Alternatively, subcutaneous injections of 5,000 to 10,000 units of heparin are given every 12 hours. Newer biologically active low molecular weight heparins (LMWHs) (eg, enoxaprin [Lovenox], Sanofi-Aventis, Bridgewater, NJ, tinzaparin [Innohep], Pharmion, Boulder, CO, dalteparin [Fragmin], Pfizer) administered subcutaneously once or twice daily are less likely to result in thrombocytopenia and bleeding complications. Protamine sulfate can rapidly reverse the anticoagulant effects of heparin.

Coumarin

Coumarin anticoagulants, which include warfarin and dicumarol (Coumadin, DuPont Pharmaceuticals, Wilmington, DE), are used for anticoagulation to prevent recurrent thromboembolic events, such as pulmonary embolism, venous thrombosis, stroke, and myocardial infarction; to treat atrial fibrillation; and in conjunction with prosthetic heart valves.[75] They slow thrombin production and clot formation by blocking the action of vitamin K. Levels of vitamin K–dependent Fs II, VI, IX, and X (prothrombin complex proteins) are reduced. The anticoagulant effect of coumarin drugs may be reversed rapidly by infusion of fresh frozen plasma (FFP) or over the course of 12 to 24 hours by administration of vitamin K. PT/INR is used to monitor anticoagulation levels. Medically indicated target ranges vary from a PT of 18 to 30 seconds/INR of 1.5 to 4.0 but are seldom above 3.5. Daily doses of 2.5 to 7.5 mg coumarin typically are required to maintain adequate anticoagulation. Patients with paroxysmal atrial fibrillation and porcine heart valves require minimal anticoagulation (INR target 1.5–2.0), and venous thrombosis is managed with intermediate-range coagulation (INR 2.0–3.0), whereas mechanical prosthetic heart valves and hypercoagulable states require more intense anticoagulation (INR target 3.0–4.0).[75]

Coumarin therapy requires continual laboratory monitoring, typically every 2 to 8 weeks, as fluctuations can occur. It has a longer duration of action, with coagulant activity in blood decreased by 50% in 12 hours and 20% in 24 hours of therapy initiation. Coagulation returns to normal levels in approximately 2 to 4 days following discontinuation of coumarin drugs. Coumarin therapy can result in bleeding episodes that are sometimes fatal. Intramuscular injections are avoided in anticoagulated patients because of increased risk of intramuscular bleeding and hematoma formation. Coumarin drugs are particularly susceptible to drug interactions. Drugs that potentially increase coumarin potency (ie, elevate the INR) include metronidazole, penicillin, erythromycin, cephalosporins, tetracycline, fluconazole, ketoconazole, chloral hydrate, and propoxyphene; those that reduce its potency (ie, decrease the INR) include barbiturates, ascorbic acid, dicloxacillin, and nafcillin.[76] Additive hemostatic effect is seen when coumarin drugs are used in combination with aspirin or NSAIDs.

▼ DISEASE-RELATED COAGULOPATHIES

Liver Disease

Patients with liver disease may have a wide spectrum of hemostatic defects depending upon the extent of liver damage.[77] Owing to impaired protein synthesis, important factors and inhibitors of the clotting and the fibrinolytic systems are markedly reduced. Additionally, abnormal vitamin K–dependent factor and fibrinogen molecules have been encountered. Thrombocytopenia and thrombocytopathy are also common in severe liver disease. Acute or chronic hepatocellular disease may display decreased vitamin K–dependent factor levels, especially Fs II, VII, IX, and X and protein C, with other factors still being normal.

Vitamin K Deficiency

Vitamin K is a fat-soluble vitamin that is absorbed in the small intestine and stored in the liver. It plays an important role in hemostasis. Vitamin K deficiency is associated with the production of poorly functioning vitamin K–dependent Fs II, VII, IX, and X.[78] Deficiency is rare but can result from inadequate dietary intake, intestinal malabsorption, or loss of storage sites due to hepatocellular disease. Biliary tract obstruction and long-term use of broad-spectrum antibiotics, particularly the cephalosporins, can cause vitamin K deficiency. Although there is a theoretic 30-day store of vitamin K in the liver, severe hemorrhage can result in acutely ill patients in 7 to 10 days. A rapid fall in F VII levels leads to an initial elevation in INR and a subsequent prolongation of aPTT. When vitamin K deficiency results in coagulopathy, supplemental vitamin K by injection restores the integrity of the clotting mechanism.

Disseminated Intravascular Coagulation

DIC is triggered by potent stimuli that activate both F XII and tissue factor to initially form microthrombi and emboli throughout the microvasculature.[79] Thrombosis results in rapid consumption of both coagulation factors and platelets while also creating FDPs that have antihemostatic effects. The most frequent triggers for DIC are obstetric complications, metastatic cancer, massive trauma, and infection with sepsis. Clinical symptoms vary with disease stage and severity. Most patients have bleeding at skin and mucosal sites. Although it can be chronic and mild, acute DIC can produce massive hemorrhage and be life threatening.

Fibrinolytic Disorders

Disorders of the fibrinolytic system can lead to hemorrhage when clot breakdown is enhanced or excessive clotting and thrombosis when clot breakdown mechanisms are retarded. Primary fibrinolysis typically results in bleeding and may be caused by a deficiency in α_2-antiplasmin or plasminogen activator inhibitors, natural proteins that turn off activation of the fibrinolytic system. Laboratory coagulation tests are normal with the exception of decreased fibrinogen and increased FDP levels. Impaired clearance of tPA may contribute to prolonged bleeding in individuals with severe liver disease. As discussed above, deficiency of F XIII, a transglutaminase that stabilizes fibrin clots, is a rare inherited disorder that leads to hemorrhage. Patients with primary fibrinolysis are treated with FFP therapy and antifibrinolytics.

Differentiation must be made from the secondary fibrinolysis that accompanies DIC, a hypercoagulable state that predisposes individuals to thromboembolism. Dialysis patients with chronic renal failure show a fibrinolysis defect at the level of plasminogen activation.[80] Reduced fibrinolysis may be responsible, along with other factors, for the development of thrombosis, atherosclerosis, and their thrombotic complications. Activators of the fibrinolytic system (tPA, streptokinase, and urokinase) are frequently used to accelerate clot lysis in patients with acute thromboembolism, for example, to prevent continued tissue damage in myocardial infarction or treat thrombotic stroke.

▼ IDENTIFICATION OF THE DENTAL PATIENT WITH A BLEEDING DISORDER

Identification of the dental patient with or at risk for a bleeding disorder begins with a thorough review of the medical history.[81,82] Patient report of a family history of bleeding problems may help identify inherited disorders of hemostasis. A patient's past history of bleeding following surgical procedures, including dental extractions, can help identify a risk. Surveying the patient for current medication use is important. Identification of medications with hemostatic effect, such as coumarin anticoagulants, heparin, aspirin, NSAIDs, and cytotoxic chemotherapy, is essential. Active medical conditions, including hepatitis or cirrhosis, renal disease, hematologic malignancy, and thrombocytopenia, may predispose patients to bleeding problems. Additionally, a history of heavy alcohol intake is a risk factor for bleeding consequences.

A review-of-systems approach to the patient interview can identify symptoms suggestive of hemostatic abnormalities (see Table 1). Although the majority of patients with underlying bleeding disorders of mild to moderate severity may exhibit no symptoms, symptoms are common when disease is severe. Symptoms of hemorrhagic diatheses reported by patients may include frequent epistaxis, spontaneous gingival or oral mucosal bleeding, easy bruising, prolonged bleeding from superficial cuts, excessive menstrual flow, and hematuria. When the history and the review of systems suggest increased bleeding propensity, laboratory studies are warranted.

▼ MANAGEMENT

Management of the patient with a hemorrhagic disorder is aimed at correction of the reversible defect(s), prevention of hemorrhagic episodes, prompt control of bleeding when it occurs, and management of the sequelae of the disease and its therapy.

Platelet Disorders

Treatment modalities for platelet disorders are determined by the type of defect. The thrombocytopenias are primarily managed acutely with transfusions of platelets to maintain the minimum level of 10,000 to 20,000/mm^3 necessary to prevent spontaneous hemorrhage. Corticosteroids are indicated for ITP, with titration governed by the severity of hemorrhagic symptoms.[49,50] Splenectomy may be necessary in chronic ITP to prevent antiplatelet antibody production and sequestration and removal of antibody-labeled platelets.[50] Plasma exchange therapy combined with aspirin/dipyridamole or corticosteroids has recently lowered the mortality rate for patients with TTP over that previously obtained by treatment with FFP infusions.[83,84] Thrombocytopenia of Wiskott-Aldrich syndrome may be managed with platelet transfusions, splenectomy, or bone marrow transplantation.[45]

Treatment of bleeding episodes in the patient with the congenital qualitative platelet defect of Glanzmann's thrombasthenia is usually not warranted unless hemorrhage is life threatening. Therapy has included periodic random platelet transfusions, which carry the risk of development of antiplatelet isoantibodies. Human leukocyte antigen (HLA)-matched platelets may be required after antibody development, to reduce the number of platelet transfusions needed for hemostasis. In the absence of satisfactorily compatible platelets, blood volume and constituents can be maintained with low-antigenicity blood products. Plasmapheresis to remove circulating isoantibodies is held in reserve for cases of severe thrombasthenia and life-threatening bleeding.

Hemophilias A and B

Therapy for hemophilias A and B is dependent upon the severity of disease, type and site of hemorrhage, and presence or absence of inhibitors. Commercially prepared Fs VIII and

IX complex concentrates, desmopressin acetate (DDAVP [1-deamino-8-D-arginine vasopressin]), and, to a lesser extent, cryoprecipitate and FFP are replacement options (Tables 6 and 7). Since partially purified Fs VIII and IX complex concentrates prepared from pooled plasma were first used in the late 1960s and 1970s, multiple methods of manufacturing products with increased purity and reduced risk of viral transmission have been developed.[85,86] Current intermediate-purity products are prepared by heat or solvent/detergent treatment of the final product. In 1987, dry heat–treated concentrates constituted approximately 90% of the total F VIII concentrate consumption in the United States.[86]

High-purity F VIII products, manufactured using recombinant or monoclonal antibody purification techniques, are preferred today for their improved viral safety.[87] However, their cost of up to 10 times more than dry-heated concentrates can be financially restrictive for uninsured patients.[86] High-purity products generally cost over $1.00 (US) per unit. F VIII concentrates are dosed by units, with one unit of F VIII being equal to the amount present in 1 mL of pooled fresh normal plasma. The plasma level of F VIII is expressed as a percentage of normal. Since one unit of F VIII concentrate per kilogram of body weight raises the F VIII level by 2%, a 70 kg patient would require infusion of 3,500 units to raise his factor level from <1 to 100%. A dose of 40 U/kg F VIII concentrate typically is used to raise the F VIII level to 80 to 100% for management of significant surgical or traumatic bleeding in a patient with severe hemophilia. Additional outpatient doses may be needed at 12-hour intervals, or continuous inpatient infusion may be established.

Highly purified recombinant and monoclonal F IX concentrates were developed in the late 1980s and early 1990s and are the treatment of choice for hemophilia B patients undergoing surgery.[88–90] F IX complex concentrates (prothrombin complex concentrate [PCC]), which contain Fs II, VII, IX, and X, are also widely used at present for patients with hemophilia B. One unit of PCC or higher-purity F IX concentrates given by bolus per kilogram of body weight raises the F IX level by 1 to 1.5%. Thus, a dose of 60 U/kg of F IX concentrate typically is needed to raise the F IX level to 80 to 100% for management of severe bleeding episodes in a patient with a severe F IX deficiency. Repeat outpatient doses may be needed at 24-hour intervals. Properly supervised home therapy, in which patients self-treat with factor concentrates at the earliest evidence of bleeding, is a cost-effective method offered to educable and motivated patients by some medical centers.[91]

Currently, cryoprecipitate and FFP are rarely the treatment of choice for hemophilias A and B because of their disadvantages of potential viral transmission and the large volumes needed to raise factor levels adequately for hemostasis. Cryoprecipitate is the cold insoluble precipitate remaining after FFP is thawed at 4°C. A typical bag (1 unit) of cryoprecipitate contains about 80 units of F VIII and vWF and 150 to 250 mg fibrinogen in a 10 to 15 mL volume. Cryoprecipitate has been used to treat selected patients with vWD and hemophilia A. FFP contains all coagulation factors

TABLE 6   Principal Products for Systemic Management of Patients with Bleeding Disorders

Product	Description	Source	Common Indications
Platelets	"One pack" = 50 mL; raises count by 6,000	Blood bank	< 10,000 in nonbleeding individuals; < 50,000 presurgical; < 50,000 in actively bleeding individuals; nondestructive thrombocytopenia
Fresh frozen plasma	Unit = 150–250 mL; 1 h to thaw Contains Fs II, VII, IX, X, XI, XII, XIII and heat-labile Fs V and VII	Blood bank	Undiagnosed bleeding disorder with active bleeding; severe liver disease; when transfusing > 10 units blood Immune globulin deficiency
Cryoprecipitate	Unit = 10–15 mL Contains Fs VIII and XIII, vWF, and fibrinogen	Blood bank	Hemophilia A, von Willebrand's disease, when factor concentrates/DDAVP are unavailable Fibrinogen deficiency
F VIII concentrate (purified antihemophilic factor)*	Unit raises F VIII level by 2% Heat treated contains vWF Recombinant and monoclonal technologies are pure F VIII	Pharmacy	Hemophilia A, with active bleeding or presurgical; some cases of von Willebrand's disease
F IX concentrate (PCC)*	Unit raises F IX level by 1–1.5% Contains Fs II, VII, IX, and X Monoclonal F IX is only F IX	Pharmacy	Hemophilia B, with active bleeding or presurgical PCC used for hemophilia A with inhibitor
DDAVP	Synthetic analogue of antidiuretic hormone 0.3 µg/kg IV or SQ Intranasal application	Pharmacy	Active bleeding or presurgical for some patients with von Willebrand's disease, uremic bleeding, or liver disease
ε-Aminocaproic acid	Antifibrinolytic 25% oral solution (250 mg/mL) Systemic: 75 mg/kg q6h	Pharmacy	Adjunct to support clot formation for any bleeding disorder
Tranexamic acid	Antifibrinolytic 4.8% mouthrinse—not available in US Systemic: 25 mg/kg q8h	Pharmacy	Adjunct to support clot formation for any bleeding disorder

DDAVP = desmopressin acetate; F = factor; IV = intravenously; PCC = prothrombin complex concentrate; SQ = subcutaneously; vWF = von Willebrand's factor.
*See Table 7 for additional factor concentrate products.

in nearly normal concentrations and may aid hemorrhage control in a patient with mild hemophilia B. In the average-size patient, one unit of FFP raises F IX levels by 3%. Postoperative bleeding in mild to moderate F X deficiency can be managed with FFP, and PCCs may be held in reserve for severely deficient patients.[92]

Desmopressin acetate provides adequate transient increases in coagulation factors in some patients with mild to moderate hemophilia A and type I vWD, avoiding the need for plasma concentrates.[93] This synthetic vasopressin analogue is now considered the treatment of choice for bleeding events in patients with these bleeding diatheses owing to its absence of viral risk and lower cost. DDAVP can be given at a dose of 0.3 µg/kg body weight by an intravenous or subcutaneous route prior to dental extractions or surgery or to treat spontaneous or traumatic bleeding episodes.[94] It results in a mean increase of a two- to fivefold rise (range 1.5–20 times) in F VIII coagulant activity, vWF antigen, and ristocetin cofactor activity, with a plasma half-life of 5 to 8 hours for F VIII and 8 to 10 hours for vWF.[93] Intranasal spray application of DDAVP (Stimate, Aventis Behring, King of Prussia, PA) contains 1.5 mL of desmopressin per milliliter, with each 0.1 mL pump spray delivering a dose of 150 µg. Children require one nostril spray, and adults require two nostril sprays to achieve a favorable response; correction of bleeding occurs in around 90% of patients with mild to moderate hemophilia A and type I vWD.[95] Time to peak levels is 30 to 60 minutes after intravenous injection and 90 to 120 minutes following subcutaneous or intranasal application.[93]

Unfortunately, DDAVP is ineffective in individuals with severe hemophilia A. A DDAVP trial or test dose response may be indicated prior to extensive surgery to evaluate the level of drug effect on assayed F VIII activity in the individual patient. DDAVP, thought to stimulate endogenous release of F VIII and vWF from blood vessel endothelial cell storage sites, is hemostatically effective provided that adequate plasma concentrations are attained.[96] Prolonged use of DDAVP results in exhaustion of F VIII storage sites and diminished hemostatic effect; hence, antifibrinolytic agents are useful adjuncts to DDAVP therapy.

Complications of factor replacement therapy, in addition to allergic reactions, include viral disease transmission (hepatitis B and C, cytomegalovirus, and human immunodeficiency virus [HIV]), thromboembolic disease, DIC, and development of antibodies to factor concentrates. Hepatitis C and non-A/non-B have been major causes of morbidity and mortality in the hemophiliac population, resulting in chronic active hepatitis and cirrhosis in a number of patients.[66] More recently, hepatitis C and HIV infection have become the most common transfusion-related infections in hemophiliacs. By the end of 1986, some centers reported that 80 to 90% of

TABLE 7 Coagulation Factor Concentrate Products

Product Category	Proprietary Name*	Manufacturer/Distributor	US Corporate Location
High-purity F VIII concentrates			
Monoclonal	Hemofil-M	Baxter Healthcare Corp.	Deerfield, IL
	Monoclate-P	ZLB-Behring LLC	King of Prussia, PA
	Monarc-M	Baxter Healthcare Corp.	Deerfield, IL
Recombinant	Kogenate	Bayer Corp.	Clayton, NC
	Recombinate	Baxter Healthcare Corp.	Deerfield, IL
	Advate	Baxter Healthcare Corp.	Deerfield, IL
	Helixate-FS	ZLB-Behring LLC	King of Prussia, PA
	Bioclate	ZLB-Behring LLC	King of Prussia, PA
	ReFacto	Wyeth Biopharma	Andover, MA
Intermediate-purity F VIII concentrates			
Pasturized	Humate-P	ZLB-Behring LLC	King of Prussia, PA
Solvent/detergent	Koate-DVI	Talecis Biotherapeutics	Clayton, NC
	Alphanate	Alpha Therapeutic Corp.	Los Angeles, CA
Porcine F VIII concentrates	Hyate-C	Ipsen, Inc.	Milford, MA
High-purity F IX concentrates			
Monoclonal	AlphaNine-SD	Alpha Therapeutic Corp.	Los Angeles, CA
	Mononine	ZLB-Behring LLC	King of Prussia, PA
Recombinant	BeneFix	Wyeth Biopharma	Andover, MA
Prothrombin complex concentrates (PCC) and F IX activated PCCs			
	Profilnine-SD	Alpha Therapeutic Corp.	Los Angeles, CA
	Proplex-T	Baxter Healthcare Corp.	Deerfield, IL
	Bebulin-VH	Baxter Healthcare Corp.	Deerfield, IL
	Konyne 80	Bayer Corp.	Clayton, NC
	FEIBA-VH	Baxter Healthcare Corp.	Deerfield, IL
	Autoplex-T	Baxter Healthcare Corp.	Deerfield, IL
F VIIa concentrate			
Recombinant:	NovoSeven	Novo-Nordisk	Princeton, NJ

F = factor.
*Product availability changes periodically.

hemophiliacs treated with F VIII concentrates and around 50% of those who had received F IX concentrates were HIV seropositive.[97] Since 1987, with viral screening of donated plasma, there have been no transfusion-related HIV seroconversions in the United States.

Use of F IX complex concentrate can result in thrombotic complications, such as deep venous thromboses, myocardial infarctions, pulmonary emboli, and DIC. Concurrent use of systemic antifibrinolytics with these products may increase the risks. DIC is believed to occur as a consequence of high levels of activated clotting factors, such as Fs VIIa, IXa, and Xa, that cannot adequately be cleared by the liver.

Development of F VIII or F IX inhibitors is a serious complication. These pathologic circulating antibodies of the IgG class, which specifically neutralize F VIII or F IX procoagulant activity, arise as alloantibodies in some patients with hemophilia.[98] A systematic review found the overall prevalence of inhibitors in unselected hemophiliac populations to be 5 to 7%.[99] The cumulative risk of inhibitor development varied (0–39%), with incidence and prevalence being substantially higher in patients with severe hemophilia.[99] Inhibitors develop in at least 10 to 15% of patients with severe hemophilia A and less commonly in patients with hemophilia

B.[100,101] Development is related to exposure to factor products and genetic predisposition.[98,100] Inhibitor level is quantified by the Bethesda inhibitor assay and is reported as Bethesda units (BU).

The inhibitor titer and responsiveness to further factor infusion (responder type) dictate which factor replacement therapy should be used. Patients with inhibitors are classified according to titer level—low (< 10 BU/mL) or high (> 10 BU/mL)—and also by responder type.[101] Low responders typically maintain low titers with repeated factor concentrate exposure, whereas high responders show a brisk elevation in titer due to the amnestic response and are the most challenging to manage.[101,102] Patients with low inhibitor titers are usually low responders and those with high titers are often high responders. Seventy-five percent of hemophilia A patients with inhibitors are high responders, whereas only 25% are low responders.[101]

For hemorrhages, hemophilia A patients with low-level low-responding inhibitors are treated with F VIII concentrates in doses sufficient to raise plasma F VIII levels to the therapeutic range. Critical hemorrhages in patients with high-responding inhibitors may be treated with large quantities of porcine F VIII; however, routine hemorrhages are often managed initially with PCCs, which provoke anamnesis in a few patients.[98] PCCs can bypass the F VIII inhibitor and are effective about 50% of the time.[103] Activated PCCs show slightly increased effectiveness (65–75%). Highly purified porcine F VIII product use can be advantageous in patients with less than 50 BU since human F VIII inhibitors cross-react less frequently with porcine products.[98] However, because of the risk of hemostatic failure, surgery should be performed under coverage of F VIII.[104] Treatment of the patient with low-level (<10 BU) F IX inhibitors requires higher doses of F IX complex concentrates to achieve hemostasis. Developed in the early 1990s, recombinant F VIIa is a novel product that provides an alternative treatment option for patients with hemophilia A or B with inhibitors by enhancing the extrinsic pathway.[105] It has been proven to effectively control bleeding in patients with high-titer inhibitors[106,107] and for dental extractions.[108,109]

Several methods have demonstrated temporary removal of high-titer inhibitors in both hemophilia A and B. Exchange transfusion or plasmapheresis produces a rapid transient reduction in antibody level, with a rate of 40 mL plasma per kilogram decreasing levels by half.[110] Although laborious, it may be attempted in cases of critical hemorrhage as an adjunct to high-dose F VIII concentrate therapy. Antibody removal by extracorporeal adsorption of the plasma to protein A Sepharose or a specific F IX–Sepharose in columns has also shown promise in hemophilias A and B.[111,112]

von Willebrand's Disease

Therapy for vWD depends on the type of vWD and the severity of bleeding. Type I is treated preferentially with DDAVP, as described above. Intermediate-purity F VIII concentrates, FFP, and cryoprecipitate are held in reserve for DDAVP nonresponders.[113] Types II and III require intermediate-purity F VIII concentrates, such as Humate-P or Koate-HS, or, rarely, cryoprecipitate or FFP. Bleeding episodes in patients with platelet-type vWD are usually controlled with platelet concentrate infusions. Other therapy is used for site-specific bleeding, such as estrogens or oral contraceptive agents for menorrhagia and local hemostatic agents and antifibrinolytics for dental procedures. Occasionally, circulating plasma inhibitors of vWF are observed in multiply transfused patients with severe disease. Cryoprecipitate infusion can cause transient neutralization of this inhibitor.[114]

Disease-Related Coagulopathies

Management of disease-related coagulopathies varies with hemostatic abnormality.

LIVER DISEASE

Hepatic disease that results in bleeding from deficient vitamin K–dependent clotting factors (Fs II, VII, IX, and X) may be reversed with vitamin K injections for 3 days, either intravenously or subcutaneously. However, infusion of FFP may be employed when more immediate hemorrhage control is necessary, such as prior to dental extractions.[115] Cirrhotic

patients with moderate thrombocytopenia and functional platelet defects may benefit from DDAVP therapy.[116] Antifibrinolytic drugs, if used cautiously, have markedly reduced bleeding and thus reduced need for blood and blood product substitution.[77]

RENAL DISEASE

In uremic patients, dialysis remains the primary preventive and therapeutic modality used for control of bleeding, although it is not always immediately effective.[117] Hemodialysis and peritoneal dialysis appear to be equally efficacious in improving platelet function abnormalities and clinical bleeding in the uremic patient. The availability of cryoprecipitate[118] and DDAVP[119] offers alternative effective therapy for patients who require shortened bleeding times acutely in preparation for urgent surgery. Conjugated estrogen preparations[120] and recombinant erythropoietin[121] have also been shown to be beneficial for uremic patients with chronic abnormal bleeding.

DISSEMINATED INTRAVASCULAR COAGULATION

It is important to expeditiously identify the underlying triggering disease or condition and deliver specific and vigorous treatment of the underlying disorder if long-term survival is to be a possibility. Although somewhat controversial, active DIC is usually treated initially with intravenous unfractionated heparin or subcutaneous LMWH, to prevent thrombin from acting on fibrinogen, thereby preventing further clot formation.[122–124] Infusion of activated protein C, antithrombin III, and agents directed against tissue factor activity are being investigated as new therapeutic approaches.[125] The dentist may be called upon to provide a gingival or oral mucosal biopsy specimen for histopathologic examination to confirm the diagnosis of DIC by the presence of microthrombi in the vascular bed. Replacement of deficient coagulation factors with FFP and correction of the platelet deficiency with platelet transfusions may be necessary for improvement or prophylaxis of the hemorrhagic tendency of DIC prior to emergency surgical procedures. Elective surgery is deferred due to the volatility of the coagulation mechanism in these patients.

▼ PROGNOSIS

The prognosis for patients with bleeding disorders depends on the appropriate diagnosis and the ability to prevent and manage acute bleeding episodes. Individuals with mild or manageable disease may have a normal life expectancy, with morbidity relating to bleeding episode frequency and severity. Acute DIC carries the highest risk of death by exsanguination. Individuals with severe liver disease may succumb to rupture of esophageal varices. Severe thrombocytopenia and other severe coagulopathies carry a higher risk of hemorrhagic stroke.

Advances in the treatment of hemophilia, from the use of cryoprecipitate in the 1960s to the introduction of plasma-derived factor concentrates in the 1970s, led to dramatic improvement in quality of life and raised the life span for hemophiliacs from 11 years in 1921 to 60 years in 1980.[126] Viral infections, such as hepatitis B, C, and G and HIV acquired from infected blood products, have since altered the prognosis for some patients.[127–131] In a Dutch study of hemophiliacs from 1992 to 2001, age-adjusted mortality was 2.3 times higher in hemophilia patients than in the general male population.[132] This was largely because of the consequences of viral infections, with acquired immune deficiency syndrome (AIDS) as the main cause of death in 26% and 22% of deaths resulting from hepatitis C.[132] In patients with severe hemophilia, life expectancy decreased from 63 (1972–1985) to 59 years (1992–2001). Exclusion of virus-related deaths resulted in a life expectancy at birth of 72 years.[132]

As discussed above, before effective virucidal methods were used in the manufacture of clotting-factor concentrates in 1985, hemophiliacs were at a very high risk of contracting bloodborne viruses from factor concentrates that exposed them to the plasma of thousands of donors. HIV seroprevalence increased to 60 to 75% of patients with hemophilia (85–90% with severe hemophilia), with HIV-associated opportunistic infections and neoplasms contributing substantially to the morbidity and mortality of hemophiliacs.[127,128,130] Oral mucosal diseases were common in hemophiliacs with HIV, particularly in those with advanced immunosuppression.[131,133] HIV protease inhibitor-containing drug combinations that resulted in improved health of some HIV-infected patients in the late 1990s have shown significant clinical and laboratory benefits when used by HIV-infected hemophiliacs.[134] Major reductions in AIDS and death rates were observed from 1997 to 2003 in hemophiliacs, with survival improvements largely attributable to decreases in AIDS-related deaths yet accompanied by increases in liver disease death rates.[135] Coinfection with viral hepatitis remains a challenge for the future. In the United States, those who received care in hemophilia treatment centers had a significantly decreased risk of death.[136]

▼ ORAL HEALTH CONSIDERATIONS

Oral Findings

Platelet deficiency and vascular wall disorders result in extravasation of blood into connective and epithelial tissues of the skin and mucosa, creating small pinpoint hemorrhages, called petechiae, and larger patches, called ecchymoses. Platelet or coagulation disorders with severely altered hemostasis can result in spontaneous gingival bleeding, as may be seen in conjunction with hyperplastic hyperemic gingival enlargements in leukemic patients. Continuous oral bleeding over long periods of time fosters deposits of hemosiderin and other blood degradation products on the tooth surfaces, turning them brown. A variety of oral findings are illustrated in Figures 4 to 6.

Hemophiliacs may experience many episodes of oral bleeding over their lifetime. Sonis and Musselman reported an average 29.1 bleeding events per year serious enough to

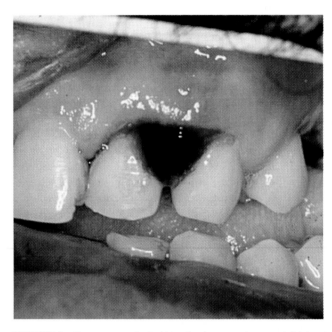

FIGURE 4 Spontaneous gingival bleeding between the upper left lateral incisor and canine and labial petechiae in a 38-year-old white male with idiopathic thrombocytopenic purpura.

require factor replacement in F VIII–deficient patients, of which 9% involved oral structures.[137] The location of oral bleeds was as follows: labial frenum, 60%; tongue, 23%; buccal mucosa, 17%; and gingiva and palate, 0.5% (Figure 7). Bleeding occurrences were most frequent in patients with severe hemophilia, followed by moderate and then mild hemophilia. They most often resulted from traumatic injury. Bleeding events may also be induced by poor oral hygiene practices and iatrogenic factors. Kaneda and colleagues reported frequency of oral hemorrhage by location in people deficient of F VIII and F IX as follows: gingiva, 64%; dental pulp, 13%; tongue, 7.5%; lip, 7%; palate, 2%; and buccal mucosa, 1%.[138] Many minor oral bleeds, such as those from the gingiva or dental pulp, can be controlled by local measures.

Hemarthrosis is a common complication in hemophiliacs' weight-bearing joints, yet it rarely occurs in the TMJ. Two TMJ cases have been reported.[139,140] An acute TMJ hemarthrosis associated with F IX deficiency was resolved with factor replacement without aspiration[139]; a chronic hemophilic TMJ arthropathy required arthrotomy, arthroscopic adhesion lysis, factor replacement, splint therapy, and physical therapy in a patient with F XI deficiency.[140]

Evaluation of dental disease patterns in children with severe hemophilia revealed a significantly lower prevalence of dental caries and lower plaque scores compared with matched, healthy controls.[141]

▼ DENTAL MANAGEMENT

Dental modifications required for patients with bleeding disorders depend on both the type and invasiveness of the dental procedure and the type and severity of the bleeding disorder.

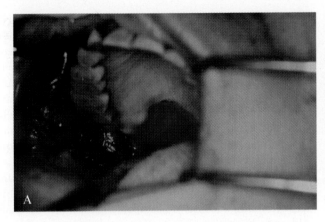 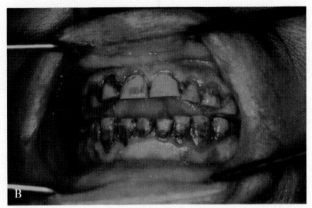

FIGURE 5 A 68-year-old female with acute myelogenous leukemia and a platelet count of 9,000/mm³. Platelet transfusion and ε-aminocaproic acid oral rinses were used to control bleeding. A, Buccal mucosa and palatal ecchymoses. B, Extrinsic stains on teeth from erythrocyte degradation following continual gingival oozing.

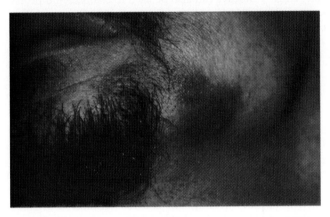

FIGURE 6 A 46-year-old male with severe liver cirrhosis due to hepatitis C infection. Shown is purpura of facial skin 1 week after full-mouth extractions.

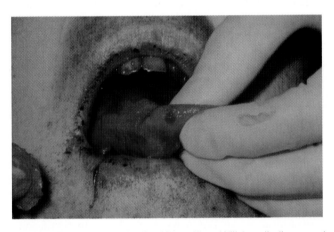

FIGURE 7 A 27-year-old male with type III von Willebrand's disease and a 2-week duration of bleeding from the tongue that reduced his hematocrit to 16%. Hemorrhage control was obtained with cryoprecipitate.

while supporting coagulation with adjunctive and/or local measures. For reversible coagulopathies (eg, coumarin anticoagulation), it may be best to remove the causative agent or treat the primary illness or defect in order to allow the patient to return to a manageable bleeding risk for the dental treatment period. For irreversible coagulopathies, the missing or defective element may need to be replaced from an exogenous source to allow control of bleeding (eg, coagulation factor concentrate therapy for hemophilia). Assessment of the coagulopathy and delivery of appropriate therapy prior to dental procedures are best accomplished in consultation with a hematologist and may involve treatment either in specialized hospital facilities or the local general dentist's office.[142]

Platelet Disorders

When medical management is unable to restore platelet counts to above the level of 50,000/mm³ required for surgical hemostasis, platelet transfusions may be required prior to dental extractions or other oral surgical procedures. The therapeutically expected increment in platelet count from infusion of one unit of platelets is approximately 10,000 to 12,000/mm³. Six units of platelets are commonly infused at a time. Patients who have received multiple transfusions may be refractory to random donor platelets as a result of alloimmunization. These individuals may require single-donor apheresis or leukocyte-reduced platelets. Local hemostatic measures are also important. The thrombasthenic patient needing dental extractions may be successfully treated with the use of hemostatic measures such as microfibrillar collagen and antifibrinolytic drugs.[43,44]

Since the antiplatelet activity of aspirin remains for the 8- to 10-day lifetime of the affected platelets, avoidance of aspirin is recommended, when possible, for 1 week prior to extensive oral surgical procedures. Aspirin is rarely withheld, however, prior to minor oral surgical procedures such as dental extractions. Other NSAIDs and antiplatelet agents have a similar but less pronounced antiplatelet effect. Adjunctive local hemostatic agents are useful in preventing postoperative oozing when aspirin therapy is in use at the

Thus, less modification is needed for patients with mild coagulopathies in preparation for dental procedures anticipated to have limited bleeding consequences. When significant bleeding is expected, the goal of management is to preoperatively restore the hemostatic system to an acceptable range time of minor oral surgery. When extensive surgery is emergently indicated, DDAVP can be used to decrease the aspirin-induced prolongation of the BT or to treat aspirin-related postoperative oozing, often eliminating the need for platelet infusion.[143]

Chemotherapy-associated oral hemorrhages, most frequently related to thrombocytopenia, are best managed by transfusions of HLA-matched platelets and FFP, together with topically applied clot-promoting agents.[58] A pilot study suggests a possible benefit of DDAVP for the prevention or treatment of bleeding in patients with thrombocytopenia associated with hematologic malignancy.[144]

Hemophilias A and B and vWD

ORAL SURGICAL PROCEDURES

Oral surgical procedures have the greatest potential for hemorrhage of all dental procedures. Hemorrhagic problems after extractions have drastically declined over the last 10 years such that only an estimated 2% of hemophilic patients experience one or more delayed bleeding episodes.[145] Appropriate precautionary measures now allow surgery to be performed safely with no significantly greater risk of bleeding than in nonhemophiliacs.[146] To make certain that preoperative factor levels of at least 40 to 50% of normal activity have been obtained, transfusion recommendations generally aim for replacement of missing coagulation factors to levels of 50 to 100% when single-bolus infusion is used for outpatient treatment. This provides greater assurance of hemorrhage control, given the problems of possible failure of factor activity to rise as high as expected and variable plasma half-lives of 8 to 12 hours for F VIII and 18 to 24 hours for F IX. Additional postoperative factor maintenance may be indicated for extensive surgery. This can be accomplished by infusion of factor concentrates, DDAVP, cryoprecipitate, or FFP, depending on the patient's deficiency state. When postsurgical bleeding occurs due to fibrinolysis, it commonly starts 3 to 5 days after surgery and can usually be controlled by local measures and use of antifibrinolytics. Continual oozing from unstable fibrinous clots may require their removal and the repacking of the extraction socket with hemostatic agents.

Determination of factor replacement requirements for surgical hemostasis and selection of plasma product or drug therapy should be accomplished in consultation with the patient's hematologist. Canadian clinical practice guidelines recommend replacement factor levels of 40 to 50% of F VIII (dose 20–25 U/kg) and F IX (dose 40–50 U/kg), used in conjunction with antifibrinolytics.[147] Gingival or dental bleeding unresponsive to antifibrinolytics requires 20 to 30% clotting F VIII or F IX.[147] The level of factor activity required for hemostasis varies in relation to local factors. Higher hemostatic factor levels are needed for large wound cavities created by extraction of multiple or multirooted teeth or when gingival inflammation, bleeding, tooth mobility, or apical lesions are present.[138] Kaneda and colleagues reported that deficient factor activity levels required for postextraction hemostasis varied from 3.5 to 25% for deciduous teeth and 5.5 to 20% for permanent teeth.[138]

Three methods of replacement therapy have been employed to maintain circulating factor levels above the 20% minimum necessary for hemostasis during surgical and healing phases. These include intermittent replacement therapy, continuous intravenous factor infusion therapy, and a single preoperative factor concentrate infusion combined with an antifibrinolytic mouthwash.[148] F VIII levels may be sufficiently raised by DDAVP in some patients with moderate to mild hemophilia A and vWD to allow dental extractions without transfusion.

Local hemostatic agents and techniques include pressure, surgical packs, vasoconstrictors, sutures, surgical stents, topical thrombin, and use of absorbable hemostatic materials. Although having no direct effect on hemostasis, primary wound closure aids patient comfort, decreases blood clot size, and protects clots from masticatory trauma and subsequent bleeding.[149] Sutures can also be used to stabilize and protect packing. Resorbable and nonresorbable suture materials have proven to be equally effective. Avitene (Davol Inc, Cranston, RI) or Helitene (Integra Life Sciences, Plainsboro, NJ), microfibrillar collagen hemostatic fleece, aids hemostasis when placed against the bleeding bony surface of a well-cleansed extraction socket. Microfibrillar collagen acts to attract platelets, causing the release phenomenon to trigger aggregation of platelets into thrombi in the interstices of the fibrous mass of the clot.[150] Topical thrombin (Thrombogen, Ethicon Inc., Somerville, NJ), which directly converts fibrinogen in the blood to fibrin, is an effective adjunct when applied directly to the wound or carried to the extraction site in a nonacidic medium on oxidized cellulose. Surgifoam (Ethicon Inc.) is an absorbable gelatin sponge with intrinsic hemostatic properties. A collagen absorbable hemostat manufactured as a 3 × 4–inch sponge (INSTAT, Ethicon Inc.) or fabricated as a nonwoven pad or sponge (Helistat, Integra Life Sciences, Plainsboro, NJ; Gelfoam, Pharmacia & Upjohn Co., Kalamazoo, MI; Ultrafoam, Davol Inc) ais also a useful adjunct. Surgical acrylic stents may be useful if carefully fabricated to avoid traumatic irritation to the surgical site. Diet restriction to full liquids for the initial 24 to 48 hours, followed by intake of soft foods for 1 to 2 weeks, will further protect the clot by reducing the amount of chewing and resultant soft tissue disturbances.

Antifibrinolytic drugs such as EACA[151] (Amicar 25% syrup, Xanodyne Pharmacal Inc, Florence, KY) and tranexamic acid (AMCA; Cyclokapron, Pharmacia Corp, Peapack, NJ) inhibit fibrinolysis by blocking the conversion of plasminogen to plasmin, resulting in clot stabilization. Postsurgical use of EACA has been shown to significantly reduce the quantity of factor required to control bleeding when used in conjunction with presurgical concentrate infusion sufficient to raise plasma F VIII and F IX levels to 50%.[148,152,153] A regimen of 50 mg/kg of body weight EACA given topically and systemically as a 25% (250 mg/mL) oral rinse every 6 hours for 7 to 10 days appears adequate as an adjunct. Tranexamic acid (4.8%) oral rinse was found to be 10 times more potent than was EACA in preventing postextraction bleeding in hemophiliacs, with fewer side effects, but it is not routinely available in the United States.[154,155] Systemic antifibrinolytic therapy can be given orally or intravenously as EACA 75 mg/kg (up to 4 g) every 6 hours or AMCA 25 mg/kg every 8 hours until bleeding stops.[147] For the treatment of acute bleeding syndromes due to elevated fibrinolytic activity, it is suggested that 10 tablets (5 g) or 4 teaspoons of 25% syrup (5 g) of Amicar be administered during the first hour of treatment, followed by a continuing rate of 2 tablets (1 g) or 1 teaspoon of syrup (1.25 g) per hour. This method of treatment would ordinarily be continued for about 8 hours or until the bleeding situation has been controlled.

Fibrin sealants or fibrin glue has been used effectively in Europe since 1978 as an adjunct with adhesive and hemostatic effects to control bleeding at wound or surgical sites.[156] Its use has allowed reduction in factor concentrate replacement levels in hemophiliacs undergoing dental surgeries when used in combination with antifibrinolytics.[157–159] Use of fibrin glue does not obviate the need for factor concentration replacement in severe hemophiliacs.[158] In the United States, extemporaneous fibrin sealant can be made by combining cryoprecipitate with a combination of 10,000 units of topical thrombin powder diluted in 10 mL saline and 10 mL calcium chloride. When dispensed over the wound simultaneously from separate syringes, the cryoprecipitate and calcium chloride precipitate almost instantaneously to form a clear gelatinous adhesive gel. The first proprietary formulation, Crosseal Fibrin Sealant (Human; Ethicon, Inc, Israel, distributed by Johnson & Johnson Wound Management, Somerville, NJ), was approved in the United States in 2003 for patients undergoing liver surgery and is derived from human plasma, so it is not completely without risk of viral transmission.

Although useful as an adjunct, a prospective study comparing the effectiveness of a 4.8% tranexamic acid mouthwash versus an autologous fibrin glue preparation to control hemostasis in patients therapeutically anticoagulated with warfarin who required dental extractions without interruption of their treatment demonstrated slight superiority of the antifibrinolytic mouthwash.[160]

PAIN CONTROL

A variety of techniques are used to control pain in individuals with coagulopathies. An assessment of the patient's pain threshold and invasiveness of the dental procedure to be undertaken allows selection of an effective management approach. Some patients opt for treatment without anesthesia. Hypnosis,[161] intravenous sedation with diazepam, and nitrous oxide/oxygen analgesia, used as adjuncts to control anxiety, drastically reduce or totally eliminate the need for local anesthesia.[162] Intrapulpal anesthesia is safe and effective following access for pulp extirpation. Periodontal ligament and gingival papillary injections can be accomplished with little risk when delivered slowly with minimal volume.[163,164] Anesthetic solutions with vasoconstrictors such as epinephrine should be used when possible. In patients with mild disease, buccal, labial, and hard palatal infiltration can be attempted for maxillary teeth, with slow injection and local pressure to the injection site for 3 to 4 minutes without

coverage.[162] If a hematoma develops, ice packs should be applied to the area to stimulate vasoconstriction, and emergency factor replacement should be administered in a hospital.

Block injections used in dentistry, including inferior alveolar, posterior superior alveolar, infraorbital, lingual, and (to a lesser extent) long buccal, require minimal coagulation factor levels of 20 to 30%. These injections place anesthetic solutions in highly vascularized loose connective tissue with no distinct boundaries, where formation of a dissecting hematoma is possible.[165] Webster and colleagues reported development of hematomas in 8% of hemophilic patients not treated with prophylactic factor replacement prior to mandibular block injection.[148] Greater risk occurred with severe disease than with mild and with hemophilia A than with B. Extravasation of blood into the soft tissues of the oropharyngeal area in hemophiliacs can produce gross swelling, pain, dysphagia, respiratory obstruction, and grave risk of death from asphyxia (Figure 8).[166–168]

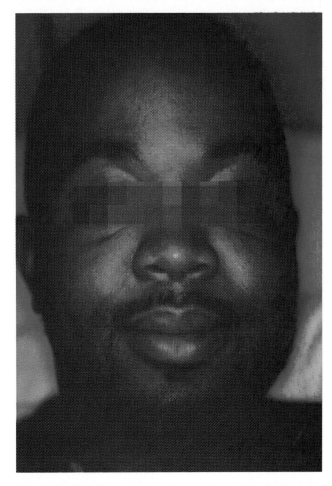

FIGURE 8 A 24-year-old male with severe hemophilia A and low-titer inhibitor, 3 days after inferior alveolar block–induced parapharyngeal hemorrhage. Patient presented with difficulty swallowing and pending airway compromise 8 hours after nerve block. Subsequent treatment with prothrombin complex concentrates over 3 days controlled the bleeding and began the resolution of facial swelling.

Dental treatment in the operating room under general anesthesia may be indicated when extensive procedures necessitate numerous expensive factor infusions, when patient cooperation or anxiety prohibits outpatient clinic or office treatment, or when the patient with an inhibitor has multiple treatment needs. Although oral endotracheal intubation provides access challenges for the dental operator, it is preferred over nasal endotracheal intubation, which carries the risk of inducing a nasal bleed that can be difficult to control. The use of aspirin and other NSAIDs for pain management is contraindicated in patients with bleeding disorders due to their inhibition of platelet function and potentiation of bleeding episodes. Intramuscular injections should also be avoided due to the risk of hematoma formation.

PREVENTIVE AND PERIODONTAL THERAPIES

Periodontal health is of critical importance for the hemophiliac for two principal reasons: (1) hyperemic gingiva contributes to spontaneous and induced gingival bleeding and (2) periodontitis is a leading cause of tooth morbidity, necessitating extraction. Individuals with bleeding diatheses are unusually prone to oral hygiene neglect due to fear of toothbrush-induced bleeding. On the contrary, oral physiotherapy can be accomplished without risk of significant bleeding. Periodontal probing and supragingival scaling and polishing can be done routinely. Careful subgingival scaling with fine scalers rarely warrants replacement therapy. Severely inflamed and swollen tissues are best treated initially with chlorhexidine oral rinses or by gross débridement with a cavitron or hand instruments to allow gingival shrinkage prior to deep scaling.[142] Deep subgingival scaling and root planing should be performed by quadrant to reduce gingival area exposed to potential bleeding. Locally applied pressure and post-treatment antifibrinolytic oral rinses are usually successful in controlling any protracted oozing.[169,170] Local block anesthesia required for scaling may necessitate raising factor levels to a minimum of 30% of normal prior to treatment.[171] Periodontal surgical procedures warrant elevating circulating factor levels to 50% and use of post-treatment antifibrinolytics. Periodontal packing material aids hemostasis and protects the surgical site; however, it may be dislodged by severe hemorrhage or subperiosteal hematoma formation.

RESTORATIVE AND PROSTHODONTIC THERAPY

General restorative and prosthodontic procedures do not result in significant hemorrhage. Rubber dam isolation is advised to minimize the risk of lacerating soft tissue in the operative field and to avoid creating ecchymoses and hematomas with high-speed evacuators or saliva ejectors. Care is required to select a tooth clamp that does not traumatize the gingiva. Matrices, wedges, and a hemostatic gingival retraction cord may be used with caution to protect soft tissues and improve visualization when subgingival extension of cavity preparation is necessary. Removable prosthetic appliances can be fabricated without complications. Denture trauma

should be minimized by prompt and careful postinsertion adjustment.

ENDODONTIC THERAPY

Endodontic therapy is often the treatment of choice for a patient with a severe bleeding disorder, especially when an inhibitor is present because extraction carries a high risk of hemorrhage, and treatment is expensive. Generally, there are no contraindications to root canal therapy, provided that instrumentation does not extend beyond the apex.[172] Filling beyond the apical seal also should be avoided. Application of epinephrine intrapulpally to the apical area is usually successful in providing hemostasis. Endodontic surgical procedures require the same factor replacement therapy as do oral surgical procedures.

PEDIATRIC DENTAL THERAPY

The pediatric dental patient occasionally presents with prolonged oozing from exfoliating primary teeth. Administration of factor concentrates and extraction of the deciduous tooth with curettage may be necessary for patient comfort and hemorrhage control. Moss advocates extraction of mobile primary teeth using periodontal space anesthesia without factor replacement after 2 days of vigorous oral hygiene to reduce local inflammation.[39] Hemorrhage control is obtained with gauze pressure, and seepage generally stops in 12 hours. Pulpotomies can be performed without excessive pulpal bleeding. Stainless steel crowns should be prepared to allow minimal removal of enamel at gingival areas.[173] Topical fluoride treatment and use of pit-and-fissure sealants are important noninvasive therapies to decrease the need for extensive restorative procedures.

ORTHODONTIC THERAPY

Orthodontic treatment can be provided with little modification. Care must be observed to avoid mucosal laceration by orthodontic bands, brackets, and wires. Bleeding from minor cuts usually responds to local pressure. Properly managed fixed orthodontic appliances are preferred over removable functional appliances for the patient with a high likelihood of bleeding from chronic tissue irritation. The use of extraoral force and shorter treatment duration further decrease the potential for bleeding complications.[174]

Patients on Anticoagulants

Management of the dental patient on anticoagulant therapy involves consideration of the degree of anticoagulation achieved as gauged by the PT/INR, the dental procedure planned, and the level of thromboembolic risk for the patient.[175] In general, higher INRs result in higher bleeding risk from surgical procedures.[176]

It is generally held that nonsurgical dental treatment can be successfully accomplished without alteration of the anticoagulant regimen, provided that the PT/INR is not grossly above the therapeutic range and trauma is minimized.[177–179] Greater controversy exists over the management of anticoagulated patients for oral surgical procedures.[76,180–182] The American Heart Association and American College of

Cardiology scientific statement recommends that for patients undergoing dental procedures, tranexamic acid or EACA (Amicar) mouthwash can be applied without interrupting anticoagulant therapy.[183] The Sixth American College of Chest Physicians (ACCP) Consensus Conference on Antithrombotic Therapy made several weak recommendations (risk/benefit unclear) as follows: (1) For patients undergoing dental procedures who are not considered to be at high risk for bleeding, ACCP recommends that warfarin therapy not be discontinued. In patients at high risk for bleeding, ACCP recommends that warfarin therapy be discontinued. (2) For patients undergoing dental procedures in whom local bleeding must be controlled, tranexamic acid or EACA mouthwash can be administered without interrupting anticoagulant therapy.[184]

Figure 9 suggests INR levels at which specific dental procedures may be safely undertaken. Preparation of the anticoagulated patient for surgical procedures depends on the extent of bleeding expected. The flow chart shown in Figure 10 graphically outlines an algorithm for assessment

Dental Treatment	Suboptimal INR Range		Normal Target INR Range			Out of Range
	<1.5	1.5 to <2.0	2.0 to <2.5	2.5 to 3.0	>3.0 to 3.5	>3.5
Examination, radiographs, impressions, orthodontics						
Simple restorative dentistry, supragingival prophylaxis						
Complex restorative dentistry, scaling & root planing, endodontics					Caution: Probably safe	
Simple extraction, curettage, gingivoplasty, biopsy				Caution: Local measures	Caution: Local measures	
Multiple extractions, removal of single bony impaction			Caution: Local measures	Caution: Local measures	Caution: Local measures	
Gingivectomy, apicoectomy, minor periodontal flap surgery, placement of single implant	Probably safe	Caution: Probably safe	Caution: Probably safe			
Full mouth or full arch extractions	Caution: Probably safe	Caution: Local measures				
Extensive flap surgery, extraction of multiple bony impactions, multiple implant placement	Caution: Probably safe					
Open fracture reduction, orthognathic surgery	Hospital procedure	Hospital procedure	Hospital procedure	Hospital procedure	Hospital procedure	Hospital procedure

Key: INR= International Normalized Ratio

Green indicates that it is safe to proceed in a routine manner (local factors such as periodontitis/gingivitis can increase the severity of bleeding; the clinician should consider all factors when making a risk assessment). Yellow, use caution, but in many instances the procedure can be safely performed with judicious use of local measures. Red, procedure not advised at current INR level; refer to physician for adjustment.

Local measures include sutures, oxidized cellulose, microfibrillar collagen hemostat, topical thrombin, and an antifibrinolytic such as: epsilon aminocaproic acid or tranexamic acid.

FIGURE 9 Safety of Outpatient Dental Treatment for Patients Receiving Comadin Anticoagulant Therapy. (adapted with permission from: Herman WW, Konzelman JL Jr, Sutley SH. Current perspectives on dental patients receiving coumarin anticoagulant therapy. J Am Dent Assoc 1997;128: 327–35.)

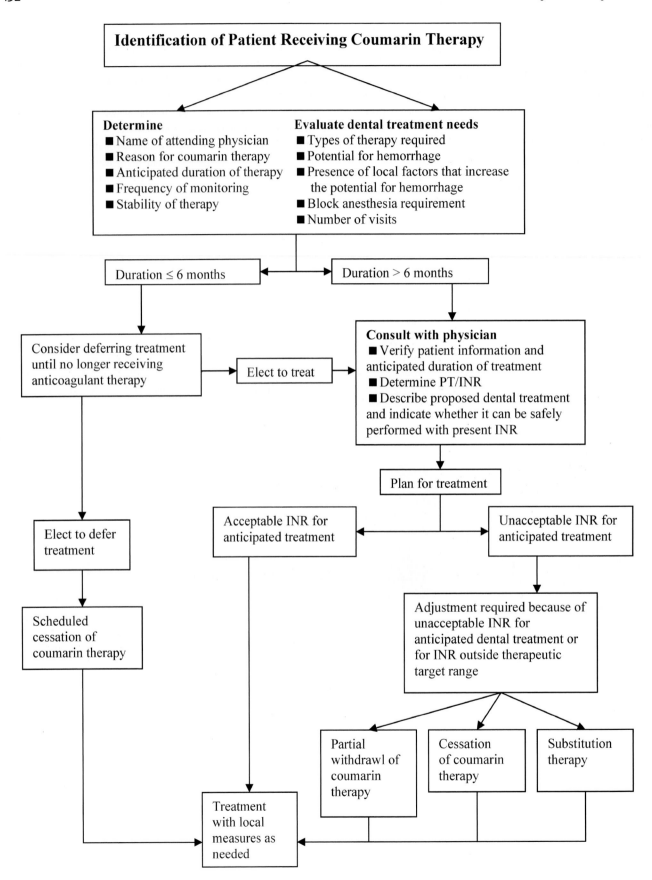

FIGURE 10   Assessment and management approaches for the dental patient on coumarin therapy.

and management of the dental patient on coumarin therapy. No surgical treatment is recommended for those with an INR of >3.5 to 4.0 without coumarin dose modification.[76,180] With an INR <3.5 to 4.0, minor surgical procedures with minimal anticipated bleeding require local measures but no coumarin modification. At an INR of <3.5 to 4.0, when moderate bleeding is expected (multiple extractions or removal of wisdom teeth), local measures should be used, and INR reduction should be considered. When significant bleeding is anticipated, as from full-mouth or full-arch extractions, local measures are combined with reduction of anticoagulation to an INR of <2.0 to 3.0.[76,185] Extensive flap surgery or multiple bony extractions may require an INR of <1.5.[76]

For surgical procedures, physician consultation is advised in order to determine the patient's most recent PT/INR level and the best treatment approach based on the patient's relative thromboembolic and hemorrhagic risks. When the likelihood of sudden thrombotic and embolic complications is small and hemorrhagic risk is high, coumarin therapy can be discontinued briefly at the time of surgery, with prompt reinstitution postoperatively.[175,186,187] Coumarin's long half-life of 42 hours necessitates dose reduction or withdrawal 2 days prior to surgery in order to return the patient's PT/INR to an acceptable level for surgery.[175,188] For patients with moderate thromboembolic and hemorrhagic risks, coumarin therapy can be maintained in the therapeutic range with the use of local measures to control postsurgical oozing.[189,190]

High-risk cardiac patients undergoing high-bleeding-risk surgical procedures may be managed most safely with a combination unfractionated heparin–coumarin method,[187] which allows maximal hemostasis with minimal nonanticoagulated time (14 to 18 hours for a 2-hour surgery, as opposed to 3 to 4 days with the coumarin discontinuation method). This technique, which requires hospitalization at additional cost, substitutes parenteral unfractionated heparin, which has a 4-hour half-life, for coumarin. Coumarin is withheld 24 hours prior to admission. Heparin therapy, instituted on admission, is stopped 6 to 8 hours preoperatively. Surgery is accomplished when the PT/INR and aPTT are within the normal range. Coumarin is reinstituted on the night of the procedure and may require 2 to 4 days to effectively reduce the patient's procoagulant levels to a therapeutic range. Heparin is reinstituted 6 to 8 hours after surgery when an adequate clot has formed. Heparin reinstitution by bolus injection (typically a 5,000 U bolus) carries a greater risk of postoperative bleeding than does gradual reinfusion (typically 1,000 U/h).

As a less costly alternative to intravenous heparin substitution therapy requiring hospital admission, LMWHs injected subcutaneously have been used as substitution therapy. Using this management technique, a LMWH (such as enoxaprin) is substituted for warfarin a few days before surgery, and it is withheld from the patient for only a few hours on the day of the surgery.[191]

Use of additional local hemostatic agents such as microfibrillar collagen, oxidized cellulose, or topical thrombin is recommended for anticoagulated patients. Fibrin sealant has been used successfully as an adjunct to control bleeding from oral surgical procedures in therapeutically anticoagulated patients with INRs from 1.0 to 5.0, with minimal bleeding complications.[192] In Europe, 4.8% tranexamic acid solution used as an antifibrinolytic mouthwash has proven effective in control of oral surgical bleeding in patients with INRs between 2.1 and 4.8.[193,194] Use of antifibrinolytics may have value in control of oral wound bleeding, thereby alleviating the need to reduce the oral anticoagulant dose.[193] Use of medications that interact with coumarin, altering its anticoagulant effectiveness as discussed above, is to be avoided.

The shorter-acting anticoagulant heparin is administered by an intravenous or subcutaneous route. The most common outpatient use of subcutaneous heparin is for the treatment of deep venous thrombophlebitis during pregnancy,[196] with the goal being regulation of the aPTT between 1.25 and 1.5 times control. In general, oral surgical procedures can be carried out without great risk of hemorrhage when local hemostatics are used in a patient receiving heparin subcutaneously; however, on consultation, the patient's physician may recommend withholding the scheduled injection immediately prior to the operation. Continuous intravenous unfractionated heparin, with greater hemorrhagic potential than LMWH delivered subcutaneously, is discontinued 6 to 8 hours prior to surgery to allow adequate surgical hemostasis. If a bleeding emergency arises, the action of heparin can be reversed by protamine sulfate. Dosage for unfractionated heparin reversal is 1 mg protamine sulfate intravenously for every 100 units of active heparin. If given within 8 hours of the LMWH injection, then the maximum neutralizing dose of 1 mg protamine/100 units of LMWH given in the last dose is used.

Susceptibility to Infection

Susceptibility to infection among patients with congenital bleeding disorders is not a significant concern. However, due to bleeding into weight-bearing joints, hemophiliacs may have had joint replacement. For these patients, antibiotic prophylaxis should be considered.[197] Should a hematoma form as a result of an anesthetic injection or other dental trauma or spontaneously, use of a broad-spectrum antibiotic is indicated to prevent infection during resolution. If bleeding results from bone marrow–suppressive systemic disease or chemotherapeutic drug use, antibiotics may be required to prevent infection from bacteremia-inducing dental procedures when production of mature functional neutrophils is substantially diminished.

Ability to Withstand Care

Patients with bleeding disorders, appropriately prepared preoperatively, are generally as able to withstand dental care as well as unaffected individuals. Consultation with the patient's physician is recommended for guidance on medical management required for higher-risk surgical dental procedures. Because of the expense of some medical management approaches to severe bleeding disorders (eg, coagulation factor replacement for severe hemophiliacs), the coumarin withdrawal–heparinization approach to extractions for patients at high risk of thrombosis, and the bleeding risk to the patient, long treatment sessions may be required to maximize treatment accomplishments while minimizing the risk and cost.

▼ SELECTED READINGS

Association of Hemophilia Clinic Directors of Canada. Clinical practice guidelines. Hemophilia and von Willebrand's disease: 2. Management. Can Med Assoc J 1995;153:147–57.

Beirne OR. Evidence to continue oral anticoagulant therapy for ambulatory oral surgery. J Oral Maxillofac Surg 2005;63: 540–5.

Bolton-Maggs PH, Pasi KJ. Haemophilias A and B. Lancet 2003;361:1801–9.

Brewer AK, Roeubek EM, Donachie M, et al. The dental management of adult patients with haemophilia and other congenital bleeding disorders. Haemophilia 2003;9:673–7.

Furie B, Limentani SA, Rosenfield CG. A practical guide to the evaluation and treatment of hemophilia. Blood 1994;84:3–9.

Greer JP, Foerster H, Lukens JN, et al, editors. Wintrobe's clinical hematology. 11th ed. Philadelphia: Lippincott Williams & Wilkins; 2004.

Hemophilia and von Willebrand's disease: 1. Diagnosis, comprehensive care and assessment. Association of Hemophilia Clinic Directors of Canada. CMAJ 1995;153:19–25.

Herman WW, Konzelman JL Jr, Sutley SH. Current perspectives on dental patients receiving coumarin anticoagulant therapy. J Am Dent Assoc 1997;128:327–35.

Lockhart PB, Gibson J, Pond SH, et al. Dental management considerations for the patient with an acquired coagulopathy. Part 2: coagulopathies from drugs. Br Dent J 2003;195:495–501.

Mannucci PM. Desmopressin (DDAVP) in the treatment of bleeding disorders: the first 20 years. Blood 1997;90:2515–21.

Mannucci PM. Treatment of von Willebrand's disease. N Engl J Med 2004;351:683–94.

Mannucci PM, Tuddenham EG. The hemophilias—from royal genes to gene therapy. N Engl J Med 2001;344:1773–9.

Martinowitz U, Schulman S, Horoszowski H, et al. Role of fibrin sealants in surgical procedures on patients with hemostatic disorders. Clin Orthop 1996;328:65–75.

Shopnick RI, Brettler DB. Hemostasis: a practical review of conservative and operative care. Clin Orthop Relat Res 1996;328: 34–8.

Todd DW. Evidence to support an individualized approach to modification of oral anticoagulant therapy for ambulatory oral surgery. J Oral Maxillofac Surg 2005;63:536–9.

For the full reference list, please refer to the accompanying CD ROM.

18

IMMUNOLOGIC DISEASES

JANE C. ATKINSON, DDS

MATIN M. IMANGULI, DDS

STEPHEN CHALLACOMBE, PhD, FDSRCS, FRCPath

▼ GENERAL PRINCIPLES OF IMMUNOLOGIC DISEASE

Immunology, once a small branch of microbiology, has evolved into a major field of biomedical research. Every month, new findings are published that further our understanding of the immune response, the genetics controlling immunity, pathology, oral biology, biochemistry, immunopathology and neuroimmunology. Multiple modern pharmaceuticals target specific immune pathways, such as antigen recognition or antigen presentation. Therefore, a good understanding of immunology is needed to treat patients receiving immunomodulating agents to comprehend their mechanisms of action and possible side effects. Basic concepts of the immune response are reviewed in this chapter. However, the reader should study more complete texts to have a better understanding of the principles of immunology.[1]

Immunity: Protection against Disease

The immune system is a multifaceted system that counteracts insults from the environment and whose main function is protection against infection.[1] It neutralizes foreign or "nonself"-antigens that are expressed by a large variety of microbial agents and some tumors. This coordinated system must be able to perceive antigens as foreign, generate activation signals, produce a variety of effector proteins that neutralize pathogens or activate other cells, and downregulate the inflammatory process once the foreign agent is eliminated.

Immune responses of vertebrates are frequently classified into two functional systems: the innate system and the specific or adaptive system. These two systems are highly coordinated with crosstalking signals. The biologic advantage of having two systems of defense is that innate immunity eliminates foreign entities in a nonspecific manner, whereas the adaptive immune response is highly specific and targeted. However, the adaptive response takes several days to develop after antigen recognition, whereas the innate response is immediate.

Innate Immunity

The innate immune response is further divided into the physical barrier, such as the skin or mucosa that is fortified by a variety of secreted antimicrobial peptides and molecules, and circulating cells that possess receptors that recognize a wide variety of pathogens. In the oral cavity, the oral mucosa covered with its mucin layer is the physical barrier. In addition to blocking penetration of pathogens, oral mucosal cells produce antimicrobial peptides that kill or limit many organisms. Saliva plays an important role in innate immunity. Several salivary proteins have antimicrobial, immunomodulatory, and anti-inflammatory properties, including histatins, beta-defensins, cystatins, cathelicidin, lactoferrin, lysozyme, and mucins.[2] Many of these proteins are highly conserved between distant species, emphasizing their evolutionary importance.[3]

The major cells of the innate immune system are the phagocytes (neutrophils, eosinophils, basophils, monocytes, and macrophages), natural killer (NK) cells, certain T cells such as gamma-delta T cells and NK T cells, and dendritic cells (DCs). Over 70 types of leukocytes have now been characterized and defined by their cluster of differentiation (CD) surface antigens. The primary phagocytic cells are tissue macrophages and neutrophils, which are derived from a common myeloid precursor in the bone marrow. The phagocyte internalizes foreign material by creating an endosome, where the potential pathogen is degraded eventually. This process is enhanced when the material is bound by specific antibody and/or complement, a process known as opsonization. Another major function of foreign material internalization is antigen processing and presentation to lymphocytes to initiate the adaptive immune response. This is predominantly the function of DCs that originate from hematopoietic precursors and migrate into the tissues, but macrophages and B cells may perform these functions.[1] Macrophages also activate T lymphocytes through the secretion of cytokines.

Neutrophils constitute about 75% of the circulating white blood cells. They are activated by bacterial products and other cytokines released during inflammation. To function appropriately, neutrophils also must possess appropriate receptors that allow them to leave the circulation and migrate to sites of inflammation. Their life span is short (on average 24 to 48 hours), and the bone marrow releases increased numbers of neutrophils in response to certain infections. NK cells account for 10 to 15% of peripheral blood lymphocytes. They lack a T- or B-cell receptor and are concentrated in the peripheral blood, spleen, and mucosal epithelia. Their primary function is to induce the cytolysis of tumor or virus-infected cells and secrete cytokines that direct DC

maturation and promote T- and B-cell functions. Their cytotoxic reactions are independent of antigen presentation in the context of the major histocompatibility complex (MHC). Another main effector arm of innate immunity is complement, which is a compilation of 30 proteins[1] with multiple functions, including pathogen lysis, opsonization of microorganisms for phagocytosis, chemotaxis and activation of leukocytes and mast cells, clearance of immune complexes, and enhancement of antigen presentation. The primary components act in a particular order and sequentially activate each other. The complement system is highly regulated to minimize host tissue damage from inflammation.

Adaptive (Acquired) Immunity

ANTIGEN PRESENTATION

A highly specific immune response develops after specific lymphocytes recognize nonself-antigens, are stimulated, and divide. Two outcomes of this process are the creation of T-cell populations that target one antigen and antigen-specific antibody production by B cells. Antigen presentation and recognition are central to this process. Antigen must be processed and bound to a class I or II MHC molecule on the surface of the antigen-presenting cell for the T cell to recognize it via the T-cell receptor. MHC molecules, expressed by most human cells, present both self-antigens and nonself-antigens to T cells. The T cell recognizes the MHC molecule as "self" and normally does not activate if no nonself-antigen is present. In addition to the primary signal through the specific receptor (T-cell receptor on T cells or surface immunoglobulin on B cells), T and B cells must receive costimulatory signals from coreceptors and cytokines to activate and proliferate.

CELL-MEDIATED IMMUNITY

After production in the bone marrow, T-cell precursors migrate to the thymus, where a functional T-cell repertoire is selected through positive selection and clonal deletion. After that, T cells populate the paracortical areas of lymph nodes and the white pulp of the spleen and constitute 70 to 80% of lymphocytes circulate in the peripheral blood. When activated, T cells produce multiple cytokines, which are pluripotential proteins that both up-regulate and down-regulate inflammation. There are two major T-cell subsets, which bear either the CD4 or CD8 coreceptor on their surface. The CD4 coreceptor binds exclusively to a MHC class II molecule of an antigen-presenting cell, and these T cells develop into T helper cells. T helper cells are further subdivided into Th1 or Th2 cells by their cytokine secretion profile. Th1 cells secrete cytokines such as interferon-γ and interleukin (IL)-2 that activate macrophages and lead to elimination of phagocytosed intracellular organisms, such as mycobacteria and certain fungi. Extracellular organisms, such as helminths and parasites, are eliminated primarily through the action of Th2 cells, which attract and activate eosinophils. Th2 cells secrete IL-4 and IL-10 in addition to other cytokines and provide costimulatory signals that allow the B cell to differentiate into a plasma cell and produce antibody. Certain antigens (notably viral and tumor) are processed in the cytoplasm by the proteosome and presented on the MHC class I molecules to CD8 T cells.[1] These cells then proliferate and become cytotoxic T lymphocytes, eventually leading to lysis of the infected or transformed host cell. Movement of leukocytes between blood and tissues is dependent on a spectrum of leukocyte-endothelial cell adhesion molecules known as selectins, integrins, and intercellular adhesion molecules. The activity of leukocytes in the tissues is modulated by cytokines, including ILs.

ANTIBODY (HUMORAL IMMUNITY)

B cells migrate from the bone marrow and populate follicles around germinal centers of the lymph nodes, spleen, and tonsils. Efficient antibody production occurs after the B cell recognizes an antigen through the surface-bound immunoglobulin receptor and receives costimulatory signals from T helper cells. Early in the humoral immune response, B cells differentiate into IgM-producing plasma cells. Further development of humoral response involves increased antibody affinity and diversity through the processes of affinity maturation and somatic hypermutation. In addition, after a series of gene rearrangements, the most B cells undergo "class switching" and produce one of the other antibody isotypes (IgG, IgA, IgD, or IgE). IgG isotypes, with lesser amounts of IgA, IgM, and IgE, are found in serum, whereas secretions such as saliva contain primarily IgA and IgM.

Each immunoglobulin has different chemical and biologic properties. IgM antibodies are macromolecules composed of five antibody monomers and are produced chiefly during the body's primary response to a foreign antigen. IgM also plays an important role in the activation of complement and in the formation of immune complexes, which are aggregates of antibody, antigen, and complement. Most IgM in the body is intravascular. IgG constitutes 75% of the serum immunoglobulins and is the major component of the secondary antibody response. IgG is also the immunoglobulin that crosses the placenta, giving protection to the newborn. It is also the main immunoglobulin in tissue fluid, and over 50% of IgG in the body is extravascular. Four primary subgroups of IgG have been identified (IgG1, IgG2, IgG3, and IgG4), which have different biologic properties. Serum IgA is the next most predominant serum immunoglobulin and is mainly monomeric. IgE binds to mast cells and basophils, triggering the release of histamine during allergic reactions such as anaphylaxis, hay fever, and asthma.

Antibodies found in secretions, such as saliva or bronchial secretions, are predominantly IgA isotypes with lesser amounts of IgM produced by resident plasma cells of mucosal tissues. The antibodies are linked to secretory component, which facilitates antibody transport through the secretory epithelium. Another important molecule of secretory immunoglobulins is the J chain, which binds terminal portions of the IgM or IgA monomers together to prevent proteolysis of the immunoglobulin molecule by secretory enzymes. Mucosal IgA is mainly dimeric and induced independently from serum IgA. It protects through virus or enzyme neutralization, aggregation of bacteria, and by preventing adherence of pathogens to the host.

PRIMARY AND SECONDARY RESPONSES

Initial antigen recognition and the subsequent adaptive immune response typically peak at 7 to 10 days, with IgM being the primary antibody produced.[1] After this first response, the sensitized specific T- and B-cell clones become antigen-specific memory cells, which can mount an adaptive immune response much more quickly when challenged by the same antigen a second time. This secondary response peaks at 3 to 5 days and is characterized by higher titers of predominantly IgG antibody.

IMMUNE SYSTEM OF THE ORAL CAVITY

Homeostasis in the oral cavity is maintained by the innate and adaptive systems in conjunction with normal oral flora and an intact oral mucosa. Components contributing to oral defenses include major and minor salivary gland saliva, salivary innate antimicrobial proteins, gingival crevicular fluid, transudating plasma proteins, circulating white blood cells, oral mucosal keratinocyte products, and proteins from microbial flora. Mucosal integrity prevents penetration of microorganisms and macromolecules in the diet and environment that might be antigenic. Different systems protect specific sites in the mouth. The crown of the tooth is protected from caries by salivary secretions, although while neutrophil number and function must be adequate to prevent aggressive periodontitis. The complexity of the oral defense system is best illustrated by studies of humans who are deficient in particular arms of the immune system.

▼ IMMUNODEFICIENCY

The term *immunodeficiency* is used to describe an individual who is not capable of mounting a normal immune response. The immunodeficiency may be hereditary, secondary to an infection such as human immunodeficiency virus (HIV), or secondary to other major diseases, such as cancer, diabetes, or alcoholism. The number of patients with significant immunodeficiencies is increasing as patients with once-fatal diseases are living longer. Organ or hematopoietic stem cell transplantation (HSCT), cancer therapy, and treatments for various autoimmune diseases can cause profound immunosuppression.

▼ PRIMARY IMMUNODEFICIENCIES

Although rare, patients with primary immunodeficiencies are studied intensively to help define the immune system of humans. Careful observations of their infections, coupled with laboratory studies of their immune cells, can help establish the specific pathways responsible for combating different types of microorganisms. In general, specific types of infections are found in different immunodeficiencies (Table 1). Therefore, when evaluating a patient suspected of having an immunodeficiency, a clinical immunologist notes the

TABLE 1 Infectious Susceptibilities and Oral Complications in Specific Immunodeficiencies

Immune Defect	Disease Example	Common Infectious Susceptibility	Oral Complications
Severe decrease in neutrophil number	Kostmann's syndrome; Severe congenital neutropenia	Intra- and extracellular bacterial infections; fungal infections	Aggressive periodontitis, often involving primary and permanent dentitions; recurrent oral ulcerations Delayed wound healing; oral candidiasis
Defective chemotaxis of neutrophils	Leukocyte adhesion deficiency	Intra- and extracellular bacterial infections; fungal infections	Aggressive periodontitis, often involving primary and permanent dentitions; recurrent oral ulcerations Delayed wound healing; oral candidiasis
Unknown	Job's syndrome	Recurrent skin and mucous membrane infections, often with Staphylococcus or Candida	Delayed exfoliation of primary teeth; midline defects of the tongue; oral candidiasis; characteristic face with broad nasal bridge
Severely decreased T- and B-cell numbers	Severe combined immunodeficiency	Infections of all types	Oral candidiasis; herpes; recurrent oral ulcerations; severe necrotizing gingival ulcerations
Decrease in T-cell number	DiGeorge syndrome	Recurrent viral and fungal infections	Oral candidiasis; recurrent herpetic infections
Abnormal T-cell function	MHC class I deficiency of CD8 T cells	Respiratory, viral, and fungal infections	Oral candidiasis; recurrent herpetic infections
	MHC class II deficiency of CD4 T cell	Respiratory, viral and fungal infections	Oral candidiasis; recurrent herpetic infections
Severely decreased B-cell numbers	Bruton's X-linked agammaglobulinemia	Recurrent respiratory and sinus infections with extracellular bacteria	Possible sepsis from odontogenic infections
Solitary immunoglobulin class deficiency	Selective IgA deficiency Selective IgG deficiency	Varied; may have no symptoms or recurrent respiratory and sinus infections	Candidiasis, oral ulcerations; others report no oral changes Possible sepsis from odontogenic infections

MHC = major histocompatibility complex.

microbiologic agent and frequency of infection. For example, a physician would suspect a T-cell defect but not a selective IgG deficiency in a patient having recurrent viral infections and oral candidiasis. Examples of different categories of primary immunodeficiencies are reviewed in this chapter.

Deficiencies in Innate Immunity: Phagocyte Deficiencies

To function correctly, neutrophils and monocytes must migrate to sites of infection, a process known as chemotaxis; phagocytize bacteria; and have the capacity to kill engulfed pathogens. Recurrent infections with staphylococci, *Pseudomonas*, *Candida*, and other fungi occur if the neutrophil number is severely decreased or the phagocyte function is very abnormal (see Table 1).[4] Diseases of neutrophil number and function are covered in Chapter 16, "Hematologic Diseases."

Deficiencies in Adaptive Immunity

COMBINED T- AND B-CELL DEFICIENCY

Severe Combined Immunodeficiency. Children born with severe combined immunodeficiency (SCID) are profoundly immunocompromised. Without treatment, most die of infection before the age of 1 year.[5] Affected children have few to no circulating B and T cells, leaving them susceptible to infection with multiple bacteria, viruses, and fungi. The genetic defects resulting in SCID can be classified into four categories: adenosine deaminase (ADA) deficiency, mutations in the γc subunit of cytokine receptors that result in X-linked SCID, mutations in the recombination-activating gene 1 or 2

(*RAG1* or *RAG2*), and mutations in the CD3δ and CD3ε chains. Mutations of these genes block T- and B-cell maturation. HSCT is the standard treatment for these children at present,[6] but many children may not have a human leukocyte antigen (HLA)-matched sibling. Ex vivo gene therapy was used successfully to correct the immunodeficiency in 20 children with ADA deficiency. Unfortunately, three children subsequently developed leukemic T-cell expansion, but new research may produce a safer gene vector for treatment of these patients.[7]

Oral complications noted in children with SCID include aphthous-like ulcerations,[6,8] candidiasis,[9] and herpetic infections.[10] Children treated with HSCT may present with multiple complications associated with transplant and graft-versus-host-disease (see Chapter 19, "Transplantation Medicine").

Wiskott-Aldrich Syndrome. Wiskott-Aldrich syndrome (WAS) is a rare X-linked disorder characterized by thrombocytopenia, microcytic platelets, eczema, recurrent infections, and an increased incidence of autoimmune disease and malignancies.[11] Clinical manifestations occurring shortly after birth include petechiae, bruising, and bloody diarrhea. Complications such as otitis media, pneumonia from bacteria, and skin infections are frequent problems. The central defect in WAS is a defect in the *WAS* gene, which is involved in transduction of signals from the cell surface of immune cells to the actin cytoskeleton. The severity of the immune deficiency in WAS varies between families, depending on the location of the mutations in this gene. The mutation affects both T and B cells, as well as platelets. Children born with

WAS initially may have normal numbers of T cells, but T-cell counts may decline as the child ages. B-cell numbers may be decreased or normal. Although WAS patients produce some antibodies, they often have impaired responses to polysaccharide antigens. Other clinical problems include an increased incidence of B-cell lymphomas.[12] Reported oral manifestations include purpura, candidiasis, and herpetic infections.

Ataxia-Telangiectasia. Ataxia-telangiectasia (AT) is an inherited, autosomal recessive, degenerative disorder characterized by cerebellar degeneration. The classic form of AT results from a mutation of the *ATM* gene, which is broadly involved in cellular responses to deoxyribonucleic acid (DNA) double-strand breaks.[13] It is estimated to occur in 1:40,000 to 1:300,000 births, affecting males and females equally.[13,14] Early clinical presentation includes deterioration of the gait between 1 and 4 years of age, with continued ataxia. Other features are ocular and facial telangiectases and a varied immunodeficiency, including sinopulmonary infections.[14,15] Telangiectases of the skin and eyes become apparent after infancy. Although not all patients with AT have immunodeficiency, up to 75% have evidence of a T-cell deficiency,[14] with 60% having decreased serum IgA, IgG2, and IgG4.[14,15] Reduced release of naive T cells by the thymus is proposed as a mechanism for the immunodeficiency in this disease.[16] Patients with recurrent infections are treated with intravenous pooled immunoglobulin. Approximately 10 to 15% of patients with AT develop cancers of lymphoid origin while in childhood.[13] Many develop opportunistic infections consistent with their T-cell deficiency, including warts, herpes simplex, molluscum contagiosum, candidal esophagitis, and herpes zoster.[15]

T-Cell Deficiencies

DECREASE IN T-CELL NUMBER

DiGeorge Syndrome (Velocardiofacial Syndrome). After production in the bone marrow, progenitors of T lymphocytes migrate to the thymus for further selection and differentiation.[1] Before entering the thymus, T lymphocytes do not express the T-cell receptor, or CD4 or CD8 markers. During their time in the thymus, T cells acquire the CD4 or CD8 molecule, and autoreactive T cells are deleted through a process of negative selection. Children with DiGeorge syndrome fail to develop a complete thymus secondary to a hemizygous deletion of 22q11.2.[17] Consequently, there is abnormal development of the facial and neural crest tissues, which ultimately leads to aberrant development of the thymus, the parathyroid glands, the great vessels of the heart, and the craniofacial complex. There may be partial or complete aplasia of the thymus. Approximately 90 to 95% of children present with a cardiac defect, hypocalcemia, and decreased numbers of circulating T cells.

DiGeorge syndrome is the prototypical classic T-cell disorder. The absence of adequate numbers of circulating T cells (both CD4 and CD8) creates an immunodeficiency characterized by an increased susceptibility to infections with viruses and fungi. The severity of the T-cell deficiency is dependent on the degree of thymic hypoplasia. Although children may present with florid candidiasis (Figure 1), some patients have very few opportunistic infections.[17] The rare patient with complete absence of the thymus may be treated with thymic transplantation.[18] Presumed long-term consequences of thymic hypoplasia include increased autoimmune disease, including idiopathic thrombocytopenia, and a possible predisposition to malignancy.[17] Craniofacial features of DiGeorge syndrome include cleft palate (up to 11%), bifid uvula, oral candidiasis, short palpebral fissures, a small mouth, prominent forehead, enamel hypoplasia, and anterior glottic webs.[17,19] Schizophrenia occurs with increased frequency in these patients.[17]

QUALITATIVE T-CELL DEFECTS

Defects in the MHC. If genes encoding the essential MHC proteins are mutated or deleted, there can be an impairment of both cell-mediated and humoral responses. The immunodeficiency associated with these defects was originally called "bare lymphocyte syndrome." Further studies established that this syndrome encompasses several diseases mediated by defects in the expression of MHC molecules. Patients unable to express MHC class I antigens correctly lack adequate presentation of antigenic peptides to CD8 T cells. This results in inadequate cytotoxic T-cell activation. Defects in MHC class II expression ultimately lead to a decrease in CD4 T cells that need these molecules for maturation. Although B-cell numbers are normal in patients with MHC defects, serum immunoglobulin levels are decreased as T cells fail to present antigen to B cells. *Candida albicans*, herpes simplex viruses, and other opportunistic pathogens can infect the oral cavity of these patients, who may die at a young age without HSCT.[20]

B-Cell Deficiencies

Inadequate B-cell number or function translates clinically into insufficient levels of circulating antibody, termed hypogammaglobulinemia.[1] Extracellular bacteria often cause respiratory and sinus infections in patients with B-cell defects, demonstrating the importance of antibodies for defense of these tissues. Decreased resistance to bacterial infections is a major feature of patients with B-cell deficiencies, so these patients may become septic from odontogenic infections.[21] There is an increased susceptibility to oral ulceration.

DECREASE IN B-CELL NUMBER

Bruton's X-Linked Agammaglobulinemia and Non-Bruton's Agammaglobulinemia. B-cell maturation and subsequent antibody production are a complex series of events with multiple steps. Initially, the precursor is produced in the bone marrow,[5] where it develops into a pro-B cell. The pro-B cell must successfully transition through the pre-B-I and pre-B-II stages before leaving the bone marrow. Two genetic primary immunodeficiencies caused by mutations in the genes involved with this process are Bruton's X-linked agammaglobulinemia and non-Bruton's agammaglobulinemia.

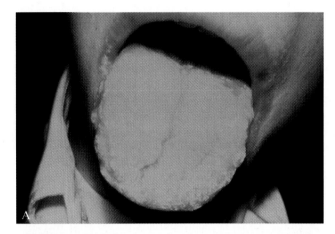

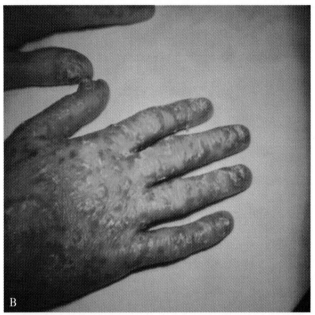

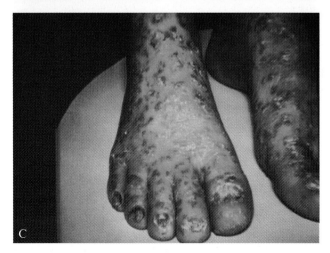

FIGURE 1 *A,* Chronic mucocutaneous candidiasis in patient with DiGeorge syndrome, with lesions of the tongue. *B,* Lesions of the same infection, on the hands. *C,* Lesions of the same infection, on the feet.

Bruton's X-linked agammaglobulinemia is a very rare disorder (estimated to occur in 1 in 200,000 births) characterized by grossly depressed numbers of circulating B cells and little or no circulating immunoglobulin.[22] Newborns with this immunodeficiency are protected initially from infection by maternal antibodies, so diagnosis may be delayed for several months or even a few years. Clinical presentation is a male child with recurrent pulmonary and sinus infections.[23] Patients have a high incidence of pneumonia, arthritis, and meningitis and may also present with diarrhea and otitis media. Organisms often involved in these infections include streptococci, staphylococci, *Pseudomonas*, and *Haemophilus influenzae*.[22,23] The primary defect in Bruton's X-linked agammaglobulinemia is a mutation of the *Btk* gene that is encoded in 19 exons at Xq22[22] and is expressed in all stages of B-cell maturation except for the plasma cell stage. Over 174 unique mutations in *Btk* have been identified from 199 families to date, but it has been difficult to relate specific mutations to clinical phenotypes.[22] With aggressive antibiotic treatment and intravenous pooled immunoglobulin transfusions, patients with Bruton's X-linked agammaglobulinemia are surviving into middle age.[22] Many patients have adequate T-cell and phagocyte function, which provides protection from many viral and fungal infections once T-cell immunity develops. HSCT has not been successful in restoring adequate numbers of circulating B lymphocytes or serum immunoglobulin levels.[22]

Non-Bruton's agammaglobulinemia is a term for a less common group of immunodeficiencies that have the same clinical presentation as Bruton's. These patients may be male or female and often have a homozygous recessive mutation in one of a number of genes involved with the maturation of pro-B cells to pre-B cells.[1,21] They do not have mutations involving *Btk*. Since non-Bruton's and Bruton's agammaglobulinemia have the same clinical course and infectious susceptibilities, they are managed similarly.

DECREASE IN CERTAIN CLASSES OF IMMUNOGLOBULINS

Common Variable Immunodeficiency. Common variable immunodeficiency (CVID) is a class of diseases characterized by an inability to produce sufficient levels of all classes of antibodies, particularly IgG and IgA.[24] Onset of clinical symptoms is varied, manifesting in both males and females sometime during early childhood to the second or third decade of life. Patients have the same infectious susceptibilities as those with Bruton's agammaglobulinemia, and many develop autoimmune disease.

Genetic mutations in several immune pathways can cause the clinical phenotype of CVID. Some of these genes regulate expression of cell surface ligands needed for T-cell–B-cell interactions.[24] Without these interactions, B cells are not stimulated to make antibody. Two such examples are mutations of the inducible T-cell costimulator gene (*ICOS*) and mutations of *TNFRSF13B*, which encodes the transmembrane activator and calcium modulator and cyclophilin ligand interactor (TACI). It is expected that future genetic studies will identify new mutations and functional deficiencies in many of these patients.

Selective Immunoglobulin Deficiencies.   Selective immunoglobulin deficiencies are characterized by an inability to produce a single class of antibody.[1] They are extremely varied in clinical presentation. Many patients have a fully functional immune system, and the deficiency is noted only if immunoglobulin levels are determined for another reason. Patients usually are healthy because immunoglobulins of the other classes provide adequate humoral defenses. Other patients present with recurrent respiratory infections, which leads to the diagnosis. Immunoglobulin isotypes, such as IgG subclasses, must be determined to make the diagnosis.

The most common immunodeficiency is selective IgA deficiency, occurring in 1 in 400 to 1 in 2,000 people.[21,25] Whereas some people are healthy, others have chronic respiratory or gastrointestinal infections.[21,25] Autoimmune diseases, such as systemic lupus erythematosus (SLE), rheumatoid arthritis (RA), and pernicious anemia are more common in this deficiency.[25,26] Developmentally, B-cell maturation in IgA deficiency is impaired. In one study, 8% of IgA-deficient individuals also were deficient for IgG2 and 27% for IgG4.[25] Since secretory IgA is the major immunoglobulin of saliva, the oral health of this patient group has been studied in detail. There is not sufficient evidence to conclude that patients with this selective immunodeficiency have an increase in dental caries or periodontal disease.[21,27] In one study, anti-streptococcus mutans salivary IgM was higher in patients without salivary IgA, suggesting that IgM compensates for the loss of IgA in this population.[28]

JOB'S SYNDROME

Hyperimmunoglobinemia E Syndrome/Job's Syndrome. This syndrome, also known as Buckley's syndrome, is a systemic disorder with multiple oral manifestations. Patients have an unknown immune deficiency, alterations in bones, and other craniofacial manifestations.[29] The genetic mutation associated with Job's syndrome is still unknown. One of the most common laboratory findings is an elevation of serum IgE,[29] but not all patients demonstrate this abnormality. Clinically, patients suffer from eczema, staphylococcal abscesses, pneumonia, and candidiasis. Oral manifestations include oral candidiasis (up to 83%), midline defects of the tongue, and delayed resorption and exfoliation of the primary teeth (Figure 2).[30] The typical Job's syndrome face is

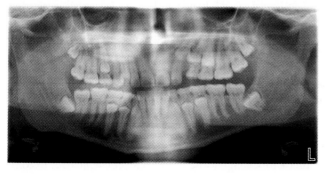

FIGURE 2   Panorex from a 22 year old male with Job's syndrome demonstrating a generalized failure in primary tooth root resorption.

characterized by a broad nasal bridge, a prominent forehead, and rough skin texture. Skeletal problems include recurrent bone fractures, hyperextensible joints, and scoliosis.[29]

▼ SECONDARY IMMUNODEFICIENCIES

Many disorders are secondarily associated with decreased numbers or function of the various components of the immune system, leading to increased incidence of infections. Just like primary immunodeficiencies, the type of infections suffered by patients with secondary immunodeficiencies depends on which particular component of the immune system is compromised, although, frequently, multiple defects are present. Secondary immunodeficiencies result either from decreased production or increased destruction of immune cells or loss of components of humoral immunity.

Innate Immune System

CELLULAR (PRIMARILY NEUTROPHILS)

Neutropenia can occur in several conditions, including hematologic malignancies, especially when the malignancy suppresses growth of myeloid precursors. Decreased neutrophil counts occur frequently during cancer chemotherapy, stem cell transplantation, aplastic anemia, and autoimmune neutropenia (see Chapter 16, "Hematologic Diseases"). There is progressively increasing risk of infection in patients with a low neutrophil count, starting at an absolute neutrophil count (ANC) of 1,000 cells/mm³. However, the majority of infections occur with counts below 500 cells/mm³ and in particular below 100 cells/mm³. Although no published evidence exists regarding the efficacy of prophylactic antibiotics prior to invasive dental procedures in neutropenic patients, many authorities recommend their use in patients with an ANC below 1,000 cells /mm³. Whenever used, basic principles of antibiotic prophylaxis should be followed; antibiotics should be given in a single dose prior to the start of the procedure. Protocols recommended by the American Heart Association (AHA) are designed to prevent bacteremia from oral sources and are the most appropriate for this purpose.[31–34]

COMPLEMENT

Acquired deficiency in complement components has been observed in advanced liver disease and is associated with an increased incidence of bacterial infections in these patients. In addition, dysfunction of the complement pathway has been demonstrated in some malignancies, such as chronic lymphocytic leukemia (CLL). The contribution of this finding to increased incidence of infections in these patients is unclear.[35,36]

ADAPTIVE IMMUNE SYSTEM

Several conditions decrease T-cell numbers (HIV) and/or function (chronic graft-versus-host disease, treatment with calcineurin inhibitors, treatment with anti–tumor necrosis factor [TNF]-α agents). Clinically, patients often present with opportunistic infections. Specific aspects of these conditions are covered in the dedicated portions of this book. Infections with intracellular bacteria and fungi (*Pneumocystis carinii*), viruses (such as herpes family viruses and papillomaviruses; Figures 3 and 4), and parasites (*Toxoplasma* and *Cryptosporidium*) are typical of T cell–deficient states. Oral candidiasis is frequently the first sign of advanced HIV infection. Herpes zoster is common in patients with CLL.[37]

HUMORAL (ANTIBODIES)

Secondary humoral immunodeficiency can be observed in conditions associated with increased loss (nephrotic syndrome) or decreased production (multiple myeloma, CLL) of immunoglobulins. Antibodies are important in combating primarily extracellular bacterial infections and, to a lesser degree, viral infections prior to cell entry. Patients with decreased blood antibody concentrations are particularly susceptible to systemic infections with encapsulated bacteria such as *Streptococcus pneumoniae*, *Klebsiella*, and *H. influenzae*.[38].

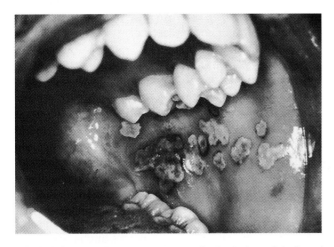

FIGURE 3 Extensive recurrent herpes simplex lesions of the buccal mucosa and palate of a patient receiving chemotherapy for leukemia.

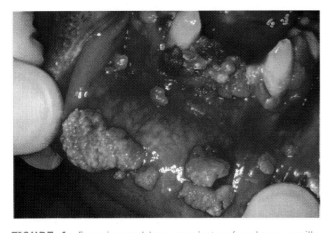

FIGURE 4 Extensive condyloma acuminatum from human papillomavirus infection in a patient receiving chemotherapy for non-Hodgkin's lymphoma.

▼ AUTOIMMUNE DISEASES

The term *autoimmune disease* refers to a disorder in which there is evidence of an immune response against self. At present, there is substantial proof that autoimmunity is central to the pathologic processes of more than 80 diseases.[1] Autoimmune diseases may be primarily due to either antibodies (autoantibodies) or immune cells, but a common characteristic is the presence of a lymphocytic infiltration in the target organ. Examples include type 1 diabetes mellitus, autoimmune thyroiditis, Sjögren's syndrome, SLE, and multiple sclerosis. Circulating antibodies can often be detected in vitro by binding to appropriate human tissue substrates. In many cases, there is clear evidence that the autoantibodies are involved in the disease pathophysiology (eg, pemphigus), but in others, these autoantibodies have undefined roles, and their presence is used primarily for diagnosis. In addition, autoantibodies are rarely specific for one autoimmune disease (Table 2). A common mechanism believed to be central to all autoimmune diseases is a failure of peripheral tolerance systems that normally control autoreactive T-cell clones.

Systemic Lupus Erythematosus

SLE is a multisystem autoimmune inflammatory disorder of unknown etiology. It is regarded as the archetypal autoimmune disease, and the main feature is the formation of antibodies to DNA, which may initiate immune complex reactions, in particular a vasculitis. In the United States, SLE has a prevalence between 12 and 64 per 100,000, with a female to male ratio of 9:1, and is more common in persons of non-European descent.[39] Women of Afro-Caribbean decent have an estimated ninefold increased risk of developing SLE. In addition to systemic and isolated cutaneous lupus (chronic discoid lupus), a distinct syndrome of drug-induced lupus is recognized. Unlike SLE, drug-induced lupus rarely affects the kidney and is reversible on discontinuation of the offending agent.

ETIOLOGY AND PATHOGENESIS

Although the exact etiology of SLE is unknown, a complex interplay of genetic and environmental factors that leads to a progressive loss of peripheral tolerance and production of autoantibodies is believed to be crucial for SLE initiation. The genetic predisposition to SLE is demonstrated by twin studies. Concordance for SLE in dizygotic twins is 2 to 5%, whereas it is up to 58% for monozygotic twins. The risk of SLE developing in a sibling of an affected person is 20 times higher than that in a general population. Genome-wide linkage and association studies have identified several gene groups strongly correlated with SLE. In contrast to many autoimmune conditions, association of MHC-related genes with SLE susceptibility is not striking. Although certain MHC class II genes, particularly *DR2*, have been associated with SLE, other polymorphisms and structural complement component variants confer a much higher risk of SLE. Genetic deficiency in complement components, although rare overall, is among the strongest risk factors for SLE. Ninety percent of persons with

TABLE 2 Autoantibody Profiles of Different Autoimmune Diseases

Autoantibody	Prevalence (% Positive)*					
	SLE	RA	Sjögren's Syndrome	Systemic Sclerosis	PM/DM	MCTD
ANA	95–100	30–60	90	90–96	60–80	>99
Anti-double-stranded DNA	40–80		5			
IgM rheumatoid factor	5–30	70–80	73	25	8	48
Anticyclic citrullinated antibody	13	65–80	1	11		
Anti-Sm	30–40	10	1	4		Rare
Anti-U1 RNP	13–23	5	2	5–11	4	100
Anti-Ro/SS-A	24–60	3–15	54–80	11	21–30	24
Anti-La/SS-B	6–35	0–2	26–42	6	13	
Anti-Scl-70				84 (in diffuse form only)		8
Anticentromere				70–80 (in CREST form only)		
Anti-Jo-1					23–36 (highest in DM)	

*Adapted from references 49, 60, 108, 114, 115, and 131 to 135.

ANA = antinuclear antibodies, which is a screening test that detects multiple autoantibodies; DM = diabetes mellitus dermatomyositis; DNA = deoxyribonucleic acid; MCTD = mixed connective tissue disease; PM = polymyositis; RA = rheumatoid arthritis; SLE = systemic lupus erythematosus.

homozygous C1q deficiency will develop SLE, and having the S structural variant of complement receptor 1 is associated with a much higher risk of SLE in Caucasians. Polymorphisms in FcγRIIA and FcγRIIIA receptors have been the most strongly associated with increased risk of SLE. Associations with cytokine genes (encoding IL-10, TNF-α, and TNF-β), genes important for immunologic tolerance (encoding CTLA-4 and PD-1) and apoptosis (encoding BCL-2 and Fas/Fas-L pathway), have been reported.[40,41]

Since the concordance in monozygotic twins is less than 100%, factors other than genetic predisposition must play a role in the development of SLE. Environmental factors, including infections, particularly with Epstein-Barr virus and other viruses, exposure to pollutants, hormonal factors, ultraviolet light, and smoking, and possibly diet have been linked to the development of SLE. Additionally, over 80 drugs, classically hydralazine, isoniazid, and procainamide, are associated with drug-induced lupus.[42]

Numerous immunologic abnormalities have been described in SLE. Processes thought to be central to the pathogenesis are immune complex formation and deposition in target organs, complement activation, attraction of effector cells, and subsequent target tissue destruction. B lymphocytes are involved at several stages in the development of lupus. Autoreactive B cells occur in normal individuals and are usually controlled by a variety of mechanisms, including clonal deletion, anergy, and regulatory T cells. In patients with SLE, autoreactive B cells escape peripheral control mechanisms and begin actively producing pathogenic autoantibodies. Autoantibody production usually precedes clinical manifestations of SLE by many years.

Other components of the immune system may participate in the pathogenesis of SLE. Efficient antibody production cannot occur in the absence of appropriate T-cell help, and T cells specific for viral antigens may provide help to autoreactive B cells and stimulate anti-DNA antibody production. Several viruses have been linked to the pathogenesis of SLE. Complement plays a dual role in the pathogenesis of SLE. Although deficiencies in certain complement components are risk factors for SLE, complement activation following immune complex deposition is the major mechanism responsible for target tissue damage in SLE, and decreases in complement components C3 and C4 correlate with flares of the disease.[43–45]

CLINICAL MANIFESTATIONS

Lupus is known as "the great mimic." Indeed, SLE can affect virtually every organ system and cause a wide spectrum of clinical symptoms. Skin is affected in up to 85% of SLE patients (Figure 5). In addition, cutaneous lupus can occur without multisystem involvement. Skin lesions of lupus can be classified into lupus-specific (having diagnostic clinical or histopathologic features) and nonspecific lesions.

Three subtypes of lupus-specific skin lesions have been described: acute, subacute, and chronic. Acute cutaneous lupus occurs in 30 to 50% of patients and is classically represented by the butterfly rash–mask-shaped erythematous eruption involving the malar areas and bridge of the nose but typically (as opposed to dermatomyositis [DM]) sparing nasolabial folds (Figure 6). Bullous lupus and localized erythematous papules also belong to the acute lupus category. Chronic cutaneous lupus occurs in 15 to 20% of cases and

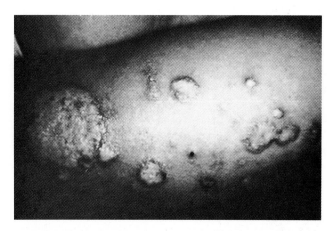

FIGURE 5 Skin lesions in a patient with systemic lupus erythematosus. (Courtesy of Dr. George Ehrlich)

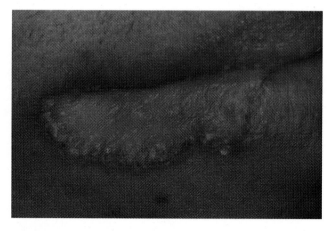

FIGURE 7 Discoid lupus lesions on the lower lip.

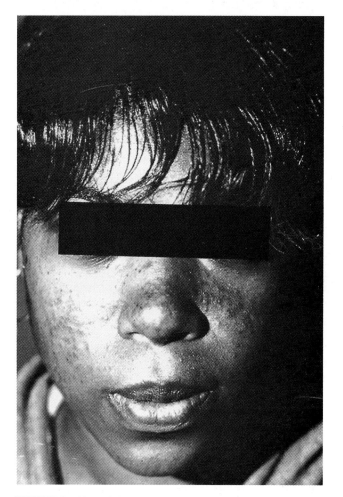

FIGURE 6 "Butterfly" rash on the face of a patient with systemic lupus erythematosus. (Courtesy of Dr. Robert Arm)

affects the skin of the face or scalp in about 80% of cases (Figure 7). The least common subtype, subacute cutaneous lupus, occurs in 10 to 15% of patients and includes papulosquamous (psoriasiform) and annular-polycystic eruptions, usually on the trunk and arms. Nonspecific but suggestive skin manifestations of lupus are common and include

alopecia (both scarring following discoid lesions and nonscarring), photosensitivity, Raynaud's phenomenon, livedo reticularis, urticaria, erythema, telangiectases, and cutaneous vasculitis.[46–48]

Renal. Kidney involvement occurs in about 50 to 75% of patients with SLE and is the primary cause of morbidity and mortality in this population. Clinically, renal disease in SLE can range anywhere from asymptomatic proteinuria to rapidly progressive glomerulonephritis with renal failure. Several histologic subtypes have been described. The severity of renal disease and its response to treatment are good predictors of overall prognosis in SLE.[49]

Musculoskeletal. Musculoskeletal manifestations occur in about 95% of patients with SLE, and arthralgia is the first presenting symptom in about 50% of cases. Nonerosive symmetric arthritis most commonly affecting the hands, wrists, and knees is typical of SLE. Fixed joint deformity (Jaccoud's arthropathy) rarely occurs and is due to ligamentous and tendon involvement. A history of temporomandibular joint–related symptoms was reported in two-thirds of SLE cases in one study.[50] Myalgias and myositis are also common. Avascular necrosis of the bones is a major cause of morbidity and is usually associated with corticosteroid therapy.[51]

Central Nervous System. Central nervous system (CNS) involvement occurs in about 20% of patients with SLE and is usually due to cerebral vasculitis or direct neuronal damage. CNS manifestations include psychosis, stroke, seizures, and transverse myelitis and are associated with poor overall prognosis.[52]

Cardiovascular. Cardiovascular involvement in SLE is classically manifested by vasculitis and pericarditis. In addition, endocardial damage (Libman-Sacks endocarditis and superimposed bacterial endocarditis), myocarditis, and conduction defects are commonly described. With increasing survival of lupus patients, accelerated atherosclerosis with coronary artery disease has become an important clinical problem.[53] In a community-based study, myocardial infarction, heart failure, and stroke were 8.5, 13.2, and 10.1 (respectively) times more likely to occur in women with SLE than in the general population.[54] Multiple defects of blood coagulation pathways have been described in SLE. Abnormalities in fibrinolysis, decreases in anticoagulant proteins (protein S), and the presence of antiphospholipid antibodies contribute to increased tendency to thrombosis in SLE. CNS and deep venous thromboses with pulmonary emboli are major causes of morbidity in these patients, requiring a high level of anticoagulation for prevention.[55]

Other Manifestations. Fatigue, depression, and fibromyalgia-like symptoms are commonly present and can be debilitating. Serositis manifested by pleuritic chest pain and auscultatory rub is one of the distinctive signs of SLE. Lupus pneumonitis, pulmonary hemorrhage, diffuse interstitial lung disease, and pulmonary hypertension occur infrequently but can have serious implications. Gastrointestinal manifestations are uncommon but can include pancreatitis, hepatitis, peritonitis, and enteritis. Premature ovarian failure is usually associated with cyclophosphamide therapy, and spontaneous abortions occur in patients with antiphospholipid syndrome. The most common ophthalmic manifestation of SLE includes keratoconjunctivitis sicca, present in up to a third of patients. Lupus retinopathy and optic neuritis are uncommon but can lead to blindness. In addition to oral lesions, other head and neck manifestations of SLE include sensorineural hearing loss, nasal ulcerations sometimes complicated by septal perforation, auricular chondritis, laryngeal ulcerations and stenosis, and vocal cord paralysis.

ORAL MANIFESTATIONS

The oral mucosa is affected in a significant percentage of lupus patients. Two predominant types of oral lesions are discoid lesions and ulcerations. Oral ulcerations are listed among the criteria for SLE diagnosis but occur in a minority of patients (Figure 8). In one study, the prevalence of oropharyngeal ulceration was 15% at the initial assessment.[56]

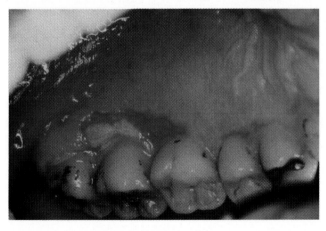

FIGURE 8 A chronic palatal lesion (the initial sign of systemic lupus erythematous in this patient).

Oral ulcerations associated with SLE cannot be easily distinguished from other common oral conditions, such as aphthous ulcers, although they occur with increased frequency on the palate and in the oropharynx and are characteristically painless. Histologically, they are characterized by lymphocytic infiltrate at the base of the ulcer and in the perivascular distribution, which is similar to that observed in discoid lesions.

Discoid oral lesions are similar to those occurring on the skin and appear as whitish striae frequently radiating from the central erythematous area, giving a so-called "brush border." Atrophy and telangiectases are also frequently present. Buccal mucosa, gingiva, and labial mucosa are the most commonly affected intraoral sites. Isolated erythematous areas are also common, especially on the palate. It may be difficult to differentiate these lesions from other common mucosal disorders, such as lichen planus, especially if there are few lesions and there is no systemic or cutaneous involvement. Histologically, both subepithelial and perivascular infiltrates are usually present. Disturbed keratinization with resulting in cellular atypia can also be observed. Direct immunofluorescent staining for immunoglobulins and complement C3 factor is a useful aid to diagnosis. Granular deposition of IgM, IgG, and C3 along the basement membrane is characteristic.[57–59]

LABORATORY FINDINGS

Anemia, leukopenia, and thrombocytopenia are among the most common manifestations of SLE. Anemia of chronic disease is the predominant type, and leukopenia (neutropenia, lymphopenia, or both) occurs in about 50% of patients. Autoimmune thrombocytopenia is also common and may be severe. Elevation of the erythrocyte sedimentation rate with normal C-reactive protein levels is characteristic of SLE.

Although over 100 different autoantibody types are associated with SLE, the best studied are directed against various nuclear components and phospholipids.[60] Antinuclear antibodies (ANAs) are present in 98% of SLE patients (see Table 2) and are the most sensitive diagnostic test for this disease. However, the ANA test may be nonspecific, being present in many other autoimmune diseases and in low titers in up to a third of the normal population. The highest value of ANA, therefore, is the exclusion of SLE in those with a negative result. Anti-double-stranded DNA antibodies are present in 50 to 60% of SLE patients and are highly specific[61]. Antibodies classically associated with Sjögren's syndrome, anti-Ro/SS-A and anti-La/SS-B, are present in SLE in 25 to 40% and 10 to 15% of cases, respectively, and are included in diagnostic criteria. Other antibodies highly specific for SLE but found in a relatively small percentage of patients are antiribosomal P, anti-Smith antigen (anti-Sm), and antinuclear ribonucleoprotein (anti-nRNP). Various autoantibody patterns are associated with distinct clinical presentations of SLE. For example, anti-Ro antibody is linked to subacute cutaneous lupus and neonatal heart block, and antiribosomal P antibody is linked to lupus psychosis and nephritis.[61]

Antiphospholipid antibodies (anticardiolipin and lupus anticoagulant) are causatively associated with many manifestations of SLE, including thrombocytopenia, thrombotic complications and recurrent abortions (antiphospholipid syndrome), and endothelial damage with accelerated atherosclerosis.[62]

DIAGNOSIS

Diagnosis of SLE is based on the compatible symptoms and signs in the presence of suggestive laboratory abnormalities. A standardized set of criteria, last modified in 1997, was proposed by the American College of Rheumatology (Table 3).[63,64] The presence of four positive findings has a sensitivity and specificity for SLE of 70 to 96% and 90 to 100%, respectively.[65]

TREATMENT

Corticosteroids remain the cornerstone of therapy in SLE and are especially useful for controlling disease flares. Although effective in a significant number of cases, long-term corticosteroid use is associated with a number of serious complications, including opportunistic infections, steroid-induced diabetes, osteoporosis, avascular necrosis, and hypertension. A pulse intravenous cyclophosphamide regimen for remission induction followed by quarterly infusions for maintenance is the mainstay of modern therapy of severe SLE, especially lupus nephritis. Despite its high level of efficacy, cyclophosphamide is toxic, with a high frequency of complications, such as hemorrhagic cystitis, bladder cancer, and ovarian failure. Recently, maintenance with other less toxic agents, such as mycophenolate mofetil (MMF) and azathioprine, has been shown to possess efficacy equivalent to that of quarterly cyclophosphamide, with fewer side effects. Targeting of B cells with rituximab, monoclonal antibody to CD20, has recently shown promise in SLE. Agents targeting costimulation pathways and B-cell activation are in the early phase trials. Nonsteroidal anti-inflammatory drugs (nsaids) are frequently used in SLE for symptomatic relief of arthritis but are of little benefit in more severe disease. Cyclosporine, tacrolimus, sirolimus, methotrexate, and intravenous immunoglobulins have also been used in SLE, but data to support efficacy are scarce. Antimalarials, such as hydroxychloroquine, are effective in cutaneous lupus with fewer adverse effects.[66–68]

DENTAL MANAGEMENT

The dental management of the lupus patient should take into account the complex pathologic manifestations of the disease, including oral aspects and complications of immunosuppressive treatment.

Risk of Infection. A complete blood count should be obtained prior to dental treatment of SLE patients. Elective oral surgical procedures with the potential for bacteremia should be delayed if the ANC is over 1,000 cells/mm^3, prophylactic antibiotics are often recommended. Although the evidence behind prophylactic antibiotics prior to dental management in neutropenic patients is scarce, current guidelines recommend prophylactic antibiotics when the ANC falls below 500 to 1,000 cells/mm^3. Since no studies have been performed regarding the efficacy of antibiotic prophylaxis in neutropenic patients prior to oral surgical procedures, the

---

TABLE 3   American College of Rheumatology Criteria of Classification of Systemic Lupus Erythematosus and Rheumatoid Arthritis

Systemic Lupus Erythematosus	Rheumatoid Arthritis
The presence of four or more	*The presence of four of seven*
Malar rash	Morning stiffness ≥ 1 h
Discoid rash	Arthritis of three or more joints (PIP, MCP, wrist, elbow, knees, ankle and MTP joints)
Photosensitivity	Arthritis of joints of the hands
Oral or nasal ulcerations	Symmetric arthritis
Nonerosive arthritis involving two or more joints	Rheumatoid nodules
Renal disorder	Serum rheumatoid factor
Neurologic disorder (seizures or psychosis in the absence of offending drugs)	Radiographic changes, including erosions or bony decalcifications
Hematologic disorder (hemolytic anemia, leukopenia, lymphopenia, or thrombocytopenia)	The first four criteria must be present for at least 6 wk, and the second through fifth criteria must be observed by a physician
Immunologic disorder (anti-DNA, anti-Sm, antiphospholipid antibodies, a positive test result for lupus anticoagulant using a standard method, or a false-positive serologic test for syphilis)	
Antinuclear antibody	

Adapted from Hochberg MC[63] and Kaplan MJ.[110]

DNA = deoxyribonucleic acid; MCP = metacarpophalangeal; MTP = metatarsophalangeal; PIP = proximal interphalangeal.

optimum regimen is unknown, but a single dose, according to the AHA endocarditis prophylaxis guidelines, is probably the most appropriate.[31,32,57,69]

In lupus patients treated by immunosuppressive medications preferentially targeting the adaptive immune system (rituximub, cyclosporine, MMF, tacrolimus), the increased risk of infection following dental procedures has not been reported and antimicrobial prophylaxis is not indicated. Patients at highest risk for infective endocarditis should be given antibiotic prophylaxis consistent with AHA recommendations.[31] In planning the dental treatment of SLE patients on dialysis, the potential for increased bleeding, infection, and decreased renal clearance of medications should be taken into account.[69] Patients should be treated on nondialysis days (see Chapter 15, "Renal Disease").

Risk of Bleeding. Traditionally, platelet transfusions have been recommended in surgical patients with a platelet count below 50,000/mm³. However, more recent data show that minor invasive procedures may be safely performed in patients with platelet counts as low as 10,000 to 20,000/mm³ and that platelet count in itself is a poor predictor of postoperative bleeding.[70] The decision for preoperative transfusion should take into account the location and extent of the surgery and potential risk if bleeding does occur, and the ability to control the bleeding by local measures rather than rely on a preset platelet count trigger. Routine platelet transfusions are associated with risks such as alloimmunization and infection transmission. Since oral surgical procedures are usually minor in extent and bleeding can be readily controlled by local measures such as pressure and application of hemostatic agents, a conservative approach to platelet transfusion should be exercised. Platelet transfusion can be performed postoperatively in patients in whom bleeding occurs despite local measures.

In patients with lupus who are receiving anticoagulants, established guidelines should be followed. In general, oral surgical procedures are safe in patients with therapeutic international normalized ratio ranges (2–3.5) and do not require discontinuation of anticoagulation.[70,71]

Adrenal Suppression. It has proved to be very difficult to estimate the risk of adrenal suppression based on the dose, duration of therapy, or time since the last dose without formal testing, such as the adrenocorticotropic hormone suppression test. Any patient treated with supraphysiologic doses of corticosteroids (7.5 mg of prednisone a day or higher) for 2 weeks or longer is at risk of adrenal suppression.[72] The duration of adrenal suppression is dependent on both the dose and duration of the treatment, with abnormal adrenal responses observed ranging from about a week (20 mg of prednisone for 5 days) to up to a year after long-term high-dose steroid administration. Although older guidelines recommended routine doubling of the steroid dose in patients at risk of adrenal suppression undergoing surgical procedures, current recommendations are based on the rational approach, taking into account the physiology of the adrenal secretion (Table 4). It has been determined that the rate of corticosteroid secretion does not exceed 200 mg of cortisol/d in patients undergoing major surgery and 50 mg/d in case of minor surgery. Given that most oral surgical procedures fall in the category of minor surgery, replacement of over 50 mg of hydrocortisone a day (12.5 mg of prednisone) is unnecessary.[72,73]

There are no reported controlled studies specifically addressing management of oral mucosal involvement in SLE. Hydroxychloroquine is commonly used for discoid lesions on the skin and mucosa. Topical steroids with antifungal agents are recommended for discoid and ulcerative lesions. Systemic agents such as dapsone, thalidomide, clofazimine, and methotrexate have also been used. Patients with secondary Sjögren's syndrome should be managed accordingly (see Chapter 8, "Salivary Gland Diseases").

Scleroderma

The term *scleroderma*, derived from the Greek words for hard and skin, is used to describe a group of clinical disorders characterized by thickening and fibrosis of the skin. The generalized form, progressive systemic sclerosis, is a multisystem connective tissue disease in which the fibrosis extends to the internal organs, including the heart, lungs, kidney, and gastrointestinal tract.[74] The prevalence is estimated to be between 18 and 20 per million, with women being affected three to four times as frequently as men.[49] There are two main forms, progressive systemic sclerosis (PSS) and localized sclerodema.

PSS is further divided into limited cutaneous scleroderma (previously called CREST syndrome for calcinosis cutis, Raynaud's phenomenon, esophageal dysmotility, sclerodactyly, and telangiectasia) and diffuse cutaneous scleroderma. Patients with limited scleroderma often have a long history of Raynaud's phenomenon before the appearance of other symptoms. They have skin thickening limited to the hands and frequently have problems with digital ulcers and esophageal dysmotility. Although generally a milder form of disease than diffuse scleroderma, limited scleroderma can have life-threatening complications. Diffuse scleroderma patients have a more acute onset, with constitutional symptoms, arthritis, carpal tunnel syndrome, and marked swelling of the hands and legs. They also characteristically develop widespread skin thickening (progressing from the fingers to the trunk), internal organ involvement (including gastrointestinal and pulmonary fibrosis), and potentially life-threatening cardiac and renal failure. Other possible variants are an overlapping syndrome with SLE, Sjögren's syndrome, RA, and DM.

Localized scleroderma refers to scleroderma primarily involving the skin, with minimal systemic features.[74] It is rare that patients with localized scleroderma progress to PSS. There are two major types of localized scleroderma, linear scleroderma and morphea. Linear scleroderma is characterized by a band of sclerotic induration and hyperpigmentation occurring on one limb or side of the face. This form of the disease develops as a thin band of sclerosis that may run the entire length of an extremity, involving underlying muscle,

TABLE 4 Guidelines for Supplementation of Patients at Risk of Adrenal Insufficiency Undergoing Dental Surgery

Dental Surgical Procedure	Previous Systemic Steroid Use	Current Systemic Steroid Use / Systemic Steroid Use	Daily Alternating Steroid Use	Current Topical Steroid Use
Routine dental procedures	None	None	None	No
Minor oral surgery lasting <1 h with local anesthetic only	Consider supplementation with 25 mg of hydrocortisone equivalent before surgery, especially if the patient is infected	Consider supplementation with 25 mg hydrocortisone equivalent before surgery, especially if the patient is infected. No need to supplement if the patient is taking over 50 mg hydrocortisone equivalent daily.	Treat on day when patient is taking steroid	No
Oral surgery with or without general anesthesia lasting >1 h	50–100 mg of hydrocortisone equivalent the day of surgery, with continuation of the dose for an additional day dependent on the amount of blood loss, the presence of infection, and the length of the surgery			No
Major oral surgery with general anesthesia lasting >1 h and having significant blood loss, such as cancer or orthognathic surgery	Usual daily dose before surgery and hydrocortisone equivalent of 50 mg hydrocortisone intravenously during surgery and every 8 h after the initial dose for up to 72 h			No

Adapted from references Axelrod L,[72] Salem M et al,[73] and Miller CS et al.[136]

bones, and joints. When the disease crosses a joint, limitation of motion is possible, along with growth abnormalities. The lesion of linear localized scleroderma of the head and face is called en coup de sabre, and these lesions may result in hemiatrophy of the face. Morphea is characterized by small violaceous skin patches or larger skin patches (guttate morphea) that indurate and lose hair and sweat gland function (Figure 9). Later in the disease, the lesion "burns out" and appears

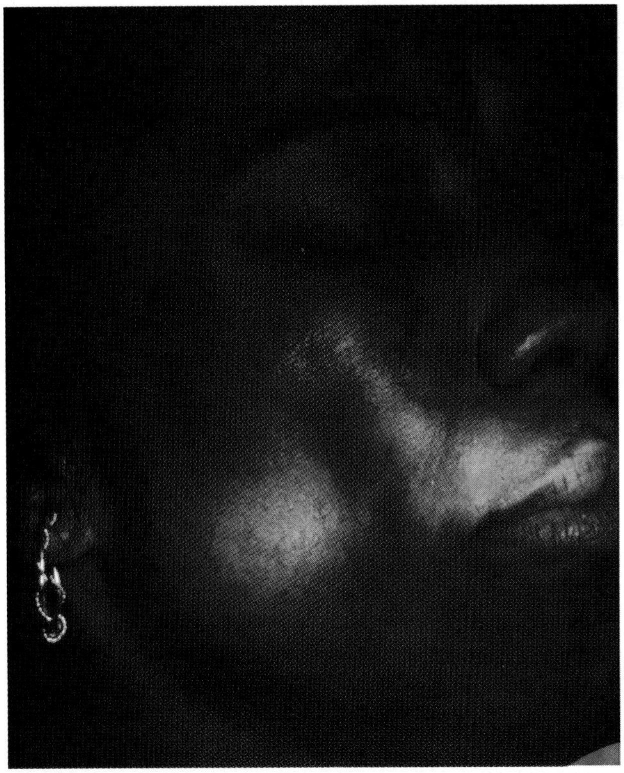

FIGURE 9 Morphea of the face.

as a hypo- or hyperpigmented area depressed below the level of the skin. A small number of patients develop numerous larger lesions that coalesce, and these patients are said to have generalized morphea (see Figure 9). Scleroderma localized to the hands is called acrosclerosis.

ETIOLOGY AND PATHOGENESIS

The etiology of PSS is unclear, but the pathogenesis is characterized by vascular damage and an accumulation of collagen and other extracellular matrix components at involved sites.[74] Biopsies of the skin in early stages demonstrate bundles of collagen in the lower dermis and upper subcutaneum in association with perivascular and interstitial mononuclear cell infiltrates. The inflammatory process precedes the deposition of collagen. Once in the tissue, T cells drive processes through secretion of cytokines such as IL-4 and IL-13 that result in vasculopathy and fibrosis.[75] These cytokines induce fibroblast production of transforming growth factor β_1, which is the main profibrotic cytokine in PSS. As the disease progresses, the rete pegs are lost and the epidermis thins.[49]

Unregulated collagen deposition is a hallmark of this disease. Cultured fibroblasts from patients synthesize more collagen in vitro that is structurally normal, although collagen degradation pathways appear to be normal.[49] The excess collagen narrows small arteries and changes the microvasculature in early stages of the disease, causing eventual pulmonary hypertension, renal disease, myocardial dysfunction, and digital gangrene.

There appears to be a small genetic predisposition to PSS.[74] Environmental exposure to pesticides, benzene derivatives, and silica has been linked to the development of scleroderma-like conditions in miners and stonemasons. Viral triggers, such as parvovirus B19, are proposed.[74]

CLINICAL MANIFESTATIONS

Patients with PSS as opposed to limited scleroderma typically have rapid skin thickening and visceral organ involvement. Severe skin and kidney complications developed in 70% of a cohort of 953 patients with diffuse cutaneous systemic sclerosis followed for more than 20 years.[76] Forty-five to 55% also had serious heart, lung, and gastrointestinal tract disease. Visceral organ involvement was significantly associated with an increase in mortality.

Raynaud's Phenomenon.   Raynaud's phenomenon is the most common initial finding of PSS. Marked initimal hyperplasia of the digital arteries of scleroderma patients narrows the vessels. Stimuli such as cold that normally stimulate vasoconstriction can cause complete obstruction of the blood flow to the fingertips.[49] More than 95% of scleroderma patients eventually experience a more severe form of the digital cyanosis, numbness, and blanching found with Raynaud's phenomenon.[77] In addition to pain, patients with severe Raynaud's phenomenon can develop digital pitting scars, nail fold infarcts, or ulcers that occasionally cause loss of the digit.[77]

Cutaneous Manifestations.   Skin thickening of PSS patients begins in the fingers and hands in almost all cases.[49] The neck and the face are usually the next sites to be involved.[49] The changes begin with pitting edema that is replaced by a tautness and hardening of the skin. This limits motion in affected areas. Hyperpigmentation, telangiectases (Figure 10),

and subcutaneous calcifications may also occur, leading to deformity and severe cosmetic problems (Figure 11).

Musculoskeletal Manifestations.   Generalized arthralgias and morning stiffness are common in PSS and may be confused with RA.[49] Clinically evident joint inflammation is uncommon, although erosions are reported in as many as 29% of patients.[49] Muscle weakness can occur from disuse

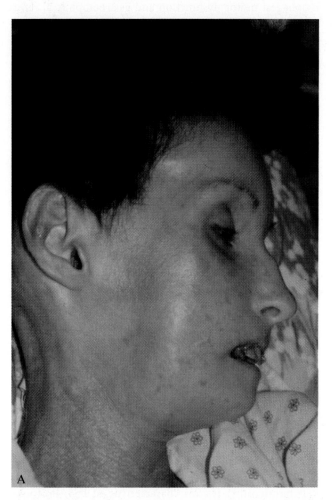

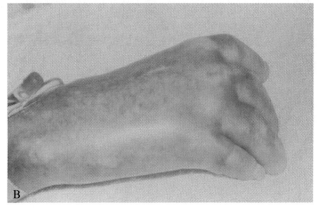

FIGURE 11   Manifestations of scleroderma. *A,* Severe tightening of the skin and narrowing of the oral aperture of a patient with scleroderma. *B,* Extensive involvement of the fingers and hand of the same patient causes a lack of mobility and the resorption of phalanges.

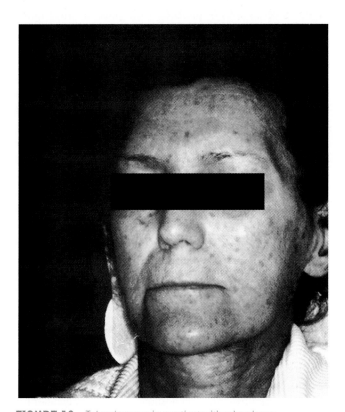

FIGURE 10   Telangiectases in a patient with scleroderma.

atrophy or from primary myopathy that is accompanied by mild elevations of serum muscle enzymes.[49]

Gastrointestinal Manifestations. Upper or lower gastrointestinal involvement is reported in up to 90% of scleroderma patients with either the progressive or limited cutaneous forms.[78] Patients may have disorders of motility and transit time, affecting any area from the esophagus to the anus. Esophageal motor dysfunction and gastroesophageal reflux disease occur in the majority of scleroderma patients. In severe forms, the intestinal fibrosis results in malabsorption.

Cardiac Manifestations. Cardiac injury in scleroderma may occur secondary to the primary pathologic processes of this disease.[79] The microvasculature is altered, and collagen production is increased in the infiltrated tissue. These processes lead to ischemic, fibrotic, and inflammatory lesions in the pericardium, myocardium, and cardiac conduction system. "Patchy fibrosis" is a term used to describe the myocardial lesions associated with PSS. Hypertension, dysrhythmias, conduction disturbances, and left ventricular hypertrophy can develop.[79]

Pulmonary Manifestations. Pulmonary complications of scleroderma are now the leading cause of death in patients with scleroderma.[49] They can be insidious in onset and resist treatment. Progressive interstitial lung disease can lead to pulmonary arterial hypertension, which is estimated to occur in 10 to 15% of patients.[80] Longitudinal studies suggest that pulmonary deterioration tends to progress once the pathologic process is established.

Renal Manifestations. Until recently, renal involvement was the most deadly complication of scleroderma. "Scleroderma renal crisis" is a syndrome characterized by malignant hypertension, rapidly progressive renal insufficiency, hyperreninemia, and evidence of microangiopathic hemolysis.[49] Pathologic changes are present in the kidney that mimic other lesions characteristic of PSS. Profound decreases in hemoglobulin and platelet counts can occur.[49] Normotensive renal failure related to arteriolar thrombosis is associated with previous glucocorticoid therapy.[49]

ORAL MANIFESTATIONS

The clinical signs of scleroderma of the mouth and jaws are consistent with findings elsewhere in the body. The lips become rigid, and the oral aperture narrows considerably.[81] Skin folds are lost around the mouth, giving a masklike appearance to the face. The tongue can also become hard and rigid, making speaking and swallowing difficult. Involvement of the esophagus may cause dysphagia.[78] Oral telangiectasia is equally prevalent in both limited and diffuse forms of PSS and is most commonly observed on the hard palate and the lips.[81]

When fibrosis involves the muscles of mastication, mandibular resorption can occur. One study reported that one-third of patients had resorption of either the angle of the mandible, the condylar heads, the coronoid process, or the digastric region. Mandibular movement may be restricted by muscular fibrosis. Linear localized scleroderma may cause hemiatrophy of face. Dental radiographic findings have been reported and widely described. Classic findings such as uniform thickening of the periodontal membrane are found in less than 10% of patients (Figure 12). Other characteristic radiographic findings include calcinosis of the soft tissues around the jaws. The areas of calcinosis will be detected by dental radiography and may be misinterpreted as radiographic intrabony lesions. A thorough clinical examination will demonstrate that the calcifications are present in the soft tissue.

Medications may reduce salivary flow rates, or patients with scleroderma may have secondary Sjögren's syndrome. Small studies have estimated the prevalence of secondary Sjögren's syndrome in patients with scleroderma to be between 21 and 44%.[81,82] Significant fibrosis was seen in the minor salivary gland biopsies of patients. Gingival hyperplasia can result from the use of calcium channel blockers; pemphigus, blood dyscrasias, or lichenoid reactions may result from penicillamine use. Xerostomia results in an increased susceptibility to dental caries and *Candida* infections (see Chapter 8, "Salivary Gland Diseases").

LABORATORY EVALUATION AND DIAGNOSIS

Circulating ANAs are present in >90% of scleroderma patients (see Table 2). Several are highly specific for the disease.[83] These include anticentromere (ACA), which is found in up to 50% of patients; antitopoisomerase I (anti-topo I); anti–ribonucleic acid (RNA) polymerase I/III; and anti-Th/To2-36. Other autoantibodies not specific to scleroderma can be detected in serum, including anti-PM-Scl, anti-U3RNP, and anti-U1RNP.[84] Autoantibodies appear to have prognostic value for patients. ACAs are strongly associated with slowly progressive, limited disease, whereas anti-topo I and anti-RNA polymerase I/III are found more frequently in patients with progressive and diffuse disease.[83] Other abnormal laboratory findings include anemia, an elevated erythrocyte sedimentation rate, and hypergammaglobulinemia. The diagnosis of systemic scleroderma is made from the presence of characteristic cutaneous skin thickening in association with Raynaud's phenomena. Proximal sclerodermatous skin changes (proximal to the metacarpophalangeal joints) in the presence of two minor criteria (sclerodactyly, digital pitting scars of fingertips or loss of the distal finger pad, or bibasilar pulmonary fibrosis) are necessary to classify a patient as having systemic sclerosis.

TREATMENT

Treatment of PSS depends on the extent and severity of skin and organ involvement. Early diagnosis and treatment are advised.[85] Calcium channel blockers are prescribed for moderate to severe Raynaud's phenomenon, and D-penicillamine is used to control skin thickening and decrease visceral

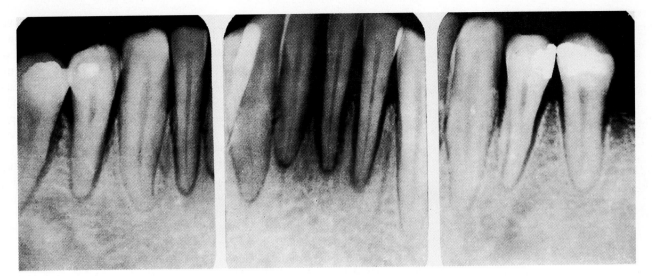

FIGURE 12 Radiographs showing thickening of the periodontal membrane in a patient with scleroderma.

involvement.[49] The latter drug interferes with collagen cross-linking and is an immunosuppressive agent. Cyclophosphamide is used to treat early lung disease with alveolitis.[85] Epoprostenol, treprostenol, bosentan, and inhaled iloprost have been shown to improve pulmonary arterial hypertension, whereas angiotensin inhibitors have greatly improved patient outcomes for those with scleroderma renal crisis.[85]

DENTAL MANAGEMENT

The most common problem in the dental treatment of scleroderma patients is the physical limitation caused by the narrowing of the oral aperture and rigidity of the tongue. Procedures such as molar endodontics, prosthetics, and restorative procedures in the posterior portions of the mouth become difficult, and the dental treatment plan may sometimes need to be altered because of the physical problem of access. The oral opening may be increased an average of 5 mm by stretching exercises. One particularly effective technique is the use of an increasing number of tongue blades between the posterior teeth to stretch the facial tissues. Mechanical stretching devices are available. If these approaches are insufficient, a bilateral commissurotomy may be necessary. Patients may have great difficulty with hygiene. Caries and plaque were associated with decreasing dexterity and strength in a study of 22 patients with scleroderma.[86] Customized toothbrush handles should be provided for patients who cannot grip an ordinary toothbrush.

When treating a patient with diffuse scleroderma, the extent of the heart, lung, or kidney involvement should be considered, and appropriate alterations should be made before, during, and after treatment. Patients with extensive resorption of the angle of the mandible are at risk of developing pathologic fractures from minor trauma, including dental extractions. Patients with Sjögren's syndrome should apply topical fluorides daily (such as 1.1% neutral sodium fluoride) and have professional hygiene appointments three to four times per year (see Chapter 8, "Salivary Gland Diseases").

Idiopathic Inflammatory Myopathies

The idiopathic inflammatory myopathies (IIMs) are a group of systemic rheumatic diseases that include adult polymyositis (PM), adult dermatomyositis (DM), juvenile DM, myositis associated with cancer or another connective tissue disease, and inclusion body myositis (IBM).[87] All are characterized by muscle weakness and nonsuppurative inflammation of the skeletal muscle. The true incidence and prevalence are difficult to ascertain because of the rarity of these diseases and the lack of consistent diagnostic criteria. Most studies have found that the incidence is higher in women, although males are reported to have a higher prevalence of IBM.[88]

SUBTYPES

PM usually has an insidious onset characterized by symmetric weakness of the limb girdle muscles and anterior neck flexors that develops into progressive muscle atrophy. Characteristic histologic changes that include necrosis of type I and II muscle fibers are present in a skeletal muscle biopsy. DM has most of the features of PM, with additional characteristic skin lesions. The most common cutaneous manifestation is a rash, termed Gottron's papules, which is a symmetric, palpable, erythematous eruption of the skin overlying the extensor surfaces of the metacarpophalangeal and interphalangeal joints of the fingers and other sites of the body (Figure 13).[89] This sign is considered pathognomonic for DM. The juvenile form typically occurs between ages 6 and 11 years, whereas the adult form develops in the fourth to sixth decades of life.[88] The most recently defined subset of the inflammatory myopathies is IBM. Clinical presentation is similar to that for PM, with the diagnosis made histologically.[49] IBM and myositis in association with malignancy commonly occur after the age of 50 years.[49]

ETIOLOGY AND PATHOGENESIS

The etiology and pathogenesis of inflammatory myositis are unknown. Evidence suggests roles for autoimmune injury,

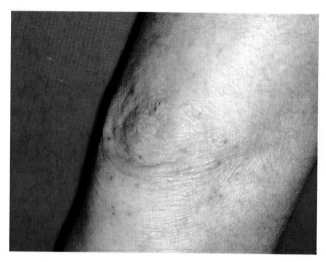

FIGURE 13 Gottron's papules on the knees of a patient with polymyositis (Courtesy of Dr. Jaime Brahim).

genetics, and the environment. Most patients will have auto-antibodies to various antigens involved in protein translation. The types of cells found at the sites of inflammation differ in the various forms of inflammatory myositis, suggesting that each has a unique etiology.[90] In PM, the endomysial inflammation is primarily T cell, with few NK cells and no B cells. In DM, the muscle infiltrate has a high percentage of B cells and CD4[+] T cells with loss of capillaries.[90]

Recent studies of a large patient cohort (571 patients) established that alleles of the 8.1 ancestral haplotype (8.1 AH) are important risk factors for the development of IIM in patients who have the autoantibodies antisynthetase/anti-Jo-1, anti-La, anti-PM/Scl, and anti-Ro in their serum. Further analyses suggested that 8.1 AH-associated alleles B*0801 and DRB1*0301 are the principal HLA risk markers.[91]

Enviromental factors suggested as cofactors for IIM are influenza, hepatitis, coxsackievirus infection, and infection with the protozoan *Toxoplasma gondii*. A recent registry report found that symptoms of rash and weakness often followed a history of respiratory or gastrointestinal complaints in juvenile DM, suggesting that the response to an infectious process is involved in its pathogenesis.[92]

No one malignancy is associated with the myositis of malignancy. Patients with ovarian, lung, pancreatic, stomach, and colorectal cancer or non-Hodgkin's lymphoma have developed DM, whereas patients with non-Hodgkin's lymphoma and lung and bladder cancers have the higher rates of PM.[88]

CLINICAL MANIFESTATIONS

Most patients present with an acute or subacute onset of weakness of the proximal muscles that is symmetric.[89] Patients may have difficulty raising their head while supine, climbing stairs, and dressing themselves. Muscle involvement may become severe enough to confine the patient to bed or to cause respiratory failure and death.

The primary classic skin lesion seen in DM is a violaceous macular erythema distributed symmetrically. Pathognomonic skin manifestations, occurring in approximately 70% of patients, are Gottron's papules (described above). The symmetric rash of DM is violaceous to dusky erythematous, sometimes with edema, involving the periorbital area and upper eyelids. Macular erythema over the lower neck, upper chest, and upper back in a shawl-like distribution, severe erythema of the palms, scaling scalp plaques, and hyperkeratosis of the palmar and lateral aspects of the fingers (mechanic's hands) are commonly seen. Periungual abnormalities, including telangiectases and cuticular overgrowth and gingival bushy loop formations, may occur in juvenile DM. Other skin changes include telangiectases and Raynaud's phenomenon.

Skin calcinosis is most commonly seen in children or young adults. Fibrosis of muscles can cause a retrognathia similar to scleroderma. Interstitial lung disease secondary to fibrosing alveolitis, cardiac conduction abnormalities, conjunctival edema, and renal damage also occur.

ORAL MANIFESTATIONS

A study of 34 patients with PM and DM found increased numbers of decayed, missing, and filled teeth; fewer teeth; poorer oral hygiene; and decreased masticatory forces in this patient group.[93] The most common mucosal lesion was telangiectasia, detected in seven cases. Fibrosis of the minor salivary glands was found in 12 patients, and interstitial-perivascular infiltration was detected in 8 cases. Dysphagia may complicate oral health. Calcinosis of the soft tissues is seen, especially in children. These calcified nodules may appear in the face and radiographs. The tongue may also become rigid due to severe calcinosis. Gingival changes with severe DM have been noted in children with juvenile DM (Figure 14).

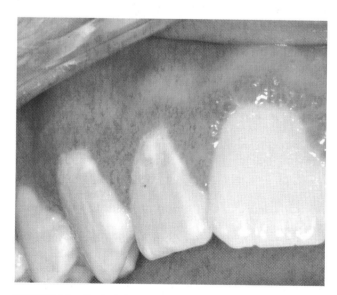

FIGURE 14 Gingival changes seen in juvenile dermatomyositis. Note the marked dilation of the capillaries of the attached gingiva.

LABORATORY EVALUATION AND DIAGNOSIS

Patients with PM demonstrate (1) symmetric weakness of the limb girdle muscles, progressing from weeks to months; (2) skeletal muscle biopsy showing necrosis of type I and II muscle fibers and other characteristic changes; (3) elevation of serum muscle enzymes (creatine kinase, aldolase, alanine aminotransferase, aspartate aminotransferase, and lactate dehydrogenase); and (4) electromyographic features of myopathy.[49] The diagnosis of DM is made if a patient has the features of PM plus a cutaneous eruption that is typical of DM. "Ragged red" fibers, angulated atrophic fibers, and characteristic intracellular lined vacuoles are additional features in a muscle biopsy of IBM. Disease subsets may be identified by their autoantibodies, but only 50% of patients with IIM will be autoantibody positive (see Table 2).[94]

TREATMENT

After exclusion of malignancy, patients are treated according to the extent of their disease. Initial therapy consists of high doses of systemic corticosteroids.[87] Other agents used for management include methotrexate, azathioprine, cyclosporine, and intravenous immunoglobulin. TNF-blocking agents have been suggested as therapies for resistant cases.[95] Physical therapy should be included in the management plan.

DENTAL MANAGEMENT

Gingival lesions should be treated with standard hygiene therapy. However, they may continue to bleed and resolve only when the systemic disease responds to immunosuppressive therapy. Precautions are necessary for all patients taking high-dose long-term steroids and other immunosuppressives (see "Dental Management" under "Systemic Lupus Erythematosus," above).

Rheumatoid Arthritis

RA is a disease characterized by symmetric, inflammatory arthritis of small and large joints.[49] It is one of the most common autoimmune diseases, estimated to affect up to 2% of the population in the United States over the age of 60 years,[96] with a higher prevalence in women. Epidemiologic studies suggest that the incidence of RA is declining in younger age groups for unknown reasons.[97] In contrast to degenerative joint disease (osteoarthritis), RA is a systemic disease with constitutional symptoms, including fatigue, weight loss, morning stiffness, low-grade fevers, and anemia.[49]

SUBTYPES

Juvenile rheumatoid arthritis (JRA) is an illness of children less than 16 years of age that is defined by two of the following symptoms: joint stiffness, decreased range of motion, pain on range of motion, or joint warmth for at least 6 weeks without another cause.[49] Like RA in adults, JRA can sometimes cause severe joint and organ damage. There are three classifications of JRA: pauciarticular (having four or fewer joints involved),

polyarticular (having more than four joints involved), and systemic (Still's disease), characterized by joint swelling, fever, rash, and organ involvement.[98] The prevalence of JRA is estimated to be as high as 1:1,000 children. Long term, these patients may have failure to thrive secondary to steroid treatment. Recent data suggest that growth hormone may reduce their deficiency in stature.[99] Etanercept, a TNF-blocking agent, has been used safely in these children.[100]

Felty's syndrome is characterized by neutropenia and splenomegaly in conjunction with RA. These patients have additional susceptibilities to bacterial infection if neutropenia is severe.[101]

ETIOLOGY AND PATHOGENESIS

The etiology of RA is unknown, but there is substantial evidence that it is a complex genetic disease. However, other factors appear to either initiate or sustain RA as the prevalence of RA has decreased in more genetically homogeneous populations, such as Pima Indians.[97]

Genetic Factors. There is strong evidence from association studies that certain genes in the HLA region of chromosome 6 increase the risk of having RA. Associations with HLA-DRB1-shared epitope haplotypes and RA are reported in several populations.[102] Another new significant finding in the area of genetics and RA is an association between a single-nucleotide polymorphism outside the HLA region, *PTPN22*, and RA.[103] The association between *PTPN22* and RA was found in five large populations from the United Kingdom, United States, Spain, and Finland.[102] This gene encodes the protein Lyp, which acts as a negative regulator of T-cell activation. Twin studies are used to calculate the contribution of genetics and environment to the development of diseases.[104] The finding of concordance in only 16% of monozygotic twins with RA suggests that the environment plays a significant role in the etiology of this disease. Smoking, environmental factors, diet, and infectious agents have all been suggested as triggers for RA.[104] A recent study examined the interactions of environment and genetics in RA. Patients with specific HLA-DRB1 genotypes that conferred a genetic susceptibility to seropositive RA had a much greater risk of developing RA if they smoked. This study demonstrated a gene–environment interaction between smoking and HLA–DRB1 genotypes.[105] The finding that the disease is much more common in women (2:1 to 4:1 female: male ratio[49]) suggests that there may be hormonal influences.

Immune Factors. The target organ of RA is the synovial tissue and the cartilage of the joint. Inflammatory cells, including T cells, infiltrate the synovium, causing an expansion of the tissue and formation of a "pannus" that overlays the articular surface of the cartilage and invades the bone.[106] Mediators of inflammation, such as the cytokine TNF-α, are released by invading cells and contribute to the destruction of the cartilage and bone. B cells, which can differentiate into plasma cells, are also found within the synovial infiltrate.[107]

These cells may participate in the pathophysiology of RA by producing cytokines and autoantibodies. The most commonly found autoantibody in RA is rheumatoid factor (RF), an antibody reactive against antigenic determinants on the Fc fragment of the IgG molecule. Approximately 80% of RA patients will have circulating RF. Typically, either IgM RF or IgA RF is found in the circulation. Both the severity and the activity of RA are correlated with RF levels. A putative role for RF in the pathogenesis of RA is that it forms large immune complexes within the synovium that subsequently bind and activate other inflammatory molecules. Newer autoantibodies described in RA that have aided in its diagnosis are anticyclic citrullinated antibodies, although these antibodies are also found in other autoimmune diseases, such as SLE.[108]

Infectious Agents. The finding that many infections produce clinical symptoms similar to RA has generated interest in the role of infectious agents in this disease. These include parvovirus, rubella virus, Epstein-Barr virus, *Borrelia burgdorferi*, and others. However, epidemiology studies have not supported a role for any one agent.[109]

CLINICAL MANIFESTATIONS

RA is a symmetric polyarthritis often involving the proximal interphalangeal joints of the fingers and metacarpophalangeal joints of the hands (Figure 15); the wrists, elbows, knees, and ankles also can be affected. In some patients, all joints may be involved, including the temporomandibular joint and the cricoarytenoid joint of the larynx. Affected joints develop redness, swelling, and warmth, with eventual atrophy of the muscle around the involved area.

The clinical course and severity of RA vary greatly between patients. Some patients may have a short course of nondisabling disease, whereas others have advancing disease that responds poorly to therapy. Those with progressive active disease develop joint destruction and deformity with time, including subcutaneous nodules and swan-neck deformities. Cervical spine disease may cause C1–C2 subluxation and spinal cord compression. Rheumatoid nodules may develop in the lungs, pleura, pericardium, sclerae, and, rarely, the heart, eyes, or brain. RA can decrease life expectancy by as much as 5 to 10 years. One long-term complication of RA is a marked increase in cardiovascular disease.[110]

ORAL MANIFESTATIONS

The treatment of RA can cause oral manifestations. The long-term use of methotrexate and other antirheumatic agents, such as D-penicillamine and NSAIDs, can cause stomatitis. Minocyline may cause hyperpigmentation intraorally. Gingival overgrowth may occur if patients are taking cyclosporine, whereas prednisone or TNF-α-blocking therapy may predispose patients to the development of opportunistic infections (Figure 16). The direct effects of the disease are also seen. Small studies of RA cohorts suggest an increased prevalence of periodontal disease in patients with RA and a

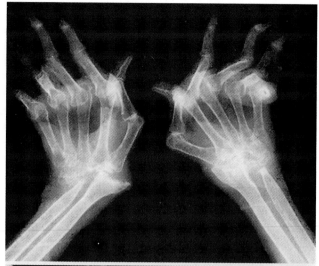
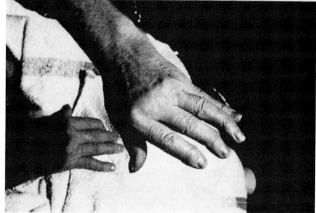

FIGURE 15 Characteristic involvement of the hands in a patient with rheumatoid arthritis. (Courtesy of Dr. George Ehrlich.)

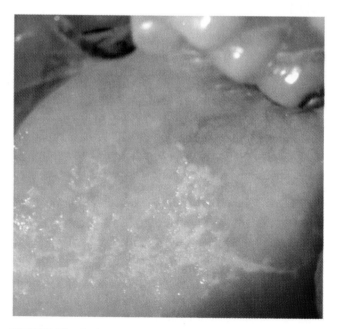

FIGURE 16 Oral candidiasis in a 24 year old female with rheumatoid arthritis and secondary Sjögren's syndrome treated with TNF-alpha blocking agents and prednisone.

similar cytokine profile in patients with RA and aggressive periodontitis.[111,112] However, the increased dental and periodontal disease in this patient population may be related to a decreased ability to maintain proper oral hygiene or to smoking habits. Secondary Sjögren's syndrome is common in RA and is the most significant oral association (see Chapter 8, "Salivary Gland Diseases"). Involvement of the temporomandibular joint in RA is common but is usually asypmtomatic (see Chapter 9, "Temporomandibular Diseases").

LABORATORY EVALUATION AND DIAGNOSIS

The initial diagnosis of RA is made primarily by observing clinical features. As with many autoimmune diseases, a list of diagnostic criteria developed by the American College of Rheumatology is used to evaluate patients (see Table 3).[113]

RF and anti-CCP antibodies are present in approximately 80% of adult patients with RA, and antiperinuclear factor antibodies are present in up to 48.5% of patients (see Table 2).[114,115] Several other autoantibodies may be detected in these patients. Although these autoantibodies are not specific to RA and are found in patients who have other conditions, such as SLE and scleroderma, a positive test for RF and anti-cyclic citrullinated proteins (CCP) antibodies adds considerable weight to the diagnosis of RA. RF, particularly in high titers, is associated with more destructive disease and a worse prognosis. Other associated laboratory findings include an elevated erythrocyte sedimentation rate and normochromic normocytic anemia.

DENTAL MANAGEMENT

When treating an RA patient, it is imperative that the dentist understand the mechanism of action of the patient's current medications, their possible side effects, and their potential interactions with drugs commonly used in dentistry. Appropriate measures should be taken with these patients prior to dental care (see "Dental Management" under "Systemic Lupus Erythematosus," above).

Methotrexate is often used as initial therapy for symmetric polyarthritis involving three or more joints.[116] This drug reduces disease activity and joint erosions and is associated with a significant long-term reduction in mortality in these patients.[117] Patients with severe disease usually are treated with combination therapy, and early aggressive therapy has been shown to be advantageous. Although high-dose prednisone therapy is not used as frequently as it was in the past, lower doses of prednisone (<10 mg/d) are still used commonly.[118] Many biologic agents, typically antibodies that block receptors or mediators of inflammation, are being developed and used as treatments for RA. The most commonly prescribed at present are etanercept and infliximab, agents that block the actions of the cytokine TNF. Anti-TNF antibody therapy is associated with an increased risk of serious infections and a dose-dependent increased risk of malignancies in patients with RA.[119] Leflunomide, which inhibits pyrimidine synthesis and may inhibit T-cell activation, may cause diarrhea, abdominal pain, allergic reactions, and elevated serum transaminases.[118]

Many patients with RA will take NSAIDS, which can cause gastric ulcerations and affect kidney function.[118] Older medications sometimes used include aspirin, which inhibits platelet function; intramuscular doses of gold salts, which may cause stomatitis; blood dyscrasias or nephrotic syndrome; azathioprine, which is associated with bone marrow suppression, hepatitis, or pancreatitis; and D-penicillamine, a drug that may cause bone marrow depression, renal toxicity, hepatotoxicity, or drug-induced pemphigus. Therefore, any patient who is taking any of these drugs should have a complete blood count and serum chemistry studies prior to invasive dental treatment.

Patients with cervical spine disease may have C1–C2 subluxation and spinal cord compression. Hyperextension of the neck must be avoided. Prolonged morning stiffness is common in RA, so later-morning appointments may be best for patients. Patients with severe RA who have prosthetic joints may require prophylactic antibiotic therapy before invasive dental procedures (Table 5). No prophylaxis is indicated for otherwise healthy patients 2 years following placement of the prosthesis. However, patients should receive prophylactic antibiotics after the 2 years if they are on immunosuppressive agents or have had postoperative joint infections. Antibiotic prophylaxis should be considered for patients who will be undergoing dental procedures that are associated with a higher incidence of bacteremia. Such procedures include dental extractions, periodontal surgery, implant placement, replacement of avulsed teeth, endodontic therapy beyond the apex, intraligamentary local anesthetic injections,

TABLE 5 Indications for 2003 Antibiotic Prophylaxis Guidelines for Dental Patients with Total Joint Replacements and Suggested Antibiotic Regimens

Dental procedures for which antibiotic prophylaxis recommended
  Dental extractions
  Periodontal procedures
  Dental implant placement
  Endodontic instrumentation beyond apex or endodontic surgery
  Initial placement of orthodontic bands (not brackets)
  Intraligamentary injections of local anesthetic
  Prophylactic cleaning of teeth or implants when bleeding is anticipated

Suggested antibiotic prophylaxis regimens
  Patient not allergic to penicillin: cephalexin, cephadrine, or amoxicillin 2 g PO 1 h before dental procedure
  Patient not allergic to penicillin and unable to take oral medications: cefazolin (1 g) or ampicillin (2 g) IM or IV 1 h before dental procedure
  Patient allergic to penicillin: clindamycin 600 mg PO 1 h before dental procedure
  Patient allergic to penicillin and unable to take oral medications: clindamycin 600 mg IV 1 h before dental procedure

Adapted from[137]
IM = intramuscularly; IV = intravenously; PO = orally.

placement of orthodontic bands, and any procedure in which bleeding is anticipated.[31] Patients with Sjögren's syndrome may require additional instruction in personal oral care and instruction on diet and dietary modifications (see Chapter 8, Salivary Gland Diseases). They should use topical fluorides such as 1.1% neutral sodium fluoride to prevent caries and have more frequent recall visits and radiography and more conservative treatment plans. Salivary stimulants such the cholinergic agonists pilocarpine or cevimeline can be prescribed for eligible patients. If the RA patient has Felty's syndrome, a complete blood count should be obtained before treatment since these patients may have neutropenia and thrombocytopenia.[101]

Mixed Connective Tissue Disease

The term *mixed connective tissue disease* (MCTD) was adopted in 1972 to describe a condition that has overlapping clinical features of SLE, PSS, and DM. The prevalence of MCTD is unknown, and there is some debate as to whether it is a distinct clinical entity.[120]

ETIOLOGY, PATHOGENESIS, AND CLINICAL MANIFESTATIONS

There are few long-term studies of patients with this disease. Most patients with MCTD are females who develop symptoms in the second or third decade of life.[49] Initial presentation usually includes polyarthritis, myositis, Raynaud's phenomenon, puffy hands or mild sclerodactyly, interstitial lung disease, and esophageal dysmotility.[120] Other inflammatory manifestations of MCTD include serositis, skin rash, arthritis, aseptic meningitis, myocarditis, myositis, lymphadenopathy, anemia, trigeminal nerve sensory neuropathy, and leukopenia.[121] In addition, patients may have scleroderma-like features, including esophageal involvement and pulmonary hypertension that can be unresponsive to corticosteroid therapy. Peripheral neuropathies, nephrotic syndrome, and severe deforming arthropathy are known to occur. Gastrointestinal manifestations of MCTD are similar to those in scleroderma. Pulmonary hypertension is the main cause of death in patients.[122]

LABORATORY FINDINGS AND DIAGNOSIS

The presence of autoantibodies against the U1 small nuclear ribonucleoprotein autoantigen (U1-snRNP) is an essential component of the classification criteria for MCTD (see Table 2).[49] Other characteristic laboratory abnormalities in MCTD cases include high titers (>1:1,000) of speckled ANAs.

ORAL MANIFESTATIONS AND DENTAL MANAGEMENT

Little has been reported concerning the oral manifestations of MCTD. Focal sialadenitis and other salivary findings supporting the diagnosis of secondary Sjögren's syndrome were present in 14 of 15 patients with MCTD in one small study.[123] Patients receiving high-dose immunosuppression should be managed appropriately (see "Dental Management" under "Systemic Lupus Erythematosus," above).

▼ ALLERGY AND HYPERSENSITIVITY REACTIONS

The modern dentist uses a wide variety of drugs to treat patients, including antibiotics, hypnotics, and anesthetics. All practitioners who use these medications must know how to manage adverse reactions triggered by these agents. A dental practitioner also uses a wide range of materials, such as impression materials, adhesives, latex, and restorative and endodontic materials that contain potential allergens. These include preservatives, coloring agents, fixatives, binding agents, flavorings, and latex.

Hypersensitivity Reactions

Immunologic reactions may be of several different types: type 1 IgE mediated (anaphylactic), type 2 antibody mediated, type 3 (immune complex mediated), and type 4 (cell-mediated or delayed hypersensitivity). Type 1 reactions are acute (eg, penicillin, latex, or peanut allergy) and require immediate recognition and action. Type 2 reactions are not usually found in response to dental materials or drugs but are found in autoimmune conditions affecting the oral cavity, such as pemphigus. Such conditions are discussed in Chapter 3, "Ulcerative, Vesicular, and Bullous Lesions." Type 3 reactions can be seen in response to dental materials but more commonly in response to viral infections, such as recurrent herpes labialis, giving rise to erythema multiforme or Stevens-Johnson syndrome (clinical manifestations are discussed in Chapter 4). Delayed hypersensitivity (cell-mediated or contact sensitivity) reactions to dental materials are very common and are usually seen in the oral cavity where an amalgam or gold restoration is in direct contact with the buccal or lingual mucosa. Stomatitis associated with allergy is discussed in Chapter 4. In this section, acute allergic reactions and their management are discussed.

Acute allergic reactions are caused by an immediate-type hypersensitivity reaction mediated by IgE and are the most serious of allergies. Reactions can occur rapidly, and full-scale anaphylactic reactions may occur and be associated with local and systemic swelling. Type 1 reactions require the presence of mast cells with attached IgE. A patient previously exposed to a drug or other antigen has antibody (primarily IgE) fixed to mast cells. When the antigen (in the form of a drug, food, or an airborne substance) is reintroduced into the body, it will react with and cross-link the cell-bound antibody. This causes an increase in intracellular calcium and the release of preformed mediators, including histamine, proteases, and newly synthetized lipid-derived mediators such as leukotrienes and prostaglandins. Cytokines are also released, which attract eosinophils and augment the inflammatory response. These substances cause vasodilation and increased capillary permeability, ultimately leading to fluid and leukocyte accumulation in the tissues and edema formation. Constriction of bronchial smooth muscle results when IgE is bound in the pulmonary region. The anaphylactic reaction may be localized, producing urticaria and angioedema, or may result in a generalized reaction, causing anaphylactic shock (Figure 17).

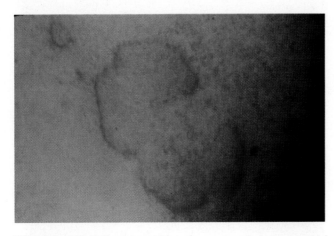

FIGURE 17 Urticaria resulting from use of a nonsteroidal anti-inflammatory drug.

LOCALIZED ANAPHYLAXIS

A localized anaphylactic reaction involving superficial blood vessels results in urticaria (hives). Urticaria begins with pruritus in the area where histamine and other active substances are released. Wheals (welts) then appear on the skin as an area of localized edema on an erythematous base. These lesions can occur anywhere on the skin or mucous membranes. There seems to be little doubt that the oral mucosa is well endowed with mast cells and that type 1 reactions can occur in the oral cavity. Urticaria of the lips and the oral mucosa occurs most frequently after food ingestion by an allergic individual. Common food allergens include chocolate, nuts, shellfish, and tomatoes. Drugs such as penicillin and aspirin may cause urticaria, and cold, heat, or even pressure may cause the reaction in susceptible individuals. Impression compounds, coloring agents and preservatives, and ingredients of mouthwashes may all cause local anaphylaxis.

Angioedema (incorrectly called angioneurotic edema in earlier literature) is characterized by rapid development of edematous swelling, particularly of the head and neck, sometimes accompanied by urticarial rashes. It occurs when blood vessels deep in the subcutaneous tissues are affected, producing a large diffuse area of subcutaneous swelling under normal overlying skin. This reaction may be caused by contact with a known allergen, but a significant number of cases are idiopathic. Many patients have short-term disfiguring facial swelling, but if the edema involves the neck and extends to the larynx, it can lead to fatal respiratory failure.

Angioedema most commonly occurs on the lips and tongue and around the eyes (Figure 18). It is temporary but not serious unless the posterior portion of the tongue or larynx compromises respiration. The patient who is in respiratory distress should be treated immediately with 0.5 mL of epinephrine (1:1,000) subcutaneously or, preferably, intramuscularly. This can be repeated every 10 minutes until recovery starts. The patient should be given oxygen, placed in a recumbent position with the lower extremities elevated unless there is a danger of shortness of breath or vomiting,

given fluids intravenously, and transported to hospital immediately. Patients may need intubation to maintain the airway.[124,125] When the immediate danger has passed, 50 mg of diphenhydramine hydrochloride (Benadryl, Pfizer, Parsippany, NJ) should be given four times a day until the swelling diminishes.

Hereditary angioedema is another life-threatening condition that is not associated with allergens.[126] It is a genetic disease with an autosomal dominant pattern of inheritance. The underlying defect is a failure to produce adequate levels of C1 esterase inhibitor, which normally acts as an inhibitor of the first component of complement and kallikrein. This inhibitor controls the degree of complement activation. Activation of kinin-like substances causes a sudden increase in capillary permeability. C4 is consumed and plasma levels fall, but C3 levels remain normal. An acquired form of angioedema in which antibody develops against C1 esterase inhibitor has also been described. Dental procedures can trigger attacks of hereditary angioedema. These attacks do not respond well to epinephrine, and diagnosed patients are usually treated with the androgen danazol, which increases C1 esterase inhibitor plasma levels. Fresh frozen plasma may be given to patients before dental procedures until recombinant C1 esterase inhibitor is available for clinical use.

GENERALIZED ANAPHYLAXIS

Generalized anaphylaxis is an allergic emergency. The mechanism of generalized anaphylaxis is the reaction of IgE antibodies to an allergen causing the release of histamine, bradykinin, and slow reactive substance of anaphylaxis (SRS-A) from mast cells and later eosinophil chemotactic factor (ECF). These chemical mediators cause the contraction of smooth muscles of the respiratory and intestinal tracts, as well as increased vascular permeability. Within dentistry, penicillin is a frequently encountered cause, but muscle relaxants, cephalosporins, sulfonamides, vancomycin, radiographic contrast media, and vaccines may also cause anaphylaxis.

The following factors increase the patient's risk of anaphylaxis: (1) a history of allergy to other drugs or food, (2) a history of asthma, (3) a family history of allergy (atopy), and (4) parenteral administration of the drug. Anaphylactic reactions may occur within seconds of drug administration or may occur 30 to 40 minutes later, complicating the diagnosis. Symptoms of generalized anaphylaxis should be known so that diagnosis and prompt treatment may be initiated. It is important to be able to differentiate anaphylaxis from syncope or a hypoglycemic event. The generalized anaphylactic reaction may involve the skin, the cardiovascular system, the gastrointestinal tract, and the respiratory system. The first signs often occur on the skin and are similar to those seen in localized anaphylaxis (eg, facial flushing, pruritis, paresthesia, or peripheral coldness). Pulmonary symptoms include dyspnea, wheezing, and asthma. Gastrointestinal tract disease, such as abdominal pain and vomiting, often follows skin symptoms. Symptoms of hypotension (loss of consciousness,

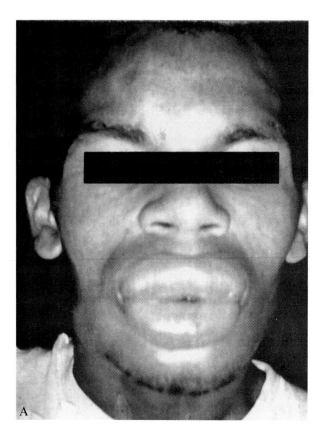

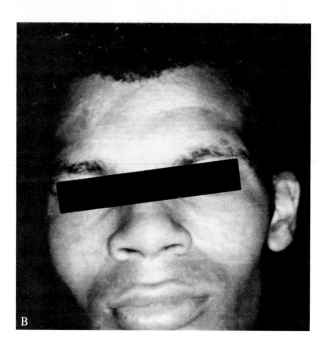

FIGURE 18 *A*, Angioedema of an allergic reaction to intramuscularly administered penicillin. *B*, Same patient 48 hours later, after therapy with epinephrine and antihistamine agents.

pallor, and a cold clammy skin) appear as the result of the loss of intravascular fluid. The pulse becomes rapid, weak, and faint. If untreated, this leads to shock. Patients with generalized anaphylactic reactions may die from respiratory failure, hypotensive shock, or laryngeal edema.

The most important therapy for generalized anaphylaxis is the administration of epinephrine. Clinicians should have a vial of aqueous epinephrine (at a 1:1,000 dilution) and a sterile syringe easily accessible. For adults, 0.5 mL of epinephrine should be administered intramuscularly or subcutaneously; smaller doses from 0.1 to 0.3 mL should be used for children, depending on their size. If the allergen was administered in an extremity, a tourniquet should be placed above the injection site to minimize further absorption into the blood. The absorption can be further reduced by injecting 0.3 mL of epinephrine (1:1,000) directly into the injection site. The tourniquet should be removed every 10 minutes. Epinephrine will usually reverse all severe signs of generalized anaphylaxis. If improvement is not observed in 10 minutes, readminister epinephrine. If the patient continues to deteriorate, several steps can be taken, depending on whether the patient is experiencing bronchospasm or edema. For bronchospasm, slowly inject 250 mg of aminophylline intravenously, over a period of 10 minutes. Too rapid an administration can lead to fatal cardiac arrhythmias. Do not give aminophylline if hypotensive shock is a part of the clinical picture. Inhalation sympathomimetics may also be used to treat bronchospasm, and oxygen should be given to prevent or manage hypoxia. For the patient with laryngeal edema,

establish an airway. This may necessitate endotracheal intubation; in some cases, a cricothyroidotomy may be necessary. Patients who have had an anaphylactic attack should carry self-injectable epinephrine.[125]

Latex Allergy

Latex allergy has been noticed with increasing frequency over the last few years. The increased use of protective gloves has led to numerous undesirable cutaneous and mucosal reactions. Dental staff and students appear to be at high risk of latex sensitization, which occurs as early as the second year of glove use. The overall prevalence of skin sensitization in dentists in a number of studies was about 10% compared with 16% in anesthetists, 5 to 8% in general hospital staff, and 9% in nurses, although this may be 30% in those reporting asthmatic symptoms. Much of the sensitization appears to have been by inhalation of the glove powder.[127]

The symptoms of latex allergy are usually those of type 1 hypersensitivity, but contact dermatitis to rubber chemicals is also well described. Allergenic proteins have been identified, but testing for them is not yet routine. Cross-reacting antigens are found in banana, kiwifruit, avocado, and chestnuts. The important concept that latex allergy can induce clinical symptoms to specific foods (food allergy) is reinforced by the demonstration of amino acid sequence homology between latex antigens and proteins in kiwifruit, avocado, tomatoes, and potatoes. Cross-reacting IgE antibodies to 33 and 37 kDa antigens shared between bananas and latex have been described.[128]

TESTING

Recently, a skinprick test reagent that contains most of the known clinically significant allergens for diagnosis of type 1 latex allergy was standardized. The protein content of the gloves correlates with immunoreactivity, and the ratio of the IgE to IgG response correlated positively with the severity of symptoms. In most studies, a history of atopy was a significant factor in latex allergy. There seems to be a reasonable correlation between in vitro IgE testing and in vivo skinprick tests.

MANAGEMENT

Patients with latex allergy may also show high levels of positive responses to certain foods, so a good medical history is imperative. Originally, urticaria, rhinitis, and eyelid edema were identified as immediate manifestations of latex allergy. Severe systemic reactions (such as asthma and anaphylaxis), which may result in permanent disability or even death, have now been recognized. In the health care setting, the two major strategies for management are the safe care of the latex allergic patient and the prevention and treatment of occupational latex allergy in employees. In managing a patient with latex sensitivity,[127] the distinction between an immediate hypersensitivity reaction to latex and an allergic contact dermatitis due to other irritants must be established. At initial evaluation, latex allergy status should be established by the history and documented clearly on the chart. Any history of an immediate hypersensitivity reaction to latex necessitates a latex-free environment for that person. The operatory should include nonlatex products; "hypoallergenic" latex gloves or latex-containing products (such as blood pressure cuffs and disposable tourniquets) should not be worn or used in the vicinity of persons who are allergic to latex. Premedication with antihistamines, steroids, and histamine H$_2$-blocking agents is sometimes carried out in operating rooms, but anaphylactic reactions have occurred despite such pretreatment. Workers who are irritated by gloves should change the type of gloves worn or change the type of soap used for scrubbing.

In addition, the use of cotton liners and emollients may effectively prevent sensitivity reactions. In cases of true latex allergy, the avoidance of all latex products is the only measure that can avert a serious allergic reaction. All persons with latex hypersensitivity should carry an epinephrine autoinjection kit and wear MedicAlert identification. Acute systemic reactions to latex should be treated in the same manner as other anaphylactic reactions are treated (ie, airway and circulation assessment, administration of oxygen, and administration of epinephrine and steroids as needed). In the course of resuscitation, all latex contact must be avoided.[129]

Oral Allergy Syndrome

Swelling of the lips, tongue and palate, and throat, along with oral pruritis and irritation, sometimes associated with other allergic clinical features, including rhinoconjunctivitis, urticaria, and even anaphylaxis, has been termed the oral allergy syndrome.[128] It seems to be precipitated by fresh foods, including apples, in people who have been sensitized to cross-reacting allergens in pollens, particularly birch.[130]

Serum Sickness

Serum sickness is named for its frequent occurrence after the administration of foreign serum, which was given for the treatment of infectious diseases before the advent of antibiotics. It is a type 3 immune complex–mediated disease. The reaction is now uncommon but still occurs as a result of the susceptible patient being given tetanus antitoxin, rabies antiserum, or drugs that combine with body proteins to form allergens. The pathogenesis of serum sickness differs from that of anaphylaxis. Antibodies form immunocomplexes in blood vessels with administered antigens. The complexes fix complement, which damages vessels and attracts leukocytes to the area, amplifying direct tissue injury. Serum sickness and vasculitis usually begin 7 to 10 days after the administration of the allergen, but this period can vary from 3 days to as long as 1 month. Unlike other allergic diseases, serum sickness may occur during the initial administration of the drug.

Major symptoms consist of fever, swelling, lymphadenopathy, joint and muscle pains, and rash. Less common manifestations include peripheral neuritis, kidney disease, and myocardial ischemia. Serum sickness is usually self-limiting, with spontaneous recovery in 1 to 3 weeks. Treatment is symptomatic; aspirin is given for arthralgia, and antihistamines are given for the skin rash. Severe cases should be treated with a short course of systemic corticosteroids, which significantly shortens the course of the disease. Although this reaction is rare, the dentist who is prescribing penicillin should be aware of the possibility of serum sickness occurring weeks after use of the drug. It is thought that penicillin binds to host proteins to form a recognizable antigen, and as antibodies form, they meet across vessel walls and give a localized vasculitis.

▼ SELECTED READINGS

Amerongen AV, Veerman EC. Saliva—the defender of the oral cavity. Oral Dis 2002;8:12–22.

Axelrod L. Perioperative management of patients treated with glucocorticoids. Endocrinol Metab Clin North Am 2003;32:367–83.

Atkinson JC, O'Connell A, Aframian D. Oral manifestations of primary immunological diseases. J Am Dent Assoc 2000;131:345–56.

Bonilla FA, Geha RS. 2. Update on primary immunodeficiency diseases. J Allergy Clin Immunol 2006;117(2 Suppl):S435–41.

Brennan MT, Valerin MA, Napenas JJ, Lockhart PB. Oral manifestations of patients with lupus erythematosus. Dent Clin North Am 2005;49:127–41, ix.

Charles C, Clements P, Furst DE. Systemic sclerosis: hypothesis-driven treatment strategies. Lancet 2006;367:1683–91.

Dooley MA, Ginzler EM. Newer therapeutic approaches for systemic lupus erythematosus: immunosuppressive agents. Rheum Dis Clin North Am 2006;32:91–102, ix.

Grimbacher B, Holland SM, Puck JM. Hyper-IgE syndromes. Immunol Rev 2005;203:244–50.

Harris ED BR, Budd RC, Firestein GS, et al. Kelley's textbook of rheumatology. 7th ed. Philadelphia: Elsevier; 2005.

Huber MA, Terezhalmy GT. Adverse reactions to latex products: preventive and therapeutic strategies. J Contemp Dent Pract 2006;7:97–106.

Lockhart PB, Brennan MT, Fox PC, et al. Decision-making on the use of antimicrobial prophylaxis for dental procedures: a survey of infectious disease consultants and review. Clin Infect Dis 2002;34:1621–6.

Mak TW, Saunders ME. The immune response. Basic and clinical principles. London: Elsevier; 2006.

Nath SK, Kilpatrick J, Harley JB. Genetics of human systemic lupus erythematosus: the emerging picture. Curr Opin Immunol 2004;16:794–800.

Oddis CV. Idiopathic inflammatory myopathy: management and prognosis. Rheum Dis Clin North Am 2002;28:979–1001.

Pisetsky DS, St Clair EW. Progress in the treatment of rheumatoid arthritis. JAMA 2001;286:2787–90.

Rus VHA, Hochberg M. Systemic lupus erythematosus. In: Silman AJ, editor. Epidemiology of rheumatic diseases. New York: Oxford University Press; 2001. p. 123–40.

Schiodt M. Oral manifestations of lupus erythematosus. Int J Oral Surg 1984;13:101–47.

Sicherer SH, Leung DY. Advances in allergic skin disease, anaphylaxis, and hypersensitivity reactions to foods, drugs, and insects. J Allergy Clin Immunol 2006;118:170–7.

Sampson HA, Munoz-Furlong A, Campbell RL, et al. Second symposium on the definition and management of anaphylaxis: summary report—second National Institute of Allergy and Infectious Disease/Food Allergy and Anaphylaxis Network symposium. Ann Emerg Med 2006;47:373–80.

Sullivan KE. The clinical, immunological, and molecular spectrum of chromosome 22q11.2 deletion syndrome and DiGeorge syndrome. Curr Opin Allergy Clin Immunol 2004;4:505–12.

For the full reference list, please refer to the accompanying CD ROM.

19
▼

TRANSPLANTATION MEDICINE

THOMAS P. SOLLECITO, DMD
ANDRES PINTO, DMD, MPH
ALI NAJI, MD, PhD
DAVID PORTER, MD

Transplantation has become the treatment of choice for the restoration of function in end-stage organ disease. Innovative surgical techniques have played a major role in enhancing the success of organ transplants, leading to improved graft and patient survival. Advances in the biology of organ preservation have led to improved cold storage of the solid organs, improving the overall quality of the transplanted organs and diminishing the damage incurred by warm ischemia, allowing optimization of the medical conditions of the donor and the recipient.[1] Furthermore, insights into the biology of immune responses to transplanted tissues have aided the development of immunosuppressive agents to prevent the rejection of the organ transplants while minimizing the morbidities associated with the chronic immunosuppression of the recipients. The main limitation to even greater use of transplantation as a treatment modality for end-stage organ damage is the shortage of organ donors.

Attempts at organ and bone marrow transplantation date back to the 1800s. In more recent history, Dr. Joseph Murray performed the first successful human renal transplantation between identical twin brothers in 1954. This procedure was well tolerated as there was no rejection by the genetically identical recipient. The first successful allogeneic (not genetically identical) transplantation was a kidney transplant between fraternal twins performed in 1959 in which the recipient was "conditioned" (immunosuppressed to prevent rejection) by total-body irradiation. In 1962, a successful cadaveric donor renal transplantation was achieved, and in 1966, a pancreas transplantation was successfully performed. In the following year, the first human liver transplantation was performed, resulting in a 13-month survival. In the same year, a heart was transplanted. In 1968, a genetically related bone marrow transplantation (today referred to as a hematopoietic cell transplantation [HCT]) was performed, and in 1973, a genetically unrelated HCT was performed. Lung transplantation has also been performed both as a single procedure and in combination with a heart transplantation. The first heart-lung transplantation in the United States was done in 1981, and the first single-lung transplantation in Canada was performed in 1983. Other organs that have been successfully transplanted include the small bowel, the skin, various limbs, and components of the human eye.

In the past 20 years, significant advances, including tissue typing and the development of immunosuppressive medications, have increased the success of transplantation. Overall, long-term patient survival has also significantly increased over the past 30 years, both in solid organ and HCT recipients. Most transplant clinicians consider the discovery of the immunosuppressive agent cyclosporine (CSA) to be the most significant advance in transplantation medicine. This medication was approved for use in 1983.[2]

Both solid organ and non–solid organ transplantations are becoming more routine throughout the world. In June 2006, nearly 100,000 patients in the United States alone were waiting for a solid organ transplant. In 2005, 28,108 solid organs were transplanted (Table 1). Presently, in the United

TABLE 1 Waiting Lists (as of June 30, 2006) and Transplanted Solid Organs (2005*) in the United States

Organ	Transplants Awaited	Transplants Performed
Liver	17,161	6,444
Kidney	67,010	16,476
Lung	2,942	1,406
Heart	2,933	2,125

Adapted from the 2005 annual report of the United States Scientific Register of Transplant Recipients, Organ Procurement and Transplantation Network.[2]

*Note that these numbers do not equal those cited in the text since other organs, including the small intestine and pancreas, are not included in this table.

States, there are over 800 transplantation programs performing various types of solid organ transplantations.[2]

As the process of solid organ transplantation expands, there is an urgent need to increase the supply of organs suitable for transplantation. The limitation of available donor organs will hopefully become less of an issue with increased awareness of organ donation and perhaps with alternative organ procurement methods, including xenografts or stem cell–derived tissue.

The likelihood of a dentist having the opportunity to treat a transplanted patient is increasing as many of these transplant recipients resume normal ways of life after the transplantation. This chapter reviews different aspects of transplantation medicine pertinent for the oral health professional.

▼ CLASSIFICATION

When describing a transplant, most clinical classification systems employ both the type of tissue transplanted and the genetic relationship of the tissue to the recipient. It is extremely important for the clinician to know exactly what type of transplantation was performed as both the management and the prognosis are intimately related. This will become evident as it is discussed later in this chapter.

Some authorities broadly divide clinical transplantations as being either a solid organ/tissue or an HCT. Virtually all types of solid organs/tissues have been transplanted, including hearts, lungs, kidneys, livers, intestines, pancreas, skin, and eye components, as well as composite tissue transplants, including the face and limbs. Another type of transplantation frequently used to treat various hematologic and nonhematologic malignancies/disorders is known as HCT. HCT uses either an autologous graft (in some cases of hematologic malignancies, autoimmune diseases, and even some solid tumors) or a donor (allogeneic graft); HCT poses special management concerns to the clinician, which are detailed in this chapter.

Classification of transplants can also be based broadly on the genetic relationship of the recipient to the donor. For the purpose of this chapter, the transplanted cell, tissue, or organ is referred to as the graft. A transplant to and from one's self (autograft) is known as an autologous transplant. A transplantation from an identical twin (identical genetic make-up) is known as an isograft, with the process of this type of transplantation known as isogeneic or syngeneic transplantation. Most transplants are from donors that are not genetically identical to the recipient (allografts). These types of transplants are known as allogeneic transplants. Finally, transplants from donors of one species to recipients of another species (xenografts) are known as xenogeneic transplants (Table 2).[3]

Due to the scarcity of isografts and the obvious limitations to autografts, allogeneic transplants are most commonly used today. The success of allogeneic transplantation relies on sophisticated mechanisms for identifying and matching specific genetic markers between the donor and the recipient, as well as suppressing the recipient's immune system to prevent transplant rejection. These are the concepts that serve as the basic foundation in transplantation medicine. In the future, these concepts may be extended and improved to allow transplantation across species. Tissue xenografts, which have been treated to reduce their immunogenicity, have been used as a successful treatment modality in some applications (ie, porcine heart valves), but whole-organ xenografts have been unsuccessful. Research regarding genetically altered xenografts is ongoing. When the important immunologic barriers to xenogeneic transplantation are eliminated, the use of animal donors may possibly alleviate the relative paucity of available organs. Of course, significant ethical questions, as well as transplant longevity and transmissible infectious diseases from animals, are questions that must be entertained before these types of transplants become commonplace.[4–6] Perhaps genetically derived tissues/organs may someday be fabricated in vitro and transplanted back into the patient.

▼ TRANSPLANTATION IMMUNOLOGY

Transplantation immunology encompasses most aspects of the human immune response to alloantigens expressed by the donor organ/tissue. When donor and recipient genetic disparities exist, the recipient mounts a specific immune response to the alloantigens expressed by the donor grafted organ/tissue. Transplantation medicine would be grossly unsuccessful if this concept were not appropriately appreciated and manipulated. To appreciate the intricacies of organ transplantation, a basic understanding of immunologic concepts is helpful.

Lymphocytes, particularly T lymphocytes (T cells), are activated after allogeneic transplantation and are critical effector populations mediating the immunologic rejection of the transplants. The major histocompatibility complex (MHC), a genetic region found on the short arm of chromosome number 6 of all mammalian cells, codes for products (antigens) that allow immune cells to identify self from nonself. In humans, the self-antigens encoded by the MHC include the human leukocyte antigen (HLA) system. Although there are many other gene products, from more than 30 histocompatibility gene loci, that can stimulate graft rejection, it is the HLA system that produces the strongest immunologic response.[3]

MHC genes are inherited from each parent; every child has components of both the mother's and the father's HLAs on their cell surfaces. The MHC/HLA system is broadly divided into regions. MHC class I and class II regions are those significantly involved in rejection. MHC class I regions include HLA-A, -B, -C, -E, -F, and -G. (The present role of the E, F, and G regions in transplantation is not well understood.) MHC class II regions include HLA-DR, -DQ, -DP, -DO, and -DN. MHC class II genes have two chains, allowing for four different gene products for each locus.

The MHC has extensive polymorphism, allowing remarkable diversity among genes of the HLA system.[7] There are over 180 different class I alleles in the HLA-B region alone and over 220 class II alleles in just one loci of the HLA-DR region that have been recognized in humans. Today, deoxyribonucleic acid (DNA)-based typing (see below) has led to a more specific and detailed classification of the transplantation genes, such that the HLA alleles are related to their DNA sequences.[7]

HLA class I antigens are expressed on most nucleated cells and on red blood cells, whereas class II antigens are expressed only on certain cells known as antigen-presenting cells (APCs). APCs include macrophages, B cells, dendritic cells, and some endothelial cells. The expression of these MHC gene products (antigens) on a cell's surface is regulated by various cytokines such as interferon-γ (IFN-γ) and tumor necrosis factor (TNF).

Transplanted foreign MHC molecules activate the immune response by stimulating the recipient's T cells to respond to foreign antigens. The interaction of the MHC of the donor cells with the recipient's T-cell receptor (TCR) initiates the immune reaction. T cells can be activated either by the donor's or the recipient's APCs, resulting in expression and production of lymphokines and cytokines that promote activation of cytotoxic T cells, activation of B cells, and activation of natural killer cell activity, as well as promote enhanced expression of MHC and increased macrophage activity. This, in turn, causes further immune reactions that result in direct tissue damage and damage to the vascular endothelium of the graft, which may ultimately result in graft rejection.

TABLE 2 Types of Transplants

Type of Graft	Procedure	Description
Autograft	Autologous	Transplant from self
Isograft	Syngeneic	Transplant between genetically identical individuals (monozygotic twin)
Allograft	Allogeneic	Transplant from a genetically different individual of the same species
Xenograft	Xenogeneic	Transplants between different species

Despite the treatment of recipients with immunosuppressive drugs, the possibility of the immunologic rejection is not entirely eliminated. The rejection may evolve as an acute process occurring within days to weeks of the transplantation surgery. This acute process is related to the primary activation of T cells and usually can be reversed by modifying or intensifying the immunosuppressive regimen.

Chronic rejection of the transplanted organ is also a significant problem leading to organ failure. This type of rejection is slow and insidious and in most cases cannot be reversed by conventional immunosuppressive drugs. It probably occurs by continued, albeit muted, cell-mediated toxicity that results in vascular endothelial damage of the transplanted organ (as well as other actions, which have not been fully elucidated), leading ultimately to graft failure.[8]

Another type of rejection is known as hyperacute rejection; this occurs within minutes to hours after a transplantation procedure. This pattern of rejection occurs in patients who have undergone previous transplantations, patients who have had multiple pregnancies, and patients who have had multiple blood transfusions. It is caused by the presence of preformed antidonor antibodies in the recipient that activate complement cascade, resulting in severe damage to the parenchymal constituents of the graft, which often cannot be reversed (Table 3).[9,10]

▼ CLINICAL INDICATIONS

The clinical indications for transplantation vary, but the disease outcome is usually fatal without the transplant (except perhaps for renal, pancreatic, eye, skin, or limb), regardless of the transplant indication. The more common indications for transplantation are listed in Table 4.

Other indications can also be added to this list when quality of life can be improved by transplantation. For example, autologous HCT may ameliorate the affects of systemic lupus erythematosus or other autoimmune disorders.[11] More recently, autologous HCT has been cited as a possible treatment for the management of various solid tumors, including metastatic breast cancer,[12] although the role in this indication remains controversial.[13] Other potential uses for stem cell therapy in various other disorders, such as diabetes and amyloidosis, are also being considered.[14–17]

TABLE 3   Rejection

Type of Rejection	Description
Acute	Usually occurs within days to weeks due to primary activation of the T-cell response
Chronic	Usually occurs months to years after transplantation; probably occurs by continued, albeit muted, cell-mediated toxicity and other unclear causes
Hyperacute	Usually occurs minutes to hours after transplantation and is caused by preformed antidonor antibodies activating complement

TABLE 4   Major Indications for Transplantation*

Type of Transplant	Indications
Kidney	End-stage renal disease Glomerulonephritis Pyelonephritis Congenital abnormalities Nephrotic syndrome
Liver	End-stage liver disease Primary biliary cirrhosis Biliary atresia (children) Chronic hepatitis Sclerosing cholangitis
Pancreas	Severe diabetes leading to renal disease
Intestinal	Massive short-bowel syndrome
Heart	Cardiomyopathy Severe coronary artery disease Congestive heart failure
Heart and lung	Multiorgan end-stage disease Congenital abnormalities Amyloidosis
Lung	Primary pulmonary hypertension COPD/emphysema Pulmonary fibrosis Cystic fibrosis
Hematopoietic cell transplantation (autologous)	Acute myelogenous leukemia, multiple myeloma and amyloidosis, lymphoma (Hodgkin's and non-Hodgkin's), possibly solid tumors (breast, germ cell, ovarian), ? SLE/autoimmune disorders
Hematopoietic cell transplantation (allogeneic)	Acute myelogenous leukemia, acute lymphoblastic leukemia, chronic myelogenous leukemia, aplastic anemia, primary immunodeficiencies, hemoglobinopathies (sickle cell, thalassemia)

COPD = chronic obstructive pulmonary disorder; SLE = systemic lupus erythematosus.
*Partial listing only.

▼ MEDICAL MANAGEMENT

Medical management of the transplant candidate focuses on successfully preventing rejection. In solid organ transplantation, when the donor and recipient tissue are genetically identical (autologous or syngeneic), the outcome of the transplantation is dependent solely upon the surgical success of the procedure. For autologous HCT, success is largely dependent on the high-dose chemotherapy or radiation used to irradicate residual malignant cells prior to HCT. When tissue from genetically different sources is transplanted, a sophisticated means of preventing rejection must be instituted to ensure graft survival, and in the setting of allogeneic stem cell transplant, methods must be used to prevent not just graft rejection but also graft-versus-host disease (GVHD), as described below. Transplantation surgeons and oncologists have mastered the surgical procedures for various transplantations; medical management to achieve longer-term successful grafts and longer-term overall patient survival has been quite successful, yet it still is fraught with complications. The success of an allogeneic transplantation relies on the ability to identify and match certain genetic markers between the donor and the recipient while suppressing the recipient's immune system in order to prevent rejection. In addition, one must also be concerned with suppressing the new donor immune system in HCT, to prevent rejection of the host, referred to as GVHD.

▼ BLOOD AND TISSUE TYPING

Blood and tissue matching is used today for all allogeneic transplants. Standard ABO and Rh±blood typing is performed to prevent red blood cell agglutination. In addition to blood typing, some method of tissue typing is usually performed (as timing allows) before solid allogeneic transplantations take place and always before allogeneic HCT. Tissue typing allows for matching of the HLA system of antigens found on donor and recipient cells. There is significant variation in HLA testing, depending on the methods employed. Furthermore, based on the type of organ to be transplanted, there is variation in the extent of testing needed to safely transplant the organ. For example, typing is mandatory in allogeneic HCT, but it may be less important in first renal transplantations and for graft survival in liver or heart transplantations.[18] Tissue typing generally can be performed by serologic or DNA-based testing methods. Serologic testing methods for HLA class I antigen identification can be performed by adding antisera of known HLA specificity with complement to a donor sample. Death of the donor cells confirms that they carried the specific HLA antigen. This test usually can be conducted in a couple of hours.[3]

Another test used to specifically determine HLA class II antigens is the mixed lymphocyte culture reaction, in which test lymphocytes are incubated with cells expressing known HLA. This results in either proliferation of the stimulated cell or no reaction if the HLA region is the same. This test is time consuming, and because of the short viability of the donor organ/tissue, it is not practical to confirm HLA compatibility in a deceased donor allogeneic transplantation.[7]

DNA-based testing for tissue typing is being used more commonly today. Polymerase chain reaction is used to identify the DNA in the HLA genes of both the donor and recipient cells. As DNA-based techniques become a more common method for tissue typing, HLA nomenclature will probably change to reflect DNA sequences rather than names that have been serologically defined previously.

Matching for all known HLA alleles is not practical. However, matching for specific MHC class I and class II antigens, especially HLA-A,-B, -C, and -DR (and perhaps -DQ), is important for transplant success in HCT and renal transplantation.

Cross-matching (crossing recipient serum with donor lymphocytes) is usually done to prevent hyperacute rejection in allogeneic solid organ transplants. This is a basic serologic test that is regarded as necessary in those allogeneic transplant recipients who have previously experienced massive immune challenges such as a prior transplantation, multiple pregnancies, or multiple blood transfusions. Since transplantation of solid organs (heart, lung, liver) often requires some expediency, time-consuming complex cross-matching or tissue typing cannot be performed. Instead, absence of antibodies to a panel of cells (defined in advance and known as panel-reactive antibodies) is usually adequate for heart and lung transplantation.[19] Interestingly, MHC compatibility in liver transplantation seems negligible in achieving better outcomes.[18] This is fortunate because the timing of liver transplantation often precludes HLA typing.[20]

▼ IMMUNOSUPPRESSION

Immunosuppressive regimens vary among transplant centers and according to the type of the transplanted organ (intestines, liver, etc.). Since tissues in allogeneic transplants are not genetically identical, medications used to control the immune response are essential for graft survival.[21,22] All allogeneic transplantations initially require immunosuppression if the transplanted organs are not to be acutely rejected. Furthermore, most allogeneic solid organ transplant recipients require lifelong maintenance immunosuppression. This is usually not the case with allogeneic HCT (and no immunosuppression is required for autologous HCT). Additionally, more intensive immunosuppressive regimens are employed later in the post-transplantation period in cases of acute rejection episodes.

Most immunosuppressive medications are nonspecific and cannot prevent a specific component of the immune response. More sophisticated and directed medications are being developed currently; these will allow for graft tolerance while allowing the body to still react to infectious and other detrimental antigens.

Arguably, the most significant advances in transplantation have been made in pharmacotherapeutic immunosuppression. As there is improved understanding of how graft rejection transpires, there is improvement in the specificity of the immunomodulator. The most frequently used contemporary medication classes are discussed in this chapter, with a brief review of some promising formulations (Table 5).

▼ CYCLOSPORINE ANALOGUES

CSA is a cyclic polypeptide macrolide medication derived from a metabolite of the fungus *Beauveria nivea*. It is indicated for the prevention of graft rejection because of its immunosuppressive effects. It specifically and reversibly inhibits immunocompetent lymphocytes in the G0 and G1 phase of the cell cycle. CSA binds with an intracellular protein, cyclophilin, and inhibits calcineurin. Calcineurin activates a nuclear component of T cells that is thought to initiate gene transcription for the formation of interleukin (IL)-2. Presumably, CSA inhibits IL-2 by preventing the expression of its gene. CSA also reduces the expression of IL-2 receptors.

TABLE 5 Major Immunosuppressive Agents*

Drug	Type	Indications	Major Side Effects[†]	Dental Implications[†]
Cyclosporine	Macrolide immunosuppressant Calcineurin inhibitor	Prophylaxis against organ rejection	Hepatotoxicity Nephrotoxicity Elevation of blood pressure	Immunosuppressant[‡] P-450 metabolized[§] Gingival hyperplasia Monitor CV system May effect renal elimination of some drugs Risk of neoplasm
Tacrolimus	Macrolide immunosuppressant Calcineurin inhibitor	Prophylaxis against organ rejection	Hepatotoxicity Neurotoxicity Nephrotoxicity Post-transplantation diabetes mellitus Elevation of blood pressure	Immunosuppressant[‡] P-450 metabolized[§] Monitor CV system May effect renal elimination of some drugs Risk of neoplasm
Sirolimus	Macrolide immunosuppressant	Prophylaxis against acute and perhaps chronic organ rejection	Hyperlipidemia Hypertriglyceremia	Immunosuppressant[‡] P-450 metabolized[§] Monitor CV system May effect renal elimination of some drugs Risk of neoplasm
Azathioprine	Antimetabolite	Prophylaxis against organ rejection	Bone marrow suppression Hepatotoxicity	Immunosuppressant[‡] Risk of neoplasm
Mycophenolate mofetil	Antimetabolite	Prophylaxis against organ rejection	Immunosuppressant[‡] Leukopenia	Absorption is altered by antibiotics, antacids, and bile acid binders Risk of neoplasm
ATG/ALG	Polyclonal antibody	Conditioning agents used prior to transplantation	Leukopenia PTLD Pulmonary edema Renal dysfunction	Immunosuppressant[‡]
Muromonab-CD3	Monoclonal antibody	Reversal of acute organ rejection, including steroid-resistant acute rejection	Cytokine release syndrome PTLD	Immunosuppressant[‡] Interacts with indomethacin
Daclizumab and basiliximab	Monoclonal antibodies	Reversal of acute organ rejection	Pulmonary edema Renal dysfunction	Immunosuppressant[‡] Risk of neoplasm
Corticosteroids	Nonspecific immunosupressant	Reversal of acute organ rejection	Multiple#	Broad nonspecific immunosuppressant[‡] Avoid NSAIDs and ASA Monitor CV system Poor wound healing Risk of neoplasm Steroid supplement may be needed with stressful procedures

ASA = acetylsalicylic acid; ATG/ALG = antithymocyte globulin/antilymphocyte globulin; CV = cardiovascular; NSAIDs = nonsteroidal anti-inflammatory drugs; PTLD = post-transplantation lymphoproliferative disease.

*Major mechanisms of action are outlined in the text.

[†]Partial listing only.

[‡]Use of an immunosuppressant results in an increased risk of infection.

[§]Dental/oral pharmacotherapeutics that are metabolized by the liver's cytochrome P-450 3A system alter this drug's serum levels. This group of medications includes, but is not limited to, erythromycin, clarithromycin, "azole" antifungals, benzodiazepines, carbamazepine, colchicines, prednisolone, and metronidazole.

T helper and, to some extent, T suppressor cells are preferentially suppressed.[23,24] This medication has some effect on humoral immunity but not on phagocytic function, neutrophil migration, macrophage migration, or direct bone marrow suppression. Absorption of this drug is variable, and frequent blood levels must be drawn to ensure that the drug is in the therapeutic range. A microemulsion formulation is used to enhance the drug's bioavailability.[25]

▼ TACROLIMUS

Tacrolimus (FK-506) (Prograf, Fujisawa Healthcare Inc, Deerfield, IL) is a macrolide immunosuppressant produced by *Streptomyces tsukubaensis* that is used to prevent organ rejection. This medication is similar to CSA in that it suppresses cell-mediated reactions by suppressing T-cell activation. Tacrolimus inhibits calcineurin by interacting with an intracellular protein known as the FK-binding protein. Consequently, T cells are not activated, and cell-mediated cytotoxicity is impeded.[24] There may be a lower incidence of rejection with the use of tacrolimus as compared with the use of CSA in liver, kidney, and lung transplantations. Overall graft and patient survival rates in kidney transplantations do not seem to differ significantly with the use of this medication.

▼ SIROLIMUS

Sirolimus (Rapamycin) (Rapamune, Wyeth-Ayerst Pharmaceuticals, Philadelphia, PA) is another macrolide immunosuppressive agent; it was discovered more than 25 years ago in the soil of Easter Island and is produced by *Streptomyces hygroscopicus*. It is used for prophylaxis against acute rejection of various organs[26–29] and may be appropriate for use in chronic rejection.[30] Sirolimus's mechanism of action is somewhat unique. Sirolimus inhibits the activation of a particular cellular kinase (target of rapamycin [TOR]), which then interferes with intracellular signaling pathways of the IL-2 receptor, thereby preventing lymphocyte activation. The response of T cells to IL-2 and other cytokines is inhibited. Specifically, the overall effect is interference of T-cell activation during the cells' G1 to S phase. Sirolimus is recommended to be used in conjunction with CSA and corticosteroids. This medication has been shown to reduce acute rejection in the first 6 months following renal transplantation, compared with rejection rates when azathioprine (AZA) is used.[31,32]

▼ AZATHIOPRINE

AZA is an antimetabolite that inhibits ribonucleic acid and DNA synthesis by interfering with the purine synthesis that results in decreased T- and B-cell proliferation. It does not interfere with lymphokine production but has significant anti-inflammatory properties. AZA can be bone marrow suppressive, leading to pancytopenia, and it can also cause significant liver dysfunction. Significant drug interactions with allopurinol[33] and angiotensin-converting enzyme inhibitors have been reported. AZA has been used for many years in conjunction with CSA and corticosteroids as triple immunosuppressive therapy. Today, mycophenolate mofetil (MMF), a newer purine analogue, is being used as an alternative to AZA as it may have a more specific action against T cells.

▼ MYCOPHENOLATE MOFETIL

MMF, an ester of mycophenolic acid, is an antimetabolite that is used for prophylaxis against graft rejection, and that may have some action in reversing ongoing acute rejection. It inhibits inflammation by interfering with purine synthesis. Both T cells and B cells, which are dependent on this synthesis for their proliferation, are prevented from reproducing. Additionally, MMF interferes with intercellular adhesion of lymphocytes to endothelial cells. It does not inhibit IL-1 or IL-2 but may inhibit medial smooth muscle proliferation. Based on a multicenter trial, it is thought that this medication can replace AZA in a triple-drug regimen in kidney and heart transplantation.[34] Although the incidence of graft rejection episodes is less with MMF, 1-year renal transplant graft and patient survival have not been significantly improved by the use of MMF.[35]

▼ MUROMONAB-CD3

Muromonab-CD3 (Orthoclone OKT-3, Ortho Biotech Products, L.P., Raritan, NJ) is a murine monoclonal antibody (IgG2A) to the CD3 receptor on mature human T cells. It is indicated for reversal of acute allograft rejection and cases of corticosteroid-resistant acute rejection. Monoclonal antibodies in general are effective immunosuppressants. They act by various mechanisms, including cell depletion (via opsonization or complement fixation) and antigenic modulation. Cell depletion occurs by phagocytosis or cell lysis. Cell surface coating acts to interfere with cell-to-cell interaction. Antigenic modulation works via redistributing antigen/antibody complexes on the cell surface by internalizing certain receptors or shedding them. OKT3 blocks the generation and function of cytotoxic/mature T cells. This drug is effective for approximately 1 week; approximately 3 days after administration, the patient has no detectable circulating mature T cells. There may be some neutralizing antibodies to OKT3.

▼ ANTITHYMOCYTE AND ANTILYMPHOCYTE GLOBULIN

Polyclonal antilymphocyte sera, antilymphocyte globulin, and antithymocyte globulin are part of the same medication class. These agents are produced by immunizing animals with human lymphoid cells; the animals then produce antibodies to reduce the number of circulating T cells. Individually, these agents affect lymphocyte immunosuppression by reacting with common T-cell surface markers and then coating (opsonizing) the lymphocyte—marking it as foreign for phagocytosis. Polyclonal antibodies are used as conditioning agents prior to transplantation.

▼ DACLIZUMAB AND BASILIXIMAB

Daclizumab and basiliximab are synthetic monoclonal antibodies used for reversal of acute organ rejection. They also have a significant role during induction immunosuppression.[36] These monoclonal antibodies bind the CD25 receptor (IL-2 receptor) on the surface of activated T cells (IL-2 receptor antagonists), preventing the expansion of CD4 and CD8 lymphocytes. They may be effective in conjunction with MMF and corticosteroids to eliminate the need for CSA use in the early post-transplantation period.[36] Anti-CD25 agents have also been reported to be efficacious in treatment of corticosteroid-resistant GVHD.[37]

Other promising targets for monoclonal antibody immunomodulation are being studied currently. The target receptors vary in their function, but development of target-specific medications will probably aid in selected immunosuppression.

▼ CORTICOSTEROIDS

Corticosteroids are consistently used in all allogeneic transplantations for prophylaxis against graft rejection and for reversal of acute rejection. The mechanism of action of this medication is extremely nonspecific as it affects the immune system in many complex ways. Steroids have anti-inflammatory effects and are able to suppress activated macrophages. They also interfere with antigen presentation and reduce the expression of MHC antigens on cells. Steroids reverse the effect of IFN-γ and alter the expression of adhesion molecules on vascular endothelium. These medications also have significant effects on IL-1 activity and block the IL-2 gene and its production.[38]

▼ OTHER CYTOTOXIC AGENTS

Cytotoxic agents that are used in conditioning bone marrow prior to HCT include medications, specifically busulfan and/or cyclophosphamide, and also total-body irradiation. They cause bone marrow suppression, resulting in pancytopenia (loss of cellular blood elements such as leukocytes and thrombocytes). Cytotoxic therapies are designed to destroy malignant cells, totally immunosuppress the recipient, and make room in the recipient's bone marrow for the HCT. As a result of these agents, the patient is not only highly susceptible to infection but is at a significantly high risk for bleeding.

▼ NEWER IMMUNOSUPPRESSIVE STRATEGIES

Novel approaches to immunosuppression are currently being developed. The definitive immunosuppressive agent would be an agent that is able to destroy only the T cells that are involved with graft rejection while leaving the remainder of the T cells and the immune system intact. Other monoclonal antibodies are currently under development, with promising immune modulation targets, including more specific T cells and natural killer cells, as well as endothelium-activated cells.[37]

FTY 720 is a new immunosuppressive compound that may cause antigen-induced apoptosis (programmed cell death)[39] of cytotoxic T cells; it is presently being studied in clinical trials.[40] This agent exhibits no inhibition on the production of IL-2 or IL-3 but seems to act synergistically with CSA. Further study of this agent's mechanism of action is warranted.[41,42]

Another promising approach to chemically induced immunosuppression is via a class of agents called the T-cell co-stimulatory pathway modifiers.[43] Studies have suggested that immune system function has significant self-regulatory capabilities. It is now well recognized that TCRs must recognize MHC-presented antigens to activate a T-cell response. However, it is also thought that TCR recognition requires two specific signals to stimulate T-cell activation—that is, recognition of both the TCR signal and a costimulatory receptor(s) such as CD28 and/or CD40 ligand, both mandatory for T-cell activation. Blocking of the costimulatory signal is the basis of this novel approach to preventing rejection of an allogeneic transplant. An engineered monoclonal antibody (Belatacept, LEA29Y) with potent costimulation blockade has been rationally designed from CTLA4-Ig-binding site modification. This monoclonal antibody has been an effective costimulatory agent in the prevention of renal transplant rejection, allowing avoidance of calcineurin inhibitor agents (tacrolimus and cyclosporine) that have nephrotoxicity.[44]

Another interesting finding that has been reported is that use of pravastatin during the early transplantation period may have some effect as an adjunct in immunosuppressive therapy via reduction in natural killer cell cytotoxicity.[45,46]

Although newer immunosuppressive agents have been developed and are being used, they have not shown any clear benefit in patient or organ survival over CSA or tacrolimus. The newer agents, however, have shown some promise in reducing the incidence and severity of rejection. These newer agents probably have a role in reducing the need for corticosteroids as well as reducing the toxic profiles of CSA or tacrolimus.[47]

Clinical studies to prove a possible synergistic interaction between sirolimus and CSA in reducing renal graft rejection may, in the future, reduce the need for steroids and CSA.[31] Thus far, sirolimus has been approved as an adjuvant to CSA.[48] Ultimately, graft and patient survival profiles coupled with side effects will determine the best antirejection "cocktail" to be used in various transplantations.

A different strategy, aimed at reducing the need for profound immunosuppression, is pretreatment of the recipient with donor blood. This procedure may extend graft survival, as evidenced in some animal models,[49] by enhancing chimerism (ability of both donor and recipient immunocompetent cells to coexist). This concept of transplantation tolerance, whereby the recipient's immune system is first significantly stimulated and then muted, was initially described by Starzl in 1963.[50] The exact mechanism is speculative, but it has been verified experimentally. Starzl described low-level leukocyte chimerism in patients who received allografts and postulated that coexisting donor and recipient leukocyte populations lead to a down-regulated immune response to donor antigens. This is not to suggest that immunosuppression is not needed during the transplantation process but, rather, that if donor immunocompetent cells are transferred with the organ, they can take residence in the recipient's bone marrow and perhaps allow for coexistence and tolerance. Protocols have been developed to infuse donor bone marrow at the time of transplantation, and they are presently being explored.[49] Nevertheless, this therapy has been extremely controversial and has shown no clear benefit.

▼ ANTIMICROBIAL MEDICATION

In addition to immunosuppressive medication regimens, antimicrobial medication regimens are important in preventing infection in the transplant recipient. These regimens vary from center to center and from program to program. Patients with a transplant usually need prophylactic antibiotic, antifungal, and, in some cases, antiviral preparations. These medications may include sulfamethoxazole-trimethoprim, nystatin, fluconazole, acyclovir, ganciclovir, and others.

The Centers for Disease Control and Prevention (CDC) has published guidelines for preventing opportunistic infections among HCT recipients based upon the quality of the evidence supporting the recommendation.[51] During the HCT process, all patients take multiple broad-spectrum antibiotics until their donated hematopoietic cells produce functional blood count levels. Additionally, most patients, especially those with a history of herpes simplex virus (HSV), take acyclovir.

Various protocols have been proposed based on the type of transplant, the time frame after transplantation, and the signs and symptoms that a transplant patient may experience.[52] Antimicrobial medication coverage has proven to be effective in prevention of some of the transplant-associated infections,[53] especially in HCT, but it still requires further study.[54,55] Some have questioned whether antimicrobial agents are overused during the perioperative period in renal transplants.[56]

The CDC also proposes guidelines for vaccination for HCT patients and for their family members/close contacts.[51] Vaccination against hepatitis B and varicella-zoster viruses is usually considered if the transplant recipient does not have antibodies to these diseases. Special consideration for vaccination must be taken into account in the pediatric population. It is of utmost importance for children to receive appropriate vaccination.[51,57]

▼ COMPLICATIONS

Complications with transplantation are still frequent and require close medical management. General complications can be broadly characterized into those caused by rejection, side effects from medication, and those induced by immunosuppression. Additionally, there are some organ-specific complications observed in certain types of transplantations.

▼ REJECTION

As previously mentioned, rejection of the transplanted organ remains a significant obstacle to long-term transplant graft and patient survival. The temporal relationship between the transplant and rejection episodes allows categorization of the particular rejection process (see Table 3). Rejection leads to end-organ damage and remanifestation of the various complications of a nonfunctioning organ. Clinically, rejection may be indicated in many ways, including an increased bleeding tendency (rejection of liver), a decreased metabolism or elimination of medications (rejection of liver/kidney), or even complete organ failure and death (rejection of lung/heart). In cases of end-organ disease (except those of kidney failure), retransplantation may be the only way to prevent death.

Rejection is continually monitored throughout the post-transplantation period. Most chronic rejections are insidious and are monitored by frequent laboratory analysis and by organ biopsy. Biopsy of tissue from the transplanted organ provides a reliable means to assess rejection. An alternative approach to monitoring rejection in a transplanted heart is the use of pacemakers to record changes in ventricular evoked response amplitude (VERA). Subtle changes in VERA have been correlated with acute rejection of heart transplants.[58]

▼ MEDICATION-INDUCED COMPLICATIONS

The medications used to produce immunosuppression and prevent graft rejection have significant systemic side effects, which pose serious complications to the transplant recipient. Some of the major side effects are listed here; however, complete drug information can be obtained through an appropriate medication reference source.

CSA, a mainstay in immunosuppression, is nephrotoxic and may alter renal function. It is associated with hypertension and is hepatotoxic. CSA is metabolized via the P-450 CYP 3A system of the liver; therefore, it has many drug interactions, including interactions with drugs frequently used in dentistry (see below).

Tacrolimus has also been associated with hypertension and hepatotoxicity. In addition, it is nephrotoxic and neurotoxic. There are many other side effects associated with the use of this medication, one of which is the development of insulin-dependent post-transplantation diabetes mellitus (PTDM). The incidence of PTDM appears to be higher with tacrolimus use than with CSA use in liver transplantations.[59] Tacrolimus is metabolized by the P-450 CYP 3A system in the liver. It is 99% protein bound and requires titration. Tacrolimus also has significant interactions with medications used in dentistry (see below).

Sirolimus is hepatotoxic and may cause liver dysfunction. Sirolimus is also associated with a high incidence of hyperlipidemia owing to elevated triglyceride and cholesterol levels.[26–28] Being a substrate for P-450 CYP 3A, sirolimus also interferes with the metabolism of other medications.

AZA may cause bone marrow suppression, resulting in pancytopenia, which leaves the patient not only susceptible to opportunistic infections but also at significant risk for bleeding.

MMF has significant drug interactions that are particularly important to the dentist. One interaction that is commonly cited occurs as a result of antibiotic regimens that can alter gastrointestinal flora, leading to dramatic changes in MMF drug levels. For example, if a patient is taking a broad-spectrum antibiotic for a dentoalveolar infection, the possibility and probability of an abnormal MMF level do exist. Other medications, such as antacids (containing magnesium or aluminum) and bile acid binders, may also interfere with absorption of MMF. MMF is usually well tolerated, without significant hepatotoxicity (although higher doses are associated with gastrointestinal symptoms of nausea, vomiting, and diarrhea) or nephrotoxicity, but hematologic alterations (mostly leukopenia) can be a side effect.

OKT3 can be associated with a severe reaction known as cytokine release syndrome. Cytokines (including TNF-α) are rapidly released, resulting in significant medical issues, including fever, chills, nephrotoxicity, vomiting, pulmonary edema, and, in a few instances, arterial thrombosis.[60] OKT3 has been reported to have interactions with indomethacin, including the potential development of encephalopathy.[61,62]

Both monoclonal and polyclonal antibodies have been associated with significant side effects (in addition to significant cytokine release), including a high risk of viral/fungal infection and an increased incidence of post-transplantation lymphoproliferative disorders (PTLDs).[37]

Corticosteroids, another mainstay used in transplantation immunosuppression, can have multiple detrimental side effects, causing various disorders (Table 6).

Cytotoxic agents such as cyclophosphamide, busulfan, and total-body irradiation cause bone marrow suppression, resulting in pancytopenia.

▼ IMMUNOSUPPRESSION-INDUCED COMPLICATIONS

Immunosuppression used to prevent rejection of a transplanted organ also can pose serious complications to the recipient, including life-threatening infections and cancer.

Infections in this population are a significant problem.[63] The type of transplant and the time that transpires since the transplantation often predict the specific infection. For example, patients who have had an HCT usually have broad immunologic defects, either due to their underlying disease or to the induction chemotherapeutic regimen, resulting in profound immunosuppression of all "branches" of the immune system. These patients are at a significantly higher risk of infection than are those patients transplanted with solid organs. Additionally, transplants of certain organs are associated with a greater likelihood of a particular infection.

Timing following the transplantation may correspond with a specific infective process.[52] Bacterial infections are usually seen in the early postoperative period (immediately after transplantation) in solid organ transplantations. The type of bacteria varies with each specific organ. Infections may include both gram-positive and gram-negative bacterial species. Drug-resistant bacterial infections have been documented, such as staphylococcal infections associated with skin wounds, upper and lower respiratory infections (pneumonia), and tuberculosis. Infective endocarditis has also been seen in transplant recipients. In this population, endocarditis is often related to *Staphylococcus* or aspergillosis.[64]

Systemic viral infections are also a common problem in immunosuppressed patients. Cytomegalovirus (CMV) and HSVs are often the etiologic viral agents involved. Other viral agents, including adenovirus, hepatitis B and C viruses, varicella-zoster virus, Epstein-Barr virus (EBV), and human parvovirus B19, have also been implicated in causing disease in a transplant population.[65] Viral infections are also related to time following transplantation. HSV infections usually occur at 2 to 6 weeks after organ transplantation, whereas CMV infections usually occur at 1 to 6 months after transplantation, and varicella-zoster virus infections usually occur between 2 and 10 months post-transplantation.[66]

Patients who are immunosuppressed are susceptible to local and systemic fungal infections. These infections vary from those of *Candida* species to deep fungal infections caused by *Aspergillus*, *Cryptococcus neoformans* phaeohyphomycosis, *Fusarium*, and *Trichosporon*. Deep fungal infections are usually seen later in the transplantation process. Systemic fungal infections are often difficult to treat in the immunosuppressed patient and require systemic antifungal agents.[52,67] Some have considered the role of macrophage colony-stimulating factor, a cytokine used to stimulate macrophages and monocytes, in the treatment of patients with fungal infections.[68–70]

Parasitic infections caused by *Toxoplasma gondii*, *Pneumocystis carinii* (now classified as a fungus species),[71] *Strongyloides stercoralis*, and others can be seen in immunosuppressed transplant recipients.

In addition to, and perhaps directly related to, infectious complications, immunosuppression renders the patient at a higher risk for the development of cancer. The immune system provides surveillance against antigens that may act as initiators or promoters of cancer. When the immune response is muted, so, too, is the surveillance system. Cancers

TABLE 6 Corticosteroid Side-Effect Profile
Induces diabetes
Induces muscle weakness
Induces osteoporosis
Alters fat metabolism and distribution
Induces hyperlipidemia
Induces electrolyte imbalances
Induces central nervous system effects, including psychological changes
Induces ocular changes—cataracts, glaucoma
Aggravates high blood pressure
Aggravates congestive heart failure
Aggravates peptic ulcer disease
Aggravates underlying infectious processes (eg, tuberculosis)
Suppresses the pituitary-adrenal axis, resulting in adrenal atrophy
Suppresses the stress response

most commonly associated with immunosuppression are squamous cell carcinomas of the skin,[72,73] lymphomas (mostly B-cell lymphomas, collectively referred to as PTLDs), and Kaposi's sarcoma.[74,75] Squamous cell carcinoma of the skin may be related to the human papillomaviruses,[76] whereas human herpesvirus 8 has been implicated in Kaposi's sarcoma[77] and EBV virus in PTLDs.[74] The incidence of PTLD is most common in lung followed by heart and then kidney transplant patients. Important factors in the development of PTLD is the level of immunosuppression and the EBV serology status.[78,79] Additionally, there seems to be a clinico-pathologic difference between those transplant recipients who are diagnosed with PTLD early (within the first year of transplantation, which are EBV + PTLD) versus those diagnosed after the first year.[80] PTLDs have been treated with decreased immunosuppression, antilymphocyte agents, conventional chemotherapy, radiotherapy, and IFN-α therapy.[81,82]

▼ SPECIFIC ORGANS/HCT COMPLICATIONS

A significant medical complication seen in patients receiving solid organ transplants is accelerated advanced cardiovascular disease, including coronary artery disease (CAD). The cause of this rapid CAD is thought to be either infectious (CMV), medication induced, or, more likely, both. Many investigators have explored the etiologic role of hypertension in CAD.[83] Probably in this population, CAD is multifactorial. For instance, steroids, CSA, and sirolimus have been associated with hyperlipidemia, a condition associated with CAD.

Hypertension is also a common post-transplantation problem, often related to the immunosuppressive medication regimen.[84] In many transplantation facilities, hypertension is being treated by calcium channel antagonists. Some clinicians note that this group of medications may raise serum levels of CSA, thus decreasing the cost of immunosuppression.[85] Caution must be exercised with any drug affecting CSA metabolism; for this reason, most clinicians prefer to prescribe medications that do not alter CSA levels. Nifedipine is one such calcium channel antagonist, but it has adverse oral effects, such as gingival overgrowth (see below).

Another significant condition associated with transplantation is post-transplantation diabetes mellitus. This disorder is a frequent consequence of allogeneic organ transplantation. Experimental and clinical observations both suggest that this phenomenon is related to the immunosuppressive agents.[86] Post-transplantation diabetes mellitus may cause both macro- and microvascular changes, which affect both graft and patient survival.[86]

Neurologic complications, such as neuropathies, can also be noted in transplant recipients.[87]

Reinfection with hepatitis C virus after transplantation is high in recipients of liver transplants. This reinfection is associated with a high mortality rate.[88]

The second most common long-term cause of morbidity and mortality (infection being the first) after lung transplantation is bronchiolitis obliterans.[89,90] This disorder is an inflammation and constriction in bronchioles. It probably is related to chronic rejection and infection and perhaps altered microvasculature.[90]

Heart transplantation is also fraught with complications. As previously mentioned, post-transplantation CAD is common in all transplants, including heart transplants. Additionally, early after transplantation, the heart is denervated such that symptoms of angina may be absent and the heart may have diminished vagal response.[91,92] There is, however, evidence of sympathetic and possibly parasympathetic reinnervation later in the post-transplantation period, suggesting that angina and heart rate changes to stress are regained.[91,93,94] Care of patients with cardiac transplants must recognize these cardiac abnormalities.[95] Mitral and tricuspid regurgitation has also been observed after heart transplantation.[96,97]

Perhaps the largest numbers of complications are those observed after an allogeneic HCT. Allogeneic transplantation often involves both administration of very high doses of myeloablative chemotherapy and total-body irradiation. The major complications of allogeneic HCT include the following:

1. End-organ damage from pretransplantation conditioning therapy
2. GVHD
3. Infections

A significant complication seen in these patients prior to HCT occurs during the conditioning regimen. Unlike solid organ grafting, HCT requires intensive chemotherapy and/or radiation to "condition"; this is required as immunosuppression of the recipient to prevent rejection but is also used to kill residual malignant cells. The conditioning therapy is typically given at myeloablative doses and is associated with high rates of organ toxicity. One such complication is known as veno-occlusive disease of the liver. This is caused by nonthrombotic occlusion of the central veins of the hepatic lobules. It is characterized by jaundice, hepatomegaly, and fluid retention. Treatment for this process is supportive, and severe veno-occlusive disease is associated with high mortality rates.[98] Another major complication is pulmonary toxicity manifested as interstitial pneumonitis or alveolar hemorrhage. Pulmonary complication of both solid organ and HCT has been reviewed in detail.[89] Techniques in allogeneic transplantation which include less toxic conditioning regimens are now being used in patients at higher risk for developing serious conditioning-related morbidity/mortality. These transplants are referred to as mini allogeneic transplants.

Perhaps the most frequently cited and unique complication associated with allogeneic HCT is GVHD, which is a complex immunologic phenomenon that occurs when immunocompetent cells from the donor are given to an immunodeficient host. The host, who possesses transplantation antigens foreign to the graft, stimulates an immune response by the newly engrafted immune cells. GVHD affects the entire gastrointestinal system, including the mouth, as well as the skin and the liver.[99] This reaction can be lethal and requires therapy with intensive immunosuppression. Chronic mucosal ulceration seen in GVHD may serve as an entry port for other infectious pathogens.[100] Chronic low-grade GVHD may be beneficial insofar as it could be considered as a graft-versus-leukemia reaction to kill persistent leukemic cells.[101]

▼ PROGNOSIS

Transplantation outcomes have improved over the past decade. In this chapter, the outcomes of patients who have received HCT are separated from outcomes of those receiving solid organ transplants. Furthermore, solid organ transplants are summarized and categorized by each specific organ. Data regarding clinical outcomes of solid organ transplantation must also be separated into graft survival as well as patient survival (Table 7). In the United States, total solid organ transplantation totaled just over 26,500 in 2004. The 1-year graft survival of renal transplantations performed in 2002–2003 was approximately 95% for a living donor transplant and 89% for a cadaveric kidney transplant. Liver transplant graft survival was 82%. Heart transplant graft survival was 87%, whereas lung and heart/lung graft survivals were 81% and 56%, respectively.[2]

One-year patient survival was 98% for those receiving a living donor renal transplant, 87% for a liver transplant, 88% for a heart transplant, and 83% for a lung transplant. Five-year graft and patient survival rates for solid organ transplants are lower. The 5-year graft survival rate (1998–2003) for cadaveric donor kidney transplants was 67%, whereas the rate for living donor kidney transplants was 80%. Five-year liver graft survival was 67%, whereas heart and lung graft survivals were 72% and 48%, respectively. Patient survival

rate at 5 years was 81% for cadaveric donor kidney transplant recipients and 90% for living transplant recipients. Five-year patient survival rates for liver, heart, and lung transplantations were 73%, 73%, and 49%, respectively.[2]

The number of patients on waiting lists for solid organ transplants continues to significantly increase. The deaths of patients awaiting kidney transplants increased from 2002 to 2004, whereas the death rates for patients awaiting heart and liver transplants decreased.

Current estimates of HCTs performed annually are 30,000 to 40,000 worldwide. The annual rate of growth of this procedure has been estimated to between 10 and 20%.[102] Improved HCT-related health care has resulted in less morbidity and lower mortality rates. Historically, HCTs for hematologic malignancies were undertaken as salvage therapy for refractory cancers, but outcomes are actually better for patients who are treated with HCT soon after diagnosis or in remission rather than after multiple relapses of hematologic disease. Outcomes have improved in both autologous and allogeneic HCTs. There are various reasons that the success of HCT has improved. In the setting of autologous HCT, hematopoietic growth factors and the use of peripheral blood stem cells rather than bone marrow stem cells have been credited in part with improving mortality by shortening the duration of neutropenia (and incidence of severe infections) after intensive chemotherapy or radiation. In addition, better supportive care, antibiotic use, and blood product support have all improved outcomes for autologous HCT. Transplant-related mortality following autologous transplantation is approximately 5%.[102] For allogeneic HCT, CSA was introduced in the 1980s as an immunosuppressive agent limiting the severity of GVHD, making donor HCT practical. Currently, CSA is often used with other medications, including methotrexate or corticosteroids, in prevention of GVHD. Both acute and chronic GVHD after HLA-matched sibling allogeneic transplantations occur in 40 to 60% of patients. Nevertheless, severe GVHD has decreased to approximately 20 to 30%.[101,102] Additionally, CMV used to account for high rates of mortality of allogeneic SCT. Today, viral transmission can be limited by using screened "CMV-free" blood products for CMV-negative patients or using leukocyte-reduced blood products for transfusions. CMV-positive patients are treated with a prophylactic or, more recently, "preemptive" strategy using new high-sensitivity assays for CMV reactivation. These procedures have decreased the mortality associated with CMV interstitial pneumonitis.[51,103] Post-transplantation cell growth factors have also been cited as improving outcomes in allogeneic HCT patients.[69] In allogeneic HCT, these advances have led to a decrease in overall mortality from 50% in 1974 to approximately 30% in 1994.[102,104] There are over 20,000 patients who have survived HCT for 5 years or greater, and the future holds even greater promise as the various transplantation techniques become further refined.

Outcomes of recipients who have received both bone marrow and solid organ transplantation have also been

TABLE 7 Outcomes of Solid Organ Transplantations

Type of Survival	Type of Transplantation				
	Renal (Living Donor)	Renal (Cadaveric Donor)	Heart	Liver (Cadaveric)	Lung
1-year graft survival (%)	95	89	87	82	81
5-year graft survival (%)	80	67	72	67	48
1-year patient survival (%)	98	95	88	87	83
5-year patient survival (%)	90	81	73	73	49

Data from the 2005 annual report of the United States Scientific Register of Transplant Recipients, Organ Procurement Transplantation Network.[2]

reviewed.[105] Some of the patients in this review by Dey and colleagues had an HCT and subsequently developed end-organ damage as a complication of some aspect of the transplantation procedure. They were later treated with a solid organ transplantation. Similarly, there were patients who received a solid organ transplant only to be subsequently diagnosed with a hematologic disorder, which was treated by an HCT. A total of 28 patients were studied: 21 had an HCT followed by a solid organ transplantation, whereas the other 7 received the solid organ transplant first. Eight patients died before they could be included in this review. None of the reported deaths were due to graft failure or rejection. Of the patients reviewed, two were cardiac transplant recipients. At the time of this review, one patient was noted to be leukemia free and free of congestive heart failure at 1 year, and the other patient was disease free at 6 months. Three lung transplant survivors after HCT were noted at 9, 14, and 15 months. Five of 10 recipients of liver transplants after HCT died. One partial liver transplant recipient was reported as "doing well." Four kidney transplant recipients were noted to be "doing well"; they each had received a transplant of a kidney from the same person who had donated bone marrow to them.

Allogeneic HCTs were performed on seven patients who had been treated with a renal or a liver transplantation. Four liver transplant recipients were noted to be "well" 2 years after their HCTs. One of three patients who underwent renal transplantation followed by HCT was "well" at 22 months post-HCT.

There are many clinical and immunologic considerations that are highlighted by reviewing this unique patient population. Further research regarding the concept of immunologic tolerance/chimerism in these patients may provide clues for future studies or for consideration of routine treatment regimens, including HCT with the transplanted solid organ. Close monitoring of these patients will allow a better understanding of the concept of chimerism and tolerance.[105]

▼ ORAL HEALTH CONSIDERATIONS

Oral Lesions

Patients who have had an organ transplantation may present to their health care practitioner with oral complaints. Often these complaints are related to oral mucosal lesions or masses. These lesions can be broadly related to an infectious process or a noninfectious process. Oral mucosal lesions and masses need to be identified, diagnosed, and treated.

Comprehensive oral examination is paramount in the transplant recipient, given the fact that the patient is more susceptible to oral infections of bacterial, viral, and fungal origins. Signs of oral infection may be muted due to a decreased inflammatory response, or, occasionally, the signs of infection may be exaggerated. The presentation of an oral infection is dependent upon the patient's level of immunosuppression and the patient's ability to mount an immune response. Oral infections must be diagnosed and treated as local infections may spread quickly, and systemic infections

may manifest orally. It is also important to remember that in severely immunocompromised hospitalized patients, the infectious agent associated with oral ulceration may be one that is normally not associated with oral infections.[106,107] Culture and sensitivity testing of all types of infections is prudent.

Bacterial infections, including dentoalveolar abscesses, may not manifest in traditional patterns. Therefore, treatment of bacterial infections requires prompt antibiotic therapy. Culture and sensitivity should be considered in severe infections or in those not responding quickly to empiric antibiotic therapy.

Dental caries, a bacterial infection, has been associated with many end-stage diseases and is presumably related to the various therapies/medications required to treat those diseases. However, the precise cause of the increased rate of caries remains somewhat questionable. Caries in the post-transplantation period has been reported. Children who have had an HCT for acute lymphoblastic leukemia have had a higher number of restored teeth.[108] Caries in limited numbers of kidney transplant recipients were studied in relation to salivary IgA. Low salivary IgA level (presumably related to immunosuppressive medications) was not associated with increased incidence of caries within 12 months post-transplantation. It should be noted that the relationship might differ in transplant recipients after the initial 12-month period, and long-term effects on caries have not been studied.[109]

Periodontal health in this patient population is often compromised. Medications and their side effects have been related to periodontal disorders, particularly gingival overgrowth. The medication-induced gingival overgrowth seen in the transplant recipient seems to be related to the immunosuppressive agent CSA (Figure 1). Furthermore, CSA-associated gingival overgrowth may be exaggerated by the coadministration of nifedipine, a calcium channel blocker often used to treat hypertension in this patient population. Nifedipine is often the drug of choice because it will not alter plasma levels of CSA, as do some other antihypertensive medications.

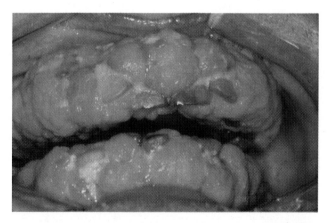

FIGURE 1 Gingival overgrowth in a kidney transplant recipient taking cyclosporine and nifedipine who also had poor oral hygiene.

Biopsy should be performed on gingival overgrowth as case reports of malignant tumors have been associated with some of these growths.[110,111] Impeccable oral hygiene has been noted to be helpful in preventing gingival overgrowth.[112] Partial reversal of CSA-induced overgrowth has been reported upon discontinuation of the medication.[113] However, treatment of severe gingival overgrowth usually requires gingivectomy.

Viral infections are a common problem in immunosuppressed patients. HSV is the most common viral pathogen cultured from oral infections. Recurrent herpes simplex infections can be both of the labial and intraoral varieties (Figures 2 to 4). Recurrent intraoral herpes may be chronic and difficult to diagnose based solely on clinical appearance (Figure 5). Varicella-zoster virus and EBV, as well as other viruses, have also been implicated in oral disease. Oral hairy leukoplakia (OHL) related to EBV has been seen in transplant recipients not infected with human immunodeficiency viruses.[114–116] In one case, OHL was identified as an earlier indicator of EBV-associated PTLD.[117] Treatment of viral infections involves the appropriate antiviral agent. Occasionally, HSV mutants not responsive to acyclovir require treatment with foscarnet (an antiviral medication with a mechanism of action different from that of

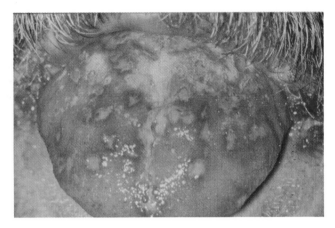

FIGURE 4   Recurrent intraoral herpes in a cardiac transplant recipient.

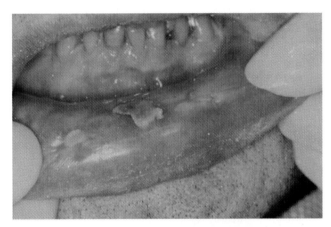

FIGURE 5   Chronic herpes simplex in a chronically immunosuppressed transplant recipient.

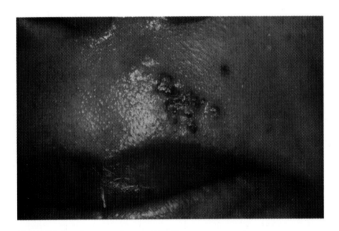

FIGURE 2   Recurrent herpes labialis.

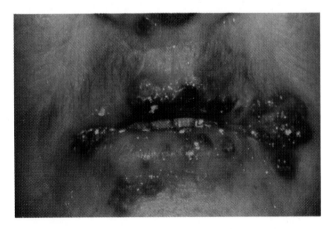

FIGURE 3   Recurrent herpes labialis in an immunocompromised patint.

acyclovir).[118] Cases are now emerging of both acyclovir- and foscarnet-resistant oral HSV. Successful treatment of multiresistant HSV infection with cidofovir has been reported.[119]

Patients who are immunosuppressed are more susceptible to fungal infections. These infections vary from those of candidal species, including pseudomembranous candidiasis, to deep fungal infections, including aspergillosis, cryptococcosis, mucormycosis, and blastomycosis (Figures 6 and 7). These infections may manifest in various presentations in the oral cavity. Candidiasis can present as the classic pseudomembranous form, or it can be atrophic or even hyperplastic (see Figures 6 to 9). Hyperplastic candidiasis is not removed by scraping the lesion and often requires biopsy for definitive diagnosis. Occasionally, candidiasis is not responsive to the typical azole-type antifungal agents[120,121] and may require treatment with amphotericin B. It is important to note that candidal hyphae have been reported in CSA-induced gingival overgrowth.[122]

Deep fungal infections involving the upper respiratory tract/sinuses may manifest as necrotic plaques in the palatal areas of recipients of HCT (see Figure 7). These fungal infections are very difficult to treat and often require intravenous

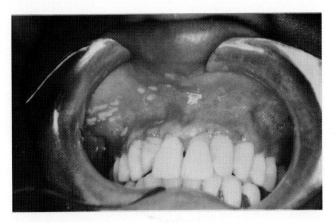

FIGURE 6 Pseudomembranous candidiasis.

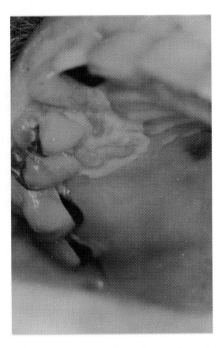

FIGURE 7 Deep fungal aspergillosis in a patient who underwent hematopoietic cell transplantation. The patient succumbed to isseminated aspergillosis shortly after this photograph was taken.

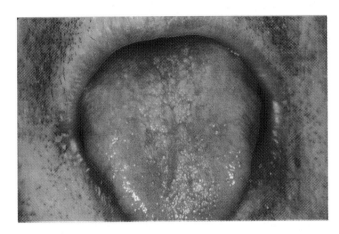

FIGURE 8 Atrophic candidiasis.

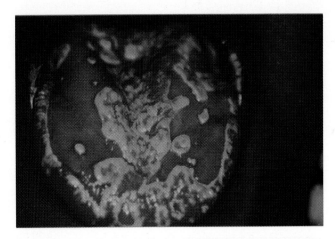

FIGURE 9 Hyperplastic candidiasis in a kidney transplant recipient. This infection did not respond to fluconazole.

antifungal agents, such as amphotericin B. In patients who are severely neutropenic, these infections may prove fatal, with the patient ultimately succumbing to a systemic deep fungal infection.

Noninfectious oral lesions are also common in the transplant recipients. Isolated case reports of oral ulceration related to MMF[123] and tacrolimus[124] have been noted. Other lesions may represent neoplasms. The transplant recipient is at a higher risk of developing lymphoma and other cancers, such as Kaposi's sarcoma and squamous cell carcinoma of the skin (see above). Lymphoma and Kaposi's sarcoma can be present in the mouth,[110,125,126] whereas epithelial malignancy often involves the lips.[127,128] One reported case describes a cutaneous squamous cell carcinoma metastasizing to the parotid gland.

Treatment of opportunistic PTLDs may include decreased immunosuppression, antilymphocyte agents, conventional chemotherapy, radiotherapy, and IFN-α therapy.[81,82]

GVHD is a unique complication of HCT. In the oral cavity, this process clinically resembles lichenoid inflammation/lichen planus. Oral GVHD appears as an area of wispy hyperkeratosis on an erythematous base in various areas of the oral mucosa. In more severe GVHD, the lesions can appear significantly eroded and may be associated with chronic mucosal ulceration (Figure 10).[129] These ulcerations may serve as a systemic port of entry for oral pathogens. GVHD not only affects the mouth but also the entire gastrointestinal system, as well as the skin and the liver. This reaction can be lethal, and in acute disease, it needs to be reversed. However, chronic GVHD may be considered somewhat beneficial if it functions as a graft-versus-leukemia reaction, an immunologic process to kill persistent leukemic cells. GVHD in the oral mucous membrane is often difficult to treat locally and often requires a change in the immunosuppressive regimen.[129] Some have used topical CSA in a bioadhesive base with good results.[130] Ultraviolet B irradiation as well as ultraviolet A irradiation with oral psoralen (PUVA) has been reported to be effective.[131,132] A novel approach for treating oral GVHD involves the use of topical AZA.[133]

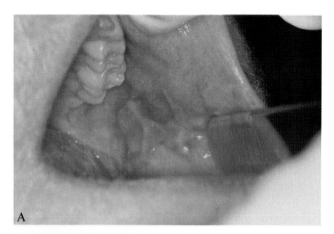

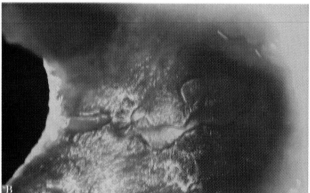

FIGURE 10 Graft-versus-host disease in a patient who had undergone hematopoietic cell transplantation. Note the clinical resemblance to erosive lichen planus.

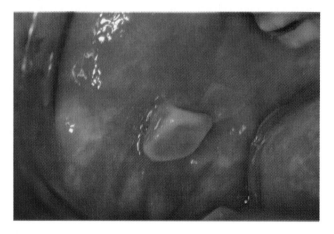

FIGURE 11 Nongingival soft tissue growth.

In addition to GVHD, a patient who has had an allogeneic HCT may also experience a nongingival soft tissue growth, presumably related to the use of CSA. These lesions can be seen in the buccal mucosa, alveolar mucosa, and elsewhere (Figure 11).[134]

Oral mucositis (OM) is a common complaint of patients who have had chemotherapy.[135] OM is a significant and dose-limiting complication of high-dose chemotherapy. Mucositis after HCT is usually related to the preconditioning regimen, and it is difficult to distinguish from an oral infection (Figure 12). Often mucositis is treated with palliative agents; a

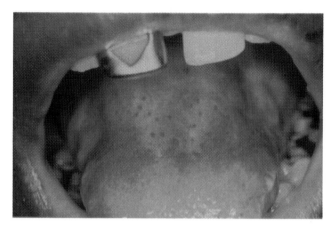

FIGURE 12 Mucositis shortly after induction chemotherapy for acute myelogenous leukemia.

mixture of an anesthetic, an antihistamine, and a coating agent is commonly used. These agents tend to provide transient relief with no significant improvement in the mucositis. Palliative treatment with lidocaine has been associated with only minor systemic absorption.[136] Some have suggested the use of topical tretinoin prophylaxis to prevent HCT mucositis.[137] Newer agents with specific antimucositis indications are presently being explored. One product, Gelclair (OSI Pharmaceuticals, Melville, NY), is a bioadhesive gel that in a noncontrolled open-label trial reduced pain scores by 30% in persons with mucositis.[138] Another recent development in mucositis prevention has focused on using growth factors to stimulate the proliferation of epithelial cells. One such growth factor, recombinant human erythrocyte growth factor 1, has been evaluated in a phase III trial and found to significantly reduce the duration and incidence of mucositis.[139] Other studies examined the use of granulocyte-macrophage colony-stimulating factor in preventing oral mucositis and found moderate evidence to suggest its efficacy.[140] The role of antibacterial topical agents, such as chlorhexidine rinses, in preventing OM is controversial.[140]

Salivary gland dysfunction is also quite common in patients after HCT. This may be acutely related to the chemotherapeutic regimens used to rid the bone marrow of leukemic cells. Patients who have chronic GVHD also have diminution of salivary flow, presumably from a lymphocytic infiltrate of salivary tissue (Figure 13).[141]

Developmental tooth defects such as altered root formation and dentofacial alterations must also be considered as they have been reported in children who have undergone HCT (Figure 14).[142] Description and follow-up of late dental effects of HCT are limited to isolated case series.

Dental Management

Dental treatment for patients who are preparing for transplantation or for those who have had a transplant should be coordinated with the performing physician. The patient may be a better candidate for elective dental treatment after the transplanted organ is stable. Often, however, the physician may consult the patient's general dentist before "listing" the patient for the transplantation. The nature of this

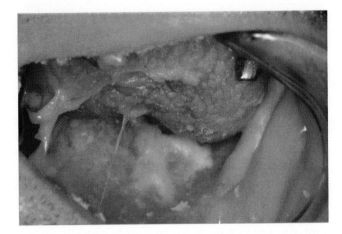

FIGURE 13 Salivary hypofunction.

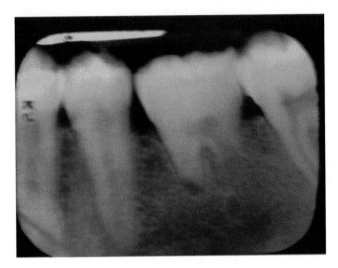

FIGURE 14 Dental root alteration as a result of childhood treatment for lymphoma.

TABLE 8 Dental Management Considerations
Pretransplantation considerations
Significantly ill patient with end-organ damage
Medical consultation required
Consider postponing elective treatment
Dental consultation prior to anticipated transplantation
Rule out dental infectious sources, definitively
Perform necessary treatment; this will require consultation with transplantation physician to determine medical risk to benefit ratio
Obtain laboratory information/supplemental information as needed
Become acquainted with specific management issues (eg, blood products, prophylactic antibiotics) that may need to be employed if treatment is rendered
Post-transplantation considerations
Immediate post-transplantation period
No elective dental treatment performed
Emergency treatment only with medical consultation and consideration of specific management needs
Stable post-transplantation period
Elective treatment may be performed after medical consultation with the transplantation physician
Issues of immunosuppression must be recognized
Oral mucosal disease must be diagnosed and treated
Supplemental corticosteroids (steroid boost) may be necessary
Consideration of antibiotic prophylaxis needed
Consideration of specific management needs
Post-transplantation chronic rejection period
Only emergency treatment
Patients are very ill as they are immunosuppressed and have organ failure

consultation is to ensure that the patient does not have any acute (or potentially acute) dental/oral infection that could complicate the transplantation process. It is prudent for a transplant candidate to be examined by the dentist in the pretransplantation period.

A dentist treating members of this unique population must be aware of certain considerations regarding the medical health of the individuals; providing dental care is often challenging. Close and detailed communication between the health care workers is essential. Dental management for this patient population can be divided into pretransplantation and post-transplantation issues (Table 8).

▼ PRETRANSPLANTATION CONSIDERATIONS

Pretransplantation concerns include the fact that these patients are critically ill and have significant end-organ damage. Specific organ damage poses unique challenges. Patients with end-stage liver disease may have difficulties with excessive bleeding due to coagulopathy. These patients may have difficulty metabolizing medications (Table 9).

Patients awaiting a kidney transplant have end-stage renal disease and are usually receiving hemodialysis. These patients may be fluid overloaded and have hypertension; therefore, monitoring of the patient's blood pressure is usually prudent. When determining the blood pressure, the cuff must not be placed on the arm used for dialysis access. Occasionally, electrolyte balance may be altered. Variation of drug metabolism and excretion must also be considered in this population as changing of the dose of various medications, including those used in dentistry, may be required (see Table 9).[143]

Patients awaiting a heart transplant are usually poor candidates for outpatient dental treatment. The majority of these patients have severe CAD or congestive heart failure. Both conditions can easily progress to life-threatening complications during invasive dental treatment. The sole effect of stress and pain can cause an adverse outcome in labile patients. The cardiovascular reserve of these patients is small, rendering them much better candidates for elective dental treatment after they have undergone transplantation. Some patients awaiting heart transplants may not be discharged from the hospital until they receive their new heart.

Patients awaiting lung transplants are also critically ill. Most are on oxygen therapy and have difficulty breathing. Dental treatment should preclude the use of combustible sources near the patient if he or she is using oxygen therapy. Inhaled anesthetics are contraindicated in these patients.

TABLE 9 Medication Considerations in Patients with Liver or Kidney Failure*

Drug	Dose Change Required?	
	Kidney Failure†	Liver Failure
Acetaminophen	–	Avoid use
Acyclovir	+	–
Amoxicillin	+	–
Cephalexin	+	–
Clavulanic acid with amoxicillin	+	–
Clindamycin	–	+
Codeine	+	+
Diazepam	+	+
Erythromycin	–	+
Ibuprofen	–	Unknown
Ketoconazole	–	+
Lidocaine	–	–
Metronidazole	+	+
Minocycline	–	+
Naproxen	+	+
Penicillin	+	–
Salicylates	+/Avoid use	Avoid use
Tetracycline	+/Avoid use	Avoid use

Adapted from Byme, BE. Therapeutics in renal hepatic disease. In: Ciancio S. editor. ADA guide to dental therapeutics. Chicago (IL): ADA publishing Co.; 1998. p. 432–40.

+ = May require a dose change and/or avoidance of use, depending on severity of renal or hepatic disease.

– = No dose change required.

*Includes only drugs commonly used in dentistry.

†Degree of function of renal system must be considered before dose change is determined.

Narcotic medications that cause respiratory depression are also contraindicated.

Patients awaiting pancreatic transplants have significant problems in glucose management; therefore, considerations of serum glucose levels prior to initiating treatment must be made. These patients may be poor wound healers and may have "brittle insulin-dependent diabetes"; that is, these patients may experience sharp alterations in blood glucose levels and be prone to both ketoacidosis and insulin shock (see Chapter 21, "Diabetes Mellitus and Endocrine Diseases"). Pancreatic dysfunction may be accompanied by hepatic failure. Hence, coagulation complications and medication/local anesthetic metabolism must be considered when performing dental procedures in these individuals.

HCT candidates are frequently also significantly ill. Most have been through induction and have endured consolidation chemotherapy to treat a hematologic malignancy. Many of these patients are pancytopenic and are prone to infections and bleeding. They are therefore considered poor candidates for routine outpatient dental treatment. Other patients may have had a significant remission of their disease with normalizing blood counts, allowing emergency dental treatment prior to the HCT.

When treating patients who are transplantation candidates, the dentist must be familiar with the underlying disorder as well as laboratory evaluations pertinent to the particular disorder. Consultation with the patient's physician is mandatory.

A dentist caring for members of the pretransplantation population must not only consider providing/withholding care after considering the underlying disorders, he or she must also consider the potential dental complications that can significantly impact the transplantation process. A detailed clinical examination of the dentition, periodontium, and oral mucosa as well as the head and neck areas, including the lymph nodes and salivary glands, is prudent. There has been some controversy as to the optimal radiographic examination regimen required to evaluate patients who will undergo HCT[144]; however, recent dental radiographs must be part of the evaluation.

Once the evaluation has been performed, a medical/dental risk assessment should be formulated. Generally speaking, elective dental treatment in patients with end-stage disease should be postponed as the patient will be more "medically stable" after the transplantation. However, whenever possible, it is important for the dentist to eliminate dental infections prior to the transplantation as the patient will be significantly immunosuppressed immediately and for some time after the transplantation. Dental treatment planning must therefore take into account the patient's laboratory evaluation, including such parameters as blood cell and platelet counts, serum chemistry to determine the degree of organ dysfunction, and coagulation studies. In addition, other tests more specific for each particular organ function must be obtained and reviewed. A medical risk assessment is necessary to determine if a patient can systemically tolerate an extraction or other dental procedure. Some HCT and heart transplant candidates cannot withstand even emergency treatment. When risk assessment favors treatment, the most definitive treatment option should be considered (often extraction). Antibiotic prophylaxis prior to the dental treatment is often warranted in patients awaiting HCT or heart or kidney transplants. Patients awaiting HCT or liver transplants may need platelets, coagulation factors, or other supportive products prior to dental treatment.

▼ POST-TRANSPLANTATION CONSIDERATIONS

Patients who have undergone transplantation also pose concerns to the treating dentist. The post-transplantation period can be divided into the immediate post-transplantation period, the stable period, and the chronic rejection period.

The immediate post-transplantation period is the time when the patient is most susceptible to both rejection and severe infection. This period of time begins immediately post-transplantation and extends to when the grafted organ is functioning appropriately. Due to increased levels of immuno-suppression used to foil rejection during this period, the dentist should not perform elective dental treatment, and emergency treatment should be provided only after consultation with the transplantation physician. Patients have shown benefit from chlorhexidine mouthrinses during this period of time.[145]

The stable post-transplantation period occurs when the grafted organ is stable. It is during this time that the problems of chronic rejection, immunosuppression, and side effects of immunosuppressive medications may become apparent. Dental treatment planning must consider these important factors. The length of time that a patient remains in this stage is variable. Generally, this period is the best time to perform elective dental treatment since the organ is functioning appropriately. In general, there are no absolute contraindications to any type of dental procedure in patients after a successful HCT without medical or oral complications.[146] Consultation with the transplantation physician is essential due to the delicate balance of rejection/immunosuppression and their implications in medical/dental risk assessment.

Antibiotic prophylaxis prior to dental treatment is often requested by the transplantation physician, although whether this is necessary requires further evidence-based research. Corticosteroid supplementation may also be required due to adrenal suppression associated with higher-dose chronic corticosteroid use. This supplementation may help avoid cardiovascular collapse during stressful procedures, and it is recommended when the stress of the procedure or the patient's perception of the stress (pain) of the procedure is increased.[147] Some have questioned the need for supplementation when treating gingival overgrowth via gingivectomy under local anesthetic.[148]

Other considerations for the dental provider during the stable post-transplantation period involve medication interactions as several antirejection immunosuppressive medications have interactions with medications that a dentist may prescribe. For example, patients who are taking CSA as one of their antirejection medications may require the use of clindamycin instead of erythromycin. CSA levels are affected by anti-inflammatory drugs such as diclofenac, sulindac, and naproxen; antifungal medications such as itraconazole, fluconazole, and ketoconazole; and antibiotics such as clarithromycin and erythromycin. Reviewing potential interactions between the medications that the transplant patient is taking and those the dentist intends to prescribe is prudent. As the trends in immunosuppression change, the dentist will need to be familiar with the newer medications and the potential risk of interactions with the various medications used in dentistry.

The stable post-transplantation period ends and the chronic rejection period starts when a grafted organ begins to fail. Laboratory parameters indicate organ function failure, and biopsies are used to confirm this process. For dentists, these patients are often the most complicated to manage since the organ is failing and the patient is immunosuppressed. Only emergency dental treatment is indicated, and the transplantation physician's input is essential. The treating dentist must consider the ramifications of organ failure and make appropriate provisions.

▼ CONCLUSION

Oral considerations in the transplantation population are vast. The dentist needs an exceptionally strong knowledge base in medicine to minimize adverse outcomes secondary to provision of oral health care. As this unique population grows, so does the need for qualified dental practitioners. It is essential that the dentist familiarize himself or herself with the special needs of these patients. Their dental health is imperative; therefore, patients who have had an organ transplantation need to have routine dental examinations. It is incumbent on the dental practitioner to expediently diagnose and treat any oral infection. Gingival health in this population is extremely important and must be monitored regularly, particularly because CSA may induce gingival overgrowth, which precludes adequate home care and encourages further periodontal breakdown.

Arguably, patients undergoing allogeneic HCT should be evaluated more frequently than the general population owing to the decreased salivary flow, which may be associated with an increased caries rate.[149] Consideration should be given to providing patients with supplemental topical fluoride applications. These patients may also have oral ulceration from GVHD. These ulcers can serve as a portal of entry for any oral pathogen to infect the immunocompromised host.

The patient's medical history should be updated with each dental appointment. Close coordination with the transplantation physician is necessary as the patient's medical condition can change quickly.

As with all dental patients, excellent oral hygiene is difficult to achieve solely by the clinician's professional service. It is extremely important to provide oral hygiene instruction and to discuss with the patient the need for appropriate hygiene to prevent oral infection. These patients can be at high risk of serious complications, even from initially minimal dental infections. The patient should also be taught to perform an oral examination and encouraged to perform it frequently at home. This procedure enables the patient to constantly monitor his or her own oral condition and to aid the health care professional in early diagnosis of pathology.

▼ SELECTED READINGS

Caillard S, Dharnidharka V, Agodoa L, et al. Posttransplant lymphoproliferative disorders after renal transplantation in the United States in era of modern immunosuppression. Transplantation 2005;80:1233–43.

Casiglia J, Woo SB. Oral hairy leukoplakia as an early indicator of Epstein-Barr virus-associated post-transplant lymphoproliferative disorder. J Oral Maxillofac Surg 2002;60:948–50.

Comenzo RL. Hematopoietic cell transplantation for primary systemic amyloidosis: what have we learned? Leuk Lymphoma 2000;37:245–58.

Crespo M, Delmonic F, Saidman S, et al. Acute humoral rejection in kidney transplantation. Graft 2000;3:12–7.

Dykewicz CA, Jaffe HW, Kaplan JE, et al. Guidelines for preventing opportunistic infections among hematopoietic stem cell transplant recipients: recommendations of CDC, the Infectious Disease Society of America, and the American Society of Blood and Marrow Transplantation. MMWR Morb Mortal Wkly Rep 2000;49:1–128.

Garrigue V, Canet S, Dereure O, et al. Oral ulcerations in a renal transplant recipient: a mycophenolate mofetil induced complication? Transplantation 2001;72:968–9.

Ghobrial IM, Habermann TM, Macon WR, et al. Differences between early and late posttransplant lymphoproliferative disorders in solid organ transplant patients: are they two different diseases? Transplantation 2005;79:244–7.

Innocenti M, Moscatelli G, Lopez S. Efficacy of Gelclair in reducing pain in palliative care patients with oral lesions: preliminary findings from an open pilot study. J Pain Symptom Management 2002;24:456–7.

Kotloff RM, Ahya VN, Crawford SW. Pulmonary complications of solid organ and hematopoietic stem cell transplantation. Am J Respir Crit Care Med 2004;170:22–48.

Stadtmauer EA, O'Neill A, Goldstein LJ, et al. Conventional-dose chemotherapy compared with high-dose chemotherapy plus autologous hematopoietic stem-cell transplantation for metastatic breast cancer. Philadelphia Bone Marrow Transplant Group. N Engl J Med 2000;342:1069–76.

Uberfuhr P, Frey AW, Reichart B. Vagal reinnervation in the long term after orthotopic heart transplantation. J Heart Lung Transplant 2000;19:946–50.

Vincenti F, Larsen C, Durrbach A, et al. Costimulation blockade with belatacept in renal transplantation. N Engl J Med 2005;353:770–81.

Worthington HV, Clarkson JE, Eden OB. Interventions for preventing oral mucositis for patients with cancer receiving treatment. Cochrane Database of Systematic Reviews 2006;(2):CD000978.

For the full reference list, please refer to the accompanying CD ROM.

20

INFECTIOUS DISEASES

Lakshman Samaranayake, Hon DSc, Hon FDSRCS(Edin), DDS(Glas), BDS, FRCPath, FHKCPath, MIBiol, FCDSHK, FHKAM(Path), FHKAM(DSurg)

Michaell A. Huber, DDS

Spencer W. Redding, DDS, MEd

The oral cavity is a portal of entry for many pathogens. Some of them, such as *Neisseria gonorrhoeae* and herpes zoster, enter the oral cavity and cause mainly localized disease, whereas others, such as *Treponema pallidum* and human immunodeficiency virus (HIV), proliferate locally in the oropharynx with or without apparent tissue damage and then gain entry into the bloodstream, causing systemic disease. A number of oral infections discussed here are rare; therefore, few clinicians will have personally examined cases or be familiar with the clinical and laboratory investigations that are required to reach a definitive diagnosis. Others have a relatively narrow geographic distribution and, although common in some parts of the world, are rarely, if ever, found in other areas. Nonetheless, due to the rapid and cheap transportation methods now available, there is an increasing likelihood of infections being imported into countries where the disease is unknown, with the attendant danger that it will not be recognized and incorrectly treated. Therefore, in this chapter, we discuss both common and rare oral infections arranged alphabetically under the following headings: bacterial, chlamydial, rickettsial, fungal, and viral infections.

▼ DIAGNOSIS OF ORAL INFECTIONS

A definitive diagnosis of oral infections requires the collection and critical assessment of a number of factors: clinical signs and symptoms; details of the past medical, dental, and social history; appropriate sampling and shipping of specimens; and correct interpretation of the laboratory results (Figure 1).

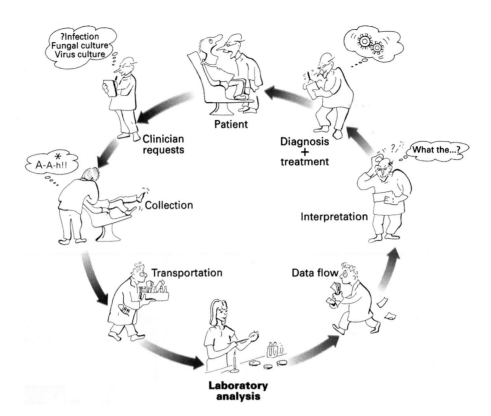

FIGURE 1 The cycle of important events in the diagnosis of an infectious disease, depicting the interaction between the clinician and the microbiology laboratory. Adapted with permission from Samaranayake LP.[1]

The oral lesion could be either a purely localized infection or a secondary manifestation of a (primary) systemic infection. In the latter situation, clues related to systemic disease, such as fever, malaise, headache, sore throat, respiratory disease, joint pain, lymph node enlargement, rash, pain, and isolated lesions on other parts of the body, should be sought. It is also important to eliminate traumatic, neoplastic, or other immunoinflammatory diseases as they may manifest as ulceration, pain, enlarged lymph nodes, trismus, or salivary gland swellings. Although the presence or absence of pain may be useful in the differential diagnosis of oral ulcers, it should be remembered that almost any ulcer in the mouth can be painful, especially if secondarily infected by the oral flora. Hence, many oral infections present with almost identical clinical presentation, and the definitive diagnosis could be obtained only through point of care rapid diagnostic methods and further laboratory investigations.

Appropriate therapy should be started as soon as a provisional diagnosis has been made. It is a matter of clinical judgment and experience how far an individual patient should be investigated at the first visit, using laboratory tests. As a general rule, if the patient fits into the 'classic' presentation of a particular disease, then laboratory tests are usually unnecessary, but if the signs, symptoms, or history suggest an atypical picture, or if the lesions are extensive and painful, then laboratory tests should be instituted as soon as possible. If at the next appointment the condition has not responded to treatment, the case should be critically reviewed, taking

into account any available laboratory results. The review may result in a change in therapy, additional tests, or referral to another clinician. Due to the large number of possible pathogens that may be involved in any given oral lesion, it is important that the differential diagnosis appears on the laboratory request form. If there is doubt about which specimens are required for an investigation, the laboratory should be contacted for advice.[1]

▼ BACTERIAL INFECTIONS

Actinomycosis

Actinomycosis is an endogenous, granulomatous disease that may occur in the cervicofacial region (most common; 60–65%), abdomen (10–20%), and lung and peripheral skin. In humans, the main infecting organism is *Actinomyces israelii*, a gram-positive filamentous branching rod that is commonly found in plaque biofilms, carious dentine, and calculus; *Actinoymyces bovis* and *Actinomyces naeslundii* may occasionally be isolated. Although most infections are monomicrobial in nature (ie, with *Actinomyces* alone causing the disease), a significant proportion of infections could be polymicrobial, with other bacteria, such as *Actinobacillus actinomycetemcomitans*, *Haemophilus* spp, and anaerobes, acting as coinfecting agents. Trauma to the jaws, tooth extraction, and teeth with gangrenous pulps may precipitate infection (eg, calculus or plaque becoming impacted in the depths of a tooth socket at the time of extraction). Actinomycosis cannot be transmitted from human to human.

ORAL CONSIDERATIONS

Cervicofacial actinomycosis is predominantly a disease of younger people, although all ages may be affected. The infection can present in an acute, subacute, or chronic form. There is usually a history of trauma, such as a tooth extraction or a blow to the jaw (Figure 2). Most infections start as an acute swelling indistinguishable on clinical grounds from a dento-alveolar abscess. The chronic form of the disease follows, due to either inadequate or no therapy or subacute infection related to trauma.

Swelling is common and is either localized or diffuse; if untreated, it may progress into discharging sinuses. Classically, this discharge of pus contains visible granules that may be gritty to touch and yellow and are known as 'sulfur granules' (a descriptive term as sulfur is not found in the granules). These granules in pus are almost pathognomonic of the disease.

The submandibular region is most commonly affected; rarely, the maxillary antrum, salivary glands, and tongue may be involved. Pain is a variable feature. Other features, depending on the site of infection, are multiple discharging sinuses, trismus, pyrexia, fibrosis around the swelling, and the presence of infected teeth.

DIAGNOSIS AND MANAGEMENT

If a fluctuant abscess is present, fluid pus can be collected by aspiration using a syringe or in a sterile container if drainage by external incision is performed. Examine the pus for the presence of 'sulfur granules' (so called due to their yellow granular appearance); Gram films are made from any part with a lumpy or granular appearance. When crushed

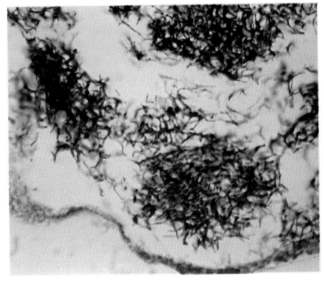

FIGURE 2 A histopathologic section from an actinomycotic lesion of the mandible showing branching filamentous mass of *Actinomyces* species infiltrating the bony cortex. Adapted with permission from Samaranayake LP.[1]

granules are cultured anaerobically, on blood agar, at 37°C for 7 days, colonies with a typical 'molar tooth' morphology appear. Pure cultures are then identified using biochemical techniques. A Gram film of a colony will reveal moderate to large clumps of gram-positive branching filaments.

Acute lesions are managed by removal of any associated dental focus, incision, and drainage of the facial abscess and a 2- to 3-week course of antibiotics, penicillin being the drug of choice. In the case of subacute or chronic lesions, surgical intervention and a longer antibiotic course, up to 6 weeks, may be necessary. If penicillin cannot be given because of hypersensitivity, erythromycin, tetracycline, and clindamycin are good alternatives as the latter drugs penetrate bony tissues. Differential diagnosis includes tuberculosis (TB), systemic mycoses, nocardiosis, periodontal abscess, dentoalveolar abscess and donovanosis.

Anthrax

Caused by *Bacillus anthracis*, anthrax is primarily a disease of animals and is now extremely rare in the West. Humans usually become infected by working with animals, eating contaminated meat, or handling animal products, such as hides, skins, bone meal, hair, or bristles. Humans can also become accidental hosts when spores enter abrasions on the skin or are inhaled. Anthrax spores can survive in soil for decades. Infection causes septicemia and death; pulmonary anthrax (woolsorter's disease) is a life-threatening pneumonia caused by inhalation of spores. The polyglutamic acid capsule of the organism is antiphagocytic. Recently, the organism has received much attention due to the likelihood of the use of the anthrax spores in biologic warfare and bioterrorism.

The skin of the arms, face, or neck is the common site of the initial lesion, the so-called 'malignant pustule.' This term is a misnomer since the lesions are neither malignant nor do they contain pus. In addition to the cutaneous form of anthrax, inhalational and gastrointestinal anthrax have been described. Septicemia and meningitis may complicate any of these. The potential for human to human transmission of anthrax through spore dissemination exists.

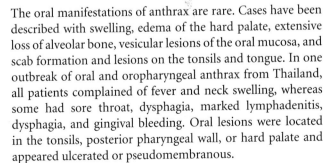

ORAL CONSIDERATIONS

The oral manifestations of anthrax are rare. Cases have been described with swelling, edema of the hard palate, extensive loss of alveolar bone, vesicular lesions of the oral mucosa, and scab formation and lesions on the tonsils and tongue. In one outbreak of oral and oropharyngeal anthrax from Thailand, all patients complained of fever and neck swelling, whereas some had sore throat, dysphagia, marked lymphadenitis, dysphagia, and gingival bleeding. Oral lesions were located in the tonsils, posterior pharyngeal wall, or hard palate and appeared ulcerated or pseudomembranous.

DIAGNOSIS AND MANAGEMENT

A swab and smear of the lesion should be taken. If the patient's occupation and the presentation and progress of the disease suggest anthrax, treatment should be started without awaiting bacteriologic confirmation. The antibiotic of choice is penicillin.[2] The patient should be isolated and the appropriate authorities notified. *B. anthracis* is susceptible to other common antibiotics.

Brucellosis

This is primarily a disease of animals caused by small gram-negative coccobacilli of the genus *Brucella*. Humans become infected either through contact with infected animals (eg, farmers and abbattoir workers) or by consuming infected milk products. The disease presents in five main forms: an acute illness characterized by fever, headache, sweating, fatigue, and joint pains; a subacute form characterized by muscle weakness and an overwhelming fatigue that reduces the patient to a state of inertia and helplessness; a chronic illness with vague, influenza-like symptoms lasting for many years and accompanied by neuropsychiatric manifestations; a latent or subclinical form with no apparent history of brucellosis; and, finally, a relapsing form that recurs at 2- to 3-month intervals with signs and symptoms similar to the acute illness.

The incubation period is about 2 to 4 weeks. *Brucella* may enter the body via the gastrointestinal tract, through small skin abrasions, or through the mucosa of the respiratory tract or conjunctiva. The organisms are carried to the regional lymph nodes, where they proliferate and then spread into the bloodstream. They are then carried round the body and localize mainly in the reticuloendothelial cells in the liver, spleen, lymph glands, and bone marrow. Contact transmission of *Brucella* from human to human is possible.

ORAL CONSIDERATIONS

Oral manifestations of brucellosis are uncommon. Cases have been reported with red and edematous gingivae and numerous small ulcers with grayish surfaces scattered around the oral mucosa.

DIAGNOSIS AND MANAGEMENT

The clinical diagnosis of acute brucellosis is not difficult if a history of exposure to the organism is present and the clinical course conforms to the classic signs and symptoms of the disease. In the absence of these features, the diagnosis is difficult and blood and emulsified biopsy material should be cultured and serum removed for serologic tests. Fluorescence polarization assays provide a valuable alternative to conventional serologic tests that are complicated by the naturally occurring *Brucella* strains. Sensitive assays, such as radioimmunoassay and enzyme-linked immunosorbent assay (ELISA), have replaced the older serologic techniques.

Treatment is symptomatic, and specific therapy consists of a combination of streptomycin and tetracycline, which has a synergistic action against *Brucella abortus*. A 3-week course of therapy is recommended to destroy organisms that are liberated into the circulation following the death of parasitized tissue cells.[3]

Granuloma Inguinale (Donovanosis)

Granuloma inguinale or donovanosis is a chronic, ulcerative, granulomatous disease that is transmitted by sexual intercourse. The causative agent is *Calymmatobacterium granulomatis*, a gram-negative bacillus with prominent polar granules. The incubation period is uncertain and ranges from 1 week to 1 year. The initial lesion is a papule or nodule in the inguinal or anogenital region that progresses to a locally destructive granulomatous ulcer. Extragenital lesions are present in about 6% of cases and are the result of autoinoculation or dissemination from the primary genital lesion. The sites commonly involved are the mucous membranes of the oropharynx and eyes, the skin, and subcutaneous tissues. Cases of donovanosis have been described in the Americas, the Far East, and Africa. The common age group affected is 20 to 40 years, and in the United States, the incidence is higher in the colored population. There is a high possibility of human to human transmission of donovanosis through unprotected sexual activity.

ORAL CONSIDERATIONS

Primary infection of the mouth is rare, and the majority of oral lesions of donovanosis are secondary to primary genital infection. In one large study of 858 patients with donovanosis inguinale, 6% of cases were found with orogenital lesions and only 2 patients had primary oral donovanosis. The oral manifestations appear a few months to years after the initial infection. Since there is commonly little pain associated with the early lesion, the patient does not present for treatment until some time later, when extensive tissue destruction has occurred. Almost any oral site may be involved, and the clinical appearance of the lesions is variable. Sites of infection include the lip, gums, cheek, palate, and pharynx, and extra-oral sites include the neck, nose, larynx, and chest. It is often misdiagnosed as actinomycosis. Three main types of donovanosis have been described: ulcerative, exuberant, and cicatricial. The ulcerative lesion is usually extensive and painful, either with a punched-out appearance and a smooth red base or covered with thick dark crusts that bleed easily. The exuberant lesion is raised with a sharply defined border and may be single and extensive or multiple and small, characteristically with a rough surface due to numerous raised projections. The cicatricial lesion appears as areas of fibrous scar tissue that are often extensive. Lesions of all three types may be present within the mouth at the same time, and the regional lymph nodes are not usually enlarged. Long-standing lesions are characterized by multiple extraoral sinuses and scar formation, and, depending on the site and extent of the disease, contraction of scar tissue may result in limitation of mouth opening and jaw movement.

DIAGNOSIS AND MANAGEMENT

Direct examination of a fragment of friable granulation tissue compressed between two slides, fixed and then stained by Giemsa's method, and examined for the presence of Donovan bodies shows a cluster of bacilli lying within leukocytes.

Complex media are needed to culture the organisms, and this is not usually necessary for routine diagnosis. Polymerase chain reaction (PCR) diagnostic methods have been described but are only available as a research tool. Currently, azithromycin is the best drug available for donovanosis in that it can be given intermittently, and directly observed therapy may be necessary.[4] Donovanosis is complicated by other coexisting sexually transmitted diseases, such as syphilis and HIV disease. In cases where gross scarring has occurred, surgery may be required to allow normal movement.

Gonorrhea

Gonorrhea is a sexually transmitted infection with a worldwide distribution that has reached epidemic proportions in some countries.[5] The causative agent, *Neisseria gonorrhoeae*, is transmitted by sexual activity, and lesions occur in the genitals, the anal canal, the oral cavity, particularly the pharynx, and in combinations of these sites. The major risk factor for gonococcal pharyngitis is orogenital sex. The disease is caused by the adherence of *N. gonorrhoeae* to either the genital or oral muscosa and subsequent penetration into the deeper tissues between the surface epithelial cells. Spread may then occur by direct continuity, by lymphatics, or hematogenously. Locally, there is an intense inflammatory reaction with the production of pus, which on microscopy reveals numerous polymorphonuclear leukocytes with intracellular gram-negative diplococci. In males, the disease is characterized by an itching and burning sensation in the urethra with associated moderate to severe pain and the presence of a yellow discharge. In females, the urethra is the main site of initial infection, but the presentation is less acute than in the male, or asymptomatic. In about 2% of patients, disseminated gonococcal infection occurs, which may lead to arthritis, periostitis, carditis, bursitis, and meningitis. It is noteworthy that an estimated 75 to 80% of female patients and 15 to 20% of male patients may be clinically asymptomatic. There is a very high likelihood of human to human transmission of gonorrhea, essentially through unprotected sexual activity.

ORAL CONSIDERATIONS

The oral mucosa is relatively resistant to infection by *N. gonorrhoeae*, but gonorrheal stomatitis is being diagnosed with increasing regularity in sexually active adults, especially in men having sex with men. The clinical presentation of primary oral gonorrhea is variable depending on the severity and distribution of the infection. The patient usually complains of a burning or itchy sensation or a dry hot feeling in the mouth, which in 24 to 48 hours changes to acute pain. The patient may also complain of a foul oral taste, the salivary flow may be increased or decreased, the breath may be fetid, and the submandibular lymph nodes are usually enlarged and painful. The patient may be febrile if the infection is severe.

Lesions have been reported on all parts of the oral mucosa and described usually as consisting of a variable mixture of the following clinical signs: inflammation, edema, vesiculation, ulceration, and pseudomembranes. The latter are white, yellow, or gray in color; easily removed by scraping; and leave a bleeding surface. In some patients, a diffuse painful stomatitis occurs in which all oral membranes become fiery red and edematous. Speech, swallowing, and simple mouth movements become extremely painful. The oral sites of primary infection that have been reported are the gingivae, the tongue, the buccal mucosa, the hard and soft palates, and the oropharynx. *N. gonorrhoeae* has also been isolated from lesions of central papillary atrophy of the tongue. The tonsils and the oropharynx appear to be the commonest site of oral infection. It is thought, but not proven, that oral mucosa anterior to the pharynx is resistant to gonococcal infection; thus, the older reports in the literature of gonorrhea in the latter locations are equivocal.

The clinical presentation is varied, ranging from asymptomatic patients to those with acute tonsillitis. Some of these infections appear to be primary in nature, but others are secondary to genital infection. It is difficult to classify cases for a number of reasons: infection of the genitalia and mouth may be simultaneous, or the oral lesion may develop later, transmission taking place by autoinoculation. In addition, oropharyngeal gonorrhea is more resistant to antibiotic therapy than genital infection, and a course of therapy for genital infection may result in viable organisms remaining in the oropharynx that cause recurrent symptomatic disease some months later. There is evidence that primary infection of the mouth can lead to disseminated lesions. Secondary gonorrheal infection of the parotid gland is rare but may occur in patients who have oral gonorrhea or carry the organisms in their oropharynx. The significance of persistent oropharyngeal carriage of gonococci in asymptomatic individuals is not clear.

Oral manifestations of disseminated gonococcal infection can take two main forms, both of which appear to be rare: septic embolic phenomena and hypersensitivity reactions. The clinical appearances of septic gonococcal lesions of the oral mucosa are varied, consisting of erythematous, purpuric, vesiculopustular, hemorrhagic, and ulcerative lesions either alone or in a number of combinations. The oral sites of infection that have been described are the gingivae, tongue, and hard and soft palates. The hypersensitivity reactions to *N. gonorrhoeae* may result in oral signs and erythematous lesions on the palate, buccal mucosa, and gingivae.

Gonococcal arthritis is one common sequel of urogenital infection. The temporomandibular joint may be occasionally involved, especially if the primary infection is in the pharynx. The clinical symptoms of gonococcal arthritis include rapid-onset fever, a migrating polyarthritis, and inflamed and swollen joints; fluid aspirates from the joint contain large numbers of polymorphonuclear leukocytes and gram-negative diplococci. In the temporomandibular joint, local manifestations include trismus due to spasm of the masseter muscles and inflammatory swelling and edema in and around the joint. Uncommon sequelae of this condition are perforation through the tympanic plate with extension of infection into the external auditory meatus and destruction of the articular cartilage with fibrous ankylosis of the joint.

It is surprising that with the high incidence of gonorrhea throughout the world, there are so few reports of gonococcal stomatitis or pharyngitis. It would seem likely that the true incidence is much higher than the literature suggests and that many oral cases have been dismissed as nonspecific stomatitis. The recognition and diagnosis of oropharyngeal gonorrhea are important for three main reasons: (1) cases may act as reservoirs for the transmission of infection in the community; (2) they are a potential source of gonococcemia, leading to arthritis, meningitis, and other septic embolic lesions; (3) they may cause significant localized tissue damage, pain, and discomfort. Differential diagnosis includes streptococcal stomatitis, herpetic infection, and candidiasis.

DIAGNOSIS AND MANAGEMENT

The only way in which a diagnosis of gonorrheal stomatitis can be made is by laboratory investigation. The examination of Gram-stained films from oral lesions is of little direct diagnostic value due to the presence of oral commensal *Neisseria* species that cannot be differentiated from *N. gonorrhoeae* microscopically. The presence of numerous gram-negative intracellular diplococci in a smear from a suspect lesion should be investigated further. Specimens are usually inoculated on to Martin-Lewis culture medium in JEMBEC plates and incubated under 5 to 10% carbon dioxide for the laboratory diagnosis of gonorrhea. A commercially available enzyme immunoassay (EIA) system for direct detection of gonococci and newer deoxyribonucleic acid (DNA) probe systems are proving popular.

The majority of gonococci are resistant to β-lactam drugs; hence, the choice is β-lactamase-stable, third-generation cephalosporins. Of all the current agents used to treat all forms of gonococcal disease, only the third-generation cephalosporins (most notably cefexime) or ciprofloxacin have retained their efficacy; however, decreased susceptibility to these antibiotics has also appeared. Prevention of gonorrhea requires the practice of 'safe sex,' health education, and contact tracing. There is a high possibility of human to human transmission of donovanosis through unprotected sexual activity.

Meningococcal Meningitis

Neisseria meningitidis is a common bacterial cause of meningitis and is transmitted by droplet infection. Human to human transmission of meningococcal meningitis through the respiratory route is relatively common.

ORAL CONSIDERATIONS

The organism initially colonizes and proliferates in the nasopharynx and then gains access to the bloodstream and is thus carried to the meninges of the brain. About half of the patients with acute meningococcal meningitis develop a petechial rash, which is found on the trunk, limbs, and face. Petechiae may also be found on the mucous membrane of the mouth and conjunctiva. The mouth lesions may involve large areas of the mucous membrane and in severe fatal forms of the disease the uvula may turn back due to submucosal hemorrhage. In one study, meningococcal pharyngitis was reported in over 80% of patients with pneumonia due to *N. meningitidis*.

Mycobacterial Diseases

The two major mycobacterial diseases that are endemic globally are TB and leprosy. These diseases are, unfortunately, highly prevalent in developing regions of the world, but developed nations also harbor a fair proportion of infected despite the availability of appropriate therapy. TB is discussed first, followed by leprosy.

TUBERCULOSIS

Epidemiology Many people in the United States feel that TB is not a serious medical problem any longer. However, on the international scene, TB remains a leading killer of young adults, with some 2 billion people infected, one-third of the world's population. TB is the second leading cause of death by infectious disease, only surpassed by HIV infection.[6] The World Health Organization estimates that over 8 million people develop active TB and that 2 million die each year worldwide. Ten percent of infected people will develop active TB at some time.[7] The potential for human to human transmission of TB through the respiratory route is extremely high.

Even in the United States, TB remains a problem. The number of active cases has dropped from over 80,000 in 1953 to 14,093 in 2005 (Table 1). However, in 2005, the Centers for Disease Control and Prevention (CDC) estimated that 10 to 15 million people had latent TB in the United States. Ethnic background is a strong risk factor for acquiring TB in the United States affecting the following groups in descending

TABLE 1 Reported Cases of Tuberculosis in the United States by Year

Year	Total Number of Cases
1953	84,304
1955	77,368
1960	55,494
1965	49,016
1970	37,137
1975	33,989
1980	27,749
1985	22,201
1990	25,701
1995	22,860
2000	16,337
2005	14,093

Adapted from World Health Organization.[7]

order: Asians, Pacific Islanders, African Americans, Hispanics, Americans Indians, Caucasians. Over half of new cases in the United States are foreign-born persons, and this group is eight times more likely to be diagnosed with TB than native-born Americans.[8] This has had a particular impact on health care workers (HCWs), who are at risk for transmitting TB to patients. In 2002, the incidence of TB in New York State was 10 times higher among foreign HCWs than among US-born HCWs.[9]

Several trends in the United States during the 1980s and 1990s resulted in an increase in TB infection rates and continue to complicate the management of the disease today. People with HIV/acquired immune deficiency syndrome (AIDS) are at significant risk of developing active TB after being exposed. As mentioned above, increased numbers of foreign-born people are coming to the United States from areas with high rates of TB, such as Asia, Africa, and Latin America. Poverty, injection drug use, alcoholism, and homelessness have contributed to the spread of TB as large numbers of these people are in crowded shelters and/or prisons, where they are chronically exposed. Elderly people in nursing homes with declining health status are at risk for reactivating TB they were exposed to earlier in life or being newly infected when immunosuppressed. Finally, people commonly do not comply with their TB treatment regimen, which makes them infectious longer and more likely to develop resistance to treatment.[10]

Diagnosis Diagnosis is initiated by performing a tuberculin skin test on the forearm with purified protein derivative (PPD), a mycobacterial antigen. If a red welt forms within 72 hours, the patient is considered to have been exposed to *Mycobacterium tuberculosis*. This screening test is recommended for certain high-risk populations (Table 2). Signs and symptoms are evaluated to look for active disease. These include productive cough, fever, chills, or night sweats. A chest radiograph is taken to look for pulmonary involvement. The final test, or acid-fast bacillus test, involves collecting patient sputum to look for the infecting organism. If present, the patient is considered to have an active infection requiring treatment.[10,11]

Pathogenesis TB is caused by the acid- and alcohol-fast bacillus *M. tuberculosis*. The organism is usually acquired by airborne transmission and grows in the pulmonary alveoli and macrophages with a local inflammatory response. In most cases, T helper cells activate macrophages through the secretion of cytokines and gamma-interferon, and the infection is suppressed permanently or may remain latent to reactivate months or years later. If the immune response is compromised and cannot prevent replication of the bacteria, active disease begins. Five to 10% of exposed patients will go on to develop active TB during their life.[12] With active infection, the following symptoms are common: chronic cough, moderate fever, night sweats, fatigue, decreased appetite, and weight loss. Occasionally, TB can spread to other parts of the body by the lymph and blood systems. Miliary (blood infection) and meningeal TB are the most serious forms of the disease, with high mortality rates.[13]

Medical Management TB is curable in most patients, but compliance with drug regimens is critical to prevent reactivation of the disease or the development of resistance. The usual course of therapy is 6 to 9 months and involves several drug regimens (Table 3). If patients fail initial therapy, they may have multidrug-resistant TB. If so, they will require special therapy with at least three drugs for up to 2 years. Even with this therapy, up to 60% of patients with multidrug-resistant TB will die of their disease.[14] The directly observed therapy regimen has been extremely successful in curing recalcitrant lowly compliant patients and also in preventing drug-resistant strains from emerging.

Prevention programs have helped reduce the incidence of TB in the United States. Where there are large populations in close proximity, adequate ventilation is the most effective measure to prevent the spread of TB. High-risk groups are screened for TB and, if positive, treated with isoniazid (INH) for 6 to 12 months to prevent active disease. Health

---

TABLE 2 High-Risk Groups Recommended for Purified Protein Derivative Testing

1. Person with signs, symptoms, and/or laboratory abnormalities suggestive of clinically active TB
2. People who interact with persons with active TB
3. Poor and medically underserved people
4. Homeless people
5. Those who come from countries with high TB incidence rates
6. Nursing home residents
7. Alcoholics and intravenous drug users
8. People with HIV or AIDS or who are otherwise immunosuppressed
9. People in jail or prison
10. Health care workers and others, such as prison guards, who work with high-risk populations.

Adapted from American Lung Association.[11]

AIDS = acquired immune deficiency syndrome; HIV = human immunodeficiency virus; TB = tuberculosis.

TABLE 3 Treatment for Tuberculosis Infection

Timing	Medications
Months 1 and 2	INH, RIF, PZA, EMB
Next 4 to 7 months depending on condition	INH, RIF

EMB = ethambutol; INH = isoniazid; PZA = pyrazinamide; RIF = rifampin (rifabutin may be substituted for rifampin).

care facilities use ultraviolet light, special filters, special respirators, and masks to reduce the spread of TB. People with active TB are isolated in rooms with controlled ventilation until they are no longer infectious.[10]

There is a vaccine for TB termed bacille Calmette-Guérin (BCG), which is made from live weakened *Mycobacterium bovis*. In countries where TB is common, this vaccine is given to children with 60 to 80% efficacy. However, the vaccine is much less effective for adults, and it results in a positive skin test, reducing the effectiveness of this test in screening for TB exposure. The vaccine is not routinely used in the United States.[15]

Oral Considerations   Oral manifestations may occur in up to 3% of patients with long-term systemic TB. Lesions occur in the oral tissues and the neck lymph nodes. The latter is termed scrofula. The oral lesions are found in various soft tissues and supporting bone.[16,17]

The risk of a dental care provider acquiring TB from a patient appears to be low, particularly in a conventional dental office.[18] However, health care settings involving the patients listed in Table 2 put dental personnel at higher risk. Hospitals, nursing homes, prisons, and clinics that treat high-risk populations are of particular concern. Patients with active TB will typically be in isolation, and dental treatment should be deferred until the patient is no longer considered infectious. Patients are no longer considered infectious if they have two consecutive negative sputum cultures or have received TB treatment for at least 2 weeks. To identify HCWs who have been exposed to TB, many hospitals require personnel to be skin-tested annually. This appears to be a reasonable practice in settings with a significant high-risk population. As mentioned previously, HCWs who have seroconverted since their last skin test are considered for 6 to 12 months of INH therapy.[10]

LEPROSY

Leprosy is a chronic, granulomatous systemic disease that is mostly prevalent in the developing world, mainly Africa and Asia, although cases of leprosy occur in other countries, especially those bordering the Mediterranean, Adriatic, and Black seas. Droplet infection is the probable mode of transmission of leprosy, the source of the infection being the nasal discharge of patients with lepromatous leprosy.

Leprosy is a chronic infectious disease of peripheral nerves, skin, and sometimes other tissues. It is caused by *Mycobacterium leprae*, which usually causes a mild or subclinical infection on initial entry to the tissues. The subsequent clinical pattern of disease depends on the type and extent of the host immune reaction and could lead to lepromatous, tuberculoid, or borderline variants. In lepromatous leprosy, a cell-mediated response to *M. leprae* does not occur, whereas the humoral response is marked, with the production of high titers of antibodies. Clinically, the infection is widespread throughout the body, and large numbers of bacilli are present in the lesions. The lepromin skin test is negative, and little or no lymphocytic infiltration is found.

In tuberculoid leprosy, cell-mediated immunity is strong, whereas little or no antibody is produced. Clinically, the disease is localized to a few sites and the lepromin test is positive. Histologically, bacilli are scanty in the lesions and there are noncaseating tuberculoid granulomas present that destroy tissue and nerves. In the third category, borderline leprosy, patients progress from a tuberculoid-like form of the disease to a more lepromatous presentation. The potential for human to human transmission of leprosy is relatively low compared with tuberculosis.

Oral Considerations   There is no record of any cases of tuberculoid leprosy affecting the oral mucosa, but the neurologic features associated with this form of leprosy may affect the mouth and face. If the trigeminal nerve is involved, hyperesthesia or paresthesia of the face, lips, tongue, palate, cheeks, or gingiva may occur, and if the facial nerve is involved, the facial muscles may be partially or completely paralyzed. The dermal lesions of tuberculoid leprosy on the face are normally single and elsewhere, if multiple, have an asymmetric distribution. The lesions consist of dry, hairless plaques with a well-defined and raised border about 2.5 cm in diameter, which on white skin are red and on dark skin are hypopigmented. The patient usually complains that the lesion is numb and on testing is anesthetic to touch and pinprick. Secondary ocular changes may occur, with subsequent corneal and conjunctival sensory loss. In borderline leprosy, oral lesions appear as focal or diffuse enanthemas, or papules, rarely forming ulcers.

Finally, in lepromatous leprosy, *M. leprae* is present in many tissues of the body, and multiple, erythematous, bilateral, and symmetric lesions are found on the skin of the face, arms, and legs. The lesions are anesthetic. Bone lesions also occur related to the hands, feet, and skull, leading to deformities in these areas. The lesions of the skull may cause atrophy of the anterior nasal spine either alone or combined with atrophy and recession of the alveolar process in the premaxillary region, with loosening of the maxillary incisor teeth (Figure 3). In addition, inflammatory changes in the superior surface of the hard palate may occur. Dental deformities in lepromatous leprosy have been noted as pink discoloration of the upper incisors due to invasion of the pulp by infected granulomatous tissue that can produce pulpitis and pulp death.

The incidence of oral lesions in lepromatous leprosy varies from 10 to 60%. Intraoral nodules have been described as yellowish-red, soft to hard, sessile, single or confluent lesions that tend to ulcerate. Healing is by secondary intention with fibrous scars. The sites most commonly involved are the premaxillary gingivae, the hard and soft palates, the uvula, and the tongue. Tongue lesions, particularly on the anterior two-thirds, consist of single or multiple nodules, giving a 'cobblestone' appearance, or in some instances may resemble a geographic tongue. In the borderline variant of leprosy, oral lesions are uncommon and may appear as papules, erythema, or ulcers. As the saliva of patients with oral lesions commonly

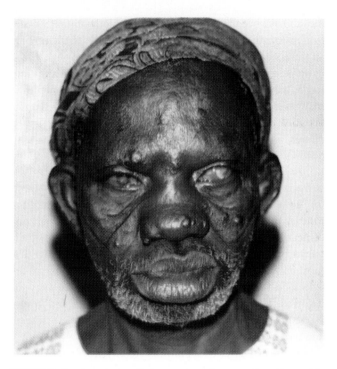

FIGURE 3 A patient with lepromatous leprosy. Note the saddle nose and associated general disfigurement and blindness. Adapted with permission from Samaranayake LP.[1]

contains *M. leprae*, this could be a possible source of infection, although the pathobiology of leprosy transmission is still a mystery.

Diagnosis and Management The diagnosis of leprosy is not usually difficult as long as the patient is carefully examined for the signs and symptoms of the disease, that is, anesthetic skin lesions and thickened peripheral nerves. In lepromatous leprosy, an incision is made into the dermis and the lesion is scraped using the blunt side of the blade. A smear is made and stained by Ziehl-Neelsen's method to demonstrate acid- and alcohol-fast bacilli. In tuberculoid leprosy, it is difficult to demonstrate bacilli, and the disease is diagnosed by histologic examination of a biopsy of skin or thickened nerve. *M. leprae* has never been cultured in vitro, but experimental infection of armadillos and thymectomized irradiated mice has been successful. The lepromin test is of little diagnostic value.

Treatment is usually undertaken by those with experience of leprosy, and advice from the Panel of Leprosy Opinion is essential in the United Kingdom. Therapy consists of the administration of long-acting diaphenylsulfone (dapsone), with rifampicin plus clofazimine or ethionamide or prothionamide. As drug resistance is a growing problem, combination therapy, as in TB, is always given. Family contacts may be given dapsone. No vaccine is available.

SYPHILIS

Syphilis is a classic disease with protean manifestations. There has been a significant rise in the prevalence of syphilis both in the developed and developing world during the past two decades, mainly as a disease associated with HIV infection and sexual promiscuity.[19] Particularly striking increases have been noted in Eastern Europe, especially in the United Kingdom, and in the United States. As the prevalence of syphilis in heterosexuals has been on the rise, there has been a proportionate increase in the number of children born with congenital syphilis. Syphilis is preventable and treatable with effective and inexpensive antibiotics; hence, its rapid diagnosis is important to prevent its late and severe sequelae. The disease is caused by *T. pallidum*, the syphilis spirochete. There is a very high likelihood of human to human transmission of syphilis through unprotected sexual activity.

Syphilis has an incubation period of 10 to 90 days (average 3 weeks) and is characterized by four main clinical stages: primary, secondary, tertiary, and late or quaternary.

Primary Syphilis After the inital exposure to infection with *T. pallidum*, the spirochetes pass through the mucous membrane or skin and are then carried in the blood throughout the body. After an incubation period of about 3 to 4 weeks, there develops, at the site of entry, an ulcerated lesion called a primary chancre: a flat, red, indurated, highly infectious ulcer with a serous exudate. The typical lesion is painless, and edema of the surrounding tissues is usually present. The regional lymph nodes become enlarged about 2 weeks after the appearance of the chancre and on examination are firm, painless, and discrete, with a rubbery consistency. The chancre disappears spontaneously within 3 to 8 weeks.

Secondary Syphilis Approximately 2 months after healing, the secondary stage of syphilis usually develops, and in about one-third of patients, the primary chancre may be present at the same time. The signs of secondary syphilis are variable: generalized skin lesions in about 75% of cases, mucosal ulcers in about 33% of cases, generalized lymphadenopathy in about 50% of cases, and systemic symptoms that are 'influenza like,' including fever, headache, malaise, and general aches and pains. The skin lesions are found predominantly on the face, hands, feet, and genitalia and appear as dull red macular or papular spots.

Tertiary Syphilis Reactivation of syphilis can occur at any time 2 or 3 years after the date of first infection, but such late lesions of syphilis are rarely seen today. The characteristic lesion is the gumma, which is usually localized, single or multiple, varying in size from a pinhead to a lesion several centimeters in diameter. Gummas develop in the skin, the mucous membranes, and bones. These lesions are not infective as the tissue damage is due to a delayed type of hypersensitivity. The other organs involved in tertiary syphilis are the cardiovascular system and the nervous system.

Late or Quaternary Syphilis This condition is seen one to two decades after primary syphilis. The two main clinical forms of late syphilis are cardiovascular syphilis and neuro-syphilis, with resultant pathology of the aorta and the nervous system, respectively.

Latent Syphilis　This may be seen in some after many years without any symptoms. The disease lies dormant, without any clinical signs (except for positive serology), and may manifest as cardiovascular or neurosyphilis.

Congenital Syphilis　*T. pallidum* is one of the few microor-ganisms that has the ability to cross the placental barrier; thus, the fetus may be infected during the second or third trimester from a syphilitic mother (either in the primary or secondary stage of syphilis). The disease will manifest in the infant as either (1) latent infection—no symptoms but positive serology; (2) early infection—lesions such as skin rashes, saddle nose, bone lesions, and meningitis appear up to the end of the second year of age; or (3) late infection—after the second year of age; lesions include Hutchinson's incisors (notching of incisor teeth), mulberry molar teeth (due to infection of the enamel organ in the fetus), interstitial keratitis, bone sclerosis, arthritis, and deafness.

Oral Considerations

Primary Syphilis　The normal site for the chancre is on the genitalia, but extragenital primary lesions occur in about 4 to 12% of patients with syphilis. A chancre of the lip is the most common extragenital lesion, accounting for about 60% of cases, and may present at the angles of the mouth.[1] Most chancres in the male tend to be located in the upper lip and in the female on the lower lip. Other sites affected are the tongue and, to a lesser extent, the gingivae and tonsillar area. Intraoral chancres are usually slightly painful due to secondary bacterial infection, as are the enlarged lymph nodes in the submaxillary, submental, and cervical regions. The lesions are infectious, and transmission may occur by kissing, unusual sexual practices, and even intermediate contact with cups, glasses, and eating utensils. The differential diagnosis of primary syphilis includes ruptured vesicles of herpes simplex, traumatic ulcers, and carcinoma.

Secondary Syphilis　Characteristic slightly raised, grayish white, glistening patches on the mucous membrane, so-called 'mucous patches,' of the tongue, soft palate, tonsil, or cheek but rarely the gingival tissues are common in the secondary stage. Lesions on the larynx and pharynx may lead to hoarse-ness. The surface of these lesions is covered with a grayish membrane, which can be easily removed and contains many spirochetes. The ulcers may coalesce to give the characteristic 'snail tracks' and mucous patches in about a third of those affected. These lesions, like the primary chancre, are highly infectious. Maculopapular eruptions have been described in the mouth and are confined mainly to the palate, but, occasionally, the entire oral mucosa may be involved. In recent years, the secondary syphilitic lesions found in the

mouth have been noted as often atypical, due, in many cases, to inadequate treatment: as a result of antibiotic therapy for an unrelated infection. Other manifestations are generalized lymphadenopathy and condylomata (warts) of the anus and vulva; rarely, periostitis, arthritis, and glomerulonephritis may be seen. The differential diagnosis of secondary syphilis includes aphthous ulcers, erythema multiforme, lichen planus, and tonsillitis. The secondary-stage lesions heal 2 to 6 weeks after the time they first appear.

Tertiary Syphilis　The representative lesion of this stage is the 'gumma,' which begins as a small, pale, raised area of the mucosa that ulcerates and rapidly progresses to a large zone of necrosis with denudation of bone and in the case of the palate may eventually perforate into the nasal cavity. The most common site for gumma formation is the hard palate, although the soft palate, lips, tongue, and face may be involved. The palatal lesions are usually midline, and in rare cases, the soft palate may be involved. Gummas are painless and have no infectivity.

Occasional cases of syphilitic osteomyelitis involving the mandible and, less commonly, the maxilla have been described. This condition represents a gummatous involve-ment of bone with extensive necrosis. The condition is characterized by pain, swelling, suppuration and sequestra-tion, and both clinically and radiographically, the condition may resemble pyogenic osteomyelitis. If the lesion ossifies, then the radiographic appearance of the affected area may be similar to that of an osteogenic sarcoma.

Atrophic or interstitial glossitis is another oral manifesta-tion of tertiary syphilis. Clinically, there is atrophy of the filiform and fungiform papillae, which results in a smooth, sometimes wrinkled lingual surface. This appearance is prob-ably due to obliterative endarteritis of the lingual vasculature, leading to circulatory deficiency. Loss of the protective papillae subjects the dorsum of the tongue to many noxious stimuli, and leukoplakia frequently develops. The relation-ship between syphilitic glossitis and carcinoma of the tongue is not clear.

Syphilis very rarely affects the salivary glands, but both secondary and tertiary lesions have been described in the parotid glands. The other main salivary glands have also been involved either on their own or together with the parotid. Patients with general paresis of the insane may have perioral tremors and fine irregular tremors of the tongue and fingers. Although an association between oral squamous cell carci-noma and syphilis has been suggested in early studies, this relationship remains unproven.

Congenital Syphilis　The dental lesions of congenital syphilis are a result of infection of the developing tooth germ by *T. pallidum*. Since the deciduous teeth are usually well devel-oped by the time the spirochetes invade the developing dental tissues, these teeth are minimally affected. The permanent teeth are at an early stage of development, and infection may result in the complete failure of development of a tooth or the production of malformed teeth. Early oral manifestations include diffuse maculopapular rash, periostitis (frontal bossing of Parrot), and rhinitis, whereas late features, manifesting at least 24 months after birth, comprise the hutchinsonian triad of interstitial keratitis of the cornea, sensorineural hearing loss, and dental anomalies. The most common dental manifestation of congenital syphilis is the so-called 'mulberry molar' teeth, which are highly suggestive of prenatal syphilis. The first permanent molar teeth are usually involved and have roughened, dirty, yellow, hypoplastic, occlusal surfaces with poorly developed cusps and are smaller in size than normal. Hutchinson's incisors are another manifestation of congenital syphilis. The upper central incisors are usually involved and have crescentic notches in the middle of their incisal edge. The tooth tends to be wider gingivally than at the incisal edge, giving a 'screwdriver' appearance. The lower incisors show similar defects, but they are affected much less often than their maxillary counterparts. Of note, the maxillary incisors are more commonly affected than the mandibular ones. Infection of the developing bones of the face may lead to permanent facial deformities, which produce an open bite and a 'dished' appearance to the face. Skin around the lips may show yellow discoloration soon after birth, leading to crack formation and eventual (Parrot's) radial scars—rhagades—of the lips. Other, less common orofacial features include atrophic glossitis and a high, narrow palatal vault.

Diagnosis and Management Exudate from primary or secondary lesions may be collected in fine capillary tubes and examined using dark-ground microscopy for typically motile *T. pallidum*. This technique has limited value in lesions affecting the mouth since the oral commensal *Treponema microdentium* closely resembles *T. pallidum*. However, specific immunofluorescence tests, if available, are helpful in diagnosis.

The laboratory diagnosis of syphilis is usually made by serology since *T. pallidum* cannot be routinely cultured in vitro. Ten milliliters of venous blood is sufficient to carry out all the serologic tests for syphilis. It is usual to carry out at least two different tests on each specimen of serum, and the interpretation of these complex test results should be left to an expert in genitourinary infections. Antigens used for syphilis serology are of two types:

- *Cardiolipin or lipoidal antigen*. Although not derived from the spirochete, it is sensitive for detecting antibody. The most popular test that uses this antibody is the VDRL (Venereal Diseases Reference Laboratory) test; it is simple and sensitive, but biologic false-positive reactions are common. As the antibody disappears after treatment, it can be used to monitor the efficacy of antimicrobial therapy.
- *Specific treponemal antigen*. Using *T. pallidum* as an antigen gives fewer false-positive reactions, and tests remain positive after treatment. The tests are *T. pallidum* hemagglutination test, fluorescent

treponemal antibody-absorption test (FTA-Abs), which detects both IgM and IgG antibody, and ELISA. The last is increasingly used as a screening test to detect IgG antibody, although some false positives may result.

Differential Diagnosis Primary and secondary syphilis include candidiasis, leukoplakia, hairy leukoplakia, lichen planus, aphthous ulcers, herpetic gingivostomatitis, erythema multiforme, TB, and trauma.

The most effective drug for syphilis is procaine benzylpenicillin. Doxycycline or erythromycin can be used in patients who are sensitive to penicillin. Follow-up with regular clinical and serologic examinations is necessary for at least 2 years, and contact tracing is recommended.

TETANUS

Although a rare disease in the developed world, tetanus remains an important cause of morbidity and mortality in the developing world, causing an estimated 800,000 to 1,000,000 deaths each year.[20] Tetanus is caused by the spore-forming gram-positive bacillus *Clostridium tetani*. The spores of the organism germinate under anaerobic conditions and produce an exotoxin, tetanospasmin, as well as a hemolysin (tetanolysin), which reaches the brainstem and the anterior horn of the spinal cord, either between fibers of the regional nerve trunks or via the bloodstream. The toxin produces increased muscle tone (rigidity), which results in muscle spasms or convulsions. The source of entry is commonly a wound made by an object contaminated with earth, manure, or dust. In about one-third of cases, the wound may be no more than a superficial abrasion and be so small as to be undetected. Deep wounds heavily infected and containing foreign bodies, for example, war wounds or injuries due to car accidents, provide the most favorable conditions for the germination of spores and the multiplication of bacilli. Tetanus has been rarely described in association with oral sepsis and after dental extractions.

The incubation period of tetanus is variable, ranging from a few days to 3 weeks, and this represents the interval between the infection of the wound, the production of toxin, and its reaction with nervous tissue. The prognosis is regarded as poor if the incubation period is less than a week, whereas a long incubation period is often associated with a mild attack. *C. tetani* may remain in the tissues for months or even years until activated by irritation or trauma. Human to human transmission of tetanus is not feasible.

Oral Considerations After a short period of nonspecific prodromal symptoms, the first manifestation of tetanus is tonic rigidity of the muscles of mastication. The patient presents with stiffness of the face followed by difficulty in chewing and swallowing. The endentulous patient may complain of an inability to insert his dentures. The spasm of the muscles of mastication often increases until the jaws are finally locked and the mouth cannot be opened. If the muscles of facial expressions are involved, the corners of the mouth are drawn back, the lips are protruded, and the forehead is wrinkled, giving the characteristic appearance of risus sardonicus. Other muscle groups become involved, for example, the trunk and the proximal parts of the limbs. The spine may become arched (opisthotonus) and the chest fixed in a state of expiration. There is often a board-like rigidity of the abdominal muscles, and as the infection develops, the patient has difficulty in swallowing and breathing is embarrassed because of restricted respiratory movements. Death occurs from exhaustion, aspiration pneumonia, or asphyxia due to respiratory muscle spasm.

There are many causes of trismus that must be eliminated before a diagnosis of tetanus can be made, and the dentist, rather than the physician, may see the patient first. The more common causes of trismus are impacted third molar teeth with pericoronitis, periapical abscesses of the posterior teeth, tonsillitis, submasseteric abscess, retropharyngeal abscess, mumps, arthritis, dislocation of the temporomandibular joint, and fracture of the mandible. A unusual form of poliomyelitis mimics tetanus by causing paralysis of the masseter muscles and dysphagia, with the true diagnosis only becoming evident postmortem.

Diagnosis and Management Laboratory investigations are not usually helpful, and the diagnosis of tetanus can usually be made from the clinical history and presentation. The treatment must be started immediately once a clinical diagnosis is made and not await microbiologic results. The isolation of *C. tetani* from the wound is often difficult and uncertain due to the small numbers of organisms present and the heavy mixed growth of other microorganisms. If there is an open wound, a swab of pus should be sent for culture and animal inoculation.

Treatment consists of the administration of antitoxin, preferably human tetanus immunoglobulin; thorough wound débridement, antibiotics, usually penicillin; and sedatives to control muscle rigidity and spasm.

TULAREMIA

Tularemia has been reported most frequently in the United States and Russia and sporadically in Canada, Mexico, Japan, and parts of Europe.[21] The causative agent is *Francisella tularensis*, which is a small pleomorphic gram-negative rod. The main reservoirs of the infection are small wild mammals such as ground squirrels, hares, and rabbits. Transmission to humans usually occurs by direct contact with infected tissue or secretions, although the bacteria occasionally enter the body through the respiratory or gastrointestinal tracts or via biting flies. The clinical types of infection can vary from ulceroglandular, glandular, oculoglandular, oropharyngeal, intestinal, and pneumonic to typhoidal. These developments are related to the route of infection and the virulence of the infecting strain. The onset of the disease is sudden, and the main symptoms include headache, fever, chills, profuse sweats, body pain, nausea, and vomiting. Fever is a prominent feature and may persist for weeks or months in untreated cases. Clinical diagnosis is supported by evidence or a history of a tick or deerfly bite, exposure to tissues of a mammalian host of *F. tularensis*, or exposure to potentially contaminated water.

Oral Considerations The oropharyngeal variant is relatively common and presents as stomatitis or pharyngitis or tonsillitis and cervical lymphadenopathy. Primary infection of the mouth usually occurs from eating infected meat, and the sites affected are the soft palate, tongue, gingiva, and angle of the mouth. The ulcer that occurs at the site of entry is initially shallow, with a whitish fibrinous pseudomembrane, but may extend more deeply due to secondary infection. The cervical lymph nodes are usually tender and enlarged and may suppurate, and cervical lymphadenopathy is seen in 5 to 6% of cases with tularemia. Oral lesions may develop secondary to infection in the lungs or other sites. Acute tonsillitis may be the presenting symptom, and the tonsils, posterior pharyngeal wall, soft palate, base of the tongue, and buccal mucosa may be covered by a grayish-white membrane simulating the appearance of diphtheria. Oral lesions heal without scarring.

Diagnosis and Management Elevated serum antibody titer(s) to *F. tularensis* antigen in a patient with no history of tularemia vaccination and detection of *F. tularensis* in a clinical specimen by fluorescent assay are diagnostic. Newer molecular biology diagnostics are currently being tested. The antibiotics of choice are streptomycin and tetracycline, either alone or in combination.[22] There is a slim possibility of human to human transmission of tularemia by direct contact with infected tissue or secretions.

▼ CHLAMYDIAL INFECTIONS

Most infections are asymptomatic, as shown by a high worldwide seroprevalence (> 50% of cases). It is a common cause of acute respiratory infections, mainly pneumonia (> 50% of cases) and other acute respiratory tract infections (25% of acute bronchitis, < 5% of sinusitis, otitis, and pharyngitis). About 10% of the community-acquired pneumonia cases have been associated with *Chlamydia pneumoniae* infection. This incidence depends on a cyclic epidemiology with a high incidence for 2 to 3 years followed by a low prevalence for 3 to 4 years. Most chlamydial infections are mild but occasionally severe, with death especially in old people. Mostly, acute infections are recurrent infections. The seroprevalence is higher in asthmatic patients; its role in acute exacerbation of chronic bronchitis is not definitely established. Extrarespiratory acute infections that are less frequent include either fever alone or cardiovascular diseases (acute myocarditis, pericarditis, and endocarditis) or neurologic manifestations (encephalitis, meningitis, or Guillain-Barré syndrome). In addition, seroepidemiologic studies have shown an association with coronary artery disease; *C. pneumoniae* was detected in coronary atheroma by immunochemistry, PCR, and electron microscopy. *C. pneumoniae* may be involved in the atherosclerotic process. To define the clinical spectrum of infection requires precise laboratory diagnosis. The most efficient tests (PCR, direct immunofluorescence, and culture) are done in specialized laboratories; serologic tests are less reliable. Macrolides, cyclines, and fluoroquinolones are the most potent antibiotics. Bacteriologic failures have been described despite the in vitro activity.

Lymphogranuloma Venereum

Lymphogranuloma venereum is a sexually transmitted disease caused by *Chlamydia trachomatis* and is common in tropical and temperate zones. Chlamydia are minute gram-negative cocci that are intracellular parasites. *C. pneumoniae* has been recently implicated in atherosclerotic processes. There is a very high likelihood of human to human transmission of lymphogranuloma venereum through unprotected sexual activity.

The primary lesion of lymphogranuloma venereum occurs in the anogenital region about 10 days after exposure and presents as a small vesicle, which ruptures and heals without scarring. About 1 week to 2 months later, swelling and tenderness of the regional lymph nodes occur, and suppuration via multiple sinuses may supervene. The large intestine may also become involved, and healing usually occurs with scar formation.

ORAL CONSIDERATIONS

Orogenital contact may result in the primary lesion of lymphogranuloma venereum occurring in the mouth. The tongue is the most frequently affected site in primary infections, and the lesion appears as a painless vesicle. As the disease progresses, the tongue may become enlarged, with areas of scarring and deep grooves on the dorsum. The grooves are intensely red, with loss of superficial epithelium, or, alternatively, grayish opaque papules may develop. Other areas of the mouth may be involved, and lesions of the lips, cheeks, tongue, floor of the mouth, uvula, and pharynx have been described. The cervical lymph nodes become painfully enlarged within 7 days to 2 months after the appearance of the initial lesions and may suppurate, forming abscesses and fistulae.

DIAGNOSIS AND MANAGEMENT

Microscopic examination of Giemsa-stained films of pus or sections from a lymph node biopsy may demonstrate minute intracellular cocci. PCR, direct immunofluorescence, and culture of aspirated pus or lymph node biopsy material could be performed in specialized laboratories as serologic tests are less reliable. Macrolides, tetracyclines, and fluoroquinolones are the most potent antibiotics.

▼ RICKETTSIAL INFECTIONS

Rickettsia are intracellular parasites that have characteristics similar to bacteria and viruses. They are bacillary or coccoid in form, about 0.3 to 1.0 μm in diameter, and highly pleomorphic. The organisms are harmless parasites for various arthropods such as mites, lice, and ticks and inhabit the lining cells of their intestines. Also, rickettsiae are found in the saliva of these arthropods and can be transmitted to humans by bites. On gaining access to the tissues of humans, the *Rickettsia* localizes and multiplies in the endothelial cells of blood vessels. The infected endothelial cells eventually rupture, and bleeding occurs into the tissues with the formation of a characteristic rash. There are a number of diseases caused by *Rickettsia*, but oral manifestations have been described only in the following: Rocky Mountain spotted fever, scrub typhus (tsutsugamushi fever), and rickettsialpox.

Rocky Mountain Spotted Fever

The causative agent of Rocky Mountain spotted fever is *Rickettsia rickettsii*. The disease is not uncommonly misdiagnosed as measles due to similarities in the onset and development of the infection. Rocky Mountain spotted fever has a sudden onset, with fever, headache, and chills; the cheeks are flushed, and the eyes are red (or injected!). A reddish macular rash appears on the wrists and ankles and spreads rapidly to cover the entire body, becoming maculopapular, petechial, or, rarely, purpuric. Necrosis may occur, especially on the digits, nose, ears, and scrotum. Rocky Mountian spotted fever cannot be transmitted from human to human.

ORAL CONSIDERATIONS

Oral lesions may involve the buccal mucosa, throat, and tongue, which become swollen and dry with prominent papillae, fissured, and coated. Thrombosis of small blood vessels is common in Rocky Mountain spotted fever, and necrosis of the soft palate as a consequence has been described.

DIAGNOSIS AND MANAGEMENT

A rapid skin biopsy using fluorescent-antibody techniques is available for diagnosing Rocky Mountain spotted fever. Tetracycline and chloramphenicol are the drugs of choice.

Scrub Typhus

Scrub typhus is caused by *Rickettsia tsutsugamushi* and is transmitted by a mite. A painless papule develops at the site of the bite, which enlarges, ulcerates, and forms an area of necrosis with dark slough. Scrub typhus cannot be transmitted from human to human.

Systemic symptoms develop suddenly and include malaise, fever, headache, hard spasmodic cough, and a cutaneous rash. About 5 days later, a rash of large reddish-brown macules or papules develops on the trunk and then the limbs.

ORAL CONSIDERATIONS

In a few instances, lesions may be found on the tongue, soft palate, and pharynx, which typically appear as tiny bright-red macules. In more developed cases, ulcers may appear on the soft palate, tongue, and fauces, and numerous small petechiae may be seen scattered bilaterally on the buccal oral mucosa. If the primary site of infection is within the drainage area of the parotid group of lymph nodes, then enlargement of this group of nodes may lead to a misdiagnosis of mumps.

DIAGNOSIS AND MANAGEMENT

Serologic and molecular diagnostic tests are available for rickettsial infections. Although drug-resistant strains have been reported, the infection usually responds to drugs such as doxycycline or chloramphenicol.

Rickettsialpox

Rickettsialpox is caused by *Rickettsia akari* and mainly occurs in New York City. At the primary site of inoculation, a firm red papule develops, which becomes vesicular and then regresses and forms a dry black eschar. The regional lymph nodes become enlarged and tender. As the disease develops, various systemic symptoms appear: fever, backache, headache, sore throat, and muscular pain with a skin rash, which is similar in type to the primary lesion. Rickettsialpox cannot be transmitted from human to human.

ORAL CONSIDERATIONS

Transient oral mucosal lesions have been described that appear at the same time as skin lesions. Characteristically, vesicles about 2 mm in diameter, surrounded by a zone of erythema, are seen on the lips, tongue, buccal mucosa, hard and soft palates, and pharynx.

DIAGNOSIS AND MANAGEMENT

The common method of laboratory diagnosis of these infections is by serology. A number of tests can be used: the Weil-Felix reaction, which measures nonspecific serum agglutinins for strains of *Proteus* species; indirect immunofluorescence; ELISA; and complement fixation tests.

▼ FUNGAL INFECTIONS

Candidal infections are the most common fungal disease in the oral cavity and manifest in various guises. These are described in detail in Chapter 4, "Red and White Lesions of the Oral Mucosa." Apart from the latter, a number of systemic mycotic diseases, once considered exotic, manifest intraorally, with increasing frequency due to the high prevalence of compromised individuals in the community.[23] These are described in the next section. For the sake of convenience, they are discussed in alphabetical order (Table 4).

Aspergillosis

Aspergillosis has been reported as second only to candidiasis as the most prevalent opportunistic mycotic infection. It is also the second most frequent orofacial fungal infection in those receiving cancer chemotherapy. *Aspergillus* species are filamentous saprophytes that live in soil and decaying vegetation, and the most common pathogen of the species is *Aspergillus fumigatus*. Human infections are also caused by the less common *Aspergillus flavus*, *Aspergillus glaucis*, *Aspergillus terrus*, and *Aspergillus niger*. Aspergillosis may present as three clinical variants: (1) saprophytic—superficial infection without invasion; (2) allergic—a hypersensitivity reaction; and (3) invasive—infection into viable tissue.

Aspergillosis is generally contracted through inhalation of spores, leading to both upper and lower respiratory tract infection—bronchopulmonary aspergillosis. Infections may then spread to the brain, bone, or endocardium. The paranasal sinuses, larynx, eyes, ears, and oral cavity may be involved in primary aspergillosis. The potential for transmission of aspergillosis from human to human is low.

ORAL CONSIDERATIONS

Orofacial aspergillosis may affect the paranasal sinuses, nasal cavity, oral mucosa, and underlying structures, as well as the skin of the face. *A. fumigatus* is the usual agent of sinus aspergillosis, whereas *A. flavus* is more common in invasive lesions in immunosuppressed individuals. Orofacial aspergillosis appears to be relatively common in patients undergoing treatment for malignancies of the blood and blood-forming organs.

In general, the lesions are yellow or black in color, with a necrotic ulcerated base, typically located on the palate or posterior tongue. The hyphal elements of the fungus may invade the oral mucosa and penetrate the walls of small- to medium-sized arteries and veins, producing thrombosis, infarction, and necrosis, finally leading to systemic spread. Aspergilloma of the maxillary antrum is not uncommon, presenting in a healthy host as a hyphal ball in a chronically obstructed sinus.

DIAGNOSIS AND MANAGEMENT

The main differential diagnoses are from *Mucor* and *Pseudomonas* oral infection. Bone erosion can be more easily detected by nuclear magnetic resonance or computed tomography, and the diagnosis can be confirmed by periodic acid–Schiff–stained smear; immunostains may be of help. Systemic amphotericin B is the choice antimycotic if the superficial infections do not resolve within 72 hours of ketoconazole or clotrimazole therapy.

Blastomycosis

Although becoming more prevalent due to the HIV pandemic, blastomycosis is a relatively uncommon fungal disease. Blastomycosis is a deep mycotic infection, caused by *Blastomyces dermatitidis*, found mainly in North America, particularly in the rural Mississippi, Ohio, and Missouri river basins as well as the Great Lakes region. In humans, blastomycosis presents as either pulmonary, disseminated, or localized cutaneous lesions. As in aspergillosis, the fungal spores are found in the soil and may initiate the disease when inhaled. Transmission of blastomycosis from human to human is unlikely and has not been reported.

TABLE 4   Uncommon Systemic Mycoses and Their Oral Manifestations

Disease and Representative Agent	Main Sites Affected	Major Oral Manifestations	Frequency of Oral Affection
Aspergillosis *Aspergillus fumigatus*	Paranasal sinuses; rarely tongue, soft palate	Plaque formation and intense local pain in oral lesions	Uncommon
Blastomycosis (North American) *Blastomyces dermatitidis*	Tongue, oral mucosa, gingivae, lip, mandibular bone	Ulceration, sessile projections, indurated swellings, actinomycosis-like draining abscesses	Rare
Coccidioidomycosis *Coccidioides immitis*	Nasolabial folds, skin	'Verrucous granulomas' resembling carcinomas	Very rare
Cryptococcosis* *Cryptococcus neoformans*	Gingiva, hard and soft palate, mucosa, tonsillar pillar	Violaceous colored nodules or granulations, swellings, ulcers	Uncommon
Geotrichosis *Geotrichum candidum*	Oral mucosa	Similar to acute pseudomembranes of candidiasis	Uncommon
Histoplasmosis† *Histoplama capsulatum* *Histoplasma duboisii*	Oral mucosa, tongue, plate, gingiva, periapical area	Nodular, indurated, or granular masses or tissue destruction with bone erosion	Common
Mucormycosis *Mucor* species	Extension from maxillary sinus through palate into the mouth	Sloughing ulcers with gray eschar and exposed bone (especially maxilla); unilateral facial pain	Common
Paracoccidioidomycosis (South American blastomycosis) *Paracoccidioides brasiliensis*	Hard and soft palate, gingiva, tongue	Papules or vesicles leading to ulcers; extensive local destruction	Common
Sporotrichosis *Sporotrichum schenckii*	Oral mucosa	Erythematous, ulcerative lesions leading to granuloma or papillomas	Uncommon

*AIDS-associated oral lesions have been described.
†May present to the dentist with initial oral manifestations.

ORAL CONSIDERATIONS

Oral lesions may arise through disseminated blastomycosis. Oral blastomycosis is uncommon and may present as single or multiple ulcerations, sessile projections, and granulomatous or verrucous lesions. In one study of 40 patients with blastomycosis, one-quarter demonstrated oral or nasal lesions and another 7 of 10 patients had nonspecific oral ulcerations in addition to systemic disease.

DIAGNOSIS AND MANAGEMENT

Diagnosis is based on biopsy, smear, or culture. Amphotericin B, ketoconazole, miconazole, and itraconazole are all effective.

Coccidioidomycosis

This condition is mainly seen in the southwest United States, Mexico, Central America, and some parts of South America. The disease is caused by inhalation of *Coccidioides immitis* spores found in soil. Antibodies to the fungus are found in 90% of the population of these endemic areas. The illness is typically an acute pulmonary disease and fever, sometimes with erythema nodosum or erythema multiforme. Chronic pulmonary disease is less common. Disseminated coccidioidomycosis is seen in pregnant women, immigrant workers, and immunocompromised individuals. Oral manifestations are almost always secondary to lung involvement.

Transmission of coccidioidomycosis from human to human is unlikely and has not been reported.

ORAL CONSIDERATIONS

Oral lesions are rare and manifest as verrucous lesions with underlying infection of the jaw.

DIAGNOSIS AND MANAGEMENT

Diagnosis is by history and examination supported by histology. The coccidioidin skin test is helpful. Management is with systemic amphotericin B supplemented with azoles if necessary.

Cryptococcosis

Cryptococcosis is a chronic fungal disease involving the lungs, the central nervous system, and, occasionally, the skin and mouth. The disease occurs worldwide, and the main source of the causative agent, *Cryptococcus neoformans*, is bird droppings. The disease is primarily a pulmonary infection and is usually subclinical, with few, if any, noticeable signs or symptoms. However, in compromised individuals, the disease may become rapidly systemic, involving the central nervous system, skin, mucous membranes, bone, and a wide variety of other tissues. Skin lesions are not uncommon in the disseminated form of the disease but rarely represent the site of primary infection. The face, scalp, and neck are the common sites of cutaneous lesions, which present in a variety of ways, such as papules, acneiform pustules, abscesses, ulcers, superficial granulomas, or sinus tracts. Cryptococcosis is unlikely to be transmitted from human to human unless in extreme situations, such as in hospitals, where infected patients are not adequately quarantined when other debilitated patients may acquire the disease nosocomially, through the pulmonary route.

ORAL CONSIDERATIONS

Oral lesions occur in patients who have the disseminated form of cryptococcosis. Lesions have been described on the gingiva, hard and soft palates, pharynx, oral mucosa, and tonsillar pillar and in a tooth socket after extraction. The lesions have been variously described as violaceous nodules of granulation tissue, swellings, or ulcers. The majority of reported cases of oral cryptococcosis have been reported in HIV-infected individuals.

DIAGNOSIS AND MANAGEMENT

Diagnosis is confirmed by microscopy. Culture and assay of serum or cerebrospinal fluid for capsular antigen are useful. Systemic amphotericin B is the drug of choice and can be supplemented with flucytosine.

Fusariosis

Fusarium species were once considered harmless, saprophytic, filamentous fungi living in soil. They, however, are now emerging as pathogens due to the high prevalence of compromised patients in the community. Fusariosis is the disseminated form of the disease. The disease is highly unlikely to be transmitted from human to human.

ORAL CONSIDERATIONS

Human *Fusarium* infections may present as local, focally invasive, or disseminated disease. Oral infections are rare and usually present as secondary lesions of disseminated disease, where they have been described as black, necrotic ulcers occurring mainly on the palate. As these lesions are similar in appearance to those of aspergillosis and mucormycosis, a definitive diagnosis should be made by histology and cultural techniques.

DIAGNOSIS AND MANAGEMENT

The management depends on the degree of invasion and the status of the patient. Superficial infections reportedly respond to local treatment; however, disseminated infections have a very poor prognosis. The infection can be managed by ketoconazole or voriconazole given for a prolonged period.

Geotrichosis

Geotrichum candidum is usually saprophytic but occasionally causes opportunistic infection in humans. The fungus has been isolated from the skin, sputum, and feces and is carried in the alimentary tract of some individuals. Infections have been described in the bronchi, lung, mouth, and intestine. Bronchial geotrichosis is the most commonly recognized form of the disease and is characterized by a persistent cough,

the production of gelatinous sputum, and the absence of fever. Disseminated infections are seen in debilitated patients or in those receiving immunosuppressive drugs. Geotrichosis cannot be transmitted from human to human.

ORAL CONSIDERATIONS

The oral lesions of geotrichosis are indistinguishable clinically from those of acute pseudomembranous candidiasis (thrush), and the reported low incidence of the disease may be due to such misdiagnosis. Other reports indicate that the clinical appearance is edematous and erythematous gingivae and ulcerations. In one study, it was the second commonest oral yeast isolated from patients with hematologic malignancies suffering from stomatitis.

DIAGNOSIS AND MANAGEMENT

Diagnosis is confirmed by histology and culture. Nystatin may be effective for localized oral lesions, whereas systemic infections respond well to itraconazole therapy.

Histoplasmosis

Histoplasma capsulatum, a dimorphic fungus, is endemic in the Mississippi and Ohio river valleys and found in Latin America, India, the Far East, and Australia. The organisms are found especially in bird and bat feces. Infection ensues when microconidiae or hyphae are inhaled into the lung and develop into yeast or when old foci of infection are reactivated. AIDS patients are particularly at risk due to impairment of cellular immunity.

Clinical presentations include acute and chronic pulmonary cutaneous histoplasmosis, with or without disseminated disease. The latter is particularly common in immunocompromised persons. Histoplasmosis is unlikely to be transmitted from human to human.

ORAL CONSIDERATIONS

Oral lesions are mostly chronic with nodular, indurated, or granular masses and ulceration; hard and soft tissue destruction may rarely occur. Up to 40 to 50% of cases with systemic histoplasmosis present with oral lesions. The major oral sites affected are the mucosa, tongue, palate, gingivae, and periapical region of the teeth. The severity of the disease in AIDS patients is greater when the CD4 count is below 200 cells/cm^2.

DIAGNOSIS AND MANAGEMENT

Diagnosis is confirmed by microscopy, culture, and serology. Amphotericin B is the first-choice drug, whereas fluconazole and itraconazole are alternatives. Relapse rates may be high as 80% for patients not placed on maintenance regimens following initial treatment with amphotericin B.

▼ MUCORMYCOSIS (ZYGOMYCOSIS, PHYCOMYCOSIS)

The term *mucormycosis* refers to a distinctive group of diseases caused by ubiquitous, saprophytic fungi of the order

Mucorales. The organisms are common inhabitants of soil and may be found in the nasal cavities of healthy individuals. Infection arises by inhalation of spores that are deposited in pulmonary alveoli. Other modes of infection include contamination of traumatized tissues and direct inoculation. The infection may present in different anatomic sites, specifically the paranasal, rhino-orbital, rhinocerebral, cerebral pulmonary, and gastrointestinal areas. It can also appear in the soft tissues of the extremities or as disseminated disease. The fungus preferentially erodes arteries, resulting in thrombosis with subsequent necrosis of the surrounding tissues. The host response is suppurative rather than granulomatous, although chronic forms of mucormycosis occasionally occur. The infection is often associated with acidosis due to diabetes, diarrhea, or uremia. Diabetic acidosis was considered to be the predisposing condition in 50 to 70% of the reported patients with mucormycosis prior to the HIV pandemic. More recently, it is commonly seen associated with HIV infection and AIDS. Other predisposing conditions are blood dyscrasis, malignant disease, hepatitis, burns, malnutrition, irradiation, TB, and the administration of corticosteroids and immunosuppressive drugs. Mucormycosis is highly unlikely to be transmitted from human to human.

ORAL CONSIDERATIONS

Symptoms involving the oral, cranial, and facial structures account for about 60% of all cases. Oral ulcerations and sinusitis and/or facial cellulitis have been described in mucormycosis. The mortality from mucormycosis is high, 50 to 100%, and there is little doubt that the fulminating nature of the infection, late diagnosis, and lack of rational therapy account for the poor prognosis. Other important symptoms include blood-tinged nasal discharge, unilateral facial pain, or numbness. Occasionally, the most significant presenting symptom is necrotic ulceration or sloughing of the maxillary or palatal mucosa.

DIAGNOSIS AND MANAGEMENT

Diagnosis is confirmed by smear and histologic demonstration of tissue invasion by hyphae. Magnetic resonance imaging may show thickening of the mucosa with patchy destruction of the antral walls in sinus infection. Management of mucormycosis comprises (1) detection of acidosis or other predisposing factors, (2) antifungal therapy using amphotericin B, and (3) surgical débridement.

Paracoccidioidomycosis (South American Blastomycosis)

South American blastomycosis caused by *Paracoccidioides brasiliensis* is a chronic granulomatous disease that primarily infects the lungs and then disseminates to form ulcerative granulomas of the oral and nasal mucosa or other organ systems. This infection cannot be transmitted from human to human.

Lymph nodes are commonly involved in mucormycosis, and local extension to skin or systemic involvement of multiple organs may occur. The disease is restricted to South and Central America, especially Brazil. The source of the infection is thought to be soil and vegetative material and is acquired by direct inhalation or by direct contact. Infection is present 10 times more commonly in males that females, especially in the 20- to 40-year-old age group. Clinical cases of South American blastomycosis can be classified in one of four categories: pulmonary, mucocutaneous, lymphangitis, or disseminated.

ORAL CONSIDERATIONS

The oral manifestations of this fungal infection are common and may present in all three forms of the disease. Primary infection of the mouth or gastrointestinal tract is thought to be rare; hence, oral lesions are mainly secondary. In the mucocutaneous form of the disease, the oral lesions may be the most apparent presenting symptom. The lesions appear initially as small papules or vesicles, which then ulcerate and appear as shallow ulcers with a rolled edge and a white exudative base studded with small hemorrhagic dots. The lesions have a granulomatous appearance and spread slowly, causing extensive local destruction. Pain is not usually a feature of early lesions but may become severe as the disease progresses, leading to cachexia as a result of acute pain on eating. In severe cases, infection may extend into bone, leading to perforation of the hard palate. Gross fibrosis and scarring may occur as a result of attempted healing. Lesions have been described in almost all parts of the mouth and pharynx, including the hard and soft palates, gingiva, tongue, and tonsils. Infections in the gingival and periodontal tissues may lead to loosening and loss of teeth. Infiltration of the oral tissues, especially the lips and cheeks, may severely reduce facial mobility and radically inhibit movement of the mandible. The face may become grossly swollen and the mouth held open with a constant escape of saliva at the angles. Regional lymph nodes draining the areas involved enlarge and often suppurate, with the formation of sinus tracts. The fluid that drains from the sinuses contains numerous fungal cells.

DIAGNOSIS AND MANAGEMENT

Diagnosis is confirmed by histology and culture. Sulfonamide or amphotericin B, alone or in combination, is the treatment of choice. The doses used and length of administration are matters for expert clinical judgment in individual cases. Ketoconazole has been successfully used in the management of paracoccidioidomycosis.

Penicilliosis

Penicillium marneffei is a yeast-like fungus and cause diseases—penicilliosis—in the normal host, as well as in immunosuppressed patients, but, significantly, it has now become a major opportunistic pathogen in HIV-infected patients in Indochina, particularly northern Thailand. Imported cases of *P. marneffei* infections have been reported from Australia, France, Italy, the Netherlands, the United

Kingdom, and the United States. Human to human transmission of penicilliosis is highly unlikely.

P. marneffei infection may either be disseminated or focal in patients who are otherwise healthy, but in HIV disease, disseminated infection is the norm. The clinical and histologic appearances of focal infection strongly resemble TB. Fungemia may be present with systemic disease, together with skin, reticuloendothelial system, lung, and gut infiltration. Patients usually present with nonspecific symptoms of fever, anemia, and weight loss.

ORAL CONSIDERATIONS

Skin lesions are usually located on the face, trunk, and extremities. The most common skin lesions are papules, often with a central necrotic umbilication with or without subcutaneous abscesses that may ulcerate. Intraorally, the lesions may be seen as papules, erosions, or shallow ulcers of varying size covered with yellow necrotic slough. The palate, gingiva, labial mucosa, tongue, and oropharynx are the most common sites involved.

DIAGNOSIS AND MANAGEMENT

Diagnosis is confirmed by histology and culture. Although itraconazole is extremely effective against *P. marneffei* infection, initial treatment is usually amphotericin B followed by oral itraconazole up to 10 weeks. As relapse is common, long-term maintenance therapy with itraconazole is recommended.

Sporotrichosis

Sporotrichosis is a chronic nodular subcutaneous mycotic disease with a worldwide distribution but is most frequently found in Central America, Brazil, and Mexico. The causative agent is *Sporotrichum schenckii*, a fungus found in moss, soil, and rotting wood, with the result that persons such as agricultural workers, florists, and miners have a higher incidence of the infection than the general population. Sporotrichosis is highly unlikely to be transmitted from human to human.

S. schenckii gains access to the subcutaneous tissues via traumatic lesions, and proliferation of the fungus leads to the appearance of a nodule or small ulcer as soon as 5 days or as long as 6 months after inoculation. The nodule becomes a bubo, which may change color from pink to purple and then ulcerate. The common site of the primary lesions is the finger, although the face can also be involved. After several weeks or months, the initial lesion tends to heal with scarring as new buboes develop in other areas. The regional lymph nodes become infected, and the spread of the fungus can be recognized by the inflammation of the lymph vessels draining the initial lesion. The infection usually becomes chronic and locally destructive or may disseminate to the skin, oral mucosa, bone, and other organs.

ORAL CONSIDERATIONS

The oral manifestations of sporotrichosis may be primary, which is rare, or secondary as a result of dissemination from the skin or lung. The lesions are initially erythematous, ulcerative, and suppurative and eventually become granulomatous, vegetative, or papillomatous. The oral lesions are usually painful, and the regional lymph nodes are hard and enlarged. The mucosal lesions usually heal without residual scarring. Oral sporotrichosis may resemble aphthous ulcers, lichen planus, or secondary cutaneous leishmaniasis. On rare occasions, the nose and sinuses may be involved, with extension of infection to the orbit.

DIAGNOSIS AND MANAGEMENT

Diagnosis is confirmed by histology and culture. Amphotericin B is the most effective drug for treating relapsed lymphocutaneous sporotrichosis or the pulmonary and disseminated forms of the disease. Itraconazole is an alternative.

▼ VIRAL INFECTIONS

Viral Hepatitis

Approximately 80% of viral hepatitis infections are caused by hepatitis A (HAV), hepatitis B (HBV), hepatitis C (HCV), hepatitis D (HDV), or hepatitis E (HEV) (Table 5).[24,25] As a consequence of their parenteral mode of transmission and ability to establish chronic infection, hepatitis types HBV, HDV, and HCV are of particular concern for oral health care professionals. HAV and HEV are predominantly spread through enteral modes and do not incur chronic disease. This section briefly reviews our current understanding of HBV, HCV, and HDV epidemiology, pathogenesis, and management. However, the etiologic viral agent remains unidentified in an estimated 20% of acute hepatitis cases, 10% of fulminant hepatitis cases, and 5% of chronic hepatitis cases.[26] Although a plethora of new putative etiologic viruses, including hepatitis G (HGV, GBV-C), the Torque Teno virus (TTV) superfamily, and NV-F, have been identified, their contribution to the etiopathogenesis of hepatitis remains an area of ongoing research and is summarized at the end of this section.[24,27,28]

EPIDEMIOLOGY

HBV, HDV, and HCV all exhibit significant genetic diversity as evidenced by traceable geographic distributions. From a

---

TABLE 5 Hepatitis Viruses

Agent	Family	Genome	Size (nm)	Incubation Periods (d)	Vaccine
Type A	Picornaviridae	ss RNA	27	15–50	Y
Type B	Hepadnaviridae	ds DNA	42	45–160	Y
Type C	Flaviviridae	ss RNA	30–60	15–150	N
Type D	Subviral satellite	ss RNA	35	15–150	Y*
Type E	Caliciviridae	ss RNA	27–34	15–60	N

Adapted from Howard CR.[24]

DNA = deoxyribonucleic acid; ds = double stranded; RNA = ribonucleic acid; ss = single stranded.

*Hepatitis B virus vaccination confers protection.

clinical perspective, genotype assessment is useful for monitoring the clinical course, directing therapeutic interventions, and, ultimately, predicting prognosis of infection.[29] For HBV, there are eight genotypes (A–H) and numerous subgenotypes and hepatitis B surface antigen (HbsAg) subtypes.[30] The predominant genotypes observed in the United States are A, D, and G. HDV is a defective virus that requires the simultaneous presence of HBV to establish infection, and three distinct genotypes are recognized (I, II, III). The predominant HDV genotype observed in the United States is type I. For HCV, there are six genotypes (1 to 6) and numerous subtypes. The predominant HCV genotype present in the United States is type 1.

These viruses are all spread via contact with contaminated blood. Vertical transmission from an infected mother to child accounts for most cases of HBV infection worldwide.[31] For children born of infected mothers who are hepatitis B e antigen (HBeAg is a serologic marker for viral replication) negative, the risk is 10 to 40%, whereas for children born of mothers who are HBeAg positive, the risk is 70 to 90%. Child to child transmission can also occur. Transmission via the aforementioned routes has decreased dramatically in the industrialized world, in large part due to the implementation of aggressive vaccination and screening programs. Other major risk factors for HBV infection include having multiple sex partners, sex with HBV-infected persons, and intravenous drug use. The risk of developing chronic HBV infection correlates well with the patient's age at initial infection. Thus, neonates, whose immune systems are immature, have a 90% chance of developing chronic HBV infection, compared with a 30% chance for children aged 1 to 5 years and a 5% chance for adults.[32]

The predominant risk factors for HDV infection are intravenous drug use, sex with an infected partner, and exposure to blood products prior to 1992.[33] Infection may occur simultaneously with an HBV infection (coinfection) or as a new infection affecting a patient with chronic HBV (superinfection). Chronicity is more likely to occur as a consequence of superinfection.

For HCV, the predominant route of transmission is intravenous drug use, accounting for 50% of cases.[34] Mother to child transmission risk is estimated to be about 4 to 7%, with a four- to fivefold increase noted if the mother is also coinfected with HIV. Other risk factors for HCV infection include exposure to blood products prior to 1992, undergoing unsanitary medical procedures, having sex with an infected partner, and household contact. Approximately 50 to 85% of patients acutely infected with HCV subsequently develop chronic infection.[35]

The worldwide disease burden of viral hepatitis is significant, and there is extensive geographic variation. Over 2 billion people have been infected with HBV, with an estimated 350 million manifesting chronic infection.[36] Chronic infection rates are highest in sub-Saharan Africa, most of Asia, and the Pacific (8–10%) and lowest in western Europe and North America (<1.0%). For HDV and HCV, the worldwide estimates for chronic infection are 10 million and 170 million people, respectively.[33–37] Most cases of HDV infection affect those living in the Eastern Mediterranean. Prevalence rates for HCV are highest in Africa and the Eastern Mediterranean (> 4.5%) and lowest in Europe (1.0%).

DIAGNOSIS

For both acute and chronic forms of viral hepatitis, many patients have either no symptoms or symptoms so mild as to be easily overlooked (fatigue, nausea, fever, abdominal pain, loss of appetite). As a consequence, hepatitis is often discovered during routine laboratory screening as part of a physical examination or voluntary blood donation. The likelihood of developing symptomatic illness is inversely related to one's age at the time of infection. The more characteristic signs and symptoms of jaundice, urticaria, dark-colored urine, light-colored stools, and an enlarged/tender liver signal the presence of more extensive liver damage. Other conditions to consider in the differential diagnosis include alcohol abuse, fatty liver, autoimmune hepatitis, primary biliary cirrhosis, hemochromatosis, Wilson's disease, and α_1-antitrypsin deficiency.[35]

Laboratory testing is essential for establishing the diagnosis, monitoring disease progression, and assessing the results of therapeutic interventions. Basic liver function tests include alanine aminotransferase, alkaline phosphatase, aspartate aminotransferase, albumin, and total protein. Although useful, liver function tests must be correlated with specific serologic tests to establish etiology. For HBV, available tests include HBsAg, HBV surface antibody (anti-HBs), HBeAg, HBV e antibody (anti-HBe), and HBV core antibody (anti-HBc and IgM anti-HBc). For HDV, HDV antigen (HDAg) and HDV antibody (anti-HD) may be obtained. For HCV, the only routinely ordered test is for HCV antibody (anti-HCV). Table 6 lists the more common serologic patterns observed in the course of HBV or HCV infection.[38,39] Viral load testing for all three viruses is available and useful in assessing disease status, as is liver biopsy.[40]

PATHOGENESIS

The pathogenic mechanisms of HBV, HDV, and HCV are only partially understood, and numerous factors, such as route of transmission, viral subtype, and the patient's age, immunocompetence, and health, influence pathogenesis. Although these viruses are hepatotropic, they do not appear to be directly cytopathic, and the severity of hepatocyte injury reflects the intensity of the host cellular immune response.[41,42] Patients who develop a vigorous cytotoxic T-cell response to infection are more likely to manifest severe, at times fulminant, liver injury, but they are at low risk of developing chronic infection. In contrast, patients who generate a less vigorous cytotoxic T-cell response to infection manifest little acute liver injury but are at much greater risk for developing chronic infection. Putative mechanisms underlying the ability of these viruses to circumvent the host immune response and establish chronic infection include the suppressive actions of

TABLE 6 Common Serologic Patterns of Hepatitis B and C Virus Infection

Serologic Result	Interpretation
HbsAg *neg*, anti-HBc *pos*, anti-HBs *pos*	Immunity from natural infection
HBsAg *neg*, anti-HBc *neg*, anti-HBs *pos*	Immunity from vaccination
HBsAg *pos*, anti-HBc *pos*, IgM anti-HBc *pos*, anti-HBs *neg*	Acute infection
HBsAg *pos*, anti-HBc *pos*, IgM anti-HBc *neg*, anti-HBs *neg*, HBeAg *pos*, anti-HBe *neg*	Chronic infection: active carrier states, high infectivity
HBsAg *pos*, anti-HBc *pos*, IgM anti-HBc *neg*, anti-HBs *neg*, HBeAg *neg*, anti-HBe *pos*	Chronic infection: inactive carrier states, low infectivity
HBsAg *neg*, anti-HBc *pos*, anti-HBs *neg*	Recovering from acute infection, *or* Distant immunity with undetectable levels of anti-HBs, *or* False-positive anti-HBc, *or* Undetectable levels of HBsAg; thus, a chronic carrier
Anti-HCV	Recovering from acute infection, *or* Chronic infection *or* Resolved infection

Adapted from Kelly D and Skidmore S[38] and Wilson TR.[39]

anti-HBc = hepatitis B core antibody; anti-HBs = hepatitis B surface antibody; HbeAg = hepatitis B e antigen; HbsAg = hepatitis B surface antigen; HCV = hepatitis C virus; IgM = immunoglobulin M.

viral antigens on the host immune system, reduced CD4 T-cell help, the suppressive effects of T-regulatory cells, and the high rate of viral mutation.[43]

Chronic infection is a dynamic process for which the outcome varies from patient to patient. Some patients manifest no symptoms throughout their lives; others manifest only occasional flares of clinical illness; and still others experience unrelenting progressive clinical illness. The two main concerns related to chronic viral hepatitis are the increased risks for developing cirrhosis and hepatocellular carcinoma (HCC). The association between chronic viral hepatitis and HCC, although strong, is poorly understood. A multitude of factors that possibly contribute to the development of HCC include direct virus-induced mutagenesis, the accumulation of genetic and epigenetic lesions associated with continuous hepatocyte necrosis and regeneration, and an increased susceptibility to the carcinogenic actions of aflatoxins and alcohol.[44] For patients with chronic HBV, the risk of developing cirrhosis or HCC is 15 to 40%.[31] Contributing factors include male sex, infection at an early age, heavy alcohol consumption, coinfection with other hepatotropic viruses or HIV, immunosuppression, and high HBV viral loads. For chronic HCV infection, 2 to 20% of patients develop cirrhosis, typically over a period of 20 to 30 years.[35] Once cirrhosis occurs, 1 to 4% of patients with chronic HCV develop HCC each year. For chronic HDV, progression to cirrhosis typically occurs within 5 to 10 years and affects 60 to 70% of patients.[33]

MEDICAL MANAGEMENT

Treatment protocols for acute viral hepatitis are supportive, and there is no consensus on the value or need to provide antiviral therapy during an acute infection. For chronic viral hepatitis, the decision on how and when to institute therapy is complex and must be based on factors such as patient interest, clinical and laboratory findings, risk of disease progression without intervention, odds of therapeutic success, risk of therapeutic adverse effects, and the overall health of the patient.[35,45] The goals of therapy are to slow the progression to cirrhosis, prevent hepatic failure, and prevent the development of HCC.[46] For patients with advanced disease, in whom medical therapy is either ineffective or contraindicated, the only remaining option is liver transplantation.[47]

Approved drug therapies to treat chronic HBV include interferon-α2b, pegylated interferon-α2a, adefovir dipivoxil, lamivudine, and entecavir. Since these drugs do not eradicate HBV, therapeutic protocols tend to be prolonged. Interferon-α2b and pegylated interferon-α2a are biologic response modifiers that enhance the host's natural immune response.[48] Adefovir dipivoxil, lamivudine, and entecavir are nucleoside analogues that inhibit HBV DNA synthesis. The emergence of resistant HBV strains is of particular concern for lamivudine, reaching 32% after 1 year and 70% after 5 years of therapy. Overall, about two-thirds of patients who qualify for antiviral therapy enter an inactive phase, marked by HBeAg seroconversion and a drop in HBV DNA viral load below $3 \log_{10}$ IU/mL.[46] However, 20% will suffer relapse later in life. Current therapeutic strategies to control chronic HDV infection are ineffective.

Drugs available for the treatment of HCV are pegylated interferon-α and ribavarin.[49] Therapeutic success results in a sustained virologic response (SVR) and is largely predicated on the HCV genotype and the pretreatment HCV viral load. SVR rates are highest for patients who are under 40 years of age, weigh less than 75 kg, have genotype 2 or 3 HCV infections, and have low pretreatment viral loads. Patients with genotype 1 HCV infection are less responsive to therapy. The overall SVR rate is about 40%.[50]

Preventive measures to reduce viral hepatitis spread include aggressive vaccination protocols (for HBV); adequate screening and handling measures for donated blood and tissues; the implementation of proven infection control measures in the health care setting; and promotional/educational efforts to reduce the practice of unsafe injection drug use and/or high-risk sexual practices. Approximately 90% of healthy adults and 95% of infants, children, and adolescents produce protective antibodies against HBV after vaccination.[51] An adequate response is defined as a serum level of anti-HBs antibody of ≥ 10 mIU/mL. Although some waning of the anti-HBs response may occur over time, clear guidelines regarding the need for booster immunization have yet to be established. Unfortunately, there exists no vaccine against HCV.

ORAL HEALTH CONSIDERATIONS

Prior to initiating therapy, the clinician should ascertain the patient's overall status with attention focused on the patient's potential for increased hemorrhage and impaired drug metabolism. In general, ambulatory patients who do not manifest signs and symptoms of active disease and are not under active medical therapy will tolerate the delivery of routine dental care. However, if there is doubt as to the patient's status, it is prudent to consult the treating physician in order to develop a treatment plan for the patient that is safe and appropriate. Pertinent laboratory testing includes complete blood count, prothrombin time, partial thromboplastin time, international normalized ratio, bleeding time, and liver function tests.[52] Clinical clues of impaired liver function include jaundice, easy hemorrhage, and the presence of petechiae, hematomas, or ecchymoses. Additional clues to the presence of liver disease include Dupuytren's contracture, palmar erythema, edema, urticaria, gynecomastia, spider nevi, and sialosis.[52,53] Patients with severe liver impairment are best managed in a hospital setting, where close monitoring and indicated supplemental therapies, such as fresh frozen plasma, may be provided. All drugs metabolized by the liver should be avoided when possible or administered cautiously to patients with severely impaired liver function. For a more extensive discussion about patients with liver disease, see Chapter 14, "Diseases of the Gastrointestinal Tract."

An association between the occurrence of oral lichen planus and HCV infection has been noted in several studies, particularly among Japanese and Mediterranean populations, where the prevalence of HCV infection is high.[54] However, other studies fail to substantiate any correlation, prompting some to postulate that these findings are more reflective of the epidemiology of HCV rather than a true causal association.

As bloodborne agents, HBV, HCV, and HDV pose serious occupational concerns for HCWs, in whom there is a risk of patient to HCW, HCW to patient, and patient to patient transmission. The risk of infection is influenced by the route of exposure, the concentration of infectious virions in the source body fluid, and the volume of infected material transferred.[55] For HBV, the risk has been reduced dramatically through HBV vaccination programs. Prior to the availability of HBV vaccination, an estimated 10,000 HCWs became infected annually in the United States. For 2002, the estimated number of cases affecting HCWs had fallen to 400. Another benefit of HBV vaccination is prevention of HDV infection since HDV requires the presence of HBV to establish infection. However, since HBV vaccination is not universally effective and there exists no vaccine for HCV, HCWs must strictly follow established infection control recommendations to minimize the risk of occupational transmission.[56,57]

For HCWs who either decline HBV vaccination or fail to seroconvert, the risk of HBV infection after a percutaneous exposure is 37 to 62% if the source is HBeAg positive and 23 to 37% if the source is HBeAg negative.[55] For such scenarios, postexposure prophylaxis with hepatitis B immunoglobulin is effective 75% of the time in preventing infection if prescribed within 1 week of exposure.[58] The risk of occupationally acquiring HCV from an infected patient appears to be much less than HBV, with reported rates of seroconversion ranging from 0.0 to 7.0% after percutaneous exposure. However, no prophylactic postexposure protocols exist.

Patient to patient transmission of viral hepatitis occurs as a consequence of cross-contamination and is unlikely to occur in the dental setting when adequate infection control measures are followed. The risk of an HCW infected with viral hepatitis cross-infecting a patient in the occupational setting is fortunately low. There have been over 51 published reports addressing this issue, and most cases occurred before the widespread implementation of contemporary infection control measures.[59] To ensure patient safety, recommendations regarding practice restrictions have been formulated but vary from country to country. In general, HBV-infected practitioners who are deemed highly infectious should not practice exposure-prone procedures. The two indicators of high HBV infectivity are the presence of HBeAg in the serum or a high viral load of HBV DNA. However, there exists a variant of HBV (precore mutant) that does not express HBeAg but is still capable of producing a high viral load of HBV DNA. As a consequence, most authorities now consider the HBV DNA viral load as the best measure of infectivity. Since the risk of HCV transmission from an infected HCW to a patient is low, most authorities do not recommend preemptive practice limitations.

HGV, GBV-C, TTV Superfamily, and NF-V

Both HGV and GBV-C represent two coincidentally discovered isolates of the same virus.[60] A member of the Flaviviridae family, it is closely related to HCV, and at least five genotypes have been discovered.[61] However in contrast to HCV, it appears to not be hepatotrophic but lymphotrophic and does not appear to represent a substantial health risk. Indeed, HGV/GBV-C coinfection with HIV has been shown to slow HIV progression. In contrast, HGV/GBV-C infection has been reported to be associated with a 10-fold increase in the development of B-cell non-Hodgkin's lymphoma.[62]

The TTV superfamily of viruses encompasses an ever-increasing number of circular single-stranded DNA viruses related to the animal virus family Circoviridae.[25,63,64] Five phylogenetic clusters (1–5) and at least 39 genotypes are recognized. Cluster 1 includes the prototype TTV (genotype 1); cluster 2 includes the PMV isolate (genotype 17); cluster 3 includes the TUS01, SANBAN, TJN01, and the eight SEN-V isolates; cluster 4 includes the YONBAN isolates; and cluster 5 contains at least three genotypes. In addition, a similar but smaller TTV variant, the torque teno mini virus (TTMV), has been described.[65] The overall pathogenic potential for the TTV superfamily remains to be determined. On the one hand, the high worldwide prevalence rates (10–90%) combined with an apparent lack of correlation between virus acquisition and the development of clinical disease lead many to dismiss its importance as a human pathogen. However, reports of members of the TTV superfamily being associated with such maladies as an increased HCC risk in HCV-infected patients,[66] an increased idiopathic pulmonary fibrosis risk,[67] an increased thrombocytopenia risk,[68] and an increased risk of systemic lupus erythematosus[69] indicate a need for further study.

Recently, a novel single-stranded DNA sequence associated with a newly proposed human hepatitis agent (NV-F) was discovered.[28] Although the pathogenic potential of NV-F remains to be determined, it appears to frequently occur in cases of HBV or HCV chronic infection.[26,70]

Human Immunodeficiency Virus (HIV)

After almost three decades, the scourge of HIV infection continues to devastate the global landscape. The first indication of a new human epidemic surfaced in 1981 with the publication of reports of the rare opportunistic infection *Pneumocyctis carinii* pneumonia and an aggressive form of Kaposi's sarcoma affecting clusters of young homosexual men in California and New York.[71,72] In September 1982, the CDC formally introduced the term *acquired immune deficiency syndrome* (AIDS) in describing the 593 cases reported to the CDC through September 15, 1982.[73] Working independently, researchers in both France and the United States announced the discovery of a virus they believed caused AIDS.[74,75] Whereas the French team referred to the virus as lymphadenopathy-associated virus (LAV) and the US team referred to the virus as human T-cell lymphotropic virus type 3 (HTLV-III), it became apparent that they were one and the same. In May 1986, the unifying name of human immunodeficiency virus (HIV) was adopted by the International Committee on Taxonomy of Viruses.[76] Current medical therapies to manage HIV disease are both expensive and compliance intense, rendering them unavailable to vast segments of the world population. This section briefly reviews our current understanding of the epidemiology, pathogenesis, and management of HIV.

EPIDEMIOLOGY

There exist two recognized types of HIV: HIV-1 and HIV-2.[77] Both have the same modes of transmission, and both may cause immunosuppression and AIDS. However, compared with HIV-1, HIV-2 rarely occurs outside Africa and tends to follow a more indolent clinical course. HIV-1 is further classified into three groups: M, N, and O. Twenty-seven forms of the HIV-1 group M are recognized, and M forms collectively account for 95% of human infections.[78] Most scientists believe that each type of HIV is a descendant of a specific simian immunodeficiency virus (SIV). SIVs are primate lentiviruses that infect at least 36 nonhuman primate species in sub-Saharan Africa.[79] Contact with nonhuman primates, such as occurs during hunting and butchering, has been shown to allow for species cross-contamination and is believed to have sparked the HIV pandemic.[80] Researchers have established that the immediate precursor to HIV-1 is SIVcpz, whose natural host is the chimpanzee of the subspecies *Pan troglodytes troglodytes*.[81] Similarly, the immediate precursor to HIV-2 is SIVsm, whose natural host is the sooty mangabey.[82]

The prime modes of transmission for HIV are (1) unprotected penetrative sex between men, (2) unprotected heterosexual intercourse, (3) injection drug use, (4) unsanitary injections and blood transfusions, and (5) mother to child spread during pregnancy, delivery, or breast-feeding.

The initial case definition for AIDS was published by the CDC in 1982 and subsequently updated and revised in 1985, 1987, and 1993 (Table 7).[73,83–85] During the 1980s, when the temporal relationship between HIV exposure and progression to AIDS was predictable, the tracking of AIDS as a surrogate marker for HIV infection was adequate. However, with advances in medical therapy significantly delaying the progression to AIDS, the statistical coupling of HIV infection and AIDS has become tenuous. Efforts to more accurately determine the actual burden of HIV infection have been undertaken.[86,87] The results must be interpreted with caution since there are no enforceable testing requirements or protocols and not all agencies who do have data choose to report.

During 2005, nearly 5 million people worldwide became infected with HIV and the cumulative number of people living with HIV disease exceeded 40 million.[88] The estimated number of people worldwide succumbing to HIV disease in 2005 was greater than 3 million, and the cumulative death toll of the epidemic exceeded 25 million.

In the United States, an estimated 1,039,000 to 1,185,000 persons were living with HIV/AIDS at the end of 2003.[89] The most recent surveillance information on HIV/AIDS in the United States is available at the CDC Web site: <http://www.cdc.gov/hiv/topics/surveillance/resources/reports/>. Through 2005, the cumulative number of reported AIDS cases in the United States and its territories reached 956,019.[90] Of the 41,983 new cases of AIDS reported in 2005, males accounted for 74% and females accounted for 26%. The cumulative death toll due to AIDS through 2005 is estimated to be 550,394. African Americans, who account for 12% of the US population, accounted for 49% of the HIV/AIDS cases diagnosed in 2005. Although the national annual rate of reported AIDS cases was 14 per 100,000, the rate varied significantly according to geographic location. For the US Pacific island of American Samoa, the reported rate was zero per 100,000, whereas for the District of Columbia, the rate was 128.4 per 100,000. Advances in the medical management of AIDS have slowed disease progression and led to a dramatic decrease in AIDS deaths and an increase in the number of persons living with AIDS.

The United Nations and the World Health Organization publish annual reports on the global epidemiology of HIV disease. This information can be accessed at <http://www.unaids.org/en/HIV_data/ and http://www.who.int/healthinfo/statistics/en/>.

DIAGNOSIS

The diagnosis of HIV infection is obtained by appropriate laboratory testing.[91] In the standard HIV-antibody test

TABLE 7   Revised Classification System for HIV Infection and Expanded Case Definition for AIDS among Adolescents and Adults

CD4+ T-lymphocyte categories
  The lowest accurate CD4+ T-lymphocyte count is used for classification, even though more recent and possibly different counts may be available.

Clinical category A
  Conditions:
  Asymptomatic HIV infection
  Persistent generalized lymphadenopathy
  Acute (primary) HIV infection with accompanying illness or history of acute HIV infection
  Conditions listed in categories B and C must not have occurred.

Clinical category B
  Symptomatic conditions in an HIV-infected adolescent or adult that are not included among conditions listed in clinical category C and that meet at least one of the
    following criteria: (a) the conditions are attributed to HIV infection or are indicative of a defect in cell-mediated immunity or (b) the conditions are considered by
    physicians to have a clinical course or to require management that is complicated by HIV infection.
  Examples of, but not limited to, the following conditions:
  Bacillary angiomatosis
  Candidiasis, oropharyngeal (thrush)
  Candidiasis, vulvovaginal; persistent, frequent, or poorly responsive to therapy
  Cervical dysplasia (moderate or severe)/cervical carcinoma in situ
  Constitutional symptoms, such as fever (38.5°C) or diarrhea lasting greater than 1 month
  Oral hairy leukoplakia
  Herpes zoster (shingles) involving at least two distinct episodes or more than one dermatome
  Idiopathic thrombocytopenic purpura
  Listeriosis
  Pelvic inflammatory disease, particularly if complicated by tubo-ovarian abscess
  Peripheral neuropathy

Clinical category C
  Conditions:
  Candidiasis of bronchi, trachea, or lungs
  Candidiasis, esophageal
  Cervical cancer, invasive
  Coccidioidomycosis, disseminated or extrapulmonary
  Cryptococcosis, extrapulmonary
  Cryptosporidiosis, chronic intestinal (greater than 1 month's duration)
  Cytomegalovirus disease (other than liver, spleen, or nodes)
  Cytomegalovirus retinitis (with loss of vision)
  Encephalopathy, HIV related
  Herpes simplex: chronic ulcer(s) (greater than 1 month's duration) or bronchitis, pneumonitis, or esophagitis
  Histoplasmosis, disseminated or extrapulmonary
  Isosporiasis, chronic intestinal (greater than 1 month's duration)
  Kaposi's sarcoma
  Lymphoma, Burkitt's (or equivalent term)
  Lymphoma, immunoblastic (or equivalent term)
  Lymphoma, primary, of brain
  Mycobacterium avium complex or *M. kansasii*, disseminated or extrapulmonary
  Mycobacterium tuberculosis, any site (pulmonary or extrapulmonary)
  Mycobacterium, other species or unidentified species, disseminated or extrapulmonary
  Pneumocystis carinii pneumonia
  Pneumonia, recurrent
  Progressive multifocal leukoencephalopathy
  Salmonella septicemia, recurrent
  Toxoplasmosis of brain
  Wasting syndrome due to HIV

Clinical Classification for HIV infection (CD4 information + Clinical category)

CD4+ counts or %	Category A Condition	Category B Condition	Category C Condition
≥ 500 or ≥ 29%	A1	B1	C1*
200–400 or 14–28%	A2	B2	C2*
< 200 or < 14%	A3*	B3*	C3*

* Expanded acquired immunodeficiency syndrome (AIDS) surveillance case definition
Adapted from Centers for Disease Control and Prevention.[85]

A = asymptomatic acute HIV or PGL; AIDS = acquired immune deficiency syndrome; B = symptomatic, no A or C condition; C = AIDS indicator condition; HIV = human
immunodeficiency virus; PGL = persistent generalized lymphadenopathy.
*Expanded AIDS surveillance case definition.

algorithm, a plasma or serum sample is subjected to an EIA; if the result is positive, a second EIA is performed; and if that result is positive, a confirmatory Western blot analysis is performed. This algorithm is highly sensitive and specific, with reported false-positive rates ranging from 1 in 130,000 to 1 in 251,000.[92] However, cases of recent HIV infection may be missed as it takes several weeks (even months) for a measurable antibody response to develop. As a consequence, several other testing methods targeting HIV antigen identification have been developed and approved by the Food and Drug Administration (FDA).[93] New testing protocols using saliva, urine, and fingerprick testing, along with rapid tests, yield tentative results in as little as 20 minutes.[94]

Determining who should be tested for HIV infection represents an area of ongoing debate.[95] In the past, only patients at high risk for exposure to HIV (ie, injection drug users, men having sex with men, sexually active men and women with multiple partners) or those presenting with signs and symptoms suggestive of HIV infection were recommended for testing.[92,96] However, recently published recommendations from the CDC advocate routine volunteer HIV testing as a normal part of medical practice for all patients aged 13 to 64 years.[97,98]

PATHOGENESIS

Although our overall understanding of the pathogenesis of HIV has improved tremendously over the past couple of decades, many unanswered questions persist. For untreated HIV infection, a common pattern of disease progression has been established consisting of three phases: (1) primary infection, (2) prolonged (median = 10 years) period of clinical latency, and (3) the appearance of clinically apparent disease.[99,100] Although the immunopathologic mechanisms have only been partially identified, the available scientific evidence clearly reveals a dynamic process in which the initial and ongoing immunologic response to HIV infection is not only unsuccessful in clearing the HIV but is paradoxically paralleled by a progressive reduction in immunocompetence and eventual development of AIDS.[101]

HIV is a spherically shaped retrovirus whose outer coat, or envelope, consists of two layers of fatty molecules called lipids.[102] These lipids are actually taken from the human cell membrane when newly formed virus particles bud from the cell. Protruding from the envelope are approximately 72 sets of a complex HIV protein known as Env. Env consists of a stem consisting of three glycoprotein (gp) molecules called gp41 and a cap consisting of three glycoprotein molecules called gp120. Both gp120 and gp41 are essential for the recognition and binding of target cells. Within the envelope is the bullet-shaped core or capsid, which consists of about 2,000 copies of the HIV protein p24. The capsid encircles two single strands of HIV ribonucleic acid (RNA) and the enzymes reverse transcriptase, integrase, and protease.[103] HIV RNA contains the three structural genes (gag, pol, env), two regulatory genes (tat, rev), and four genes for accessory proteins (nef, vif, vpr, vpu) that constitute the virus's nine genes.[102,104]

For example, env codes for a protein called gp160, which is further processed by viral enzymes to produce the aforementioned gp41 and gp120.

The predominant portal of entry for HIV is through blood and/or mucosal exposure. The virus can enter through various mucosal surfaces, including the linings of the vagina, vulva, rectum, penis, or, rarely, oral cavity. Infection is enhanced in scenarios where the mucosal tissues are ulcerated or inflamed. Dendritic cells within the mucosa, which normally process and present antigen to immune cells, express a molecule called DC-SIGN, which has a high affinity for HIV gp120.[103,104] HIV virions bound to DC-SIGN are compartmentalized and, upon migration of the dendritic cells to the lymph nodes, subsequently regurgitated and presented to T cells. In this fashion, dendritic cells appear to act as a Trojan horse to facilitate infection.

HIV targets cells expressing the CD4 molecules, especially CD4[+] T lymphocytes, monocytes, and macrophages. Viral gp120 molecules bind tightly to the CD4 molecules, resulting in conformational changes in the gp120, which, in turn, allows it to bind to a second "coreceptor" molecule on the host cell surface. The most notable of these coreceptors is called CCR5, but others, such as CXCR4, have been identified.[103,105] CCR5 specifically binds macrophage-tropic, non–syncytium-inducing isolates of HIV (R5 strain), whereas CXCR4, which is exclusive to T cells, binds a more pathogenic syncytium-inducing variant of HIV (X4 strain).[104,106]

Upon initial infection, a rapid sequence of virologic, immunologic, and clinical events occurs within the first 4 to 8 weeks of infection (ie, primary infection). There is a rapid rise in plasma viremia and seeding of the virus in lymphoid tissues throughout the body.[106] A firestorm of immunologic activity occurs during this period, highlighted by the production of an estimated 10 billion virions per day (half life ≈ 1.6 days) combined with the destruction and replacement of about 2 billion CD4[+] lymphocytes per day.[107,108] Although many individuals experience minimal symptoms, an estimated 40 to 90% experience an acute viral syndrome characterized by varying degrees of fever, fatigue, maculopapular rash, headache, lymphadenopathy, pharyngitis, myalgia, arthralgia, gastrointestinal distress, night sweats, and oral or genital ulcers.[106] Unlike most infections, the normal immune response associated with HIV infection produces confounding detrimental effects since (1) newly generated CD4[+] lymphocytes represent new targets for HIV infection and (2) increased production of proinflammatory cytokines (ie, tumor necrosis factor α and interleukin-6) may promote viral expression.[101]

Eventually, a virus-specific cell-mediated immune response (CD8[+] lymphocyte) acts to partially dampen the viremia.[101] The cellular response is subsequently followed by the production of HIV-neutralizing antibody.[109] The dampening of viremia to a lowered viral setpoint corresponds to the beginning of the period of clinical latency. However, although the level of viral burden in peripheral blood-mononuclear cells is reduced, it remains 1,000 times higher in the lymphoid tissue.[110] In general, the higher the viral setpoint, the more rapid the progression to AIDS.[106] However, the overall variability regarding the rate of natural disease progression is high. An estimated 10% of patients develop AIDS within 2 to 3 years of exposure to HIV, whereas 10 to 17% of HIV-infected patients may not develop AIDS even 10 years after exposure.[111] The manner in which HIV successfully persists and ultimately overwhelms the host's immune system likely results from a multitude of factors, such as host genetic predisposition, viral pathogenicity, high viral mutation rates, perturbations of antigen processing and presentation, immunologic sanctuary, and proviral latency.[104]

MEDICAL MANAGEMENT

Tremendous strides in terms of medical management have largely turned this once almost universally fatal infection into a manageable chronic illness. A review of current therapeutic recommendations may be found at the AIDSinfo Web site: <http://AIDSinfo.nih.gov>. The initial patient workup of the HIV-infected patient should identify the state of current infection (acute or chronic) and the presence of comorbidities. It consists of a complete medical history, physical examination, and laboratory evaluation. Essential laboratory tests include HIV antibody testing, CD4$^+$ count, and plasma HIV RNA (viral load). Medical therapy is essentially two pronged, targeting the opportunistic infections associated with immunosuppression and the HIV itself. This chapter limits its discussion to the antiretroviral arm of therapy. The decision to initiate antiretroviral therapy is primarily based on the baseline CD4$^+$ count and viral load. In general, antiviral therapy is recommended for any patient with a history of an AIDS-defining illness, regardless of CD4$^+$ counts, or any asymptomatic patient with a CD4$^+$ count < 200 cells/mm^3.[112] The efficacy of antiretroviral therapy is determined by frequent monitoring of both the CD4$^+$ count and the viral load.

Available antiretroviral drugs target structural and functional differences between viral and human proteins. Four classes exist: (1) fusion inhibitors, (2) nucleoside reverse transcriptase inhibitors (NRTIs), (3) non-nucleoside reverse transcriptase inhibitors (NNRTIs), and (4) protease inhibitors (PIs).[112,113] The fusion inhibitor enfuvirtide (T20) is an anti-HIV peptide structurally similar to HIV gp41 and competitively inhibits viral entry into host cells. NRTIs mimic deoxyribonucleoside triphosphate, the natural substrate for reverse transcriptase. As they become incorporated into the growing DNA chain, they terminate elongation and decrease or prevent HIV replication in infected cells. NRTIs include abacavir (ABC), didanosine (ddI), emtricitabine (FTC), lamivudine (3TC), stavudine (d4T), tenofovir disoproxil fumarate (TDF), zalcitabine (ddC), and zidovudine (AZT, ZDV). NNRTIs bind near the catalytic site of reverse transcriptase and inhibit a crucial step in the transcription of the RNA genome into a double-stranded retroviral DNA. NNRTIs include delavirdine (DLV), efavirenz (EFV), and nevirapine (NVP). PIs block the cleavage of viral proteins during assembly and maturation, a process essential for the newly formed virus to become infectious. PIs include amprenavir (APV), atazanavir (ATV), fosamprenavir (f-APV), indinavir, lopinavir + ritonavir (LPV/r), nelfinavir (NFV), ritonavir (RTV), saquinavir (SQV, SQV-sge), and tipranavir (TPV).

The treatment of HIV infection requires combination therapy known as highly active antiretroviral therapy (HAART). Antiretroviral regimens currently recommended for the treatment of naive patients may be NNRTI based (1 NNRTI + 2 NRTIs), PI based (1 or 2 PIs + 2 NRTIs), or triple NRTI based (3 NRTIs).[112] The treatment of patients with acute HIV infection, HIV-infected adolescents, injection drug users, HIV-infected women of reproductive age and pregnant women, and patients with coinfections (HBV, HCV, and tuberculosis) requires special antiretroviral regimens. Although HAART can dampen viremia, delay disease progression, and thus prolong and improve the quality of life for the HIV-infected patient, it is not curative and not a panacea to address the worldwide HIV burden. Furthermore, HAART drugs are expensive, rendering them unavailable for much of the infected population; they often incur significant toxicity and serious adverse drug interactions; their use is frequently compliance intense; and the emergence of drug resistance remains a serious concern. Potentially serious or life-threatening adverse reactions associated with antiretroviral therapy are usually drug specific and include bleeding episodes, bone marrow suppression, hepatoxicity, hepatic necrosis, hypersensitivity reactions, lactic acidosis, nephrolithiasis, nephrotoxicity, pancreatitis, and Stevens-Johnson syndrome/toxic epidermal necrolysis.[114,115]

Although HAART usually results in improved CD4$^+$ counts and decreased viral load, a subset of patients experience a paradoxical condition termed immune reconstitution inflammatory syndrome (IRIS).[116,117] In these patients, HAART-induced immune recovery results in a spectrum of presentations ranging from clinical worsening of established opportunistic infection and the appearance of new opportunistic infections to autoimmune disorders. Most cases of IRIS manifest themselves within the first few months of HAART, and those at highest risk are patients with low baseline CD4$^+$ counts and/or an underlying opportunistic infection when HAART is initiated.

There are no oral lesions that are specific to HIV-infected patients. However, numerous oral lesions have been documented to occur in association with the HIV-induced immunosuppression.[118,119] The most recently published formal listing categorized oral lesions as either (1) strongly associated with, (2) less commonly associated with, or (3) simply seen with HIV infection.[120] The most strongly associated lesions in adult patients are candidiasis (erythematous, pseudomembranous), hairy leukoplakia, Kaposi's sarcoma, non-Hodgkin's lymphoma, and periodontal disease (linear gingival erythema, necrotizing ulcerative gingivitis, necrotizing ulcerative periodontitis). For pediatric patients, the most strongly associated lesions are candidiasis (erythematous, pseudomembranous, angular cheilitis), herpes simplex infection, linear gingival erythema, parotid enlargement, and recurrent aphthous stomatitis (minor, major, herpetiform). The risk of developing these lesions is inversely related to the CD4[+] counts. Thus, these lesions often serve as good clinical markers signaling a loss in therapeutic efficacy of HAART.[121,122]

ORAL HEALTH CONSIDERATIONS

Dental practitioners should anticipate that HIV-infected patients will seek care either for their routine dental concerns or oral conditions associated with their underlying disease.[123,124] Prior to initiating therapy, the clinician should ascertain the patient's immune status, presence of comorbidities, current medication profile, and prognosis. In this regard, it may be necessary to obtain permission from the patient to liaise with his or her physician in order to adequately determine the patient's medical status. The most pertinent criteria related to the provision of oral health care are the CD4[+] count, HIV viral load, neutrophil count, platelet count, and the medications the patient is taking.

As with other medically complex patients, significant concerns for the HIV-infected patient are impaired hemostasis, susceptibility to dentally induced infection, adverse drug effects/interactions, and the patient's ability to tolerate the stresses associated with the delivery of dental care. In general, HIV-infected patients presenting in the outpatient dental setting are sufficiently healthy to tolerate the full spectrum of modern dental services.[125–127] The goals of therapy should be to optimize oral hygiene and function, establish a recall schedule, monitor for and manage HIV-associated oral lesions, and monitor for and manage drug-induced oral side effects, such as xerostomia.

There are no evidence-based studies demonstrating either a need or justification for the routine use of antimicrobial prophylaxis to reduce the occurrence of a bacteremia arising from routine dental procedures in the HIV-infected patient.[127] An indication where antimicrobial prophylaxis is empirically recommended is neutropenia (ie, neutrophil counts $<500/mm^3$). Patients with low platelet counts (ie, $<50,000$ cells/mm^3) are at risk for increased bleeding and should be managed accordingly. The medication profile for the HIV-infected patient is typically complex, reinforcing the obligation of the dental practitioner to routinely monitor for adverse drug effects/interactions. Common side effects that may require modification of routine dental protocols include hepatotoxicity, hyperglycemia, and an increased susceptibility for coronary artery disease. HAART appears to modulate, but not eradicate, the risk of oral lesions in the HIV-infected patient.[128,129] It is postulated that an increased occurrence of some oral conditions, such as oral warts, salivary gland enlargement, and dry mouth, may represent the oral consequences of IRIS.[130] Management protocols for a specific oral lesion or condition are discussed elsewhere in the text.

The transmission of HIV infection from patients to health care personnel (HCP) may occur after percutaneous (cut with a sharp instrument or needle stick) and, infrequently, mucocutaneous exposure to blood and other body fluids containing blood. A retrospective case-control study found that the risk of infection among HCP following percutaneous exposure to HIV-infected blood was more likely (1) in the presence of visible blood on the instrument before injury; (2) if the injury involved a needle, which was placed directly into the patient's vein or artery; (3) if the injury caused by the contaminated instrument or needle was deep; or (4) if the source patient has an increased viral load, that is, was terminally ill.[131] Prospective studies of HCP estimate that the average risk for HIV infection after percutaneous and mucous membrane (eyes, nose, mouth) exposure to HIV-infected blood is approximately 0.3 and 0.09%, respectively.[132,133] The transmission of HIV infection after nonintact skin exposure is estimated to be less than the risk following mucous membrane exposure.[134] Similarly, the risk of transmission after exposure to fluids or tissues other than HIV-infected blood is probably considerably lower than the risk following exposure to blood.[132] As of 2002, occupational exposure to HIV was confirmed in 57 HCP, and of these, none were oral HCP.[135] Clearly, when adequate infection control precautions are observed, the risk of HIV transmission in the oral health care setting is extremely low.

▼ SELECTED READINGS

Bell DM. Occupational risk of human immunodeficiency virus infection in healthcare workers: an overview. Am J Med 1997;102 Suppl 5B:9–15.

Cutler SJ, Whatmore AM, Commander NJ. Brucellosis—new aspects of an old disease. J Appl Microbiol 2005;98:1270–81.

Driver CR, Stricof RL, Granville K, et al. Tuberculosis in health care workers during declining tuberculosis incidence in New York State. Am J Infect Control 2005;33:519–26.

Frieden TR, Sterling TR, Munsiff SS, et al. Tuberculosis. Lancet 2003;362:887–99.

Golla K, Epstein JB, Cabay RJ. Liver disease: current perspectives on medical and dental management. Oral Surg Oral Med Oral Pathol Oral Radiol Endod 2004;98:516–21.

Hammer SM. Clinical practice. Management of newly diagnosed HIV infection. N Engl J Med 2005;353:1702–10.

HIVDENT. An Internet based resource addressing oral heath care and HIV disease. Available at: http://www.hivdent.org/. HIVDENT site accessed February 12, 2007.

Howard CR. Hepatitis viruses: a Pandora's box? J Gastroenterol Hepatol 2002;17 Suppl:S464–7.

Kelly D, Skidmore S. Hepatitis C-Z: recent advances. Arch Dis Child 2002;86:339–43.

Kohn WG, Collins AS, Cleveland JL, et al. Guidelines for infection control in dental health-care settings–2003. MMWR Recomm Rep 2003;52(RR-17):1–61.

O'Farrell N. Donovanosis. Sex Transm Infect 2002;78:452–7.

Peterlin BM, Trono D. Hide, shield and strike back: how HIV-infected cells avoid immune eradication. Nat Rev Immunol 2003;3:97–107.

Samaranayake LP. Essential microbiology for dentistry. 3rd ed. Edinburgh: Churchill Livingstone Elsevier; 2006.

Scully C, de Almeida OP. Orofacial manifestations of the systemic mycoses. J Oral Pathol Med 1992;21:289–94.

Sherrard JS, Bingham JS. Gonorrhoea now. Int J STD AIDS 1995;6:162–6.

Swartz MN. Recognition and management of anthrax—an update. N Engl J Med 2001;345:1621–6.

Tramont EC. Syphilis in the AIDS era. N Engl J Med 1987;316: 1600–1.

For the full reference list, please refer to the accompanying CD ROM.

21

DIABETES MELLITUS AND ENDOCRINE DISEASES

SUNDAY O. AKINTOYE, BDS, DDS, MS

MICHAEL T. COLLINS, MD

JONATHAN A. SHIP, DMD

▼ DIABETES MELLITUS

Diabetes mellitus (DM) is a clinically and genetically heterogeneous metabolic disease characterized by abnormally elevated blood glucose levels (hyperglycemia) and dysregulation of carbohydrate, protein, and lipid metabolism. The primary feature of this disorder is chronic hyperglycemia, resulting from either a defect in insulin secretion from the pancreas or resistance of the body's cells to insulin action, or both. Sustained hyperglycemia has been shown to affect almost all tissues in the body and is associated with significant complications of multiple organ systems, including the eyes, nerves, kidneys, and blood vessels. These complications are responsible for the high degree of morbidity and mortality seen in the diabetic population. Clinical presentation of DM covers a wide spectrum from acute onset to asymptomatic cases discovered only during routine screening. The oral health care professional is a crucial part of the health care team in screening for and monitoring of patients with diabetes mellitus.

Epidemiology

Worldwide prevalence of DM in 2000 was similar in both males and females at 0.19% in individuals 20 years of age and younger, 8.6% in those over 20 years, and 20.1% in those older than 65 years. In the United States, 20.8 million people or 7.0% of the population have DM, of which 6.2 million are still undiagnosed.[1] An estimated 14.4% of the population aged 20 years and above as well as 33.6% of those aged 60 years and above have either diagnosed diabetes, undiagnosed diabetes, or impaired fasting glucose according to the National

509

Health and Nutrition Examination surveys (NHANES) 1999–2000.[2] In 2005, 1.5 million new cases of DM were diagnosed in individuals at least 20 years old. The incidence of DM rises as the population ages and prevalence of obesity increases. Based on US prevalence data, an "average" medical practice will have between 60 and 70 diabetic individuals for every 1,000 patients, and 50% of these patients will be undiagnosed.[3]

Classification

The classification of DM was formerly based on age at onset and type of therapy. It has been revised by the American Diabetes Association since each type of DM extends across a clinical continuum of hyperglycemia and insulin requirements (Table 1).[4] The new classification uses four categories: (1) type 1 (formerly juvenile diabetes, insulin-dependent diabetes, or type I), (2) type 2 (formerly adult-onset diabetes, non–insulin-dependent diabetes, or type II), (3) "other specific types," and (4) gestational diabetes. Arabic numbers are used instead of Roman numerals, thereby eliminating the confusion of type II as number 11. It is also based on the pathophysiology of DM and not the management regimen since both insulin-dependent and non–insulin-dependent diabetic individuals may take insulin as part of their management regimen. Type 1 patients are truly dependent on insulin therapy, whereas type 2 patients may benefit from insulin therapy but are not dependent on it for survival. Other types of DM may occur in individuals with certain genetic disorders, pancreatic diseases, infections, injuries to the pancreas, and endocrine diseases. Drug therapy with certain agents may also induce a diabetic state. However, gestational DM occurs during pregnancy and usually resolves after delivery.

TABLE 1   Etiologic Classification of Diabetes Mellitus by the American Diabetes Association (1997)[4]

Classification	Characteristics
Type 1 diabetes mellitus	Beta cell destruction, usually leading to absolute insulin deficiency Immune mediated Idiopathic
Type 2 diabetes mellitus	Insulin resistance with relative insulin deficiency
Other specific types of diabetes mellitus	Heterogeneous group in which etiology is established or partially known Genetic defects of beta cell function Genetic defects in insulin action Diseases of exocrine pancreas Endocrinopathies Drugs or chemical induced Infections Uncommon forms of immune-mediated diabetes Other genetic syndromes sometimes associated with diabetes
Gestational diabetes mellitus	Any degree of glucose intolerance with onset or first recognition during pregnancy

Pathophysiology

Pathophysiology of DM is mediated by alterations of carbohydrate metabolism and insulin action.[5] After a meal, breakdown of carbohydrates leads to elevation of blood glucose levels. Hyperglycemia stimulates insulin secretion from pancreatic beta cells because insulin is needed by most cells to permit glucose entry. Insulin binds to specific cellular receptors and facilitates entry of glucose into the cell, which uses the glucose for energy. The end result is a lowered blood glucose level and ultimate decrease in insulin secretion. If insulin production and secretion are altered by disease, blood glucose dynamics will also change. If insulin production is decreased, glucose entry into cells will be inhibited, resulting in hyperglycemia. The same effect ensues if insulin is secreted from the pancreas but is not used properly by target cells. A rise in insulin secretion may cause blood glucose levels to become very low (hypoglycemia) as large amounts of glucose enter tissue cells and little remains in the bloodstream. Following meals, the amount of glucose available from carbohydrate breakdown often exceeds the cellular need for glucose. Excess glucose is stored in the liver in the form of glycogen, which serves as a ready reservoir for future use. When energy is required, glycogen stores in the liver are converted into glucose via glycogenolysis, elevating blood glucose levels and providing the needed cellular energy source. The liver also produces glucose from fat (fatty acids) and proteins (amino acids) through the process of gluconeogenesis. Glycogenolysis and gluconeogenesis both serve to increase blood glucose levels. Thus, glycemia is controlled by a complex interaction between the gastrointestinal tract, the pancreas, and the liver. Multiple hormones also affect glycemia. Insulin is the only hormone that lowers blood glucose levels. Counterregulatory hormones such as glucagon, catecholamines, growth hormone (GH), thyroid hormone, and glucocorticoids all act to increase blood glucose levels, in addition to their other effects.

TYPE 1 DM

Type 1 DM is characterized by idiopathic autoimmune destruction of pancreatic beta cells, usually leading to absolute insulin deficiency.[4] It comprises 5 to 10% of all DM cases, has a sudden onset, and develops over a period of a few days to weeks. Type 1 DM occurs before the age of 25 years in 95% of affected persons but may occur at any age. Although it affects both sexes equally, it is more prevalent in Caucasians. The risk of developing type 1 DM is increased by a family history of type 1 DM, gluten enteropathy (celiac disease), or endocrine disease.

There are two distinct subclasses of type 1 DM. The immune-mediated form of type 1 DM is a chronic disease with a subclinical prodromal period characterized by cellular-mediated autoimmune destruction of the insulin-producing beta cell in the pancreatic islets. This may be triggered by an environmental event such as a viral infection[6] but may be associated with autoimmune disorders, such as

Hashimoto's thyroiditis, Addison's disease, vitiligo, or pernicious anemia. The idiopathic form is not associated with autoantibodies, and the cause of beta cell destruction is not understood. It is prevalent among people of African or Asian origins and strongly inherited but not associated with histocompatibility genes.[7]

The risk of type 1 DM is reflected in the frequency of high-risk human leukocyte antigen (HLA) alleles among ethnic groups in different geographic locations. Most type 1 DM individuals are of normal weight or are thin in stature. Since the pancreas no longer produces insulin, a type 1 DM patient is absolutely dependent on exogenously administered insulin for survival. People with type 1 DM are highly susceptible to diabetic ketoacidosis. Because the pancreas produces no insulin, glucose cannot enter cells and remains in the bloodstream. To meet cellular energy needs, fat is broken down through lipolysis, releasing glycerol and free fatty acids. Glycerol is converted to glucose for cellular use. Fatty acids are converted to ketones, resulting in increased ketone levels in body fluids and decreased hydrogen ion concentration (pH). Ketones are excreted in the urine, accompanied by large amounts of water. The accumulation of ketones in body fluids, decreased pH, electrolyte loss and dehydration from excessive urination, and alterations in the bicarbonate buffer system result in diabetic ketoacidosis. Untreated diabetic ketoacidosis can result in coma or death. Many patients with type 1 DM are initially diagnosed with the disease following a hospital admission for diabetic ketoacidosis. In a known diabetic patient, periods of stress or infection may precipitate diabetic ketoacidosis. More often, however, diabetic ketoacidosis results from poor daily glycemic control. Patients who remain severely hyperglycemic for several days or longer due to inadequate insulin administration or excessive glucose intake are prone to developing diabetic ketoacidosis.

TYPE 2 DM

Type 2 DM is the most common type, comprising 90 to 95% of DM cases. It is characterized by insulin resistance in peripheral tissue and defective insulin secretion by the pancreatic beta cells. The etiology of type 2 DM is multifactorial, including genetic predilection, advancing age, obesity, and lack of exercise. About 90% of diabetic Americans have type 2 DM.[2] It is more prevalent in African Americans, Native Americans, Hispanics, and Pacific Islanders than in Caucasians. Most type 2 DM patients are overweight, and most are diagnosed as adults. The genetic influence in type 2 DM is greater than that seen in type 1 DM. Whereas concordance rates between monozygous twins for type 1 DM are about 30 to 50%, the rate is approximately 90% for type 2 DM; however, no single genetic defect has yet been associated with type 2 DM.[8]

The underlying pathophysiologic defect in type 2 DM does not involve autoimmune beta cell destruction but rather is characterized by the following three disorders: (1) peripheral resistance to insulin, especially in muscle cells; (2) increased production of glucose by the liver; and (3) insulin

secretory defect of the beta cells.[5] Increased tissue resistance to insulin generally occurs first, followed by impaired insulin secretion. The pancreas produces insulin, yet insulin resistance prevents its proper use at the cellular level. Glucose cannot enter target cells and accumulates in the bloodstream, resulting in hyperglycemia. The high blood glucose levels often stimulate an increase in insulin production by the pancreas; thus, people with type 2 DM often have excessive insulin production (hyperinsulinemia). However, over several years, pancreatic insulin production usually decreases to below normal levels.

In addition to hyperglycemia, patients with type 2 DM often have a group of disorders called "insulin resistance syndrome" or syndrome X that comprises hyperglycemia, hypertension, dyslipidemia, central or abdominal obesity, and atherosclerosis.[9] Despite the strong association of type 2 DM with genetic factors, the etiology of type 2 DM is considered heterogeneous with environmental and lifestyle factors superimposed on genetic predilection. Obesity contributes greatly to insulin resistance, even in the absence of DM, and may explain the dramatic increase in the incidence of type 2 DM among young individuals in the United States in the past 10 to 20 years and worldwide in general. Intra-abdominal fat is the site that conveys the highest risk of type 2 DM. Other risk factors include advancing age, high caloric intake, sedentary lifestyle, and low birth weight. People with impaired glucose tolerance, impaired fasting glucose, and gestational DM have a high risk of developing type 2 DM in the future; these conditions are considered preclinical stages of type 2 DM.

The onset of type 2 DM is usually slow; it may remain undiagnosed for years because about 50% of affected people are unaware of their disease. Unfortunately, the insidious nature of the disease allows prolonged periods of hyperglycemia to begin exerting negative effects on major organ systems. By the time many type 2 DM patients are diagnosed, diabetic complications have already begun. Type 2 DM patients do not require exogenous insulin for survival since they still produce insulin. However, insulin injection is often an integral part of medical management for type 2 DM. Unlike patients with type 1 DM, those with type 2 DM are generally resistant to diabetic ketoacidosis because their pancreatic insulin production is often sufficient to prevent ketone formation. Severe physiologic stress may induce diabetic ketoacidosis in those with type 2 DM. Long periods of severe hyperglycemia may result in hyperosmolar nonketotic acidosis. Hyperglycemia results in the urinary excretion of large amounts of glucose, with attendant water loss. If fluid is not replaced, the dehydration can result in electrolyte imbalance and acidosis.

OTHER SPECIFIC TYPES OF DM

Approximately 1 to 2% of DM cases are in this category. It is caused by various specific genetic defects of beta cell function and insulin action, diseases of the exocrine pancreas, endocrinopathies, pancreatic dysfunction induced by drugs, chemicals, or infections. Other genetic syndromes sometimes associated with DM include Turner's syndrome, Down syndrome, Wolfram syndrome, Klinefelter's syndrome, Friedreich's ataxia, Huntington's chorea, Laurence-Moon-Biedl syndrome, myotonic dystrophy, porphyria, and Prader-Willi syndrome.[4] Thus, the etiology of this category of DM is heterogeneous because the abnormal glucose tolerance may be secondary to the precipitating condition or it may be apparently causal in a manner that still remains unclear.

GESTATIONAL DM

Gestational DM includes development of type 1 DM or discovery of undiagnosed asymptomatic type 2 DM during pregnancy.[4] It does not include women with DM before pregnancy, which is referred to as "pregestational diabetes mellitus." Approximately 2 to 5% of pregnant women in the United States develop a mild degree of fasting hyperglycemia or glucose intolerance during the third trimester, which significantly increases perinatal morbidity and mortality. As with type 2 DM, the pathophysiology of gestational DM is associated with increased insulin resistance. High incidence of gestational DM is found in older women, overweight women, and women of minority ethnic groups, but age has the highest correlation with incidence. Most patients with gestational DM return to a normoglycemic state after parturition; however, about 30 to 50% of women with a history of gestational DM will develop type 2 DM within 10 years.

Clinical Presentation

Type 1 DM is of sudden onset, whereas type 2 DM is often present for years without overt signs or symptoms. Patients with undiagnosed DM may present with one or more signs and symptoms of hyperglycemia that include polydypsia, polyphagia, polyuria, and acute manifestations of hyperglycemia (Table 2). Patients may complain of unexplained weight loss, poor wound healing, blurred vision, gingival bleeding, and high susceptibility to infections and may be easily fatigued. When complications of poor glucose control develop, patients complain of visual impairment; neurologic symptoms such as numbness, dizziness, and weakness; chest pain; gastrointestinal symptoms; genitourinary symptoms, especially urinary incontinence; and sexual dysfunction.

Diagnosis and Monitoring

The diagnosis of DM is based on specific laboratory findings, as well as the presence of clinical signs and symptoms (Table 3). Diagnostic guidelines include fasting glucose and casual (nonfasting) glucose levels, with restricted routine use of the oral glucose tolerance test. Diagnosis is not made until the patient has exceeded threshold glucose levels on two separate occasions. Urinary glucose analysis is no longer used for diagnostic purposes.

Both the fasting and casual plasma glucose tests provide a determination of glucose levels at a single moment in time (at the time the blood sample is collected). It is often useful to

TABLE 2 Signs and Symptoms of Undiagnosed Diabetes Mellitus

Clinical Features	Type 1 Diabetes Mellitus	Type 2 Diabetes Mellitus
Polydipsia (excessive thirst)	++	+
Polyuria (excessive urination)	++	+
Polyphagia (excessive hunger)	++	−
Unexplained weight loss	++	+
Weakness, malaise	++	+
Nocturnal enuresis	++	−
Irritability	++	+
Dry mouth	++	+
Chronic skin infections	++	+
Ketoacidosis	++	+
Periodontal diseases	++	+
Changes in vision	+	++
Vulvovaginitis or pruritus	+	++
Paresthesia, loss of sensation	+	++
Impotence	+	++
Postural hypotension	+	++
Initially asymptomatic	−	++

++ = more common; + = less common; − = rare.

TABLE 3 Diagnostic Criteria for Diabetes Mellitus*[4]

	Normal	Impaired Fasting Glucose	Diabetes Mellitus
Fasting glucose[†]	< 110 mg/dL	110–126 mg/dL	≥ 126 mg/dL
2 h postprandial plasma glucose	< 140 mg/dL	140–200 mg/dL	≥ 200 mg/dL
OGTT[‡] (not recommended for routine clinical use)			Plasma glucose at 2 h ≥ 200 mg/dL

*These criteria should be confirmed by repeat testing on a different day.
[†]Fasting = no caloric intake for at least 8 hours.
[‡]OGTT = oral glucose tolerance test performed using an oral load of 75 g anhydrous glucose dissolved in water.

assess the long-term control of glycemia, especially in known diabetic patients.

The glycosylated hemoglobin assay (or glycohemoglobin test) allows the determination of blood glucose status over the 30 to 90 days prior to collection of the blood sample. As glucose circulates in the bloodstream, it becomes attached to a portion of the hemoglobin molecule on red blood cells. The higher the plasma glucose levels are over time, the greater is the percentage of hemoglobin that becomes glycosylated. There are two different glycosylated hemoglobin assays: the hemoglobin A_1 (HbA_1) test and the hemoglobin A_{1c} (HbA_{1c}) test. Because these tests measure two different portions of the hemoglobin molecule, the normal ranges for the test results differ.[10] The normal HbA_1 value is less than 8%, whereas the normal HbA$_{1c}$ value is less than 6.0 to 6.5%. These tests are not currently standardized across all laboratories; therefore, glycosylated hemoglobin values must be interpreted in the context of normal ranges for the specific laboratory performing the test. The American Diabetes Association recommends that individuals with DM attempt to achieve a target HbA$_{1c}$ value of less than 7%, whereas an HbA$_{1c}$ value of more than 8% suggests that a change in patient management may be needed to improve glycemic control.[4] The glycosylated hemoglobin assay is not currently recommended as a screening tool or as an initial test for the diagnosis of DM. It is used to monitor glycemic control in patients with previously diagnosed DM.

Another assay that can be used to determine long-term glucose control is the fructosamine test.[11] This test is not used as widely as the glycosylated hemoglobin assay but is often helpful in managing women with gestational DM. The fructosamine assay assesses glycemic control over the 2 to 4 weeks preceding the test. The normal range for fructosamine is 2.0 to 2.8 mmol/L. This test may become more widely used in the future since at-home testing is now available. Self–blood glucose monitoring has revolutionized patient management of DM.[12] The development of small handheld glucometers has allowed the diabetic individual to take much greater control of his or her disease. Glucometers use a small drop of capillary blood from a finger-stick sample to assess glucose levels within seconds. Almost all insulin-using patients (and many who are on oral agents) have glucometers. There are many different glucometers available, and frequency of use depends on a patient's individual treatment regimen.

Complications

The major cause of the high morbidity and mortality rate associated with DM is a group of microvascular and macrovascular complications affecting multiple organ systems (Table 4). People with DM have a greatly increased risk of blindness, kidney failure, myocardial infarction, stroke, the need for limb amputation, and a host of other disorders. These complications are linked to sustained hyperglycemia, which can dramatically alter the function of multiple cell types and their extracellular matrix and thereby cause structural and functional changes in the affected tissues. Other disorders, such as hypertension and dyslipidemia, commonly seen in people with DM increase the risk of microvascular and macrovascular complications. The vascular complications result from atherosclerosis and microangiopathy. Increased lipid deposition and atheroma formation are seen in the larger blood vessels, along with increased thickness of arterial walls. Proliferation of endothelial cells, alterations in endothelial basement membranes, and changes in the function of endothelial cells induce microvascular damage. The pathophysiology of diabetic complications is complex. There is considerable heterogeneity within the diabetic population in regard to the development and progression of diabetic complications (Figures 1 to 3). Although poor

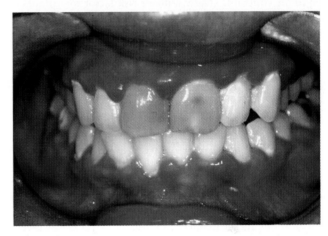

FIGURE 1 Generalized gingivitis in a patient with poorly controlled type 2 diabetes mellitus. The swollen, erythematous marginal gingival tissue was exacerbated by poor oral hygiene and plaque accumulation.

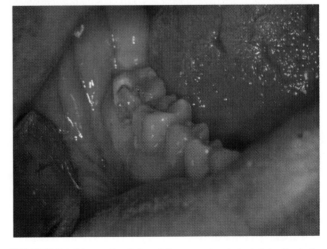

FIGURE 2 Advanced periodontal disease and periodontal abscess in the mandibular right first molar that developed in a patient with uncontrolled type 2 diabetes mellitus.

TABLE 4	Complications of Diabetes Mellitus
Site	**Presentation**
Eyes	Retinopathy, cataracts, blindness
Kidney	Nephropathy, renal failure
Nervous system	Sensory: peripheral neuropathy, cranial neuropathy affecting cranial nerves III, IV, VI, VII
	Autonomic: gastroparesis; changes in cardiac rate, rhythm, and dysfunction; postural hypotension; gastrointestinal neuropathy; urinary bladder atony; and impotence
Skin and oral mucosa	Unusual infections, delayed wound healing
Periodontium	Gingivitis and periodontal diseases
Cardiovascular system	Macrovascular disease (accelerated atherosclerosis) leading to peripheral vascular disease, coronary artery disease and cerebrovascular disease, ischemic ulcers, and gangrenous feet

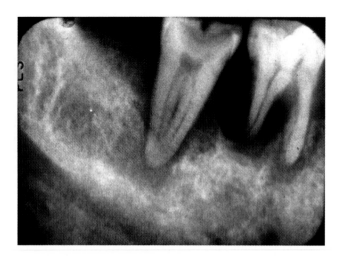

FIGURE 3 Periapical radiograph demonstrates extensive bone loss in the mandibular right first molar in the patient with type 2 diabetes illustrated in Figure 2. This resulted from a combination of delayed healing, chronic periodontitis, and a protracted periodontal abscess.

TABLE 5 Oral Agents for Management of Diabetes Mellitus

Class	Agent	Generic name
Oral agents	Sulfonylurea/First generation	Chlorpropamide
		Tolazamide
		Tolbutamide
		Acetohexamide
	Sulfonylurea/Second generation	Glyburide
		Glipizide
		Glimeperide
	Meglitinides	Repaglinide
		Nateglinide
	Biguanides	Metformin
	Thiazolidinediones	Rosiglitazone
		Pioglitazone
	A-glucosidase inhibitors	Acarbose
		Miglitol
Injectable	Amylin analogues	Pramlintide
	Glucagon-like peptide-1 analoges	Exanatide

glycemic control is clearly a major risk factor for complications, not all poorly controlled diabetic patients develop complications. Conversely, some individuals develop complications despite relatively good glycemic control.

Management

Primary treatment goals for DM are achieving blood glucose levels that are as close to normal as possible and prevention of diabetic complications.[13] Other goals are normal growth and development, normal body weight, the avoidance of sustained hyperglycemia or symptomatic hypoglycemia, the prevention of diabetic ketoacidosis and nonketotic acidosis, and the immediate detection and treatment of long-term diabetic complications. Diet, exercise, weight control, and medications are the mainstays of diabetic care. Obesity is very common in type 2 DM and contributes greatly to insulin resistance. Weight reduction and exercise improve tissue sensitivity to insulin and allow its proper use by target tissues. The primary medication used in type 1 DM is insulin, on which these patients are dependent for survival. Type 2 DM individuals frequently take oral medications, although many also use insulin to improve glycemic control.

Several oral agents are available for treating DM; most of these are taken by those with type 2 DM (Table 5). The first-generation sulfonylureas have been replaced with second-generation agents that are more potent, have fewer drug interactions, and produce less significant side effects. Sulfonylureas stimulate pancreatic insulin secretion. The increased quantity of secreted insulin helps counteract the qualitative decrease in tissue sensitivity to insulin, allowing greater glucose entry into target cells and thereby lowering blood glucose levels. Sulfonylureas have a relatively long duration of action (12–24 hours), depending on the drug, and are taken once or twice per day. Hypoglycemia is a major side effect of sulfonylureas. In patients taking these agents, food intake must be adequate to prevent glucose levels from falling too low.

Repaglinide stimulates pancreatic insulin secretion; however, its pharmacodynamic properties and mechanism of action are different from those of the sulfonylureas. Repaglinide is rapidly absorbed, reaches peak plasma levels in 30 to 60 minutes, and is then rapidly metabolized. The drug is taken with meals and lowers the peaks of postprandial plasma glucose to a greater degree than the sulfonylureas.

Metformin is a biguanide agent that lowers plasma glucose mainly by preventing glycogenolysis in the liver. Metformin also improves insulin use, counteracting the insulin resistance seen with type 2 DM. Because metformin does not stimulate increased insulin secretion, hypoglycemia is much less common with this drug.

The thiazolidinedione agents (troglitazone, rosiglitazone, pioglitazone) increase tissue sensitivity to insulin, thus increasing glucose use and decreasing blood glucose levels. These drugs also decrease hepatic gluconeogenesis. Like metformin, the thiazolidinediones generally do not cause hypoglycemia.

Acarbose has a mechanism of action that is unlike that of the other agents used in DM management. Acarbose is taken with meals; it slows the digestion and uptake of carbohydrates from the gut and is unlikely to cause hypoglycemia.

All patients with type 1 DM use exogenous insulin, as do many with type 2 DM. Insulin is taken via subcutaneous injection, most often with a syringe.[13] Insulin infusion pumps deliver insulin through a subcutaneous catheter. There are a variety of insulin preparations available; they vary in their onset, peak, and duration of activity and are classified as long-, intermediate-, short-, or rapid-acting (Table 6). Although beef and pork insulin species are still available, most individuals use human insulin preparations today. Ideally, the use of exogenous insulin provides an insulin profile similar to that seen in a nondiabetic individual, with a continuous basal level of insulin availability augmented by increased availability following each meal. There is no single insulin preparation that can achieve this goal with only one

TABLE 6   Types of Insulin

Type	Classification	Onset of Activity (h)	Peak Activity (h)	Duration of Activity (h)
Insulin glargine	Long-acting	onset 2 h	no peak	20 to >24 h duration
Insulin detemir	Long-acting	onset 2 h	no peak	6 to 24 h duration
Ultralente	Long acting	6–10	12–16	20–30
Lente	Intermediate acting	3–4	4–12	16–20
NPH	Intermediate acting	2–4	4–10	14–18
Regular	Short acting	0.5–1.0	2–3	4–12
Lispro	Rapid acting	0.25	0.5–1.5	<5
Inhaled insulin	Rapid-acting	onset 0	2–0.4 hr	peak 30–90 min

NPH = Neutral Protamine Hagedorn.

or two injections per day. Combinations of different insulin preparations taken three or more times daily or the use of a subcutaneous infusion pump more closely approximate the ideal profile, but even with such regimens, blood glucose levels are often unstable.

Ultralente insulin is the longest-acting insulin. Commonly called "peakless" insulin, Ultralente has a very slow onset of action, minimal peak activity, and a long duration of action. It is usually taken to mimic the basal metabolic rate of insulin secreted from a normally functioning pancreas. The intermediate-acting insulins (Lente and Neutral Protamine Hagedorn [NPH]) take several hours after injection to begin having an effect. Peak activity varies among individuals and sites of injection but generally occurs 4 to 10 hours after injection. Thus, a patient who injects intermediate-acting insulin in the early morning will reach peak plasma insulin levels at about lunchtime. Regular insulin is short-acting, with an onset of activity at 30 to 60 minutes after injection and a peak activity at 2 to 3 hours. The rapid-acting insulin (lispro insulin) is rapidly absorbed, becomes active about 15 minutes after injection, and is at peak activity at 30 to 90 minutes. Rapid- and short-acting insulins are usually taken just prior to or during meals. Thus, regular insulin taken prior to breakfast will peak at about midmorning; when taken prior to lunch, it will peak during the midafternoon. Some examples of common insulin regimens are given in Table 7.

The most common complication of insulin therapy is hypoglycemia, a potentially life-threatening emergency.[5] Although hypoglycemia may occur in patients who are taking oral agents such as sulfonylureas, it is much more common in those who are using insulin. Intensified treatment regimens for DM increase the risk of hypoglycemia. Thus, the long-term benefit of reduced diabetic complications seen with intensive treatment must be weighed against the increased

TABLE 7   Common Insulin Regimens

Description	Characteristics
Single injection of intermediate-acting insulin (early morning)	Peak insulin activity at midday Can provide enough insulin for mid-day meals only Hyperglycemia common upon rising and following breakfast and dinner
Single injection of mixture of intermediate-acting and regular or lispro insulin (early morning)	Peak insulin activity at both midmorning (from regular or lispro insulin) and midday (from intermediate-acting insulin) Can provide enough insulin for breakfast and midday meals Hyperglycemia common upon rising and from late afternoon until next morning
Twice-daily injection of intermediate-acting insulin (prior to breakfast and dinner)	Peak insulin activity at both midday (from morning injection) and late evening (from dinner injection) Can provide enough insulin for lunch and sometimes dinner; often prevents early-morning high blood glucose levels Hyperglycemia common after breakfast and shortly after dinner
Twice-daily injection of mixture of intermediate-acting insulin and regular or lispro insulin (prior to breakfast and dinner)	Peak insulin activity after breakfast (from morning regular or lispro insulin), after lunch (from morning intermediate-acting insulin), after dinner (from dinnertime regular or lispro insulin), and late evening or early morning (from dinnertime intermediate-acting insulin) Can provide enough insulin for all meals; often prevents early-morning high blood glucose levels
Three daily injections of regular or lispro insulin (prior to each main meal) and one injection of intermediate-acting insulin (bedtime)	Peak insulin activity after breakfast, lunch, and dinner (from regular or lispro insulin before each meal) and late evening or early morning (from dinnertime intermediate-acting insulin) Can provide enough insulin for all meals; often prevents early-morning high blood glucose levels Often provides better glycemic control than once- or twice-daily injection regimens
Three daily injections of regular or lispro insulin (prior to each masin meal) and one injection of Ultralente insulin (morning)	Peak insulin activity after breakfast, lunch, and dinner (from regular or lispro insulin before each meal); insulin activity in late evening or early morning (from morning Ultralente insulin) Can provide enough insulin for all meals; often prevents early-morning high blood glucose levels; often provides better glycemic control than once- or twice-daily injection regimens
Use of insulin infusion pump with regular or lispro insulin; basal metabolic rate set to provide continuous delivery of small amounts of insulin (bolus of insulin programmed prior to each meal)	Provides on-demand insulin with meals Basal metabolic rate most closely mimics normal pancreatic function Often (but not always) provides better glycemic control than any injection regimen

risk of symptomatic low blood glucose. One-third of severe hypoglycemic episodes result in seizure or loss of consciousness and 36% of the episodes occur with no warning symptoms for the diabetic patient. The phenomenon known as "hypoglycemia unawareness" is more common in diabetic patients with good glycemic control than in those with poor control.[14] Hypoglycemia unawareness is characterized by an inability to perceive the warning symptoms of hypoglycemia until the blood glucose drops to very low levels. Signs and symptoms of hypoglycemia are most common when blood glucose levels fall to <60 mg/dL, but they may occur at higher levels in diabetic patients with chronic poor metabolic control.[12] In people with hypoglycemia unawareness, glucose levels can fall to 40 mg/dL or lower before an individual "feels" hypoglycemic.

An emerging therapeutic option for type 1 DM is transplantation of the whole pancreas or pancreatic islet cells.[15,16] Both are still complicated by major side effects and are thereby performed in patients who have already developed significant morbidity from DM. The use of glucagon-like peptide 1, a potent insulin secretagogue, may prove useful in the future for type 2 DM. Also in the advanced stages of clinical trials are inhaled insulin and insulin analogues.[17,18] Complications of DM may be reduced by the use of aminoguanidine, an inhibitor of the formation of advanced glycosylation end products, and use of protein kinase C inhibitors.[19–22] With the development of continuous glucose-monitoring technology, it may now be possible to use closed-loop pumps that infuse the correct amount of insulin in response to changing blood glucose levels.

Oral Manifestations of DM

There is a plethora of oral manifestations in patients with DM, many related to the degree of glycemic control. Mucosal conditions include oral dysesthesia, including burning mouth, altered wound healing, increased incidence of infection,[23] and candidal infections (particularly acute pseudomembranous candidiasis of the tongue, buccal mucosa, and gingiva).[24] Xerostomia and bilateral generalized salivary gland enlargement or sialadenitis (especially in the parotid glands) can occur (Figure 4), and both are often related to poor glycemic control.[25,26] Medications taken by DM patients for related or unrelated systemic conditions may produce salivary hypofunction. Thus, the xerostomia seen in these patients may result more from medications than from the diabetic condition itself. Dry mucosal surfaces caused by insufficient salivary output are easily irritated, causing minor mucosal ulcerations, oral burning sensations, and increased likelihood of overgrowth of fungal organisms. Neuropathy of the autonomic system can also cause changes in salivary secretion since salivary flow is controlled by the sympathetic and parasympathetic pathways.[27] The high incidence and severity of dental caries in diabetes mellitus patients have been associated with xerostomia, increased gingival crevicular fluid glucose levels, and increase in dental plaque accumulation.[28,29]

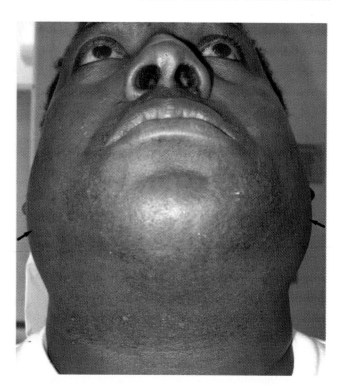

FIGURE 4 Bilateral parotid gland enlargement (sialadenitis or sialosis) in a patient with poorly controlled type 2 diabetes mellitus. *Black arrows point to enlarged parotid glands.*

DM is also an established risk factor for the prevalence and severity of gingivitis and periodontitis.[30] Depending on the level of glycemic control, DM promotes gingival inflammation in response to bacterial plaque to a greater extent than seen in well-controlled DM or nondiabetic individuals.[31] Hyperglycemia increases glucose levels in gingival crevicular fluid. This may alter periodontal wound healing significantly by changing the interaction between cells and their extracellular matrix within the periodontium.[32] Vascular changes seen in the retina, glomerulus, and perineural areas of poorly controlled DM patients also occur in the periodontium; hence, progressive destructive periodontitis is more common in patients with poor glycemic control.[30] In addition to hyperglycemia, poor oral hygiene and smoking contribute to the increased incidence and severity of periodontitis in DM. All of these factors must be considered in the dental management of patients with DM.

Dental Management

OVERALL DENTAL MANAGEMENT OF THE PATIENT WITH DM

In general, adults with well-controlled DM have similar risks for oral disease progression and respond similarly to most dental procedures as nondiabetic individuals.[33] However, a DM patient's response to dental treatment depends on factors that are specific to each individual. These include glycemic control, concomitant medical problems, diet, oral hygiene, and habits such as excessive use of alcohol and tobacco.[34] For example, the patient with DM, poor oral hygiene, a history of smoking, sporadic dental checkups, and high fermentable-carbohydrate intake is more likely to experience oral diseases such as caries and periodontitis. This patient will likely encounter delayed treatment responses compared with a DM patient without these factors.[35]

Glycemic control plays a role in the response of DM patients to periodontal surgery. Poorly controlled diabetics are highly susceptible to dentoalveolar infections[36]; they respond less favorably to both surgical and nonsurgical periodontal therapy, and short-term improvements in periodontal health are frequently followed by regression and disease recurrence. Therefore, it is imperative that dentists have an updated assessment of each patient's level of glycemic control prior to initiating treatment and maintain a close working relationship with the patient's physician.[37] A patient presenting with signs and symptoms of undiagnosed or poorly controlled DM (see above) should be referred to a physician for diagnosis and treatment. Antibiotic prophylaxis may be indicated if a patient's HbA1c level is very high (>11–12%) and there are signs of recurrent intraoral bacterial infections. Oral health practitioners should also be familiar with the common tests (see above) used to diagnose and monitor DM. They should have in-office glucose monitoring devices or glucometers to readily obtain immediate information about glycemic status if needed. These devices can provide rapid results within a few seconds.[38] This is particularly important when a stressful, surgical, or long dental procedure is scheduled so that the dentist can help avoid a hypoglycemic event (see below for management recommendations). It is also useful to determine if glucose levels are at the low range of normal during a procedure so that oral carbohydrates can be given to help prevent a hypoglycemic event.

The first step in treating the dental patient with DM is determining the type of DM (see above), methods of treatment (diet, oral hypoglycemics, insulin, a combination of these), level of control, and presence of DM complications (see Table 2).[39] This may require consultation with the patient's physician. Diabetes-associated medical complications require assessment since they could impact the provision of dental care. For example, hypertension, cardiovascular disease, and renal insufficiency require blood pressure monitoring and modification of anticoagulant drugs (eg, aspirin) before and after oral surgery. If the patient has renal insufficiency, potentially nephrotoxic drugs (eg, acetaminophen, acyclovir, aspirin, nonsteroidal anti-inflammatory drugs [NSAIDs]) should be avoided or dosages revised. Patients on hemodialysis or peritoneal dialysis are immunocompromised and at risk of endarteritis and endocarditis.

Dentoalveolar and oral-surgical procedures should be carefully planned to reduce the risk of hypoglycemia and nutritional deficiencies. Glucometers are extremely useful to check blood glucose levels prior to these procedures. If glucose levels are generally below 60 mg/dL, specific modifications to treatment are required (see below), dental procedures may have to be rescheduled, and medical consultation should be requested. Patients undergoing periodontal or oral surgery procedures other than single, simple extractions should be given dietary instructions after surgery; these instructions should be established with input from the patient's physician and nutritionist. The total caloric content and the protein/carbohydrate/fat ratio of the diet should remain identical so that proper glycemic control is maintained. If there is an acute oral infection, particularly in poorly controlled DM, antibiotics should be prescribed and appropriate modifications may be required in the patient's medications. For example, it may be necessary to increase the insulin dose to prevent hyperglycemia related to the pain and stress of infection; however, any changes in medications should be made by the patient's physician.

Appointment scheduling is often determined by the individual's medication regimen.[40] Traditionally, it was recommended that medically complex patients, including those with DM, receive dental treatment in the morning to reduce stress, but this may not be true for some patients with DM. The release of endogenous epinephrine from stress can have a counterregulatory effect on the action of insulin, leading to hyperglycemia. Therefore, the dentist must review with the patient the diabetes medications, foods, and fluids taken before the dental procedure.[41]

Generally, the best time for dental treatment is either before or after periods of peak insulin activity. This reduces the risk of perioperative hypoglycemic reactions, which occur most often during peak insulin activity. For those who take insulin, the greatest risk of hypoglycemia will therefore occur about 30 to 90 minutes after injecting lispro insulin, 2 to 3 hours after regular insulin, and 4 to 10 hours after NPH or Lente insulin. For those who are taking oral sulfonylureas, peak insulin activity depends on the individual drug taken. Metformin and the thiazolidinediones rarely cause hypoglycemia. The main factor to consider in determining appointment times is the peak action of insulin and the amount of glucose being absorbed from the gut following the last food intake. The greatest risk would occur in a patient who has taken the usual amount of insulin or oral hypoglycemic agent but has reduced or eliminated a meal prior to dental treatment. For example, if the patient takes the usual dose of regular insulin before breakfast but then fails to eat or eats less than the usual amount, the patient will be at increased risk of hypoglycemia during a morning dental appointment. Patients with poor long-term glycemic control and patients with a history of severe hypoglycemic episodes are at greater risk of future hypoglycemia. Often it may not be possible to plan dental treatment in a way that will avoid peak insulin activity. This is particularly true for patients who take frequent insulin injections; these patients have greater risks of developing perioperative hypoglycemia. Pretreatment blood glucose level can be measured with a glucometer, and there should be a readily available source of carbohydrates in the dental office. A final general recommendation for the patient with DM is that the dentist must help in modifying a patient's health destructive habits. These include cigarette smoking, poor eating habits, improper use of diabetes medications, infrequent glucose monitoring, inadequate visits to physicians, and insufficient oral hygiene and exercise.

SPECIFIC MANAGEMENT GUIDELINES FOR THE PATIENT WITH DM

Use of Epinephrine. Under stressful situations, endogenous production of epinephrine and cortisol increases. These hormones can elevate blood glucose levels and interfere with glycemic control. Therefore, during dental treatment, adequate pain control and stress reduction are paramount. Epinephrine is not contraindicated in these patients because it helps promote better dental anesthesia and significantly lowers the amounts of endogenous epinephrine released in response to pain and stress.[42] However, in a patient with concomitant cardiovascular or renal disease, the levels of epinephrine may need to be reduced to two or fewer carpules of local anesthetic containing 1:100,000 epinephrine.

Oral Candidiasis. Oral fungal infections can signify uncontrolled DM[43] and can manifest in the presence of salivary hypofunction. Treatment of oral fungal infections in the patient with DM is similar to standard regimens except that topical antifungal medications should be sugar free. If topical antifungal therapy is not successful after 7 to 10 days, systemic antifungal agents may be required (see Chapter 2, Pharmacology).

Management of Recurrent Herpes Simplex Virus Infections. Treatment of recurrent orofacial herpes simplex virus infection should be initiated early, if possible in the prodromal stage, to reduce the duration and symptoms of the lesion. Oral acyclovir, famciclovir, or valacyclovir can be used therapeutically or prophylactically, depending on the duration and intensity of recurrent herpetic episodes (see Chapter 2, Pharmacology). If the DM patient also has renal insufficiency or renal failure, nephrotoxic antiviral drugs (acyclovir, famciclovir, valacyclovir) will require dose modifications.

Management of Burning Mouth Syndrome. In uncontrolled DM, xerostomia and candidiasis can contribute to the symptoms associated with burning mouth. In addition to treating both conditions, an improvement in glycemic control is essential to alleviate the burning sensations. Treatment guidelines for burning mouth syndrome are well detailed in Chapter 10. Interestingly, amitriptyline, a drug used for burning mouth symptoms, has also been used to treat autonomic neuropathy in DM.[44]

Surgical Considerations and Periodontal Management. Prior to any oral surgical procedure, the oral health care provider must review any previous history of surgical complications, assess glycemic control, and update concurrent DM management. Following the oral surgical procedures, it is critical that patients maintain a normal diet to avoid hypoglycemia. In general, the well-controlled adult DM patient may not require antibiotics during and following surgical procedures, whereas antibiotics should be considered for orofacial infections and oral surgical procedures in the poorly controlled DM patient.[41] The decision to administer antibiotics should be based on multiple factors that include the current level and duration of glycemic control, extent of surgical procedures planned, presence of underlying infections, concurrent medical problems, anticipated level of postoperative pain and stress, and estimated healing period. The antibiotic coverage selected should be based on type and scope of infection, microbial sensitivity, and specificity results and prescribed in consultation with the patient's physician.

Periodontal disease has been referred to as the sixth complication of DM, and the longer the duration of DM, the greater the likelihood of developing severe periodontal disease.[33,45] Severe periodontitis has also been suggested to be a risk factor for poor glycemic control.[46,47] Since glycemic control is connected to periodontal disease and alveolar bone loss progression,[48] periodontal treatment must be conducted in parallel with DM treatment.[38,39,41,49,50] Primary treatment of periodontal diseases in DM patients is usually nonsurgical since surgical procedures may require modification of the patient's medications before and after treatment and could result in prolonged healing. Periodontal infections may also develop depending on the degree of glycemic control[51]; therefore, antibiotics should be considered.

The combination of nonsurgical débridement and systemic antibiotics in DM patients with advanced periodontitis has been shown to enhance treatment of periodontitis[52] and produce a potential positive influence on glycemic control.[50] In controlled clinical trials, a combination of tetracycline or doxycycline with scaling and root planing resulted in better periodontal control compared with scaling and root planing alone.[53] Similar results have also been demonstrated in patients who received topic intrasulcular doxycycline. The mechanism proposed for the additional therapeutic benefit from tetracyclines and doxycyclines is that these antibiotics inhibit human matrix metalloproteinases (eg, collagenase, gelatinase), which are connective tissue–degrading enzymes, For example, a low subtherapeutic dose of doxycycline has been shown to inhibit human gingival crevicular fluid collagenase, which significantly eliminated the risk of bacterial resistance.[54] These tetracycline-based drugs can therefore function as inhibitors of bone resorption or bone loss, a property that is independent of their antimicrobial activity.[55]

If periodontal surgery is necessary, several factors should be considered depending on the extent of the surgery, anticipated level of postsurgical pain and stress, and level of glycemic control. These include use of antibiotics, nutritional counseling, and changes in DM medications. Supportive periodontal therapy should also be provided at relatively close intervals of 2 to 3 months.

Oral Disease Management with Corticosteroids. Corticosteroid therapy for oral vesiculobullous conditions (see Chapter 2, Pharmacology) can increase glucose levels. Corticosteroids should be used with caution in collaboration with the patient's physician. If systemic corticosteroids are required, an adjustment of DM drugs may be necessary. Regular monitoring of glucose levels will be paramount to ensure good glycemic control.

MANAGING THE DIABETIC EMERGENCY IN THE DENTAL OFFICE

The most common emergency related to DM in the dental office is hypoglycemia, a potentially life-threatening situation that must be recognized and treated expeditiously.[49,56,57] Signs and symptoms include confusion, sweating, tremors, agitation, anxiety, dizziness, tingling or numbness, and tachycardia. Severe hypoglycemia may result in seizures or loss of consciousness. Prevention starts with the practitioner being familiar with the general medical risks for hypoglycemic events (Table 9) and assessing the patient's risk for developing hypoglycemia (Tables 8 and 10). Every dental office that treats DM patients should have readily available sources of oral carbohydrates (eg, fruit juice, nondiet soda, hard candy). As soon as a patient experiences signs or symptoms of possible hypoglycemia, the patient or the dentist should check the blood glucose with a glucometer, which has a typical response time of less than 15 seconds. If a glucometer is unavailable, the condition should be treated presumptively as a hypoglycemic episode (Table 11). Rapidly absorbed oral carbohydrates are preferable, particularly if the dentist is not trained or adequately equipped to administer intravenous, intramuscular, or subcutaneous glucagons or dextrose. Following treatment, the signs and symptoms of hypoglycemia should resolve in 10 to 15 minutes, and the patient should be carefully observed for 30 to 60 minutes after recovery. A second evaluation with a glucometer should be done to ensure that a normal blood glucose level has been achieved before the patient is released.

A medical emergency from hyperglycemia is less likely to occur in the dental office since it develops more slowly than hypoglycemia. Care is initiated by activating the emergency medical system, opening the airway, and administering oxygen. Circulation and vital signs should be maintained and monitored, and the patient should be transported to a hospital as soon as possible. However, under some instances, severe hyperglycemia may present with symptoms mimicking hypoglycemia. If a glucometer is not available, these symptoms must be treated as hypoglycemia, as described

TABLE 9   Factors that Increase Risk of Hypoglycemia

Skipping or delaying food intake

Injection of too much insulin

Injection of insulin into tissue with high blood flow (eg, injection into thigh after exercise such as running)

Increasing exercise level without adjusting insulin or sulfonylurea dose

Alcohol consumption

Inability to recognize symptoms of hypoglycemia

Anxiety, stress

Denial of warning signs or symptoms

Past history of hypoglycemia

Hypoglycemia unawareness

TABLE 10   Determining Risk of Hypoglycemia: Questions for the Dental Patient

1. Have you ever had a severe hypoglycemic reaction?

2. How often do you have hypoglycemic reactions?

3. How well controlled is your diabetes?

4. What diabetic medication(s) do you take?
    Did you take them today?
    When did you take them?
    Is that the same time as usual?
    How much of each medication did you take?
    Is this the same amount you normally take?

5. What did you eat today before you came to the dental office?
    What time did you eat?
    Is that when you normally eat?
    Did you eat the same amount you normally eat for that meal?
    Did you skip a meal?

TABLE 8   General Management Considerations for the Patient with Diabetes

Assess level of glycemic control

Refer patients with signs and symptoms suggestive of undiagnosed or uncontrolled diabetes to physician for diagnosis and treatment

Obtain medical consultation if systemic complications are present

Use a glucometer to help avoid emergencies related to diabetes

Treat aggressively acute oral infections

Place patients on frequent recall visits to monitor and treat oral complications and maintain optimal oral hygiene and diet

Adapted from Vernillo AT.[38]

TABLE 11   Treatment of Hypoglycemia in the Dental Office

Patient Condition	Treatment
Patient is awake and able to take food by mouth	Give 15 g oral carbohydrate 4–6 ounces (125–175 mL) fruit juice or soda (nondiet) 3–4 tsp (equivalent to 15–20 mL) table sugar Hard candy Cake frosting
Patient is unable to take food by mouth and intravenous line is in place	Give 25–30 mL D50 (50% dextrose solution) or 1 mg glucagon
Patient is unable to take food by mouth and intravenous line is not in place	Give 1 mg glucagon subcutaneously or intramuscularly at almost any body site

above. If it is an actual hyperglycemic event, the small amount of extra glucose delivered will not have any deleterious effect. However, emergency measures that will elevate serum glucose should not be delayed or withheld from a DM patient even if hyperglycemia is wrongly suspected in a patient who is actually hypoglycemic. This delay may result in severe adverse outcomes. The best strategy for determining the true nature of a glucose-related emergency is to check the blood glucose level with a glucometer.

▼ ENDOCRINE DISEASES

Hormones are substances released from cells that circulate and affect distant organs. The main physiologic functions of hormones are growth, maintenance of homeostasis, and reproduction.

Growth

Multiple hormones and nutritional factors mediate the complex phenomenon of growth. Short stature may be caused by growth hormone (GH) deficiency, hypothyroidism, Cushing's syndrome (excess cortisol), precocious puberty (excess sex steroids), malnutrition or chronic illness, or genetic abnormalities that affect the epiphyseal growth plates. Understanding the interaction of these hormones is essential for proper management of growth abnormalities.

Maintenance of Homeostasis

To some extent, all hormones affect some aspect of homeostasis. For example, thyroid hormone controls approximately 25% of basal metabolism in most tissues; insulin maintains glucose level in the blood; parathyroid hormone (PTH) regulates calcium and phosphorus levels; vasopressin regulates serum osmolality by controlling renal water clearance; and aldosterone controls vascular volume and serum electrolyte (Na^+, K^+) concentrations.

Reproduction

Hormones play a central role in sexual development. Perhaps no other endocrine system changes as much as the reproductive system over the human life span. They function at different stages, including sex determination during fetal development, sexual maturation during puberty, conception, pregnancy, lactation, child-rearing, and menopause, when reproductive capability ceases. Many hormones are involved in reproduction, and some include the pulsatile secretion of estrogen and progesterone from ovaries during monthly menstrual cycles. During pregnancy, the increased production of prolactin, in combination with placentally derived steroids (estrogen and progesterone), prepares the breast for lactation. The nervous system and oxytocin mediate the suckling response and milk release during breast-feeding.

Hormonal Feedback Regulatory Systems

Feedback control, either negative or positive, is a fundamental feature of endocrine systems to maintain hormone levels within a relatively narrow range. This system of one hormone stimulating a second, which, in turn, stimulates a third, and the ability of both the second and the third to feed back on the first, allows for exquisitely sensitive and precise regulation of a hormone (or mineral or ion) within a very narrow physiologic range (Figure 5). It also allows for either positive or negative amplification of any given signal. Undoubtedly, these multilevel positive and negative feedback systems can complicate the understanding of an endocrine pathway. Assessing the level of a hormone should be within the larger context of the feedback loop within which it exists. For example, a small reduction in thyroid hormone level by the thyroid gland triggers a rapid increase of thyrotropin-releasing hormone (TRH) from the hypothalamus and thyroid-stimulating hormone (TSH) from the pituitary. This results in thyroid gland stimulation and increased thyroid hormone production. When the thyroid hormone reaches a normal level, it feeds back to suppress TRH and TSH (negative feedback), and a new steady state is attained. Thus, very small changes in thyroid hormone result in large changes in TSH (see Figure 5)

Hormonal Rhythms

Circulatory hormonal changes are not only influenced by the feedback mechanisms discussed above but also adapt to environmental changes and fluctuate in response to known but poorly understood biologic rhythms. Seasonal changes, daily occurrence of the light-dark cycle, sleep, meals, and stress are examples of many environmental events that affect hormonal rhythms. The menstrual cycle is under control of intrinsic biologic "clocks" within the brain that very precisely regulate the timing of pulses of hypothalamic hormones over the 28-day menstrual cycle. In addition, many hormones are under the control of "24-hour clocks" and generate reproducible patterns that are repeated approximately every 24 hours. For example, serum cortisol levels peak in the early morning, wane throughout the day, and reach their lowest level or nadir at night.

The recognition and understanding of these rhythms are important for endocrine testing and treatment so that appropriate hormonal replacement strategies that mimic diurnal production will be instituted. For example, cortisol is administered as a larger dose in the morning than in the afternoon. Some endocrine rhythms occur on a more rapid time scale because many peptide hormones are secreted in discrete bursts every few hours. These intermittent pulses of many hormones are required to maintain target organ sensitivity, whereas continuous exposure will cause desensitization. In clinical practice, it is important to collect 24-hour urine to assess overall cortisol level, whereas the amount of insulin-like growth factor 1 (IGF-1) released by the liver in response to GH is a surrogate biologic marker for the integrated level of GH action. Similarly, the percentage of blood HbA_{1c} is an index of long-term (weeks to months) glycemic control in a patient with diabetes.

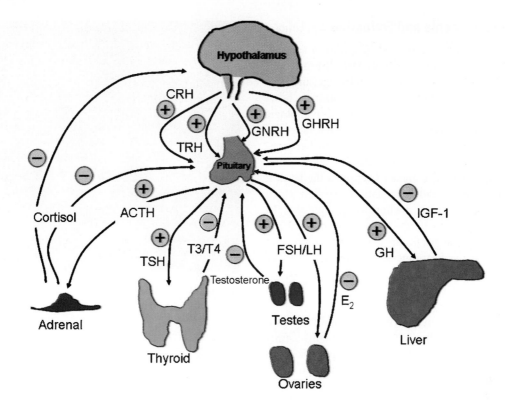

FIGURE 5 Regulation of hormonal levels by multiple endocrine feedback loops. The hypothalamus at the base of the brain is the source of many of the "releasing" hormones: corticotrophin-releasing hormone (CRH), thyrotropin-releasing hormone (TRH), gonadotropin-releasing hormone (GNRH), and growth hormone–releasing hormone (GHRH). These hormones act on the pituitary gland to stimulate the synthesis and secretion of the "trophic" or "stimulating" hormones: adrenocorticotropic hormone (ACTH), thyroid-stimulating hormone (TSH), follicle-stimulating hormone (FSH), luteinizing hormone (LH), and growth hormone (GH). These hormones act on their respective end-organs (labeled), which stimulate the synthesis and secretion of the active hormones: cortisol from the adrenal, the thyroid hormones triiodothyronine (T_3) and thyroxine (T_4), the sex steroids testosterone from the testes and estradiol from the ovaries, and insulin-like growth factor 1 (IGF-1) from the liver. Besides having effects on multiple tissues, these end-organs feed back as indicated in an inhibitory fashion at either the level of the pituitary and/or the hypothalamus.

Furthermore, hormone levels must be interpreted in the context of other hormonal results. For example, the level of PTH, which acts to raise blood calcium levels, must be interpreted in the context of the blood calcium level. A high PTH level may be appropriate in the setting of a low blood calcium level, and, conversely, a low PTH may be appropriate in the setting of a high blood calcium. In conclusion, the interpretation of any given hormone level may be impacted by the developmental stage of the patient, time of day the hormone level is measured, and point of action of the particular hormone within the feedback loop.

Mechanisms of Endocrine Diseases

Syndromes of hormone excess can be caused by neoplastic growth of endocrine cells (eg, overgrowth of cortisol-producing adrenal cells causing Cushing's syndrome) or autoimmune disorders in which activating antibodies mimic trophic hormones (eg, Graves' disease of the thyroid gland).

Most examples of hormone deficiency can be attributed to glandular destruction caused by autoimmunity, surgery, infection, inflammation, infarction, hemorrhage, or tumor infiltration. Autoimmune damage to the thyroid gland (Hashimoto's thyroiditis) and pancreatic islet cells (DM type 1) is a common example. Less common endocrine disorders can be caused by "hormone resistance," in which an endocrine gland is resistant to the action of the hormone, usually due to molecular defects in hormone receptors or molecules in the downstream signaling pathway. These disorders are characterized by defective hormone action, despite the presence of increased hormone levels. In complete androgen resistance, for example, mutations in the androgen receptor cause genetic (XY) males to have a female phenotypic appearance, even though luteinizing hormone (LH) and testosterone levels are increased. In addition to these relatively rare genetic disorders, more common acquired forms of functional hormone resistance include insulin resistance in DM type 2.

Hormone Measurements and Endocrine Testing

Hormonal tests should be interpreted in a clinical context. The normal range for most hormones is relatively broad, and interpretation depends on the patient's gender, age, and time of the day the specimen was taken. It is not uncommon, however, for baseline hormone levels associated with pathologic endocrine conditions to overlap with the normal range. In this circumstance, dynamic testing is useful to further separate the two groups. Dynamic testing includes "suppression tests," in which an attempt is made to suppress the level of the hormone in question, and "stimulation tests," in which attempts are made to stimulate the hormone in question. In general, stimulation tests are used when it is presumed that a hormone level is pathologically low, whereas suppression tests are used when the hormone level is presumed to be elevated.

Pituitary Gland

The pituitary gland, located in the sella turcica, is divided into two anatomically, functionally, and developmentally distinct structures, the anterior pituitary or adenohypophysis and posterior pituitary or neurohypophysis. The posterior pituitary is a group of neural cells, an extension of the hypothalamus, which have secretory capacity. The posterior pituitary secretes two hormones, arginine vasopressin (AVP, also known as antidiuretic hormone [ADH]), and oxytocin. The anterior pituitary is a mixture of cells that produce the following hormones: GH, adrenocorticotropic hormone (ACTH), TSH, LH, follicle-stimulating hormone (FSH), and prolactin. ACTH, TSH, FSH, and LH are all intermediaries in endocrine axes; each responds to a specific hypothalamic hormone and, in turn, acts upon an end-organ gland to bring about the endocrine response.

The primary physiologic functions of the posterior pituitary hormone oxytocin include contraction of the myoepithelial cells of the alveoli of the mammary gland, which is important during lactation as part of the "let-down response," and contraction of the uterus during child birth and immediately postpartum. AVP is a hormone important in water balance. A decrease in total body water causes high serum sodium (hypernatremia); this increases thirst and release of AVP from the posterior pituitary and prevents free water loss from kidneys.

The only established role for the anterior pituitary hormone prolactin is for the initiation and maintenance of lactation. Prolactin levels are increased during pregnancy, breast-feeding, nipple stimulation, stress, and chest wall injury and by medications with antidopaminergic properties (eg, antipsychotics). Prolactin release is under inhibitory control by dopaminergic neurons.

HORMONAL EXCESS

Overgrowth of any of the cell types in the pituitary gland can result in adenomas (Figure 6). Pituitary adenomas have been classified based on size and the cells of origin. Lesions smaller than 1 cm are microadenomas, and those greater than

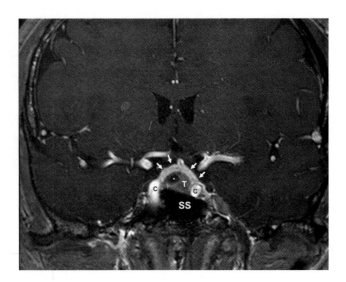

FIGURE 6 Pituitary macroadenoma. Shown is the post contrast MRI study of the pituitary of a 54 year-old man with acromegaly. The study demonstrates a large pituitary adenoma with a central area of necrosis. The sphenoid sinus (SS) and carotid arteries (C) are indicated. The gland is enlarged and replaced by a large tumor (T) with an area of necrosis in the tumor (*). The remaining normal pituitary has been compressed and displaced superiorly. The normal pituitary tissue is represented by the cup-shaped area of bright, enhancing tissue partially encircling the adenoma and necrotic area and is outlined by the white arrows.

1 cm are macroadenomas. Pituitary adenomas can result in increased secretion of the hormone(s) produced by the cells represented in these lesions and/or decreased secretion of other hormones due to compression of other cell types. Symptoms related to the physical enlargement of the adenoma are usually visual impairment or headache. Occasionally, these are detected incidentally as a finding on a magnetic resonance imaging (MRI) or computed tomography (CT) scan performed for an unrelated purpose (see Figure 6). Visual impairment is caused by extension of the adenoma in the superior direction compressing the optic chiasm. It presents as visual field defects, usually loss of peripheral vision, and less often as diminished visual acuity. The course of the visual deficit is usually very gradual, so many patients are undiagnosed for months or years. Pituitary apoplexy (infarction of the pituitary), on the other hand, has a dramatic manifestation. It presents as sudden and severe headache, often with diplopia. Apoplexy results from sudden hemorrhage within the tumor. Extension of the tumor inferiorly is rare but can result in cerebrospinal fluid leak through the nose (rhinorrhea) and meningitis. Evaluation of masses within the sella turcica includes anatomic description by MRI (see Figure 6) and evaluation of the hormonal profile for loss of function. Hormonal assessment of different axes is described in the relevant sections for each hormone.

HYPERPROLACTINEMIA

Hyperprolactinemia can be caused by hyperplasia of the so-called lactotroph cells (prolactinomas) or decreased tonic dopaminergic inhibition of prolactin secretion (eg, compression by a central nervous system tumor).[58] Prolactinomas can cause hypogonadism by suppressing gonadotropin secretion. In women, hypogonadism results in low serum estrogen levels that can present as oligomenorrhea, amenorrhea, infertility, and osteoporosis. In men, hypogonadism causes low serum testosterone concentrations that result in decreased libido and energy, decreased need for shaving, loss of muscle mass, and osteoporosis. Hyperprolactinemia in men may also be associated with impotence even when the serum testosterone concentration is normal. It can cause galactorrhea (leakage of milk from the breast other than during lactation in women), but this occurs very rarely in men.

Prolactinomas are relatively common, accounting for 30 to 40% of all clinically recognized pituitary adenomas. The diagnosis is made more frequently in women than in men, especially between the ages of 20 and 40 years, presumably because hyperprolactinemia disrupts menses. However, the adenomas that occur in men are usually larger, due in part to the lack of symptoms or delay in seeking medical attention. Serum prolactin levels in patients with prolactinomas can range from minimally elevated to very high.

Prolactinomas can be treated with dopamine agonists, such as cabergoline or bromocriptine. These drugs have the dual effect of decreasing hormone secretion and tumor size. If the adenoma does not respond to increasing doses of these medications or there is imminent visual loss, transsphenoidal surgery is indicated.

GH EXCESS

GH is of vital importance for normal growth and development. The pituitary cells that make GH are referred to as somatotrophs, and its release is under positive regulation by the hypothalamic peptide GH-releasing hormone. GH is the primary tropic factor responsible for postnatal growth. Although many cells have GH receptors and may respond to GH, the vast majority of the growth-stimulating effects of GH are mediated by IGF-1. GH is released from the pituitary in a pulsatile fashion, with the peaks of secretion at night. The pattern of GH release changes across the life cycle, but the largest area under the curve for its release is during the peak growth periods of childhood and adolescence. Thus, serum GH values vary considerable over the course of a 24-hour period, and a "spot" or randomly drawn level may not be a reliable indicator of the status of the GH axis. The serum levels of IGF-1, on the other hand, are relatively constant over the course of the day, so IGF-1 measurement any time of the day reflects the individual's GH status fairly well. In normal growth, IGF-1 values vary considerably across the life cycle, with the highest levels in childhood and low levels in advanced age.

GH excess leads to gigantism if it occurs before completion of linear growth; however, acromegaly results if it occurs after the growth plates have fused.[59] The mean age at diagnosis is 40 to 45 years. The progression of disease is usually very slow, so the interval from the onset of symptoms until diagnosis is often as long as 12 years. Acral overgrowth is

manifested with a classic facial appearance (Figure 7), including coarse facies, macrognathia, macroglossia, increased spacing between teeth (Figure 8), and enlargement of the nose and frontal bones (frontal bossing). Soft tissue edema leads to a "doughy" feel to the hands and feet, as well as an increase in shoe, hat, glove, and ring sizes. This swelling is

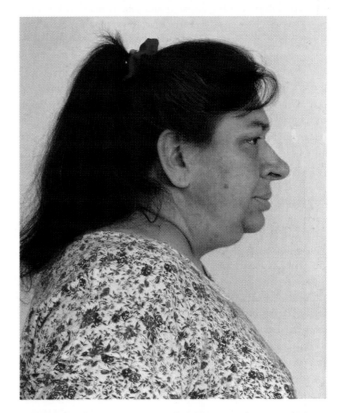

FIGURE 7 Characteristic coarse facial features of acromegaly: large, "acral" structures, broad nose, large ears, thickened lips, and slight frontal bossing. She also has a large cranium that is partially masked by the hair style. (Her dentition is illustrated in Figure 8.)

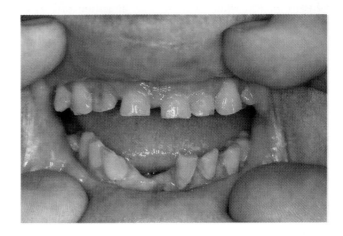

FIGURE 8 Dental characteristics of acromegaly (same patient illustrated in Figure 7). The maxilla and mandible are enlarged, producing large spaces between the teeth. The excessive thrust of the enlarged tongue (macroglossia) caused anterior displacement of incisors (the fingers shown in the picture are those of the patient).

probably due to a direct effect of GH on sodium retention. It has often been said that acromegaly can be diagnosed at the first meeting by the sweaty, doughy feel of the handshake and the appearance of the hands. Acromegaly has many symptoms, including increased sweating, enlargement of synovium and cartilages, deepening of the voice due to enlargement of the thyroid cartilage and vocal cords, hypertrophic arthropathy (of knees, ankles, hips, spine, and other joints), back pain, hypertension, left ventricular hypertrophy, skin tags, nerve compression (causing paresthesia of the hands, as in carpal tunnel syndrome), enlargement of the soft tissues of the pharynx and larynx (which can lead to obstructive sleep apnea), increased risk of uterine leiomyomata, colonic polyps, and visceromegaly (including the thyroid, heart, liver, kidneys, and prostate). Cardiomyopathy is the single aspect of acromegaly that is associated with increased mortality. In spite of these, patients seldom seek care on their own because the acral changes are so insidious. It is often a relative or friend who has not seen the patient for sometime who notices the typical changes described above.

Gigantism is the childhood version of GH excess. The rapid linear growth of gigantism can be distinguished from that of precocious puberty by the fact that in gigantism, the growth occurs in the absence of early secondary sexual characteristics. In fact, pituitary tumors that lead to GH excess often crowd out and replace the other pituitary hormones, such as TSH, FSH, and LH, leading to rapid growth without any sexual development. Mild to moderate obesity commonly accompanies tall stature in these patients. Progressive macrocephaly is also seen in children with gigantism and may constitute the presenting complaint, particularly during early childhood.

The serum IGF-1 is the best single test for the diagnosis of GH excess. Unlike GH, serum IGF-1 concentrations do not vary during the day. However, diagnosis requires confirmation by dynamic testing using an oral glucose tolerance test. In normal individuals, serum GH concentrations will fall to 1 ng/mL or less within 2 hours after ingestion of 75 g of glucose.

Surgical resection through a transsphenoidal approach is the treatment of choice for most patients with somatotroph adenomas. Medical therapy consists of somatostatin receptor analogues (octreotide and lantreotide) or a new clinically approved GH receptor antagonist, pegvisomant. Somatostatin analogs can inhibit GH secretion and decrease tumor size. External beam irradiation can be used in patients whose disease is not controlled by surgery or medical therapy.

DISORDERS OF ADH

Disorders of ADH are disorders of water. Too little ADH (diabetes insipidus [DI]) is a syndrome of the inability to hold on to free water by the kidneys.[60] It can be caused by inadequate pituitary production of ADH or resistance to ADH by the kidneys. The primary presenting symptom is polyuria (> 3 L/d), and resultant hypernatremia. Diagnosis of DI is made by a water deprivation test, which should be done under appropriate medical supervision. Improvements in assays for ADH in recent years have increased the utility of ADH measurements as part of the diagnosis.

Excessive ADH (syndrome of inappropriate antidiuretic hormone [SIADH]) is a syndrome of too much total body water and manifests as hyponatremia.[61] The primary clinical manifestation is a change of mental status that can lead to seizures and death if undetected. Major causes of SIADH include central nervous system disturbances such as stroke, infection, trauma, and hemorrhage. Other causes are medications, critical illness (especially in the elderly), and some types of cancer.

Oral Manifestation of Pituitary Disorders

Patients with GH excess have a characteristic coarse facial appearance because of the thick rubbery skin, enlarged nose, and thick lips. They have macrocephaly, macrognathia, disproportionate mandibular growth manifesting as mandibular prognathism, and generalized diastemata (see Figure 8). They also have anterior open bite and malocclusion because of the macrognathia and tooth migration. Intraorally, excessive soft tissue growth usually presents as macroglossia and hypertrophy of the pharyngeal and laryngeal tissues, making the patient susceptible to sleep apnea. Dental radiographs may demonstrate large pulp chambers (taurodontism) (Figure 9) and excessive deposition of cementum on the roots (hypercementosis).[62]

Individuals with GH deficiency present with disproportionate delayed growth of the skull and facial skeleton, giving them a small facial appearance for their age. Tooth formation and growth of the alveolar regions of the jaws are abnormal and may be disproportionately smaller than adjacent anatomic structures, leading to tooth crowding and malocclusion. Eruption of primary and secondary dentition and shedding of deciduous teeth are delayed. Due to the dental anomalies and crowding, there is a high tendency for plaque accumulation, and patients have difficulty maintaining good oral hygiene. Therefore, these patients may be prone to gingivitis and periodontal disease.[63] The dental concern for patients with DI is that excessive polydypsia and polyuria

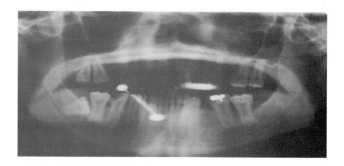

FIGURE 9 Panoramic radiograph demonstrating the characteristic taurodontism seen in a patient with growth hormone excess. All the permanent molars display excessively large pulp chambers. Radiograph kindly provided by Dr. Arthur Kuperstein, Department of Radiology, School of Dental Medicine, University of Pennsylvania.

can lead to excessive consumption of optimally fluoridated water to the point that affected individuals can develop dental fluorosis and enamel defects.[64]

Dental Management

Fifty percent of GH excess patients develop hypertension, 10% develop cardiomegaly and overt heart failure, and 30% develop insulin resistance or DM type 2. The dental management of these patients must consider these complications and should be conducted in consultation with their physician. Patients with GH deficiency will require correction of dental and skeletal malocclusions. If a DI patient requires major dental treatment that will be performed under general anesthesia, the anesthetist should balance the fluid and electrolyte intake because the urine of DI patients is mainly solute-free water.[65] The clinician should also avoid or reduce the use of high-dose glucocorticoids in DI patients since glucocorticoids can increase renal loss of water and further complicate DI.

Adrenal Gland and Its Disorders

The adrenal gland and its hormones are broadly divided into the cortex, secreting cortisol and aldosterone, and the medulla, secreting epinephrine and norepinephrine. Cortisol is the active and end hormone in the hypothalamic-pituitary-adrenal (HPA) axis. It is produced in response to the pituitary hormone ACTH, which is generated by response to the hypothalamic hormone corticotrophin-releasing hormone (see Figure 5). Cortisol is a steroid hormone that is essential, especially in states of stress, for the maintenance of blood pressure and gluconeogenesis (thus its moniker as a glucocorticoid). It has a diurnal pattern of secretion: very low levels are secreted overnight, and they begin to rise in the early morning, with peaks at about 8 am.

Aldosterone is another hormone produced by the adrenal cortex. It is also a steroid hormone, and its physiologic role is confined to maintenance of blood pressure by intravascular volume expansion via retention of the mineral sodium (thus its moniker as a mineralocorticoid). Volume expansion is accomplished by production of the enzyme renin by the kidneys in response to low renal arterial blood flow. Renin converts angiotensinogen to angiotensin I, which, in turn, is converted to angiotensin II, a vasoactive and potent stimulator of aldosterone production.

The primary hormone produced by the medulla is epinephrine (adrenaline). The adrenal medulla usually acts in response to, and in conjunction with, activation of the sympathetic nervous system. It is central in the "fight-or-flight" response, and its primary product, the catecholamine epinephrine, acts through the array of adrenergic receptors (α_1, α_2, β_1, and β_2) that are specifically expressed on a given tissue. Surprisingly, the adrenal medulla is not essential for life, and its absence is not associated with a specific disease state.

CORTISOL EXCESS

One of the most clinically relevant disorders of the adrenal gland is that of excess cortisol secretion by the adrenal glands or Cushing's syndrome.[66] Patients have a round (moon) face due to fullness in the cheeks and temporal fat pads, with a plethoric appearance that is often associated with acne and/or hirsutism (Figure 10). Since cortisol acts on almost every tissue in the body, the effects of excess cortisol are protean and include fat accumulation in the temporal-supraclavicular and dorsocervical areas ("buffalo hump"), increased abdominal fat with proximal muscle wasting in the arms and legs ("a lemon on sticks"), loss of skin integrity with easy bruising and purple striae (Figure 11), osteoporosis, menstrual irregularities, and mood disturbance (depression or mania). Untreated, Cushing's syndrome is fatal. When the cause of cortisol excess is specifically due to a pituitary adenoma overproducing ACTH (and thus cortisol), it is known as Cushing's disease, after the famous neurosurgeon and Pulitzer Prize–winning

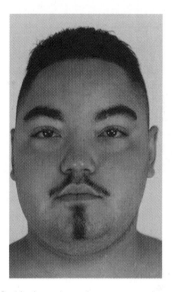

FIGURE 10 Cushing's syndrome features appearing as a round (moon) face caused by excessive fat deposition in the temporal fossae. The face is plethoric with fullness in the supraclavicular area.

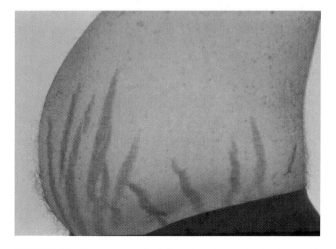

FIGURE 11 The presence of wide purple striae on the skin is an additional feature of Cushing's syndrome. The purple hue is due to the proximity of the underlying blood vessels to the surface from thinning of the skin by excess glucocorticoids.

TABLE 12 Diagnosis of Endocrine Disorders

Gland/Disease	Hormonal Problem	Diagnosis
Adrenal		
Cushing syndrome	Excess cortisol	24 h urinary free cortisol, 1 mg dexamethasone suppression test, midnight serum (or salivary) cortisol
Addison's disease	Low cortisol (and aldosterone)	ACTH stimulation test
Aldosteronism	Excess aldosterone	Plasma renin activity after posture or furosemide test, 24 h urinary aldosterone, saline infusion
Pheochromocytoma	Excess epinephrine and/or norepinephrine	Plasma catecholamines
Thyroid		
Hyperthyroidism	Excess T_4 and/or T_3	Suppressed TSH (most sensitive test)
Hypothyroidism	Low T_4 and/or T_3	Elevated TSH (most sensitive test)
Gonads		
Male—hypogonadism	Low serum testosterone	Low serum free testosterone levels
Male—hypergonadism	Androgen excess	Elevated serum free testosterone (or other androgen) levels
Female—ovarian failure	Loss of ovarian estradiol	Elevated serum gonadotropins (FSH and LH)

author Harvey Cushing. Many of the other features, including obesity, hypertension, and glucose intolerance, are common in patients who do not have adrenal hyperfunction, but glucocorticoid excess should be suspected when several of these symptoms develop simultaneously and continue to increase in severity.

The best single test for the diagnosis of Cushing's syndrome is the measurement of urinary free cortisol, which is unbound to cortisol-binding globulin (Table 12). However, 24-hour urine collections are cumbersome and often inaccurate. Therefore, a relatively simple and accurate test is the 1 mg overnight dexamethasone test. One milligram of dexamethasone is administered in the evening and the serum cortisol is measured in the morning. In patients with cortisol oversecretion, cortisol will not be suppressed, as it should be in a normal physiologic state, and the morning cortisol will be > 50 nmol/L. An elevated 24-hour urine cortisol excretion associated with a high-normal or high ACTH concentration usually indicates a corticotroph adenoma, resulting in Cushing's disease. Occasionally, the ACTH production is "ectopic," that is, from a tumor other than a pituitary adenoma, often a bronchial carcinoid tumor. If the ACTH is suppressed or undetectable, adrenal gland hyperplasia or an adrenal gland tumor is the cause.

The primary treatment for Cushing's syndrome is surgery. Transsphenoidal surgery is performed for Cushing's disease, and adrenalectomy is indicated if the cortisol excess is of adrenal origin. If surgery is not possible, a number of medications are able to block adrenal steroidogenesis, including ketoconazole and mitotane.

ADRENAL INSUFFICIENCY

Adrenal insufficiency is known as Addison's disease.[67] Cortisol deficiency leads to loss of appetite, weight loss, low energy, and hypotension and in stressful situations can lead to cardiovascular collapse and death. Adrenal insufficiency can be due to loss of pituitary function (ACTH). It is also

commonly caused by loss of adrenal tissue due to autoimmune destruction (also associated with oral candidiasis, especially in children as part of a polyglandular autoimmune failure) or replacement of the adrenal gland by a number of infiltrative processes (tumor, tuberculosis, sarcoidosis, hemochromatosis). Hyperpigmentation, including the oral mucosa, occurs because compensatory hypersecretion of ACTH by the pituitary gland causes a similar increase in pituitary secretion of melanocyte-stimulating hormone. Diagnosis of Addison's disease can be confirmed by a lack of glandular response as demonstrated by low serum cortisol (< 20 µg/dL) 1 hour after an intravenous injection of synthetic ACTH (cosyntropin 0.25 mg) (see Table 12).

PHEOCHROMOCYTOMA

Pheochromocytomas are tumors that produce epinephrine, norepinephrine, or some combination thereof. Patients are often hypertensive and have episodes of headache, sweating, tachycardia, palpitations, and pallor. Occasionally, these can be syndromal as part of multiple endocrine neoplasia syndrome type 2B (MEN2B) presenting as marfanoid habitus, high arched palate, neuromas (of the tongue, buccal mucosa, lips, conjunctivae, and eyelids), and corneal nerve thickening. The diagnosis of pheochromocytoma is confirmed by measuring urinary and plasma metanephrines and catecholamines, but diagnostic levels vary according to the specific assay.[68]

Oral Manifestations of Adrenal Gland Disorders

HYPERADRENOCORTICISM (GLUCOCORTICOID EXCESS OR CUSHING'S SYNDROME)

The primary orofacial feature of Cushing's syndrome is a round, moon face due to muscle wasting and accumulation of fat. Surface capillaries in the face and other skin regions become fragile, rendering them readily susceptible to hematomas after mild trauma. Facial skin has a ruddy color that simulates glowing health; acne and excessive facial hair (hirsutism) are common. Long-standing Cushing's syndrome produces delayed growth and development, including skeletal and dental structures. Many of the systemic findings of Cushing's syndrome are similar to those seen in patients on moderate- to high-dose glucocorticoid therapy, and these patients are considered to be immunosuppressed. Therefore, oral signs and symptoms of immunosuppression can be seen, including oral candidiasis, recurrent herpes labialis and herpes zoster infections, gingival and periodontal diseases, and impaired wound healing.

HYPOADRENOCORTICISM (GLUCOCORTICOID DEFICIENCY OR ADDISON'S DISEASE)

The primary orofacial feature of Addison's disease is unusual skin pigmentation, most intensely over sunexposed areas. On the face, freckles and moles become more intense, as well as the appearance of a tan-like complexion, except that the increased pigmentation will not disappear. The mucocutaneous junctions undergo increased pigmentation, including the lips, but it can also occur on intraoral mucosal surfaces such as the gingival margins, buccal mucosa, palate, and lingual surface of the tongue. The oral pigmentations appear as irregular spots that range from pale brown to gray or black. The treatment of Addison's disease includes administration of corticosteroids. This increases the risk of immunosuppression with concomitant susceptibility to oral candidiasis, recurrent herpes labialis and herpes zoster infections, gingival and periodontal diseases, and impaired wound healing.

Dental Management of Patients with Adrenal Gland Disorders

HYPERADRENOCORTICISM (CUSHING'S SYNDROME)

Dental management of the patient with Cushing's syndrome must take into consideration concomitant medical conditions that include easy bruising, impaired wound healing, osteoporosis, hypertension, heart failure, DM, immunosuppression, and depression or psychosis. Patients with Cushing's syndrome and those on long-term moderate- to high-dose glucocorticoid therapy are considered to be immunocompromised and are more susceptible to infections. Antibiotic coverage should be considered for dentoalveolar infections or any scheduled oral surgery, but this decision should be based on the underlying oral conditions and not solely on glucocorticoid therapy.

Assessment of the ability to withstand stress is an essential component of dental management of patients with Cushing's syndrome and other patients who have been on long-term moderate- to high-dose glucocorticoid therapy. Stress may be induced by an invasive surgical procedure, the onset of infection, an exacerbation of an underlying disease, or a serious life event, such as the death of a family member.[69] When normal individuals undergo stress, the plasma cortisol levels may double, suggesting an inherent ability of the adrenal glands to increase cortisol production by 100%. In a patient with adrenal insufficiency, adrenal function is inadequate

to produce adequate cortisol in response to stress, and the patient may experience severe hypotension, nausea, cardiovascular events, stroke, coma, and death. Patients with established severe adrenal insufficiency usually require premedication with oral or intramuscular glucocorticoids before an invasive procedure. Dosages must be agreed upon with the patient's physician; a frequent regimen is to double the daily dose of oral glucocorticoids the day before the surgery and on the day of surgery.

HYPOADRENOCORTICISM (GLUCOCORTICOID DEFICIENCY OR ADDISON'S DISEASE)

Dental management is similar to that for the patient who has taken long-term moderate to high doses of glucocorticoids (see above) since Addison's disease is frequently treated with exogenous glucocorticoids. The oral health practitioner must be able to recognize and provide initial management of an acute adrenal crisis (intramuscular or intravenous hydrocortisone) when treating these patients.[69]

Thyroid Gland and Its Disorders

The relevant hormones made by the thyroid gland are thyroxine (T_4) and triiodothyronine (T_3). Ninety percent of the hormone made by the gland is T_4, and approximately 10% is T_3. Since T_3 is the active hormone that binds to the thyroid hormone receptor and brings about the many physiologic actions of thyroid hormone, T_4 must be converted to T_3. The majority of circulating thyroid hormones are bound to a protein (thyroid-binding globulin), so the concentration of "free" or unbound hormone is clinically relevant. Thyroid hormone secretion is under the regulation of the pituitary hormone TSH, which, in turn, is under the regulation of the hypothalamic hormone TRH (see Figure 5). With very few exceptions, every tissue in the body has thyroid hormone receptors and responds to the action of thyroid hormone, primarily with increased oxygen consumption and heat production. The effect of this phenomenon is dependent upon the normal physiologic function and role of the end-organ.

THYROID HORMONE EXCESS

The manifestations of hyperthyroidism are protean.[70] The hyperthyroid patient is hot when others are cool, is hungry and eating all the time but losing weight, has thinning hair, is anxious and jittery, and has a fine tremor and tachycardia. The most common causes of excess production of thyroid hormone are TSH-stimulating autoantibodies (Graves' disease) and thyroid hormone–secreting nodules (toxic nodules). The classic feature of Graves' disease or hyperthyroidism is a "stare" with proptosis caused by deposition of glycosaminoglycans in the orbital musculature (Figure 12). In these patients, there is often periorbital edema, and the thyroid gland is diffusely enlarged and smooth. A rare complication of Graves' disease is Graves' dermopathy or pretibial myxedema, characterized by asymmetric or symmetric nonpitting edema of the anterior and lateral aspects of the lower leg (Figure 13). An increase in size of the midline pyramidal

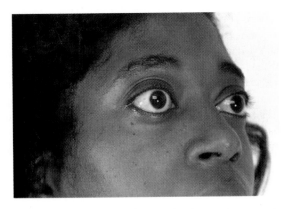

FIGURE 12   This patient has the 'stare' and proptosis commonly seen in Graves' disease.

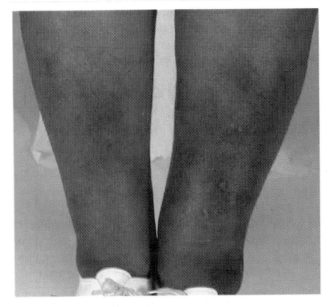

FIGURE 13   This patient has the less commonly seen Graves' dermopathy on the anterior lateral aspect of both legs.

lobe of the gland is diagnostic of Graves' disease. Enlarged asymmetric thyroid nodules are also associated with MEN2B syndrome.[71]

DIAGNOSIS

Since the vast majority of cases of hyperthyroidism are caused by primary thyroid gland dysfunction with overproduction of T_4 and/or T_3, and resultant suppression of pituitary TSH, a suppressed TSH is the most sensitive diagnostic test for hyperthyroidism (see Table 12). Therefore, a low TSH is the single best test for the diagnosis of hyperthyroidism. After primary hyperthyroidism is diagnosed, the clinician must identify the exact cause, which could be stimulating antibodies, autonomous nodule(s), or gland destruction with hormone release. This is done by assessing the uptake and pattern of diagnostic radioactive iodine by the thyroid gland; it is diffuse in Graves' disease, patchy in autonomous nodules, and little or none in gland destruction.

TREATMENT

The treatment of hyperthyroidism depends on the severity of the disease and the underlying cause. The initial step is to ameliorate the symptoms. This usually involves β-blockers (for tachycardia) and antithyroidal medications (thionamides), which block hormone synthesis by the gland. Definitive treatment is variable; radioactive iodine (^{131}I) is the treatment of choice in the United States, whereas surgery is recommended more commonly elsewhere. Thionamides are sometimes used chronically. If the cause is a TSH-secreting adenoma, transsphenoidal surgery is recommended.

HYPOTHYROIDISM

The hypothyroid patient is the mirror image of the hyperthyroid patient.[72] Patients are chronically fatigued, cold when others are comfortable, gaining weight without eating more, constipated, and bradycardic, with slowed reflexes. A slowed relaxation phase on the Achilles tendon reflex is an accurate physical sign of hypothyroidism. As the disease progresses, mental slowing, depression, and hypothermia can develop. The most common cause of hypothyroidism is autoimmune destruction of the gland (Hashimoto's thyroiditis). It is more common in women and may often be found in the context of a family or personal history of other autoimmune diseases. Hypothyroidism may also result from the loss of the TSH-producing cells of the pituitary gland (secondary hypothyroidism). Although less common, it can be caused indirectly by a large, nonfunctioning pituitary adenoma.

DIAGNOSIS

As with hyperthyroidism, since the vast majority of the cases of hypothyroidism are primary (thyroid gland) in nature, and since the pituitary response is to increase TSH secretion, an elevated TSH is the single best test for the diagnosis of hypothyroidism. This is accompanied by a low T_4 or free T_4. However, in the rare cases of secondary (pituitary) disease, the low thyroid hormone levels are accompanied by a low TSH. As in secondary hyperthyroidism, this is usually caused by a nonfunctioning pituitary tumor.

TREATMENT

Treatment of hypothyroidism involves replacement of the missing hormone. T_4 has a long half-life, can be administered once per day, and is inexpensive. T_4 acts as a prohormone that is converted at the tissue level to the active T_3.

Oral Manifestations of Thyroid Gland Disorders

OVERVIEW

As part of a routine head and neck examination, the oral health practitioner should palpate the thyroid gland. During a screening, the thyroid gland is examined with the patient's head extended to one side.[73] The examiner uses the fingers of both hands to palpate the thyroid gland. Next, the patient is instructed to swallow while the examiner evaluates the anatomic extent of the lobules using the last three fingers of one hand. In healthy patients, the right lobule is usually larger

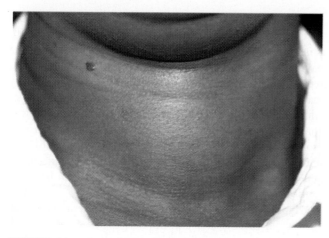

FIGURE 14 Asymmetric thyroid gland enlargement was observed in this patient during a routine dental examination. She was referred to her physician for further follow-up.

than the left, and the outline of the relaxed gland cannot be easily observed. The presence of an asymmetric thyroid gland enlargement (Figure 14) on routine examination should be referred for follow-up by an internist or endocrinologist. This is particularly true for the patient with a history of hyperthyroidism or hypothyroidism.

HYPERTHYROIDISM

Hyperthyroidism can exacerbate the patient's response to dental pain and anxiety. Routine examination of the head and neck may disclose signs of thyroid disease, including changes in oculomotor function, protrusion of the eyes, excess sweating, enlargement of the thyroid or the tongue, lingual thyroid tissue, and difficulty in swallowing. Patients may have increased susceptibility to dental caries and periodontal diseases.

HYPOTHYROIDISM

In hypothyroidism, orofacial findings include facial myxedema, an enlarged tongue (macroglossia), compromised periodontal health, delayed tooth eruption, delayed wound healing, and a hoarse voice. Salivary gland enlargement, changes in taste, and burning mouth symptoms have also been reported.[74,75] Hashimoto's thyroiditis has been associated with xerostomia and impaired salivary output.[76,77]

Dental Management of Thyroid Gland Disorders

OVERVIEW

The first concern in treating the patient with thyroid disease is the level of metabolic control and the second concern is concomitant medications. Well-controlled hyperthyroidism and hypothyroidism should not present major risks to the patient undergoing dental care. A complete history and physical examination are necessary to define the particular thyroid disease and assess its level of control. If the thyroid disorder is undiagnosed, untreated, or unstable, the patient's physician should be consulted to determine possible risks associated

with use of local anesthetics, infection, bleeding, wound healing, and ability to withstand stress. Inquiry about cardiovascular status, coagulation factors, level of disease control, and a history of other disease complications are important aspects of medical consultations. Drug interactions may result from the increased metabolic rate associated with hyperthyroidism or the decreased metabolic rate associated with hypothyroidism. Before prescribing any medications for a poorly controlled patient with hyperthyroidism or hypothyroidism, the clinician should consult with the patient's physician to determine the appropriate medication, dosage, and delivery schedule.

Patients with a history of thyroid cancer have probably undergone surgery or radiation therapy to the neck that would have affected regional hard and soft tissues. Salivary gland dysfunction is one of the most common side effects of high-dose ^{131}I therapy for thyroid cancer.[76,78] ^{131}I targets the salivary glands where it is concentrated and secreted into saliva. Dose-related damage to the salivary parenchyma results from the ^{131}I irradiation and causes parotid swelling, pain, and hypofunction.[79–81] As with the complications of other head and neck cancer therapies, postsurgical or postradiation complications may require special oral health care measures, depending on the patient's presentation. Tooth loss, diminished mandibular bone density, decreased salivary flow, dysgeusia, dysphagia, and skin and mucosal ulcerations are potential complications of radiation therapy.[82]

Patients with autoimmune thyroid diseases (Hashimoto's thyroiditis) may also be susceptible to other autoimmune connective tissue disorders, including Sjögren's syndrome. Antinuclear antibodies (ANAs) are found in one-third of patients with autoimmune thyroid disorders, and Sjögren's syndrome is found in nearly one-tenth of ANA-positive patients with autoimmune thyroid disorders.[83] The most common additional autoimmune disease identified in patients with primary Sjögren's syndrome has been identified as hypothyroidism[84]; also, there is a 7 to 17% prevalence of detectable thyroid antibodies in patients with primary and secondary Sjögren's syndrome and rheumatoid arthritis.[85] Therefore, the thyroid patient who presents with signs and symptoms of xerostomia and xerophthalmia should be evaluated further for evidence of Sjögren's syndrome.[86] Similarly, a patient with Sjögren's syndrome should be monitored for the risk of developing thyroid disease.[87] Oral health complications resulting from salivary hypofunction should be prevented in all patients who have received head and neck radiotherapy or ^{131}I treatment or those with autoimmune thyroid diseases. They must be counseled on their increased risk of developing dental caries, gingival and periodontal problems, oral candidiasis, dysgeusia, difficulty wearing dentures, and dysphagia.

HYPERTHYROIDISM

The most important concern in treating the patient with hyperthyroidism is the risk of development of thyrotoxicosis or a "thyroid storm," which includes symptoms of extreme irritability and delirium, hypotension, vomiting, and diarrhea.[88] It can be triggered by surgery, sepsis, and trauma. Emergency medical treatment is required for this condition. Epinephrine is contraindicated, and elective dental care should be deferred for patients who have hyperthyroidism and exhibit signs or symptoms of thyrotoxicosis. In general, stress management and short appointments are recommended in these patients, and treatment should be discontinued if signs or symptoms of a thyrotoxic crisis develop.

Patients who have hyperthyroidism are susceptible to cardiovascular diseases, including atrial dysrhythmias, tachycardia, and hypertension. Patients with high arteriolar pressures may require increased attention and a longer duration of local pressure to stop bleeding. Consultation with the patient's physician is required to document these and other organ system problems and to ascertain the level of control of hyperthyroidism.

Due to chronic medication use for hyperthyroidism and the risk of developing polypharmacy problems, the oral health practitioner should be familiar with the patient's current medications. Increased susceptibility to infection may develop as a drug side effect since one commonly used drug (propylthiouracil) can cause agranulocytosis or leukopenia. Propylthiouracil can also cause sialolith formation and can increase the anticoagulant effects of warfarin. Certain analgesics must be used with caution in these patients. Aspirin and NSAIDs may cause increased levels of circulating T_4, leading to thyrotoxicosis. NSAIDs can also decrease the effect of β-blockers. However, pain can complicate cardiac function in patients who have hyperthyroidism and should be treated by a multidisciplinary team with an emphasis on accurate diagnosis and reduction of risks associated with polypharmacy.

The use of epinephrine and other sympathomimetics requires special consideration when treating hyperthyroid patients and those taking nonselective β-blockers.[73] Epinephrine acts on α-adrenergic receptors, causing vasoconstriction, and on β2 receptors, causing vasodilation. Nonselective β-blockers eliminate the vasodilatory effect, potentiating an α-adrenergic increase in blood pressure. This pathophysiology is applicable to any patient taking nonselective β-blockers and those with hyperthyroidism due to concurrent cardiovascular complications.

HYPOTHYROIDISM

Lethargy is a common finding in the patient with uncontrolled hypothyroidism, and the oral health practitioner should be aware of lethargy, which could indicate a poorly controlled condition. Lethargy could become a concern due to a diminished respiratory rate and increased risk of aspiration of dental materials.

These patients are susceptible to cardiovascular diseases; therefore, consultations with medical providers are required to ascertain a patient's cardiovascular status. Patients who have atrial fibrillation may be taking anticoagulants and may also require antibiotic prophylaxis before invasive

procedures, depending on the severity of the arrhythmia. Coagulation tests (prothrombin time, partial thromboplastin time, international normalized ratio) are required when the patient is taking an oral anticoagulant and thyroid hormone replacement therapy. The presence of cardiac valve pathology may also require antibiotic prophylaxis. Intraoral use of epinephrine is not contraindicated if hypothyroidism is well controlled, but in patients who have cardiovascular disease (congestive heart failure, atrial fibrillation) or who have uncertain control of their thyroid disease, local anesthetic and retraction cord with epinephrine should be used cautiously.

Hypothyroidism patients are sensitive to central nervous system depressants and barbiturates, so these medications should be used carefully, with input from the patient's physician. For postoperative pain control, narcotic use should be limited since there is greater susceptibility to these agents in patients with hypothyroidism.

Patients with long-standing hypothyroidism may experience increased bleeding after trauma or surgery. Subcutaneous mucopolysaccharide deposition is increased in these patients due to its decreased degradation. The presence of excess subcutaneous mucopolysaccharides may decrease the ability of small vessels to constrict when cut and may result in increased bleeding from the infiltrated tissues, including mucosa and skin. Extended application of local pressure should control the small vessel bleeding in most cases.

Patients with hypothyroidism may have delayed wound healing due to decreased metabolic activity in fibroblasts. Delayed wound healing may increase the risk of infection because of the longer exposure of the unhealed tissue to pathogenic organisms. However, this may also relate to the level of disease control because a study of well-controlled primary hypothyroid patients treated with dental implants demonstrated no differences in the risk of implant failures when compared with matched controls.[89] Therefore, hypothyroid patients are not considered to be immunocompromised, but the health care practitioner must assess the level of disease control when planning oral surgical procedures.

Gonads and Gonadal Dysfunction

The gonads, like most other endocrine organs, are incorporated into an endocrine axis: the hypothalamic-pituitary-gonadal (HPG) axis. The physiologic function and regulation of the HPG axis, especially in the female, are complex and change dramatically over the life cycle. The hypothalamic hormone in the HPG axis is gonadotropin-releasing hormone (GnRH). GnRH is released in a complicated pulsatile fashion that varies widely over the life cycle and is different between men and women. The general principles of stimulation and feedback inhibition apply to the HPG axis (see Figure 5); however, this axis is complicated by two issues: GnRH is pulsatile, and the pituitary makes two hormones, LH and FSH. In the male, LH stimulates testosterone production from the Leydig cells of the testicles, and FSH stimulates sperm production by the Sertoli cells. In females, FSH stimulates maturation of the follicle, and LH causes "luteinization," or maturation of the follicle into a corpus luteum, as well as the production of ovarian estradiol.

In both males and females, the HPG axis is relatively dormant before the onset of puberty. The onset of puberty in girls occurs approximately 2 years before boys. In girls, the average age at which breast development starts is 10.5 years, and menses starts at about 12 years of age. In boys, the peak growth rate and beginning of voice change are about the age of 14 years, whereas facial hair appears on average at the age of 15 years. In men, from late puberty until about age 60 years, the serum testosterone levels are relatively constant and begin to decline gradually thereafter. In women, serum estradiol levels vary widely over the course of the menstrual cycle, but after menopause (average age is 50 years), serum estradiol levels become very low and gonadotropin (LH and FSH) levels are elevated.

PRECOCIOUS PUBERTY, DELAYED PUBERTY, AND HYPOGONADISM

In both males and females, precocious puberty, delayed puberty, and hypogonadism are clinical diagnoses, made by early or late signs of secondary sexually differentiation or loss of sexual characteristics.[90] Pubertal development is measured clinically by a staging system developed by Tanner.[91] This assesses the development stage of breasts and pubic hair in girls and the pubic hair, testes, and penile length in boys. Puberty is generally considered precocious in boys if it starts before age 10 years and in girls before age 8.5 years or delayed if there are no signs of sexual development by the age of 13 years in girls and 14 years in boys.

Once a clinical diagnosis of gonadal dysfunction is established (see Table 12), the next step is to determine if the pathophysiologic process is in the gonads (primary), pituitary (secondary), hypothalamus (tertiary), or, in the case of precocious puberty, an ectopic (or exogenous) source of hormone. Gonadal testing usually involves measuring the appropriate sex steroid (testosterone or estradiol) and the pituitary gonadotropins LH and FSH. The most common cause of precocious puberty in boys and girls is early onset of pituitary hormone production, central precocious puberty. If the end-organ hormones are elevated, and the gonadotropins are suppressed (gonadotropin-independent precocious puberty), this suggests primary (autonomous) gonadal dysfunction. Finally, the adrenal gland also produces androgens that can lead to early puberty in boys and masculinization in girls.

Premature ovarian failure is the onset of menopause, often including hot flashes, before the age of 40 years. The most common associated problem is cessation of menstrual cycles. Hypogonadism in men presents with a loss of libido and decreased growth rate of facial hair and can lead to osteoporosis and fractures. Premature ovarian failure is diagnosed by the early loss of menstrual cycles in the setting of an elevated serum FSH. Hypogonadism in men is diagnosed by a low serum testosterone level.

Replacement of the primary gonadal steroid (testosterone or estradiol or one of its analogues) in men and women is straightforward. However, replacement of the missing hormone will not return fertility, which is often a major issue. If the gonad is still functional but loss of pituitary hormones led to loss of function, the pituitary hormones can be replaced using a very sophisticated treatment approach.

Oral Manifestations of Gonadal Disorders

Hypersecretion of female sex hormones commonly occurs in pregnancy. Several unusual oral manifestations may occur in a pregnant woman, such as bilateral brown facial pigmentation (melasma), which disappears after delivery of the newborn baby. High levels of female sex hormones cause increased capillary permeability, making them susceptible to gingivitis (pregnancy gingivitis), gingival hyperplasia, and pyogenic granuloma (pregnancy tumor). These factors may complicate preexisting periodontal disease. A decrease in gonadal hormones at menopause is associated with a decrease in salivary flow and salivary composition. These may predispose individuals to dental caries, glossodynia, dysgeusia, unpleasant metallic taste, and oral candidiasis. Gingival tissues become atrophic; there is a higher tendency for plaque accumulation and increased risks of gingivitis and periodontitis. After dental extractions, unrestored edentulous ridges rapidly undergo resorption. Postmenopausal women have increased susceptibility to osteoporosis, so dental radiographs may demonstrate hypocalcified bone. There is also an increase in the incidence of several systemic disorders, including Sjögren's syndrome, pemphigus vulgaris, burning mouth syndrome, and trigeminal neuralgia, but the direct relationship of these with gonadal insufficiency has not been established.[92]

Dental Management

The specific dental management concerns in patients with gonadal disorders are focused on the associated secondary disorders. The pregnant patient is susceptible to gestational diabetes since insulin action is antagonized by estrogens and progesterone. The dental care practitioner should consult with the patient's physician if dental care is required and determine if the patient has been diagnosed with gestational diabetes. Elective and stressful dental procedures should be avoided during the first trimester and the last half of the third trimester. The second trimester is the safest period to provide dental care during pregnancy. During this time, emphasis should be on prevention, maintenance of optimal oral health, and treatment of dental concerns that may lead to complications in late stages of pregnancy.[93] Injudicious use of medications should be avoided in pregnancy; choice of medication should be guided by Food and Drug Administration pregnancy classifications for prescription drugs to avoid those with possible teratogenic effects.[94] It is also important to carefully evaluate panoramic radiographs for the presence of a carotid atheroma in postmenopausal women; if found, the patient should be promptly referred for further evaluation.[95]

Parathyroid Gland and Metabolic Disorders

PTH is secreted by four parathyroid glands closely associated with the thyroid gland in the neck region. Secretion of the

PTH is in response to the level of serum ionized calcium. Low serum ionized calcium stimulates PTH secretion, whereas high serum ionized calcium suppresses PTH secretion. Another major regulator of PTH is the active form of vitamin D_3 (1, 25-dihydroxyvitamin D_3 or calcitriol). It suppresses PTH synthesis by its ability to promote intestinal calcium absorption. PTH protects the body from chronic low serum calcium (hypocalcemia); therefore, an individual with hypocalcemia and vitamin D deficiency may develop parathyroid gland hyperplasia.

HYPERPARATHYROIDISM

Hyperparathyroidism is chronic excessive secretion of the PTH by the parathyroid glands. It results in uncontrolled chronic high serum calcium (hypercalcemia). The condition occurs in 0.1% of adult patients, is more common within the third to fifth decades of life, and is three times more prevalent in women than men. The vast majority (90%) of patients with hypercalcemia have either primary hyperparathyroidism or hypercalcemia of malignancy. Modern immunoradiometric and chemiluminometric assays can distinguish between the two since PTH is usually elevated or normal in primary hyperparathyroidism but suppressed when hypercalcemia is caused by a malignancy unrelated to the parathyroid glands.

When excessive PTH secretion arises from one or more parathyroid glands, it is referred to as primary hyperparathyroidism. It is usually caused by a solitary adenoma (80% of cases), whereas 15% are due to hyperplasia and 1% are due to carcinoma of the parathyroid glands. Postmenopausal women are more commonly affected by primary hyperparathyroidism. The amount of PTH secreted usually correlates with the size of glandular enlargement. However, pathologic parathyroid gland enlargement may affect more members of the same family, resulting in familial hyperparathyroidism. This type may also be associated with the MEN syndrome types 1, 2A, and 2B or the hyperparathyroid jaw tumor syndrome (HPT-JT). HPT-JT is a rare autosomal dominant disorder consisting of parathyroid cystic adenomas or carcinomas, multiple ossifying fibromas of the mandible and maxilla, and renal disorders that may include cysts, hamartomas, and Wilms' tumors. The risk of developing parathyroid carcinoma is much higher in HPT-JT syndrome. Another condition, secondary hyperparathyroidism, may also occur due to compensatory glandular enlargement in response to unusual hypocalcemia induced by metabolic disorders such as renal failure, deficiency of 1,25-dihydroxyvitamin D or malabsorption of calcium found in rickets, and some forms of osteomalacia. PTH secretion from enlarged parathyroid glands may become autonomous (secreting without control or response to feedback inhibition), leading to tertiary hyperparathyroidism.

The pathophysiology of hyperparathyroidism is related to the tight control of ionized calcium in the extracellular fluid by PTH and vitamin D and the central role of extracellular calcium in both cellular physiology and regulation of metabolism. Specifically, the PTH can be referred to as the body's defense against hypocalcemia. It binds specific receptors on the surface of PTH-responsive cells such as osteoblasts and renal tubular cells. PTH acts on osteoblastic cells to express RANKL (receptor activator of nuclear factor κB ligand), an inducer of osteoclastic bone resorption. To further maintain normal serum calcium, PTH stimulates renal tubular reabsorption of calcium and magnesium while inhibiting renal tubular reabsorption of phosphate and bicarbonate. This allows elimination of phosphates released from bone during osteoclastic bone resorption so as not to bind to serum ionized calcium. In the kidneys, PTH activates 1-α-hydroxylase, an enzyme that converts inactive vitamin D (25-hydroxyvitamin D) to the active form, 1,25-dihydroxyvitamin D. Active vitamin D acts to promote intestinal absorption of calcium. Therefore, excessive PTH secretion causes diffuse bone resorption, hypercalcemia, and excessive renal excretion of calcium and phosphate. The severity of hypercalcemia increases calcium in the glomerular filtrate, a process that eventually leads to hypercalciuria and formation of kidney stones. Chronic bone resorption eventually results in patchy cystic bone lesions and pathologic fractures.

Many cases of hyperparathyroidism may be asymptomatic and only detected by serum analysis during routine serologic evaluations. Clinically, the patients have manifestations of skeletal and renal disorders and hypercalcemia. They complain of bones, stones, abdominal groans, psychic moans, and psychic overtones.

Skeletal presentations include bone demineralization that manifests as reduction in bone mass. Patients complain of bone pains and arthralgia and may develop pathologic fractures. Bone radiographs show well-circumscribed unilocular or multilocular radiolucent lesions known as "brown tumor" of hyperparathyroidism, but brown tumors are now rare occurrences in modern medicine because of early detection. If brown tumors occur, they contain abundant hemorrhagic tissue and hemosiderin, which give it a characteristically dark reddish-brown color. Degeneration of brown tumor leads to patchy osteoclastic bone resorption, cystic lesions, and replacement of bone with abundant vascular cellular fibrous tissue. This transformation is referred to as "osteitis fibrosa cystica." In addition, skull radiographs show patchy regions of demineralization ("salt and pepper" appearance). Due to routine screenings and early detection of hypercalcemia, skeletal presentation is now commonly osteopenia without the classic features of brown tumor and osteitis fibrosa cystica. Brown tumors may be seen in developing countries and in patients with parathyroid carcinoma. In patients with HPT-JT syndrome, the multiple fibro-osseous jaw tumors and parathyroid adenomas can occur in isolation. However, unlike brown tumors of hyperparathyroidism, jaw tumors of HPT-JT are distinct because they do not resolve after parathyroidectomy.

Renal presentations include polyuria and polydypsia as a result of hypercalcemia-induced DI, and 10 to 15% of patients may develop kidney stones consisting of calcium phosphate or calcium oxalate. Nonspecific presentations of hypercalcemia include "abdominal groans" of constipation, indigestion, weight loss, nausea, vomiting, peptic ulcer, and pancreatitis, as well as "psychic moans" of lethargy, fatigue, depression, loss of memory, paranoia, neuroses, change in personality, confusion, stupor, and coma. Metastatic calcium precipitation in the cornea may cause keratitis and conjunctivitis, and if in soft tissues, it may cause calciphylaxis.

The most common laboratory finding is high alkaline phosphatase in patients with bone lesions. Serum calcium is elevated (>10.5 mg/dL), but phosphate may vary from low-normal (<3.5 mg/dL) to low (<2.5 mg/dL). Serum PTH is often elevated, and the level of 1,25-dihydroxyvitamin D may also be high due to the stimulatory effect of PTH on 1-α-hydroxylase. Imaging techniques are required for assessment of a parathyroid adenoma. For symptomatic primary hyperparathyroidism, definitive treatment is surgical parathyroidectomy, which has a 95% success rate. Medical management may involve use of vitamin D when associated with vitamin D deficiency, as well as bisphosphonates and calcimimetics that compete with PTH to decrease its secretion. Medical treatment of hyperparathyroidism also includes the use of the calcium-sensing receptor agonist cinacalcet (Sensipar).

Since postmenopausal women are commonly affected by hyperparathyroidism, high-dose estrogen replacement therapy is often needed to treat bone lesions and reduce serum calcium, but it does not reduce the PTH level.

Hypoparathyroidism and Hypocalcemia

Hypoparathyroidism is a deficiency in the production, secretion, or action of PTH and the most common cause of hypocalcemia. It usually results when parathyroid glands are surgically removed to correct primary hyperparathyroidism or during thyroidectomy. Hypoparathyroidism can also result from cell-mediated autoimmune glandular destruction associated with mutations of the autoimmune regulator (*AIRE*) gene. It can also occur when there is activating mutations of the calcium-sensing receptor (autosomal dominant hypocalcemia). Radiation to the neck, metastatic cancer, infection, and magnesium deficiency are other unusual causes of hypoparathyroidism. Damage to the parathyroid glands by heavy metals (eg, copper in Wilson's disease, iron in hemochromatosis) and transfusion hemosiderosis are other unusual causes of hypoparathyroidism. Parathyroid glands may be underdeveloped or completely absent in DiGeorge syndrome, a developmental abnormality of the third and fourth pharyngeal pouches. *Pseudohypoparathyroidism* is a term used to describe a group of disorders that cause hypocalcemia as a result of renal resistance to PTH despite high levels of PTH. Other causes of hypocalcemia in addition to hypoparathyroidism are vitamin D deficiency, hyperphosphatemia, malabsorption of calcium, and chronic renal failure.

Hypocalcemia is often asymptomatic; however, acute hypocalcemia produces symptoms that result from neuromuscular irritability or excitability. This leads to muscular and mental manifestations that include paresthesia of hands, feet, and circumoral muscles; electroencephalographic abnormalities; anxiety; confusion; and depression. A positive Chvostek's sign may be elicited if tapping on the facial nerve in the preauricular region causes twitching of the facial muscles. Patients may develop tetany characterized by tonic-clonic seizures, carpopedal spasm, and severe laryngospasm. In DiGeorge syndrome, tetany is usually noticed in infancy but may remain undetected until adulthood.

Laboratory findings are low PTH and low serum calcium levels, but serum phosphate is elevated and alkaline phosphatase is normal. Most patients with hypocalcemia can be treated with oral calcium and vitamin D supplements, although acute cases may require intravenous calcium infusions.

Oral Manifestations of Parathyroid Gland Disorders

HYPERPARATHYROIDISM

The primary clinical orofacial signs and symptoms of hyperparathyroidism are reflections of the systemic effects of hypercalcemia. Long-standing hypercalcemia causes generalized osteoporosis, which is visible on dental radiographs. Patients develop cortical resorption and rarefactions, loss of trabeculation presenting as "ground-glass" appearance, partial or total loss of lamina dura, lytic lesions, and metastatic calcifications.[96] The rarefactions occur secondary to generalized osteoporosis when fine trabeculae disappear later in the disease process, leaving a coarse pattern. Alveolar bone is particularly sensitive to increased levels of PTH from either primary or secondary hyperparathyroidism.[97] Thinning and eventual loss of the cortical bone of the maxilla and mandible may occur, especially on the lower border of the mandible. Severe cases result in spontaneous mandibular fracture.

The lytic jaw lesions or brown tumors[98] can increase in size, causing the bony cortex to expand, ultimately becoming destroyed.[99] These tumors rarely expand into the periosteum but can produce gingival swelling. Biopsy of the lytic lesion is necessary for definitive diagnosis; however, they are histologically similar to central giant cell tumors and giant cell reparative granulomas.[100] Fully developed teeth are not affected except that they appear more radiopaque. Due to bony changes, the teeth become mobile, drift, and cause malocclusion. With gradual loosening of the dentition, periradicular radiolucencies develop, with increased periodontal pocketing, root resorption, and dental pain.

HYPOPARATHYROIDISM

In hypoparathyroidism, hypocalcemia produces increased muscular and peripheral nerve irritability that may be mistaken for a seizure disorder. Painful muscular spasms affect oral and laryngeal muscles. Despite low serum calcium levels, the maxilla and mandible are abnormally dense, with well-calcified trabeculae. If the hypoparathyroidism is part of an autoimmune polyendocrinopathy syndrome, oral mucocutaneous candidiasis may be present in an acute or chronic form.

If hypoparathyroidism occurs when teeth are still developing, there will be abnormalities in the appearance and eruption pattern. There may be enamel hypoplasia, single or parallel horizontal bands on the enamel, and poorly mineralized dentin. Other dental findings include malformed teeth, anodontia, short blunt root apices, elongated pulp chambers (some occluded by pulp stones, even in the primary dentition), impacted teeth, and mandibular exostoses. If hypoparathyroidism occurs after dental development, there are no abnormalities seen in erupted teeth.

Dental Management of Patients with Parathyroid Gland Disorders

HYPERPARATHYROIDISM

Clinicians must be careful to avoid iatrogenic jaw fractures during oral surgical procedures due to the presence of lytic bone lesions and cortical bone loss. Following successful treatment of hyperparathyroidism, recalcification of the skeleton occurs and serum calcium levels return to normal. Surgical intervention of giant cell tumors is not necessary except to correct large deformities or remove displaced or resorbed teeth.

HYPOPARATHYROIDISM

Low serum calcium levels may precipitate cardiac arrhythmias, convulsions, laryngospasm, or bronchospasm. Therefore, consultation with the patient's physicians is required to ascertain level of metabolic control and update serum calcium and phosphate levels as well as the PTH level. Patients with dental abnormalities require frequent oral examinations due to increased caries risk associated with hypoplastic teeth. Periodic dental radiographs are required to screen for dentigerous cysts that may develop at sites of impacted teeth.

Rickets, Osteomalacia, and Vitamin D Deficiency

Rickets is failure of mineralization of endochondral new bone formed at the growth plates in children, whereas osteomalacia is failure of mineralization of newly formed organic bone matrix (osteoid mineralization) at sites of bone turnover. Therefore, osteomalacia is usually found in adults, whereas rickets and osteomalacia may coexist in children whose growth plates have not fused. Rickets/osteomalacia and osteoporosis are referred to as metabolic bone diseases because they cause generalized decrease in bone density (osteopenia) and bone strength. Unlike osteoporosis, which is characterized by a decrease in bone matrix and minerals, the bone matrix is normal in rickets/osteomalacia. Abnormalities in vitamin D metabolism or resistance to the actions of vitamin D can cause rickets or osteomalacia because the primary actions of vitamin D are to increase absorption of calcium and phosphate from the intestine.

Ergocalciferol or vitamin D_2 derived from plants is insufficient in major food items, so the human daily requirement is supplemented by formation of cholecalciferol or vitamin

D_3 in the skin. Dermal synthesis of vitamin D can be impaired by inadequate sunlight in geographic regions of extreme latitude or in cultural regions that wear extensive clothing to cover the whole body. Hepatic and renal disorders can also affect vitamin D metabolism.

Clinical and radiologic presentations of rickets are skeletal pain, fracture of abnormal bone, bone deformity such as bowing of the long bones, scoliosis, bell-shaped thorax, and basilar invagination of the skull. Patients with osteomalacia also experience diffuse skeletal pain, especially the weight-bearing areas. The radiographic presentations are usually nonspecific but may include osteopenia, poorly defined trabecular bone, and masking of the junction between the cortical and trabecular bone. It is common to observe bilateral and symmetric pseudofractures called Looser's zones on several bones (femur, pelvis, ribs, and scapula). Although bone biopsy is usually not necessary for diagnosis, these microfractures are also visible in undecalcified histologic bone sections (Figure 15).

Clinical and radiologic presentations of rickets are usually obvious in children, but diagnosing and identifying the cause of osteomalacia are more challenging. The serum calcium level is usually low to normal and serum phosphorus is low, but serum alkaline phosphatase and PTH levels are elevated because of secondary hyperparathyroidism and increased bone resorption. A low level of 1,25-dihydroxyvitamin D_3 confirms vitamin D deficiency, but sometimes the vitamin D level is normal. Bone biopsy and histomorphometric analysis may be necessary but not required to diagnose osteomalacia.

Vitamin D deficiency is treated with vitamin D and calcium supplements at doses dependent upon the severity

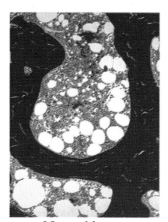
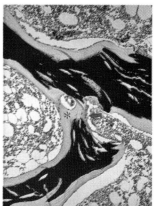

Normal bone   Osteomalacic bone

FIGURE 15 Undecalcified, plastic embedded sections of normal and osteomalacic bone stained with Giemsa (blue) and Von Kossa (black) reveal histological features of osteomalacia. The normal bone (left panel) demonstrates complete mineralization of the trabeculae (black) whereas osteomalacic bone (right panel) is poorly mineralized as demonstrated by a thick layer of un-mineralized osteoid (stained blue, red star) around irregular bone trabeculae. There is smooth continuity of normal bone trabeculae compared with irregular discontinuous trabeculae or microfracture in osteomalacic bone (red arrow).

of the disorder and other associated medical conditions. Patients with malabsorption syndrome or those taking barbiturates or phenytoin will require higher doses. Barbiturates and phenytoin cause resistance to 1,25-dihydroxyvitamin D and also accelerate its metabolism.

Oral Manifestations and Dental Management

Children with rickets/osteomalacia may present with delayed tooth eruption, loss of lamina dura, and enamel and dentine hypoplasia that may progress to periapical infections. Malocclusion and hypoplastic teeth increase the risks of dental caries; therefore, regular oral health evaluation is necessary to monitor dental and periodontal health.

▼ SELECTED READING

Akintoye SO, Lee JS, Feimster T, et al. Dental characteristics of fibrous dysplasia and McCune-Albright syndrome. Oral Surg Oral Med Oral Pathol Oral Radiol Endod 2003;96:275–82.

Antonelli JR, Hottel TL. Oral manifestations of renal osteodystrophy: case report and review of the literature. Spec Care Dentist 2003;23:28–34.

Arnaldi G, Angeli A, Atkinson AB, et al. Diagnosis and complications of Cushing's syndrome: a consensus statement. J Clin Endocrinol Metab 2003;88:5593–602.

Centers for Disease Control and Prevention. Prevalence of diabetes and impaired fasting glucose in adults-United States, 1999-2000. MMWR Morb Mortal Wkly Rep 2003;52:833–7.

Fox RI, Stern M, Michelson P. Update in Sjögren's syndrome. Curr Opin Rheumatol 2000;12:391–8.

Gomez-Perez FJ, Rull JA. Insulin therapy: current alternatives. Arch Med Res 2005;36:258–72.

Leroith D, Taylor SI, Olefsky JM. Diabetes mellitus: a fundamental and clinical text. 3rd ed. Philadelphia: Lippincott Williams & Wilkins; 2004.

Little JW. Thyroid disorders. Part I: hyperthyroidism. Oral Surg Oral Med Oral Pathol Oral Radiol Endod 2006;101:276–84.

Mandel L, Patel S. Sialadenosis associated with diabetes mellitus: a case report. J Oral Maxillofac Surg 2002;60:696–8.

Mandel SJ, Mandel L. Radioactive iodine and the salivary glands. Thyroid 2003;13:265–71.

Mealey BL, Oates TW. Diabetes mellitus and periodontal diseases. J Periodontol 2006;77:1289–303.

Melmed S, Casanueva F, Cavagnini F, et al. Consensus statement: medical management of acromegaly. Eur J Endocrinol 2005;153: 737–40.

Pinto A, Glick M. Management of patients with thyroid disease: oral health considerations. J Am Dent Assoc 2002;133:849–58.

Report of the Expert Committee on the Diagnosis and Classification of Diabetes Mellitus. Diabetes Care 2003;26 Suppl 1:S5–20.

Schlechte JA. Clinical practice. Prolactinoma. N Engl J Med 2003;349:2035–41.

Ship JA. Diabetes and oral health: an overview. J Am Dent Assoc 2003;134:4S–10S.

Singer I, Oster JR, Fishman LM. The management of diabetes insipidus in adults. Arch Intern Med 1997;157:1293–301.

Suresh L, Radfar L. Pregnancy and lactation. Oral Surg Oral Med Oral Pathol Oral Radiol Endod 2004;97:672–82.

Taylor GW. Periodontal treatment and its effects on glycemic control: a review of the evidence. Oral Surg Oral Med Oral Pathol Oral Radiol Endod 1999;87:311–6.

Uwaifo GI, Ratner RE. Novel pharmacologic agents for type 2 diabetes. Endocrinol Metab Clin North Am 2005;34:155–97.

For the full reference list, please refer to the accompanying CD ROM.

22

NEUROMUSCULAR DISEASES

ERIC T. STOOPLER, DMD
DAVID A. SIROIS, DMD, PhD

Diseases affecting the neuromuscular system have a collective lifetime prevalence rate of 3 to 5%. Thus, every oral health care provider will encounter a patient who has had, or presently has, a neuromuscular disease diagnosis. The signs and symptoms as well as the complications and implications of these disorders or their treatment can have significant impact on oral health as well as dental management decisions. This chapter focuses on the most common neuromuscular diseases, or those with greater impact on the orofacial region and/or dental treatment.

▼ CEREBROVASCULAR DISEASE

Epidemiology and Etiology

Cerebrovascular disease refers to disorders that result in damage to the cerebral blood vessels leading to impaired cerebral circulation. A cerebrovascular accident (CVA), or complete stroke, is a sudden impairment in cerebral circulation resulting in death or a focal neurologic deficit lasting more than 24 hours.[1,2] Neurologic events related to CVA include transient ischemic attack (TIA), defined as a reversible, acute, short-duration, focal neurologic deficit ("mini stroke") resulting from transient (reversible within 24 hours) and localized cerebral ischemia; reversible ischemic neurologic defect (RIND), defined as a reversible, acute, focal neurologic deficit due to transient and localized cerebral ischemia but resulting in neurologic deficits that last more than 24 hours; and stroke in evolution, defined as progressive worsening of stroke symptoms.[1–3]

CVAs are the third leading cause of death and leading neurologic cause of long-term disability in the United States and Europe, with over 750,000 strokes and more than 150,000 stroke-related deaths each year in the United States.[4–7] From 1950 to 2004, the age-adjusted incidence of first stroke per 1,000 person-years for all adults decreased from 7.6 to 5.3 in men and 6.2 to 5.1 in women. The overall lifetime risk at age 65 years decreased from 19.5% to 14.5% in men and from 18.0% to 16.1% in women. Risk for stroke increases with age, with a crude age-adjusted rate per 1,000 persons of 0.5 for ages 18 to 44 years, 2.5 for ages 45 to 64 years, 6.9 for ages 65 to 74 years, and 12.4 for ages 75 years and older.[4,6] The 30-day mortality rate following stroke over the past 50 years has decreased significantly in men from 23% to 14% but only from 21% to 20% in women.[4–6] As the population ages, it is expected that morbidity and mortality due to stroke will increase, with some estimates of doubling by 2020.[3,5,7]

Impaired cerebral blood flow leading to ischemia and energy failure is the common pathogenic mechanism for stroke. A 50% decrease in blood flow to the brain for as few as 3 to 4 minutes can result in irreversible brain injury. Following infarction, edema and excessive neurotoxic excitation contribute to further regional tissue injury and death. Approximately 15% of strokes result from hemorrhagic events leading to infarction, most often related to hypertension, trauma, substance abuse, or aneurysmal rupture.[1] Eighty-five percent of strokes result from ischemia due to atherosclerotic disease, thromboembolic events, and occlusion of cerebral blood vessels, with neurologic deficits related to the loss of neural function in tissues distal to the event.[1] Three major types of ischemic stroke syndromes have been described: small vessel (lacunar), large vessel (cerebral infarction), and brainstem stroke.

Lacunar strokes result from obstruction of the small (< 5 mm diameter) penetrating arterioles supplying the basal ganglia, anterior limb of the internal capsule, and (less commonly) deep cerebral white matter. Age and uncontrolled hypertension are the greatest predisposing factors. Symptoms usually include unilateral motor or sensory deficit without visual field changes or disturbances of consciousness or language. The prognosis for recovery from lacunar infarction is fair to good, with partial or complete resolution usually occurring over 4 to 6 weeks.

Cerebral (large vessel) infarction is characterized by extensive downstream ischemia, usually due to a thromboembolic event along the distribution of the internal carotid artery and cerebral arteries. Emboli often originate from the heart after acute myocardial infarction or in hyperdynamic conditions such as chronic atrial fibrillation. Hypertension is an important risk factor in the development of thrombosis, particularly at the carotid bifurcation, and treatment of severe hypertension is essential for the prevention of stroke. High-level brain functions are affected, and the prognosis is poor.

Brainstem infarction results from occlusion of small or large vessels supplying the brainstem, resulting in variable deficits ranging from motor and sensory deficits to death when respiratory centers are affected.

Clinical Manifestations

The clinical manifestations of stroke vary depending on the size and location of the affected brain region. The most common signs and symptoms include sensory and motor deficits, changes (paresis) in extraocular muscles and eye movements, visual defects, sudden headache, altered mental status, dizziness, nausea, seizures, impaired speech or hearing, and neurocognitive deficits such as impaired memory, reasoning, and concentration.[1,8]

Diagnosis

Stroke should be considered whenever a patient experiences the clinical manifestations described above. Other causes for these signs and symptoms, particularly when focal, may include seizures, hypoglycemia, intracranial tumors, trauma, infection, encephalitis, multiple sclerosis (MS), and prolonged migrainous aura.[8] In addition to a thorough neurologic and cardiovascular examination, anatomic and functional brain imaging is central to the diagnosis of stroke. Cerebral angiography and brain magnetic resonance imaging (MRI) (more accurate than computed tomography [CT]) are the most effective techniques for localizing the stroke site.[9–11] Laboratory evaluation of the stroke patient includes compete blood count, comprehensive metabolic panel, urinalysis, coagulation profile, and, when indicated, blood culture, echocardiography, and lumbar puncture.[8]

Treatment

The outcome of stroke and related TIAs and RIND is significantly affected by the timeliness of treatment. Early intervention is critical to prevention, treatment, and recovery. TIAs and RIND are treated by reduction in hypertension (lifestyle changes such as diet, exercise, smoking cessation, and stress reduction; medical therapy for hypertension; and anticoagulant or antiplatelet medications).[11,12] The reader is referred to the chapters in this textbook that describe more thoroughly anticoagulant and antihypertensive therapies.

Management of acute stroke includes medical therapy to reduce bleeding or thromboembolic occlusion, medical therapy to reduce brain edema and neurotoxicity/nerve injury, and surgical interventions (revascularization, hemorrhage control).[8,13] Thrombolysis with intravenous tissue plasminogen activator (t-PA) within 3 hours of a stroke can improve reperfusion,[14] although only a small percentage of acute stroke victims receive t-PA due to delays in detection, diagnosis, and arrival at a treatment facility. Extensive investigation continues to develop and test new neuroprotective drugs to minimize neurotoxicity, reduce edema, and correct ischemia, mostly among excitatory amino acid antagonists, free radical scavengers, and cytokine inhibitors.[14,15]

Oral Health Considerations

Following stroke, patients may experience several oral problems, including masticatory and facial muscle paralysis, impaired or lost touch and taste sensation, diminished protective gag reflex, and dysphagia. These problems can lead to impairment of food intake, poor nutrition, and weight loss due to diminished taste satisfaction, chewing capacity, and swallowing; choking; and gagging.[16–18] Diminished motor function of masticatory and facial muscles may also reduce food clearance from the mouth and teeth and alone or combined with the presence of diminished dexterity of the arms or hands may adversely affect oral hygiene and increase the risk for caries and periodontal disease.[18,19] Creative and effective use of adjuvant oral hygiene techniques and devices (oral antimicrobial rinse, oral irrigation, floss holders) represents an important approach to oral health promotion and disease prevention, supported by frequent recall examination and prophylaxis. Replacement of missing teeth and adequacy of removable and fixed prostheses are essential to effective chewing and diet. Finally, one provocative study recently reported improved oral function and stereognosis with the diligent use of a removable prosthesis among edentulous patients with stroke or Parkinson's disease.[20]

Dental management of the patient with a history of TIA, RIND, or stroke presents several challenges.[2,18] Stroke prevention through routine monitoring of blood pressure is an important step in hypertension risk detection and reduction through referral and effective management. Prior history of TIA or stroke increases the risk of a future or second stroke, with the highest risk during the first 90 days,[21,22] leading to the recommendation that elective dental treatment be deferred for 6 months following a stroke or for a patient with active TIAs or RIND.[18]

Use of antiplatelet and anticoagulant medications is common in patients with a history of stroke, TIA, and RIND. This includes oral aspirin, oral antiplatelet drugs such as ticlopidine and clopidogrel, subcutaneous low molecular weight heparin, and, less commonly, warfarin. These medications taken in therapeutic dosages, and for warfarin with an international normalized ratio (INR) ≤ 3.5, rarely require dose modification before routine dental and minor oral surgical treatment.[23–27] For additional information regarding management of patients taking antiplatelet and anticoagulant medications, the reader is referred to the chapter in this textbook that describes altered hemostasis more thoroughly. Concomitant use of nonsteroidal anti-inflammatory drugs (NSAIDs) may increase the risk for bleeding, and their long-term use may reduce the protective effect of aspirin. Potential drug interactions of note include but are not limited to use of metronidazole, erythromycin, and tetracycline, which may alter the bioavailability of warfarin.

Stress reduction and confidence building for the patient during dental visits are important behavioral goals to make the patient comfortable and minimize anxiety-related elevation in blood pressure. Pre- or perioperative inhalation N_2O-O_2 or oral anxiolytic medication can aid in reducing treatment-related stress and anxiety.

Use of epinephrine-containing local anesthetics is not strictly contraindicated, but they should be used minimally and generally follow guidelines recommended for patients with cardiovascular disease; epinephrine-containing impression cord should not be used.[18] Blood pressure should be monitored at every visit and within a visit if long and stressful.

▼ MULTIPLE SCLEROSIS

Epidemiology and Etiology

MS is characterized by multiple areas of central nervous system (CNS) white matter inflammation, demyelination, and gliosis (scarring).[28] Myelin is critical for propagation of nerve impulses, and when it is destroyed in MS, slowing and/or complete block of impulse propagation are manifested by abnormal muscular and neurologic signs and symptoms. In Western societies, MS is second only to trauma as a cause of neurologic disability in early to middle adulthood.[29] The clinical course of MS varies from a benign, asymptomatic disease to a rapidly progressive and debilitating disorder.

The age at onset is typically between 20 and 40 years; rarely does MS appear clinically before the age of 10 or after age 60.[28] MS is more common among women than men (2:1 ratio); however, in patients with later onset of MS, the sex ratio tends to be more even. The geographic distribution of MS is uneven; in general, the prevalence of MS increases with increasing distance from the equator.[29] When racial differences are correlated with prevalence rated for MS worldwide, white populations are at greatest risk and both black and Asian populations have a low risk of disease.[28]

Although the cause of MS is unknown, genetic susceptibility to MS clearly exists, and it is thought that an initial trigger leads to autoimmune mechanisms causing demyelination. The major histocompatibility complex (MHC) on chromosome 6p21 has been identified as one genetic determinant for MS.[30] The MHC encodes the genes for the human leukocyte antigen (HLA) system, and susceptibility to MS lies with the class II alleles, particularly the class II haplotypes DR15, DQ6, and Dw2.[28] Other genetic regions implicated in MS susceptibility are located on chromosomal regions 19q35 and 17q13.[29,30]

Substantial evidence suggests that autoimmune mechanisms are involved in the pathogenesis of MS.[31] Myelin basic protein (MBP) is an important T-cell antigen that is critical in the development of experimental allergic encephalomyelitis (EAE) in animals. Certain forms of EAE are pathologically similar to MS, and activated MBP-reactive T cells are often found in the blood or cerebrospinal fluid (CSF) of MS patients, supporting the autoimmune theory of MS pathogenesis.[29] Increased levels of immunoglobulin G (IgG) and cytokines such as tumor necrosis factor are commonly detected in the CSF of patients with MS.[32,33]

Epidemiologic evidence supports the role of an environmental exposure in MS, and the two most common infectious agents to be implicated in the pathogenesis of this disease are Epstein-Barr virus and human herpesvirus 6.[34] Other viruses that have been implicated in the pathogenesis of MS include measles, mumps, rubella, *Chlaymidia pneumoniae*, parainfluenza, vaccinia, and human T-lymphotropic virus 1.[28,34]

MS lesions or "plaques" vary in size and are characterized by perivenular cuffing with inflammatory mononuclear cells, predominantly macrophages and T cells, that is generally limited to the white matter and periventricular areas of the CNS.[35] Plaques may be found in both the brain and spinal cord, and within the plaques, there is variable destruction of myelin and neuronal axons with preservation of the ground structure.[28] Uniform areas of incomplete myelination are called shadow plaques and may be evident in chronic lesions of MS.[29]

The major clinical type of MS that affects nearly 85% of those suffering from the disease is termed relapsing/remitting multiple sclerosis (RRMS).[36] This is characterized by discrete attacks that generally evolve over days to weeks and often follows with complete recovery from symptoms. RRMS may evolve into secondary progressive multiple sclerosis (SPMS), which is characterized by a steady deterioration in function unassociated with acute attacks. Approximately 50% of patients with RRMS will develop SPMS after 15 years.[29] Other minor forms of MS include primary progressive multiple sclerosis (PPMS), in which patients display steady functional decline from disease onset without attacks, and progressive/relapsing multiple sclerosis (PRMS) that features clinical characteristics of both PPMS and SPMS.

Clinical Manifestations

The onset of MS may be insidious or abrupt, and symptoms range from trivial to severe. The clinical course of disease generally extends for decades, but a rare few cases are fatal within a few months of onset. The clinical manifestations of MS depend on the areas of the CNS involved, and frequently affected areas include the optic chiasm, brainstem, cerebellum, and spinal cord.[28,36] The sudden onset of optic neuritis (diminished visual acuity, dimness, or decreased color perception), without any other CNS signs or symptoms, is often considered the first symptom of MS. Other common visual signs in patients with MS include diplopia, blurring, nystagmus, gaze disturbances, and visual field defects.[36]

Limb weakness is characteristic of MS and can manifest as loss of strength or dexterity, fatigue, or gait disturbances.[37] Spasticity associated with painful muscle spasms is often observed in the legs of patients with MS and may interfere with a patient's ability to ambulate. Ataxia may affect the head and neck of MS patients and may result in cerebellar dysarthria (scanning speech). Bladder dysfunction and bowel dysfunction frequently coexist and are present in >90% of MS patients. MS patients often demonstrate sensory impairment, including paresthesia and hyperesthesia. Fatigue, depression, and cognitive dysfunction are often observed in patients with MS.[37]

Patients with MS often experience exacerbation of neurologic symptoms in response to an elevation of the body's core temperature. This is referred to as Uhthoff's symptom and is often seen in response to increased physical activity.[29] MS patients frequently complain of electric shock–like sensations that are evoked by neck flexion and radiate down the back and into the legs. This is referred to as Lhermitte's symptom and is generally self-limiting but may persist for years.[29]

Diagnosis

There is no definitive diagnostic test for detection of MS. Clinical criteria for MS include two or more episodes of symptoms and two or more signs of pathology affecting white matter tracts of the CNS. MRI demonstrates characteristic abnormalities of MS in >95% of patients.[29] MS plaques are visible as hyperintense focal areas on T_2-weighted images that are characteristic of chronic lesions. T_1-weighted images reveal hypointense areas that are usually indicative of active MS lesions.[29] Evoked potentials measure CNS electrical potentials, and abnormalities are detected in up to 90% of patients with MS. CSF is often analyzed in patients suspected of having MS, and positive findings include an increase in total protein and mononuclear white blood cells. In addition, there is often an increase in intrathecally synthesized IgG in patients with MS.[32]

Treatment

Therapy for MS can be divided into three categories: (1) treatment of acute attacks, (2) treatment that reduces the biologic activity of MS, and (3) symptomatic therapy.[29] Glucocorticoids are used to manage both initial attacks and acute exacerbations of MS. Intravenous methylprednisolone is administered at a dose between 500 and 1,000 mg/d for 3 to 5 days to reduce the severity and length of an attack.[36] Agents that reduce the biologic activity of MS include interferon (IFN)-β1a (Avonex, Rebif), IFN-β1b (Betaseron), and glatiramer acetate (Copaxone). All four pharmacologic agents slow progression of relapsing disease and reduce the annual relapse rate by 20 to 40%.[37] Mitoxantrone (Novantrone) is a chemotherapeutic agent administered intravenously that is effective in reducing neurologic disability and frequency of clinical relapses in patients with SPMS, PRMS, and worsening RRMS.[31] Common agents employed for management of MS symptoms include potassium channel blockers for weakness, lioresal for spasticity, propantheline for bladder dysfunction, and amantadine for fatigue.[29]

The prognosis for the individual patient with MS is variable. The majority of cases are chronic, and in patients with mild MS, little permanent effect is noted, and patients have a normal life span.[38] Most patients with MS experience progressive neurologic disability, and greater than 80% of patients with MS will require assistance with ambulation 25 years after onset of the disease. Mortality as a direct consequence of MS is uncommon, and death usually results from a complication of the disease, such as pneumonia.

Oral Health Considerations

Individuals may present to the oral health care provider with signs and symptoms of MS. Trigeminal neuralgia (TGN), which is characterized by electric shock–like pain, may be an initial manifestation of MS in 0.3% of cases.[38,39] MS-related TGN is similar to idiopathic TGN, and the reader is referred to the chapter in the textbook that describes idiopathic TGN more thoroughly. Features of MS-related TGN include possible absence of trigger zones and continuous pain with lower intensity.[38] Medications often used to manage TGN are similar to those used for treatment of idiopathic TGN, and the reader is referred to the chapter that describes these medications and alternative therapies.

Patients with MS may also demonstrate neuropathy of the maxillary (V2) and mandibular branches (V3) of the trigeminal nerve, which may include burning, tingling, and/or reduced sensation. Neuropathy of the mental nerve can cause numbness of the lower lip and chin.[38] Myokymia may be seen in patients with MS and consists of rapid, flickering contractions of the facial musculature secondary to MS lesions affecting the facial nerve.[40] Facial weakness and paralysis may also be evident in MS patients. Dysarthria that results in a scanning speech pattern is often seen in patients with MS. If MS is suspected, oral health care professionals should carefully evaluate cranial nerve function. If cranial nerve abnormalities are detected upon examination, the individual should be referred to a neurologist for further evaluation.

It is recommended to avoid elective dental treatment in MS patients during acute exacerbations of the disease due to limited mobility and possible airway compromise.[18,37,41] Clinicians must evaluate the level of motor dysfunction of patients with MS as this may affect provision of dental care. Patients with significant dysfunction may require dental treatment in an operating room under general anesthesia due to the inability to tolerate treatment in an outpatient setting. In addition, electric toothbrushes and oral hygiene products with larger handles may be necessary for completing oral hygiene in patients with significant motor impairment.

▼ ALZHEIMER'S DISEASE

Epidemiology and Etiology

Dementia is defined as an acquired deterioration in cognitive abilities that impairs the successful performance of activities of daily living.[42] Memory is the most common cognitive ability lost with dementia; other mental faculties affected include problem-solving skills, judgment, visuospatial ability, and language. Alzheimer's disease (AD) is the most common form of dementia in Western countries, accounting for 50 to 60% of new cases.[42,43] The clinical features of AD were first described in 1906 by Alois Alzheimer[44]; more than 100 years later, the molecular basis of AD has been greatly elucidated, and enhanced diagnostic modalities have enabled clinicians to visualize neurologic changes secondary to AD.

AD is characterized by neuritic plaques and neurofibrillary tangles coupled with a degeneration of neurons and synapses. The most severe pathology associated with AD is usually found in the medial temporal lobe structures and cortical areas of the brain.[43] Neuritic plaques contain a central core of amyloid β (Aβ) peptide derived from amyloid precursor protein (APP), a transmembrane protein that has neurotrophic and neuroprotective effects. An imbalance between the production and clearance of Aβ in the brain, termed the amyloid cascade hypothesis, is thought to be the disease-initiating event that ultimately leads to neuronal degeneration and

dementia.[43] Amyloid is deposited around meningeal and cerebral vessels, termed *amyloid angiopathy*, and may lead to cerebral lobar hemorrhages.

Neurofibrillary tangles are twisted neurofilaments in neuronal cytoplasm that represent abnormally phosphorylated tau protein and appear as paired helical filaments by electron microscopy.[42] Tau protein is thought to aid in assembly and stabilization of the microtubules that convey cell organelles and glycoproteins through the neuron. In AD, tau becomes hyperphosphorylated and leads to sequestration of normal tau and other microtubule-associated proteins, thus impairing axonal transport and normal neuronal function. In addition, tau becomes prone to aggregation into insoluble fibrils that develop into tangles, further compromising neuronal function.[43]

The genetic basis of AD has been studied extensively, and specific genetic mutations have been implicated in both the familial and sporadic forms of the disease. Familial AD is an autosomal dominant disorder with onset typically prior to age 65 years. Mutations in the *APP* gene on chromosome 21 were the first to be identified as the cause of familial AD; subsequent investigations have demonstrated mutations in the presenilin 1 and 2 genes (*PSEN1* and *PSEN2*, respectively) that account for the majority of familial AD cases.[45] The most commonly reported gene associated with sporadic AD is apolipoprotein E (*APOE*) on chromosome 19, which is involved in cholesterol transport.[42,43,45] The ε4 allele accounts for most of the genetic risk in sporadic AD.[43]

Clinical Manifestations

AD is a slowly progressive disorder, with the typical clinical course ranging from 8 to 10 years. The initial phase usually consists of mild cognitive impairment, specifically, the inability to remember newly acquired information. This may initially go unrecognized or be viewed as forgetfulness; however, as the disease progresses, memory loss begins to affect performance of daily activities, including following instructions, driving, and normal decision making. In the middle stages of AD, the individual is often unable to work, gets confused and lost easily, and may require daily supervision. Language impairment, loss of abstract reasoning skills, and visuospatial deficits begin to interfere with simple, routine tasks. Late-stage AD is characterized by loss of cognitive abilities, agitation, delusions, and psychotic behavior. Patients may develop muscle rigidity associated with gait disturbances and often wander aimlessly. In end-stage AD, patients often become rigid, mute, incontinent, and bedridden.[43] Help is needed for basic functions, such as eating and dressing, and patients may experience generalized seizure activity. Death often results from malnutrition, heart disease, pulmonary emboli, or secondary infections.[42]

Diagnosis

Diagnosis of AD is based on an individual's medical history together with the clinical and neurologic examination findings. Criteria for the clinical diagnosis of AD include a history of progressive deterioration in cognitive ability in the absence of other known neurologic or medical problems.[46] Definite AD is reserved only for autopsy-confirmed disease. If there is no associated illness, the condition is called probable AD; possible AD refers to those who meet the criteria for dementia but have another illness that may contribute to the neurologic status, such as hypothyroidism or cerebrovascular disease.[45]

Generally, there are no specific changes seen on routine laboratory examination of a patient with suspected AD. CSF may show a slight increase in tau protein and a lower concentration of Aβ peptide compared with healthy individuals or those with other dementias. Electroencephalographic (EEG) studies typically demonstrate generalized slowing without focal features. Neuroimaging is important in evaluating suspected AD to exclude alternative causes of dementia, such as cerebrovascular disease, subdural hematoma, or brain tumor. MRI and CT typically reveal dilatation of the lateral ventricles and widening of the cortical sulci, particularly in the temporal regions.[45] Volumetric MRI uniformly demonstrates shrinkage in vulnerable brain regions, especially the entorhinal cortex and hippocampus.[45] Positron emission tomography, using ^{18}F-fluorodeoxyglucose, can identify areas of hypometabolism in the temporal, parietal, and posterior cingulated cortices and has a high ability to differentiate AD from other dementias.[43] Slowly progressive decline in memory and orientation, normal results on laboratory tests, and neuroimaging showing only diffuse or posteriorly predominant cortical and hippocampal atrophy are highly suggestive of AD.[42]

Treatment

There is no cure for AD, and therapy is aimed at slowing the progression of the disease. Cholinesterase inhibitors are approved by the US Food and Drug Administration (FDA) to treat mild to moderate cases of AD and are considered the standard of care.[47] The four types of cholinesterase inhibitors currently available are tacrine, donepezil, rivastigmine, and galantamine; tacrine is now rarely used due to its hepatotoxic effects. These medications decrease the hydrolysis of acetylcholine released from the presynaptic neuron into the synaptic cleft by inhibiting acetylcholinesterase, resulting in stimulation of the cholinergic receptor.[45] Common side effects of these medications include nausea, vomiting, diarrhea, weight loss, bradycardia, and syncope.[47] Recently, memantine received FDA approval for treatment of moderate to severe AD. This agent is a noncompetitive N-methyl-D-aspartate (NMDA) receptor antagonist that is believed to protect neurons from glutamate-mediated excitotoxicity.[47] Most clinicians reserve this medication for patients with advancing disease who are not responding to cholinesterase inhibitors. Antidepressants, such as selective serotonin reuptake inhibitors (SSRIs), are commonly used to treat depression, which is often seen in the mild to moderate stages of AD.[43,48] Antipsychotic agents are used for those patients who display aggressive behavior and psychosis, especially in the later stages of the disease. Other agents that have been reported to be of clinical value in the treatment of AD include antioxidants, such as selegiline and α-tocopherol (vitamin E),

cholesterol-lowering drugs, anti-inflammatories, and herbal remedies.[43,47] Caregivers of patients with AD must be involved in the overall treatment as they are responsible for maintaining the patient's general health and ensuring a meaningful quality of life; it is often necessary to provide educational, emotional, and psychological support to these individuals as the task for caring for patients with AD can be extremely challenging.

Oral Health Considerations

Oral and dental health is a major issue in patients with AD because significant deterioration in oral health status is commonly observed with advancing disease.[49] Oral health care providers should be able to recognize symptoms of AD and refer patients for further medical evaluation, if necessary. Patients with AD can become frustrated and irritable when confronted with unfamiliar circumstances or with questions, instructions, or information that they do not understand.[49] The oral health care provider must approach AD patients with empathy and explain all procedures and instructions clearly. Patients with AD should be placed on an aggressive preventive dentistry program, including an oral examination, oral hygiene education, prosthesis adjustment, and a 3-month recall.[50] It is recommended to complete restoration of oral health care function in the earliest stages of AD because the patient's ability to cooperate diminishes as cognitive function declines.[49] Time-consuming and complex dental treatment should be avoided in persons with severe AD.[51]

Medications used to treat AD can cause a variety of orofacial reactions and potentially interact with drugs commonly used in dentistry. Cholinesterase inhibitors may cause sialorrhea, whereas antidepressants and antipsychotics are often associated with xerostomia. In addition, dysgeusia and stomatitis have been reported with use of antipsychotic agents.[49] Antimicrobials, such as clarithromycin, erythromycin, and ketoconazole, may significantly impair the metabolism of galantamine, resulting in central or peripheral cholinergic effects.[49] Anticholinesterases may increase the possibility of gastrointestinal irritation and bleeding when used concomitantly with NSAIDs.[49]

Mercury has been implicated as a causative agent for the development of AD.[52,53] Elevated levels of mercury have been detected in the brain regions of patients with AD, and this element has been described as a neurotoxin.[54] Dental amalgam contains significant amounts of mercury, and this restorative material has been suggested in the pathogenesis of various neurologic diseases, including AD.[55] Present data suggest that the presence of dental amalgam does not increase the risk of developing AD,[52,54–57] and further investigation is required to further clarify the relationship of mercury and AD.

▼ SEIZURE DISORDERS

Epidemiology and Etiology

A seizure is a paroxysmal event due to abnormal, excessive, hypersynchronous discharges from neuronal aggregates in the CNS.[58] The term *epilepsy* describes a condition in which a person has recurrent seizures due to a chronic, underlying process. The incidence of epilepsy in developed countries is approximately 50 per 100,000 people per year and is higher in infants and elderly people.[59]

The International League Against Epilepsy (ILAE) developed a classification system of the epilepsies and epileptic syndromes based on the clinical features of seizure activity and associated EEG changes.[60] A revised classification scheme proposed by the ILAE in 2001 has taken into consideration other factors in classifying epileptic syndromes, such as genetics, age at onset, and pathophysiologic mechanisms of disease.[61] Partial, generalized, and unclassified seizures are the three major categories of seizure activity used in clinical practice.

Partial seizures are those in which the seizure activity is restricted to focal areas of the cerebral cortex; clinical manifestations of these seizures depend on the site of origin. Partial seizures are characterized by two concurrent activities in an aggregate of neurons: high-frequency bursts of action potentials and hypersynchronization.[58] Generalized seizures arise from both cerebral hemispheres simultaneously and have distinctive clinical features that facilitate diagnosis.[58] The underlying pathophysiology of generalized seizures is attributed to abnormal neuronal excitability and is poorly understood. Absence seizures (petit mal) are a type of generalized seizure that is characterized by sudden, brief lapses of consciousness without loss of body tone and may be attributed to abnormal oscillatory rhythms generated during sleep by circuits connecting the thalamus and cortex.[58] Tonic-clonic (grand mal) seizures are generalized seizures that present with dramatic clinical features, most notably, tonic contracture and uncoordinated clonic muscular movements.[59] Other types of generalized seizures include atypical absence, atonic, and myoclonic seizures. Those seizures that cannot be classified as either partial or generalized are termed unclassified seizures; the most common type of unclassified seizures is neonatal seizure activity.

Onset of seizure activity may occur at any point throughout an individual's life, and etiology usually varies according to patient age. The most common seizures arising in late infancy and early childhood are febrile seizures without evidence of associated CNS infection; these usually occur between 3 months and 5 years of age and have a peak incidence between 18 and 24 months.[58,62] Isolated, nonrecurrent, generalized seizures among adults are caused by multiple etiologies, including metabolic disturbances, toxins, drug effects, hypotension, hypoglycemia, hyponatremia, uremia, hepatic encephalopathy, drug overdoses, and drug withdrawal.[59,63] Cerebrovascular disease may account for approximately 50% of new cases of epilepsy in patients older than 65.[64] Other etiologies for epilepsy include degenerative CNS disease, developmental disabilities, and familial/genetic factors.[59,64]

Clinical Manifestations

PARTIAL SEIZURES

Simple partial seizures reflect neuronal discharge from a clinically recognizable cortical locus not associated with impaired consciousness, such as the motor cortex of the frontal lobe. Simple partial seizures consist of clonic activity, which are rapid jerks that also can be accompanied by somatosensory phenomena, visual changes/distortions, and auditory, olfactory, and gustatory symptoms.[58] These seizures can spread over a progressively larger region of the motor cortex, resulting in Jacksonian march, a phenomenon characterized by sequential involvement of the muscles in an extremity.

Complex partial seizures result in either a loss or impairment of consciousness. Many of these seizure foci originate within the temporal and inferior frontal lobes, causing patients to appear confused and to experience visual or auditory hallucinations. The seizures frequently begin with an aura (a warning of impending seizure activity) that may consist of a sense of fear, detachment, and/or intense odors/sounds. The patient displays automatisms during the seizure, which are involuntary automatic behaviors that vary from chewing and lip smacking to violent behavior.[65]

GENERALIZED SEIZURES

Absence seizures are characterized by seconds of unconsciousness with no loss of body tone.[66] In addition, subtle facial twitching and rapid eye blinking are often observed without generalized clinical muscular activity. Patients suffering from absence seizures appear to be "daydreaming," although they often have the ability to continue performing a previously started motor or intellectual activity after cessation of the seizure activity. There is generally no postictal confusion in patients experiencing absence seizures.

Tonic-clonic seizures characteristically begin abruptly and may or may not be preceded by an aura. The patient loses consciousness, while the entire musculature contracts forcibly, lasting between 20 and 40 seconds.[66] Contraction of the muscles of the larynx and forced expiration can produce a loud moan, often termed "epileptic cry." Patients often become cyanotic during the tonic phase secondary to forceful closing of the mouth accompanied with forced continued expiration. The clonic phase follows with the entire body rhythmically jerking for a period that usually lasts no longer than 1 minute. In the postictal phase, the patient may be unresponsive for minutes to hours, awakening gradually, often with no memory of the event.[66] Physical injury from falling or muscular convulsions and evidence of bladder emptying, tongue biting, or aspiration pneumonia are often experienced during the postictal phase.[67] Patients gradually regain consciousness and often complain of fatigue and headache after a tonic-clonic seizure. Generalized tonic-clonic seizures may not abate spontaneously or may recur without the patient regaining consciousness. This condition is referred to as generalized convulsive status epilepticus and is considered a medical emergency due to the number of serious sequelae of this condition, including bodily injury, cardiorespiratory dysfunction, metabolic derangements, and irreversible neurologic damage.[68]

Photosensitivity epilepsy is characterized by seizure activity induced by visual stimuli, such as stroboscope illumination, flickering sunlight, and high-contrast black and white patterns.[69] Photosensitive epilepsy has been shown to induce generalized tonic-clonic, partial, myoclonic, and atypical absence seizures.[69]

Diagnosis

The goals of evaluating a patient with new onset of seizure activity are threefold: (1) to establish whether the reported episode was a true seizure, (2) to determine the cause of the seizure by identifying possible risk factors and precipitating events, and (3) to determine the need for anticonvulsant therapy in addition to treatment of any underlying illness.[58] An in-depth history and physical examination are critical as the diagnosis of a seizure may be based on clinical findings only. A complete neurologic examination is required for all patients with suspected seizure activity, including testing of cranial nerve function, assessment of mental status, and testing of motor function. Blood studies, such as a complete blood count, electrolytes, glucose, magnesium, and calcium, are performed routinely to identify metabolic causes of seizure activity. Other useful screening tests include toxin screens to identify seizure activity due to drugs and lumbar puncture to rule out any infectious etiologies.

All patients with a possible seizure disorder are referred for brain imaging to determine underlying CNS structural abnormality and/or pathology. MRI is the diagnostic modality of choice for the detection of hippocampal sclerosis, malformations of cortical development, vascular malformations, tumors, and acquired cortical damage, all of which are common etiologies for seizure disorders.[70] Newer MRI methods, such as fluid-attenuated inversion recovery (FLAIR), have increased the sensitivity for detection of abnormalities of cortical architecture. CT is valuable for investigating intracranial calcification, skull fractures, and suspected CNS infection, which may not be as readily apparent on an MRI.[70]

An EEG is mandatory for patients with suspected seizures and is critical for classifying seizure disorders as well as helping to determine the type of anticonvulsant medication, if indicated.[63] The EEG measures the electrical activity of the brain, and the presence of abnormal, repetitive, rhythmic electrical activity having an abrupt onset and termination during the clinical event establishes the diagnosis of seizures.[58]

Treatment

For patients with recurrent seizures without identifiable causative pathology, pharmacologic therapy is initiated. The goal of pharmacologic therapy is to choose a medication that is most appropriate for the specific type of seizure activity and to administer it in the proper dose to achieve control of seizure activity with minimal side effects.[62]

Lamotrigine, carbamazepine, or phenytoin is currently the initial drug of choice for the treatment of partial seizures, including those that secondarily generalize.[59] Phenytoin has a long half-life and is dosed less frequently than carbamazepine and lamotrigine, leading to increased patient compliance. Phenytoin is associated with gingival overgrowth, hirsutism, and coarsening of facial features. Carbamazepine can cause hepatotoxicity, leukopenia, and aplastic anemia, whereas

lamotrigine has been associated with skin rash. Additional add-on therapies for patients with partial seizures include topiramate, gabapentin, and oxcarbazepine.

Currently, the best initial choice for treatment of generalized tonic-clonic seizures is valproic acid.[59] Valproic acid may cause bone marrow suppression and hepatotoxicity, requires laboratory monitoring, and should be avoided in patients with preexisting bone marrow or liver disease. Lamotrigine, carbamazepine, and phenytoin are suitable alternative treatments for generalized tonic-clonic seizures. Ethosuximide has been shown to be particularly effective for the treatment of uncomplicated absence seizures.

Discontinuation of pharmacologic therapy is considered when seizure control has been achieved. The following patient characteristics yield the greatest chance of remaining seizure free after discontinuation of drug therapy: (1) complete medical control of seizures for 1 to 5 years; (2) single seizure type; (3) normal neurologic examination, including intelligence; and (4) a normal EEG.[58] Many patients are often withdrawn successfully from medication after an interval of at least 2 years without seizures who meet the above criteria and who clearly understand the risks and benefits.

In patients with refractory epilepsy, it often becomes necessary to use a combination of antiepileptic medications to attempt seizure control. Patients may use three or more drugs to successfully treat refractory epilepsy; however, up to 20% of patients are resistant to all medical therapies. Surgical procedures may be indicated for these patients, including limited removal of the hippocampus and amygdala, temporal lobectomy, or hemisperectomy.[58] Those patients who are not candidates for resective brain surgery may benefit from vagus nerve stimulation, which involves placement of an electrode on the left vagus nerve that receives intermittent electrical pulses from an implanted generator. Stimulation of vagal nuclei has been shown to lead to widespread activation of cortical and subcortical pathways and an associated increased seizure threshold.[71]

Oral Health Considerations

Patients with seizure disorders are routinely treated in the outpatient dental setting. A complete evaluation of a patient's seizure disorder is necessary prior to initiation of any dental treatment to determine the stability of the condition and an appropriate venue for treatment. Important features for the clinician to assess include the type of seizures, etiology of seizures, frequency of seizures, known triggers of seizure activity, presence of aura prior to seizure activity, and history of injuries related to seizure activity. If a patient demonstrates signs of poorly or uncontrolled seizure disorder, consultation with the patient's physician and/or neurologist is recommended. Patients with poorly or uncontrolled seizure disorder may not be suited for private dental offices and should be referred to a hospital setting for routine dental care. Patients with implanted vagus nerve stimulators do not require antibiotic prophylaxis prior to invasive dental procedures.[72]

While providing dental care, it is prudent to avoid any known triggers of the patient's seizure activity. Patients with poorly controlled seizures often present with signs of intraoral trauma, such as fractured teeth and/or soft tissue lacerations.[72] Patients with poorly controlled disease or stress-induced seizures may require sedative medications prior to treatment; this should be determined in consultation with the patient's physician.[72] To minimize the risk of injury and aspiration during dental treatment, use of dental floss–secured mouth props (which are easily retrievable) and a rubber dam is recommended. Placement of metal fixed prostheses is recommended rather than removable prostheses to decrease the risk of displacement and aspiration risk during seizure activity.[38]

Anticonvulsant medications can induce significant blood dyscrasias that can affect provision of dental care. Phenytoin, carbamazepine, and valproic acid can cause bone marrow suppression, leukopenia, thrombocytopenia, and secondary platelet dysfunction, resulting in an increased incidence of microbial infection, delayed healing, and both gingival and postoperative bleeding.[73] Patients taking these medications may require laboratory evaluation prior to dental treatment, including a complete blood count with differential to assess white blood cell and platelet counts and coagulation studies to assess clotting ability. Patients on long-term carbamazepine should have serum blood levels evaluated prior to initiating dental treatment as insufficient doses may result in inadequate seizure control and excessive doses have been associated with hepatotoxicity.[73] Aspirin and nonsteroidal anti-inflammatory medications should be avoided for postoperative pain control in patients taking valproic acid as they can enhance the possibility of increased bleeding.[73] There are no contraindications to local anesthetics, when used in proper amounts, in patients with seizure disorders.[74]

Gingival overgrowth is a significant oral complication among seizure disorder patients taking anticonvulsant medications, most notably phenytoin.[74] The prevalence rate of gingival overgrowth varies and has been reported in up to 50% of individuals taking phenytoin.[75] The anterior labial surfaces of the maxillary and mandibular gingivae are most commonly affected and may be seen within 2 to 18 months after starting the medication. Historically, this condition has been attributed to an increased number of fibroblasts in gingival connective tissue.[38] Recent studies have shown that phenytoin alters molecular signaling pathways that control collagen degradation by gingival fibroblasts and accumulation of collagen leads to clinically evident gingival overgrowth.[75,76] Inflammation can exacerbate this condition; therefore, frequent professional cleanings and use of an electric toothbrush are recommended to maintain optimal oral hygiene. Some clinicians advocate the use of chlorhexidine and/or folic acid rinses to minimize gingival inflammation among seizure disorder patients with gingival overgrowth.[77] Surgical reduction of gingival tissue may be necessary if significant overgrowth exists. In addition to gingival overgrowth, other oral side effects of phenytoin include development of intraoral lesions that clinically resemble lupus lesions and lip enlargement.[72,78]

Xerostomia may result from the use of antiseizure medications, and oral health care providers may observe increased dental caries and oral candidiasis in patients using these agents. Topical fluoride should be considered for patients with seizure disorders who are at increased risk of developing dental caries, and antifungal agents should be prescribed if oral candidiasis develops.

▼ PARKINSON'S DISEASE

Epidemiology and Etiology

Parkinson's disease (PD) is a chronic, progressive, neurodegenerative disorder characterized by resting tremor, cogwheel rigidity (feeling of periodic resistance to passive movement owing to co-contraction of agonist and antagonist muscle pairs), and bradykinesia (slow intentional movements). Secondary symptoms include change in speech, difficulty in swallowing, pain, confusion, depression, fatigue, and constipation; postural instability develops in later stages of the illness. PD has an estimated prevalence of 31 to 328 per 100,000 persons worldwide and afflicts more than 1% of the population over age 65 and more than 1 million adults in the United States.[80] Prevalence and incidence increase with age.[79] There may be a small increased risk for PD among men compared with women, and all races and ethnic groups are affected equally. The risk for PD increases with age, and mortality among elderly PD patients is two to five times that of age-matched controls. The public health burden for PD is significant and growing as the population ages, with an annual estimated cost of 26 billion dollars in the United States.[80]

PD results from idiopathic degeneration of the dopaminergic cells in the pars compacta of the substantia nigra, leading to depletion of the neurotransmitter dopamine in the basal ganglia (caudate nucleus and putamen). The relative contributions of genetic versus environmental factors regarding the cause of PD have been hotly debated. Most agree that the pathogenesis is multifactorial, with environmental factors acting on genetically susceptible individuals.[81–83] The discovery in a small number of patients of genetic forms of PD demonstrated conclusively that PD can occur through inheritance, and several genes have been found to be associated with inherited PD: α-synuclein, parkin, pink1, and UCH-L1[84–86]; clinical genetic testing is now available for the parkin and pink1 genes. Environmental toxins, particularly pesticides, likely play an important role in the risk for PD, and the protoxin n-methyl-4-phenyl-1,2,3,6-tetrahydropyridine (MPTP) has been shown to cause parkinsonism in both humans and nonhumans.[87]

Clinical Manifestations

The four cardinal signs of PD are resting tremor (in hands, arms, legs, jaw, and face); rigidity or stiffness (limbs and trunk), bradykinesia (slowness of movement), and postural instability or impaired balance and coordination. Secondary symptoms include change in speech, difficulty in swallowing, pain, confusion, depression, fatigue, and constipation. As symptoms become more pronounced, patients may have difficulty in walking, talking, or completing other simple tasks. PD usually affects people over the age of 50, although it can occur at any age, and earlier cases occur more commonly in the familial forms of PD. Early manifestations of PD are subtle and insidious, although for some, the disease progresses more quickly.

Diagnosis

There are currently no laboratory tests with specificity for PD.[79] Clinical genetic markers are available for risk assessment where hereditary patterns of PD exist. Therefore, the diagnosis is usually based on the health history and a neurologic examination; when symptoms are subtle and the presentation is incomplete, the diagnosis can be difficult. Anatomic and functional brain imaging, CSF evaluation, and laboratory testing are often necessary to exclude other diagnoses.

Treatment

At present, there is no cure for PD, but a variety of medications and procedures provide dramatic relief from the symptoms. The most common pharmacologic treatment is dopamine replacement therapy using levodopa (used by neurons to synthesize dopamine) combined with carbidopa (delays the conversion of levodopa into dopamine until it reaches the brain). Levodopa initially helps about 75% of patients, but not all symptoms respond equally to the drug; bradykinesia and rigidity respond best, whereas tremor may be only marginally reduced and impaired balance and other symptoms may not be alleviated at all. Additionally, levodopa often has the unwanted side effect of increasing dyskinesias. Anticholinergics such as scopolamine may help control tremor and rigidity. Dopamine agonists such as bromocriptine, pergolide, pramipexole, and ropinirole, alone or in combination with levodopa, may control PD symptoms and improve daily functioning better than treatment with levodopa alone.[79] Several studies of neuroprotective agents such as selegiline and vitamins E and C have not shown any consistent benefit.

Surgical management of PD is more often selected in younger patients with advanced PD or intolerable medication side effects. Surgical procedures to reduce symptoms include pallidotomy, thalamotomy, and deep brain stimulation of the substantia nigra and basal ganglia. Embryonic stem cell research to provide transplantation, implantation, and gene therapy is an area of active investigation.

Oral Health Considerations

Patients with PD present several challenges to the dental health care team and to the patient related to both the illness and its treatment.[18] Patients with PD often must be treated in a relatively upright position, making complex dental procedures in the maxillary arch or posterior oral cavity a challenge. Resting tremors and drug-related dyskinesia can complicate procedures, and behavioral techniques to reduce anxiety as well as gentle cradling techniques can help. Dysphagia and impaired gag reflex increase the risk for aspiration of oral and irrigation fluids, and high-speed evacuation of fluids is important in reducing the risk for aspiration pneumonia. Some patients experience sialorrhea, making maintenance of a dry field difficult for some operative and surgical procedures.

Pharmacologic treatment for PD has implications of importance to dentistry. Levodopa and dopamine agonists can lead to both orthostatic hypertension and, rarely, severe hypertension; other side effects of particular importance to the dental team include oromandibular and facial dyskinesia, xerostomia, arrhythmia, and blood dyscrasias. Careful consideration and management include monitoring of blood pressure; correct positioning and repositioning during and after treatment; xerostomia and caries risk reduction through hygiene, sealants and fluorides when indicated; impact of oromandibular dyskinesia on the design of dental prostheses; and periodic evaluation of the complete blood count to detect drug-related hematologic adverse effects.

▼ MYASTHENIA GRAVIS

Epidemiology and Etiology

Myasthenia gravis (MG) is a chronic neuromuscular disease caused by autoimmune destruction of the acetylcholine receptor (AChR), disrupting cholinergic neuromuscular neurotransmission. The illness is characterized by weakness of the skeletal muscles that increases during periods of activity and improves after periods of rest. Extraocular muscles and diplopia; eyelid drooping; and weakness in the muscles of facial expression, masticatory muscles, and muscles used for swallowing and speech are the most common initial signs; limb weakness affects only 10% of patients, and respiratory muscles can be affected and present a significant risk. The estimated prevalence rate for MG is 15 to 20 cases per 100,000 population, with an estimated 60,000 affected patients in the United States.[88] However, the rate of MG diagnoses has increased every year for the past 50 years and probably remains underdiagnosed and underreported.[88–90] Historical accounts of the age at onset and sex distribution reported that women are more commonly affected than men, with an onset in the second and third decades. However, more recent data reveal that the most common age at onset is the second and third decades in women and the seventh and eighth decades in men, and as the population ages, males are more often affected than females, and the onset of symptoms is usually after age 50.

Ten percent of patients with MG have a thymic tumor and 70% have hyperplastic changes that indicate an active immune response. Removal of the tumor can improve symptoms dramatically. However, it is still unclear whether the role of the thymus in the pathogenesis of MG is causal or secondary.

Clinical Manifestations

Two-thirds of patients with MG present with a complaint of specific muscle weakness in the eyes (with associated diplopia) and/or drooping eyelids. Oropharyngeal muscle weakness, difficulty in chewing, swallowing, or talking, is the initial symptom in one-sixth of patients and limb weakness in only 10%. The severity of weakness fluctuates during the day, usually best in the morning and worse as the day progresses. The clinical course of disease is variable but usually progressive.[90] Many patients will experience weakness restricted to the ocular muscles, and about half of patients experience progressive weakness during the first 2 years that involves oropharyngeal and limb muscles. Spontaneous improvement frequently occurs early in the illness. After 10 to 15 years of fluctuating disease activity, weakness often becomes more fixed and associated with muscle disuse atrophy. Factors that worsen MG symptoms include stress, systemic illness (especially viral respiratory infections), hypothyroidism or hyperthyroidism, pregnancy, and menses.

Diagnosis

The clinical examination and history are highly suggestive of MG. A diagnosis is confirmed by serologic evidence of auto-antibodies to the AChR, although there are reports of MG without anti-AChR.[91,92] CT or MRI of the chest is highly accurate in detecting thymoma, and every patient with MG should be screened for thymoma. Although less commonly used today, a Tensilon (edrophonium) challenge test can be useful in assessing MG and in distinguishing myasthenic crisis from cholinergic crisis. A positive response is not specific for MG.

Treatment

Anticholinesterase drugs such as neostigmine and pyridostigmine bromide increase acetylcholine availability and receptor binding and provide symptomatic benefit without influencing the course of the disease. Patients with thymus tumors may have dramatic improvement following thymectomy. Patients with more severe symptoms or poor response to treatment have treatment directed at reducing autoantibody production using corticosteroids (oral or intravenous pulse therapy), plasmapheresis to remove autoantibodies, and high-dose intravenous immunoglobulin.[93,94]

Oral Health Considerations

Orofacial signs and symptoms are an important presenting feature of MG, and the dental provider may be in the position to recognize and refer for diagnosis. Difficulty with prolonged opening and swallowing presents challenges in dental treatment delivery and the ability to tolerate treatment, and difficulty in chewing can affect diet and the design of prostheses. Aspiration risks can be high and can be reduced by adequate suction and the use of a rubber dam. The MG patient may also be at risk for a respiratory crisis from the disease itself or from overmedication; if this is a substantial risk and the dental treatment is necessary, dental treatment in a hospital should be considered where endotracheal intubation can be performed. Avoid prescribing drugs that may affect the neuromuscular junction, such as narcotics, tranquilizers, and barbiturates. Certain antibiotics, including tetracycline, streptomycin, sulfonamides, and clindamycin, can affect neuromuscular activity and should be avoided or used with caution.

▼ SELECTED READINGS

Blennow K, de Leon MJ, Zetterberg H. Alzheimer's disease. Lancet 2006;368:387–403.

Carandang R, Seshadri S, Beiser A, et al. Trends in incidence, lifetime risk, severity, and 30-day mortality of stroke over the past 50 years. JAMA 2006;296:2939–46.

Collins NS, Shapiro RA, Ramsay RE. Elders with epilepsy. Med Clin North Am 2006;90:945–66.

Duncan JS, Sander JW, Sisodiya SM, Walker MC. Adult epilepsy. Lancet 2006;367:1087–1100.

Fatahzadeh M, Glick M. Stroke: epidemiology, classification, risk factors, complications, diagnosis, prevention, and medical and dental management. Oral Surg Oral Med Oral Pathol Oral Radiol Endod 2006;102:180–91.

Fox RJ, Bethoux F, Goldman MD, Cohen JA. Multiple sclerosis: advances in understanding, diagnosing, and treating the underlying disease. Cleve Clin J Med 2006;73:91–102.

Goldman MD, Cohen JA, Fox RJ, Bethoux FA. Multiple sclerosis: treating symptoms and other general medical issues. Cleve Clin J Med 2006;73:177–186.

Levine CB, Fahrbach KR, Siderowf AD, et al. Diagnosis and Treatment of Parkinson's Disease: A Systematic Review of the Literature. Evidence Report/Technology Assessment Number 57. (Prepared by Metaworks, Inc., under Contract No. 290-97-0016.) AHRQ Publication No. 03-E040. Rockville, MD: Agency for Healthcare Research and Quality. June 2003.

Little JW. Dental management of patients with Alzheimer's disease. Gen Dent 2005;53:289–96.

Palace J, Vincent A, Beeson D. Myasthenia gravis: diagnostic and management dilemmas. Curr Opin Neurol 2001;14:583–9.

Phillips LH II. The epidemiology of myasthenia gravis. Ann N Y Acad Sci 2003;998:407–12.

Saperstein DS, Barohn RJ. Management of myasthenia gravis. Semin Neurol 2004;24:41–8.

Straus SE, Majumdar SR, McAlister FA. New evidence for stroke prevention: scientific review. JAMA 2002;288:1388–95.

Vincent A, Palace J, Hilton-Jones D. Myasthenia gravis. Lancet 2001;357:2122–8.

Williams AC, Smith ML, Waring RH, Ramsden DB. Idiopathic Parkinson's disease: a genetic and environmental model. Adv Neurol 1999;80:215–8.

For the full reference list, please refer to the accompanying CD ROM.

23

Basic Principles of Human Genetics: A Primer for Oral Medicine

Harold C. Slavkin, DDS

Mahvash Navazesh, DMD

Pragna Patel, PhD

Humans have known for several thousand years that heredity affects health. However, it was only 150 years ago when Gregor Mendel first described the mechanism by which genotype results in phenotype. It was less than 100 years ago when Garrod began to apply genetic knowledge to human diseases and disorders. Ironically, for most of the twentieth century, clinicians viewed genetics as a somewhat esoteric academic specialty until rather recently with the completion of the Human Genome Project in October 2004.[1–3]

Despite enormous public interest in "genomics" and the thousands of articles published about the completion of the human genome, neither medicine nor dentistry would abruptly change or transform. Medicine and dentistry have not been "gene free" for the last 100 years. Increasingly, a growing and evolving body of knowledge and information has significantly expanded how we think about and how we use human genetics in medicine and dentistry to address epidemiology, public health and risk assessment, single and multiple predictive and prognostic gene-based diagnostics, and pharmacogenomics and pharmacogenetics with customized drug selection specific for individualized metabolism. We are experiencing an expanding knowledge base for Mendelian inheritance, complex human diseases (multifactorial diseases and disorders), and bioinformatics.[4–12]

This chapter is a primer for the emerging field of human genetics with oral medicine. The authors and readers acknowledge that the pace of transformation for oral medicine and clinical dentistry in general is limited not only by the pace of scientific discovery but also by the need to educate practicing dentists and allied health professions and our patients about the uses and shortcomings of human genetic knowledge and information. Human genetic variation is associated with many, if not all, human diseases and disabilities, including the common chronic diseases of major public health impact. Genetic variation interacts with environment and sociocultural influences to modify the risk of disease.

As we look into the future, we must anticipate the logical advances of human and microbial genetics. This extraordinary progress is already shaping how we consider the etiology and progression of diseases and disorders, how we reach diagnostically useful information, and even how we select therapeutics for particular patients and communities. In tandem, these advances will also become integrated into the continuum of dental and medical education—predoctoral, doctoral, postdoctoral, residency, and lifelong continuing professional education.

▼ BASIC HUMAN GENETIC PRINCIPLES

The general principles of genetics have been appreciated since the dawn of agriculture some 10,000 years ago when ancient farmers engaged in domestication of plants and animals. The British biologist William Bateson gave the science of inheritance a name—genetics—as recently as 1909. More recently, the use of cytogenetic techniques heralded the technology that enabled cells, intracellular organelles, and chromosomes to be visualized using light microscopy with specific histopathology stains. Karyotyping enabled visualization of the number and fidelity of human chromosomes, and this enabled better diagnostics for chromosomal disorders such as trisomy 21 or Down syndrome.

In the early 1950s, James Watson and Francis Crick discovered the molecular structure of deoxyribonucleic acid (DNA).[4] Thereafter, it became increasingly evident that DNA was arranged in a double-helical structure as an exceedingly long chain of only four units called nucleotides or bases (adenosine, A; thymidine, T; cytosine, C; and guanosine, G). Three of these nucleotides form codons (eg, UUA for leucine; U (uracil) substitutes for T, thymidine, in ribonucleic acids [RNAs]) and thereby represent the information or code for the ordering of amino acids into forming polypeptides; the so-called *genetic code* was established.

During the last three decades of the twentieth century, the fundamental science of DNA accelerated and applications of human genetics rapidly advanced so that a "genetic paradigm" for human diseases and disorders was embraced to a limited extent in many US medical and dental schools.[5–12] Terms such as *susceptibility* versus *resistance* were readily incorporated into the language of health professionals engaged in patient care. Simultaneously, there was also a major acceleration in the study of genes, proteins, and their functions during the human lifespan.[1–12]

The Human Genome Project was initiated in 1988 and was completed as of October 2004.[1,2,8] Exhaustive analyses of the enormous database (the "instruction book" of life) representing the Human Genome Project revealed that humans contain 20,000 to 25,000 genes within the nucleus of each somatic cell and another 9 genes that are encoded within mitochondria found in all human cells. Genes are discrete units of information encoded within DNA, which, in turn, is localized within chromosomes found in the nucleus of each somatic cell or within mitochondria dispersed through the cytoplasm of all cells. Each cell contains 3.2×10^9 nucleotide pairs per haploid genome in the nucleus and 16,569 nucleotide pairs in each mitochrondrion.[1–3,8]

Even before a gene's function in disease is fully understood and treatment is available, diagnostic applications can be useful in minimizing or preventing the development of health consequences. The discovery of mutations in the *BRCA1* gene associated with early breast cancer is such an example.[7] The DNA tests used for the presence of disease-linked mutations are proving to be very useful for clinicians. Such tests can assist in the correct diagnosis of a genetic disease, foreshadow the development of disease later in life, or identify healthy heterozygote carriers of recessive diseases. Testing for genetic diseases can be performed at any stage in the human life span.

Importantly, the Mendelian rules that govern the inheritance of many human traits are useful for rare human diseases with highly penetrant changes in a single gene. What is much more difficult is to tease out of the human genome are the multiple genes that are functionally related to complex human diseases such as diabetes, heart disease, oral cancer, periodontal disease, most cleft lip and palate patients, autoimmune disorders (eg, Sjögren's syndrome), and psychiatric conditions. The challenge is to find multiple, low-penetrance variants, which in the aggregate account for the vast majority of chronic diseases and disorders. This requires new strategies of conceptualizing multifactorial diseases.

There are 46 chromosomes found in every nucleus of every diploid somatic cell in the human body. These chromosomes contain approximately 6 feet in length of the double-stranded DNA and associated proteins (histones and nonhistone chromosomal proteins). These chromosomal proteins insulate and regulate genes and gene expression during the human life span. Specifically, methylation, acetylation, and deacetylation of these proteins are significant post-translational mechanisms that regulate gene functions.

Of the 46 chromosomes that contain DNA, 44 are termed autosomes that exist in homologous pairs (numbered 1 to 22, with 1 being the largest and the remaining chromosome pairs numbered in descending order of size) and the remaining 2 chromosomes (designated X and Y) are termed sex chromosomes. In addition, the maternally inherited mitochondria also contain mitochondrial deoxyribonucleic acid (mtDNA), as mentioned.

In either case, whether it is chromosomes in the nucleus of every somatic cell or mtDNA localized within mitochondria, DNA is a polymer macromolecule that is composed of recurring monomeric units called *nucleotides* or *bases*. There are 3.2 billion nucleotides in the haploid genome.[1,2,8] Each monomer or base has three components: (1) a phosphate group linked to (2) a five-carbon atom cyclic sugar group, which, in turn, is joined to (3) a *purine* or *pyrimidine* nucleotide or base. The four nucleotides are the purines adenosine (A) and guanosine (G) and the pyrimidines thymidine (T) and cytosine (C). Permutations and combinations of the four nucleotides constitute the DNA sequence within which the genetic code is embedded. Permutations and combinations of A, C, T, and G result in a DNA sequence, and this sequence becomes highly informative within regulatory or structural regions of human genes. Interestingly, only 1 to 2% of the entire human genome encodes 20,000 to 25,000 genes, with the vast majority being apparently noninformative expanses of nucleotides that include repetitive DNA sequences, pseudogenes, and additional DNA whose function is yet unknown.

The analysis of x-ray diffraction patterns of purified DNA led James Watson and Francis Crick, based on earlier data from Rosalind Franklin on adenoviral DNA, to build three-dimensional models of DNA that represented a right-handed double helix.[4] They showed that the best fit of the data would be two antiparallel chains in a structure that resembles a spiral staircase. Further, they asserted that within these two strands of DNA, A binds to T and C to G—so-called base pairing or hybridization. These rules apply to DNA found within all living organisms, such as microbes (virus, bacteria, and yeast), plants, animals, and people. Watson and Crick conclude:

> "It has not escaped our notice that the specific pairing we have postulated immediately suggests a possible copying mechanism for the genetic material.[4]"

Genes contain the information for proteins. Genes represent hereditary blueprints. All hereditary information is transmitted from parent to offspring through the inheritance of genes, which are identified as the nucleotide sequences within DNA that produce a functional protein product. The largest genetic variance has been determined to be 0.1% between any two people on Earth (or 3 million nucleotides of 3.2 billion found in the haploid human genome), or, from a different perspective, any two humans show 99.9% genetic identity or homology.[1,2]

Genetic variation has phenotypic relevance when considering the impact of this variation on the protein sequence encoded. When comparing protein sequences (of two functionally related proteins or those from two different species), the term *homology* implies that the corresponding amino acid residues in homologous proteins are also homologous. They are derived from the same ancestral residue and, typically, inherit the same function. If the residue in question is the same in a set of homologous sequences, it is assumed that it is evolutionarily conserved. Importantly, protein structure is conserved during evolution much better than protein sequence. For example, lysozyme, the enzyme that hydrolyzes bacterial cell walls, shows little sequence similarity across

species but readily adopts similar protein structures, contains identical or related amino acid residues in the bioactive site of the enzyme, and retains a similar catalytic mechanism.[13] Such shared features support the concept that despite low sequence similarities, such proteins are homologous.

With the completion of the Human Genome Project in October 2004,[1,2] numerous other species were also sequenced with subsequent sequence analysis, comparisons, and interpretations related to structure, function, and evolutionary conservation.[14] For example, vertebrates such as chimpanzee,[14] rat,[15] mouse,[16] chicken,[17] and dog[18] were completed, as were invertebrates such as microbes,[19] malarial parasites,[20] *Anopheles* mosquito,[21] roundworm,[22] fruit fly,[23] and mustard plant.[24] Genomic comparisons between human and fruit fly sequences demonstrated that 60% of the human disease genes are conserved between fruit flies and humans.[25] Curiously, two-thirds of the human genes known to be involved in cancers have counterparts in the fruit fly. It would seem counterintuitive that the fruit fly animal organism offers unique opportunities to explore the onset and progression of many human diseases and disorders such as early-onset Parkinson's disease.[26,27]

It is now accepted that profound similarities or homology exists among genomes of the earth's organisms—microbes (virus, bacteria, yeast), plants, animals, and humans—and that genomes can differ by variations in nucleotide sequences and through duplications or deletions of DNA, through combinations that rearrange the order of genes, and/or by insertions of DNA that may be derived from microbes.[28–37] In humans, the process of sexual reproduction generates new combinations of genes across multiple generations, constituting the fundamental process of evolution.

Surveys of the human genetic code reveal approximately 2 to 3 million variations of nucleotides encoded within the DNA found in human chromosomes—about 0.1% variation between two people. Millions of single nucleotide polymorphisms (SNPs) have been well characterized and enable scientific assessment of extremely small variations between people in health and in disease.[38,39] SNPs and haploid maps enable genetic linkage with specific diseases and disorders. These human genetic variants are closely linked with many diseases and disorders, a person's susceptibility or resistance to disease, and individual responses to therapeutics.[38–40] For example, nucleotide variants within genes encoding opioids and opioid receptors can explain why people differ in their responses to pain or pain stimuli.

Briefly, genes function through a complex series of processes. First, encoding sequences of DNA are *transcribed* to messenger ribonucleic acids (mRNAs). These are, in turn, *translated* into proteins. Another class of RNAs termed transfer or tRNAs are guided and instructed by DNA-derived specific mRNAs to assemble amino acids into the correct sequence to produce the functional protein on the ribosomes located in the cytoplasm of cells.

A generic gene (sequence of nucleotides A, C, T, and/or G) begins with a "start sequence" in which the mRNA transcription begins. The region before or "upstream" from this site or location contains the "switches" that turn on the gene and also constitute the gene's promoter *sequence.* Further upstream in a region, typically 2,000 nucleotides in length, there are additional control elements that regulate the rates, amplitudes, or quantity of transcription. These elements can be enhancers or repressors that respond to DNA-binding proteins, hormones, certain types of vitamins such as retinoic acid, or growth factors. The body of the gene contains discrete coding sequences that give rise to a protein product; these are called *exons.* These are separated by noncoding sequences termed *introns.* Genes terminate with a "stop sequence." DNA can be transcribed into RNAs (mRNA) by RNA polymerase II enzyme or can be replicated by DNA polymerase enzyme into copy strands of DNA (as required in mitosis or cell division). These two major processes, *transcription of DNA* into mRNA or *replication of one strand of DNA to a copy strand of DNA*, are enormously important for biologic activities (Figure 1).

A process termed *alternative splicing* can modify or alter significantly the gene sequence that is transcribed into mRNAs by producing splices and rearrangements between exons that result in as many as 8 to 10 different isoforms or variants of the gene. Alternative splicing is a regulatory mechanism by which variations in the incorporation of exons encoded within DNA into mRNAs during transcription can produce different isoforms of the same protein. About 15% of human genetic diseases appear to be caused by point mutations at or near splice junctions located within or between introns and exons that control the fidelity of alternative splicing.

Nucleic acid sequences that encode genes within DNA represent *structural proteins* (eg, genetically different types of collagens, multiple genes for keratins, globins, amelogenins, enamelins, metalloproteinases, albumins, dentin sialoglycoproteins, dentin phosphoproteins) or *regulatory proteins* (eg, transcriptional factors, signal transduction–related proteins, growth factors).

How Genes Function

How is the information encoded in DNA—sequences of nucleotides—converted into a protein with bioactivity? The process begins with several events: (1) combinations of multiple transcription factors bind to one another (ie, protein-protein binding) and through binding to DNA (ie, protein-DNA binding); (2) methylation of cytosine within nucleic acid sequences is highly informative for transcription; and (3) an enzyme, RNA polymerase II, attaches to a specific sequence within DNA and is then followed by the transcription process (DNA to mRNA), followed eventually by translation (mRNA to protein amino acid sequence) on ribosomes physically located within the cytoplasm of cells.

Transcription defines the process by which genes encoded within the DNA template are copied into mRNAs that, in turn, leave the nucleus and migrate into the cytoplasm. The number and variation of transcripts from a single discrete gene are created by alternative splicing. In addition, genes

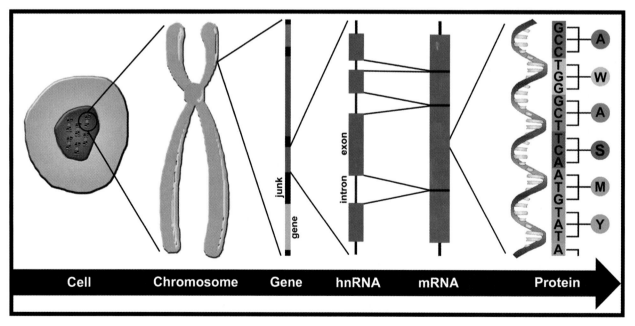

FIGURE 1   From gene to protein. Chromosomes are found in the nucleus of the cell. Comprised of DNA, these chromosomes contain thousands of genes (colored blocks) which are separated by non-coding, or "junk", DNA (black blocks). Each gene is comprised of both exons (coding DNA; red) and introns (non-coding DNA; blue) which are copied, or transcribed (expressed), for the purposes of constructing the protein it codes for, or encodes. There is an intermediary stage between the gene and the protein, where a temporary copy of the gene blueprint is produced as a heterogeneous ribonucleic acid molecule, or hnRNA. The hnRNA consists of both the exons, which are pieced together to form the messenger RNA, or mRNA, and the introns, which are discarded. The mRNA is used as the template for the synthesis of the protein from amino acid building blocks. For this, the DNA is read in three letter blocks, called codons, each of which signifies a single amino acid (colored circles).

that encode ribosomal RNA and tRNA are transcribed and also migrate to the cytoplasm, where they participate in the process of protein synthesis.

For example, tooth formation is a complex developmental process that results from a sequence of epithelial-mesenchymal interactions.[40–45] Mutations in one or more transcription factors (eg, *MSX1, MSX2, DLX5, PAX9*) may inhibit, arrest, or retard tooth development, and these are clinically diagnosed as tooth agenesis (oligodontia or hypodontia).[45–49] Mutations in regulatory genes such as growth factors and their cognate receptors related to signal transduction and/or transcription factors cause a wide variety of abnormalities in tooth number, position, and shape.[45–49]

Translation is the process that defines mRNA being translated into a precise sequence of amino acids termed *polypeptide* or *protein*. Genetic information is stored as the *genetic code*. Each member of the genetic code consists of three bases or nucleotides that represent a *codon* designating a specific amino acid. The three nucleotides within the codon are determined from four possibilities (A, C, T, and G). Therefore, there are 4^3 or 64 different codons, and all but three specify an amino acid. The functional codons designate 20 different amino acids. Since the alternative splicing of the human 20,000 to 25,000 genes is common, the proteome that reflects the human genome is measured in many thousands of different proteins beyond the size of the number of genes in the genome.

For example, dentin formation during tooth development represents secretory odontoblasts engaged in the synthesis, translation, and post-translation (eg, glycosylation, phosphorylation) of a number of structural proteins that form the extracellular matrix and control the process of tissue-specific biomineralization. Odontoblasts synthesize and secrete type I collagen and a number of noncollagenous and highly specialized glycoproteins and phosphoproteins. These extracellular matrix structural proteins control the size, shape, and structure of the minerals that engage in biomineralization. The dentin sialophosphoprotein gene (*DSPP*) is located on chromosome 4 (4q21.3) and encodes two different noncollagenous proteins: (1) dentin sialoprotein and (2) dentin phosphoprotein.[50,51] Mutations in type I collagen and/or *DSPP* produce five different patterns of inherited dentin defects termed *dentinogenesis imperfecta* types.[50,51]

Regulation of Gene Expression

The central problem in human genetics is the temporal and spatial expression of the 20,000 to 25,000 genes—the organization of the two-dimensional DNA encoded genetic information into the dynamic three-dimensional morphogenesis and development, cell determination, cell fate, and cytodifferentiation (ie, growth, development, maturation, senescence). It is unknown if there are "master regulatory genes" that control the geometry of body forms.

The most significant level for control is at the level of mRNA production termed *transcriptional control*. Transcriptional control is performed by proteins that bind to DNA, either by modifying cytosine methylation or by *transcription*

factors binding to a specific sequence or motif within DNA. A complex of multiple transcription factors often binds to the *TATA box* (a sequence of 8 to 10 T and A bases) physically located upstream to the formal start sequence of the gene. Other regulatory units encoded within the nucleic acid sequence include the *CAAT box* (a sequence of C, A, and T) and the *GC box* (GGGCGG). Promoters define when and where genes will be expressed, and enhancers define the levels of expression (ie, copies of mRNA per unit time per cell). In addition to these molecular tools for regulation, steroids, lipophilic vitamins, and trace elements also function to control protein-protein and protein–nucleic acid interactions.[6,7]

A number of morphoregulatory or master genes have been identified that are highly conserved from fish to humans. These genes encode highly conserved transcription factors such as *HOX* genes, *PAX* genes, and *T-Box* genes.[41–43] Each of these three types of gene clusters encodes master control genes that regulate the body plan for invertebrates and all vertebrates, including humans.[40–43] Further, each of these three types of transcription factors is transcribed and translated into DNA-binding proteins with high affinities for specific nucleic acid sequence motifs.

For example, two of the morphoregulatory genes are the *FOXC1* and the *PITX2* homeobox genes (Figure 2). Mutations in either of these contribute to Axenfeld-Rieger syndrome (ARS), an autosomal dominant developmental disorder that represents a spectrum that involves anomalies of the anterior segment of the eyes, iris hypoplasia, tooth anomalies, craniofacial dysmorphogenesis, cardiac defects, limb anomalies, pituitary anomalies, mental defects, and neurosensory defects.[52] Mutations in the *PITX2* gene or the *FOXC* gene have been identified in 40% of ARS.[52]

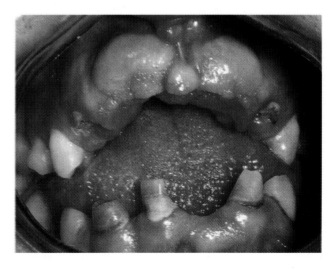

FIGURE 2 Mutations in PITX2 (pituitary homeobox transcription factor 2) and/or FOXC1 (forkhead box transcription factor C1) results in Axenfeld-Rieger Syndrome (ARS) which represents a spectrum of diseases and disorders including those of the dentition (i.e. extreme dental hypoplasia as shown in this figure.) Courtesy of Dr. Carl Allen.

Epigenetic controls, molecular controls that are not intrinsic to the nucleic acid sequence within DNA, provide the multiple gene-gene and gene-environment regulatory influences of the human condition. During embryogenesis, fetal development, infancy, childhood, adolescence, and thereafter, multiple combinations of genes are transcribed and translated into protein products that inform, regulate, and build the human organism.[40–43]

Cell Division

The cell cycle is the process by which the somatic cell divides to form two daughter cells. This process maintains the 46 chromosomes. A complete cell cycle consists of four phases: G_1, S, G_2, and M (mitosis). Progression through these phases is energy dependent and requires phosphorylation and dephosphorylation steps mediated by kinase enzymes. Gene products called cyclins regulate each of these four phases by specific interactions with kinase-phosphatases. Loss of cell-cycle controls is the signature for carcinogenesis and many birth defects. One of the major conceptual advances in the last decade is the recognition that cancer is largely a genetic disease and that neoplastic cells display a diverse array of genetic rearrangements, point mutations, and gene amplifications.

▼ MUTATION AND GENETIC HETEROGENEITY

Mutation is defined broadly as any change in the sequence of nucleic acids within DNA. Mutations or *misspellings* can be silent without clinical symptoms or can be profound, such as a single point mutation in a single nucleotide within one of the codons found in one of the exons for the globin gene that can result in sickle cell anemia. In humans, the mutation rate ranges from 1 to 10 million per gene per cell cycle. Importantly, mutations can be fundamental drivers for evolution as organisms adapt to various environs, or they can become clinically relevant as they delete, inhibit, or truncate specific gene expression during human development from conception through senescence.

Mutations can cause disease by a variety of means. The most common is *loss of function mutations*, resulting in a decrease in the quantity or function of a protein. Other mutations cause disease through *gain of function mutations*, such as the dominantly inherited Huntington's disease.

Single-Gene Mutations

Point mutations affect only one nucleotide with the substitution of one for another (Figure 3) (eg. GAG is codon for glutamic acid in the sixth exon of the β-hemoglobin gene; a point mutation or substitution of the *A* for a *T* in the codon changes meaning to valine and results in sickle cell anemia). *Missense mutation* describes a point mutation that results in the change of a codon, resulting in a change in the primary structure of the protein product resulting from translation.

This is clinically observed in select examples of hemoglobinopathies such as sickle cell anemia (globin), craniosynostosis (eg, fibroblast growth factor receptor), osteogenesis imperfecta (collagen), and amelogenesis imperfecta (AI; amelogenin). *A silent mutation* is a point mutation that has no effect on transcription or translation.

Mutations that abolish protein expression or function are termed *null alleles*. Mechanisms that produce null alleles include mutations that interfere with transcription in general, termination of transcripts, or mutations within splice sites related to alternative splicing. Human carriers of a null allele are often asymptomatic or can have clinical phenotypes if and when the mutations directly inhibit structural protein structure and function.

Chromosomal Mutations

Mutations that involve large alterations in chromosome structure are readily visible microscopically by karyotypic analysis. These macromolecular mutations include deletions, duplications, inversions, and translocations from one chromosome to another. These chromosomal mutations affect large numbers of genes encoded in specific regions of DNA.

▼ GENETIC DISEASES AND DISORDERS

Approximately 2 to 3% of all newborns are born with a serious congenital anomaly, and an additional 2 to 3% of infants and children are found to have birth defects by the age of 5 years. Genetics plays a role in 40 to 50% of childhood deaths, 5 to 10% of common cancers, and > 50% of the older population's medical problems. About 4% of human genes contribute to disease in a major way. Of the over 5,000 genetic syndromes known, over 700 have dental-oral-craniofacial defects and over 250 have associated clefting.[40–45,50–60] Facial clefting is a clinical phenotype associated with Mendelian gene inheritance (single-gene mutation), and facial clefting is also presented in complex human diseases that are polygenic, involving multiple genes and multiple environmental factors.[61,62] Mutations in many different classes of genes cause craniofacial-dental-oral defects, and these genes include those encoding transcription factors, hormone receptors, cell adhesion molecules, growth factors and their receptors, G proteins, enzymes, transporters, and collagens.[40–45,50–62]

Genetic disorders are broadly categorized as (1) single-gene or Mendelian disorders that are typically rare and familial (eg. hemophilia); (2) chromosomal anomalies that are typically sporadic (eg. Down syndrome); (3) multifactorial disorders or complex human diseases in which multiple genes are involved with a role played by environmental factors (eg. many congenital craniofacial malformations, arthritis, hypertension, many cancers, diabetes, osteoporosis, temporomandibular disorders); and (4) acquired somatic genetic disease (eg. many cancers) (Tables 1 and 2).

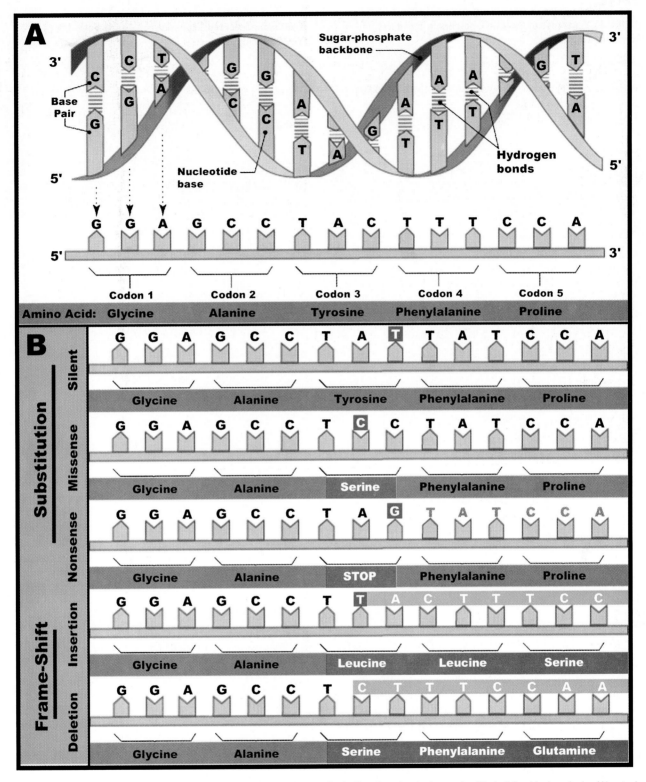

FIGURE 3 (*A*) The structure of deoxyribonucleic acid (DNA), which is comprised of just four chemical, or nucleotide, building blocks; adenine (A), cytosine (C), guanine (G) and thymine (T). Adenine always associates with thymine whilst guanine always associates with cytosine. To form individual genes, these nucleotide bases are placed in a unique order, or sequence, upon a poly-sugar backbone that determines their unique characteristics. This is sectioned into triplet nucleotide groups, called codons, which code for the different amino acids. (*B*) The five major types of mutation. Silent mutations cause no change in the encoded amino acid sequence due to redundancy in the codons. Missense mutations lead to a single change in the encoded amino acid sequence. Nonsense mutations result in the formation of one of the three translation stop codons (TAA, TAG and TGA) that result in truncation of the encoded amino acid sequence. Frame-shift mutations (insertions or deletions) result in a change in the encoded amino acid sequences from the point of the mutation as they shift the nucleotide positions in each triplet codon such that they form different codons. Mutated nucleotides are highlighted in red, affected nucleotides are highlighted in yellow and affected amino acids are highlighted in pink.

TABLE 1 Examples of Genetic Disorders in Newborn Screening Programs

Genetic Disorder	Screening Method	Treatment
Phenylketonuria	Guthrie bacterial inhibition assay Fluorescence assay Amino acid analyzer Tandem mass spectrometry	Diet restricting phenyl alanine
Congenital hypothyroidism	Measurement of thyroxine and thyrotropin	Oral levothyroxine
Hemoglobinopathies	Hemoglobin electrophoresis Isoelectric focusing High-performance liquid chromatography Follow-up DNA analysis	Prophylactic antibiotics immunization against *Diplococcus pneumoniae* and *Haemophilus influenzae*
Galactosemia	Beutler test Paigen test	Galactose-free diet
Maple syrup urine disease	Guthrie bacterial inhibition assay	Diet restricting intake of branched-chain amino acids
Homocystinuria	Guthrie bacterial inhibition assay	Vitamin B_{12} Diet restricting methionine and supplementing cystine
Biotinidase deficiency	Colorimetric assay	Oral biotin
Congenital adrenal hyperplasia	Radioimmunoassay Enzyme immunoassay	Glucocorticoids Mineralocorticoids Salt
Cystic fibrosis	Immunoreactive trypsinogen assay followed by DNA testing Sweat chloride test	Improved nutrition Management of pulmonary symptoms

All of these genetic screening tests for newborn infants are well established. Tests are offered throughout the United Sates. The other tests are available in a limited number of states.

TABLE 2 Selected Examples of Genetic Tests for Neurological, Connective Tissue, Cancer, and Renal Diseases*

Condition	Genes	Testing Utility
Neurologic		
Spinocerebellar ataxias	SCAI, SCA2, SCA3, SCA6, SCA7, SCAI0, DRPLA	Diagnostic, predictive
Early-onset familial Alzheimer's disease	PSENI, PSEN2	Diagnostic, predictive
Canavan's disease	ASPA	Diagnostic, prenatal
Nonsyndromic inherited congenital hearing loss (without other medical complications)	GJB2	Diagnostic, prenatal
Fragile X syndrome	FMRI	Diagnostic, prenatal
Huntington's disease	HD	Diagnostic, predictive, prenatal
Neurofibromatosis type 1	NFI	Prenatal
Neurofibromatosis type 2	NF2	Predictive, prenatal
Connective tissue		
Ehlers-Danlos syndrome, vascular type	COL3AI	Diagnostic, prenatal
Marfan's syndrome	FBNI	Diagnostic, prenatal
Osteogenesis imperfecta types I–IV	COLIAI, COLIA2	Diagnostic, prenatal
Oncologic		
Familial adenomatous polyposis	APC	Diagnostic, predictive
Hereditary nonpolyposis colorectal cancer	MLHI, MSH2, PMS2, MSH3, MSH6	Diagnostic, predictive
von Hippel-Lindau disease	VHL	Diagnostic, predictive
Li-Fraumeni syndrome	TP53	Diagnostic, predictive
Hematologic		
β-Thalassemia	β-Hemoglobin (HbB)	Carrier detection, prenatal diagnosis
Hemophilia A	F8C	Prognostic, carrier detection, prenatal
Hemophilia B	F9C	Carrier detection, prenatal
Renal		
Nephrogenic diabetes insipidus	AVPR2, AQP2	Diagnostic, carrier detection, prenatal
Polycystic kidney disease (autosomal dominant and autosomal recessive)	PKDI, PKD2, PKHD I	Predictive, prenatal

* This table is intended to be illustrative, not exhaustive. Most entries are based on information from GeneTests-GeneClinics at <http://www.geneclinics.org>. This Web site includes a comprehensive list of available molecular genetic tests and further clinical information about these and other genetic conditions.

Mendelian Diseases and Disorders

The **O**nline **M**endelian **I**nheritance of **M**an (OMIM) catalogues approximately 11,000 monogenic or Mendelian traits. These inherited human diseases, typically caused by a mutation in a single gene, can be transmitted within families in a dominant or recessive mode. A dominant disease results if one copy of the two copies of a given gene bears a deleterious mutation. Examples of dominant diseases include achondroplasia (or short-limb dwarfism), myotonic dystrophy, and neurofibromatosis. Certain forms of hypodontia involving molar or premolar teeth also display autosomal dominant inheritance.[45–49] Even though one copy of the gene is normal, the abnormal copy of the gene is able to override it, causing disease. Dominant diseases can be traced through family pedigrees and appear to spread vertically because everyone carrying a dominant mutant allele (form of the gene) generally shows the disease symptoms. Individuals with disease are present in successive generations. There are an equal number of males and females with disease, and each affected individual has only one parent with disease. Individuals mating with an unaffected individual rarely have an affected offspring. Over 200 autosomal dominant diseases are known and can manifest in any organ system and occur at different frequencies.

A disease displays a recessive inheritance pattern when two abnormal copies of the gene are present for the individual to be affected. Over 900 autosomal recessive diseases that manifest in a wide range of organs are known. Examples of recessive diseases include phenylketonuria, cystic fibrosis, Tay-Sachs disease, and Gaucher's disease. Recessive diseases that are rare are seen more often in communities in which consanguineous marriages are quite common since there is a high probability of mating between two carriers of the mutant gene. Parents of the affected individual show no symptoms even though they carry one mutant copy of the gene. If both parents are carriers of the gene, the child has a 1 in 4 chance of receiving a recessive allele from each parent and inheriting the disease. The distinctive features of an autosomal recessive disease are unaffected parents having affected offspring, equal numbers of affected males and females, all offspring being affected when both parents are affected, and, frequently, the presence of consangunity or origin of the population from a small group of founders.

Common population traits can be recessive, such as the blood group O; it may be brought into a pedigree by two parents independently and may appear dominant, but it is really pseudodominant and is a recessive trait. Therefore, it occurs in successive generations. Many dominant diseases may appear to skip a generation owing to a phenomenon referred to as nonpenetrance. Thus, even though a dominant disease should be apparent in all gene carriers, this is true only when the disease is 100% penetrant. The molecular basis of incomplete penetrance is unclear but is likely due to the effect of modifier genes that have an impact on the disease-causing mutation. Many psychiatric diseases, such as schizophrenia and bipolar mental disease, show incomplete penetrance owing to the effect of environmental factors and modifier genes. Late-onset diseases such as spinocerebellar ataxias demonstrate an age-related penetrance, with gene carriers being symptom free until midlife. This is the result of

slow cell death—the inability to restore the normal cellular state on environmental damage or accumulation of a toxic product over time. In contrast to penetrance, which refers to the all-or-one state with respect to disease phenotype, variable expressivity is the variable expression of the disease phenotype within the same family. Many dominant diseases (eg, Charcot-Marie-Tooth disease, neurofibromatosis) display variable expressivity, and the phenomenon is attributed to the effect of modifier genes since each member of the family who carries the same disease mutation can have a unique complement of genes other than those related to the disease that do interact with the disease gene.

Clinicians know that a major feature of gingivitis and periodontitis is the destruction of the collagenous matrix of the connective tissues by microbe-derived and/or host enzymes. Proteolytic cathepsins B, D, and L are biomarkers for the progression of disease.[63] What was quite surprising to many clinicians was the discovery that cathepsin C mutations appear to cause Papillon-Lefèvre syndrome.[64]

Sex-linked or X-linked diseases arise when there is a mutation in 1 of more than 285 genes that are located on the X chromosome. In X-linked dominant disease, both males and females are affected, although the females are usually less severely affected. This is because females have two X chromosomes, and during development, one of the two X chromosomes is selected at random and inactivated to allow X-chromosome gene dosage between males and females to be balanced. Thus, in some cells of the body, the X chromosome carrying the disease allele is inactivated, and in others, the "normal" X chromosome is inactivated. An example of an X-linked dominant disease is anhidrotic ectodermal dysplasia characterized by the absence of sweat glands, abnormal teeth, and sparse hair.[40] X-linked dominant inheritance can manifest in either sex, with more affected females than males. Females are more mildly affected than males. All female children of an affected male are affected, and all children of an affected female have a 50% chance of being affected. Most importantly, there is no male-to-male transmission of the disease since males receive their only X chromosome from their mother.

In X-linked recessive inheritance, only males are affected. Females are typically carriers with no symptoms or very mild symptoms. Affected males are usually born to unaffected parents, and the mother is normally an asymptomatic carrier. There is no male-to-male transmission of the disease. Occasionally, females may be affected if by misfortune most cells in a critical tissue have inactivated the normal X (referred to as nonrandom X-inactivation). Examples of such diseases are Duchenne muscular dystrophy and fragile X syndrome.

One example of a clinical phenotype that appears to be caused by either X-linked or autosomal inherited mutations is AI. There are three types of this genetic disorder: (1) type 1, hypoplastic AI; (2) type 2, hypocalcified AI; and (3) type 3, hypomaturation AI.[53–60] The prevalence of these disorders ranges from 1 in 700 people in northern Sweden to 1 in 14,000

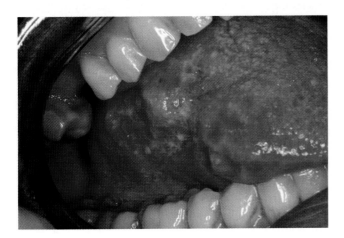

FIGURE 4 Multiple mutations in multiple genes, genes often associated with cell cycle regulation during mitosis and/or tumor suppressor genes, are implicated in squamous cell carcinoma as presented in numerous head and neck cancers (i.e. advanced oral cancer as shown in this figure.) Courtesy Dr. Parish Sedghizadeh.

people in the United States. Mutations in three structural genes cause AI: (1) the *AMELX* gene (amelogenin), the most prevalent protein in forming enamel extracellular matrix with genes located on both the X and Y chromosomes[60]; (2) the *ENAM* gene (enamelin) located on chromosome 4 (4q11-q21) and the second most prevalent protein in the forming enamel matrix; and (3) the *MMP20* gene (metalloprotease enzyme), which provides time- and position-specific protein degradation related to calcium hydroxyapatite crystal formations.[57–60] *ENAM* and *MMP20* mutations, often generated by splice-site mutations related to alternative splicing during transcription, show an autosomal recessive pattern of inheritance, with two copies of the gene in each ameloblast cell being altered. *AMELX* mutations are inherited as X-linked (represent 5% of all AI); in most cases, males with X-linked AI are more severely affected than affected females.

Y-linked inheritance implies that only males are affected. An affected male transmits his Y-linked trait to all of his sons but none of his daughters. Deletions of genes on the Y chromosome have been linked to infertility owing to azoospermia (or absence of sperm in semen) in males.

Chromosomal Diseases and Disorders

Chromosomal disorders are categorized into three general areas. The first is incorrect chromosomal number such as trisomy 21 (Down syndrome) of chromosome 21; this type is termed *aneuploidy*. Trisomies of chromosomes 13 and 18 are additional examples. Turner's syndrome occurs in women who acquire only one X chromosome. Klinefelter's syndrome occurs in men who receive two X chromosomes in addition to one Y chromosome. The second type is large chromosomal structural defects, including microdeletions. DiGeorge syndrome is characterized by T-cell immunodeficiency and cardiac anomalies and is caused by a microdeletion of chromosome 22. The third type of anomaly is uniparental disomy, which refers to the presence of two copies of a chromosome (or part of a chromosome) from one parent and none from the other parent. One example of an adverse outcome of a uniparental disomy is the consequence of genetic imprinting. This term is used to describe when a genetic trait is inherited only when transmitted by the mother in some diseases, such as in Beckwith-Wiedmann syndrome, or the father in others, such as glomus tumors. Genetic imprinting can be described as "parent of origin differences" in the expression of inherited genetic traits. Other examples of such genetic imprinting are presented with Prader-Willi and Angelman's syndromes, caused by a deficiency of paternal and maternal contributions, respectively, to a segment of the long arm of chromosome 15.

Mitochondrial Diseases and Disorders

Mitochondria are exclusively inherited from the mother since only maternal mitochondria are transmitted to the forming zygote in early embryogenesis. mtDNA is a small circular piece of DNA consisting of 16,569 nucleotides that encodes nine genes. Each mitochondrion normally contains multiple copies of mtDNA, whose total amount per cell is typically in the range of 40 to 2,000 copies. Most of these genes encode information for oxidative phosphorylation and energy production for the individual somatic cell type. Mitochondria contain a small fraction of the genes required for mitochondrial functions. Therefore, the remainder of genes are those found within the nucleus. Curiously, several codons are used for mtDNA differently from codons used for nuclear DNA.

Mitochondrial diseases frequently affect organs that are dependent on relatively high levels of energy, such as the nervous system, muscle, and beta cells in the pancreas. Each somatic cell contains different mixtures of mutant or partially deleted mitochondria that exist along with normal mitochondria. This interesting condition is known as heteroplasmy. The hallmark of mitochondrial inheritance, aside from maternal origin, is a broad spectrum of symptoms within a family segregating the same mitochondrial mutation, extreme variability in severity, and delayed onset with age. Examples of mitochondrial genetic diseases include mitochondrial encephalomyopathy or myoclonic epilepsy with ragged red muscle fibers, Leber's hereditary optic neuropathy with bilateral loss of central vision, and Kearns-Sayre syndrome, which presents retinal disease and cardiac disease (Tables 3 and 4).

Complex Human Diseases and Disorders

Complex human diseases or *multifactorial genetic disorders* are the most common forms of human genetic disease; they do not present a well-delineated Mendelian pattern of inheritance but "tend to run in families." These disorders include many types of craniofacial malformations, tooth decay, periodontal disease, atherosclerosis, cardiovascular disease, osteoporosis, autoimmune disorders, hypertension, emphysema, diabetes, peptic ulcers, numerous mental diseases, and numerous birth defects, such as clefting, spina bifida, limb deformities, and congenital heart disease (Figure 4).[7,12] These conditions are caused by multiple genes with environmental factors and appear to cluster in families over multiple generations. Further, these examples are more prevalent in females versus males or males versus females, depending on the specific disease or disorder. For example, autoimmune diseases (eg, Sjögren's syndrome, lupus) are more prevalent in females. These and other areas of interest have led to the emerging field of "gender biology" and "gender medicine."

This section of this chapter focuses on selected examples of complex human diseases and disorders that demonstrate multigene and multigene-environment interactions and that are of importance to oral health care providers in the everyday practice of dentistry.

MULTIFACTORIAL DISEASES AND DISORDERS

The etiology, pathogenesis, manifestations, management, and treatment outcomes of *complex human diseases* or *multifactorial genetic disorders* represent a dynamic interplay between regulatory and structural genes and environmental and behavioral factors. The results from international, multicenter studies of cleft lip and/or palate suggest that many genes (eg, *MSX1*, interferon regulatory factor 6 [*IRE6*]) and

TABLE 3 Craniofacial Dysmorphology Associated with Chromosomal Abnormalities

Syndrome	Chromosomal Defects	Craniofacial Features
Disorders affecting the autosomes		
Down syndrome	Trisomy 21	Mongolism, brachycephaly, mental retardation, upslanting palpebral fissures, epicanthus, iris brushfield spots, small mouth, protruding tongue, small ears, folded helix, short nose, flat nasal bridge, short neck
Edwards' syndrome	Trisomy 18	Prominent occiput, small chin, narrow palpebral fissures, occasional cleft lip, mental defect
Patau's syndrome	Trisomy 13	Cleft lip and palate, broad nasal bridge, sloping forehead, mental retardation, microcephaly, occasional holoprosencephaly, microphthalmia, forehead hemangiomas
Partial trisomy 22	Trisomy 22, partial	Microcephaly, hypertelorism, epicanthus, coloboma, preauricular pits and tags, mental retardation
9p Trisomy	Trisomy 9p	Microcephaly, small deep-set eyes, thin protruding upper lip, bulbous nose, mental retardation
Killian-Pallister mosaic syndrome	Mosaic tetrasomy of short arm of chromosome 12	Coarse facial features, broad forehead, hypertelorism, saggy cheeks, droopy mouth, prominent upper lip, sparse hair, mental retardation
Wolf-Hirschhorn syndrome	Deletion of short arm of chromosome 4	Frontal bossing, high hairline, prominent glabella, short prominent philtrum, occasional cleft lip, mental retardation
13q Syndrome	Deletion of long arm of chromosome 13	Minor dysmorphic face, trigonocephaly, microcephaly, broad nasal root, mental retardation, retinoblastoma
18q Syndrome	Deletion of long arm of chromosome 18	Midface hypoplasia, deep-set eyes, preauricular pits, short philtrum, carp-shaped mouth, narrow or atretic external auditory canal
Disorders affecting the sex chromosomes		
Turner's syndrome	45(XO)	Minor dysmorphic face, narrow maxilla, small chin, curved upper lip, straight lower lip, prominent ears, neck webbing
Females with multiple X chromosomes	47 (XXX) 48(XXXX)	Resemble Down syndrome features, broad flat nose, hypertelorism, epicanthus, prominent jaw, mental retardation

their expression are coupled with several environmental factors.[62] Protein-calorie malnutrition, vitamin deficiencies such as those related to folic acid and retinoic acid, and alcohol and tobacco consumption are a few of the environmental factors that relate to specific sets of genes essential for morphogenesis.[7,12,40–43]

The sex chromosomes were previously assumed to be the determinants of the sex of a child. Currently, it is believed that gender identity vis-à-vis sex chromosomes not only influences gender sexuality but also has profound influences on multigene and complex human disorders. Individual gene expression, multiple gene-gene interactions, and multigene-environment interactions are fundamentally different between men and women.

Gene networks that regulate metabolism, drug absorption, and drug use differ between genders. Gene circuits in the immune and endocrine systems show gender variance. These emerging observations may also reflect physiologic effects influenced by genes encoded within the two X chromosomes of the female, albeit with only one of the two active in any given cell, versus the one X and one Y chromosome of the male. Multiple gene-gene and gene-environment interactions demonstrate significant differences in many aspects of growth, development, maturation, and senescence between genders. As increasing numbers of men and women live longer within industrial nations, data are emerging that demonstrate gender differences in the prevalence and incidence of many complex conditions, such as cardiovascular diseases, diabetes, periodontal diseases, osteoporosis, and pulmonary diseases. Risk factors such as diet, lack of exercise, and stress seem to have different influences on the incidence, onset, and progression of cardiovascular diseases between men and women. Examples involve relationships such as low birth weight premature infants and periodontal diseases,[65,66] osteoporosis, and cardiovascular diseases.[67–69] Women's diseases are no longer viewed as those limited to diseases of the reproductive system and related hormones (eg, estrogen and progesterone).

The function of multiple genes encoded within both sex chromosomes and autosomes, the specific gender of the individual (ie, XX versus XY), and multiple environmental influences serve as the foundation for increased susceptibility to different manifestations of diseases. Further, gender-based genetic differences are also implicated in pharmacogenomics and individual responses to the absorption, diffusion, use, and metabolism of many therapeutics, including analgesics for pain management.[70,71] Gender differences in analgesic absorption, diffusion, and binding to specific sets of receptors suggest strong gender-specific differences, and these are important in oral medicine and other disciplines. Collectively, these and many other scientific discoveries herald the new fields of "gender biology" and "gender medicine." A primer in modern human genetics for health professionals must include "gender oral medicine."

RESPIRATORY DISEASES

Asthma is an inflammatory disease of the small airways of the lung. Adult-onset asthma is more commonly seen in women than in men. In the United States, since 1990, mortality from chronic lower respiratory diseases remained relatively stable for men, whereas it increased for women. Genetic susceptibility and environmental factors weigh equally in

TABLE 4   Selected Examples of Craniofacial-Oral-Dental Mendelian Genetic Diseases and Disorders

Type	Gene Name	Gene Symbol	Chromosomal Location	OMIM Number for Gene	Syndrome	OMIM Number for Syndrome	Inheritance	Description of Craniofacial-Oral-Dental Features*
ECM	Collagen, type I, alpha-1 chain	COL1A1	17q21.31-q22.05	120150	Osteogenesis imperfecta, type I	166200	AD	Hypoplasia of dentin and pulp, translucent teeth with yellow or blue-gray coloration, delayed tooth eruption, irregular placement of teeth, susceptibility to caries, wormian bones, occasional deafness, otosclerosis, blue sclerae
					Osteogenesis imperfecta, type III	259420	AR	Dentinogenesis imperfecta, macrocephaly, trianglar facial appearance, wormian bones, occasional deafness
					Osteogenesis imperfecta, type IV	166220	AD	Dentinogenesis imperfecta, multiple caries, wormian bones, occasional hearing loss, otosclerosis
					Ehlers-Danlos syndrome, type VII	130060	AD	Narrow maxilla, small mandible, occasional hypodontia and microdontia, wide nasal bridge, epicanthus
ECM	Collagen, type I, alpha-2 chain	COL1A2	7q22.1	120160	Osteogenesis imperfecta, type I	166200	AD	Hypoplasia of dentin and pulp, translucent teeth with yellow or blue-gray coloration, delayed teeth eruption, irregular placement of teeth, susceptibility to caries, wormian bones, occasional deafness, otosclerosis, blue sclerae
					Osteogenesis imperfecta, type III	259420	AR	Dentinogenesis imperfecta, macrocephaly, triangular facial appearance, wormian bones, occasional deafness
					Osteogenesis imperfecta, type IV	166220	AD	Dentinogenesis imperfecta, multiple caries, wormian bones, occasional hearing loss, otosclerosis
ECM	Collagen, type III, alpha-1 chain	COL3A 1	2q31	120180	Ehlers-Danlos syndrome, type IV	130050	AD	Narrow maxilla, small mandible, occasional hypodontia and microdontia, wide nasal bridge, epicanthus, large eyes, pinched nose, thin lips
ECM	Collagen, type VII, alpha-1 chain	COL7A 1	3p21.3	120120	Epidermolysis bullosa dystrophica	226600	AR	Defective tooth enamel, lingual adhesions, microstomia, bullae of conjunctiva and cornea
ECM	Collagen, type XI, alpha-2 chain	COL11A2	6p21.3	120290	Stickler syndrome, type II	184840	AD	Cleft palate, micrognathia, glossoptosis, severe myopia, flat facies, dental anomalies, deafness
ECM	Keratin 16	KRT16	17q12-q21	148067	Pachyonychia congenita, Jadassohn-Lewandowsky type	167200	AD	Oral leukoplakia, neonatal teeth, early loss of secondary teeth
ECM	Keratin 17	KRT17	17q12-q21	148069	Pachyonychia congenita, Jackson-Lawler type	167210	AD	No oral leukoplakia, neonatal teeth, early loss of secondary teeth
ECM	Amelogenin	AMELX	Xp22.3-p22.1	301200	Amelogenesis imperfecta 1, hypoplastic type	301200	XD	Hypoplastic-type amelogenesis imperfecta, very hard enamel, thin enamel, small teeth, rough tooth surface
ECM	Dentinogenesis imperfecta 1 gene	DGI1	4q13-q21	125490	Dentinogenesis imperfecta 1	125490	AD	Dentinogenesis imperfecta, blue-gray or amber brown opalescent teeth, enamel splitting, teeth have bulbous crowns, narrow roots with small or obliterated pulp chambers and root canal

TABLE 4   Selected Examples of Craniofacial-Oral-Dental Mendelian Genetic Diseases and Disorders (Continued)

Type	Gene Name	Gene Symbol	Chromosomal Location	OMIM Number for Gene	Syndrome	OMIM Number for Syndrome	Inheritance	Description of Craniofacial-Oral-Dental Features*
ECM	Fibrillin 1	*FBN1*	15q21.1	134797	Marfan's syndrome	154700	AD	Dolichocephaly, high arched palate, narrow palate, crowded teeth, micrognathia
					Shprintzen-Goldberg syndrome	182212	AD	Craniosynostosis, microcephaly, maxillary and mandibular hypoplasia, palatal shelf soft tissue hypertrophy, cleft palate, prominent nose, narrow palpebral fissures
ENZ	Alkaline phosphatase, liver/bone/kidney type	*ALPL*	1p36.1-p34	171760	Hypophosphatasia, infantile	241500	AR	Generalized lack of ossification, craniostenosis, microcephaly, leptomeningeal hemorrhage, absent bony cranial vault, poorly formed teeth
ENZ	Iduronate 2-sulfatase	*IDS*	Xq28	309900	Mucopolysaccharidosis, type II (Hunter's syndrome)	309900	X	Scaphocephaly, macrocephaly, frontal bossing, coarse facies, enlarged tongue, deafness
ENZ	Galactosamine (*N*-acetyl)-6-sulfate sulfatase	*GALNS*	16q24.3	253000	Mucopolysaccharidosis, type IVA (Morquio's syndrome)	253000	AR	Dense calvarium, broad mouth, wide- spaced teeth, thin enamel
IS	Guanine nucleotide-binding protein, alpha-stimulating activity polypeptide 1	*GNAS1*	20q13.2	139320	Pseudohypoparathyroidism, type Ia	103580	AD	Round face, low nasal bridge, short neck, cataracts, delayed tooth eruption, enamel hypoplasia
					McCune-Albright syndrome	174800	AD	Cranial foramen impingement, craniofacial hyperostosis, facial asymmetry, prognathism
IS	Retinoblastoma 1	*RB1*	13q14.1-q14.2	180200	Retinoblastoma	180200	AD	Cleft palate, high forehead, prominent eyebrows, broad nasal bridge, bulbous tip of the nose, large mouth with thin upper lip, long philtrum, prominent earlobes
IS	Cyclin-dependent kinase inhibitor 1C	*CDKN1C*	11p15.5	600856	Beckwith-Wiedemann syndrome	130650	AD	Coarse facial features, linear earlobe creases, posterior helical indentations, macroglossia, midface hypoplasia
NP	Small nuclear ribonucleoprotein polypeptide N	*SNRPN*	15q12	182279	Prader-Willi syndrome	176270	AD	Narrow bitemporal head dimension, thin upper lip, down-turned corners of mouth, viscous saliva
NP	Werner's syndrome gene	*WRN*	8p12-p11.2	277700	Werner's syndrome	277700	AR	Wide face, prematurely aged face, beaked nose
NP	CREB binding protein	*CREBBP*	16p13.3	600140	Rubinstein-Taybi syndrome	180849	AD	Microcephaly, hypoplastic maxilla, beaked nose, slanted palpebral fissures, hypertelorism, short upper lip, pouting lower lip
SEC	Sonic hedgehog	*SHH*	7q36	600725	Holoprosencephaly, type 3	142945	AD	Cyclopia, ocular hypotelorism, proboscis, midface hypolasia, single nostril, midline cleft upper lip, premaxillary agenesis
NP	Eyes absent 1 gene	*EYA1*	8q13.3	601653	Branchio-otorenal syndrorne	113650	AD	Branchial cleft fistulae; external, middle, and inner ear rnalformations; hearing loss
TM	Fibroblast growth factor receptor 1	*FGFR1*	8p11.2-p11.1	136350	Pfeiffer's syndrome	101600	AD	Mild craniosynostosis, flat facies, acrocephaly

TABLE 4   Selected Examples of Craniofacial-Oral-Dental Mendelian Genetic Diseases and Disorders (Continued)

Type	Gene Name	Gene Symbol	Chromosomal Location	OMIM Number for Gene	Syndrome	OMIM Number for Syndrome	Inheritance	Description of Craniofacial-Oral-Dental Features*
TM	Fibroblast growth factor receptor 2	FGFR2	10q26	176943	Crouzon's craniofacial dysostosis	123500	AD	Craniosynostosis, parrot-beaked nose, short upper lip, hypoplastic maxilla, relative mandibular prognathism, shallow orbit
					Jackson-Weiss syndrome	123150	AD	Craniosynostosis, midfacial hypoplasia
					Apert's syndrome	101200	AD	Craniosynostosis, brachysphenocephalic acrocephaly, flat facies, high narrow palate
					Pfeiffer's syndrome	101600	AD	Mild craniosynostosis, flat facies, acrocephaly
					Beare-Stevenson cutis gyrata syndrome	123790	AD	Craniosynostosis, cloverleaf skull, cleft palate or uvula, craniofacial anornalies
TM	Fibroblast growth factor receptor 3	FGFR3	4p16.3	134934	Achondroplasia	100800	AD	Frontal bossing, megalencephaly, midfacial hypoplasia, low nasal bridge
					Hypochondroplasia	146000	AD	Normocephaly or occasional brachycephaly, mild frontal bossing
					Thanatophoric dysplasia	187600	AD	Megalencephaly, small foramen magnum, cloverleaf skull, depressed nasal bridge
					Crouzon's disease with acanthosis nigricans	134934	AD	Craniosynostosis
					Craniosynostosis, nonsyndromic	134934	AD	Craniosynostosis
TM	Insulin receptor	IR	19p13.2	147670	Leprechaunism, insulin-resistant diabetes mellitus with acanthosis nigricans	147670	AD	Bitemporal skull narrowing, supernumerary teeth, severe premature caries, prominent lower canines and upper incisors, thickened lips, prominent ears
TM	Parathyroid hormone receptor	PTHR	3p22-p21.1	168468	Metaphyseal chondrodysplasia, Murk Jansen type	156400	AD	Sclerosis of cranial base, wide cranial sutures, supraorbital hyperplasia, prominent supraorbital ridges, frontonasal hyperplasia, micrognathia, high arched palate, deafness
TM	RET oncogene	RET	10q11.2	164761	Neuromata, mucosal, with endocrine tumors	162300	AD	Neuromata of lips and tongue, conjunctival and nasal mucosa neuromas, diffuse lip hypertrophy, high arched palate, coarse facies
TM	Ectodermal dysplasia gene, anhidrotic	EDA	Xq12.2-q13.1	305100	Ectodermal dysplasia, anhidrotic	305100	X	Absent teeth, small pointed incisors, saddle nose, sparse hair, prominent forehead, prominent lips
TM	Patched	PTC	9q22.3	601309	Basal cell nevus syndrome (Gorlin's syndrome)	109400	AD	Macrocephaly, broad facies, frontal and biparietal bossing, mild mandibular prognathism, odontogenic keratocysts of jaws, misshapened and/or carious teeth, cleft lip and palate, ectopic calcification of falx cerebri
TF	Msh homeobox homolog 1	MSX1	4p16.1	142983	Tooth agenesis, familial	142983	AD	Hypodontia
TF	Msh homeobox homolog 2	MSX2	5q34-q35	123101	Craniosynostosis, type 2	123101	AD	Craniosynostosis, forehead retrusion, frontal bossing, turribrachycephaly, Kleeblattschaedel deformity (cloverleaf skull, trilobular skull anomaly)

TABLE 4 Selected Examples of Craniofacial-Oral-Dental Mendelian Genetic Diseases and Disorders (Continued)

Type	Gene Name	Gene Symbol	Chromosomal Location	OMIM Number for Gene	Syndrome	OMIM Number for Syndrome	Inheritance	Description of Craniofacial-Oral-Dental Features*
TF	Microphthalmia-associated transcription factor	MITF	3p14.1-p12.3	156845	Waardenburg's syndrome, type IIA	193510	AD	Wide nasal bridge, short philtrum, cleft lip or palate, deafness
TF	GLI-Kruppel family member 3 oncogene	GLI3	7p13	165240	Greig's cephalopoly-syndactyly syndrome	175700	AD	Peculiar skull shape, expanded cranial vault, high forehead and bregma, frontal bossing, macrocephaly, hypertelorism
					Pallister-Hall syndrome	146510	AD	Short nose, flat nasal bridge, multiple buccal frenula, microglossia, micrognathia, cleft palate, malformed ears
TF	Paired box homeotic gene 3	PAX3	2q35	193500	Waardenburg's syndrome, type I	193500	AD	Wide nasal bridge, short philtrum, cleft lip or palate, occasional deafness, dystopia canthorum
					Waardenburg's syndrome, type III	148820	AD	Microcephaly, wide nasal bridge
					Craniofacial-deafness-hand syndrome	122880	AD	Flat facial profile, hypertelorism, hypoplastic nose and maxilla, slitlike nares, hearing loss
TF	Solurshin	RIEG	4q25-q26	601542	Rieger's syndrome, type I	180500	AD	Maxillary hypoplasia, mild prognathism, protruding lower lip, short philtrum, microdontia, hypodontia, cone-shaped teeth
TF	Core-binding factor, runt domain, alpha subunit 1	CBFA1	6p21	600211	Cleidocranial dysplasia	119600	AD	Brachycephaly, frontal and parietal bossing, wormian bones, persistent open anterior fontanel, midfacial hypoplasia, delayed eruption of deciduous and permanent teeth, supernumerary teeth
TF	Twist	TWIST	7p21	601622	Saethre-Chotzen syndrome	101400	AD	Craniosynostosis, acrocephaly, brachycephaly, flat facies, thin long pointed nose, cleft palate, cranial asymmetry, ptosis, malformed ears
UNK	DiGeorge's syndrome chromosome region	CATCH22	22q11	188400	DiGeorge's syndrome	188400	AD	Low-set ears, short ears, small mouth, submucous or overt palatal cleft, cleft lip, bulbous nose, square nasal tip, short philtrum, micrognathia
					Velocardiofacial syndrome	192430	AD	Pierre Robin syndrome, cleft palate, small open mouth, myopathic facies, retrognathia, prominent nose with squared-off nasal tip
UNK	Treacle	TCOF1	5q32-q33.1	154500	Treacher Collins mandibulofacial dysostosis	154500	AD	Malar hypoplasia, cleft palate, mandibular hypoplasia, macrostomia, malformed ears, sensorineural deafness, coloboma of lower eyelid

AD = autosomal dominant; AR = autosomal recessive; ECM = extracellular matrix protein; ENZ = enzyme; IS = intracellular signaling protein; NP = nuclear protein; SEC = secretory protein; TF = transcription factor; TM = transmembrane protein; UNK = unknown; X = X-linked; XD = X-linked dominant.
*The following description is a summary of the craniofacial-oral-dental features of the diseases and disorders. For detailed information regarding defects in other affected tissues and organs, refer to Online Mendelian Inheritance in Man (OMIM) at <http://www.ncbi.nlm.nih.gove/omim/>.

contributing to this finding. Asthma affects one child in seven in some societies and approximately 15 million individuals worldwide. Although identification of all asthma genes is incomplete, five asthma suscepitility genes have been identified by positional cloning: *ADAM33*, *PHF11*, *DPP10*, *GRPA*, and *SPINK5*. Approximately a third of the genetic predisposition to asthma has been uncovered. Genetic findings will lead to the development of new therapy and new treatments for individuals with severe asthma who do not respond to commonly available steroid inhalers.[72–75]

CARDIOVASCULAR DISEASES

Cardiovascular disease is one of the leading causes of death in the world. The 2002 World Health Report demonstrated a higher prevalence and incidence of cardiovascular diseases (rheumatic heart disease, hypertension, cerebrovascular disease, and inflammatory heart disease) in women than in men.[76] The risk for cardiovascular diseases also increases with age at a faster rate in women than in men. Genetic and environmental factors and biologic and anatomic differences have been considered as possible contributory factors to these differences. A genetic predisposition to cardiovascular disease results from gene mutations that alter the biologic function expressed by the original gene(s) and increase an individual's risk for cardiovascular diseases. A region on chromosome 13 in Caucasians and on chromosome 19 in African Americans has been linked to hypertension and stroke.[77–79]

In addition to gene mutations that directly increase susceptibility, there are multiple genes that indirectly increase the risk of cardiovascular diseases. These indirect predispositions are in the form of genes that are related to unhealthy behaviors, such as metabolic pathways related to tobacco use and alcohol consumption. For example, the complications associated with the angiotensin-converting enzyme (*ACE*) gene in ischemic cerebrovascular disease were investigated in smoking and nonsmoking patients. The *ACE* gene mutation was a risk factor only in individuals who smoked but did not appear to behave as a risk factor in those individuals who did not smoke.[80,81]

ENDOCRINE DISEASES

Oral diseases and disorders are associated with systemic diseases.[82–84] Oral infections are closely linked with diabetes, and management of diabetes is related to the management of oral infections.[67–69,82–84] At present, there is evidence that more than 20 regions of the genome may be involved in susceptibility to type 1 diabetes.[85] The genes in the human leukocyte antigen region of chromosome 6 are currently considered to have the highest influence on susceptibility to type 1 diabetes. To date, more than 50 genes have been studied for their possible association with type 2 diabetes in different populations worldwide. The most noteworthy genes are *PPAR8*, *ABCC8*, *KCNJ11*, and *CALPN10*.[85–87] For more information on diabetes, see Chapter 21, "Diabetes Mellitus and Endocrine Diseases."

AUTOIMMUNE DISEASES

Women are 2.7 times more likely than men to acquire an autoimmune disease. Women have enhanced immune systems compared with men, which increases women's resistance to many types of infection but also makes them more susceptible to autoimmune diseases.[88–90] Men appear to have higher levels of natural killer cell activity than women. This difference in bioactivity may be associated with reduced levels of autoimmune disease in men. The plasma activity level of phospholipase A_2, a key enzyme in causing chronic inflammatory diseases, is significantly higher in Caucasian and Asian Indian women than in their male counterparts.[91–93] A molecule involved in reducing the inflammatory response, interleukin-1 receptor II, is present in higher concentrations in blood fractions from men than from women.[88–93]

The most striking sex differences for complex human diseases are observed in Sjögren's syndrome, lupus, autoimmune thyroid disease (Hashimoto's thyroiditis, Graves' disease), and scleroderma; these represent a spectrum of diseases in which the patient population is greater than 80% female. In rheumatoid arthritis, multiple sclerosis, and myasthenia gravis, the sex distribution is 60 to 75% female.[88–90,94]

In addition to increased susceptibility to autoimmune disorders, women experience certain viral infectious conditions that affect their immune system disproportionately when compared with men.[94,95] For example, human immunodeficiency virus (HIV) infection that was more prevalent in men in the early 1980s is currently affecting women at an alarming rate.[96] Women account for almost 50% of the 40 million people living with HIV-1 worldwide, with an even higher percentage in developing countries. In the United States, the estimated number of acquired immune deficiency syndrome (AIDS) cases increased 15% among women and only 1% among men from 1999 to 2003.[96] The major burden of the disease was in young women, particularly African American and Hispanic women.[96]

Heterosexual transmission is now the most commonly reported mode of HIV transmission in women. Women's increased susceptibility has been linked to physiologic factors such as hormonal changes, vaginal microbial ecology, and a higher prevalence of sexually transmitted diseases. These factors, in combination with other factors, such as gender disparities, poverty, cultural and sexual norms, lack of education, and sexual and domestic violence, make women vulnerable to this and other viral infections.[95,96]

Women develop signs and symptoms of AIDS, including oral manifestations, at a lower HIV viral load than men.[97] They also seem to benefit from the initiation of antiretroviral therapy at a lower HIV viral load than men.

CANCER

The role of genetics in cancer is widely recognized. The prevalence of cancer is projected to increase 50% worldwide within the next 20 years. According to the World Cancer Report, 10 million new cancer cases are diagnosed annually. Cancer contributes to 12.6% of the global mortality rate.[98] All cancers have genetic determinants. Cancers are usually caused by a sequence of multiple genetic mutations, and this is highlighted by neoplastic diseases of the head and neck.[99–104] There are three categories of cancer: inherited, familial, or sporadic. *Inherited* cases of a dominant type are often caused by direct mutations of genes that are passed successively from parents to offspring throughout generations. These are often regulatory genes required for the control of the cell cycle and cell division, as well as genes that regulate tumor suppression. *Familial* cases involve mutations of multiple susceptibility genes that increase an individual's risk for cancer (so-called multigene-gene and gene-environment interactions). *Sporadic* cancer cases are those in which an individual randomly develops cancer in the absence of any familial pattern, such as chronic exposure to carcinogenic substances.

Three of the most studied cancers with susceptibility genes are breast, colorectal, and prostate cancer. *BRCA1*, *BRCA2*, *TP53* (breast cancer), *hMLH1*, *hMLH2*, *IGF2* (colorectal), *BRCA1*, *BRCA2*, *hMLH1*, *hMLH2* (ovarian), *CYP1A1* (lung), and *HPC2* (prostate) are among the genes of interest.[105–107]

Tumor suppressor genes are involved in regulating the cell cycle and activate cell apoptosis or cell death.[99,100] The gene mutation results in the production of altered protein that is no longer capable of initiating apoptosis. Although great progress is being made in the discovery of genetic susceptibility to cancer, little attention had been paid to gender and sex disparities in cancer. For most common cancers, men seem to have a higher incidence than women. Men and women are predisposed to different anatomic, biochemical, and genetic features, and these factors may play a role in the susceptibility to and onset of cancer. Men and women respond differently to stress-inducing environments, which may make them more susceptible to certain behaviors (eg, tobacco use and alcohol consumption) that might enhance their susceptibility to neoplastic diseases, such as oral and pharyngeal cancers (see Figure 4).[100–104]

NEURODEGENERATIVE DISEASES AND MENTAL DISEASES

Research in neurodegenerative and mental diseases and disorders is focusing on tracing positions of gene mutations coupled with environmental factors that lead to the causes of these profound chronic disease conditions. Alzheimer's disease constitutes about two-thirds of all cases of dementia. Alzheimer's disease is a progressive neurologic disease that results in irreversible loss of neurons, particularly in the cortex and hippocampus.[108,109] There are missense mutations in three genes in families with early-onset autosomal dominant Alzheimer's disease: beta-amyloid on chromosome 21, presenelin 1 on chromosome 14, and presenilin 2 located on chromosome 1. The *APOE* gene on chromosome 19 has been linked to late-onset Alzheimer's disease, which is the most common form of the disease. This gene has three different forms: *APOE2*, *APOE3*, and *APOE4*. *APOE3* is the most common form in the general population. *APOE4* occurs in 40% of all late-onset Alzheimer's disease patients but is not limited to those whose families have a history of Alzheimer's disease. Patients with no known family history (sporadic

Alzheimer's disease) are also more likely to have an *APOE4* gene.

Parkinson's disease is the second most common neurodegenerative disorder after Alzheimer's disease. The exact cause of Parkinson's disease remains unknown, but genetic factors have been identified as potential contributing factors in the onset and severity of the disease.[110] Studies with monozygotic twins show a very high level of concordance in the early-onset (before age 50 years) type of Parkinson's disease. The early-onset version appears to be autosomal dominant in families of the Mediterranean and German regions and has several missense mutations in the gene coding for α-synuclein located on chromosome 4q21.

Genetics studies are also contributing toward enhanced understanding of mental diseases and disorders. For example, men are more likely to express depression or severe unhappiness through an "externalizing pathway" of physical behaviors, including drinking, drug abuse, and violence, whereas women are more likely to "internalize," leading to depression and anorexia. This sex difference is more prominent during puberty. Epidemiologic studies have shown that in families of women with bulimia, the men often have alcoholism and other addictions. Men may cope with disasters by drinking. In some cultures, it is not acceptable for women to drink, and they may cope with disasters by developing anxiety disorder and depression. More than half of all female suicides worldwide take place in China.[105–107,111]

It has been have proposed that sex hormones are responsible for a higher incidence of mental disorders in women.[112] A comprehensive evaluation of women's mental health is currently ongoing in 28 countries as part of an epidemiologic study sponsored by the World Health Organization.[76] New emerging information by genetic epidemiologists reveals a number of structural and functional differences between men's and women's brains. Men's brains are more lateralized, whereas women's brains are not. This makes it more likely for women than for men to overcome language deficits resulting from strokes in the left hemisphere, where language is centered. This structural difference has also been linked to the lower likelihood of childhood developmental and mental disorders in girls than in boys. Sex differences are also present in substance abuse. Female substance abusers are more likely to report psychiatric symptoms before the onset of substance abuse, whereas male substance abusers are more likely to report depression and other psychiatric symptoms after chronic substance abuse. Recently, bioimaging studies have provided information about the neural processes underlying differences in the manifestations of substance abuse.[106,107,111]

▼ GENETICS, GENDER, AND TREATMENT RESPONSES (PHARMACOGENOMICS)

Human genetic variance, the 200 to 300 million base differences (SNPs) between human genomes, can explain why all patient responses to therapy are not always the same.[9,70,71] For example, despite appropriate management of hypertension and accomplishment of target blood pressure, some hypertensive patients still develop myocardial infarction or stroke, and, despite appropriate management of these conditions, some patients survive and some do not. Similarly, not all patients respond to behavioral modifications in the same way. It is known that regular exercise alleviates hypertension in some patients but not all. In summary, human genetic variations contribute to these differences. Recent investigations have identified five sources of genetic variation between multiple families receiving medications for the management of cardiovascular diseases.[113]

The birth and evolution of pharmacogenetics and pharmacogenomics have contributed significantly to a better understanding of individual variations in therapeutics. The genetics of pharmacokinetics and pharmacodynamics and physiologic regulation that is influenced by ethnicity, age, and gender all affect an individual's discrete response to a drug therapy. Men and women may respond to the same drug differently. For example, intake of certain antibiotics, antihistamines, antiarrhythmics, and antipsychotics places women at a higher risk than men for drug-induced arrhythmias.[114,115]

The differences in responses to drugs have been missed in the past because women were not always included in clinical trials; if they were, the data were not broken down by sex.[116,117] Recently, based on a long-term clinical trial, it was shown that aspirin, which protects men against heart attack but not stroke, has exactly the opposite effect in women. Evidence shows that men and women differ in the activity of liver enzymes that metabolize drugs. Women are, on average, smaller in size and have a higher percentage of body fat. Therefore, women may absorb and/or excrete drugs more slowly or may retain fat-soluble drugs longer than men. Furthermore, women were reported to have a significantly higher likelihood than men of being admitted to a hospital as a direct consequence of adverse drug reactions.[118]

Traditionally, health care providers have used a combination of history, clinical evaluation, and diagnostic tests as a basis for their diagnoses and patient management. Often multiple patients who presented with similar histories and had similar clinical and laboratory findings received the same treatment. Today, with the availability of different genetic tests, the level of risk for or susceptibility to different diseases can be identified. This will change the practice of medicine and dentistry in the future because risk factors will be the driving force for treatment selection, not merely the clinical signs and symptoms. Patients with clinical risk factors will be treated differently even though the presenting signs and symptoms are the same.

Advances in genomics and molecular tests for assessments and diagnoses, as well as pharmacogenomics and pharmacogenetics, will change the future of the practice of medicine and dentistry.[5,7,11,12,41–45,50–62,65–70,83,119–121] Efforts should be made to incorporate "genomic" information in continuing education programs for current practitioners and in medical and dental school curriculums for future health care providers.[99,122,123] The interpretation of genetic test results, the provision of appropriate counseling, and the solutions to potential ethical and confidentiality-related issues need adequate training and expertise involving all health care providers.

▼ PHENOTYPIC AND GENETIC HETEROGENEITY IN GENETIC DISEASES AND DISORDERS

Human disorders are heterogeneous as the result of complex interactions between multiple genetic loci and environmental factors during the life span. This interpretation is true for human diseases that segregate as simple Mendelian traits as well as for nonmendelian multifactorial conditions. There are many examples of single gene disorders in which identical mutations result in widely different clinical phenotypes, referred to as variable expressivity. For example, monozygotic twins, two siblings with identical genetic inheritance, show phenotypic heterogeneity with age and varying environments.[124] This nonintuitive realization has become the rapidly advancing field of *epigenetics*, which refers to the alteration of gene function without altering DNA.

Single-gene mutations can have pleiotropic or multiple effects. For example, patients who present with xeroderma pigmentosum are unusually sensitive to sunlight, and patients with α_1-antitrypsin deficiency often have a predisposition to developing emphysema and are more sensitive to tobacco smoke.[125] Single-gene mutations may also be associated with serious and inappropriate responses to certain therapeutics. Mendelian and nonmendelian multifactorial diseases may also present clinical complexities with drug use, absorption, and metabolism.[9,12,38,39,70,71] For example, glucose-6-phosphate dehydrogenase deficiency is inherited as an X-linked recessive disorder and can induce hemolytic anemia in response to various drug therapies.[126] Mendelian and nonmendelian multifactorial and pharmacogenomics are remarkably linked to genetic variations in drug metabolism in a growing array of patients. Distinct alleles of the cytochrome P-450 network of genes that function in drug metabolism have an impact on drug efficacy and toxicity.[70,71,127]

In addition to genetic heterogeneity resulting from gene-gene and gene-environment interactions, other factors serve to enhance or increase the phenotypic heterogeneity of human disorders, such as *penetrance*. The varying degree of severity and incomplete penetrance of gene expression need to be appreciated by all clinicians. Many autosomal dominant diseases often display varying severity owing to variable expressivity and incomplete penetrance. Examples of disorders with reduced penetrance are tuberous sclerosis and Marfan's syndrome.

It is important to recognize the phenomenon of locus heterogeneity wherein mutations in different genes can cause remarkably similar clinical phenotypes. One classic example is that forms of hemophilia can be caused by genetic mutations in either the gene for factor VIII (so-called "classic hemophilia") or the gene for factor IX ("Christmas disease"). Both of these two genes are located on the X chromosome, and both of these diseases or conditions are inherited as X-linked recessive disorders. Similarly, the enamel disorder AI can be caused by mutations in *AMELX*, *ENAM*, or *MMP20*.[53–60] In addition, different point mutations in the same gene can result in very different clinical phenotypes. One example is the gene fibroblast growth factor receptor 2 (*FGFR2*). Different point mutations in *FGFR2* result in very different craniofacial dysmorphogenesis syndromes with craniosynostosis.[41–43,122,125] Similarly, severe mutations within the dystrophin gene, such as deletion of large portions of the gene, result in Duchenne muscular dystrophy, whereas milder mutations, such as certain point mutations, result in the milder Becker dystrophy.

▼ PROSPECTUS: HUMAN GENETICS AND ORAL MEDICINE

Genetics will continue to dominate dental and medical education in the twenty-first century. Human and microbial genomics, proteomics, and metabolomics, coupled with pharmacogenomics, will continue to shape the future in the health professions.[119–123,125,127–129] Mendelian and nonmendelian patterns of inheritance are clinically important. Genetic screening assays for individual and multiple genes as found in multifactorial conditions will become more specific, more sensitive, faster, and cheaper.

Diagnosis will encompass the cardinal features of the clinical phenotype, differential diagnosis, and sensitive and specific tests for one or more genes and/or gene products. Risk assessment will increasingly be used, coupled with patient and family and community patterns of disease, environmental insults, and carrier detection within individuals and populations. Molecular epidemiology will emerge as increasingly useful for diagnosis. Genetic counseling will encompass psychosocial management issues. Legal and ethical issues will continue to surface related to genetic screening, privacy and confidentiality, disclosure of unexpected and unwanted findings, and obligations to identify and communicate difficult issues.

The field of genetics should no longer be limited to syndromes of the head and neck as a chapter in a textbook. It should be considered as the essential primer for all aspects of health care and should become encoded within medicine, dentistry, pharmacy, nursing, and the allied health professions and beyond. Oral medicine specialists are instrumental in closing the gap between medicine and dentistry. These specialists serve as a resource to the medical and dental communities in the detection, prevention, and management of conditions that affect systemic and oral health. Greater interaction is necessary among all health professionals in planning systemic and oral care for patients.

Molecular microbial studies led to the emergence of the concept of biofilm formation on tooth surfaces, mucosal surfaces, stents, catheters, medical and dental implants, and even water lines.[128] Biofilms contain microbial species within a three-dimensional structure. Immunology and targeted pharmaceutical developments must address antimicrobial resistance within biofilms, coupled with an aging population in the industrial nations of the world.[127] DNA microarray technology is useful for the purposes of disease diagnosis and drug development.[129] The emerging information on molecular epidemiology will facilitate the assessment of an individual's risk profile based on the host's susceptibility genotype and risk behaviors (smoking, drinking, diet), as well as exposure to common pathogens (bacterial, viral, fungal) and other environmental factors (heavy metals, allergens).

An individual's response to foreign chemicals (xenobiotics) is genetically controlled. This explains why some individuals are at risk for oral conditions such as oral cancer, dental caries, periodontal disease, and soft tissue disorders. Understanding the molecular pathogenesis of squamous cell carcinoma will provide the basis for improved risk assessment, as well as diagnostic and therapeutic approaches.[129,130] Infectious pathogens and dietary factors influence dental caries and periodontal diseases, but genetic variance also contributes to host susceptibility in different populations. Tooth morphology, tooth structure, salivary composition, response to microbial pathogens, and response to fluoride and other anticaries products, as well as susceptibility to head and neck cancers and cardiovascular, respiratory, and autoimmune disorders, are all genetic in nature. Recent studies analyzing the genetic and epigenetic changes in preneoplastic head and neck squamous cell carcinoma (HNSCC) indicated that 46% of HNSCC tumors demonstrate mutations in mtDNA.[131]

Except for monozygotic twins, each person's genome is unique. All dentists and physicians need to understand the concept of genetic variability, its interactions with the environment, and its implications for patient and population health care. In the near future, genomics will enhance prevention, diagnostics, and therapeutics.

▼ SUGGESTED READINGS

Brady KT, Randall CL. Gender differences in substance use disorders. Psychiatr Clin North Am 1999;22:241–52.

Chambers DA. editor. DNA: the double helix: perspective and prospective at forty years. New York: New York Academy of Sciences; 1995.

Collins FS, McKusick VA. Implications of the Human Genome Project for medical science. JAMA 2001;285:540–4.

Collins FS, Patrinos A, Jordan E, et al. New goals for the U.S. Human Genome Project: 1998-2003. Science 1998;282:682–9.

Davey ME, O'Toole GA. Microbial biofilms: from ecology to molecular genetics. Microbiol Mol Biol Rev 2000;64:847–67.

DeAngelis CD, Glass RM, editors. Women's health. [Theme Issue] JAMA 2006;295:1339–474.

DeAngelis CD, Winker MA, editors. Women's health. [Theme Issue] JAMA 2001;285:1399–536.

Guttmacher AE, Collins FS, Drazen JM, editors. Genomic medicine: articles from the *New England Journal of Medicine*. Baltimore: The Johns Hopkins University Press; 2004.

Hart TC, Marazita ML, Wright JT. The impact of molecular genetics on oral health paradigms. Crit Rev Oral Biol Med 2000;1:26–56.

International Human Genome Sequencing Consortium. Finishing the euchromatic sequence of the human genome. Nature 2004;431:931–45.

Kuo WP, Whipple ME, Sonis ST, et al. Gene expression profiling by DNA microarrays and its application to dental research. Oral Oncol 2002;38:650–6.

Lander ES, Linton LM, Birren B, et al. Initial sequencing and analysis of the human genome. Nature 2001;409:860–921.

Mark S. Sex- and gender-based medicine: Venus, Mars, and beyond. Gend Med 2005;2:131–6.

Mendelsohn ME, Karas RH. Molecular and cellular basis of cardio-vascular gender differences. Science 2005;308:1583–7.

Pemberton TJ, Gee J, Patel PI. Gene discovery for dental anomalies: a primer for the dental professional. J Am Dent Assoc 2006;137: 743–52.

Quinn TC, Overbaugh J. HIV/AIDS in women: an expanding epidemic. Science 2005;308:1582–3.

Ross MT, Grafham DV, Coffey AJ, et al. The DNA sequence of the human X chromosome. Nature 2005;434:325–37.

Schmutz J, Wheeler J, Grimwood J, et al. Quality assessment of the human genome sequence. Nature 2004;429:365–8.

Shum L, Takahashi K, Takahashi I, et al. Embryogenesis and the clas-sification of craniofacial dysmorphogenesis. In: Fonseca R, editor. Oral and maxillofacial surgery. Vol 6. Philadelphia: WB Saunders; 2000. p. 149–94.

Venter JC, Adams MD, Myers EW, et al. The sequence of the human genome. Science 2001;291:1304–51.

Watson JD, Crick FH. Molecular structure of nucleic acids. A structure for deoxyribose nucleic acid. Nature 1953;171:737–8.

▼ WEB-BASED RESOURCES

The reader is encouraged to access the expanding human, animal, plant, and microbial genomic databases using the Internet:

American Society of Human Genetics
http://www.ashg.org/genetics/ashg/ashgmenu.htm

Arachaea and *Eubacteria* microbial genome projects sorted by taxonomic groups, present in GenBank, annotation in progress and "in progress"
http://www.ncbi.nlm.nih.gov/Taxonomy/

Ethical, legal, and social implications of genome research on privacy/confidentiality http://www.ornl.gov/hgmis/elsi/elsi.html

GenBank, current status of human, animal, plant, and microbial genomics http://www.ncbi.nlm.nih.gov/Genbank/index.html

Gene expression in teeth
http://bite-it.helsinki.fi/

Human Genome Map compiled by the National Center for Biotechnology Information http://www.ncbi.nlm.nih.gov/gen-emap/

Genome Programs of the US Department of Energy Office of Science
http://www.doegenomes.org/

National Coalition of Health Professional Education in Genetics
http://www.nchpeg.org

OMIM, Online Mendelian Inheritance in Man
http://www.ncbi.nlm.nih.gov/entrez/query.fcgi?db=OMIM

Agency for Healthcare Research and Quality
http://www.ahrq.gov

Centers for Disease Control and Prevention
http://www.cdc.gov

GeneTests-GeneClinics
http://www.genetests.org/

National Human Genome Research Institute
http://www.nhgri.nih.gov

National Institute of Dental and Craniofacial Research
http://www.nidr.nih.gov

National Institutes of Health
http://health.nih.gov

National Center for Biotechnology Information projects with Cancer Genome Anatomy Project data
http://www.ncbi.nlm.nih.gov/ncicgap/

For the full reference list, please refer to the accompanying CD ROM.

INDEX